Neuromuscular Diseases

A Practical Approach to Diagnosis and Management

Springer-Verlag London Ltd.

Michael Swash and Martin S. Schwartz

Neuromuscular Diseases

A Practical Approach to Diagnosis and Management

Third Edition

With 219 Figures

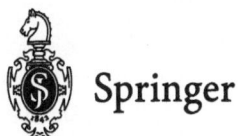 Springer

Michael Swash MD, FRCP, FRCPath
Professor of Neurology and Consultant Neurologist, St Bartholomew's and The
Royal London Hospital School of Medicine and Dentistry at Queen Mary Westfield
College, and The Royal London Hospital, London E1 1BB, UK

Martin S. Schwartz MD, FRCP
Consultant Clinical Neurophysiologist, Atkinson Morley's Hospital, London SW20
ONE, UK, and Honorary Consultant Neurologist, St George's Hospital, London
SW19 0RE, UK

ISBN 978-1-4471-3836-5

British Library Cataloguing in Publication Data
Neuromuscular diseases : a practical approach to diagnosis and management. – 3rd ed.
1. Neuromuscular diseases
I. Swash, Michael, 1939–   II. Schwartz, Martin S. (Martin Samuel)
616.7′44
ISBN 978-1-4471-3836-5   ISBN 978-1-4471-3834-1 (eBook)
DOI 10.1007/978-1-4471-3834-1

Library of Congress Cataloging-in-Publication Data
Neuromuscular diseases : a practical approach to diagnosis and
management / Michael Swash and Martin S. Schwartz (eds.). — 3rd ed.
p.   cm.
Rev. ed. of : Neuromuscular diseases / Michael Swash, Martin S. Schwartz. 2nd ed. c1988.
Includes bibliographical references and index.
ISBN 978-1-4471-3836-5
1. Neuromuscular diseases.   I. Swash, Michael.   II. Schwartz, Martin S. (Martin Samuel), 1941–
[DNLM: 1. Neuromuscular Diseases—diagnosis.   2. Neuromuscular Diseases—therapy.   WE 550
N4943 1997]
RC925.S95   1997
616.7′44—dc21
DNLM/DLC
for Library of Congress   96–39564

© Springer-Verlag London 1981, 1988, 1997
Originally published by Springer-Verlag Berlin Heidelberg New York in 1997
Softcover reprint of the hardcover 3rd edition 1997

Typeset by EXPO Holdings, Malaysia

28/3830–543210 Printed on acid-free paper

We dedicate this the third edition of this monograph to the memory of Michael Jackson, publisher, whose enthusiasm in 1980–1981 first encouraged us to write this book.

Preface to the Third Edition

Nine years have elapsed since the second edition of this book was published. In this time the principal advances in neuromuscular diseases have been in the application of molecular genetics to understanding the aetiology and pathogenesis of this group of disorders. As a result many previously unrecognised disorders have been characterised. Some clinical syndromes, such as the limb girdle dystrophies, have become better defined. In many such instances the new genetic information has led to major advances in knowledge of the biology of cell structures, for example, the membrane structural and channel proteins. The clinical syndromes themselves, and their pathological and electrophysiological characteristics, however, remain as important as ever, since they constitute the clinical problem itself and, indeed, the database from which all other concepts emerge.

Knowledge of the pathogenesis, genetics, and molecular biology of neuromuscular disorders is essential both in developing and applying new therapies and preventive measures, and in formulating genetic and prognostic advice. However, this information does not necessarily always define clinically useful syndromes. Myotonia, for example, is an electrophysiological finding in some syndromes in which it is undetectable by clinical examination, although the phenomenon itself was originally defined as a clinical entity. The limb girdle muscular dystrophy syndromes can be defined by severity, distribution of weakness, age of onset, sex distribution and other characteristics and many of these can be better understood by study of the underlying defect in cell structural proteins. For the patient, however, what is required is prognostic and, when relevant, genetic advice and, ultimately, relief of symptoms by therapy. These aims and expectations are mutually compatible, but knowledge is acquired unevenly and they cannot all be realised at once. Similar concepts underlie the application of the new knowledge concerning the Charcot–Marie–Tooth syndromes in clinical practice.

The aims of this new edition remain unchanged; indeed, we conceive it to be more important than ever to correlate the different categories of information about neuromuscular diseases into an account that allows clinicians to understand their patients' problems, and to plan appropriate investigation and management. Each category of information needs to be integrated into the clinical database. In this edition there has been extensive revision and rewriting to take account of new knowledge. Nonetheless, the basic plan of the book is unchanged. We have added many new references, and have deleted some of the older ones that no longer seem relevant; the references include papers published through the summer of 1996.

We hope that this book will continue to provide a convenient source of practical and theoretical information that will be useful in managing patients with neuromuscular problems, and that it will stimulate many of our readers to become involved in research, whether in clinical or basic science aspects, in this field of knowledge.

London, 1997   *Michael Swash*
                                                                               Martin S. Schwartz

Preface to the Second Edition

In the seven years since the first edition of this book was published there have been many important developments in knowledge of neuromuscular diseases. These are reflected in this new edition. We have taken the opportunity to add much new clinical and scientific material to the book, particularly in relation to metabolic myopathies and neuropathies, and to include more information on genetic aspects of neuromuscular diseases, quantitative electromyographic techniques, plexus and root lesions and cardiomyopathies. The aim of the book remains unchanged, but we have rearranged some of the material so that there are several new chapters. The illustrations have also been extensively revised and there are many new references. We hope that it will continue to provide a convenient source of practical and theoretical information that will not only be useful in managing patients with neuromuscular diseases, but will stimulate research.

London, May 1987

Michael Swash
Martin S. Schwartz

Preface to the First Edition

Neuromuscular diseases are common in clinical practice. Patients with these disorders may be referred to neurologists, rheumatologists, orthopaedic surgeons, paediatricians or to general physicians, and their investigation, utilising electromyography (EMG) and muscle biopsy, often requires the help of the clinical neurophysiologist and of the pathologist. Investigation must be co-ordinated and interpreted in relation to the clinical findings, but it is rare for the clinical neurophysiologist, pathologist and referring physician to confer together in considering diagnosis and management – an attitude which reflects an underlying fragmentation of opinion and of research. This is evident, also, in most textbooks dealing with neuromuscular disorders, which conventionally emphasise either physiological, pathological or clinical aspects of these diseases. As a result of this restricted approach EMG and pathological investigation are often only used to establish a diagnosis, and their potential value in assessing the functional and structural disturbance in affected muscles remains unrealised. Neuromuscular disorders affect different muscles, or groups of muscles, in varying degrees, and they may progress at different rates in individual patients. Since electrophysiological investigations can be repeated with comparatively little discomfort during the course of a neuromuscular disorder and its treatment, EMG and nerve conduction studies are particularly useful in assessing the distribution and rate of progress of any given disorder. Pathological studies, particularly nerve and muscle biopsy, can be repeated less frequently, although the advent of needle muscle biopsy may enable this investigation, like EMG, to be repeated in the quadriceps and perhaps in the biceps.

Electromyographic and pathological studies can therefore be used not only to indicate the diagnosis itself, but also to assess the overall distribution of the disease process, the effectiveness of compensatory processes and, therefore, the prognosis. Further, in some disorders, for example in polymyositis, myasthenia gravis and certain polyneuropathies, they may be used to assess the effectiveness of treatment. However, they cannot be used as a substitute for careful clinical evaluation.

It is the purpose of this book to describe and correlate the clinical, electromyographic, pathological and, when relevant, the biochemical features of neuromuscular disorders. Particular attention is paid to variations in these features during phases of progression or improvement. The effects of treatment, and of the various compensatory factors, such as reinnervation by axonal sprouting, muscle fibre regeneration, and myopathic changes in chronic neurogenic disorders, are described since these produce important and clearly recognisable changes in the course of these disorders. The role of EMG and pathological studies in this approach is emphasised since if investigation of patients with neuromuscular problems is planned as a logical progression, management becomes more effective.

Both of us have a particular interest in neuromuscular disorders. In addition to experience in clinical neurology one of us (M.S.) has a special interest in muscle and nerve pathology and the other (M.S.S.) in clinical neurophysiology. In our clinical practice and research we have approached neuromuscular problems jointly so that it has been possible for us to compare the EMG and pathological data. This approach is used in this book to show how the problems of individual patients can be assessed clinically, physiologically and pathologically. This combined approach can provide an overall understanding of the mechanisms of damage and repair of tissues in neuromuscular disorders.

London, June 1981

Michael Swash
Martin S. Schwartz

Acknowledgements

The production of a book requires the help of many people. We are grateful to the many friends and colleagues who have helped us in the production of this, the third edition. The histological preparations were made, over several years, by Ms Kathleen Fox, Ms Margaret Sargeant, Ms Elaine Cox, and Mr Geoff Vowles at the Institute of Pathology, The Royal London Hospital, and by Mr Peter Dalton at the Department of Pathology, St George's Hospital. Most of the illustrations were prepared by Mr Ivor Northey in the Photographic Department at the St Bartholomew's and The Royal London Hospital School of Medicine and Dentistry. Other illustrations were given us by colleagues in Britain and abroad. We particularly acknowledge Dr K.-G. Henriksson, Linkoping, Sweden, Professor M. B. Pranesh, University of Coimbatore, India, and Professor F. Hentati, Tunis, Tunisia for illustrations of patients seen while visiting their institutions. The manuscript was once again faultlessly prepared by Mrs Adrienne Raine.

Our sustained interest in neuromuscular disorders has been supported by grants from The Wellcome Trust, The Medical Research Council, The London Hospital Research Fund, the St Mark's Research Foundation, The Motor Neurone Disease Association and The Amyotrophic Lateral Sclerosis Association (USA). In addition we have been fortunate to receive benefactions from a number of individuals for which we are particularly grateful. A number of the illustrations are taken from our previous publications in *Brain, Journal of the Neurological Sciences, Journal of Neurology, Neurosurgery and Psychiatry, Neuropathology and Applied Neurobiology, Annals of Neurology, Muscle and Nerve, Clinical Neuropathology, Neuromuscular Disorders, British Journal of Surgery*, and in *Muscle Biopsy Pathology* (second edition published by Chapman and Hall 1991).

We especially thank all the staff at the London office of Springer-Verlag, especially Mr Nick Mowat, Mr Roger Dobbing and Dr Gerald Graham. They have unfailingly supported us in the task of rewriting this book. To Caroline and Lee we express our special thanks; without support at home no task such as this would ever be accomplished.

Contents

1   Clinical Assessment and Measurement 1

General Aspects 1

Onset and Progression 1

Clinical Findings 2

The Application of Genetics to Neuromuscular Disease 11

The Approach to Investigation 12

Biochemical Tests 12

Imaging in Neuromuscular Disorders 15

2   Electromyography, Nerve Conduction and Other Neurophysiological Techniques 19

Electromyographic Assessment 19

Recording Electrodes 19

Concentric Needle Electromyography 22

Single-Fibre EMG 33

Macro EMG 34

Scanning EMG 35

Multi-electrode studies 35

Repetitive Stimulation 36

Surface EMG 36

Nerve Conduction Studies 36

3   Muscle and Nerve Biopsies 43

Muscle Biopsy 43

The Normal Nerve 63

Nerve Biopsy 64

4   Pathophysiological Correlations and Compensatory Mechanisms 69

Pathophysiological Correlations 69

Compensatory Mechanisms 76

5   Classification of Neuromuscular Diseases 85

Main Headings Used in the WFN Classification of Neuromuscular Diseases 85

Classification of Neuromuscular Diseases 85

6   Diseases of Anterior Horn Cells 89

The Spinal Muscular Atrophies 89

Clinical Investigation of Spinal Muscular Atrophies 95

Motor Neuron Disease 103

Other Anterior Horn Cell Disorders 117

7   A Clinical Approach to the Neuropathies... **121**
Clinical Features of Neuropathies 122
Pathological Correlation in Peripheral Neuropathies 124
Positive and Negative Symptoms in Neuropathies................................... 126
Clinical Investigation of Polyneuropathy 129
Principles of Management of Polyneuropathies 131

8   Nerve Entrapment and Compression Syndromes and Other
Mononeuropathies... **133**
Injuries to Nerves.. 133
Upper Limb Syndromes 139
Lower Limb Syndromes... 151
Double-Crush Syndrome.. 155
Adequate Electrophysiological Studies in Entrapment Neuropathies............. 156
Other Mononeuropathies... 156
Mononeuritis Multiplex and Multiple Mononeuropathies 160

9   Nerve Root and Plexus Lesions **161**
Cervical Root Lesions 161
Brachial Plexus Lesions 164
Lumbo-Sacral Root and Plexus Lesions... 167

10   Genetically Determined Neuropathies **173**
The Syndrome of Peroneal Muscular Atrophy.. 174
Hereditary Sensory and Autonomic Neuropathies................................... 184
Other Neuropathies Associated with Genetic Diseases 188
Hereditary Neuropathies with Specific Metabolic Defects....................... 189

11   Acquired Polyneuropathies **201**
Diabetic Neuropathy... 201
Uraemic Neuropathy 207
Hepatic Neuropathy 209
Neuropathies Associated with Alcoholism, Malnutrition, Hypovitaminosis and
    Malabsorption 209
Tropical Ataxic Neuropathy 213
Hypothyroid Neuropathy... 213
Acromegalic Neuropathy 213
Neuropathies Associated with Malignant Disease and Dysproteinaemias........ 214
Neuropathies Associated with Monoclonal Gammopathies...................... 218
Neuropathy Associated with Myeloma 220
Other Neuropathies Associated with Paraproteinaemia............................ 222
Neuropathies Associated with Collagen Vascular Disease......................... 222
Inflammatory Polyradiculoneuropathy... 225
Multifocal Motor Neuropathy 236
Neuropathies Due to Infection 237
Drug-Induced and Toxic Neuropathies.. 247
Drug-Induced Peripheral Neuropathies 250
Peripheral Neuropathy Due to Toxic Chemicals and Metals.................... 252

12   Myasthenia Gravis and Other Myasthenic Syndromes **257**
Myasthenia Gravis 257

Penicillamine-Induced Myasthenia Gravis 275
Lambert–Eaton Myasthenic Syndrome 276
Congenital Myasthenic syndromes 279
Botulism 280
Toxins and Drugs Affecting Neuromuscular Transmission 282

13   Inflammatory Myopathies and Related Disorders 285
Idiopathic Inflammatory Myopathies 285
Aetiology of Inflammatory Muscle Disease 291
Clinical Variants of Inflammatory Myopathy 300
Clinical Criteria for Diagnosis of Polymyositis 301
Treatment and Prognosis 302
Viral Myositis 303
Bacterial Infections and Infestations of Muscle 305
Drug-Induced Inflammatory Myopathies 306
Polymyalgia Rheumatica and Giant Cell Arteritis 306
Graft Versus Host Myositis 306

14   Muscular Dystrophies 307
X-Linked Muscular Dystrophies 307
Limb-Girdle Muscular Dystrophy 325
Congenital Muscular Dystrophy 331
Facio-Scapulo-Humeral Muscular Dystrophy 332
Scapulo-Peroneal Muscular Dystrophy 335
Distal Myopathies 336
Ocular Myopathies 338

15   Myotonic Syndromes 343
The Phenomenon of Myotonia 343
Myotonic Dystrophy 346
Non-Dystrophic Myotonic Syndromes 355
Treatment of Myotonic Syndromes 360
Schwartz–Jampel Syndrome 361
Drug-Induced Myotonia 361
Muscle Contracture Induced by Exercise 362

16   Childhood Myopathies 363
Central Core Disease 363
Multicore Disease 365
Management of Central Core and Multicore Disease 366
Nemaline Myopathy 366
Myotubular (Centronuclear) Myopathy 369
Congenital Fibre-Type Disproportion 371
Other Rare Syndromes 372

17   Inherited Metabolic Myopathies 377
Glycogen Storage Disease 377
Myoadenylate Deaminase Deficiency 386
Mitochondrial Myopathies and Related Disorders 387
Periodic Paralysis 402
Malignant Hyperpyrexia Syndrome 407

Neuroleptic-Malignant Syndrome 410
Myoglobinuria and Rhabdomyolysis 411

18   Endocrine Myopathies 415
Thyroid Myopathies 415
Parathyroid Disorders 419
Adrenal Disorders and Steroid Myopathy 420
Pituitary Disorders 421
Carcinoid Myopathy 423

19   Drug-Induced, Toxic and Nutritional Myopathies 425

20   Cardiomyopathy in Neuromuscular Disorders 433
Primary Diseases of Muscle and Cardiomyopathy 434
Neurogenic Disorders with Cardiomyopathy 438
Endocrine Myopathies 439
Skeletal Muscle in Primary Cardiomyopathies 439
Conclusions 440

21   Miscellaneous Disorders 441
Stiff Man Syndrome 441
Continuous Muscle Fibre Activity Syndrome (Isaacs' Syndrome) and
     Neuromyotonia 442
Rippling Muscle Disease 444
Restless Legs Syndrome 444
Chronic Fatigue Syndrome 444
Primary Fibromyalgia and Overuse Syndrome 446
Disuse 447
Cachexia 447
Ageing 448

References 451

Subject Index 529

Chapter 1

Clinical Assessment and Measurement

Neuromuscular diseases have become better understood as knowledge of the basic processes of neuromuscular function, especially transmission of nervous impulses, the function of the neuromuscular junction and the physical and biochemical processes of muscular contraction, has increased. Indeed, some neuromuscular disorders have themselves led to insights into these basic mechanisms. Huxley (1986) has reviewed the historical background of discoveries in relation to muscular contraction.

General Aspects

In general, neuromuscular disorders cause a limited number of clinical symptoms. Of these, the most prominent are weakness and sensory disturbances. Sensory disturbances occur frequently in patients with peripheral neuropathies. In many neuromuscular disorders other organ systems are involved, giving important clues to diagnosis. For example, the violaceous skin rash of dermatomyositis is particularly associated with this disorder. Muscular pain, cramps, undue fatiguability, muscular atrophy or hypertrophy, fasciculation and stiffness are other major presenting symptoms of neuromuscular disease.

Onset and Progression

The onset and mode of progression of the illness may also suggest a particular diagnosis. Most neuromuscular disorders begin insidiously but some, for example Guillain–Barré syndrome, may present with rapidly progressive proximal weakness. Some disorders are commoner at particular ages; for example Duchenne muscular dystrophy usually presents in early childhood. In other conditions, such as myotonic dystrophy, the clinical presentation differs in infants and in adults. The distribution of symptomatic weakness at the onset may also be important in diagnosis. Diplopia occurring as an isolated symptom in a young woman is a common presentation of myasthenia gravis. However, a single localised symptom or sign such as this is not diagnostic, and diplopia may occur in many different neurological diseases. In myasthenia, however, diplopia is more marked in the evening when the patient is tired and it may be associated with other symptoms or signs of excessive muscular fatigue. Testing for exercise-induced weakness is thus an important part of the assessment of patients with a history of weakness. Sometimes the onset of a neuromuscular disease is associated with another illness. Immobilisation following an accident may bring to light an occult muscular disorder because disuse during bed rest leads to loss of power and to a rapid deterioration of a patient's adaptation to their disorder. Presentation with cardiomyopathy may be the first presentation of certain neuromuscular diseases, e.g. Becker muscular dystrophy, myotonic dystrophy or mitochondrial disease. A febrile illness may herald the onset of polymyositis, or of myasthenia gravis. Most neuromuscular diseases are progressive but some enter a non-progressive phase, usually through compensatory mechanisms rather than arrest of the disease; this phase may last many years. Other disorders may show remissions and relapses, as in myasthenia gravis, chronic relapsing polyradiculoneuritis and polymyositis.

Clinical examination alone may not only fail to establish a cause for a patient's weakness or sensory disturbance, but in some instances of familial disorders early cases may be missed altogether. Minor clinical signs of neuromuscular disease, for example pes cavus, scoliosis and other skeletal deformities, and retinitis pigmentosa, may give important clues to diagnosis and to the occurrence of a familial disorder. Recognition of the early stages of neuromuscular disorders is not always easy, even when the pattern of familial involvement is known from other cases within the family. The clinical features of genetically determined disorders are often modified by factors such as incomplete penetrance and variable age of onset. Ascertainment of affected members of a family must be completed by searching for more specific genetic or biochemical markers and electrophysiological abnormalities, such as a raised creatine kinase level in carriers of Duchenne muscular dystrophy, a raised serum phytanic acid level in those with presymptomatic Refsum's disease, or slowed nerve conduction velocity in the dominantly inherited form of Charcot–Marie–Tooth disease. Electromyography may demonstrate myotonia in siblings of patients with myotonic dystrophy, who otherwise show few stigmata of the disease.

Clinical Findings

Weakness

In assessing the complaint of weakness it is important to look at the patient's strength in relation to the severity, distribution and temporal relationships of the symptom. For example, a "frozen" shoulder secondary to trauma or disuse may lead to weakness and atrophy of the periscapular and deltoid muscles, which is unrelated to local or generalised neuromuscular factors. In myasthenia gravis, weakness may not be apparent at first, becoming evident only when exercise provocation is used. In this condition, particularly, weakness may be ascribed to psychogenic factors unless careful clinical and laboratory investigations are carried out (see Sneddon 1980).

It is tempting to simplify and to regard proximal weakness and atrophy affecting pectoral and pelvic girdle musculature as due to primary muscle disease (myopathy) and distal weakness and atrophy as due to neural causes (neurogenic). Some of the latter cases will be associated with sensory symptoms and signs, leading to a diagnosis of peripheral neuropathy. Neurogenic atrophy from primary degenerative disease of the anterior horn cells in adults often presents as distal atrophy, but in some patients proximal weakness is the major presenting feature. Similarly, acute polyradiculoneuritis usually presents with proximal involvement. Most of these disorders produce symmetrical clinical features, but variable degrees of asymmetry are frequent, even in biochemically determined disorders such as acid maltase deficiency.

Proximal weakness is most frequently noticed first in the legs. The patient complains of difficulty in walking, either because of unexpected fatigue or because of difficulty climbing stairs or walking on rough ground or over obstacles. Sometimes the postural adjustment associated with entering buses and trains leads to difficulty because one leg must be lifted onto a high step and then this limb must be used as a fulcrum to raise the body weight up onto the step. Low chairs pose a particular problem and patients with proximal weakness learn to avoid them because they cannot get up from them without assistance. Similarly it is difficult for patients with proximal weakness to get into or out of a bath without assistance. Most patients with longstanding proximal weakness learn to adapt their lives to their disability. Gowers, in 1879, described a characteristic manoeuvre by which the patient with Duchenne muscular dystrophy rises from the sitting position on the floor by first turning over onto hands and knees, then straightening the legs and arching the back before rising to the upright position by "climbing up" the thighs, pushing with the hands and arms. Variations of this manoeuvre are often used by patients with severe proximal weakness when getting up from a chair. Many such patients push with their arms on their thighs just above the knees to help knee extension (Fig. 1.1).

Most patients with proximal weakness have an abnormal gait. This is wide-based and waddling in character, because the glutei and paraspinal muscles are unable to stabilise the pelvis when one foot is taking a step so that the load of the body weight is taken on one side of the pelvis. The lumbar spine becomes excessively lordotic in the erect position, as a compensatory response, bringing the centre of gravity forward to stabilise the gleno-humeral joints. This change in centre of gravity alters the stresses on other joints, particularly the knee joints, which often become hyperextended (genu recurvatum). In time this leads to instability of the knees, an additional factor leading to difficulty in walking. In advanced cases, especially those beginning in childhood, thoracic scoliosis develops, due to paraspinal muscular weakness, and the consequent deformity may lead to additional disabilities.

Inability to run or jump is often an early symptom of proximal weakness of the legs. Watching the patient jumping or hopping is a very useful clinical test. Even when the patient's legs appear relatively

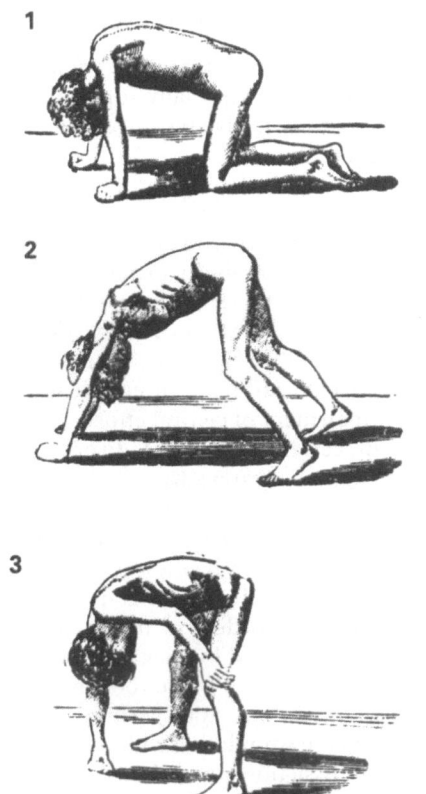

Fig. 1.1. Gowers' manoeuvre. Three stages in rising from the floor in a patient with Duchenne muscular dystrophy. The child seems to "climb up his legs" in order to compensate for the effects of weakness of the hip extensors (from Gowers 1886).

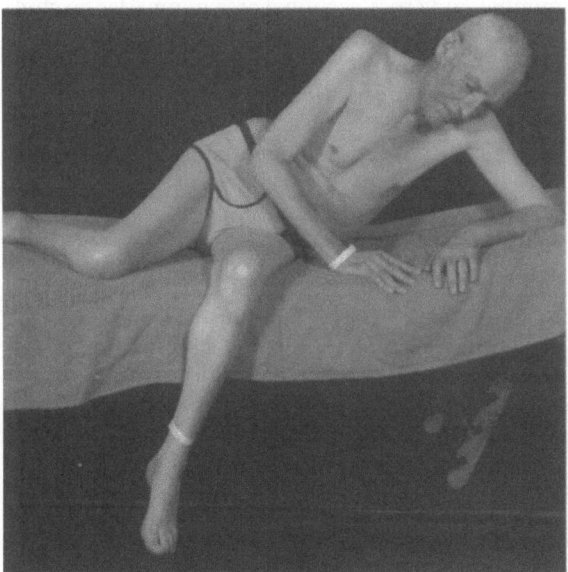

Fig. 1.2. This man with life-long proximal weakness, due to multicore myopathy, has adapted to his disability, as in this method of rising from a couch to the sitting position.

strong on formal examination, hopping and jumping may be performed poorly. It is particularly important to watch for instability of the pelvis and to notice whether the patient's heel touches the floor as he lands during hopping. In adults the ability to sit up from the supine position (Fig. 1.2), the arms remaining folded, is a useful test of the axial and pelvic musculature. In children this test is usually performed from the lying or sitting position, on the floor, when it forms a test based on Gowers' description of the typical functional disability of Duchenne muscular dystrophy. Rising from a low chair should be observed, and any assistance from arm pressure on the chair's arms should be noted. Shortening of the Achilles tendon, a feature of Duchenne muscular dystrophy and of various motor neuropathies, especially slowly progressive heredo-familial neuropathies, leads to inability to place the heel squarely on the floor so that the patient tends to walk on the ball of the foot. This may be associated with a pes equino-varus or pes cavus deformity. In spinal muscular atrophies, on the other hand, pes planus is common, the feet being placed in an everted position (Dubowitz 1995).

Weakness of neck muscles is a common component of proximal weakness and can be tested directly. Sometimes a patient may notice weakness of these muscles by loss of the ability to lift the head from the pillow without help. This is often particularly marked in myasthenia gravis and is an important sign in management of this disease because it is often accompanied by weakness of respiratory muscles. In myotonic dystrophy the neck flexor muscles are also particularly affected.

In the arms proximal weakness results in inability to lift the arms above the shoulders so that the patient cannot reach up to objects on high shelves, hang clothes on a line to dry, use a hairbrush or reach the back in dressing. Weakness of arm extension and abduction can easily be tested, and the deltoids may be very atrophic. When there is weakness in this distribution, weakness of the periscapular and serratus anterior muscles is usually also present; this can be shown by the prominence of the scapulae at rest and by the marked scapular winging that develops when the arms are outstretched, or when the patient is asked to push the outstretched arm against resistance. Weakness of biceps and triceps muscles is usually less severe and since these muscles are not of such great functional importance as the deltoid, functional deficits are not as great. In addition, most patients learn to compensate for weakness in these muscles by developing "trick" movements.

Facial muscle weakness and atrophy may easily be missed if it is symmetrical (Fig. 1.3). The facial

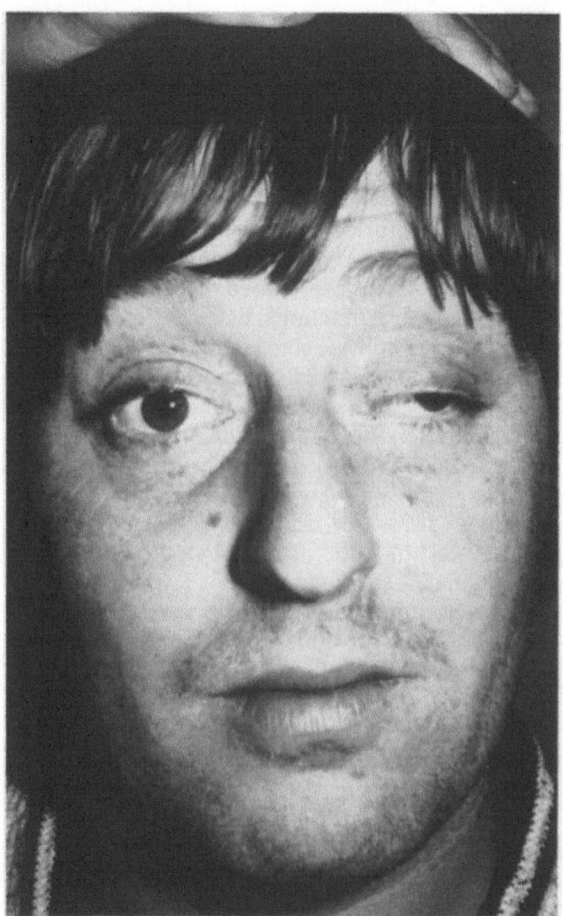

Fig. 1.3. Myasthenic facies. There is asymmetrical ptosis, with an external strabismus (exophoria) and bilateral facial weakness causing flattening of the nasolabial folds and a weak smile.

expression becomes less mobile, the lips tend to be parted and more prominent, and the tongue may protrude a little. Ptosis occurs as part of an external ophthalmoplegia in patients with neuromuscular disorders involving external ocular muscles, especially in myasthenia gravis.

Weakness can arise from neural or myopathic disease. Neural weakness can be due either to an upper motor neuron disturbance due to inadequate activation of spinal motor neurons or due to lower motor neuron disease, involving anterior horn cells, lower motor neuron axons or motor end-plate disorders. The degree of upper motor neuron weakness can be determined by comparing force generated by electrical excitation of peripheral nerve, e.g. a tetanic stimulus, with that generated by voluntary activity. The latter will be limited not only by the biology of the system but by "functional" factors related to perceived effort (Haughton et al. 1994).

Quantitative Assessment of Muscular Strength

With the advent of treatments for some neuromuscular diseases, and especially for clinical trials of new treatments, objective measurement of muscular force is essential.

Any assessment of force production in muscle must be interpreted in the context of the overall clinical problem. Patients with spasticity, sensory loss, restriction of joint mobility or joint pain will often not be able to develop full force and the contribution of muscle weakness due to motor system disease needs to be carefully considered. In addition patients may not develop full force in muscle groups when there is impairment of central effort, e.g. in depression or in certain functional disorders, such as chronic fatigue syndrome. Neuromuscular diseases, of course, commonly present with weakness or fatigue, the major *impairments of function*.

Voluntary contraction assesses the whole neuromuscular system including sensory feedback. The contribution of disorders of motor cortex can be qualitatively evaluated by magnetic stimulation of the cortex, disorders of nerve roots by electrical or magnetic stimulation and peripheral nerves by peripheral nerve stimulation with recording of compound muscle action potentials, F wave latencies and motor nerve conduction velocity. Neuromuscular transmission can be assessed by repetitive nerve stimulation and single fibre EMG. The contractile properties of muscle fibres and the propagation velocity of individual fibres can also be studied. Force production is dependent, finally, on the number and cross-sectional area of muscles, excluding fatty and fibrous tissue; but in neurogenic disorders non-innervated muscle fibres are not available for contraction. Computed tomography, magnetic resonance imaging and ultrasound have all been used for assessment of muscle bulk.

The Medical Research Council Scale. The MRC scale (Medical Research Council 1943, 1983) is much used and has the advantage of simplicity, although it is clearly ordinal, rather than linear (Table 1.1). It is sometimes helpful to further subdivide Grade 4 MRC strength on a simple proportionate basis, for example grade 4.50 or 50% of normal strength.

Table 1.1. Medical Research Council scale

Grade 0	No contraction visible
Grade 1	Flicker or trace of contraction only
Grade 2	Active movement at a joint possible with gravity eliminated
Grade 3	Active movement possible against gravity
Grade 4	Active movement possible against gravity and resistance
Grade 5	Normal strength

The MRC scale is weighted for assessment of minimal clinical activation of a muscle because it was devised for use in patients with peripheral nerve injuries sustained in wartime. The rapid development of even a flicker of movement in such patients was of great prognostic importance. The MRC scale is a poor instrument for detecting mild to moderate weakness in powerful muscles. Beasley (1956) found that clinically normal knee extensor strength was in fact reduced by up to 50% in children with polio when tested by dynamometry. Furthermore, the ability to overcome gravity requires different muscular strengths in different muscle groups. Van der Ploeg et al. (1984) found that 3% of the force output of the biceps brachii is represented in MRC Grades 0–3, but 99% is represented by Grades 4–5, illustrating the non-linear structure of this instrument.

The MRC scale can be adapted to test defined movements of a joint, rather than strength of individual muscles. Other functional scales have been devised, principally for use in assessing children with muscular dystrophy (Vignos et al. 1963). In a clinical study of the course of Duchenne muscular dystrophy 34 different movements were evaluated using the MRC scale and the reproducibility of this method between examiners was found to be excellent (Brooke et al. 1981).

Dynamometry. Quantitative measurements of isometric muscle strength provide valuable data. Much of the apparatus used for these measurements is complex, requiring special transducers and rigs to be applied to limbs under test (Edwards et al. 1977), and measurements of torque output during *maximal* voluntary contraction of a muscle, e.g. quadriceps (Tornvall 1963; Scott et al. 1982). A simpler method employs a hand-held myometer (Edwards and McDonnell 1974; Hosking et al. 1976; Scott et al. 1982). This instrument, the Hammersmith myometer, consists of a small displacement transducer and a battery-powered amplifier providing a digital readout of force expressed as kilograms. The myometer is especially useful in clinical practice since it can measure very small forces, and it is easily held interposed between the examiner's arm and the muscle group to be tested during the ordinary process of clinical examination. As a consequence serial measurements of strength in various selected muscles can be made during the course of a disease and its treatment (Edwards et al. 1979, 1986). This technique has the advantage that the examiner has the opportunity directly to assess the patient regarding hesitancy of contraction, slowness of contraction as in extrapyramidal disease, and the presence of other factors, e.g. pain, spasticity,

sensory defect or undue fatigue. The muscle tested should be tested to the point that its isometric force is "broken" by the examiner's arm strength.

Van der Ploeg et al. (1991) described reference values for hand-held dynamometry in 13 muscle groups, using standardised dynanometer placements. Each muscle group was tested three times, at 10-second intervals. The reproducibility of the test results was high, particularly in testers with long experience (Goonatilleke et al. 1994). The mean isometric strength in women is about two-thirds that of men. Van der Ploeg and Oosterhuis (1991) pointed out that in patients with functional weakness the "make" contraction force was about 20% less than the "break" contraction force, a result confirming the recognised clinical observation. Hand-held dynamometry was validated by Wiles et al. (1990) in a study of 19 patients with myositis. Dynamometry carried out in a fixed test rig, e.g. a rigid chair, has also been shown to be reliable in the clinical evaluation and follow-up of patients with neuromuscular disorders (Wiles and Karni 1983).

The Tufts Quantitative Neuromuscular Examination (TQNE). A somewhat different approach to measurement of strength was taken by Munsat and colleagues at the Tufts New England Medical Center. Multiple assessments, involving measurements of pulmonary function, oropharyngeal function, timed hand activities, isometric arm strength and isometric leg strength at several joints, were used to derive a composite score, called the "megascore", that would be useful in within-patient and across-patient comparisons, and so for use in clinical trials. This was developed with the particular aim of evaluating patients with amyotrophic lateral sclerosis (ALS), thus accounting for the inclusion of pulmonary and oropharyngeal tests (Table 1.2).

The isometric muscle strength is measured by taking the maximum voluntary isometric contraction (MVIC) force as the end-point of assessment. This has been extensively studied in men and women of different ages. Men are stronger than women after the second decade of life, and hamstring strength decreases after the fifth decade in both sexes. Quadriceps strength tends to decrease in women after the second decade. The MVIC has been used by a number of different observers, and normal data are available for at least 10 different muscles in the arm, and another 10 muscles in the leg (Jones 1947; Beasley 1961; Edwards et al. 1977; Shaunak et al. 1987). The technique now commonly used utilises a fixed rig for isometric strength testing with strain gauges and computer data storage and analysis (Brooks et al. 1991; Brooks et al. 1994). The method and its statistical manipulation using a Z

Table 1.2. TQNE protocol, assessed in studies of motor neuron disease (ALS)

		Abbreviation		No. of tests
A	*Pulmonary function*			
	Forced vital capacity	FVC		1
	Maximal voluntary ventilation	MVV		1
B	*Oropharyngeal*			
	Time to repeat "pa" 20 times	pa		1
	Time to repeat "pata" 15 times	pata		1
C	*Timed hand activities*			
	Time dialling telephone number	phone	R/L	2
	Number of pegs placed in a Purdue pegboard in 30 seconds	pegbd	R/L	2
D	*Isometric arm strength*			
	Shoulder extension	Shdext	R/L	2
	Shoulder flexion	Shdflex	R/L	2
	Elbow extension	Elbext	R/L	2
	Elbow flexion	Elflex	R/L	2
	Grip strength	Grip	R/L	2
E	*Isometric leg strength*			
	Hip flexion	Hipflex	R/L	2
	Hip extension	Hipext	R/L	2
	Knee extension	Kneext	R/L	2
	Knee flexion	Kneflex	R/L	2
	Ankle dorsi flexion	Dorsifl	R/L	2
			Total	28

Both sides of the body tested.
"Best of 2 trials" was used in all tests for data analysis.
An electronic strain-gauge tensiometer was used to assess strength.
Grip strength was assessed by a Jamar dynamometer.

transformation has been discussed by Andres et al. (1986, 1988).

The Z score represents the raw data score, minus the population mean score, divided by the population standard deviation of the score. In deriving an overall "megascore" the mean of the two scores for individual subtests is used to compare data over time in individual patients (the "megaslope") using a least squares regression analysis. The megascore thus represents averaged, smoothed data, and there is controversy as to whether this statistical manipulation has value in clinical assessment of deterioration or improvement in a clinical situation or trial, since it hides marked variance in individual data points. MVIC measurements in arm and leg muscle have been used in the assessment of several different neuromuscular diseases, and may prove useful in clinical trials, although the statistical treatment of the raw data used in such trials needs further critical study.

Functional Rating Scales. Rating scales are attractive to clinicians and physiotherapists since they may measure functional ability. It must be recognised that such scales take no account of the manner in which a task is performed, for example, a patient may get up from a chair in a very abnormal or unusual fashion, but still be capable of this function and thus "pass the test". Dubowitz et al. (1986)

found that myometry and MRC scores have a greater statistical power in Duchenne dystrophy than walking times, time to loss of ambulation or motor ability tests. Intervals to events such as these are finite, and do not change continuously in time, leading to an indirect relationship between strength and function.

Timed tests often used in neuromuscular disorders include a timed walk, climbing and descending stairs, rising from a chair or from lying supine, and peg board tests (Louwerse et al. 1990). Disability scales include measures of self-care, physical activity and role activities both in the social and working environments. These are often termed Activities of Daily Living (ADL) scales. Dressing, grooming, bathing, toileting, walking, climbing stairs, transferring from bed to chair, feeding and continence are usually included, e.g. in the Barthel scale (Mahoney and Barthel 1965), an index much used in cerebro-vascular disease (Wade and Langton-Hewer 1987; Wade 1993). Many other scales have been used, e.g. the Rankin scale, the Kurtzke scale in multiple sclerosis research, and various scales in Parkinson's disease. In motor neuron disease the Norris scale and the Appel scale, both composite indices including parts of the neurological examination, strength measurements and performance indices have been used in clinical trials. These scales, of course, are non-linear, ordinal measures that are subject to certain interpretational and statistical limitations.

Functional grading using a modified disability scale has been used in assessment of Duchenne muscular dystrophy. Different scales of functional disturbance were used for arms and shoulders, and hips and legs respectively (Brooke et al. 1983). This scale is too detailed for ordinary use but provides a basis for quantitative clinical evaluation of other neuromuscular disorders (Table 1.3).

Timed functional tests: measurements can be made of the time taken to stand from the supine position, to climb a set number of stairs or to run or walk a set distance (e.g. 10 metres), as well as of the time needed for other appropriate tasks such as dressing (Brooke et al. 1981, 1983).

Pulmonary function tests can be adapted to the assessment of neuromuscular diseases, particularly since normal values are available for subjects of different age, sex and body habitus (Griggs et al. 1981; Swash et al. 1985). The vital capacity, consisting of inspiratory capacity and expiratory reserve volume, is the simplest and most reliable measure (Macklem 1986) and this can be used as a sensitive index of progress in patients with weakness of the respiratory musculature. When vital capacity is less than 13–15 ml/kg body weight mechanical ventilation

Table 1.3. Functional grades used for assessment of Duchenne muscular dystrophy in clinical trials

Arms and shoulders	Hips and legs
1. Starting with arms at the sides, patient can abduct the arms in a full circle until they touch above the head	1. Walks and climbs stairs without assistance
2. Can raise arms above head only by flexing the elbow (i.e. shortening the circumference of the movement) or by using accessory muscles	2. Walks and climbs stairs with aid of railing
3. Cannot raise hands above head but can raise a 250 g glass of water to mouth (using both hands if necessary)	3. Walks and climbs stairs slowly with aid of railing (over 12 seconds for four standard stairs)
4. Can raise hands to mouth but cannot raise 250 g (8 oz) glass of water	4. Walks unassisted and rises from chair but cannot climb stairs
5. Cannot raise hand to mouth but can use hands to hold pen or pick up pennies from table	5. Walks unassisted but cannot rise from chair or climb stairs
6. Cannot raise hands to mouth and has no useful function of hands	6. Walks only with assistance or walks independently with long leg braces
	7. Walks in long leg braces but requires assistance for balance
	8. Stands in long leg braces but unable to walk even with assistance
	9. Is in wheelchair
	10. Is confined to bed

From Brooke et al. (1983).

should be instituted. Peak flow measurements are much less reproducible. Weakness of respiratory muscles is especially important in Guillain–Barré syndrome, myasthenia gravis and botulism; it may also be relevant in chronic disorders, such as acid maltase deficiency, motor neuron disease and the muscular dystrophies, and in these conditions evaluation of ventilation during sleep may be useful.

Fatiguability

Fatigue is a normal phenomenon, well known to everyone. Fatigue, nonetheless, is an elusive experience, difficult to measure, treat, describe or prevent (Rabinbach 1991). It consists of failure to generate the required or expected force during sustained or repeated contraction (Edwards 1986). It is most striking in myasthenia gravis, in which it is the cardinal symptom (Chap. 12). Fatigue may also occur in diseases of anterior horn cells, e.g. motor neuron disease, in disorders of peripheral nerves and in diseases of the muscle fibres themselves. The latter may be due to metabolic disturbances of energy utilisation, as in McArdle's myophosphorylase deficiency, or to disturbances of excitation–contraction coupling, as in disorders of mitochondrial oxidation. It is also prominent in hypocalcaemia, as in nutritional osteomalacia, in which muscle fibre excitation is disturbed. In the latter disorders, patients are weak and easily fatigued, but in some metabolic disorders initial muscular contractions develop normal force but fatigue sets in rapidly, as in myasthenia gravis, and in metabolic disorders of muscle. Fatigue also occurs when many muscle fibres have been destroyed, and there is a smaller reserve of muscle tissue available for force generation. The remaining muscle fibres are required to work more or less at their metabolic limits (Edwards et al. 1982b).

Exercise and training can modify the development of fatigue during exertion, and this effect is accompanied by changes in muscle enzyme content (see Chap. 2). In most instances of muscular fatigue in everyday life muscle contraction will occur with normal force when evoked by tetanic electrical stimulation of a peripheral nerve, at a time when the subject feels subjectively fatigued and tired, illustrating the importance of central factors in this subjective complaint (Bigland-Ritchie and Woods 1984). *Subjective fatigue* is a sense of weariness due to bodily or mental exertion; *objective fatigue* is a decline in muscle force resulting from exertion.

In fatigued muscle, tension is maintained by recruiting motor units additional to those normally required to maintain tension. There is thus a regrouping of motor unit discharges so that a greater proportion of units fire nearly synchronously. A course tremor may thus appear in fatigued muscle. Type 1 motor units are relatively better adapted to continued activity and must be called on during continual activity leading to fatigue.

In neuromuscular diseases fatigue may result from the same factors as in normal subjects, but the fundamental abnormalities associated with individual diseases will determine the cause and outcome of the fatigue (Table 1.4). Weak muscles are almost always abnormally fatiguable, and fatigue is therefore a feature of almost all neuromuscular disorders. The importance of fatigue as a symptom lies

Table 1.4. Causes of fatigue

Reduced central drive
    Psychogenic disturbances
    Brain lesions, e.g. stroke
    Multiple sclerosis, Parkinson's disease
Peripheral neuropathy
Disturbances of neuromuscular transmission
Metabolic muscle disease
Loss of muscle fibres, or cachexia
Chronic fatigue (effort) syndrome

in its place as the cardinal feature of disorders of neuromuscular transmission, especially myasthenia gravis, but it is also a major feature of certain metabolic myopathies, for example McArdle's disease and the mitochondrial myopathies, and it may be an important symptom in some patients with motor neuron disease. Fatiguability can usually be described by patients in terms of their exercise tolerance in repetitive tasks, and it is often useful to examine individual muscles in such tasks. Climbing stairs, repeated extension or abduction movements of the arm against resistance, repeated clenching of the fist, or maintained maximal upward gaze are useful clinical manoeuvres. Such tests can be used as standardised measures of the progress of a disease or of a patient's response to treatment. Bigland-Ritchie and Woods (1984) have defined neuromuscular fatigue as any reduction in force-generating capacity, regardless of the force required in the given situation. It has been noted (Editorial 1981) that the intensity of the perception of fatigue is not predictable from any simple physiological tests; it derives partly from the actual weakness and partly from a discrepancy between perceived effort and outcome, and perhaps also from something about fatigued muscles that can be sensed, even when they are not in use (see Chap. 4).

Fatigue can be measured by reduction in force or work capacity during exercise (Bigland-Ritchie et al. 1986), and is accompanied by a shift in the EMG power spectrum, with slowed mean frequency of EMG activity and slow conduction velocity in individual muscle fibres. In addition, hydrogen ion, lactate and other metabolites, such as ammonia, accumulate in fatigued muscle (Hakkinen and Komi 1983; Bigland-Ritchie and Woods 1984; Eberstein and Beattie 1985).

In normal subjects, highly motivated to exercise physiology, fatigue is not due to failure of neuromuscular transmission (Merton et al. 1981) or to failure of central drive (Belanger and McComas 1981), but is probably due to reduction or inequality in the rate of adenosine triphosphate (ATP) and phosphocreatine supply in relation to metabolic needs (Wilkie 1981) and the accumulation of lactic acid leading to intracellular acidosis (Berzelius 1848; Arnold et al. 1984). During fatigue slowing of muscle contraction speed shifts the force/frequency relation to a lower range, allowing all motor units to remain activated despite a substantial reduction in motor neuron firing rates, and preventing supratetanic effects that would result if the initial frequency was maintained (Bigland-Ritchie and Woods 1984). Reduction in discharge rates also safeguards against failure of neuromuscular transmission in fatigue. Clearly, if any of these mechan-

isms is disturbed, by disease of muscle cells, by biochemical abnormalities in energy metabolism causing reduced ATP and phosphocreatine production, e.g. McArdle's disease, by impaired neuromuscular transmission, e.g. in myasthenia gravis, or in other slowly progressive motor disorders such as motor neuron disease, or by abnormalities in motor transmission in the central or peripheral nervous system excessive fatigue will result. At some of the vulnerable steps in force generation, especially impaired neuromuscular transmission, effective treatment is possible. Training may be useful in improving the biochemical performance of oxidative metabolism, and of degradation of metabolic products in muscle fibres, and may not only improve force generation in normal subjects, but also in patients with neuromuscular diseases. Improvement in cardiovascular status is part of this response to training.

In *metabolic fatigue* the force produced by maximal isometric voluntary contracture declines by 80% within a few minutes, but returns nearly to normal after about 10 minutes' rest. This rapidly reversible fatigue is related to the metabolic disturbance of the contractile process resulting from continuous maximal activity. This correlates fairly well with increasing intracellular acidosis and of diprotonated phosphate (H_2PO_4) levels that interfere with the generation of force by myofilaments (Miller et al. 1987; Boska et al. 1990).

Wasting and Hypertrophy

There is no invariable correlation between atrophy of a muscle and weakness. In some instances wasting may be pronounced before the patient recognises that weakness is significant. This is a particular feature of neurogenic disorders, in which individual muscles may be involved relatively selectively, neighbouring muscles being virtually spared. Other compensatory factors, such as fibre hypertrophy and collateral reinnervation (Chap. 4), are important. In other disorders, such as myasthenia gravis and osteomalacic myopathy, weakness may be severe although muscle bulk is virtually normal. Muscle atrophy is rapid, and may be severe, after joint immobilisation, e.g. after a limb fracture, or after a period of prolonged bed rest.

In severe systemic illnesses, such as cachexia associated with malnutrition, tuberculosis or cancer, pronounced muscular wasting may occur. This is associated with reduction in subcutaneous fat, so that the general shape of individual muscles, although they are thinner than normal, is preserved. Further, most such patients show little or no mus-

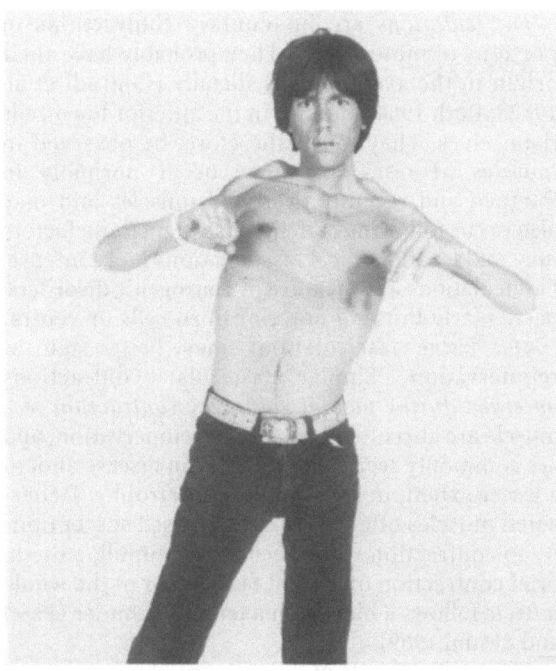

Fig. 1.4. Proximal muscle wasting, with riding up of scapulae and abnormal stance, in facio-scapulo-humeral muscular dystrophy.

cular weakness on formal testing. In proximal weakness due to neuromuscular disease, affected muscles are often atrophic (Fig. 1.4), but in some disorders hypertrophy or pseudohypertrophy may be found. Pseudohypertrophic muscles feel rubbery and firmer than normal, and on contraction do not change shape and tension in the same way as a normal muscle or a muscle with true hypertrophy. Further, they are often markedly weak. Pseudohypertrophy is a feature of Duchenne, Becker and limb-girdle muscular dystrophies. It is also seen in hypothyroid myopathy. In Duchenne dystrophy the calves, deltoids and vastus lateralis are particularly likely to show this abnormality. Histological examination of pseudohypertrophic muscle shows replacement of muscle fibres by fatty and fibrous tissue, although some of the remaining fibres may be hypertrophied.

Rarely, there may be congenital absence of individual muscles; the inferior part of the pectoral muscle is frequently affected, often unilaterally. Hypertrophy of muscles occurs with exercise, and studies of humans and other species have shown that this work-induced muscle hypertrophy is due to hypertrophy of individual fibres, with increased numbers of myofibrils in the hypertrophied fibres, but without increase in the number of fibres in the hypertrophied muscle (Denny-Brown 1960; Edstrom and Grimby 1986). Hypertrophy is also a feature of congenital myotonic disorders. Hypertrophy of individual muscles, e.g. calf muscles, may occur uncommonly in patients with root lesions, and sometimes also in spinal muscular atrophy.

Tone and Reflexes

Although muscle tone is usually somewhat reduced in patients with weakness from neuromuscular disease, this observation is of no great importance in diagnosis. In children reduced tone has been used as a major feature of a group of disorders – the "floppy infant syndrome" – but here also reduced tone has proved to be non-specific since it may occur in cerebral palsy, neuropathies, myopathies, neurogenic disorders and in ligamentous disorders such as Ehlers–Danlos syndrome.

The tendon reflexes are generally preserved, if somewhat reduced, in myopathies. However, in Duchenne muscular dystrophy the reflexes are lost in the arms and at the knees, though retained at the ankles, and in spinal muscular atrophy of infantile onset they are usually absent. In adult spinal muscular atrophy they are usually present. The finding of increased tendon reflexes in an atrophic muscle suggests combined upper and lower motor neuron lesions, a feature of motor neuron disease. In polymyositis, osteomalacic myopathy and myasthenia gravis the tendon reflexes are usually preserved, even when weakness is severe, but in Guillain-Barré syndrome (acute infective polyradiculoneuritis) the reflexes are characteristically absent even when weakness is only slight.

In peripheral neuropathies, distal tendon reflexes, especially the ankle jerks, are usually absent. This is especially true of axonal neuropathies; in demyelinating neuropathies all the tendon reflexes may be reduced or absent. In the elderly the ankle jerks are often reduced but this may have no pathological significance.

In hypothyroidism the tendon reflexes may show a characteristic prolongation of their relaxation phase.

Pain and Cramps

It is useful to differentiate between muscular pain at rest and on exercise. Muscular pain at rest is usually a dull discomfort or ache, which may be accompanied by tenderness on palpation. It occurs in polymyositis and in viral infections but may also occur in neurogenic disorders such as Guillain-Barré syndrome and, in the arms, as a presenting feature of neuralgic amyotrophy. In polymyalgia rheumatica pain, tenderness and stiffness, usually principally affecting the shoulder, are major features. Muscle pain may be focal or diffuse. Focal muscle pain, as in "fibrositis" or in chronic fatigue syndrome, rarely has a definable cause, although Bartels and Danneskiold-Samsøe (1986) reported an excess of reticulin and elastin fibres, constricting muscle fibres.

Muscular pain on exertion occurs mainly in certain myopathies. The commonest cause, however, is intermittent claudication from peripheral vascular disease. Radicular and low back pain, with aching, numbness and weakness in the distal parts of the legs, occurs in claudication of the cauda equina in people with lumbo-sacral canal stenosis. Exertional muscular pain, often associated with cramps, may be the major feature of certain metabolic myopathies, e.g. McArdle's disease (myophosphorylase deficiency), and in hypothyroidism. These symptoms often become more severe with continued exercise. In a study of 70 patients with weakness, fatigue or cramp the ischaemic exercise test revealed three cases of myophosphorylase deficiency, one of - myoadenylate deaminase deficiency and one of mitochondrial myopathy (Coleman et al. 1986). Myoglobinuria may occur in some such patients.

Cramp consists of painful involuntary spasm, involving part or the whole of a muscle. Cramps may be triggered by exercise or muscle contraction, but nocturnal cramp often appears to arise spontaneously. Although cramps may occur in normal people, they are unusually prominent in neurogenic disorders, and in metabolic disturbances, especially hypothyroidism, hyponatraemia and uraemia. They are usually associated with high-frequency electromyographic (EMG) activity in the affected muscle fascicles, but in McArdle's myophosphorylase deficiency cramps are electrically silent. The site of origin of cramps is uncertain but Denny-Brown (1953) suggested they arise in the distal part of intramuscular nerve terminals (Layzer 1985a). Most cramps are self-limited, and can be relieved by passive stretch of the affected muscle. Prolonged cramps may cause myoglobinuria, and elevation of the creatine kinase (CK) level. Layzer (1994) has reviewed the pathophysiology of cramp.

Fasciculation, Myotonia, Myokymia and Myoedema

Involuntary muscular contraction in neuromuscular disease must be distinguished from involuntary movement disorders associated with diseases of the central nervous system, that is, from chorea, myoclonus, etc.

Fasciculations are involuntary contractions of portions of motor units. They probably have their origin in the axon, usually distally (Conradi et al. 1982a; Roth 1984) and not in the anterior horn cells themselves. They must, therefore, be observed in muscles *at rest*. They may occur normally in fatigued and recently exercised muscles and may also occur following caffeine ingestion; these factors may make pathological fasciculations more intense. Fasciculations are a feature of neurogenic disorders, particularly those of anterior horn cells or ventral roots. Large fasciculations may be a sign of reinnervation. Similar fascicular contractions *observed during partial voluntary contraction* of a muscle are also often evidence of reinnervation, and are commonly seen in motor neuron disease and, to a lesser extent, in spinal muscular atrophy. Denervated muscles often show an increased susceptibility to contraction with mechanical stimuli; a brisk, brief contraction of several fasciculi or of the whole muscle follows a blow with a tendon hammer (Patel and Swami 1969).

Myotonia consists of impairment of normal muscular relaxation following voluntary contraction, or electrical or mechanical stimulation. It can be demonstrated by slowness of relaxation of muscles after contraction: for example, by slowness of relaxation of the grip, or by persistence of eye closure. Sometimes percussion of a muscle with a tendon hammer may evoke a persistent dimple of myotonic contraction in the muscle. Myotonia is a feature of myotonia congenita and of myotonic dystrophy. It also occurs in periodic paralysis. Electromyographically it must be differentiated from complex repetitive discharges and from neuromyotonia.

Neuromyotonia consists of continuous muscle fibre activity causing continuous muscle rippling and stiffness. It may be generalised or localised to a particular group of muscles, and can be so severe as to cause permanent joint deformity.

Myokymia is involuntary, repeated, worm-like or quivering contraction of part of a muscle. It occurs in many different disorders, most of which have a neurogenic basis, including neuropathies, but may be benign, not signifying disease.

Myoedema is a ridge-like elevation, preceded by a depression, occurring at the site of percussion and lasting several seconds. It is found in cachectic states and in myxoedema.

Sensory Disturbances in Neuromuscular Disorders

Sensory disturbances are a characteristic feature of peripheral neuropathy, and they are often the first and the presenting complaint. In most neuropathies there is distal impairment of all sensory modalities and this is typically found in a "glove and stocking" distribution. In some neuropathies *paraesthesiae* (pins and needles sensations) may be experienced in this distribution; this sensation may be uncomfortable (*dysaesthesiae*), especially when the feet or fingers make prolonged contact with hard surfaces, or even painful (*hyperpathia*). Certain neuropathies have characteristic sensory abnormalities, e.g. the burning, painful feet of alcoholic neuropathy. In mononeuropathies sensory disturbance is found in the distribution of the nerve affected; the anatomical distribution of sensory nerves must be carefully distinguished from the dermatomes mapped out by the individual nerve roots.

Quantitative methods for sensory testing have been devised, using threshold determinations for mechanical and temperature (heat and cold) stimuli (Dyck 1993), in order to provide continuous data from clinical examination during the natural history or treatment of neuropathies (Fowler et al. 1987; Verdugo and Ochoa 1992). Large fibre function can be assessed by mechanical and vibration thresholds and by sensory conduction studies and EMG, and small fibre function by warming and cooling thresholds. Autonomic nervous system function can be assessed by specific assessment.

Examination of Peripheral Nerves

In patients with peripheral neuropathies, or mononeuropathies, it is important to examine the nerves themselves. The ulnar nerve may be palpated in the olecranon groove, the superficial branch of the radial nerve can be felt as it passes over the head of the radius at the wrist, the common peroneal nerve is superficially located at the head of the fibula, the sural nerve is palpable on the upper part of the Archilles tendon and sometimes also on the lateral aspect of the foot, and small cutaneous branches of the greater auricular and digital nerves of the dorsal surfaces of the hands can also sometimes be felt if enlarged. Nerve hypertrophy occurs particularly in leprosy, and in other demyelinating neuropathies, e.g. Charcot–Marie–Tooth syndrome (HMSN Type 1); localised nerve lesions, as in ulnar neuritis, may be accompanied by localised nerve enlargement. In von Recklinghausen's disease multiple peripheral neuromata may be palpable on the peripheral nerves. The nerves are characteristically diffusely and focally enlarged in leprosy, and in this disease depigmentation and pigmentation of skin is also a feature.

Localised trauma to a peripheral nerve, whether due to external injury, to nerve compression or entrapment may be demonstrated by eliciting Tinel's sign: light percussion with a finger at the point of nerve damage, or at the site of a regenerating nerve trunk, results in an electric, shooting sensation in the distribution of the nerve. The sign is particularly useful in nerve regeneration but, since it can often be elicited at sites of potential entrapment in normal subjects, it is an unreliable test in patients with chronic entrapment syndromes.

Involvement of Other Systems

In many neuromuscular disorders other organ systems may be involved. This may occur as a primary manifestation, such as cardiomyopathy in Friedreich's ataxia or Duchenne muscular dystrophy; as a manifestation of an underlying causative disorder, such as diabetes mellitus in a patient with peripheral neuropathy, or rheumatoid arthritis in the carpal tunnel syndrome; or as a secondary effect, such as the contractures and deformities found in patients with muscular dystrophy.

The Application of Genetics to Neuromuscular Disease

Recent advances in genetics have led to more accurate diagnosis of, for example, Becker muscular dystrophy, the myotonic syndromes, and the hereditary motor and sensory neuropathies. Prior to the development of knowledge concerning the genetic localisation of these disorders, and the availability of precise DNA-based tests for the genetic defect, the various clinical syndromes were poorly understood and, often, inappropriately classified. These advances have therefore not only concerned improved understanding of the underlying pathophysiology and molecular biology, but also more accurate diagnosis.

This is particularly important in genetic counselling, in which the first task must always be to establish the diagnosis beyond all reasonable doubt. Genetic analysis is also important for carrier detection, and for prenatal diagnosis. Older investigations, such as measurement of CK levels in the detection of carrier status in Duchenne muscular dystrophy, about which there is a very extensive literature have been entirely superseded by the newer techniques of molecular genetics, which allow direct detection of abnormalities in the dystrophin gene at Xp 21.

Carrier detection, or recognition of disease at an early, subclinical stage, can be achieved by:

1. DNA analysis for gene deletions, or by restriction fragment length polymorphisms (RFLP) for unique changes in gene structure
2. Biochemical tests based on the primary defect, e.g. enzyme deficiency or protein defect
3. Biochemical tests based on secondary defects, e.g. elevated blood CK levels in dystrophies
4. Cytogenetic studies, in the recognition of microdeletion syndromes or chromosome translocations
5. Physiological tests, e.g. EMG studies
6. Microscopy of tissue specimens, e.g. nerve or muscle biopsy
7. Radiological or clinical studies

In the clinical assessment of patients with neuromuscular disease it is important to consider the possibility of genetic disease and, when relevant, to construct an accurate family tree. This may not be easy, since it depends on access to a family member with appropriate knowledge of the family, and acquisition of data about consanguinity in the present or previous generations, together with full knowledge of paternity. Frequently, the occurrence of the neuromuscular disorder in earlier generations or in distant relatives will be difficult to establish with certainty. The family tree will establish recessive, dominant or X-linked patterns of inheritance, and will be useful in calculation of risks to future generations, even when accurate biological testing by DNA analysis is not possible.

In many disorders the genetic risk can, as yet, be assessed only when samples are available, for example for RFLP analysis, from several members of the family in at least two generations but, as direct genomic testing becomes available for more and more genetic disorders, this limitation will become less important.

The Approach to Investigation

The objective of investigation is to amplify the clinical findings in terms of the diagnosis, and also the distribution and severity of the disease process, and the effectiveness of compensatory and adaptive processes. The clinical findings may themselves suggest a definite diagnosis, for example in myotonic dystrophy, but often do not and investigation must then be planned so as to reveal the underlying physiological and pathological processes leading to the clinical expression of the disorder. Sometimes these investigations may themselves lead directly to diagnosis; for example the muscle biopsy in polymyositis is often characteristically abnormal. However, in other patients investigation may clarify the problem without providing a definite answer. Further, in some instances physiological (EMG) and pathological (biopsy) investigations may provide apparently contradictory results (Black et al. 1974).

Biochemical Tests

An overall assessment of the patient's general status is often useful, including haematological and biochemical evaluation, and relevant radiological examinations. Other tests, such as blood lactate or carnitine measurements, or urinary myoglobin assays, may be indicated in some patients. Generally, however, the most useful biochemical test in patients with neuromuscular disorders is measurement of the blood creatine kinase levels.

Blood Creatine Kinase Levels

The enzyme creatine kinase (CK) is present in large quantities in muscle. When muscle fibres are damaged it leaks into the circulation, so that the normal circulating CK level (26–170 IU/l in men; 26–150 IU/l in women) is increased. The enzyme is important in the catalysis of the reversible transfer of the terminal phosphate group of adenosine triphosphate (ATP) to creatine to form phosphocreatine. Phosphocreatine is part of the muscle's normal energy store that is used to provide a continuous supply of ATP for excitation/contraction coupling. CK is present in other tissues but these isomers of the enzyme can be recognised biochemically. Thus the predominant CK found in skeletal muscle is CK_{MM}, in cardiac muscle CK_{MB} and in brain CK_{BB} (see Nanji 1983). The slightly higher level of circulating CK found in men has been attributed to their greater muscle mass (Hughes 1962). The highest levels of CK in normal subjects are found in the first, second and seventh decades of life (Griggs et al. 1985), and after severe exercise (Griffiths 1966; Shumate et al. 1979). The CK level is slightly raised at puberty; it is decreased in pregnancy by as much as 30% (Smith et al. 1979). The CK in black men is higher than in white men: the CK in white males is similar to that of black females, but higher than in white females. The mean CK in white males was 59% that of black males (Meltzer and Holy 1974). This difference is important in clinical practice since it is necessary to recognise that a slightly raised CK in a black male is not necessarily abnormal.

The CK level may be raised immediately after exercise, but it reaches a peak value about 24–48 hours later in most subjects; however, in some people the peak level may not be reached for several days. Generally, the more severe the exercise the higher the level of CK, and the more delayed is the peak level (Brooke et al. 1979; Newham et al. 1983). Griffiths (1966) reported a 24-fold increase following a 53-mile walk, and marked changes have been reported after cycling, marathon running and long-distance skiing (Hansen et al. 1982). This effect of exercise on the CK level is more marked in untrained compared with trained subjects, and generally does not result in a more than fourfold rise above resting levels (Newham et al. 1983). Newham et al. (1983) found that eccentric exercise, that is the slow release of muscle contraction under a lengthening load as in walking downstairs, produced marked elevation in CK in normal subjects, even reaching 34 500 IU/l in one subject exercised to the point of painful fatigue. Exercise has a much less pronounced effect on CK levels in women than in men; moderate exercise raises the CK level in men, but has no effect in women (Shumate et al. 1979).

In addition to exercise, the CK may be raised in normal subjects for several other reasons unrelated to neuromuscular diseases (Table 1.5). In some patients with elevated CK levels without evidence of neuromuscular disease, an unsuspected and subclinical neuromuscular disorder may be recognised on investigation. In these patients the CK is CK_{MM} type. Alcoholism, hypothyroidism, the carrier status

Table 1.5. Causes of elevated CK levels not associated with neuromuscular disease

Muscle origin (CK_{MM})
Trauma, surgery, burns, muscle haematoma
Intramuscular injection
Vigorous exercise in previous 24–72 hours
Idiopathic?
Septic shock
Acute psychosis

CNS origin (CK_{BB})
Cerebral infarction
Head injury
Subarachnoid haemorrhage
Bacterial meningitis
Metastatic tumours (see Nanji 1983)

Cardiac origin (CK_{MB})
Acute myocardial infarction
Electrical cardioversion

Modified from Layzer (1985b).

of Duchenne muscular dystrophy, malignant hyperthermia trait and McLeod's syndrome are the most frequent examples of this uncommon finding. Some patients with recognised systemic disease, for example mixed connective tissue disease, may have raised CK levels with little or no clinical evidence of muscular weakness. The CK level may be *lower* than normal in steroid therapy (Hinderks and Frohlich 1979), hyperthyroidism and prolonged bed rest. The term "hyper CK aemia" has been used to describe a raised CK of undetermined, idiopathic cause.

Creatine Kinase Levels in Neuromuscular Diseases

The creatine kinase level is raised when there are necrotic or regenerating muscle fibres, and is thus not an indication of the relative predominance of either of these related phenomena. When there is extensive regeneration, as in certain stages of Duchenne muscular dystrophy, the proportion of CK_{MB} present may be greater than normal. Thus a raised CK_{MB} fraction is not necessarily indicative of cardiac involvement (Silverman et al. 1976).

The CK level is raised in most myopathies. The highest values are found in Duchenne muscular dystrophy, but very high levels may be found in any disorder in which necrosis of muscle occurs, as in severe active polymyositis, rhabdomyolysis associated with malignant hyperpyrexia, and McArdle's syndrome. In many metabolic myopathies, e.g. osteomalacic myopathy, steroid myopathy and mitochondrial myopathies, in which muscle destruction is not a feature, the CK level may be normal. It is also usually normal in peripheral neuropathies and other neurogenic disorders. However, in some severe chronic neurogenic disorders, such as Kugelberg–Welander syndrome, the CK level may be moderately raised (see Chap. 6).

The elevation of CK level that may follow exercise, even in normal subjects, has been utilised in the diagnosis of McArdle's syndrome. In this disorder the patient may be normal after a period of rest, but exercise provokes muscle fibre damage leading to a transient rise in CK level. Similarly, exercise provocation tests have been used in the detection of the carrier state in Duchenne muscular dystrophy; carriers of the gene are more likely to show a brief rise in CK level after exercise. Abnormal CK levels are a feature much more of younger carriers than of older women known to be carriers (Griggs et al. 1985). Even the trauma of the EMG electrode or muscle biopsy will cause a rise in the CK blood levels and CK measurements should therefore always be carried out in resting subjects before these other investigations are undertaken.

The CK level can be used to follow the progress of myopathic disorders, and as an indication of effective treatment in polymyositis. In Duchenne muscular dystrophy it falls as the disease progresses and activity declines. Although the CK level is generally higher in heavily muscled subjects (Garcia 1974), levels of CK are not directly related to changes in muscle bulk; in cachexia the CK is normal and even rapid neurogenic atrophy is not usually associated with a rise in the CK level.

Other Serum Enzyme Tests

The levels of aldolase, lactate dehydrogenase, aspartate dehydrogenase and pyruvate kinase may also be raised in destructive myopathies but these enzyme tests are less sensitive than CK levels (Aston et al. 1984) and are unlikely to reveal abnormalities in other, less active myopathies or in chronic neurogenic disorders with associated secondary myopathic features. The lack of sensitivity of these enzyme levels in neuromuscular disease is probably a reflection of the much greater concentration of CK than of these enzymes in muscle fibres.

Carbonic anhydrase III (CAIII) is a muscle-specific enzyme that is present in both fetal and adult skeletal muscle fibres (Jeffery et al. 1980). This enzyme, like CK, leaks from damaged muscle cells into the circulation. It is present in particularly high concentration in Type I fibres (Shima et al. 1983) and, like CK, its blood level is raised in muscular diseases (Heath et al. 1983; Hibi et al. 1984). In myotonic dystrophy the CAIII level is also raised, probably reflecting Type 1 fibre involvement in this disease (Mokuno et al. 1986).

Mokuno et al. (1984) have reported that levels of muscle-specific enolase, particularly those forms containing the β subunit found in skeletal and cardiac muscle, are elevated in muscular dystrophies and in other neuromuscular diseases, including spinal muscular atrophy, but not in myotonic dystrophy. The pattern of abnormality resembled that of CK levels in these diseases, probably because the two enzymes have similar molecular weights (88 000 and 82 000 daltons respectively) and thus similar diffusion characteristics through the muscle fibre membrane.

The usefulness of these various enzyme assays in diagnosis is probably also related to whether or not the enzymes are bound to other proteins. CK and muscle-specific enolase are unbound cytoplasmic enzymes, but lactate dehydrogenase, pyruvate kinase and aldolase are all bound to actin, thus limiting their potential for mobilisation from muscle (Clarke and Masters 1976).

Other Biochemical Tests on Blood

Myoglobin levels are raised in blood and urine when there is muscle fibre destruction. The serum myoglobin level is normally lower in women than in men, but is not raised at puberty or decreased in pregnancy as is that of CK. In addition the serum myoglobin level is constant with increasing age (mean level 24 μg/l in women; 36 μg/l in men; upper limit of normal 80 μg/l) (Nicholson and Walls 1983). Estimation of serum myoglobin levels is not generally useful in diagnosis, although it has been used in assessing progress in patients with polymyositis (Kiessling et al. 1981), and in the ascertainment of the carrier state in Duchenne muscular dystrophy.

In patients with mitochondrial myopathies blood lactate levels may sometimes be raised at rest, and may be considerably increased, compared with control subjects, following exercise (Morgan-Hughes 1982). The relation between venous blood lactate and ammonia produced during exercise is decreased in glycogen pathway disorders because lactate production is decreased while ammonia production from purine nucleotide metabolism is unaffected (Sinkeler et al. 1985). In McArdle's syndrome the lactate level does not rise during ischaemic exercise.

The levels of glycogen pathway enzymes can be measured in circulating white blood cells, and serum carnitine levels can be helpful in elucidating the cause of certain lipid storage diseases. The levels of vitamins, especially vitamin E in neuropathies associated with malabsorption, and B group vitamins in malnutrition, can provide useful information. The immunological abnormalities characteristic of myasthenia gravis, and of mixed connective tissue and other autoimmune disorders, form characteristic features of the clinical abnormality. Red blood cells show morphological abnormalities in blood films in some patients with spinocerebellar degeneration, McLeod's syndrome and Duchenne muscular dystrophy, but this is rarely of practical use in patient management. Fibroblast cultures can be used for characterisation of specific biochemical enzymatic abnormalities.

Urinary Protein Excretion Tests

In Duchenne muscular dystrophy myofibrillar synthesis is decreased (Rennie et al. 1982) and myofibrillar catabolism is increased. Similarly, muscle protein catabolism is increased in polymyositis, thyrotoxicosis, steroid myopathy and motor neuron disease (Elia et al. 1981). Protein excretion has been assessed approximately, using the 24-hour urinary creatine excretion, usually expressed as the urinary creatine/creatinine ratio (Pennington 1981). The creatine excretion is dependent on muscle mass so that changes in creatinine excretion with disease activity are sometimes difficult to interpret and this method is not now generally used in practice. An added difficulty is the dependency of the result on an accurate 24-hour collection of urine.

3-Methylhistidine, a product of myofibrillar protein breakdown, is excreted unchanged in the urine, and this property has been used as an index of muscle catabolism (McKeran et al. 1979). Elia et al. (1981) used the ratio of urinary 3-methylhistidine to creatinine excretion and found that it was increased in hyperthyroidism, malignant disease, osteomalacia, steroid myopathy and motor neuron disease; but in Duchenne muscular dystrophy the results were variable. On the other hand, Mussini et al. (1984) found a markedly increased excretion of 3-methylhistidine in patients with Duchenne muscular dystrophy. Rothig et al. (1984), in a study controlled for non-skeletal muscle contributions to 3-methylhistidine excretion, found that only in neurogenic disorders was excretion of this protein clearly increased. It thus appears that this technique is not, at present, of practical value in the clinical assessment of neuromuscular disease.

Protein synthesis in muscle has been assessed by using the incorporation of radiolabelled leucine into muscle following infusion. A reduced rate of uptake of isotope into muscle, implying decreased protein synthesis, has been reported in Duchenne muscular dystrophy (Rennie et al. 1982) and in cachectic patients with cancer (Emery et al. 1984).

General Laboratory Tests

The white blood count, haemoglobin, erythrocyte sedimentation rate (ESR), liver function tests, serum electrolytes, blood calcium, serum proteins and immuno-electrophoretic pattern will all be important in some patients, particularly in the investigation of peripheral neuropathies and immune-mediated inflammatory myopathies. Special investigations, e.g. thyroid function tests and other endocrinological studies, vitamin E and B_{12} folate levels, and investigation of porphyrin metabolism, are sometimes important. Immunological investigations, e.g. autoantibody screening tests, paraprotein electrophoresis, and specific antibody studies such as anti Hu and Purkinje cell antibodies, antinuclear antibodies, rheumatoid factor, and specific antibody tests, in Sjogren's syndrome and other autoimmune disorders are relevant in some patients. Antibodies are also useful in the diagnosis of Lyme disease. Specific biochemical tests are useful in some metabolic disorders, e.g. certain ganglioside storage disorders and Refsum's disease. Genetic tests for DNA polymorphisms, deletions or mutations give specific information in many inherited neuromuscular syndromes. In some patients with acute Guillain-Barré syndrome there is evidence of exposure to infection with mycoplasma, *Campylobacter* or Epstein–Barr virus as a preceding event.

Imaging in Neuromuscular Disorders

Computed tomography (CT) scanning of muscle has been used to characterise the distribution and severity of abnormality in both neurogenic (Bulcke and Baert 1982) and myopathic disorders (De Visser and VerBeeten 1985; Calo et al. 1986). Selective involvement of certain muscle groups has been recognised, especially in myopathies (Hawley et al. 1984; Schwartz et al. 1988). Before the advent of CT imaging other imaging methods were sometimes used, usually either to allow quantification of muscle size and density, e.g. ultrasound imaging (Heckmatt et al. 1988) or to detect inflammation, e.g. radionuclide scanning of muscle. Ultrasound scanning is particularly sensitive in detecting fatty infiltration. Radionuclide scanning, e.g. with ^{99m}technetium diphosphorate given intravenously shows increased isotope uptake, because of increased blood/muscle permeability in the presence of muscle damage, e.g. polymyositis (Siegel 1977; Vita and Harris 1981). Comparison of CT imaging, ultrasound scanning and magnetic resonance imaging (MRI) has been reported in myotonic dystrophy (Schedel et al. 1992).

CT imaging (Fig. 1.5) provides additional clinical information in the diagnosis and management of neuromuscular disorders, but the diagnosis can only rarely be made by CT alone (Vliet et al. 1988). In general a rough distinction between myopathic and neurogenic disorders can be made: neurogenic disorders tend to show a diffusely distributed abnormality or, in the case of neuropathies, have a pronounced distal involvement, and myopathic disorders, particularly Duchenne, facio-scapulo-humeral muscular dystrophy, and myotonic dystrophy, show more specific involvement of certain muscle groups, and sparing of the gracilis muscle (Bulcke and Baert 1982; Serratrice et al. 1985; Schwartz et al. 1988; Vliet et al. 1988). A standard imaging paradigm, involving five transverse

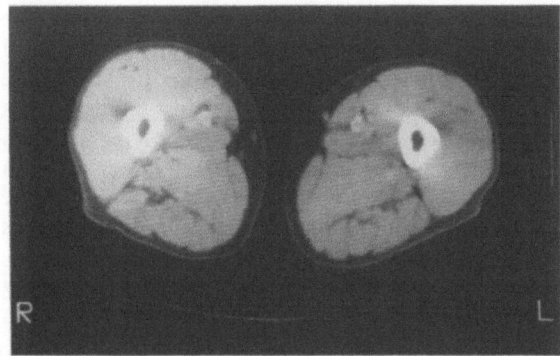

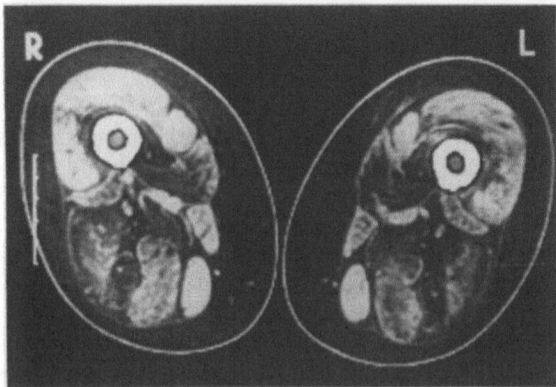

Fig. 1.5. Transverse CT scans at mid-thigh level to show muscles. **a** Normal adult thigh muscle (scale in cm). All the muscles show similar attenuation. **b** Limb-girdle muscular dystrophy, in a patient aged 43 years (scale in cm). There is selectively decreased attenuation in the lateral flexor muscles (hamstrings) with relatively less abnormality in the gracilis muscles, and in the vastus lateralis muscle although the vastus medialis muscles are abnormal. The decreased attenuation zones probably represent fat replacement of muscle. There is a thick layer of subcutaneous fat.

planes, i.e. pectoral, lumbar, pelvic, transfemoral and below-knee planes, enables a large number of proximal, axial and distal muscles to be assessed. A window setting of 250 Hounsfield units centred at 50 units is used (Schwartz et al. 1988). Vliet et al. (1988) assessed the value of CT imaging in a series of 30 patients suspected of having neuromuscular disease and found an overall diagnostic accuracy of 85% when compared with muscle biopsy using the needle technique. Serratrice et al. (1985) noted a hypodense perifemoral crescent in myotonic dystrophy, but this was not confirmed by others (Swash et al. 1995). Rickards et al. (1982) noted more fatty infiltration in more advanced cases of myotonic dystrophy. DeVisser and Verbeeten (1985) recorded characteristic differences between Becker dystrophy and spinal muscular atrophy (see also Hawley et al. 1984). Hawley et al. (1984) graded the images as

Grade 1 (normal), Grade 2 (early moth-eaten change with scattered areas of reduced attenuation), Grade 3 (discrete areas of reduced attenuation and some confluent zones of abnormality, and Grade 4 (washed-out appearance). Schwartz et al. (1988) noted a relationship between the degree of CT abnormality and the fibre density in single fibre EMG recordings. Swash et al. (1995) compared CT imaging with clinical features using MRC gradings of strength, in a double-blind study, and found that CT imaging detected more abnormality than clinical examination in neurogenic disorders, including spinal muscular atrophy and peripheral neuropathy, myopathies and polymyositis. Striking asymmetry, often unexpected, was revealed by CT in all these disorders.

MRI has also been used in the investigation of neuromuscular disorders. Fisher et al. (1986) evaluated MRI in normal and diseased muscle. Fleckenstein et al. (1988) showed that normal muscles had an increased proton density after exercise and Fisher et al. (1990) and Shellock et al. (1991) demonstrated that eccentric contraction produced more marked T2 intensity than concentric contraction. Suput et al. (1993) confirmed the selective involvement of muscles in Duchenne muscular dystrophy and noted a more homogeneous infiltration with fatty tissue in Duchenne dystrophy compared with Type III spinal muscular atrophy. In adult-onset polymyositis MRI was abnormal in 99% of patients with oedema in the acute phase. In dermatomyositis fatty infiltration was more prominent than oedema. In the chronic phase there was marked atrophy of the quadriceps muscle. In the legs the tibialis anterior was the principal abnormal muscle in dermatomyositis and inclusion body myositis, but in polymyositis the gastrocnemius showed the highest signal intensity (Reimers et al. 1994). These studies all suggest that imaging could be used in the selection of muscles for biopsy.

MRI has also found application in imaging peripheral nerves, e.g. in carpal tunnel syndrome, and in trauma to the brachial plexus. It is also useful in the diagnosis of root and plexus lesions associated with neoplastic infiltration or disc herniation.

Magnetic Resonance Spectroscopy

Nuclear magnetic resonance spectroscopy (MRS) has been used to study phosphorus metabolism (^{31}P MRS), and thus the levels of phosphocreatine (PCr), ATP and inorganic phosphate (Pi), both in vivo and in vitro. The intracellular pH of muscle can also be derived from the spectroscopy signal (Lundberg et al. 1990). The first application of this technique was in a patient with McArdle's disease, in whom no change towards a low muscle pH occurred during ischaemic exercise, implying reduced lactate production because of failure of glycogenolysis (Ross et al. 1981). The related glycogen pathway disorders of phosphofructokinase deficiency (Edwards et al. 1982) and phosphoglycerate kinase deficiency can also be studied by this method (Edwards et al. 1986). In mitochondrial myopathies increased PCr utilisation and slowed recovery of energy stores during oxidative recovery following exercise have been demonstrated, together with unusually high intracellular pH values during exercise (Gadian et al. 1981; Edwards et al. 1986). In Duchenne muscular dystrophy only non-specific changes have been reported (Griffiths et al. 1985).

During exercise in normal muscle there is a fall in the PCr peak, and a rise in the Pi peak due to the net flux of adenosine diphosphate (ADP) phosphorylation via the creatine kinase reaction. There is an accompanying decrease in muscle pH. These features allow muscle glycogenolysis to be monitored directly, together with oxidative phosphorylation (Arnold et al. 1984; Taylor et al. 1986).

Chapter 2

Electromyography, Nerve Conduction and Other Neurophysiological Techniques

The neuromuscular system can conveniently be investigated by electrophysiological methods. These provide quantitative data which can be used both in diagnosis and in measuring the effects of treatment. The scope of these methods includes:

- electromyography
- motor and sensory nerve conduction
- the measurement of the latencies of late responses, particularly F and H wave responses
- the assessment of repetitively evoked compound muscle action potentials (decrement testing) in disorders of neuromuscular transmission
- evoked potential tests
- somatosensory evoked responses
- brainstem evoked responses
- blink reflex latencies
- motor conduction time, using electrical or electromagnetic stimulation of the central nervous system (CNS)

Various special applications of these techniques, e.g. macro EMG, scanning EMG and the use of surface and monopolar electrodes, are available, but are used relatively infrequently in routine clinical work.

Electromyographic Assessment

Electromyography (EMG) is a useful technique in the diagnosis of myopathic and neurogenic disorders. Needle electrode sampling of proximal and distal muscles in arms and legs is particularly useful in assessing the distribution and severity of involvement of different muscle groups. The motor unit potentials themselves can be quantified in terms of amplitude, area, phases, firing rates and stability. Neuromuscular transmission can be assessed by repetitive nerve stimulation or single-fibre EMG techniques (see Chap. 12). Motor and sensory nerve conduction velocity measurements are valuable in the assessment of patients with peripheral nerve and root disorders.

Recording Electrodes

Several different types of electrode are used in clinical EMG studies, depending on the application.

Surface Electrodes

Recordings of summated motor unit action potential activity can be accomplished from surface recordings using metal plate electrodes approximately 1 cm × 1 cm. They are usually constructed of silver or platinum. The skin should be carefully cleansed, and saline-based electrode jelly applied between the skin and the electrode surface. One electrode is placed over the belly of the muscle to be recorded (the active lead) and an indifferent electrode is placed over the tendon of the muscle. These electrodes are mainly used for recording muscle and nerve action potentials, but they are also used for kinesiological recordings, for muscle action potential propagation velocity studies (Masuda and Sadoyama 1986) and in motor unit counting procedures.

Surface electrodes are not used to record single motor unit activity because high-frequency components are attenuated, and activity in nearby muscles may interfere with the recording. However, surface electrode recording is useful in some circumstances. For example, it can be used to determine the presence of voluntary or electrically induced activity in an atrophic muscle when selecting a muscle for

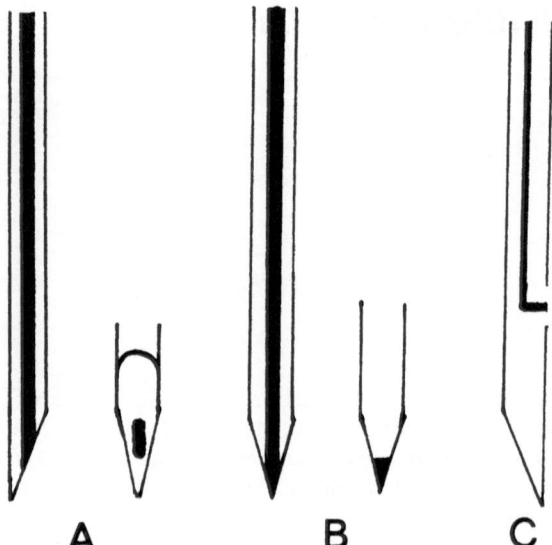

Fig. 2.1.   Needle EMG electrodes showing the leading-off surfaces from which action potentials in the uptake area are recorded. A, Concentric needle EMG electrode; the recording surface is (150 μm × 600 μm) 0.09 mm^2 in area. B, Monopolar needle EMG electrode; the recording surface is 0.14 mm^2 in area. C, Single-fibre EMG electrode; the recording surface is 25 μm in diameter (0.0005 mm^2 in area).

motor conduction studies by nerve stimulation, or when selecting a muscle for needle EMG, particularly, as in children, when a limited examination is necessary. Some useful information can be obtained by surface recording in superficial, small muscles such as the extensor digitorum brevis and abductor pollicis brevis.

Surface electrodes are also useful when searching for fasciculations, since the activity of several muscles can be recorded simultaneously on separate channels of the EMG apparatus.

Concentric Needle Electrodes

For muscle sampling concentric needle electrodes are commonly used. These electrodes consist of a steel wire, 0.1 mm in diameter, contained within a thin, pointed cannula resembling a hypodermic needle 0.3 mm in outer diameter (Fig. 2.1A). The wire electrode is separated from the cannula (needle) by an insulating resin. The recording surface consists of the oval bare tip of the wire electrode 0.9 mm^2 in area and the reference electrode is the exterior of the cannula itself (Adrian and Bronk 1929). Thin electrodes are available for studies of facial and extraocular muscles. Standard concentric electrodes vary in length. The electrical characteris-

tics of commercial electrodes show consistent differences, particularly with regard to impedance (Dorfman et al. 1985). These characteristics can be temporarily improved, when necessary, by passing a small current through the electrode (electrolytic treatment) in a saline bath (Stålberg and Trontelj 1994). The recording consists of the potential difference between the central wire leading off the surface of the electrode face and the shaft in its non-insulated terminal portion. Noise levels are relatively low because the impedance is low (about 50 k ohm).

Monopolar Electrodes

Monopolar electrodes consist of steel needles 0.8 mm in diameter insulated to just proximal to the tip with a Teflon coating (Fig. 2.1B). Recording of motor unit potentials is made using a surface or subcutaneous needle reference electrode. A separate surface plate acts as a ground electrode. The monopolar electrode has a high impedance, introducing more noise into the recording, but the potential recorded is larger and monopolar recordings are especially useful when searching for spontaneous activity, e.g. fibrillations and fasciculations. The curved symmetrical sharp tip of the monopolar electrode causes less pain during insertion than concentric electrodes, and monopolar electrodes are less expensive. The high impedance of monopolar electrodes can be reduced somewhat by soaking them in saline before use (Kimura 1989), improving the resolution of low amplitude signals. The inherent differences in motor unit amplitude and noise associated with monopolar electrodes, compared with concentric needle electrodes are caused by the wide separation of the needle tip from the surface reference electrode. Chan and Hsu (1991) compared motor unit potential (MUP) parameters between monopolar and concentric needle electrodes. They found that in monopolar recordings the MUPs had a significantly higher amplitude (2.05 times greater), a larger area (2.64 times greater) and a longer duration (1.86 times longer) than the concentric recordings. There was no difference in the mean number of phases and turns in the quantitative MUP analysis (see below), indicating that the description of neurogenic or myopathic units will be similar in monopolar and concentric recordings.

Single-Fibre EMG Electrodes

In order to record action potentials from single muscle fibres extracellularly, special electrodes have been developed. The recording surface of the most commonly used "single-fibre" needle electrode is smaller (25 μm diameter) than in conventional concentric electrodes and is situated on the shaft of the electrode cannula, opposite the bevelled sharp point (Fig. 2.1C). A variety of multi-lead electrodes with small leading-off surfaces of this type have been used in research (Ekstedt 1964). Single-fibre EMG electrodes are particularly valuable in measuring the neuromuscular jitter, e.g. in myasthenia gravis, and in fibre density measurements.

The single-fibre EMG electrode can be used with a concentric needle electrode in the *scanning EMG technique* (Stålberg and Antoni 1980; Stålberg and Droszeghy 1991), in which recordings are made from the concentric needle electrode as it is pulled through the muscle with a step-motor.

Macro EMG Electrodes

In this technique, utilised to try to record from the whole extent (all the muscle fibres) of individual motor units, a modified single-fibre EMG electrode is used in which the single-fibre EMG part is located 7.5 mm from the tip of the electrode, and recordings are made from the cannula of the electrode itself (Stålberg 1980, 1982b).

Wire Electrodes

Flexible platinum wire electrodes insulated except at their tips can be inserted into muscles for longer recordings, as in kinesiological studies (Basmajian 1978). The wire electrode is inserted into the muscle through a hypodermic needle, and the latter is then withdrawn, leaving the wire in the muscle. The wire is hooked over the tip of the needle and its position in the muscle can be adjusted by pulling it slightly. A specialised bipolar wire electrode has been developed for selective recordings from 3–5 fibres (Nelson and Soderberg 1983). These wire electrode recordings have not been standardised in the quantitative methodologies applied to more conventional needle electrode recordings.

Sterilisation of EMG Electrodes

All needle electrodes used in clinical EMG studies must be sterile. This can be achieved by heat sterilisation in a boiling pot or by autoclaving. The possibility of transmission of slow or latent viruses, or of other virus infections such as hepatitis or HIV or prion diseases such as Creutzfeldt–Jakob disease, by contaminated electrodes has led to more stringent recommendations for adequate sterilisation of needle electrodes. It is recommended that autoclaving at 134 °C and 30 lb/in^2 pressure for 3 minutes is adequate to inactivate hepatitis B and HIV virus particles.

In the case of EMG recordings made in patients with dementia, or suspected Creutzfeldt–Jakob disease the American Association of Electrodiagnostic Medicine (1992) recommends that needle electrodes should be destroyed after use by incineration to prevent possible contamination. Although no case of transmission of Creutzfeldt–Jakob disease has occurred following EMG examination, the use of disposable needle electrodes has become the preferred option not only when examining such patients but in all examinations in which the possibility of viral or prion disease exists. In many laboratories disposable electrodes are used in all EMG examinations and, although expensive, this is gradually becoming the norm (Evans et al. 1993).

Signal Amplification

Signals picked up from these electrodes, ranging in amplitude from about 20 μV to more than 15 mV, are amplified and displayed on an oscilloscope and, simultaneously, on a loudspeaker. The amplifier should have a low input capacitance and an input impedance much greater than that of the electrode. Capacitance-coupled amplifiers are always used and the amplifier must be adequately shielded and connected to a common ground with the patient. The frequency response of the amplifier should be flat between 2 Hz and 10 000 Hz. In some special electromyographic applications, such as single-fibre EMG, a low-frequency filter setting of 500 Hz or even higher is used. Variable amplifications and sweep speed settings are used during EMG examinations.

The trigger-delay line (Nissen-Petersen et al. 1969) is indispensable in the isolation of individual potentials. In principle, a DC level is established below which the oscilloscope will not be activated. Potentials of greater amplitude than this preset level (which can be varied as required) trigger the oscilloscope and are displayed from the beginning of the sweep. The delay circuit enables the earliest components of this triggering potential to be displayed. The delay is itself variable as required. It is useful to display both the undelayed and the delayed signal in order to be certain which component of any given motor unit action potential (MUAP) is triggering the sweep (Fig. 2.2). Interference from mains artefact, usually from unshielded power lines, or from

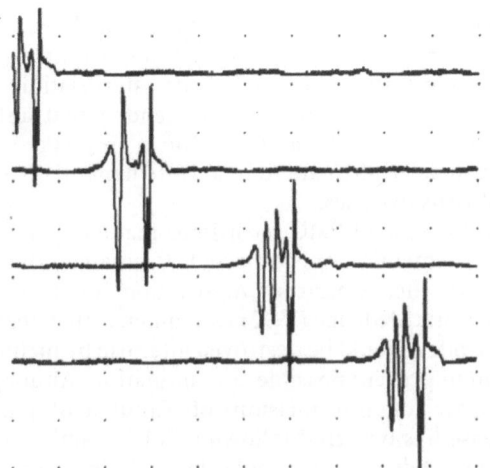

Fig. 2.2. Chronic neurogenic disorder. Concentric needle EMG showing four consecutive MUAPs, representing two different motor units. Both are of increased amplitude, and are polyphasic. 10 ms/division and 0.2 mV/division.

fluorescent lights, can be alleviated by ensuring good contact between skin and ground electrode, and that the ground is connected to a well-constructed ground system.

Modern oscilloscopes often have an inbuilt storage function so that potentials can be stored successively on the screen. This enables variations in individual potentials to be studied. A storage oscilloscope can easily be linked to standard EMG equipment in order to provide this function. Motor unit potential analysis and other complex derivations from the analogue signal can be derived by computer analysis of the digitised signal.

Concentric Needle Electromyography

Clinical Technique

When needle electromyography is to be performed it is important to have the patient confident and relaxed, in a warm room. Shivering produces unwanted EMG activity and cold limbs can result in erroneous data. The patient is best allowed to lie in a semi-recumbent position facing the EMG apparatus and oscilloscope. Individual examiners use different techniques. For example, the examiner may sit on the patient's right, thus also facing the oscilloscope. The examiner's right hand is then available to adjust the controls of the EMG apparatus, and his left can be used to manipulate the EMG electrode

itself. A more commonly used method is to use the right hand to manipulate the EMG electrode, and the left to operate the controls of the machine, so that the examiner sits facing the patient, and the EMG machine.

The skin should be adequately cleansed with a sterilising agent, as for venepuncture, and the electrodes must be sterile. A ground lead must always be attached to the patient, preferably on the limb to be investigated.

After cleansing the skin, the concentric needle electrode is inserted into the muscle with a single, rapid thrust. This should cause the patient little discomfort. It is best to insert the needle deeply into the body of the muscle; repeated small, forward movements of the needle are painful, but gradually withdrawing the electrode during the recording is usually painless. The investigation should be carefully planned, and its scope explained to the patient before it is begun.

The number of muscles examined varies according to the clinical problem. For example, in amyotrophic lateral sclerosis the study should focus on clinically involved limbs and muscles and distal and proximal muscles should be sampled. Several muscles innervated by different nerves and nerve roots, in at least three limbs, should be examined. In myopathies, muscles should be studied in at least two limbs, including a distal and a proximal muscle in a clinically affected limb. Thus relatively few muscles need be studied for diagnostic purposes in this group of diseases. In mononeuropathies and peripheral neuropathies EMG is less important than nerve conduction studies, but EMG sampling to establish the distribution of denervation and extent of denervation is valuable. EMG in disorders of neuromuscular transmission is useful if jitter and blocking are assessed. Paraspinal muscle EMG is especially useful to establish the differential diagnosis of intervertebral disk or plexus disease and, also, in the assessment of patients with polymyositis. In children the EMG examination must often be restricted to only a few muscles. In the latter, it is clearly of paramount importance to select an appropriate muscle; as a general rule the quadriceps muscle is often the most appropriate because its activation can be easily controlled and it is involved in most neuromuscular diseases.

EMG Activity in Relaxed Muscle

In the relaxed non-contracted muscle a number of EMG phenomena may be recorded. In normal subjects this activity differs from that found in patients with neuromuscular diseases.

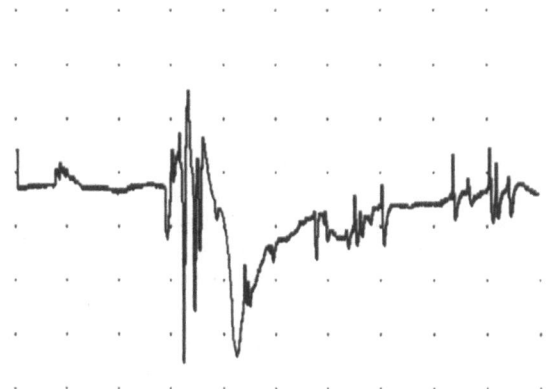

Fig. 2.3. Normal insertional activity, on advancing the concentric EMG electrode. Filters: 100 Hz and 10 kHz. Bar 20 ms.

Insertional Activity

In normal muscle insertion of the electrode results in a very brief burst of potentials, lasting less than 500 ms. These potentials are of shorter duration and smaller amplitude than motor unit action potentials. This activity is due to the movement of the electrode during insertion, probably indicating muscle fibre injury (Weichers et al. 1977), and further movements of the electrode will result in similar short bursts of insertional activity (Fig. 2.3). Increased insertional activity, as regards both amount and duration, is particularly a feature of myopathic disorders, but also occurs in denervation and myositis. Abnormally prolonged insertional activity indicates instability of muscle fibre membranes (Kugelberg and Petersen 1949).

Insertional Positive Waves

These consist of runs of positive waves at 3 to 30 Hz, lasting for seconds or even minutes on needle insertion or movement. They are found in acute denervation, or in polymyositis. Although the pattern of activity resembles pseudomyotonia the discharges consist of single positive potentials without the waxing and waning characteristic of true myotonia (Wiechers and Johnson 1979).

End-Plate Noise

Sometimes, in certain regions of a muscle, monophasic negative potentials, 10 to 50 μv in amplitude, lasting for 1–2 ms, will be recorded. These occur in short runs of high-frequency activity. They are usually found associated with painful needle placements. These potentials have been correlated with recordings made from the end-plate region and it has been suggested that they represent miniature end-plate potentials (Wiederholt 1970).

End-Plate Spikes

A second type of activity found in this region consists of larger (100–200 μV) biphasic potentials of 3–4 ms duration. The initial phase is negative. They discharge at 5–50 Hz. These potentials, which discharge at a slower rate than end-plate noise, have been thought to arise in small intramuscular nerve fibres in the innervation zone, but synchrony of miniature end-plate potentials might produce a similar finding (Buchthal and Rosenfalck 1966). It is important to recognise these potentials, a feature of normal muscle, as they may be confused with fibrillation potentials. Pickett and Schmidley (1980) described small positive potentials which represent cannula-recorded end-plate spikes. With slight movement of the electrode, end-plate noise and spikes disappear; fibrillation potentials are usually found more widely in a muscle (Heckman and Ludin 1982). Partanen and Nousrainen (1983) suggested that end-plate spikes represented activity of intrafusal muscle fibres, derived from action potentials of these muscle fibres that could be coactivated by voluntary effort.

Fibrillation Potentials

Fibrillation potentials are biphasic potentials 20–300 μV in amplitude and 1–5 ms in duration (Fig. 2.4) that are rarely found in normal muscle. They originate from a single muscle fibre (Ekstedt 1964) and can be recorded only with needle electrodes. They are usually recorded immediately after insertion of the needle electrode into the muscle, and may have either a positive or a negative initial phase (Buchthal and Rosenfalck 1966). They do not vary in amplitude or shape if recorded over a period of time. They are indicative of abnormal muscle if recorded from at least two different sites in a muscle. They usually occur at frequencies of 1–10 Hz (Conrad et al. 1972) but rarely at faster rates (Buchthal and Rosenfalck 1966). Irregularly firing fibrillation potentials may be found in normal muscle, but regularly firing fibrillations are indicative of denervation (Stohr 1977) as suggested by Denny-Brown and Pennybacker (1938). Although a particular characteristic of neurogenic disorders, fibrillation potentials may also occur in myopathies. They are more prominent in acute denervating dis-

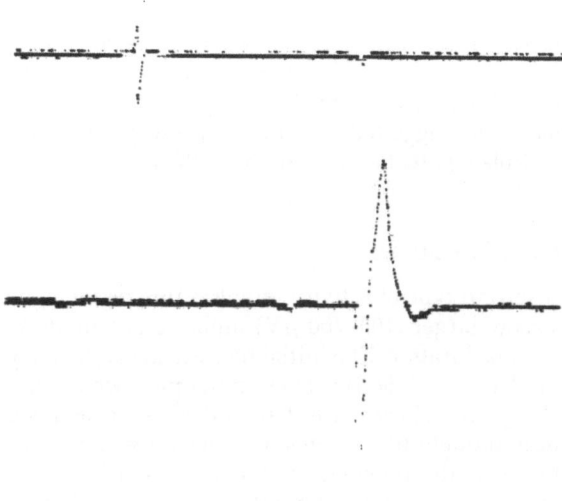

Fig. 2.4. Fibrillation and fasciculation potentials: the fasciculation potential is much larger and more complex than the fibrillation potential. Concentric needle EMG. Filters: 100 Hz and 10 kHz. Bar 20 ms.

eases but after nerve section they do not generally appear for a week or more, the delay depending on the length of nerve degenerating; the shorter the distance between the site of a nerve injury and the muscle, the shorter the time interval before fibrillations appear. Unless reinnervation occurs, fibrillations will persist, although their amplitude gradually decreases (Kraft 1990). Fibrillation potentials arise because of changes in membrane depolarisation sensitivity (stability) due to denervation, to localised muscle fibre damage, or to focal loss of innervation from separation of part of a muscle fibre from its end-plate region.

The precise point of origin of fibrillation potentials in denervated muscle has been studied by stimulation experiments in which it was shown that denervated muscle fibres, probably corresponding to the small angulated fibres typically found in biopsies of patients with neurogenic disorders, contained discrete, low-threshold sites at which the fibres could be activated electrically (Trontelj and Stålberg 1983a). At these sites ephaptic activation from other fibres occurred, giving rise to paired discharges – a common finding in spontaneous fibrillations in chronic partial denervation.

A very irregular firing pattern usually represents discharges (fibrillations) arising from more than one fibre, firing at rates varying from 0.1 to 25 Hz with intervals of several seconds silence. These may arise at multiple sites of depolarisation on abnormal denervated muscle fibres associated with increased sodium conductance. These irregular fibrillations

may be augmented by catecholamines and by sympathetic stimulation (Caswell et al. 1978).

Fasciculation Potentials

Unlike fibrillation potentials, fasciculation potentials can be recorded with both needle and surface electrodes. These potentials represent spontaneous firing of individual motor units (Denny-Brown and Pennybacker 1938) and they are therefore identical in shape to motor unit action potentials (Fig. 2.4). Denny-Brown and Pennybacker (1938) also noted that many fasciculating motor units can be activated by voluntary effort, an observation confirmed in motor neuron disease in recent times by Guiloff and Modarres-Sadighi (1992). They are most commonly found in anterior horn cell diseases, but also occur in root lesions. They are less common in peripheral neuropathies. Their firing rate is irregular, varying from 1 to 50/min. Trojaborg and Buchthal (1965) have described "malignant" fasciculations in motor neuron disease, in which the mean interval between successive fasciculation potentials was 3.5 s (SD 2.5), and "benign" fasciculations, found in patients with nerve root lesions and in some normal subjects, in which the mean interpotential interval was 0.8 s (SD 0.8). However, Hjorth et al. (1973) have challenged this distinction, and reported no predominance of slow or fast repetition rates of fasciculation potentials in motor neuron disease. Many fasciculations recorded by EMG cannot be recognised clinically since they occur in deeper parts of the muscle. Fasciculations occurring spontaneously in recordings made from muscles at rest are due to firing of parts of motor units (Conradi et al. 1982a; Roth 1984) that can be activated voluntarily. Fasciculations occurring in resting muscle arise from distal axonal sites (Roth 1982, 1984). Contraction fasciculations consist of rhythmic discharges of motor units that can be controlled voluntarily; these consist of individual motor units, or groups of motor units and these motor units are of longer duration than normal, and hence imply reinnervation.

Fasciculations at rest may occur in normal subjects ("benign fasciculations"; Reed and Kurland 1963). As many as 70% of normal people admit to having experienced muscle twitches (Reed and Kurland 1963) and these are identical by EMG criteria to fasciculations found in neurogenic disorders. However, in neurogenic disorders many fasciculations may be highly polyphasic (see Chap. 6). Therefore, fasciculation potentials by themselves are not necessarily abnormal, unless associated with fibrillation potentials or positive sharp waves, the pathognomonic features of denervation.

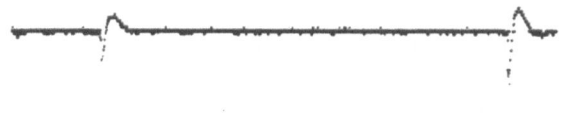

Fig. 2.5. Positive sharp waves: biphasic potentials with an initial positive deflection followed by a slow negative decay. Concentric needle EMG. Filters: 100 Hz and 10 kHz. Bar 10 ms.

Positive Sharp Waves

Another finding typical of denervation is a potential with a sharp, positive initial deflection about 120 μV in amplitude (Buchthal and Rosenfalck 1966), and a slow decay towards the baseline (Fig. 2.5), giving a characteristic "saw tooth" appearance. The duration of these positive sharp waves is about 4 ms (Buchthal and Rosenfalck 1966), but many are of longer duration. Their firing rate is similar to that of fibrillation potentials. The origin of positive sharp waves is uncertain but it has been suggested that, like fibrillation potentials, they originate from single muscle fibres; the initial positive deflection is due to current flow passing outward through an unexcited and damaged membrane, while the absence of a negative component implies failure of excitability of the membrane.

Positive sharp waves are associated with acute or rapidly progressive neurogenic disorders, and may appear before fibrillation potentials after nerve section (Wiechers et al. 1977). Both positive sharp waves and fibrillation potentials occur more commonly in peripheral nerve disorders than in lesions near to or in the anterior horn cells. Positive sharp waves are not found in normal muscle. They may occur, however, in polymyositis and in muscular dystrophy.

Complex Repetitive Discharges

This activity, also termed *bizarre high-frequency potentials* and *pseudomyotonia*, consists of continuous trains of spikes, of simple or complex patterns, repeated at a regular frequency of 5–150 Hz, having an abrupt onset and termination. Occasionally complex repetitive discharges occur at low firing rates, as low as 0.3 Hz (Trontelj and Stålberg 1983b). They are most common in neurogenic disorders but are also found in myopathic disorders. They have been recorded in the external urinary sphincter (Dyro et al. 1983; Fowler et al. 1985) in patients with difficulty initiating micturition.

Complex repetitive discharges are usually triggered by electrode movement. They are thought to originate from spontaneous activity in a single muscle fibre, which activates one or more adjacent muscle fibres ephaptically. This secondarily activated fibre then acts as a co-pacemaker producing an excitatory loop with the initially excited fibre (Trontelj and Stålberg 1983b). Since the number of fibres activated in this process may vary at any given time, the morphology of the discharge may also vary during a sequence of discharges (Fig. 2.6). Nerve blocks and curarisation fail to inhibit these complex repetitive discharges, illustrating the absence of any central factor or of neurotransmission at the motor end-plate in the initiation and continuation of this activity (Stöhr 1978). These discharges show a very low interpotential jitter (Stålberg and Trontelj 1982; Fowler et al. 1985), further indicating the absence of end-plate activity in their causation. The individual components of the repetitive discharging potential, often consisting of 10 or more distinct unit potentials, may be separated by intervals ranging from less than 0.5 ms to more than 200 ms (Trontelj and Stålberg 1983b).

In the external urethral sphincter the pattern of activity of complex repetitive discharges differs from that found in skeletal muscle in that many complexes show a gradual increase or decrease in interdischarge interval. This feature, termed *decelerating bursts*, resembles that of neuromyotonia and is not ordinarily associated with the phenomenon of complex repetitive discharges as recorded in limb muscles (Fowler et al. 1985). However, the interpotential jitter of the latter phenomenon is also less than 5 μs, indicating that the pathogenesis of this activity is similar to that of complex repetitive discharges. Willison (1982) has pointed out that ephaptic transmission from fibre to fibre in skeletal muscle is ordinarily prevented by the absence of adjacent simultaneously depolarising muscle fibres, because of the pseudorandom nature of the distribution of the motor unit. When this relationship is disturbed by reorganisation of the motor unit in neurogenic and, to a lesser extent, in myopathic diseases, cross-firing of adjacent muscle fibres is more likely.

Pseudomyotonia occurs most frequently in Duchenne muscular dystrophy, spinal muscular atrophy and Charcot–Marie–Tooth disease, but also in a large number of chronic denervating disease, including motor neuron disease, polyneuropathies and radiculopathies, hypothyroidism and Schwartz–Jampel syndrome (Emeryck et al. 1974).

Myokymia

The phenomenon of myokymia may be apparent clinically as an involuntary, irregular, quivering or

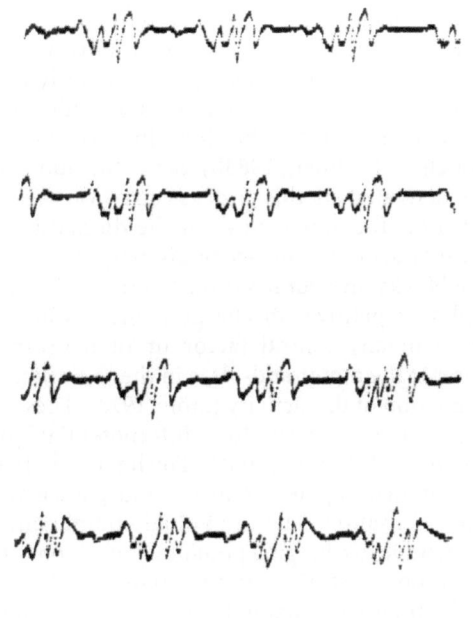

Fig. 2.6. Myokymia: spontaneous polyphasic activity at a frequency of 40 Hz. Myokymia does not show the waxing and waning of amplitude and frequency which characterises true myotonia (see Fig. 2.7). Concentric needle EMG in a patient with alcoholic myopathy. Filters: 100 Hz and 10 kHz. Bar 20 ms.

rippling contracture of parts of a muscle. It is most commonly noted in the periorbital or other components of the facial musculature. This phenomenon was recognised in limb muscles by Schultze (1895).

Myokymia in limb muscles consists of bursts of EMG activity, containing multiple spikes, at 2–60 Hz and lasting for up to 8 s, but usually for about 1 s (Albers et al. 1981), followed by a few seconds of silence. It disappears, unlike neuromyotonia, during sleep. There may be a characteristic rhythmicity to the discharge pattern (Auger 1994).

Facial myokymia is similar, although continuous and discontinuous forms have been described (Radu et al. 1975). It is unaffected by voluntary activation of an affected muscle or by sleep (Hughes and Matthews 1969), but is abolished by xylocaine block of the nerve innervating the affected muscle (Albers et al. 1981). The continuous form, consisting of high-frequency bursts recurring every 10 seconds occurs in multiple sclerosis, whereas the discontinuous form discharges faster, in shorter duration bursts that recur more frequently. These have been associated with brain stem glioma (Matthews 1966; Tenser and Corbett 1974; Radu et al. 1975). However, myokymia is more frequently noted in Guillain–Barré syndrome, multiple sclerosis and radiation plexopathies (Gutmann 1991).

Myokymia thus probably consists of bursts of motor unit activity induced by abnormal excitation occurring in motor nerve fibres, perhaps representing ephaptic transmission at sites of focal demyelination, whether central or peripheral. Hemifacial spasm is a variety of myokymia (Nielsen 1984a).

Neuromyotonia

Neuromyotonia differs from myokymia in that there is *continuous* activation of motor units, sustained for variable periods. It may produce clinical features resembling myokymia, as in generalised or facial myokymia, but in its severe form fixed postures may occur as in stiff man syndrome. In limb muscles neuromyotonia may be indistinguishable from the disorder termed continuous muscle fibre activity by Isaacs (1961). EMG recordings show activity resembling motor unit potentials, but sometimes appearing to consist of fewer components, firing at very rapid rates (up to 300 Hz). This activity is continuous even with sleep or barbiturate sedation, and resembles EMG activity found in stiff man syndrome, tetanus and Schwartz–Jampel syndrome (Ludin 1980). It is abolished by curare, indicating that neuromuscular transmission is involved, and is modulated by phenytoin and carbamazepine. It probably originates in distal motor nerve twigs rather than in more proximal parts of the peripheral nerve, as in myokymia, and probably does not arise from ephaptic transmission. Unlike myokymia, the EMG bursts do not recur repetitively and rhythmically. They may develop spontaneously or be initiated by needle movement, voluntary effort or nerve percussion.

Myotonia

True myotonia is the EMG correlate of the clinical phenomenon of impaired relaxation of a voluntarily or mechanically induced contraction of a muscle. It consists of a high-frequency repetitive discharge, with a waxing and waning of amplitude and frequency (50–150/s) producing the well-known "divebomber" sound, the most distinctive sound in EMG. The discharge represents rapid firing of single muscle fibres (Fig. 2.7). The amplitude of the discharge depends on the proximity of the recording electrode to the active muscle fibre. True myotonic discharges are ordinarily found only in myotonic dystrophy and the congenital myotonic syndromes, associated with channel disorders leading to repetitive firing of muscle fibres. The quantity of myotonic activity varies in different muscles, but is

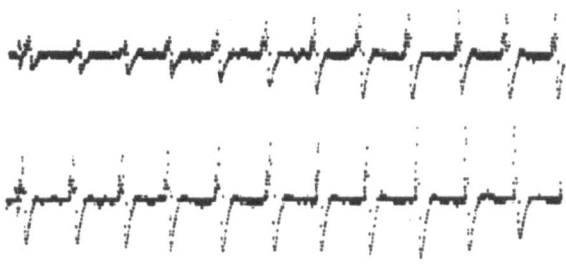

Fig. 2.7. Myotonia in myotonic dystrophy. The single-fibre activity gradually increased in amplitude during the recording. Single-fibre EMG recording. Bar 10 ms.

usually most prominent in the intrinsic hand muscles (Streib and Sun 1983).

Motor Unit Potential Analysis

Insertional activity, end-plate noise, fibrillations and fasciculation potentials are all studied with concentric needle EMG while the muscle is at rest. Motor unit potentials can only be studied during voluntary activation of the muscle and this is the next part of the concentric needle EMG study of a muscle. Voluntary activation is studied in a graded manner so that individual units can be analysed.

The most important parameters in the study of motor unit action potentials are *amplitude, duration, number of phases, area* and *firing rate* (Table 2.1). In addition satellites consisting of small potentials, probably single fibres time-locked to the main potential, may be recorded. They can be detected most easily when a trigger-delay line is used.

Table 2.1. Motor unit action potential (MUP) measurements

Peak-to-peak amplitude
Duration
Complexity
Phases
Turns
Baseline crossings
Rise time
Area
Variability of MUP morphology
Area
Jitter and blocking in single-fibre EMG recordings
Firing rate

Because needle electrodes have a limited uptake area, dependent on the size of their leading-off surface and on volume conduction effects within the muscle (Rosenfalck 1969), these parameters will vary according to the position of the electrode within the territory of individual motor units. The best studied parameter in motor unit potential analysis is turns analysis (Willison 1964; Rose and Willison 1967; Dorfman and McGill 1988).

Amplitudes

The amplitude of a motor unit potential is measured peak-to-peak. It is determined by the number and size of active muscle fibres forming part of the whole motor unit within about 500 μm of the concentric needle recording electrode (Nandedkar et al. 1988a,b). Spike-triggered MUPs are used for quantitative analysis. These are biased toward the highest amplitude and first-recruited units, and thus may be unrepresentative of the total population. However, this also means that the method is particularly sensitive in neurogenic disorders in which reinnervated large units may be recruited early (Stålberg et al. 1994).

Duration

Duration is affected also by the diameter of these muscle fibres and by their temporal dispersion. It is usually determined by the activity of 2–8 such muscle fibres (Nandedkar et al. 1986). The duration of a motor unit potential is measured between the take-off of the initial component of the motor unit, usually a positive-going waveform, and the return to baseline. These two points are often difficult to delineate precisely and in automatic analyses a combination of slope and baseline intercepts is used. Duration is determined by active muscle fibres within about 2.5 mm from the recording electrode (Nandedkar et al. 1985; Stålberg et al. 1986). The positive-going components represent activity recorded from the shaft of the electrode; the negative components represent activity recorded from the electrode tip, and therefore from a smaller uptake area. Satellite components are not usually included in duration measurements. The *area* of a motor unit potential is calculated by integrating the rectified motor unit potential activity for each potential, defined by its duration. It represents activity of 15–20 muscle fibres within 1.5 mm of the electrode core (Stålberg et al. 1986). Nandedkar et al. (1988b) found that the area/amplitude ratio was least affected by noise or inter-operator differences.

For measurements of amplitude, duration and phase the recording electrode should be in close proximity to the active muscle fibres because volume conduction effects will themselves modify these parameters when recordings are made at a distance (Rosenfalck 1969). The major criteria for proximity of a recording electrode to an active

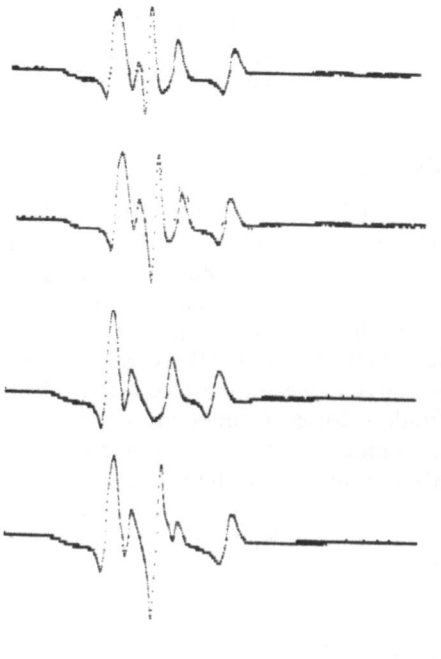

Fig. 2.8. A polyphasic motor unit action potential recorded during voluntary activity with a concentric needle EMG using a trigger-delay line and 500-Hz low-frequency filter. Four consecutive potentials are shown. The variation in configuration reflects instability of the unit. This potential has 7 phases (number of baseline crossings minus 1). Bar 2 ms.

muscle fibre are a fast rise time (<500 μs) and an adequate amplitude (>120 μV). The shape of the fast, rising phase of the motor unit action potential is determined by the proximity of the nearest 1–3 muscle fibres of the motor unit (Ekstedt 1964; Griep et al. 1982). Motor unit potentials tend to be larger in both amplitude and area in men. In children motor unit action potentials are smaller and of shorter duration than in adults (do Carmo 1960). For example the mean duration of motor unit action potentials in the biceps brachii at age 3 years is 8.2 ms; at age 30 years it is 10.6 ms; and at age 70 years, 12.4 ms (Rosenfalck 1975). More recent studies have contradicted this linear increase in MUP duration with age in adults. Bischoff et al. (1994) found no change in MUP duration or amplitude between ages 25 years and 60 years.

Complexity

A potential with more than four phases is termed a polyphasic motor unit potential. Buchthal (1977) has defined a *phase* as that part of the motor unit potential which lies between two crossings of the baseline. Those parts of the potential between the onset and the first crossing, and the last crossing and the end of the potential, are also considered separate phases (Fig. 2.8). Reversals of polarity that do not cross the baseline are termed *turns*. The number of turns increases with age, but the number of phases remains constant (Falck 1983). The number of turns is correlated with amplitude, but the number of phases does not correlate with amplitude.

Normal skeletal muscle recordings may contain up to 12% polyphasic motor unit potentials (Caruso and Buchthal 1965). However, up to 25% polyphasic potentials may be seen in the normal deltoid muscle (Buchthal 1977). It is important to recognise that when motor unit potentials are studied with a trigger-delay line, and displayed successively on the oscilloscope, the duration and number of phases in the motor unit is often at variance with those estimated in a free-running trace. The technique of recording with a trigger-delay line allows late units (units seen 15 ms or more after the first part of the motor units potential) to be recognised. Without the trigger-delay line these late units will usually be regarded as activity arising in other motor units (Fig. 2.9). Further, it is important to remember that both the amplitude and duration of motor unit potentials are modified by different filter settings (Fig. 2.10).

During contraction of increasing force additional motor units are recruited (Fig. 2.11). This recruitment occurs in an orderly fashion (Hannerz 1974). The first motor units to be activated are Type 1 units, which consist of slow-contracting oxidative fibres, resistant to fatigue (Burke et al. 1971). The first motor units activated on volition are of relatively low amplitude, about 150 μV in adults. With increasing force of contraction the firing rate of these early-activated units increases, and other units appear. The latter are usually of higher amplitude. During maximal isometric contraction electrical activity from the motor unit activity should fill the oscilloscope screen. The maximal amplitude of this activity should exceed 0.5 mV at age 5 years and 2 mV at age 15 years (Rosenfalck 1975). This constitutes a *full interference pattern.* During maximum isometric contraction only a proportion, perhaps as little as a third, of the motor units in an individual muscle are activated. Fuller activation can be produced by sudden, phasic contraction against a heavy load, but for most electromyographic purposes varying degrees of isometric contraction are more useful.

Recruitment

The graded increase in force often used in everyday tasks is accomplished by two basic mechanisms:

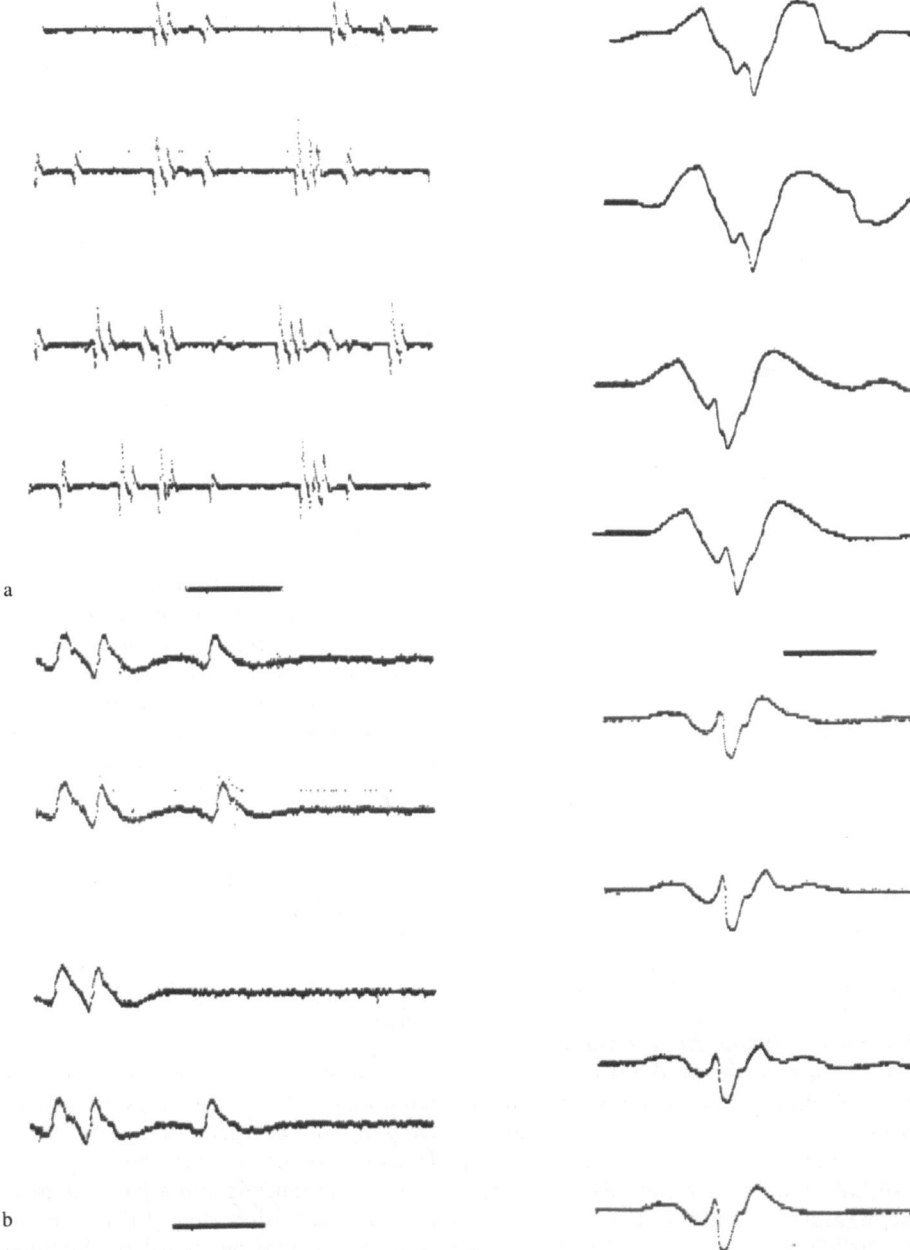

Fig. 2.9. **a** Concentric needle EMG recording during partial voluntary activation in a patient with a neurogenic disorder (motor neuron disease). A polyphasic motor unit action potential is seen; its last component can be seen more clearly to be related to its two initial components in b. Filters: 100 Hz and 10 kHz. Bar 20 ms.

b The late component can be seen in constant relationship to the two earlier components when the trigger-delay line is used. The potential has changed its configuration because the sweep speed is faster, and a 500-Hz low-frequency filter has been used. In the third of these consecutive traces the late unit is not seen. This is an example of *neuromuscular blocking*. Bar 2 ms.

Fig. 2.10. The effect on potential shape of changing the low-frequency filter from 100 Hz (**a**) to 500 Hz (**b**). The 500-Hz filter accentuates components with faster rise times. Bar 2 ms.

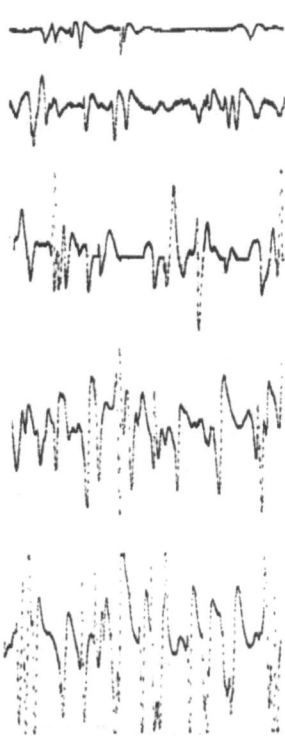

Fig. 2.11. Concentric needle EMG recording during increasing force of voluntary activation in a normal subject. The lowermost recording is a full interference pattern. With increasing force larger motor units are recruited. Filters: 100 Hz and 10 kHz. Bar 20 ms.

recruiting additional motor units and increasing the firing frequency of units that are already active (Buchthal and Schmalbruch 1980). At low force levels recruitment of new units is the predominant mechanism (Person and Kudina 1972), but at higher force levels increasing firing frequency is more important (Milner-Brown et al. 1973). Motor units recruited at low threshold tend to fire initially at 5–8 Hz, whereas the highest-threshold units commence firing at 15–20 Hz (Freund et al. 1975; Grimby et al. 1979; Freund 1983). This orderly recruitment of units of different physiological characteristics during contraction of increasing force has been correlated with histochemical studies; the first-recruited, slower-firing units are Type 1, tonic units and the later-recruited, faster-firing units are Type 2, phasic units (Grimby and Hannerz 1970; Hannerz 1974). Henneman et al. (1965) showed in the cat that the first-recruited units originate from smaller alpha motor neurons, and the later-recruited units from larger anterior horn cells. Tanji and Kato (1973) reported similar observations in humans. This concept of orderly recruitment of

units from specific types of anterior horn cells is termed Henneman's size principle. Edstrom and Grimby (1986) have shown that these relationships are maintained during physical training. During the development of fatigue, however, the firing rate of high-threshold units decreases. Low-threshold, tonic units are more resistant to fatigue although their firing rate slowly decreases as fatigue develops (Grimby et al. 1981)

Abnormal Recruitment

In patients with myopathies more units are activated during slight voluntary effort than in normal subjects and a full interference pattern develops with less than maximal voluntary contraction. This early recruitment (Petajan 1991) may be due to mismatch between force generated by the weakened muscle and the central programme in the brain previously matched to muscle afferents related to given levels of central motor drive. In myopathies individual muscle fibres, scattered among many motor units, cease to function. Neurogenic disorders produce different physiological abnormalities. In upper motor neuron disorders the firing frequency of motor units is reduced, and in lower motor neuron disorders inappropriately rapid firing rates may occur and large motor units are activated earlier. The early recruitment of large units indicates the presence of reinnervated units of larger size than normal. These units may fire irregularly (Halonen et al. 1981).

Double Discharges

Sometimes a motor unit shows repetitive firing during voluntary activity. Such potentials often appear as pairs of identical or nearly identical potentials, with 2–20 ms or occasionally up to 30 ms between the two potentials and a pause before the next potential is recorded (Fig. 2.12). Sometimes triplets or multiplets may be recorded. The innervation rate thus become irregular (Partanen and Lang 1978). The phenomenon is most commonly found in neurogenic disorders, particularly radiculopathies (Partanen 1978). Double discharges may occur in normal subjects at the beginning and at the cessation of voluntary contraction (Partanen and Lang 1978), but this is unusual and double discharges are usually a feature of polyneuropathies or root syndromes (Partanen and Lang 1978; Partanen 1978). They probably originate distally in the lower motor neuron from presynaptic excitation or ephaptic stimulation in peripheral motor axons (Partanen and Lang 1978; Roth 1985).

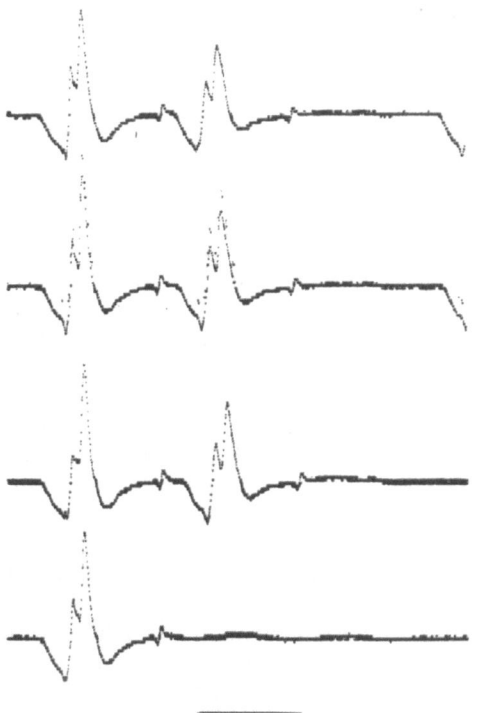

Fig. 2.12. Double discharges in syringomyelia, recorded with single-fibre EMG. In the first three traces the whole motor unit action potential fires twice in 5 ms, including the small late component. Double discharges may be seen in a number of neurogenic disorders, and also in myotonic dystrophy.

Quantitative Concentric Needle EMG Studies

Quantitative analysis of EMG potentials can be accomplished manually, but a number of automatic or computer-based methods are also available, and are becoming more important in clinical electromyography as the basic technology improves. These depend on measurements of *duration, amplitude, number of phases* and *number of turns* of motor unit action potentials. Since the characteristics of units recorded from a muscle depend on the type of unit recruited it is important, in these studies, to specify the degree of activity of the muscle examined and force measurements have been used to accomplish this. In addition, the position of the recording site relative to the end-plate zone, co-operation of the patient, and the muscle chosen for examination are all relevant variables in these studies (Buchthal and Pinelli 1953; Rosenfalck 1975; Stålberg et al. 1983; Liguari et al. 1992a,b). Nissen-Petersen et al. (1969) used the trigger-delay line to isolate individual motor unit potentials for analysis and thus improved the capacity for measurement of motor unit potential duration, amplitude and number of phases in measurements made on the oscilloscope screen, thus improving on the earlier attempts by Buchthal and colleagues to determine the characteristic parameters of individual motor unit potentials.

Automatic Analysis of Motor Unit Potentials

Computer-based methods can be used to analyse motor unit potential duration, amplitude and number of phases. Units may be collected manually or by automated methods for computer analysis. The analysis itself can be carried out using template recognition techniques or by various types of trigger-delay methodology (Lang and Falck 1980). In the template method the computer chooses a motor unit potential and pattern recognition methods are used, derived from digitised, averaged potentials, for the analysis (Tanzi et al. 1979; Stålberg and Antoni 1983). These automated methods are dependent on the accuracy of the recognition technique for individual motor unit potentials employed in the computer and on the type and degree of selection of the potentials used for analysis (Dorfman and McGill 1988). They are generally limited by the necessity for a noise-free background, and by technical limits for potential duration, and for on-line or off-line analysis determined by computer memory and by the capacity of digitisation in the system.

Automatic MUAP analysis requires that the computer recognises individual potentials when they recur during the maintained contraction. The EMG record is analysed by using an amplitude trigger, or by a template recognition technique. The latter (Bergmans 1971) uses an amplitude threshold of 20–50 μV during epochs. Potentials that recur 2–10 times, recognised by their waveform or area, are accepted for analysis. Andreassen's method (Stålberg et al. 1986) uses an amplitude trigger and sorts potentials derived in 100 ms epochs into bins according to their template. Three matched potentials are averaged for analysis. Toulouse et al. (1985) used a more complex definition of suitable potentials, involving measurement of duration, amplitude, phases and turns to identify MUAPs. The computer decides whether each MUAP is normal or abnormal by reference to a set of criteria for normality. These methods use partial or threshold contraction. Decomposition analysis (Dorfman and McGill 1988; Bischoff et al. 1994) has been used to define motor unit potential amplitude, rise time and shape from freely contracting muscle using defined values of these parameters for identification. Large numbers of potentials of low and high threshold obtained from the same site can be obtained from a short recording, using automatic rather than manual methods.

Automatic Analysis of the Interference Pattern

Individual motor unit potentials can be identified and analysed only during slight contraction, thus limiting this technique to small, fatigue-resistant Type 1 units. Analysis of the interference pattern, on the other hand, offers the possibility of evaluating the EMG during maximal or submaximal effort. These methods are based on spectral analysis of the EMG signal (Walton 1952; Larsson 1975; Lindstrom and Petersen 1983), turns analysis (Willison 1964; Hayward 1983; Fuglsang-Frederiksen et al. 1985) or pattern recognition of motor unit potentials (Guiheneuc et al. 1983).

Spectral analysis uses the Fourier transformation to provide a measure of the power spectrum of the electrical signal. The latter depends primarily on the amplitudes and durations of the motor unit potentials. In normal subjects the energy of the signal is concentrated at 100 Hz and in patients with myopathies the power is mainly at higher frequencies (400 Hz). In neurogenic disorders this is shifted to lower frequencies. Kopec and Hausmanowa-Petrusewicz (1976, 1983) used a computer-based method that utilised both motor unit potential analysis and the mean frequency of intervals between successive negative peaks in the EMG.

Turns analysis (Willison 1964; Hayward and Willison 1977) measures the number of potential reversals per unit time and the mean amplitude between turns in the EMG signal. In the original method force was set, without consideration of the strength of the muscle tested, but in subsequent modifications (Fuglsang-Frederiksen et al. 1976; Stålberg et al. 1983) the relationship of turns and mean amplitude has been used, since this index is relatively independent of force of contraction (Cenkovich et al. 1982; Fuglsang-Frederiksen et al. 1985). In myopathies the turns count is increased, and the mean amplitude decreased, but in neurogenic disorders the converse obtains (Rose and Willison 1967). The maximum value of the ratio of turns to mean amplitude (peak ratio) and the number of time intervals between turns (time intervals) have been used to differentiate myopathy and neuropathy. In myopathies there is an increase in both peak ratio and number of time intervals between 0 and 1.5 ms, and in neurogenic disorders the converse was found (Liguari et al. 1992b). In myopathies this method had a higher yield than individual MUAP analysis.

Motor Unit Counts

The EMG signal consists of the summated electrical activity of motor units recorded from the uptake area of the concentric needle or other electrode. Attempts have been made to establish methods for counting motor units in individual muscles by using graded electrical stimulation of the mixed motor nerve and attempting to identify increments in the electrical activity recorded with a surface electrode from the muscle under test using either manual or computerised template recognition techniques (McComas et al. 1971a; Ballantyne and Hansen 1974a). The original method was criticised on several grounds, but especially because of the possibility of different thresholds for different motor axons, the difficulty in recognising large motor units, and problems in establishing the comparability of recordings in test/re-test experiments (Brown and Milner-Brown 1976; Kimura 1983). A review of the technique of motor unit number estimation (MUNE) sets out the methodological difficulties (McComas 1995).

In the original manual method the stimulus intensity is gradually increased. The stepped increase in amplitude reflects activation of additional motor units. The mean difference of 10 consecutive incremental responses measured peak to peak is divided into the maximum M wave, giving a number that is an estimate of the number of functioning motor units in the muscle (McComas et al. 1971a). This method was originally applied to the extensor digitorum brevis muscle. This manual method was automated by Ballantyne and Hansen (1974a) who used template recognition in a computer to establish the increments resulting from increasing stimulus intensities. This method is relatively easy to use, but tends to produce a lower estimate of motor units since it eliminates alternating excitation of motor axons by template recognition (McComas 1995). Kadrie et al. (1976) used a multiple point stimulation technique, stimulating the motor nerve at different sites. This method requires a superficial, long motor nerve, and is time consuming (Docherty and Brown 1993). Brown et al. (1988) used a spike-triggered averaging method, that involves a needle EMG to trigger recording from a surface electrode. This method results in a high MUNE, but is tedious to perform. Stashuk et al. (1994) suggested that F waves could be used for analysis since they represent single motor units. Daube (1988) employed a Poisson quantal analysis to estimate motor unit numbers.

In the human thenar muscle these different methods give MUNE ranging from 135 to 342 units, the lowest being derived from spike-triggered averaging and the highest from the manual incremental method. Each method has a moderately large inherent variance, limiting their usefulness in practice.

Interpretation of the significance of reduced numbers of motor units in a neuromuscular disorder

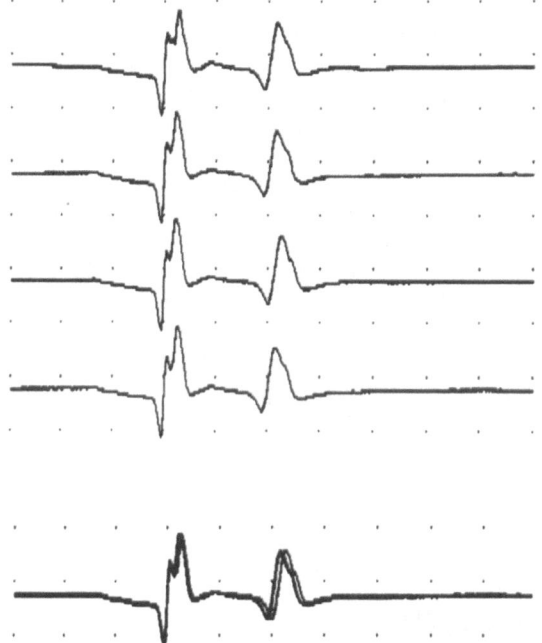

Fig. 2.13. Single-fibre EMG recording of a potential pair in a normal subject. The neuromuscular jitter is normal (<50 μs).

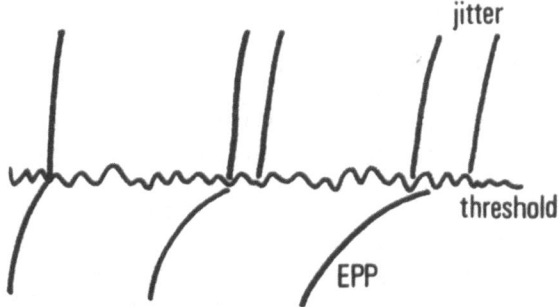

Fig. 2.14. Diagrammatic representation of increased jitter, with impulse blocking, resulting from variations in rise time of the end-plate potential (EPP). The jitter increases with increasing rise time of the EPP.

is not as simple a matter as might be supposed. For example, reduced motor unit numbers have been reported in muscular dystrophy, upper motor neuron lesions and hyperthyroidism. The technique of MUNE measures the number of functioning motor units and this concept may, in part, explain this seeming paradox. Bromberg et al. (1993) compared MUNE, isometric strength and EMG measures (including fibre density, macro EMG, turns analysis and muscle action potential amplitude) in patients with amyotrophic lateral sclerosis. They found a poor correlation between MUNE and all EMG measures, reflecting the effect of collateral reinnervation which masks the extent of motor neuron loss. Strength was also not correlated with MUNE.

Single-Fibre EMG

With concentric needle electrodes, action potentials of individual muscle fibres cannot usually be recognised within the motor unit action potential. Such action potentials can be recorded, though, using an electrode with a small leading-off surface (25 μm diameter) and an amplifier with a 500 Hz low-frequency filter setting and a trigger-delay line.

When more than one single-fibre action potential is recorded within the uptake radius of the electrode (about 270 μm; Stålberg et al. 1976a) the variability in the time interval between the triggering potential and the other potential or potentials belonging to the same motor unit recorded in this uptake can be measured (Fig. 2.13). This is called the *neuromuscular jitter* (Ekstedt 1964).

The jitter is mainly due to variation in the times of onset of the action potentials generated by the end-plate potentials of the two fibres recorded. The latter normally shows slight variability in the slope of its rise phase and when, as in some diseases such as myasthenia gravis or other structural disorders of end-plates, the slope of the end-plate potential is more variable than normal there may be a variable delay in the onset of the propagated muscle action potential (Fig. 2.14), causing an increased neuromuscular jitter (Elmqvist et al. 1964; Stålberg et al. 1976b). This jitter is usually expressed as the mean consecutive difference (MCD) between individual potentials and, in normal subjects, is less than 50 μs, although there are variations between different muscles (Gilchrist et al. 1992). The MCD can be calculated on-line by using computer-aided methods (Davis et al. 1983; Stålberg and Trontelj 1994).

The MCD can be approximated by measuring the maximum variability of the non-triggered component of a potential pair during five consecutive discharges. Half this value approximates the jitter as expressed by the MCD. In the case of four recordings the MCD approximates this value divided by 0.55 (Ekstedt et al. 1974). This is most easily done by displaying four or five consecutive potentials either on a storage oscilloscope or on a paper write-out.

In normal subjects each component of the MUAP recorded during single-fibre EMG appears with each discharge, i.e. there is no *impulse blocking*. Twenty different MUAPs are usually studied. Occasionally one of these shows an excess jitter, representing abnormal neuromuscular transmission, or abnormal activation of the muscle fibre.

The mean duration of MUAPs, consisting of more than one component, recorded by single-fibre EMG is <8 ms. In the normal extensor digitorum communis muscle the motor unit potential duration recorded by single-fibre EMG did not exceed 4 ms in 95% of recordings (Stålberg and Trontelj 1994).

The *fibre density* in single-fibre EMG recordings is the mean number of single muscle fibre action potentials recorded within the uptake area of the single-fibre EMG electrode in 20 different positions within the muscle (Stålberg and Thiele 1975). In normal subjects the fibre density in most muscles is less than 2.0 (Stålberg and Trontelj 1994), although after the age of 60 years this value increases slightly (Gilchrist et al. 1992). In the extensor digitorum communis muscle the upper limit (95% CI) of fibre density was 1.8 at the age of 30 years, 2.0 at 60 years and 2.5 at 90 years.

Single muscle fibre action potentials can be recorded with ordinary concentric needle electrodes (Payan 1978), particularly the electrodes used for facial muscle recordings, by using suitable filter settings but only a proportion of the potentials recorded in this way are, in fact, single muscle fibre action potentials. This is because the uptake area of concentric needle electrodes is too great to allow isolation of less than a few single muscle fibre action potentials from the summated activity of nearby muscle fibres belonging to the same motor unit. These electrodes should not be used, therefore, for fibre density measurements. The fibre density is a useful quantitative measure which can be used in follow-up single-fibre EMG studies. Yu and Murray (1984) found the sensitivity of single-fibre EMG was greater (93%) than concentric needle EMG (83%) in 30 patients with a variety of neuromuscular disorders.

Different Activation Procedures in Single-Fibre EMG

The usual method of recording muscle activity in single-fibre EMG utilises weak voluntary activation to induce a low level of continuous muscle contraction. This activation method is dependent on patient cooperation, and selects first-activated, low-threshold, tonic units. Fatigue and disease often result in poor activation and difficulty in completing adequate recordings. Electrical stimulation of motor axons in peripheral nerve branches in the muscle has been developed to obviate the necessity for voluntary activation. A monopolar stimulating catho-

dal electrode, insulated to its tip, is inserted into the muscle near the motor point and electrical pulses of 30 V or less (10 mA) and of short duration (5 μs) are used to stimulate an axon. A surface anode is used, and a recording is made from motor units in the muscle using a single fibre EMG electrode. The rate of stimulation can be varied from slow rates to a rapid tetanus. However, accurate fibre density measurements cannot be obtained because the technique is highly selective, and only part of the terminal axonal arborisation may be stimulated (Stålberg et al. 1992). Direct nerve stimulation, with surface electrodes is less selective, but may be useful in demonstrating blocking potentials (Schwartz and Stålberg 1975a). The main value of stimulation single-fibre EMG is in the diagnosis of myasthenia gravis and myasthenic syndrome.

Macro EMG

The technique of macro EMG can be used to study the electrical activity from a much larger portion of the motor unit than can be assessed with concentric or single-fibre EMG electrodes. In macro EMG the recording is made from the cannula of a modified single-fibre EMG electrode which is insulated except for the distal 15 mm. A single-fibre EMG recording surface located at the mid-point of this distal, uninsulated portion of the cannula (Stålberg 1980, 1983) is used to locate a single motor unit. This unit is then utilised to trigger an averaged recording from the uninsulated cannula. The averaged signal thus represents the electrical activity recorded from the motor unit by the 15 mm cannula traversing the muscle. The amplitude of this response is dependent on the number of muscle fibres active in the unit recorded, and this amplitude is increased when there is reinnervation (Stålberg and Fawcett 1982). Individual peaks in amplitude in the waveform represent the distribution of motor end-plates related to the motor unit (Nandedkar and Stålberg 1983). Motor units recruited at higher thresholds tend to be of greater amplitude (Stålberg and Fawcett 1982; Nandedkar and Stålberg 1983).

In muscular dystrophy of various types Hilton-Brown and Stålberg (1983b) found that macro EMG potentials were of normal or slightly reduced amplitude, a finding consistent with loss of functional muscle fibres from motor units. In acute denervation there is also reduced amplitude. In computer simulations of macro EMG Nandedkar et al. (1985) have estimated that the normal macro EMG potential represents up to 100 muscle fibres, but in reinnervation as many as 200 fibres contribute to the motor unit potential recorded with this technique. Bauermeister and Jabre (1992) noted that the MUP area recorded by macro EMG correlated with the area of concentric needle recordings made from the same unit, using a specially constructed dual electrode, implying that the 10–15 muscle fibres sampled by concentric needle EMG represented a good sample of fibres in the motor unit. No significant additional information was obtained in macro EMG recordings in neurogenic and myopathic disorders (Gan and Jabre 1992).

Scanning EMG

Scanning EMG provides a cross-sectional electrophysiological assessment of the distribution of muscle fibres belonging to single motor units in a muscle (Fig. 2.15). A concentric needle electrode is fitted into a small step-motor which allows the needle to be drawn through a muscle through multiple stations 50 μm apart, using a computer-controlled program. A separate single-fibre EMG electrode, placed nearby in the muscle, is used to generate a signal trigger for the motor unit under investigation in the scanning recording. This method allows visualisation of the distribution of fibres belonging to a single motor unit in the uptake area of the scanning electrode, and is useful in identifying fragmentation and multiple small groupings of fibres within motor units (Stålberg and Antoni 1980; Hilton-Brown and Stålberg 1983a,b; Stålberg and Droszeghy 1991).

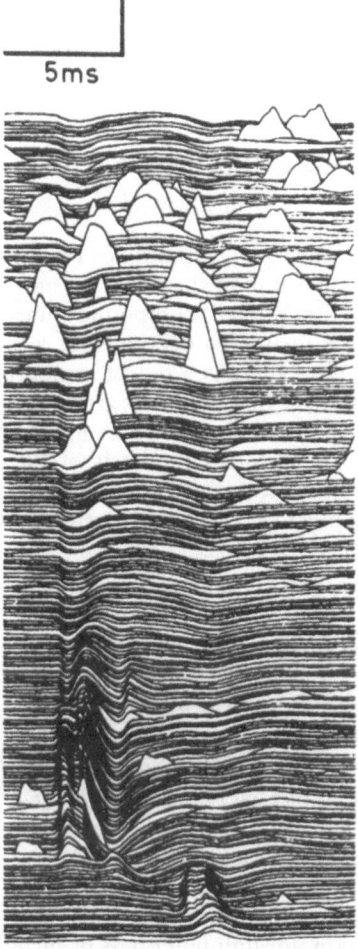

Fig. 2.15. Scanning EMG, using concentric needle electrode, in a normal tibialis anterior muscle, showing the distribution of the motor unit in the lower half of the consecutive recording. The large peaks at the top represent portions of other motor units. (From Stålberg and Antoni 1980.)

Multi-electrode Studies

Concentric needle electrodes containing multiple (up to 12) recording electrode surfaces aligned on the cannula of the electrode were used by Buchthal et al. (1957) to study volume conduction and territory of the motor unit. Stålberg et al. (1976a) adapted this concept by constructing a 14-lead single-fibre electrode array contained within a single needle electrode to study propagation velocity in single muscle fibres. An electrode with a single row of single-fibre EMG recording surfaces was used to re-examine the concept of a motor unit territory and to study the distribution of fibres in the recording areas of these electrode surfaces in normal subjects (Stålberg et al. 1976a) and in reinnervated muscle (Schwartz et al. 1976b). Lang and Falck (1980) constructed a two-channel electrode, consisting of a conventional concentric needle EMG electrode with a single-fibre EMG recording surface located adjacent to it, or with concentric and single-fibre EMG recording surfaces mounted on opposite sides of the cannula, near its tip (Falck 1983). This electrode has enabled theoretical concepts of the generator potential, the distribution of fibres (dispersion) making up the spike component, and the amplitude and duration of the MUAP to be examined (Falck 1983). Bauermeister and Jabre (1992) evaluated macro EMG and concentric needle EMG using a multi-electrode constructed for the purpose (see above).

Repetitive Stimulation

When a motor nerve is stimulated repetitively using supramaximal stimuli at a slow rate, and the amplitudes of the evoked compound muscle action potentials measured, a decremental response may be observed if there is a defect in neuromuscular transmission, as in myasthenia gravis, and an incremental response in the Eaton–Lambert myasthenic syndrome. This forms the basis of the standard, commonly used test of neuromuscular transmission in clinical practice (Oh 1988) described in Chap. 12 .

Surface EMG

Quantitative methods for evaluation of surface EMG recordings have been developed (Cioni et al. 1985). This technology is potentially applicable to the study of both central and peripheral motor system disorders and is especially attractive because it obviates the necessity for needle insertion (Tanzi and Taglietti 1981). However, it is very difficult to isolate individual motor unit potentials in surface recordings with current technological limitations, and surface recordings are therefore used regularly only in kinesiological studies, as in gait analysis (Larsson 1985). The filtering effect of skin and fat makes motor unit potential analysis of surface recorded EMG impracticable.

Nerve Conduction Studies

Motor and sensory nerve conduction measurements are invaluable in the assessment of peripheral nerve lesions. With modern methods both proximal and distal segments of the peripheral nerves can be studied. In studying motor nerve conduction it is convenient to utilise the evoked muscle response occurring after nerve stimulation, a method introduced by Helmholtz (1850) and Piper (1909). This is a large potential. In sensory conduction studies the sensory nerve action potential (SAP) recorded by surface electrodes is of low amplitude and may only

be identifiable with averaging techniques (Dawson 1954).

Nerve conduction measurements (Shahani 1985) are particularly useful:

1. To demonstrate that a disorder affects peripheral nerve rather than the muscle or the neuromuscular junctions
2. To localise entrapment or compressive lesions of nerves
3. To differentiate *axonal* from *demyelinating* neuropathies
4. To monitor the course of peripheral nerve diseases, and the response to treatment.

In general, sensory conduction studies are more sensitive than motor conduction investigations.

Conventional nerve conduction techniques are limited in scope by two factors:

1. Only the fastest conducting motor and sensory nerve fibres are assessed
2. Proximal segments of the peripheral nervous system, including the spinal roots, are accessible to study only special techniques, such as H reflexes, F responses, somatosensory evoked response and central motor stimulation techniques. Motor roots can be stimulated directly by transcutaneous or needle electrode techniques.

General Principles of Nerve Conduction Velocity Studies

Motor and sensory nerve conduction studies are usually carried out with surface stimulating and recording electrodes. In children smaller electrodes of this type are necessary. Needle recording electrodes are used in some laboratories for recording SAPs but with modern digital averaging techniques needle electrodes are not usually necessary. The stimulus duration required is usually between 0.1 and 0.3 ms. Care must be taken in motor conduction velocity studies to use supramaximal stimuli. Measurements of the applied stimulus current give a measure of the stimulus threshold of the nerve and these values are sometimes useful in detecting slight abnormalities, particularly when comparison is made between sensory thresholds in opposite limbs. It is particularly important to ensure that the limb studied is warm during nerve conduction velocity studies; in normal nerve between 29 °C and 38 °C (Ludin et al. 1977) the nerve conduction velocity decreases linearly by 2 m/s for each degree centigrade the limb is cooled. When the skin temperature is less than 34 °C the limb should be warmed. It should be routine practice to measure sensory and motor nerve conduction velocity in at least one nerve in all patients referred for electromyography because some, including those with proximal weakness, may thus be shown to have a neuropathy, for example Guillain–Barré syndrome, rather than other myopathic or neurogenic disorders.

Motor Conduction Velocity

Motor nerve conduction velocity can be easily calculated. The latency of a distal supramaximal stimulus applied to a motor nerve and the beginning of the evoked muscle action potential (the M (muscle) response, Fig. 2.16) is measured. The stimulus is then applied to a more proximal site and the difference in latency between the two responses measured in milliseconds. This, divided by the distance between the two points of stimulation measured in centimetres, gives the motor conduction velocity, usually expressed in metres per second.

In adults, motor nerve conduction velocity is inversely proportional to the height of the individual (Lang et al. 1977). In the newborn, motor nerve conduction velocity is about half that in adults (Baer and Johnson 1965). It increases rapidly in the first year of life and adult conduction velocity is attained by the age of 3–5 years. Adult conduction velocities are attained in the legs rather later in development than in the arms (Wagner and Buchthal 1972; Rosenfalck 1975; Lang et al. 1985) and are slower in the legs than in the arms. Maximal motor nerve conduction velocity normally exceeds 50 m/s in the arms and 40 m/s in the legs. In the more proximal part of the nerve, conduction is usually slightly faster. Lang et al. (1985) noted that nerve conduction tended to become slightly slower in adolescence, and it has been suggested that this might be due to tapering of the distal parts of motor axons in long limbs (Campbell et al. 1981), although this has not been thoroughly verified histologically. During ageing there is a slight slowing of motor conduction velocity. This is first apparent after the fourth decade, and by the age of 60 years amounts to a reduction of no more than 10 m/s (Mayer 1963).

Motor Conduction Block

Motor nerve conduction is particularly slowed in entrapment neuropathies and in acquired demyelinating neuropathies, i.e. when there is damage to Schwann cell myelin. In localised entrapment lesions conduction is slowed across the damaged segment,

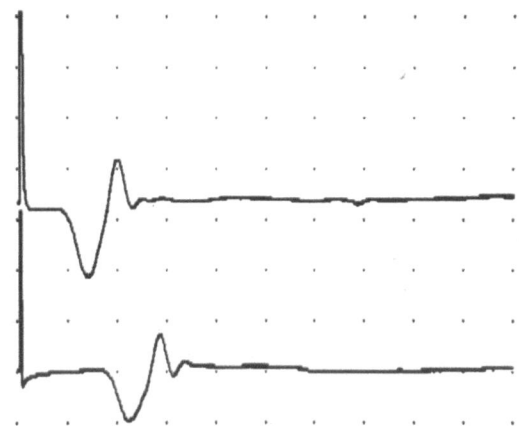

Fig. 2.16. Motor nerve conduction, using proximal (elbow) and distal (wrist) stimulation of the median nerve. The distal motor latency from the distal stimulation site is shown in the upper trace.

and the amplitude of the compound muscle action potential (CMAP) is larger with distal than with proximal stimulation. This is due to *conduction block* in nerve fibres in the damaged segment resulting in excitation in a reduced number of motor units in the muscle after proximal compared with distal stimulation. In addition, the proximal response may be dispersed because of the variable change in conduction in different, fast-conducting fibres traversing the damaged segment.

Kimura (1993) considered the clinical criteria for conduction block. He noted that the standard criteria required a reduction of the CMAP amplitude or area in proximal compared with distal stimulation of 20%–40%. Cornblath et al. (1991) noted that a reduction criterion of 20%–60% had been suggested by others, and noted that rather than discussing this disagreement (Brown and Bolton (1993) stated that a 20% difference in peak to peak amplitude should be the accepted criterion) three other points should be remembered.

First, an abrupt change in amplitude or area over a short (2–4 cm) segment, particularly in entrapment neuropathies, is important evidence of conduction block. Second, using concentric needle EMG the presence of units activated by distal, but not by proximal stimulation, suggests conduction block. Third, reconstitution of the CMAP using recordings of individual surface recordings from voluntary activity, using the template recognition technology devised for motor unit counting can be used to demonstrate blocked potentials. This method is technically complex and time consuming.

Kimura (1993) pointed out that a more than 20% increase in duration of the CMAP elicited by proxi-

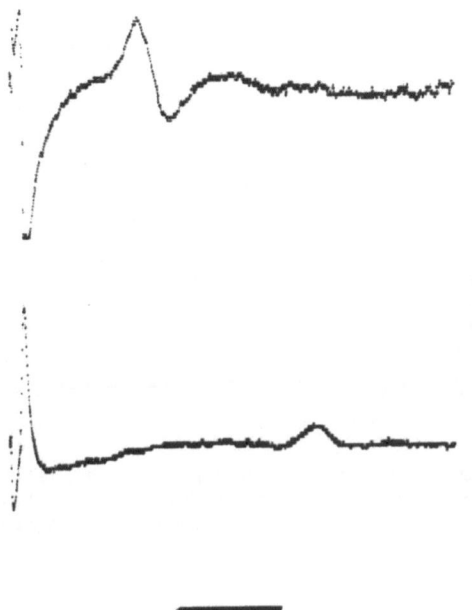

Fig. 2.17. Normal subject. Sensory nerve action potential (SAP) recorded from the median nerve at the wrist and elbow with surface electrodes after stimulation of the digital nerves of the index finger. The SAP is smaller at the elbow. Bar 2 ms.

mal stimulation was consistent with conduction block (Kimura et al. 1988). Slowed F wave latencies, large distal CMAPs despite marked weakness (Kimura 1993) and reduced number of voluntarily activated motor unit potentials (Cornblath et al. 1991b) are also associated features consistent with conduction block.

Sensory Conduction Studies

Sensory action potentials (SAPs) can be relatively easily recorded from sural, radial, median and ulnar nerves, although digital averaging may be necessary, particularly in abnormal nerves and in elderly subjects. The ulnar and median nerves are often damaged at points of compression, but the radial and sural nerves are less vulnerable to this form of occult injury, and are therefore particularly useful for sensory action potential studies. The amplitude of the SAP diminishes with age. Low-amplitude potentials may only be recorded with near-nerve needle electrodes (Rosenfalck 1975). SAPs are generally larger in women than in men.

Sensory nerve conduction velocity can be determined *orthodromically* by stimulating digital nerves and recording the SAP from median or ulnar nerves. This technique utilises only a single site of stimulation, rather than two as in motor conduction velocities. A converse electrode placement can be used to measure sensory conduction velocity *antidromically*. The antidromic response is often easier to elicit and can be useful in clinical practice.

The sensory conduction velocity is normally faster than 42 m/s in the sural nerve of adults (Burke et al. 1974b). There is no significant change with age (>40 m/s; Burke et al. 1974). However, in neonates median sensory conduction velocity is 25–30 m/s (Miller and Kuntz 1986). The adult range is reached by age 1 year. Sensory conduction in the radial nerve is faster than in the sural nerve, being >50 m/s in normal subjects (Shahani et al. 1967). In normal subjects more proximally recorded SAPs are of lower amplitude than those recorded distally (Fig. 2.17). This is a consequence of the loss of slower conducting fibres from the visible envelope of the SAP (Kimura et al. 1988).

In axonal neuropathies the first change in sensory conduction is a reduction in amplitude of the SAP, but in demyelinating neuropathies slowing of conduction is more characteristic. In mild disturbances of peripheral nerve function a small or delayed SAP may be the only abnormality. Needle electrode recordings may be especially useful in neuropathies since results can be obtained when surface recordings, even using averaging techniques, fail to disclose the SAP; for example, in patients with distal oedema. The slower conducting sensory fibres, revealed by the dispersion of the SAP, may be recognised more readily with this method. In root lesions the SAP is unaffected, indicating a lesion proximal to the dorsal root ganglion.

Mixed Nerve Action Potential Recording

When stimulating a mixed nerve a nerve action potential is propagated and can be recorded at another point along the nerve, and its conduction velocity calculated (Fig. 2.18). This technique is particularly useful in the assessment of entrapment syndromes, when it may give information about local slowing of nerve conduction and loss of nerve fibres. Sensory fibres normally conduct slightly faster than motor nerve fibres, and provide the main contribution to the potential.

H Reflex Studies

The H reflex (named after Hoffmann) is a monosynaptic reflex (Fig. 2.19), usually only obtainable in humans in the soleus muscle after stimulation of the medial popliteal nerve, and from the forearm

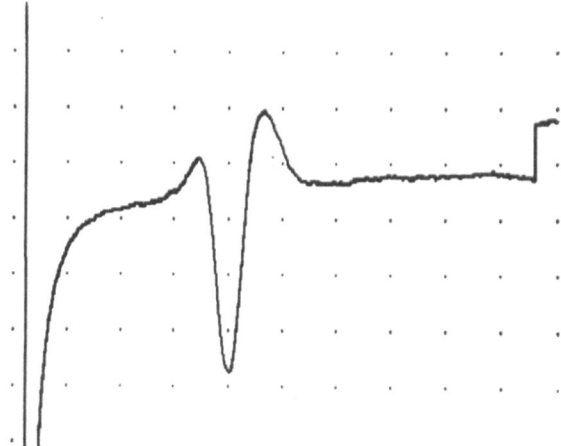

Fig. 2.18. Normal nerve action potential, recorded from the ulnar nerve at the elbow following stimulation at the wrist. Calibration signal 10 mV to right of trace.

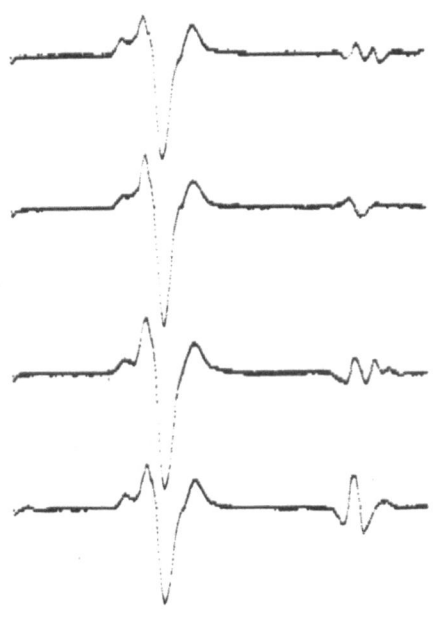

Fig. 2.20. Normal F response. Stimulation of common peroneal nerve at the fibular head; recording with surface electrodes over the extensor digitorum brevis muscles. The M response is seen at 12 ms and the first deflection of the F wave at 37–40 ms. The latency and configuration vary with successive stimuli, which were made at 1-s intervals in this recording. In measurements of the F wave latency the fastest of at least 10 responses is accepted. Bar 10 ms.

flexors after median nerve stimulation at the elbow (Deschuytere et al. 1976; Jabre 1981). Within these limitations of segmental localisation the H reflex can be useful in assessing proximal lesions in the S1/S2 and C7 roots, since it provides a measure of proximal conduction, utilising both afferent and efferent pathways. H reflex excitability curves, obtained by a double stimulation technique, have been used in the assessment of motor neuron excitability (Magladery et al. 1951) and, in the assessment of spasticity using the ratio of M wave and H reflex amplitude (Angel and Hoffmann 1963). Trontelj (1973) recorded H reflexes in single motor units, using single-fibre EMG recordings, and examined the variability in excitability of motoneurons in

individual motor unit pools. the recruitment curve of the H reflex amplitude has been used to assess this aspect of motor neuronal excitability.

The F Response

The F response (Foot and Finger) (Fig. 2.20) can be recorded from a muscle after stimulation of its nerve (Magladery and McDougal 1950). The response represents the electrically evoked firing of anterior horn cells induced by the retrogradely conducted impulse in the motor axon from the point of stimulation in the peripheral nerve. The F response is therefore recorded in a muscle *after* the M response, and its latency represents conduction in the motor nerve from the point of stimulation to the anterior horn cells and back, beyond this point of stimulation, to the muscle innervated by this motor nerve (Fig. 2.20). F responses can be recorded in *all* muscles and are therefore especially useful in the assessment of proximal conduction in motor nerve fibres. Sensory afferent fibres are not involved in the F response.

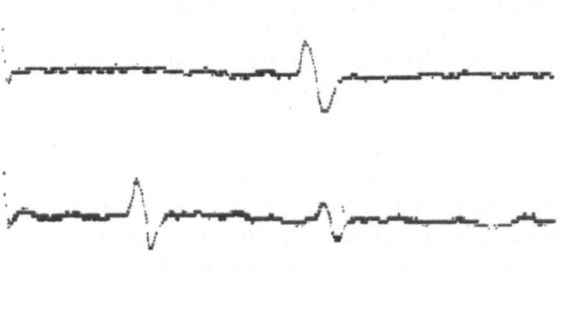

Fig. 2.19. Normal H reflex. Stimulation of medial popliteal nerve and recording with surface electrodes over the soleus muscle. At low stimulus intensity only an H reflex is seen, but at higher intensities the earlier M response is also recorded, and the H reflex amplitude becomes smaller. Bar 20 ms.

The F response conduction may be expressed as its *latency* or, indirectly, a *conduction velocity* can be calculated. The ratio of proximal (F wave) to distal motor latency is also used (Kimura 1974, 1978). The fastest F wave of at least 10 recordings should be used. *Dispersion* and *persistency* of responses are also important.

In order to calculate the *F wave conduction velocity* the distance from the stimulating electrode to the anterior horn cell must be estimated. Although this cannot be done directly, an approximation can be obtained in the upper limb by measuring the distance from the stimulating electrode to the spinous process of C7 and, in the lower limb, from the stimulating electrode to the spinous process of L2. The F wave conduction velocity (proximal motor conduction) can be calculated from the formula (Kimura 1978):

$$\text{F velocity (m/s)} = \cfrac{\text{Distance from stimulating electrode to spine of C7 or L2 (cm)}}{\left[\cfrac{\text{F wave latency} - \text{M (motor) latency}}{2} - 1\ \text{ms} \right]}$$

(1 ms is allowed for a central delay due to the time taken for the anterior horn cells to fire in response to the stimulus)

For most clinical purposes the *F wave latency*, in any limb, can be related to standing height (Lachman et al. 1980). For example, in a subject of height 150 cm the F wave latency in abductor pollicis brevis lies between 22 and 28 ms (Lachman et al. 1980). The interlimb difference in F responses in the upper limb is not more than 2 ms, and in the legs not more than 3 ms (Lachman et al. 1980; Tang et al. 1988). In general, the F max latency (upper limit of normal) is less than 30 ms in median and ulnar nerves, 48 ms in deep peroneal and 53 ms in posterior tibial nerves (Zappia et al. 1993). There is an increase in latency with increasing height, and a decrease with age. The interval between the earliest and latest F wave in any muscle is due to differences between fastest and slowest conduction velocities. This interval, termed *F wave chronodispersion* (Panayiotopoulos 1979), is a useful index of abnormal conduction in the whole length of a nerve, especially in the proximal segment; the F wave chronodispersion is usually less than 4 ms (maximum 7 ms) (Panayiotopoulos 1979; Tang et al. 1988).

The F response amplitude is normally about 5% that of the M response, suggesting that it represents the activity of a select group of motoneurons (Kimura et al. 1984). The F response amplitude is increased in spastic limbs (Fisher 1983). Zappia et al. (1993) reported that in the median nerve 70% of stimuli produced an F response, in the posterior tibial nerve 77%, and in the deep peroneal nerve only 37% persistency was recorded. The number of stimuli applied has varied in different reports, even to as many as 200 stimuli. Zappia et al. (1993) found that no further information was obtained from more than 10 consecutive stimuli compared with 20 or 50 consecutive stimuli.

Motor Nerve Conduction Velocity Distribution

Conventional motor conduction tests measure conduction in the fastest motor fibres. Several attempts have been made to devise practicable methods for estimating conduction velocity in the whole range of motor nerve fibres innervating motor units in a muscle (Meyer and Hilfiker 1983). These methods depend on the collision principle in which a distal stimulus is allowed to collide with a delayed proximal stimulus (Hopf 1962), the interval between the two increasing during the experiment so as to allow the collision point to move towards the proximal site. The refractoriness underlying this distal site at known interstimulus intervals allows the fastest and slowest conduction velocity limits to be established, and the increasing size of the CMAP is an index of the remaining fibres of intermediate conduction velocity. The collision method is limited by a number of technical problems (Dorfman 1984; Ingram et al. 1987a). Modifications involving double stimuli (Ingram et al. 1987a) suggest that it may have particular application in the assessment of the clinical course and of the effect of treatment in patients with axonal and demyelinating neuropathies. The different techniques currently used indicate a lower range of motor conduction velocities in the population of motor fibres in a nerve of 12–24 m/s (Dorfman 1984), but a value of only 8 m/s was found using the more accurate technique devised by Ingram et al. (1987a).

In diabetic neuropathy, Dorfman et al. (1983) found a shift of the distribution towards slower conduction velocities with preferential involvement of the largest, fastest-conducting fibres. There are few studies of other disorders using this technique.

Motor and Sensory Nerve Refractory Period Studies

Measurements of motor and sensory nerve refractory period, which are also dependent on a collision

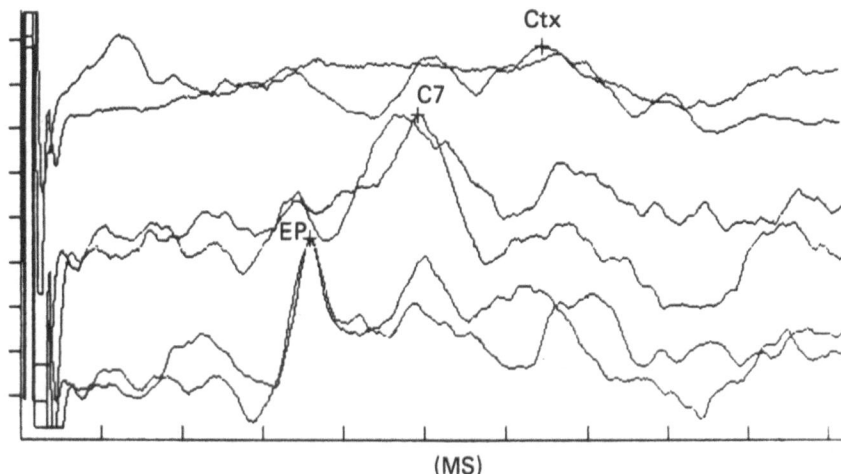

Fig. 2.21. Somatosensory evoked potential (3 ms divisions). The latency of the N13 component (C7) is increased in this patient with a cervical root lesion. EP, recording at Erb's point; C7, recording at C7 spine; Ctx, recording from contralateral sensory cortex.

technique (see Ingram et al. 1987b), are of largely theoretical interest. The sensory refractory period in whole nerve is increased in demyelinating neuropathies, including localised Schwann cell damage in entrapment neuropathy (Tackmann and Lehmann 1974a,b).

Blink Reflex

In the electrical blink reflex an electrical stimulus applied to one supraorbital nerve induces an early response in the ipsilateral orbicularis oculi muscle (R1) with a latency <13 ms, and a later bilateral response in this muscle (R2) with a latency <40 ms (Kimura 1975, 1983). The inter-side difference in the R1 latencies should not exceed 1.2 ms.

The blink reflex is useful in the assessment of Bell's palsy, in the diagnosis of peripheral neuropathies, e.g. Guillain–Barré syndrome, and in the diagnosis of multiple sclerosis (Kimura 1975). Separation of afferent and efferent lesions can be determined by utilising both R1 and R2 latency measurements (see Kimura 1983). The most important parameter in all these applications is the inter-side difference in the R1 latency, or the absolute latencies of R1 on the two sides.

Somatosensory Evoked Responses

Averaging the responses generated over the scalp, cervical and lumbar spine, and in the case of upper limb stimulation, Erb's point, following a train of

stimuli at about 1–5 Hz applied to medial popliteal, median or ulnar nerves, provides latencies to response peaks representing sensory potentials generated in the brachial plexus, dorsal root, cervical cord, thalamus and cortex. This method was initially applied to the diagnosis of multiple sclerosis (Matthews et al. 1974; Small et al. 1978). Similar responses of different latency can be produced by dermatomal stimulation of the skin itself (Pratt et al. 1979a,b).

The somatosensory evoked response (Fig. 2.21) consists of muscle afferent and cutaneous components (Burke et al. 1981), and is therefore generated by spino-cerebellar, dorsal column and spino-thalamic input in the CNS. However, it arises mainly from large, myelinated fibres so that only the former two CNS components are important in clinical practice. The technique is valuable in assessing brachial plexus and nerve root lesions (Jones et al. 1981), in cervical and lumbar spondylosis (El-Negamy and Sedgwick 1979; Eisen et al. 1983b), and in degenerative disorders such as hereditary spastic paraplegia and Friedreich's ataxia (Pedersen and Trojaborg 1981).

A limitation of somatosensory evoked potential studies is that the responses are often normal in single root lesions, because the stimulated nerves traverse several roots *en route* to the spinal cord (Syne 1986). Evoked potential studies have become especially popular in the investigation of patients with multiple sclerosis but their value in doubtful cases of this disease was overemphasised in earlier studies (Chiappa and Young 1985). In studies of the peripheral nervous system evoked potentials are of proven value in the management and evaluation of

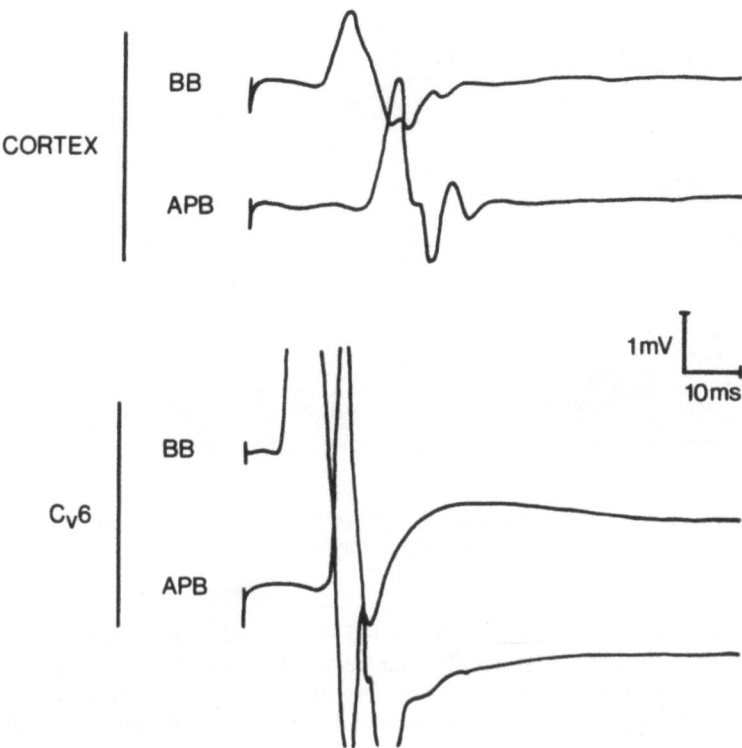

Fig. 2.22. Central motor stimulation using electrical stimulation of motor cortex (upper traces). The latencies of the responses to biceps brachii (BB) and abductor pollicis brevis (APB) are shown. In the lower traces, the latencies from root stimulation at C6 level to these muscles are shown. Subtraction of the cortical and C6 motor latencies gives *central motor conduction time* in the motor pathways subserving these muscles.

brachial plexus lesions (Yiannikas et al. 1983) and cervical and lumbar root lesions (Eisen et al. 1983b). Halliday (1992) and Kimura (1993) have reviewed the limitations of evoked potential studies in different disorders.

Stimulation of Central Motor Pathways

The proximal parts of the peripheral motor system are difficult to assess using conventional electrophysiological tests. Only F wave studies, or direct needle stimulation of motor roots, have been available until recently, but with the introduction of transcutaneous stimulation of the CNS (Fig. 2.22) it has become possible to test motor conduction in central motor pathways in the brain (Merton et al. 1982) and spinal cord (Snooks and Swash 1985), and in the motor roots at their exit foramina (Mills and Murray 1986) or in the cauda equina (Snooks and Swash 1986).

Two stimulators have been developed, one utilising electric shocks of fast rise time (50 μs), high voltage (up to 750 V) and rapid exponential delay (Merton and Morton 1980), and the other utilising a brief high-intensity magnetic field in the form of a coil. This magnetic pulse induces electrical current in the tissues and can be used to stimulate brain,

cervical nerve roots and peripheral nerves in the limb (Polson et al. 1982; Barker et al. 1986). Cervical stimulation has been used in the detection of conduction block in proximal parts of the peripheral nervous system in diseases such as Guillain–Barré syndrome (Mills and Murray 1985). A slight voluntary contraction shortens the latency by about 3 ms, and increases the amplitude of the evoked muscular response. Central motor conduction time, derived by subtracting the latency from an arm muscle recording, e.g. biceps brachii, from the latency derived from motor cortex stimulation, with the magnetic coil placed over the vertex, is often used (Cowan et al. 1984). The normal central motor conduction time is about 5 ms (less than 8 ms) and the latency from cortex to abductor digiti minimi is usually less than 22 ms (Claus 1990; Kimura 1993). Graded cortical stimuli can be used to evoke responses in single motor units, and these follow Henneman's size principle.

This technique is of value in the assessment of the excitability of the motor system in central motor disorders, and in the detection of slowed central conduction in various lesions of the nervous system such as multiple sclerosis (Cowan et al. 1984; Snooks and Swash 1985; Hess et al. 1986), radiation myelitis (Snooks and Swash 1985) and motor neuron disease (Ingram and Swash 1987).

Chapter 3

Muscle and Nerve Biopsies

The pathology of muscle and nerve is an important aspect of neuromuscular disease. Both muscle and nerve are readily accessible to biopsy. Although many muscles can be biopsied the choice of nerve is restricted, since it is important that the procedure should not result in disability. Thus nerve biopsy is virtually restricted to the sural nerve, a sensory nerve. Muscle is a surprisingly complex organ and, since muscle biopsy is a selective procedure, it is important to sample a muscle that is representative of the disease under study. Since there are variations in composition of different muscles it is also important to take diagnostic biopsy samples from muscles for which normal data are available. In most laboratories the need for these correlations implies that deltoid, biceps brachii, triceps, vastus lateralis or tibialis anterior are the usual choices for the biopsy site.

Muscle Biopsy

Selection of the appropriate muscle for biopsy is important. The muscle selected should not be very wasted since end-stage fibrosis and fatty replacement may then be found and may obscure any diagnostic features. Proximal muscles are generally the most useful since they usually show diagnostic features in both myopathic and neurogenic disorders, and are less likely to be affected by changes due to trauma, vascular disease or unrelated neuropathy. Generally triceps, biceps or deltoid in the upper extremity, or vastus lateralis in the lower extremity are preferred, since these muscles are relatively large and easy to biopsy. The biceps brachii is particularly suitable since it contains approximately equal proportions of Type 1 and Type 2 fibres. In both deltoid and vastus lateralis there are variations in fibre-type composition in different parts of this muscle. Occasionally, a muscle may be selected for biopsy because it is known from clinical, EMG, ultrasound or CT studies that it is particularly involved by the

disease process (Schwartz et al. 1988; Heckmatt et al. 1988). The cosmetic results of biopsy are particularly important in upper limb biopsies of women.

Ordinarily it is only possible to biopsy a single muscle. Muscles previously used for electromyography (EMG) should not be biopsied because of the possibility that the trauma resulting from penetration of the muscle by a needle electrode might be mistaken for features consistent with a myopathy – the so-called needle myopathy (Engel 1967). However, if the muscle is biopsied immediately after EMG, artefactual changes may not have had time to develop (Warmolts and Engel 1972a). Correlation of EMG results and muscle biopsy is possible in many disorders by performing EMG in a muscle in one limb, and muscle biopsy in the same muscle of the contralateral limb.

Needle Biopsy

Needle biopsy (Bergström 1962; Edwards 1971; Edwards et al. 1983) is a useful and relatively atraumatic technique for obtaining small muscle samples suitable for histochemical examination from the quadriceps femoris muscle, although it can be used for biopsy of other muscles (Fig. 3.1). It is a particularly useful technique for following progress and assessing the efficacy of treatment in polymyositis, since it allows repeated biopsy of the same muscle without the necessity for repeated skin incisions and sutures. We have also used needle biopsy of the quadriceps in conjunction with open biopsy of an arm muscle, e.g. biceps brachii, to assess differences in the severity and pattern of abnormality in the arm and leg in the same patient. The technique of needle biopsy of the quadriceps is, perhaps, most useful in children or frightened adults, since a biopsy can be obtained quickly and relatively painlessly as an out-patient procedure without the necessity of return visits for removal of sutures (Heckmatt et al. 1984). Heckmatt (1990) reported an overall failure rate for needle muscle biopsy in children of only 2.6%, although in spinal muscular

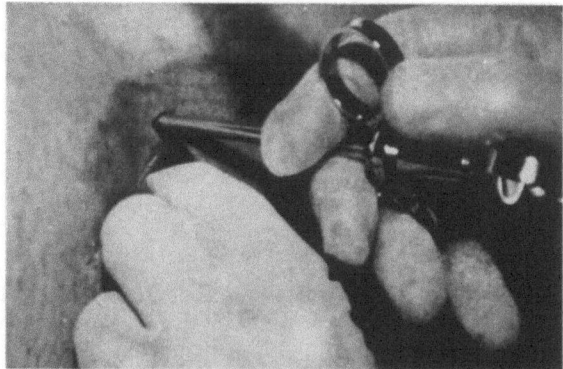

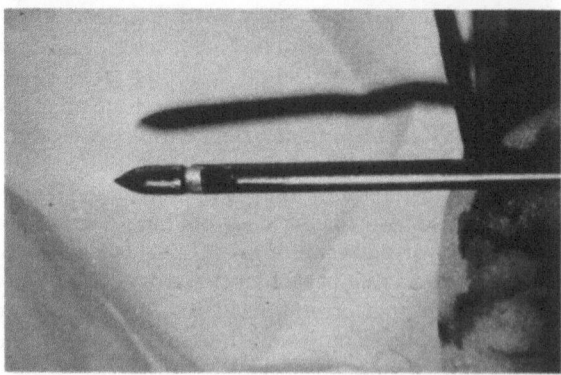

Fig. 3.1. Needle muscle biopsy using a modified Bergström biopsy needle. **a** The biopsy needle is inserted into the lateral part of the quadriceps muscle through a small (less than 1 cm) skin incision under local anaesthesia. **b** The biopsy specimen can be seen in the cavity of the needle close to the cutting edge. Sufficient muscle is usually available for enzyme histochemical and ultrastructural studies. The technique is also useful for obtaining muscle for biochemical studies.

atrophy it was 5.2% and in congenital muscular dystrophy it was 16% (Heckmatt et al. 1984).

Conchotome Biopsy

This technique is also performed by a minimally invasive method through a small skin incision that does not require suturing. The biopsy is taken from the superficial layer of the muscle and is almost painless. A wider range of muscles can be biopsied than with the Bergström technique, although it is not very suitable for quadriceps biopsies (Henriksson 1979; Heckmatt 1990).

Open Biopsy

Conventional open biopsy, however, retains certain advantages. The specimen is larger and easier to orientate for sectioning in horizontal and longitudinal planes. A long specimen can be obtained so that several blocks of tissue can be prepared, and serial sections can be studied. The specimen is large enough to provide a sufficient number of fibres for quantitative data on fibre size and fibre-type distribution to be obtained, and for the distribution of abnormality within individual fascicles to be observed. There may be sufficient muscle tissue available for quantitative biochemical and enzymatic investigations to be carried out if these are shown to be indicated by standard enzyme histochemical studies. Further, since the biopsy is taken under direct observation it is unusual for an open biopsy to consist of an unrepresentative sample of muscle. Another advantage of open biopsy is that EMG recordings can be made from the site of the biopsy, thus allowing direct correlation to be made between the electrophysiological and histological findings (Warmolts and Engel 1972a; Schwartz et al. 1976a).

If the surface of the muscle is stimulated during the biopsy procedure, the motor point, i.e. the end-plate region, can be located. Biopsies from this region are likely to contain motor end-plates and with this technique motor point biopsy intravital methylene blue impregnations can be used to study the morphology of the terminal innervation in neuromuscular diseases (Coërs and Woolf 1959). However, this method of biopsy is very time-consuming and does not provide sufficient additional information to justify its routine use in diagnosis.

Preparation of the Biopsy

Fixation in formol-saline, with subsequent paraffin-embedding, is now little used in diagnostic work on muscle biopsies. The availability of unfixed frozen material allows the use of enzyme histochemical and immunohistochemical techniques. With these methods subcellular organelles can be studied by light microscopy, and different fibre types can be identified. In addition, the classical histological staining methods, adapted for use in frozen material, can still be employed. Many of these techniques produce permanent results so that slides can be stored for future study. The blocks of frozen tissue can themselves be stored indefinitely in liquid nitrogen, or in a suitable refrigerator (at about –70 °C). The resin-embedded block, taken for electron microscopy, can also be stored indefinitely.

There are several techniques for snap-freezing muscle (see Dubowitz 1985; Swash and Schwartz 1991). In order to avoid artefact it is important to take particular care to prepare small cylindrical blocks of tissue (about 4 mm × 2 mm) from the fresh biopsy specimen. The muscle should be kept moist in buffered saline or Ringer's solution to avoid drying artefact before freezing. It is preferable to freeze the tissue, attached to a small disc of cork by a blob of Tissue-Tek or other adhesive, in isopentane cooled to near its freezing point in a flask of liquid nitrogen. When cutting sections in the cryostat, sudden changes in temperature such as would be caused by a warm cryostat knife or warm slides must be avoided, in order to prevent the development of ice crystal artefact. This artefact can sometimes be cleared from a block by allowing it to thaw at room temperature and then re-freezing it, although this manoeuvre usually results in the loss of some enzyme activity. A series of 6–12 transverse sections, each 5–8 μm thick, should be cut. Longitudinal sections, which are difficult to produce because of imperfect orientation of the muscle fibres, are only rarely useful. During each biopsy small pieces of fresh tissue should be fixed in glutaraldehyde so that sections can be prepared in resin for light and electron microscopy.

Histological Methods

The *haematoxylin and eosin* method provides general information about the biopsy. The *elastin-van Gieson* stain is sometimes useful, particularly in assessing connective tissue changes. The *modified Gomori trichrome* stain is much used since it enables delineation of nuclei, fibrous tissue, myofibrillar material (bluish) and the intermyofibrillar substance (red). These stains also usually differentiate two muscle fibre types, the red and pale fibres described by earlier workers, but this is not always very obvious.

A variety of enzyme histochemical reactions are available for histological work, and in most laboratories a routine series is used. This series should provide a clear differentiation of fibre type and should yield a variety of organelle-specific reaction products so that mitochondria, sarcoplasmic lipid droplets, myofibrils, cell membranes and sarcoplasmic glycogen, and perhaps also ribonucleic acid and acid phosphatase, can be identified by light microscopy. The *nicotine adenine dinucleotide tetrazolium reductase (NADH-tr)* technique is particularly useful as it produces a permanent preparation of good contrast which allows fibre-type differentiation to be recognised. The reaction product is localised in mitochondria and, nonspecifically, in the tubular system of the intermyofibrillar sarcoplasm. *Succinic dehydrogenase (SDH)* is located only in mitochondria but the reac-

tion product is often less easily visualised than that of the NADH-tr method.

Fibre typing is conventionally performed in *myofibrillar adenosine triphosphatase (ATPase)* preparations (see Dubowitz 1985). This reaction produces different results depending on the pH of the buffer used for preincubation. Standard preincubations are carried out at pH 9.4, 4.5 and 4.3. In good preparations there should be a pattern reversal between the pH 9.4 and pH 4.3 preincubations, fibres which are dark in the former (Type 2 fibres) being pale in the latter. In the preincubation at intermediate pH (4.5) some Type 2 fibres show an intermediate reaction product density (Type 2B fibres).

Myophosphorylase, located at the cross bridges of the actin component of the myofilament, can also be demonstrated, but this method does not produce permanent results. Neutral lipid droplets are most satisfactorily demonstrated by the *oil red O method*; a counter-stain of *Ehrlich's haematoxylin* enables basophilic fibres and sarcolemmal nuclei to be recognised. A number of other methods for neutral lipid, e.g. *Sudan black*, can be used, but they are generally less satisfactory. Glycogen granules and cell membranes, together with other myofibrillar membranous structures, can be demonstrated by the *periodic acid Schiff (PAS)* method. Predigestion with *diastase* allows proof of the presence of glycogen in the untreated sections. The sections should be fixed on the slides with alcohol for the most uniform results. *Acid phosphatase* localised in lysosomes can be demonstrated in abnormal fibres, particularly in those undergoing autolysis. A summary of the enzyme histochemical reactions in fibres of different histochemical types is given in Table 3.1.

Table 3.1. Histochemical reactions and staining intensity of fibres of different types (modified from Banker and Engel 1994)

Stain or reaction	Type 1	Type 2A	Type 2B	Type 2C
ATPase pH 9.4	+	+++	+++	+++
ATPase pH 4.6	+++	0	++	++
ATPase pH 4.3	+++	0	0	++
NADH/SDH	+++	++	+	++
Cytochrome oxidase	+++	++	+	+
PAS (glycogen)	+	+++	++	++
Myophosphorylase	+	+++	+++	+++
Esterase	+++	+	+	+
Myoadenylate deaminase	++	++	++	++
Neutral lipid	++	+	+	+
H and E	++	+	+	+
Gomori trichrome	+++	++	++	++
Physiological characteristics	Slow Fatigue resistant	Fast Fatigue resistant	Fast Rapidly fatiguing	–

In mitochondrial disorders a double stain for cytochrome oxidase (COX) and succinic dehydro-

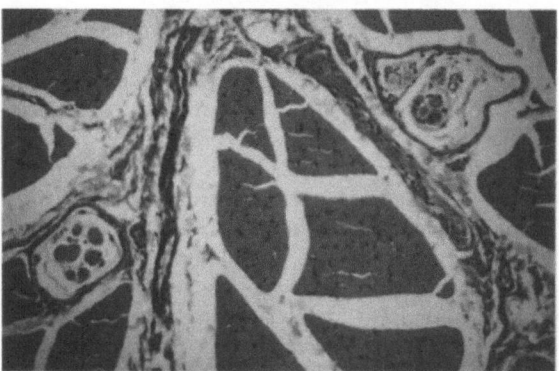

Fig. 3.2. Low-power view of two muscle spindles showing their relationship to neighbouring fascicles of muscle fibres and blood vessels. Elastin-van Gieson.

genase (SDH) is useful. The mosaicism of the mitochondrial deletion is demonstrated; there is a mosaic of light- and dark-brown COX positive fibres and blue COX negative fibres. Ragged-red fibres are usually COX-negative and show accumulations of intensely staining SDH-positive mitochondria (Bonilla et al. 1992). The role of other, less commonly used histochemical techniques is illustrated in Table 3.1. Immunoperoxidase preparations for demonstration of vimentin and desmin reactivity are used in many laboratories to pick out regenerating fibres, which express vimentin in the early phase of the regeneration reaction (Thornell et al. 1980). These proteins are intermediate filaments that are specific components of the cytoskeleton of striated muscle fibres (Bornemann and Schmalbruch 1992). Specific monoclonal antibody methods for demonstrating cell surface markers are useful in demonstrating B and T lymphocytes and T cell subtypes, and also in recognising macrophages. Monoclonal antibodies

raised against components of the dystrophin molecule, and against spectrin are useful in the diagnosis of Duchenne and Becker muscular dystrophies, and other cell membrane antigens have been investigated in certain other muscular dystrophies, e.g. certain dystrophin-associated glycoproteins in Maghreb myopathy (Mizuno et al. 1994; Yamanuchi et al. 1995). A combined acetylcholinesterase and silver impregnation method has been developed for the demonstration of motor end-plates, the terminal motor axon and the subneural apparatus by Pestronk and Drachman (1978). It is useful in motor point biopsies but is not of routine value in diagnostic work. In fresh *unfrozen* muscle, motor end-plates and the terminal innervation can be demonstrated by supravital methylene blue staining (Coërs and Woolf 1959).

Structure of Skeletal Muscle

In any muscle biopsy only a limited sample of tissue is available for study. This consists of several fascicles of muscle fibres bounded by perifascicular collagen and fibrous tissue. Fat cells, several small nerve fibre bundles, arterioles, capillaries and venules, and occasionally a muscle spindle, may also be seen. All these structures should be considered in the evaluation of a muscle biopsy. Individual muscle fibres are closely applied to each other and in a normal biopsy there is very little endomysial fibrous tissue. In transverse sections, fascicles contain variable numbers of muscle fibres, often more than 100. Each fascicle is bounded by collagenous tissue. The neuromuscular bundle, consisting of small arteries or arterioles, veins, nerve fibre bundles and sometimes a muscle spindle, is situated at the junction of two or more fascicles (Fig. 3.2). The fibrous tissue surrounding this neuromuscular bundle merges with that of the fascicle itself. Sometimes a Pacinian corpuscle may also be found at this site (Fig. 3.3). Some muscle biopsies, particularly those taken from quadriceps, contain tendinous insertions of muscle fibres in which Golgi tendon organs may be found (Fig. 3.4).

Muscle Fibres

Within each fascicle individual muscle fibres are closely applied to each other. Each muscle fibre is surrounded by several capillaries. These are particularly found in the small spaces between adjoining fibres (Carry et al. 1986). Occasionally small nerve fibre bundles can be recognised between muscle fibres and rarely an end-plate eminence (Doyère

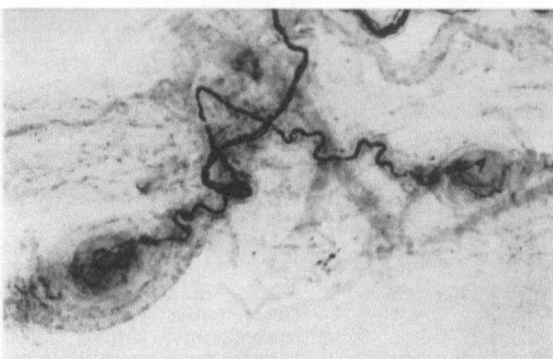

Fig. 3.3. Two Pacinian corpuscles. Silver block impregnation; teased preparation. Pacinian corpuscles are found near muscle spindles in human muscle.

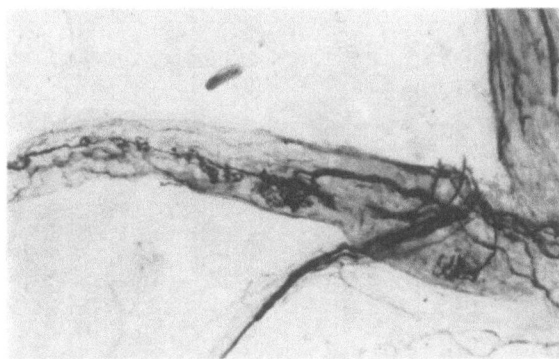

Fig. 3.4. Golgi tendon organ. Ranvier's gold chloride block impregnation; teased preparation. Note the complex ramification of the sensory nerve terminals.

eminence) may be seen (Fig. 3.5). Fat cells are not ordinarily found within fasciculi. Each muscle fibre contains one or more peripherally located "subsarcolemmal" nucleus. These nuclei are small, elongated in shape and basophilic. Centrally located nuclei are found in less than 3% of normal muscle fibres, and normal muscle fibres contain fewer than eight nuclei (Greenfield et al. 1957). Each muscle fibre is surrounded by a sarcolemmal membrane, well seen with NADH-tr and PAS stains. With the electron microscope this is seen to consist of a plasma membrane and an external layer of basement membrane (Fig. 3.6). The fine structure of muscle is only detectable in electron micrographs.

Some of the subsarcolemmal nuclei represent satellite cells. These consist of a nucleus, surrounded by sparse granular sarcoplasm, containing abundant free ribosomes, Golgi apparatus, endoplasmic reticulum and mitochondria, but usually devoid of myofilaments. The satellite cell is limited by a layer

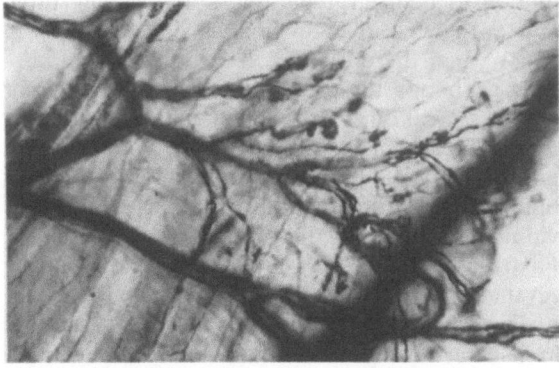

Fig. 3.5. The terminal innervation, showing motor end-plates and the terminal axonal branches. Ranvier's gold chloride; teased preparation.

of plasma membrane, but is situated beneath the basement membrane of the muscle fibre itself. Satellite cells are important in regeneration after injury.

Fibre Types and Motor Units

It has long been known that muscle consists of fibres of different colour: the red and the white fibres (Ranvier 1873). This is less obvious in man than in other species, for example birds, but both haematoxylin and eosin and Gomori preparations differentiate fibres of two types in human biopsies by their coloration and by the relative intensity of staining of their intermyofibrillar substance. Although many fibre types have been distinguished in human muscle in studies using a variety of different enzyme histochemical techniques, fibre typing is now usually based on the myosin ATPase reactions, after preincubations at pH 9.4, 4.5 and 4.3 (Brooke and Kaiser 1970). This results in a classification of fibres into two types: Type 1 and Type 2 fibres. Type 2 fibres can be further subclassified into Types 2A, 2B and 2C; this classification is useful in diagnosis in some cases, especially in neurogenic disorders. The histochemical reactions of fibres of these different types are summarised in Table 3.1. Slow myosin and fast myosin show different heavy chain and light chain compositions and slow myosin is expressed earlier in fetal life. A fetal-specific myosin ceases to be expressed during development (Pons et al. 1986). Myotubes are segregated into three distinct lineages to form a particular fibre type (Sanes 1987).

Each motor unit consists of fibres of uniform histochemical type. This has been shown in the rat (Kugelberg and Edstrom 1968; Edstrom and Kugelberg 1968) by a technique in which the fibres of a single motor unit were identified by glycogen depletion, induced by repetitive stimulation of single nerve fibres in a nerve root. These muscle fibres were found to have the same SDH reaction. The physiological properties of motor units allow classification into slow and fast contracting fibres. Burke et al. (1971, 1977) have further subdivided these physiological fibre types in the cat into slow (S), fast and resistant to fatigue (FR) and fast, rapidly fatiguing (FF) fibres and have suggested that these motor units correlate with motor units consisting of Type 1, Type 2A and Type 2B fibres in the myosin ATPase-based histochemical classification (see Table 3.1). Fast and slow myosins can be identified with monoclonal antibodies but correspondence to the ATPase-based classification of fibre types is inexact. Type 2 fibres can be subtyped into Type 2A and 2B with myosin antibodies, but

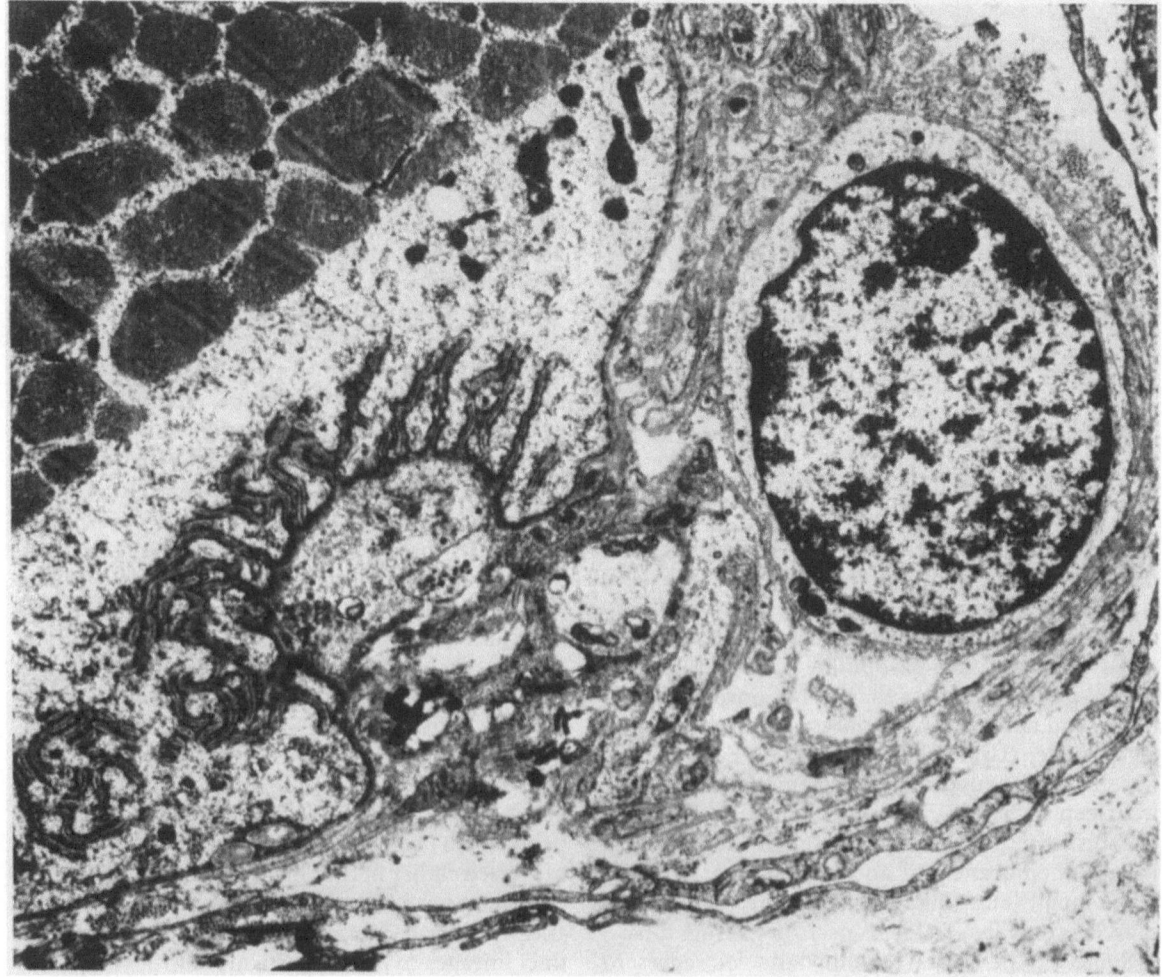

Fig. 3.6. Electron micrograph of a normal motor end-plate.

Type 2C fibres contain both 2A and 2B myosins (Pierobon-Bormioli et al. 1981; Fitzsimons and Sewry 1985).

Distribution of Muscle Fibres

In human muscle biopsies Type 1 and Type 2 fibres are distributed in a random chequerboard pattern (Fig. 3.7). The apparent randomness of this mosaic distribution varies in different muscles and is dependent on the relative predominance of fibres of each histochemical type.

Within individuals there is no consistent difference between homologous muscles on the two sides of the body in terms of fibre size or fibre type composition (Blomstrand and Ekblom 1982; Blomstrand et al. 1984). Further, repeated biopsies of the same muscle contain similar proportions of Type 1 and

Type 2 fibres (Blomstrand et al. 1984). When more than 70% of fibres in a biopsy consist of fibres of one histochemical type, these fibres will often appear to be grouped together. A similar effect will occur when there is marked atrophy of one fibre type. Although the presence of fibres of different histochemical types in a biopsy indicates that different fibres belong to different motor units, it is not possible to recognise individual motor units in biopsies. The different fibres making up an individual motor unit are distributed in many fascicles. Edstrom and Kugelberg (1968) have shown in the rat that the fibres of a single motor unit are distributed, on average, over 17% of the cross-sectional area of a muscle. These fibres tend to be more densely distributed toward the centre of the territory of the motor unit, but as many as 70% of these fibres are not in apposition to another fibre of the

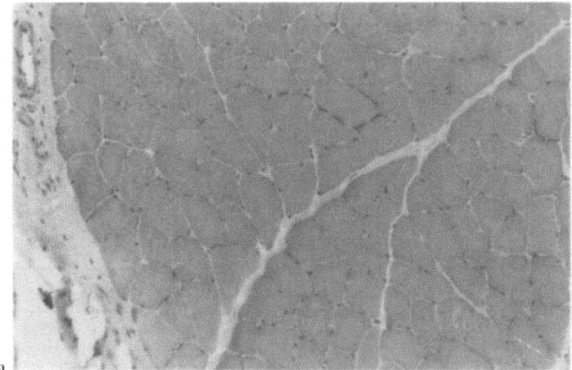

a

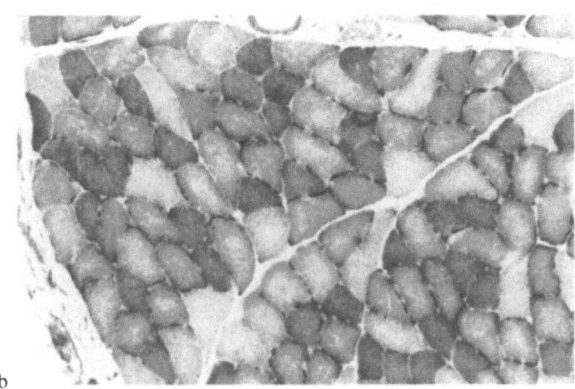

b

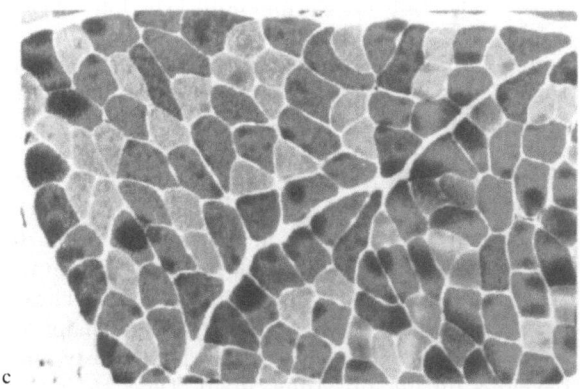

c

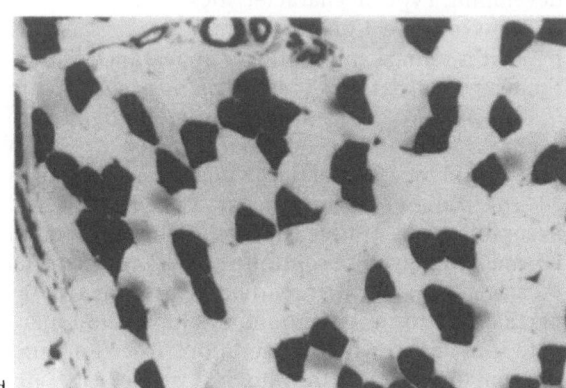

d

same motor unit (Edstrom and Kugelberg 1968). The fibres making up individual motor units are thus intermingled in many fascicles in normal muscle. The co-dispersion of fibres of different histochemical types with respect to each other, expressed as the codispersion index and calculated using a nearest-neighbour algorithm, has been suggested as a useful index of randomness of the fibre-type distribution (Lester et al. 1983). Normal muscle fibres adopt an approximately six-sided configuration in order to fit into the least cross-sectional area. This relationship implies that groups of six fibres are unlikely to occur; biopsies of normal subjects do not contain enclosed fibres, i.e. fibres surrounded by fibres of the same histochemical type, since this would necessitate the aggregation of at least seven fibres of the same type (Jennekens et al. 1971; Willison 1980; Swash and Schwartz 1984). An alternative measure of randomness is measurement of "mean cluster size" of fibres of similar type (Howel and Brunsddon 1987).

Effects of Training and Exercise

Athletic training produces a number of morphological changes in muscles. Weight-lifters and sprinters show clinical enlargement of muscles and this is accompanied by an increase in the diameter of Type 2 fibres (Saltin et al. 1976), especially of Type 2B fibres. Hypertrophy is less marked in Type 2A and Type 1 fibres in this short-duration pattern of exercise.

Endurance training does not result in such marked muscle hypertrophy, as can be seen by comparing the physique of a long-distance runner with that of a weight-lifter. Indeed the muscle fibres of endurance-trained athletes may be slightly smaller than normal (Houston et al. 1979). However, there is a quantitative change in the distribution of fibre subtypes in the trained muscles of these subjects, so

---

Fig. 3.7. Normal muscle. Serial transverse cryostat sections to show Type 1 and Type 2 fibres. × 140. **a** H and E. The close interdigitation of the muscle fibres is clearly seen. The muscle fibre nuclei are nearly all subsarcolemmal, and the fibres are arranged in fascicles. **b** NADH-tr. A mosaic arrangement of fibres of various staining intensities is seen. Type 1 fibres are darkly stained and Type 2 fibres are relatively paler, but this distinction is clearer in myosin ATPase preparations. Type 2A fibres tend to be darker than Type 2B fibres. The intermyofibrillar substance has a finely granular appearance. Arteriolar walls also stain positively. **c** ATPase, pH 9.4. Type 1 fibres are pale and Type 2 fibres are dark. Fibres showing an intermediate reaction are usually Type 1. **d** ATPase, pH 4.3. The mosaic pattern is reversed. Type 1 fibres are dark and Type 2 fibres are very pale.

that there is a relative increase in the proportion of Type 2A fibres (Edstrom and Grimby 1986). Type 2A fibres are relatively more dependent on oxidative metabolism than Type 2B fibres (Jansson and Kaijser 1977). In addition there is an increase in the number of capillaries surrounding individual fibres in the muscles of endurance-trained subjects (Andersson and Henriksson 1977). Endurance athletes tend to have more Type 1 fibres than the general population (Gollnick et al. 1972, 1973), a characteristic that is probably inherited rather than acquired, as shown from twin studies (Komi et al. 1977), since training does not influence fibre-type predominance (Dons et al. 1979; Salmons and Henriksson 1981).

The activities of enzymes involved in energy metabolism, and the capillarisation of skeletal muscle respond rapidly to altered functional demands, but there is no evidence of interconversion of Type 1 and Type 2 fibres during training (Larsson and Ansved 1985). Disuse tends to reverse the effects of training and, in extreme instances, as in a limb constrained in a plaster cast, fibre atrophy will occur.

Effects of Age

Fibre size, usually expressed as the lesser transverse diameter, increases with age. At 1 year of age the mean fibre diameter is 16 μm, and at age 10 years, 40 μm. It increases by 2 μm for each year to age 5 years and then by 3 μm for each year to age 9 years (Brooke and Engel 1969d). Adult diameters (40–80 μm in men; 30–70 μm in women) are reached between the ages of 12 and 15 years (Brooke and Engel 1969a).

Differences in size between Type 1 and Type 2 fibres are only minimal in childhood. However, in adult women Type 1 fibres are larger than Type 2 fibres, and in adult men Type 2 fibres are larger than those of Type 1 (Brooke and Engel 1969a). Normal values for the biceps muscle are shown in Tables 3.2 and 3.3. The mean diameters of Type 1 and Type 2 fibres have been studied in 36 muscles in an autopsy study by Polgar et al. (1973). Type 2 fibres were larger than Type 1 fibres in 90% of the muscles studied, but this difference was often not statistically significant. Type 2B fibres are markedly smaller in women than men; these are the fibres that undergo hypertrophy with phasic exercise.

The relative predominance of Type 1 and Type 2 fibres found in normal human muscle varies from muscle to muscle and even in different parts of the same muscle, for example in the superficial and deep parts of the deltoid muscle. There are generally more Type 2 fibres at the periphery of a fascicle than

Table 3.2. Mean fibre diameter (μm) in adult biceps brachii

	Type 1	Type 2
Males	64	73
Females	57	47

From Brooke and Engel (1969a).

Table 3.3. Mean diameters (μm) of Type 1, 2A and 2B fibres in human biceps muscle

Type 1		Type 2A		Type 2B	
Males	Females	Males	Females	Males	Females
61	53	69	52	62	42

From Dubowitz (1985)

in its central portions (Sjostrom et al. 1986). Data are available from an autopsy study of 36 different adult human muscles (Johnson et al. 1973). In adult biceps brachii and vastus lateralis muscles there are normally twice as many Type 2 as Type 1 fibres. There are approximately equal numbers of Type 1, Type 2A and Type 2B fibres (Brooke and Engel 1969a; Dubowitz and Brooke 1973). In young children, however, Type 1 and Type 2 fibres are present in approximately equal numbers (Brooke and Engel 1969d). With ageing, after the sixth decade, the proportion of Type 1 fibres increased from 36% to 55% in vastus lateralis muscle and both Type 1 and Type 2 fibres were smaller in the older than in the younger subjects (Larsson 1978, 1982). Lexell and Downham (1991) reported a tendency for fibre-type grouping to be found in subjects older than 60 years, a feature of reinnervation perhaps due to age-related loss of functioning motor units (Stålberg et al. 1989). Oertel (1986) found type 2 atrophy with minor neurogenic changes in subjects older than 70 years. In the newborn 20% of fibres are undifferentiated (Type 2C) fibres (Colling-Saltin 1978). These fibres differentiate by the age of 1 year, the majority developing into Type 1 fibres. Type 2 sub-typing develops during this time, many Type 2A fibres developing Type 2B characteristics.

Transverse sections of normal muscles usually present a remarkably uniform appearance. Sometimes a few small fibres (<40 μm in men and <30 μm in women) may be seen nesting in close proximity to a nearby fibre of normal size (Tang and Swash 1986), and occasional large fibres, greater than 80 μm in diameter, may occur. Degenerative and basophilic regenerative changes are never found in normal muscle. Fibre splitting is a feature of normal muscle fibres near their tendinous insertions and is particularly commonly found in biopsies of bipennate muscles in which a tendinous insertion runs through the length of the muscle.

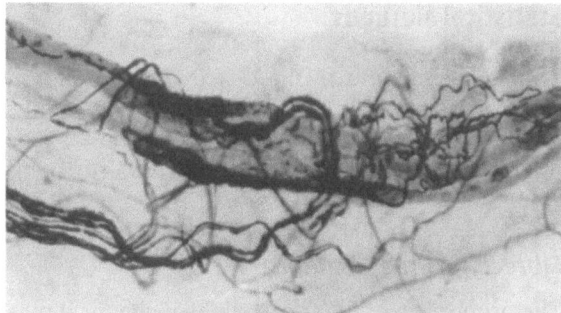

Fig. 3.8. The muscle spindle has a rich innervation, consisting of both sensory and motor nerve fibres (see Swash and Fox 1972). Ranvier's gold chloride; teased preparation.

Muscle Spindles

Muscle spindles occur in all human skeletal muscles, except facial muscles and the diaphragm. They consist of a fibrous capsule enclosing 4–14 intrafusal muscle fibres, in a mucopolysaccharide-containing periaxial space (Swash and Fox 1972). These intrafusal muscle fibres are smaller than adult extrafusal fibres, but are somewhat larger than extrafusal muscle fibres in children. The intrafusal muscle fibres have complex enzyme histochemical reactions (Kucera and Dorovini-Zis 1979). They are specialised stretch-sensitive sensory receptors, receiving a rich motor and sensory innervation (Fig. 3.8). Pacinian corpuscles are often found in close relation to muscle spindles. Since the region of the tendinous insertion is usually avoided, Golgi tendon organs are rarely present in muscle biopsies. They cannot be easily recognised in muscle biopsies unless silver or methylene blue stains are used (Fig. 3.9). Motor end-plates are rarely found in sections of normal muscle unless the biopsy is taken from the motor point. The motor point is a localised band about 1 cm wide in the biceps muscle, but in the tibialis anterior muscle the end-plates are superficially placed along the whole length of the muscle (Aquilonius et al. 1984). Further data on motor point anatomy are available in anatomical studies (Christenssen 1959; Coërs and Woolf 1959).

Indications for Muscle Biopsy

Muscle biopsies are useful in the evaluation of several different types of clinical problem, and as an investigative method for certain theoretical problems in biology. The main indications for muscle biopsy in clinical practice are shown in Table 3.4. in some disorders, e.g. polymyositis, the treatment is potentially hazardous and it is important to verify

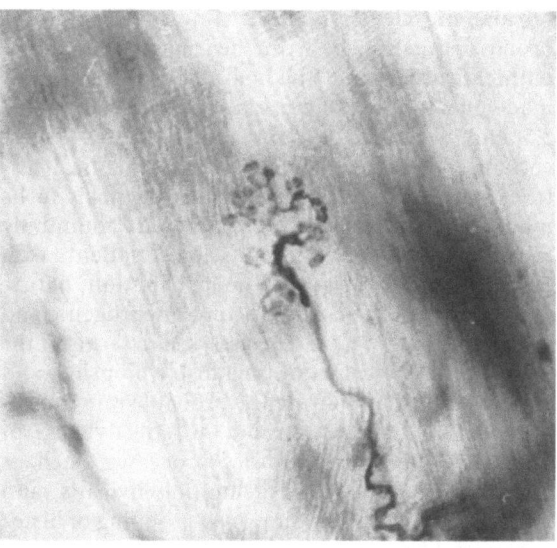

Fig. 3.9. Methylene blue impregnation of normal motor end-plate.

Table 3.4. Indications for muscle biopsy

1. Inflammatory muscle disease; and to exclude treatable disorders
2. Proximal muscle weakness of uncertain cause, whether myopathic or neurogenic, in adults and children, including "floppy baby" syndromes
3. Hereditary myopathies and muscular dystrophies
4. Suspected metabolic myopathies, particularly in patients with muscle cramps, stiffness or tenderness
5. Autoimmune vasculitis, especially polyarterities nodosa, even in the absence of muscular symptoms
6. Other systemic disorders, e.g. sarcoidosis, infestations
7. To assess the effects of steroid treatment, e.g. in polymyositis, especially when steroid myopathy is suspected
8. Occasionally in carrier detection in female siblings or other close female relatives of boys with Duchenne muscular dystrophy
9. Diagnosis of malignant hyperpyrexia syndrome by in vitro test
10. Research: e.g. exercise physiology, pathological, biochemical and immunological studies

the diagnosis by biopsy and, often, to repeat the biopsy if the response to treatment is unsatisfactory.

Muscle Biopsy Pathology

Histological examination of a muscle biopsy, using enzyme histochemical techniques, has several aims.

First, is the muscle normal or abnormal? This is usually not a difficult decision; sometimes in biopsies taken from muscles only mildly affected or even apparently not clinically affected, only very slight abnormalities (for example minor changes in fibre size or central nucleation) may be present. Such abnormalities are not themselves significant since they so closely resemble the limits of variability of normal muscle. *Second*, in abnormal muscles a broad distinction between neurogenic and myopathic disorders must be made. This distinction is made on a number of criteria summarised in Table 3.5 and described in more detail below. *Third*, certain specific histological or histochemical features may enable a more definite diagnosis to be made; for example ragged-red fibres are commonly found in biopsies of limb muscles of patients with ocular myopathy. *Finally*, the distribution, nature and severity of the changes in both neurogenic and myopathic disorders can be assessed in terms of the degree of involvement of the muscle biopsied, and so can be used to indicate the probable rate of progression of the disease, and the effectiveness of reparative and compensatory processes, such as regeneration of fibres in acute polymyositis, and effective reinnervation, shown by grouping of histochemical fibres of near-normal size. The latter factors should be considered in parallel with information derived from the EMG assessment described in Chap. 2.

Table 3.5. Comparison of the histological features of myopathic and neurogenic disorders

Myopathic	Neurogenic
Prominent degenerative and regenerative changes in individual fibres	Fibre-type grouping
Increased variability in fibre size	Fibre-type atrophy
Fibrosis may be prominent	Clusters of small pointed fibres, often dark in NADH-tr and non-specific esterase preparations
Architectural changes prominent	Target fibres or core fibres
Various specific morphological abnormalities	Type 1 hypertrophy (and predominance)
Type 2 fibre atrophy	Degenerative changes are rare
Perifascicular atrophy	Architectural changes are uncommon
Blood vessels abnormal in inflammatory myopathies	Little fibrosis
Fibre-type grouping uncommon	Blood vessels normal

From Swash and Schwartz (1991).

It is important to relate the distribution of weakness in any patient to the muscle biopsied. Generally, weaker muscles show more severe abnormalities on biopsy and very weak muscles may show such severe, endstage abnormalities that it is difficult to glean any useful diagnostic information from them. Further, in some disorders, for example Duchenne dystrophy, certain muscles are preferentially involved. In this disorder quadriceps biopsies usually show more advanced changes than biceps brachii biopsies, and any attempt at prognosis must take these factors of selection into account.

Statistical Methods

The changes found in the distribution, predominance and size of Type 1 and Type 2 fibres can be described by simple statistical methods. The myofibrillar ATPase preparations are, by convention, used for this purpose.

Fibre-Type Predominance

The proportion of fibres of each histochemical type varies in different muscles (Brooke and Engel 1969a; Johnson et al. 1973; Blomstrand and Ekblom 1982). Changes in the proportion of Type 1 and Type 2 fibres are termed fibre-type predominance. The normal ratio of Type 2 to Type 1 fibres in vastus lateralis and biceps brachii is 2 : 1 (Dubowitz and Brooke 1973). In the deltoid, Type 2 fibres are present in slightly greater numbers. In vastus lateralis and biceps brachii muscles Type 1 fibre predominance is present when more than 55% of fibres in the biopsy are Type 1 fibres, and Type 2 fibre predominance when more than 80% of fibres are Type 2 fibres. If Type 2A or Type 2B fibres represent more than 55% of fibres in the biopsy these subtypes are predominant. Fibre-type predominance occurs both in neurogenic and myopathic disorders. In general, Type 1 fibre predominance is associated with myopathies, particularly Duchenne dystrophy.

Fibre Size

Atrophy and hypertrophy of muscle fibres are difficult to assess subjectively and it is useful to calculate the means of the lesser diameters of at least 200 fibres, including fibres of both histochemical types, in order to compare these with normal values (Polgar et al. 1972; Dubowitz and Brooke 1973). Diameters should be measured in several different microscope fields within the biopsy; all the fibres in each microscope field must be measured in order to avoid selection bias. We usually use an eyepiece micrometer with a magnification of ×10 and a ×10 lens for this purpose, giving a final magnification of ×100. It is only necessary to categorise each fibre into successive 10 μm bins. Various semi-automatic electronic aids (Green et al. 1979; Round et al. 1982; Sanstedt et al. 1982b; Slavin et al. 1982; Mahon et al. 1984) have been developed but these are expensive and complicated and, with only a little practice, 200 or 300 fibres can be measured with the eyepiece micrometer in a few minutes. This procedure gives valuable quantitative information and it should be part of the routine evaluation of most biopsies. Measurement of Type 2A and Type 2B fibres is a more time-consuming task.

In normal adult women most muscle fibres are between 30 μm and 70 μm in diameter; in men they are between 40 μm and 80 μm in diameter. Brooke and Engel (1969b) devised a rating scale giving increasing weight to very small or very large fibres in order to determine the presence of atrophy and/or hypertrophy of Type 1 and Type 2 fibres in a biopsy. When there is increased variability in fibre size the standard deviation of the fibre diameter will be increased, although the mean diameter may still be normal. The standard deviation should not normally exceed 25% of the mean diameter (Dubowitz and Brooke 1973). Increased variability in fibre size is a feature of myopathies. In neurogenic disorders the combination of groups of atrophic fibres and the presence of other fibres of normal or near-normal size, produces a double peak in the histogram of fibre size.

Fibre area measurements, for different fibre types, can be calculated relatively easily with modern automated equipment, using television-enhanced images, digitised in a dedicated computer. However, such area measurements are dependent on technical excellence in the histological preparation and, most frequently, this proves impossible to attain in daily pathological work. Manual methods are also available, using graphics tablet or drawing tube, but these are relatively time-consuming and less accurate, and do not add significantly to the diagnostic process, although they are useful in research (Lexell and Taylor 1991).

Fibre-Type Atrophy

Selective Type 2 atrophy is common (Fig. 3.10); it is a feature of disuse atrophy of any cause and may therefore occur in patients immobilised in bed for orthopaedic procedures, in cachexia, in corticospinal lesions, in myasthenia gravis and in arthropathies. It may also occur in collagen-vascular diseases (Engel 1965) and in steroid myopathy and osteomalacia. Selective Type 1 atrophy is less common. It is particularly a feature of myotonic dystrophy (Engel and Brooke 1966; Brooke and Engel 1969c) and it also occurs in several congenital myopathies. Atrophy of both fibre types is uncommon, although it occurs in cachexia. Sargeant et al. (1977) have reported that after immobilisation due to fractures of tibia and fibula, both fibre types become atrophic in the quadriceps muscle. In collagen-vascular diseases, such as dermatomyositis, atrophy of fibres of both histochemical types may occur at the periphery of the fascicles; perifascicular atrophy. This is probably due to capillary shutdown from arteriolar or capillary involvement, leading to ischaemia of the periphery of the fascicle and so to

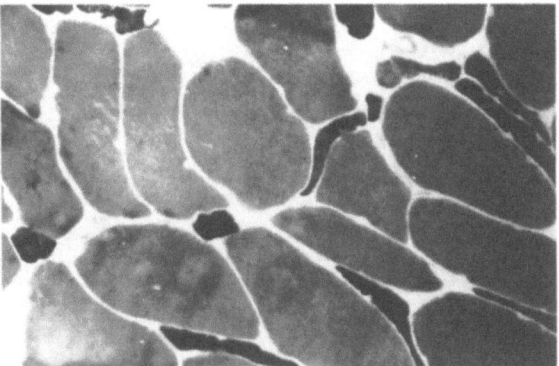

Fig. 3.10. Myosin, ATPase, pH 9.5. × 360. Disuse atrophy. The dark Type 2 fibres are atrophic. Type 1 fibres are also somewhat smaller than normal.

atrophy or even necrosis of these fibres (Carpenter et al. 1976).

Fibre Hypertrophy

Muscle hypertrophy is a normal phenomenon in trained athletes. Endurance training tends to lead to hypertrophy of Type 1 fibres (Gollnick et al. 1973), but repetitive brief exercise, as in weightlifting, tends to lead to hypertrophy of Type 2 fibres, especially Type 2B fibres. In neuromuscular disease hypertrophy of Type 1 fibres occurs in longstanding neurogenic disorders, for example chronic neuropathies. It also occurs in Werdnig–Hoffman disease. Type 2 fibres are often hypertrophied in motor neuron disease. In the dominant form of myotonia congenita there is marked muscular hypertrophy and both fibre types may show fibre enlargement (Fig. 3.11). Scattered very large fibres may be found both in myopathies and in chronic neurogenic disorders (Fig. 3.12). In the latter they are often Type 1

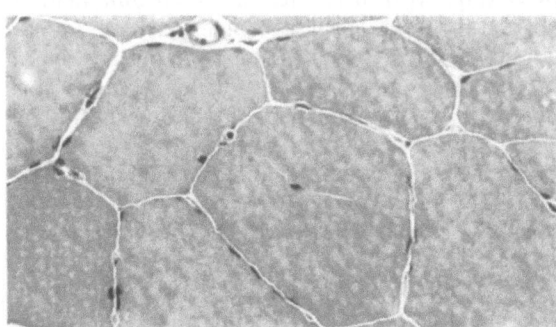

Fig. 3.11. H and E. × 140. Fibre hypertrophy in a patient with dominantly inherited myotonia congenita. Fibre splitting with a central nucleus is present.

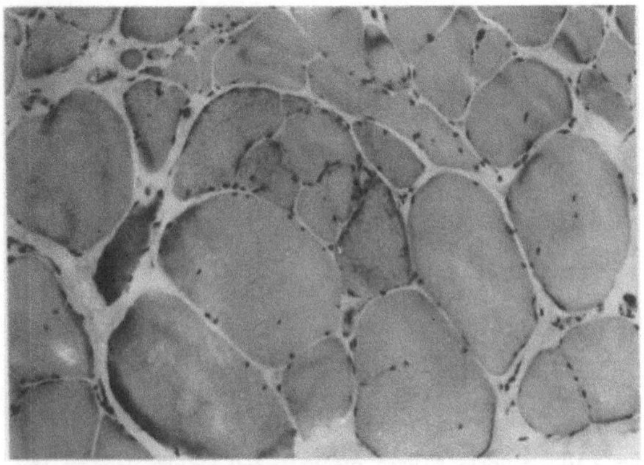

![img_1]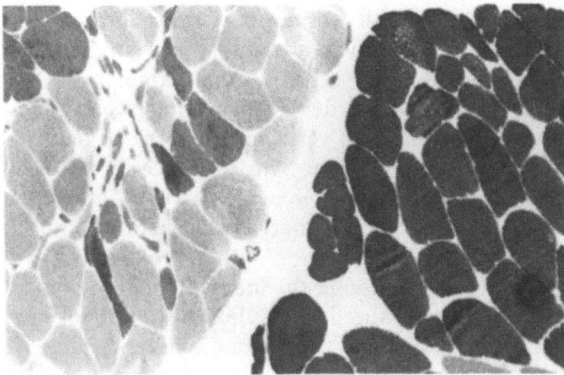

Fig. 3.12. H and E. × 140. Kugelberg–Welander disease. Several greatly hypertrophied fibres, greater than 120 μm in their lesser diameter, are present. Central nucleation, fibre splitting and increased endomysial fibrous tissue are also features of this biopsy.

Fig. 3.13. Myosin ATPase, pH 9.5 × 140. Motor neuron disease, with a slowly progressive course. There are large groups both of Type 1 and Type 2 fibres, indicating effective collateral reinnervation. A small cluster of pointed, atrophic, denervated fibres is also present.

fibres but in myopathies, especially in Duchenne muscular dystrophy, such fibres are difficult to classify histochemically since they show features of both fibre types. Fibre hypertrophy is frequent in limb-girdle muscular dystrophies, but the biopsy also contains many small fibres.

Fibre-Type Grouping

Fibre-type grouping is present when two or more fibres of one histochemical type are enclosed at all points on their circumference by other fibres of the same histochemical type. This usually means that there are at least 10 fibres in the group but, clearly, this depends on fibre size.

Fibre-type grouping is evidence that reinnervation of denervated fibres has occurred, probably by collateral sprouting from nearby axons. Small groups of fibres can be formed in a few weeks, perhaps in less than a month, but the finding of large groups (>25 fibres) implies a neurogenic disorder of some chronicity (Fig. 3.13); it is a feature of chronic neuropathies and of Kugelberg–Welander disease. The greater the degree of fibre-type grouping, the fewer the number of motor axons remaining innervating the muscle (Karpati and Engel 1968). In experimental reinnervation, following sciatic nerve crush in the rat, an increased number of intermediate (Type 2C) fibres was found at 4 weeks but fibre-type grouping was not observed before 6 weeks (Warszanski et al. 1975).

When fibre-type predominance exceeds about 80%, enclosed fibres will become frequent without necessarily implying that fibre-type grouping is present (Johnson et al. 1973). However, fibre-type predominance is itself a factor which should lead to

suspicion of a neurogenic disorder, particularly in biopsies taken from muscles normally consisting of approximately equal numbers of Type 1 and Type 2 fibres, as in the biceps and vastus lateralis. Small biopsies, as with the needle biopsy technique, taken from muscles with large fibre-type groups may give a false impression of the fibre-type distribution and predominance within the biopsy. It is important to use grouping of *both major fibre types* as the criterion for reinnervation in order to exclude bias from fibre-type predominance.

Groups of small, pointed fibres of similar histochemical type, often containing dark, pyknotic nuclei, indicate that irreversible denervation has occurred. When such groups contain large numbers of fibres, even occupying most or all of a fascicle, it is probable that denervation of a group of fibres reinnervated by collateral sprouting from a single motor unit has occurred (Fig. 3.14). This phenomenon, called *grouped denervation atrophy*, is most frequently found in motor neuron disease, when it represents death of individual anterior horn cells. Clusters of three to six small, angular fibres (*disseminated neurogenic atrophy*) typically occur in more rapidly progressive neurogenic disorders, in which reinnervation by collateral sprouting has been ineffective.

Fibre-type grouping is uncommon in myopathic disorders, but is found in chronic polymyositis (Swash et al. 1978a). When fibres arranged in groups of similar histochemical type are found in myopathies, or in muscular dystrophy, it is often found that they are difficult to classify since they show histochemical features of fibres of both histochemical types, and the significance of this apparent fibre-type grouping is uncertain (Schwartz et al. 1976a).

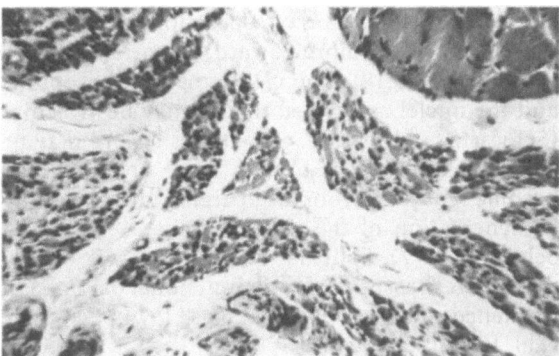

Fig. 3.14. H and E. × 140. Motor neuron disease. Paraffin-embedded hypothenar muscle obtained at autopsy. Several fascicles consist of atrophic fibres containing dark pyknotic nuclei; these are the features of grouped denervation atrophy, indicating irreversible denervation of muscle.

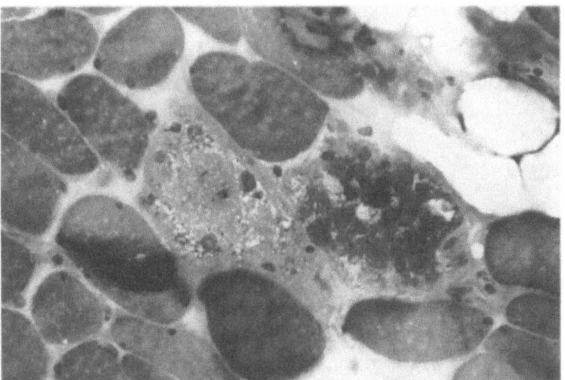

Fig. 3.16. Gomori trichrome. Two necrotic fibres; one contains a macrophage.

Central Nucleation

Central nucleation is frequently found in hypertrophied fibres, and as a feature associated with fibre splitting (Fig. 3.12). It also occurs in regenerating fibres. It is especially prominent, however, in centro-nuclear myopathy and in myotonic dystrophy, although it also occurs in other myopathies (Fig. 3.15).

Histological Features

Degenerative Changes

A number of histological changes, classified as degenerative, are found in muscle fibres in neuromuscular disorders. Some of these changes are relatively specific to Type 1 or Type 2 fibres (Table 3.6). The basic fibre changes are more universal.

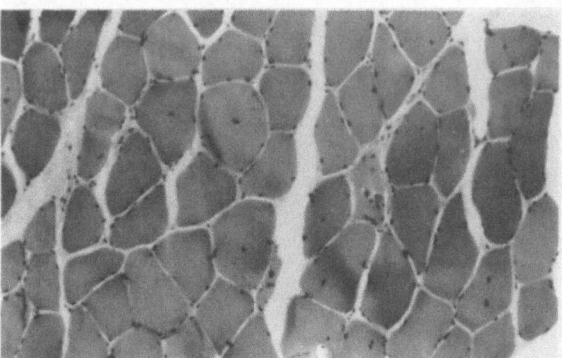

Fig. 3.15. H and E. × 140. Myopathy associated with familial hypokalaemic periodic paralysis. Central nucleation is prominent. One fibre is undergoing necrosis.

Table 3.6. Predilection of involvement of fibre-types in neuromuscular disease

Type 1 fibres	Type 2 fibres
Targets	Tubular aggregates
Rods (nemaline myopathy)	Sarcoplasmic masses (myotonic dystrophy)
Central cores	Cylindrical spirals
Mitochondrial aggregates	Polyglucosan storage (Lafora disease)
Lipid droplet accumulation	
Central nuclei in centro-nuclear myopathy	
Glycogen storage in acid maltase deficiency	
Atrophy in:	*Atrophy in:*
Fibre type disproportion	Disuse, including rheumatological and neurological disorders
Werdnig–Hoffmann disease	
Myotonic dystrophy	
	Cachexia
	Steroid effect
	Myasthenia gravis

From Karpati and Carpenter (1992).

Necrosis. Necrotic fibres (Fig. 3.16) are a common feature of the myopathies, but they may also be found in biopsies from patients with chronic neurogenic disorders (Cazzato 1970; Schwartz et al. 1976a). With haematoxylin and eosin they appear pale and hyaline. Later they lose their eosinophilic character, become pale and patchily stained, and begin to undergo phagocytosis. Sometimes an endomysial cellular reaction occurs around them, consisting of endothelial capillary nuclei and sarcolemmal nuclei. Necrotic fibres usually contain prominent acid phosphatase-positive material (Fig. 3.17). If the blood supply to a region of fibre necrosis is impaired, the endomysial tubes and basal lamina scaffold may remain intact, despite necrosis of the muscle fibres themselves, producing an appearance of rings of empty endomysial tubes, an

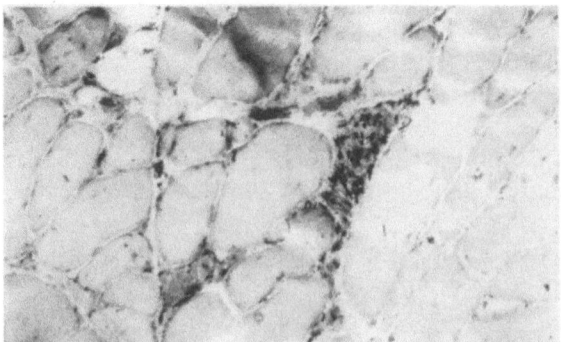

Fig. 3.17. × 140. Acid phosphatase activity in a necrotic fibre.

appearance termed *subendomysial necrosis*. This appearance occurs particularly in polymyositis (Swash and Schwartz 1977) and in other acute necrotising myopathies (Urich and Wilkinson 1970). In polymyositis muscle fibre necrosis is accompanied by expression of Class II major histocompatibility complex (MHC) antigen, a process that may enable T helper lymphocytes to recognise susceptible fibres (Engel and Arahata 1986). A similar mechanism for organ-specific autoimmune disease, as in thyroiditis, has been proposed by Foulis (1986).

Fibre Splitting. Fibre splitting is particularly a feature of muscular dystrophy, e.g. Duchenne dystrophy (Bell and Conen 1968), but is also common in chronic neurogenic disorders, such as intermediate spinal muscular atrophy. In the latter disorder it particularly affects hypertrophied Type 1 fibres. Splitting usually begins from the periphery of

affected fibres, the line of separation running into the centre of the fibre toward a centrally placed nucleus (Fig. 3.18). The cleft is usually basophilic and the nuclei associated with it may be vesicular (Schwartz et al. 1976a). Sometimes a fibre may be split into multiple fragments, some of which may become separated from the "parent" fibre, resulting in denervation of the split fragment (Swash and Schwartz 1977). Splitting of this type is probably due to stress associated with functional overload of weakened muscles (Hall-Craggs 1970; Schwartz et al. 1976a).

The fibre-splitting found in Duchenne dystrophy (Bell and Conen 1968), limb-girdle myopathies and polymyositis (Swash et al. 1978a) may have a similar origin, but could also result from defective regeneration (Schmalbruch 1976). Splitting may be important in functional compensation (Swash and Schwartz 1977); in chronic neurogenic disorders it may lead to the presence both of fibre necrosis and regeneration, with variability in fibre size and central nucleation, an appearance called secondary "myopathic" change (Drachman et al. 1967; Schwartz et al. 1976a). Fibre-splitting is a normal phenomenon near musculo-tendinous insertions (Bell and Conen 1968) and it must not be confused with subendomysial regeneration (Fig. 3.19) occurring after fibre necrosis (Schmalbruch 1976; Swash et al. 1978a).

Moth-eaten Fibres. These (Brooke and Engel 1966) are fibres in which the normally regular intermyofibrillar network seen in the oxidative enzyme preparations is disturbed. Type 1 fibres are preferentially affected. The abnormality often consists of a whorled appearance (Fig. 3.20) and areas of non-reactivity to NADH are often present near these

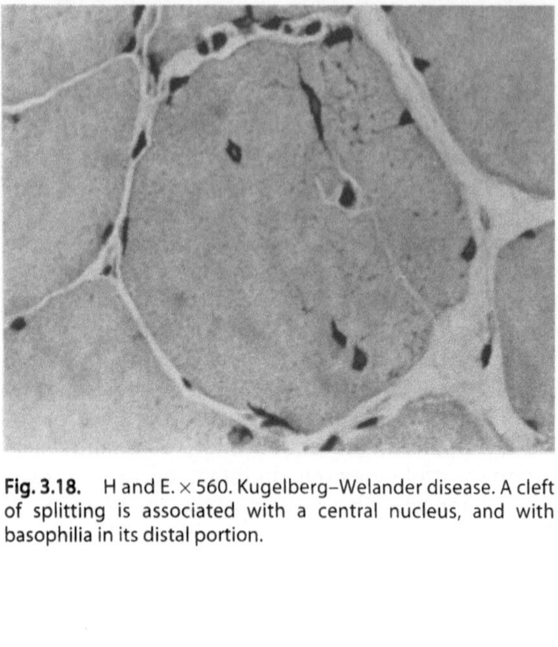

Fig. 3.18. H and E. × 560. Kugelberg–Welander disease. A cleft of splitting is associated with a central nucleus, and with basophilia in its distal portion.

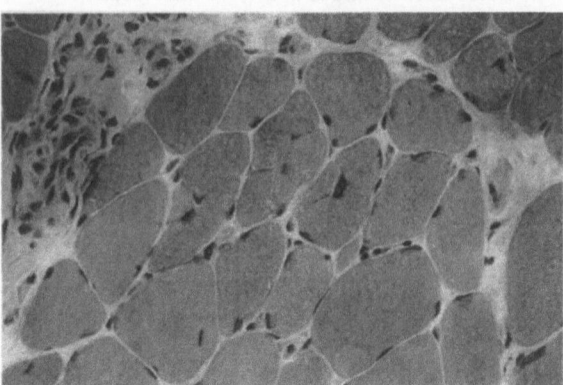

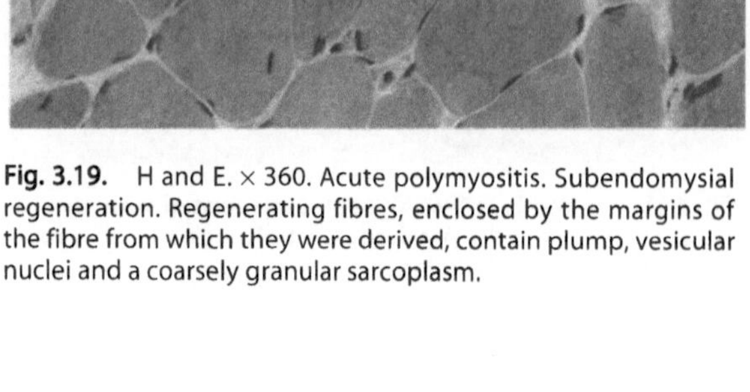

Fig. 3.19. H and E. × 360. Acute polymyositis. Subendomysial regeneration. Regenerating fibres, enclosed by the margins of the fibre from which they were derived, contain plump, vesicular nuclei and a coarsely granular sarcoplasm.

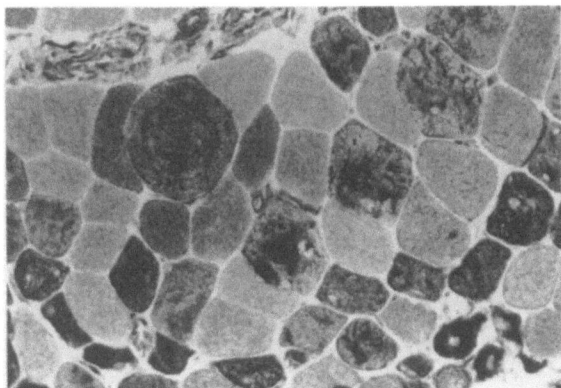

Fig. 3.20. NADH-tr. × 360. Acute dermatomyositis. Many of the darkly reacting Type 1 fibres show a moth-eaten or whorled appearance, with areas of decreased and increased reactivity in their intermyofibrillar network.

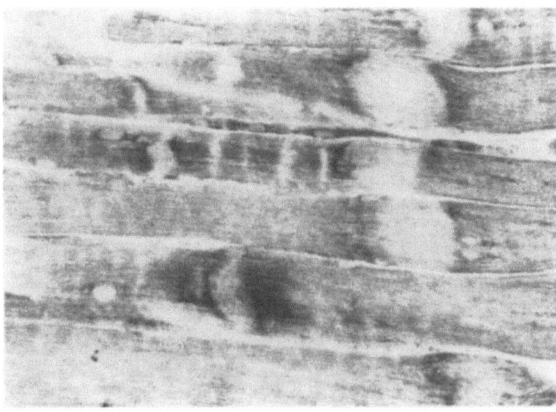

Fig. 3.22. Cores in longitudinal section. NADH. × 560. Core-like zones of non-reactivity are present. These contain degenerate myofibrils, and mitochondria are absent. In central core disease this abnormality extends through long segments of affected fibres, but in this case the abnormality is discrete. The latter is more typical of multicore disease. The slit-like zones of non-reactivity are termed "focal loss of cross striations".

whorls. This change is not specific to any single disorder but is particularly associated with inflammatory myopathies.

Target Fibres. Targets (Engel 1961) are best seen in ATPase and NADH-tr preparations (Fig. 3.21). These fibres contain a central unstained zone, surrounded by a densely stained intermediate zone and a third, relatively normal outer zone. Most affected fibres are Type 1 fibres. Target fibres are usually associated with denervation, especially that associated with neuropathies, but they have been produced experimentally by tenotomy (Engel et al. 1966).

Central Cores. Cores (Fig. 3.22) are often difficult to distinguish from target fibres. A distinction has been drawn between fibres with structured (ATPase-positive) and unstructured cores (Neville and Brooke 1973) but it is doubtful if this is useful

in practice. The latter are sometimes called core-targetoid fibres, a term which illustrates these difficulties (Schmitt and Volk 1975).

Rod Bodies. Nemaline rods are best seen in the Gomori preparation. They consist of small rod-like bodies, scattered in the sarcoplasm of affected fibres (Fig. 3.23), or found in a subsarcolemmal location. The rods are faintly visible as basophilic structures in H and E stains. They were first described in a familial non-progressive myopathy with hypotonia

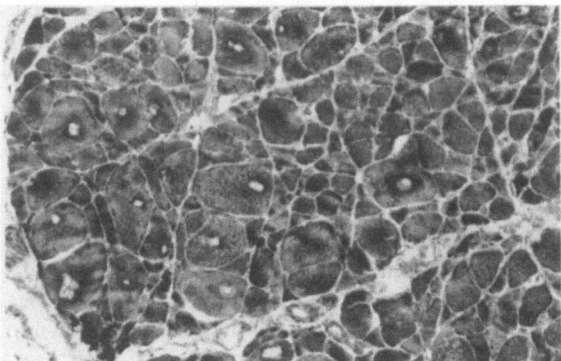

Fig. 3.21. NADH-tr. × 140. Target fibres in a biopsy from a patient with a nerve injury. The biopsy shows disseminated neurogenic atrophy and targets are seen principally in Type 1 fibres.

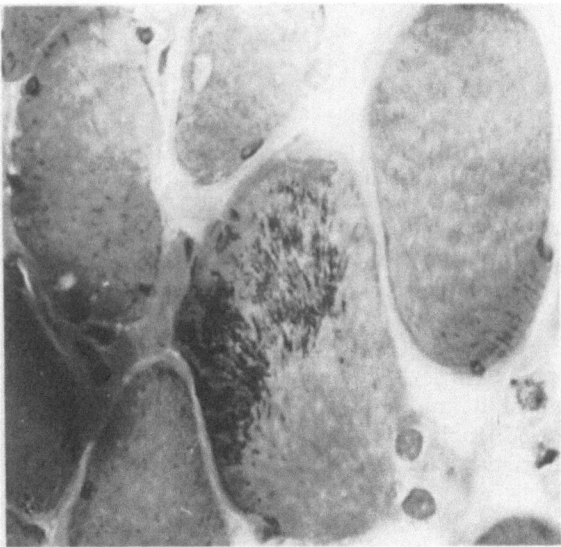

Fig. 3.23. Gomori trichrome. × 560. Nemaline bodies.

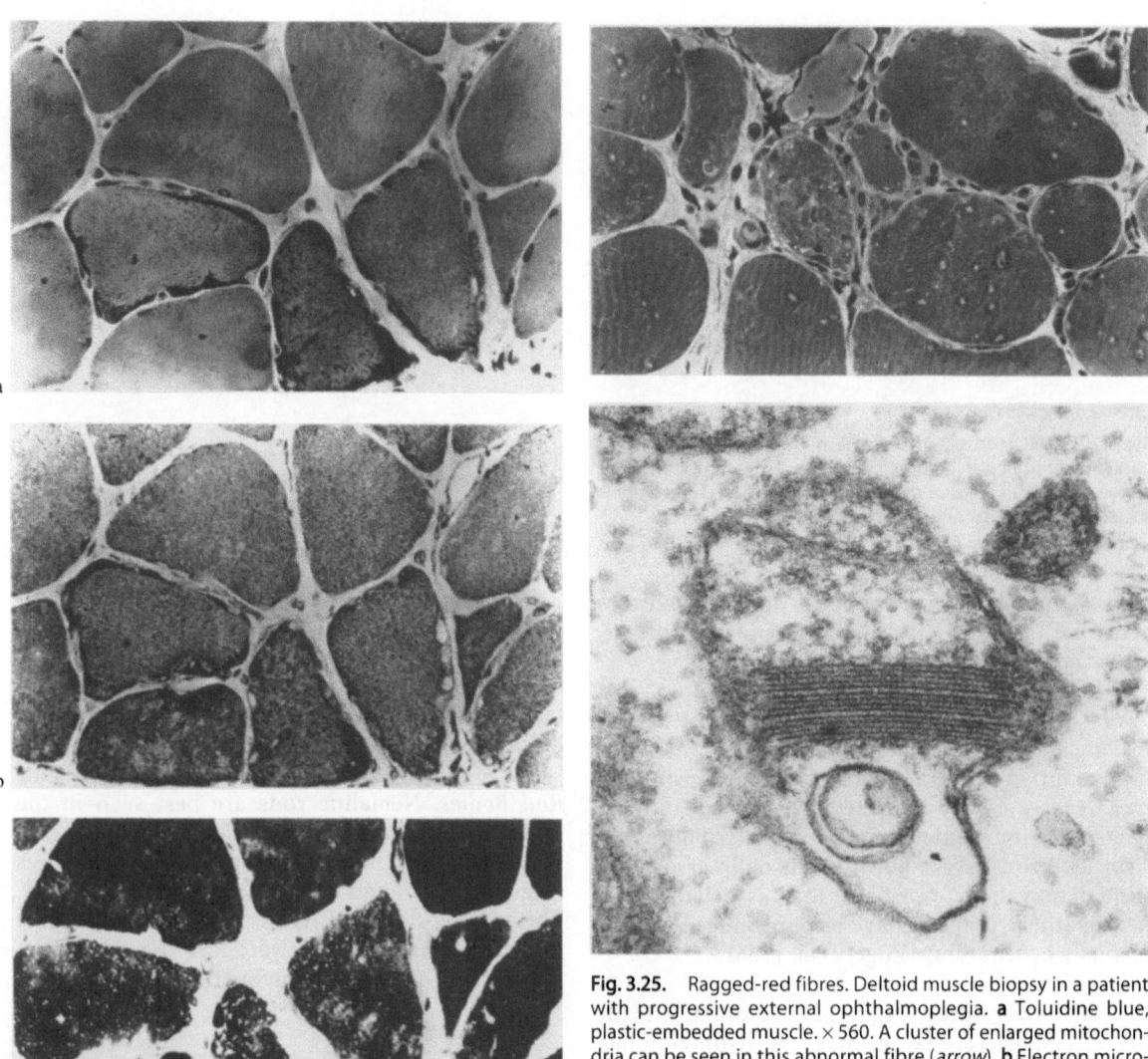

Fig. 3.24. Ragged-red fibres. × 600. **a** Gomori trichrome. There is a peripheral zone of stain, which appears red in the microscope. **b** NADH. The peripheral abnormality contains positive and negative zones of reactivity. **c** ATPase, pH 4.3. The peripheral, abnormal part of the affected fibres does not react.

Fig. 3.25. Ragged-red fibres. Deltoid muscle biopsy in a patient with progressive external ophthalmoplegia. **a** Toluidine blue, plastic-embedded muscle. × 560. A cluster of enlarged mitochondria can be seen in this abnormal fibre (*arrow*). **b** Electron micrograph. × 90 000. Abnormal mitochondrion from a ragged-red fibre, showing the typical paracrystalline inclusions.

by Shy et al. (1963), who called it nemaline myopathy. However, rod bodies have also been reported in adult limb-girdle myopathies (Engel and Resnick 1966), polymyositis (Sato et al. 1971) and in a variety of other disorders.

Ragged-red Fibres. Ragged-red fibres appear coarsely granular in haematoxylin and eosin preparations. The granular material is faintly basophilic and is unevenly distributed in the sarcoplasm; it is particularly prominent at the periphery of affected fibres. This material stains red in the Gomori trichrome preparation, is dark in NADH-tr and SDH preparations and does not stain in ATPase preparations (Fig. 3.24). Affected fibres are almost always Type 1 fibres. In addition, this material is usually faintly basophilic and is often associated with droplets of neutral lipid. Ragged-red fibres were first recognised as an isolated phenomenon in patients with progressive ophthalmoplegia (Engel 1971) associated with a mild proximal myopathy, but they are now known to be a characteristic feature of a group of mitochondrial disorders in which there is defective mitochondrial oxidation (Petty et al. 1986a). With the electron microscope the granular appearance is seen to result

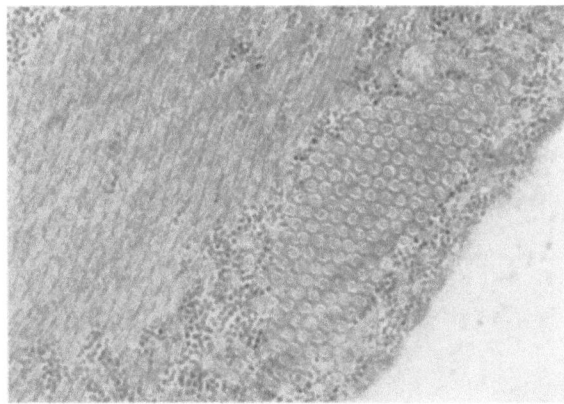

Fig. 3.26. Electron micrograph. × 54 000. Tubular aggregates seen in transverse and oblique section. The stacked tubules arise from a dilated tubule of the sarcoplasmic reticulum, in a patient with polymyositis. Note that the tubules contain a central, hollow core.

from accumulations of mitochondria, which may show morphological abnormalities, and contain osmiophilic bodies and paracrystalline material (Fig. 3.25).

Tubular Aggregates. Aggregates of tubular inclusions are limited to a peripheral segment of affected fibres. They are found in Type 2B fibres and although the abnormal zones are darkly stained in preparations of oxidative enzymes, they are negative in SDH preparations. Electron microscopy demonstrates the characteristic stacked tubules derived from sarcoplasmic reticulum (Engel et al. 1970) (Fig. 3.26). They may be empty or contain one or more thin inner tubules. They do not communicate with the exterior of the muscle fibre. Although in itself a highly characteristic finding, tubular aggregates are not specific for any particular disorder (Dubowitz and Brooke 1973). Nonetheless, some patients with this abnormality have been reported as "myopathy with tubular aggregates".

Cytoplasmic Bodies. These consist of small eosinophilic, PAS-positive zones within otherwise normal muscle fibres and are particularly associated with collagen-vascular disease such as dermatomyositis (Fig. 3.27) but when present in small numbers their significance is doubtful.

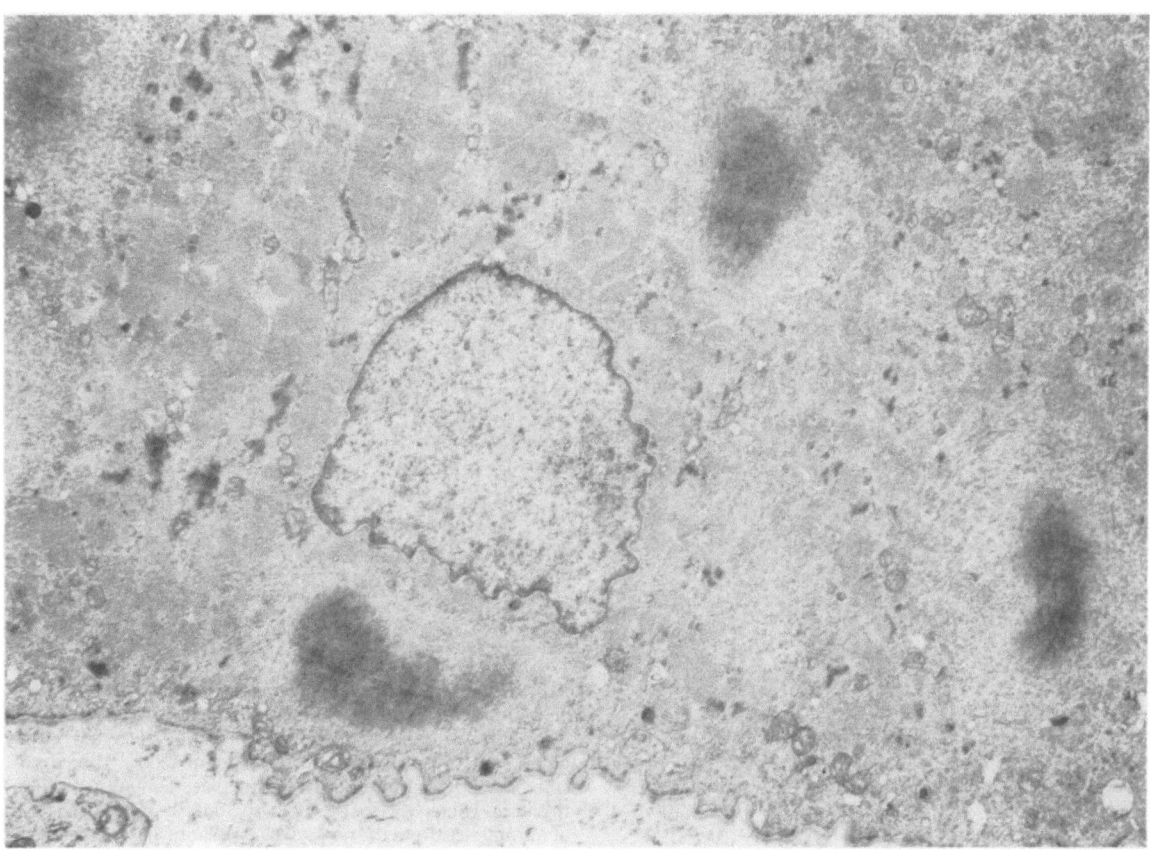

Fig. 3.27. Electron micrograph. × 15 000. Cytoplasmic bodies in dermatomyositis.

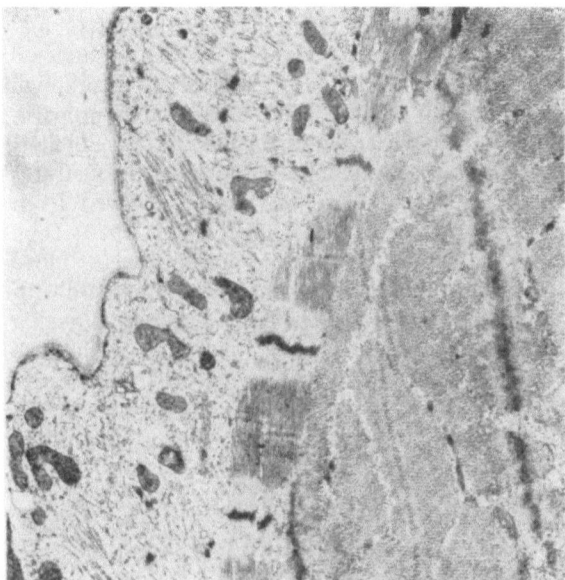

Fig. 3.28. Electron micrograph. × 30 000. Myotonic dystrophy. Ring fibres consist of fibres in which a displaced myofibril, or group of myofibrils, is situated at the periphery of the fibre. In this fibre there is a peripheral sarcoplasmic mass containing myofibrillar debris.

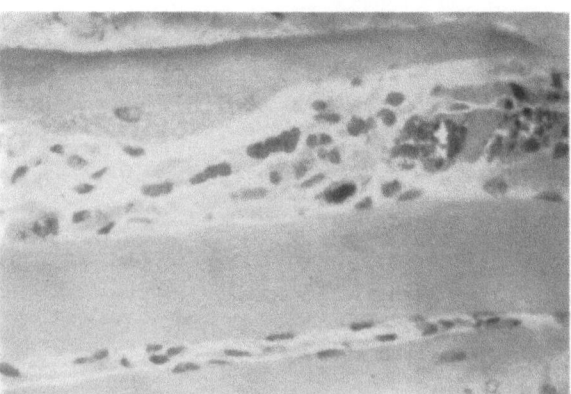

Fig. 3.30. H and E. LS. Regeneration is occurring in a necrotic fibre. Debris is in process of removal from one part of the fibre (right of the picture) and a regenerating myoblast, consisting of a short segment of sarcoplasm containing dark, enlarged nuclei, is present in another part of the fibre (left of the figure). A sub-endomysial lens-shaped mass of foamy sarcoplasm, containing a single active nucleus, represents a very early stage of regeneration from a subsarcolemmal satellite cell.

as in acid maltase deficiency, are found with lysosomal diseases, often associated with lipid storage (Carpenter and Karpati 1986).

Regenerative Changes

Regeneration occurs after necrosis or injury in most tissues of the body; muscle fibres, which are particularly suspectible to injury in everyday life, have considerable regenerative potential. Regenerating fibres

Ring Fibres. These (Fig. 3.28), although formerly associated with myotonic dystrophy, may occur in many other chronic disorders. Nonetheless, they are more frequently encountered in myotonic dystrophy and are then often associated with *sarcoplasmic masses*. Ring fibres (ringbinden) consist of fibres in which a displaced myofibrillar strand has taken up a spiral position around the periphery of the fibre. Sarcoplasmic masses consist of peripheral zones of sarcoplasm, devoid of myofibrils and of other cell particles (Klinkerfuss 1967). Acid phosphatase-positive vacuoles, sometimes containing glycogen

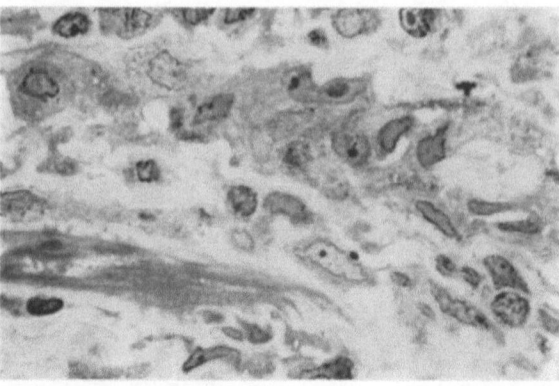

Fig. 3.31. Regeneration. **a** Toluidine blue. × 1360. Plastic-embedded section. Part of a regenerating fibre, showing several myoblasts, and their enlarged vesicular nuclei. **b** Electron micrograph. TS. × 15 000. An immature regenerating fibre. The subsarcolemmal smaller fibre, separated by plasma membrane from the larger fibre, will fuse with it to form a single new fibre of normal size. Note the enlarged vesicular nuclei and the fragments of regenerating tissue in the space between the two fibres.

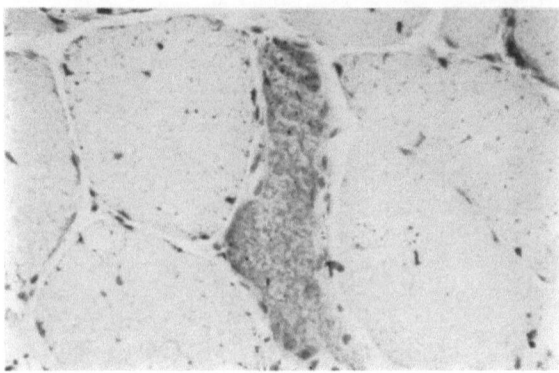

Fig. 3.29. Oil red O and haematoxylin. × 360. A basophilic regenerating fibre.

can be recognised by their sarcoplasmic basophilia in haematoxylin and eosin stains. They are usually smaller than surrounding fibres and contain central, enlarged, vesicular nuclei, with prominent nucleoli (Fig. 3.29). They are sometimes vacuolated and show increased sarcoplasmic RNA content in special stains. Vimentin and desmin intermediate filaments are upregulated in the sarcoplasm during the early phase of regeneration (Thornell et al. 1980). Serial transverse sections, or longitudinal sections, show that the early stages of regeneration co-exist with phagocytosis of necrotic remnants of the damaged segment in which regeneration is occurring (Fig. 3.30). Regeneration can thus occur

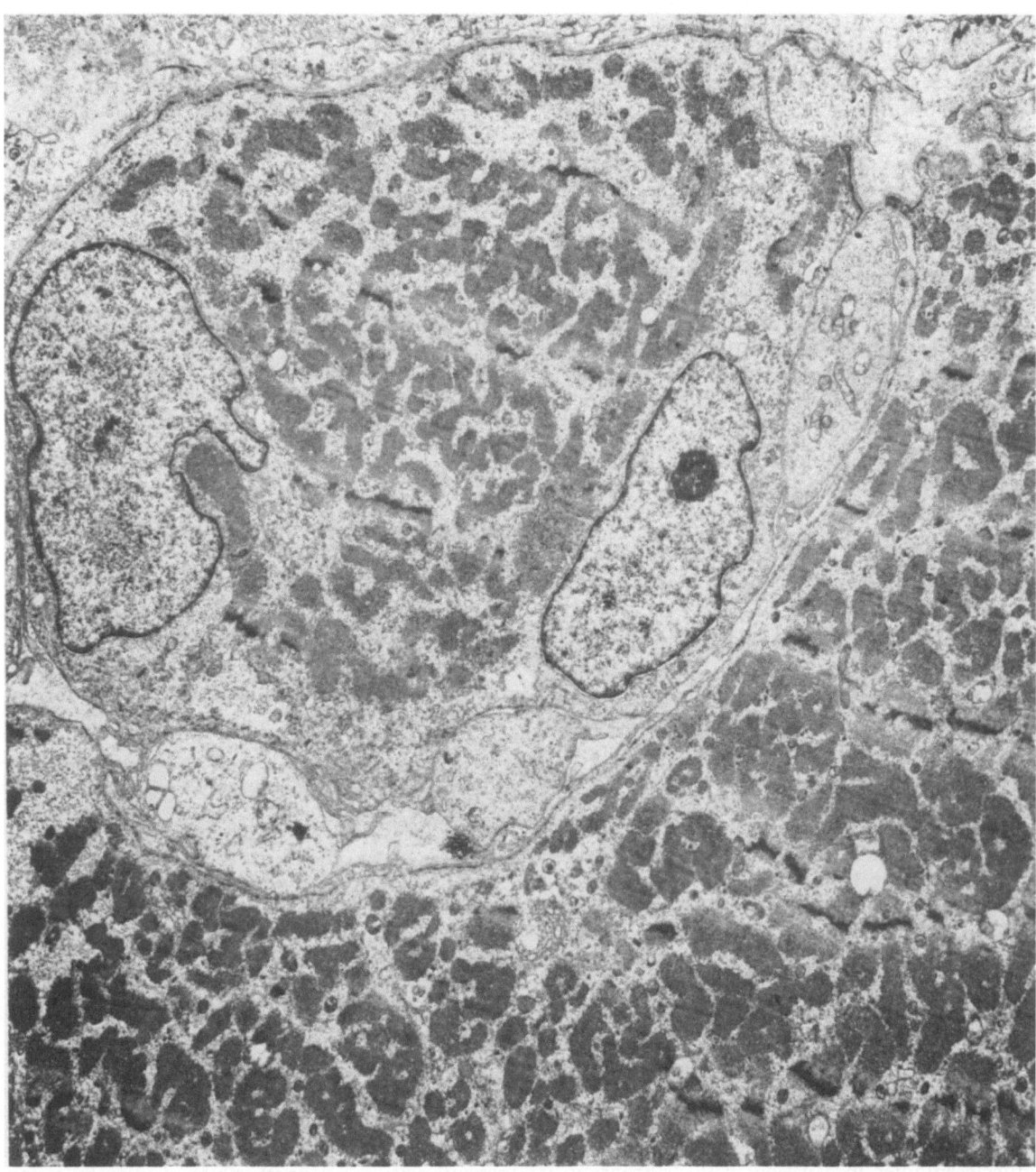

Fig. 3.31b.

either in continuity with the undamaged portions of the fibre ("continuous" repair) or from myoblast formation in the necrotic segment itself ("discontinuous" repair).

Myoblasts arise by segregation of nuclei from the damaged myofibre itself, by activation of satellite cells (Mauro 1961) pre-existing in the sarcolemmal sheath, or by metaplasia from circulating mesenchymal cells. The weight of evidence favours the first and second of these suggestions (Reznik and Engel 1970; Reznik 1973). The numbers of satellite cells are increased after injury (Reznik 1973) and after denervation (Ontell 1974). They are also found in increased numbers in the early stages of Duchenne dystrophy (Mastaglia et al. 1970b; Teresawa 1986). Satellite cells (see Ishimoto et al. 1983) are present in large numbers in infancy, but decrease in number with developing maturity (Schmalbruch and Hellhammer 1976). Reznik (1973) has reviewed the ultrastructural sequence of changes found in these cells giving rise to myoblast formation during regeneration after cold-induced injury (Fig. 3.31). The process of regeneration from myoblasts to myotube formation and then fusion to form new muscle fibres requires metabolic activity. It is accompanied by basophilia and by other features of protein synthesis, and it will not occur unless the tissue is sufficiently well capillarised (Allbrook 1981; Carlson 1986).

Muscle Spindles

Muscle spindles undergo characteristic changes in myotonic dystrophy (Fig. 3.32). These consist of fragmentation of intrafusal muscle fibres, proliferation of the motor and sensory innervation and thickening of the motor and sensory innervation and thickening of the spindle capsule (Swash and Fox 1972, 1975a,b). In Duchenne dystrophy intrafusal muscle fibres undergo necrosis and the spindles become fibrosed in the late stages of the disease (Swash and Fox 1976). In the earlier stages they appear less affected than the extrafusal fibres. Muscle spindles often appear unusually prominent in neurogenic disorders, especially in childhood, because their fibrous capsules remain, or become thickened, while extrafusal muscle fibres become atrophic, but both motor and sensory denervation also leads to changes in the innervation and morphology of the polar and equatorial parts of the intrafusal muscle fibres respectively (Swash and Fox 1974). Krugliak et al. (1978) reported absence of muscle spindles in a patient with arthrogryposis multiplex congenita.

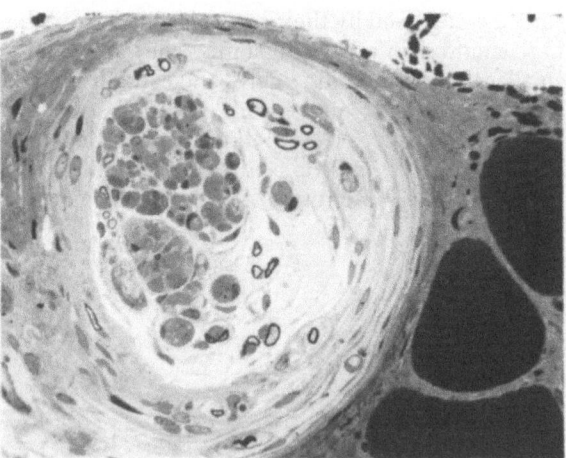

Fig. 3.32.   Toluidine blue. × 560. Muscle spindle in myotonic dystrophy. The intrafusal fibres are fragmented and the spindle capsule is thickened. Normal spindles contain fewer than 14 intrafusal muscle fibres.

Terminal Motor Innervation

Axonal sprouting occurs in neurogenic disorders and abnormalities in the subterminal apparatus of the motor end-plates in myasthenia gravis. Axonal sprouting also occurs in myotonic dystrophy.

Motor End-Plates

Motor end-plates are not commonly seen in routine muscle biopsies unless motor point biopsy is undertaken. Abnormalities occur in myasthenia gravis and in other neuromuscular disorders, including neurogenic and myopathic disorders. About 5% of control subjects show some abnormalities (Engel 1994).

Blood Vessels

Abnormalities in blood vessels are uncommon, except in polymyositis, polyarteritis nodosa and other autoimmune disorders. In these disorders, necrosis of the arteriolar wall, hyaline change, thrombosis and, more frequently, infiltration by small round cells and plasma cells may occur. Ultrastructural changes occur in some cases of polymyositis. Capillaries are difficult to study in human muscle, but they are reduced in number in inflammatory myopathies (Carry et al. 1986). Internal vascularisation of muscle fibres occurs in chronic neurogenic, or myopathic disease. Sulaiman and Kinder (1989) found this abnormality in 5% of

1091 cases surveyed, especially in neurogenic disorders, apparently in relation to degenerative change in hypertrophic fibres.

The Normal Nerve

Peripheral nerves consist of bundles of myelinated and unmyelinated nerve fibres, arranged in fascicles surrounded by connective tissue, collagen and perineural cells (Fig. 3.33). The endoneurial space contains small blood vessels. The peripheral nerves tend to be associated with arteries and veins, forming neurovascular bundles. Even small nerve branches situated in muscles show this relationship. Almost all peripheral nerves contain both motor and sensory fibres.

The *epineurial sheath*, consisting of an outer layer of connective tissue, binds the nerve fascicles together. Each nerve fascicle is surrounded by a layer of basement membrane; tight junctional complexes and pinocytotic vesicles are prominent features of these cells. These *perineurial* cells form a permeability barrier between the endoneurial space and other extracellular tissue compartments. In the nerve roots the perineurial layer is continuous with the arachnoid cellular layer that surrounds the central nervous system, and the cerebrospinal fluid and endoneurial space are thus potentially in continuity. The *endoneurium* contains nerve fibres Schwann cells and blood vessels. These cellular septa, fibroblasts and longitudinally orientated collagen fibrils are also found in the endoneurial space. Bundles of randomly orientated collagen fibrils, fibroblasts and acid mucopolysaccharide ground substance, called Renaut bodies, are also found in the endoneurium. Their function is obscure (Asbury 1973).

The proportions, diameters and numbers of myelinated and unmyelinated nerve fibres vary in different peripheral nerves, but normal values are available for several human nerves, including the sural nerve, which is the most commonly biopsied nerve (Ochoa and Mair 1969) In this nerve unmyelinated fibres (30 000/mm^2) are four times more numerous than myelinated fibres (8000/mm^2). Unmyelinated fibres in this nerve range from 0.5 to 3.0 μm in diameter and myelinated fibres range from 2.0 to 17.0 μm in diameter, with bimodal peaks of diameter at 5.0 μm and 13.0 μm. There are slight variations from these figures in very young children and in elderly subjects. Myelinated fibre density, especially that of large myelinated fibres,

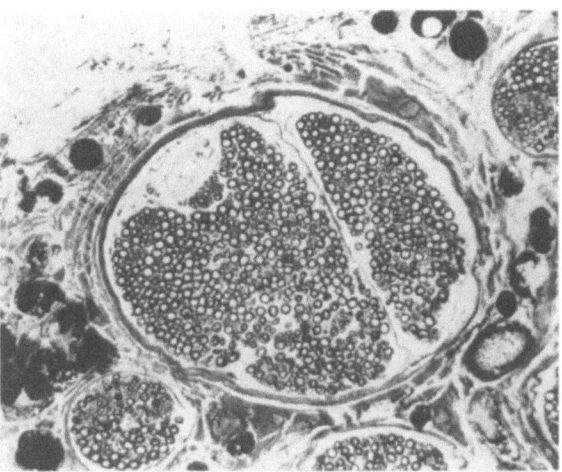

Fig. 3.33. TS. × 140. Normal median nerve, showing the normal distribution of myelinated nerve fibres. The largest axons are the most thickly myelinated. Flemming's osmium method of myelin.

decreases with age. The frequency of fibres showing segmental demyelination and remyelination, and axonal degeneration and regeneration also decrease with age (Dyck et al. 1985b).

Myelin is formed by layers of Schwannian membranes wrapped concentrically around the axon (Fig. 3.34). The numbers of Schwann cells associated with individual nerve fibres is determined in fetal life; during development these cells elongate to take account of increasing axonal length. The gap between individual Schwann cells, called the node of Ranvier, is specialised to allow electrolyte exchange during the process of saltatory conduction of the nervous impulse. The thickness of the myelin sheath is related to axonal diameter (Thomas et al. 1993).

Axons of myelinated nerve fibres can be demonstrated for light microscopy by silver impregnation. With the electron microscope they consist of a lucent cytoplasm containing neurofilaments and more peripherally located neurotubules, and surrounded by a layer of plasma membrane. Mitochondria and smooth endoplasmic reticulum can usually be recognised (Fig. 3.35). These structures and myelin itself are associated with specific cytoskeletal proteins that can be demonstrated immunocytochemically (see Landon 1985). The Schwann cells are closely invested by a layer of basement membrane, which enables them to be distinguished from fibroblasts. Several axons may be myelinated by a single Schwann cell. The ultrastructure of Schwann cells, with their nodes of Ranvier and Schmidt-Lanterman incisures, is complex (Fig. 3.36).

Unmyelinated nerve fibres (Fig. 3.36) are also associated with Schwann cells, but myelin lamellae are not present and individual Schwann cells are

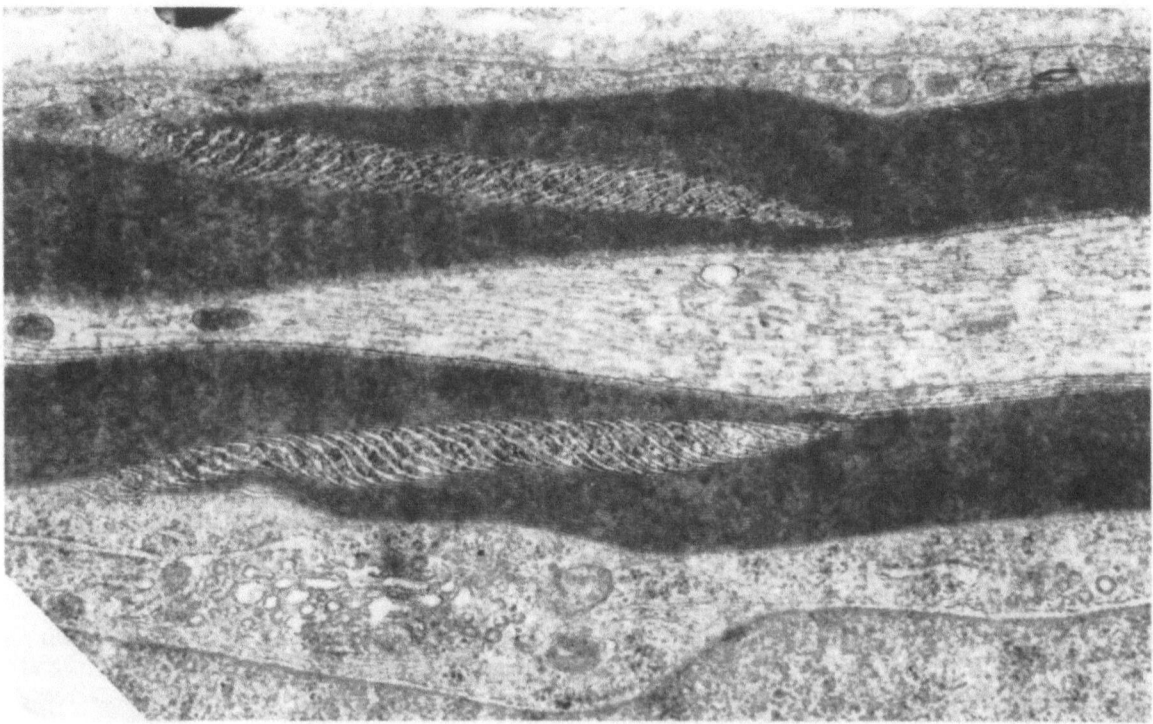

Fig. 3.34.   Electron micrograph. LS. × 35 000. Normal myelinated nerve fibre. Schmidt–Lanterman incisure. This normal structure consists of Schwann cell-filled separations of the myelin lamellae.

associated with groups of unmyelinated axons. Metabolic materials are transported along axons both towards and away from the cell body at slow and fast rates, probably utilising the neurofilamentous and neurotubular system within the axon (Wilson and Stone 1979; Tytel et al. 1981; see Dyck and Thomas 1993 for review).

Nerve Biopsy

Generally the sural nerve is biopsied. This is a sensory nerve, supplying only a small area of skin on the dorsolateral surface of the foot and ankle. The nerve is easily accessible for biopsy, being situated subcutaneously in the lower calf overlying the insertion of the soleus muscle into the Achilles tendon; small branches of the nerve can sometimes be biopsied on the lateral surface of the foot itself, particularly when they are hypertrophied and easily identified. The superficial branch of the radial nerve near the wrist is also sometimes biopsied. Occasionally in severe longstanding neuropathies it is justifiable to biopsy a fascicle of a larger, mixed sensory

and motor nerve but this can only be undertaken when there is no reasonable expectation of functional recovery from the neuropathy since, when a short length of a nerve has been removed, regeneration will inevitably be incomplete.

At biopsy it is important not to squeeze or apply tension to the nerve because this leads to artefactual tearing and even disruption of myelin lamellae. Even cutting the nerve with scissors may result in significant artefact. A 1.5 to 2.5 cm length of nerve should be removed. Small pieces of this biopsy can then be prepared for light and electron microscopy after fixing them in glutaraldehyde and embedding them in epoxy resin. Toluidine blue stains of semithin sections are particularly useful. It is helpful to snap-freeze a small piece of the nerve biopsy in isopentane-liquid nitrogen so that histochemical stains for amyloid, complement and serum immunoglobulins can be employed. Haematoxylin and eosin, elastin-van Gieson, and solarchrome cyanin (for myelin) stains are useful methods in this frozen material, both in longitudinal and transverse sections. The fresh nerve can be treated with osmium tetroxide and then teased in glycerine to study the distribution of nodes of Ranvier along a length of individual fibres but this technique is very time-consuming and is not much used in routine diag-

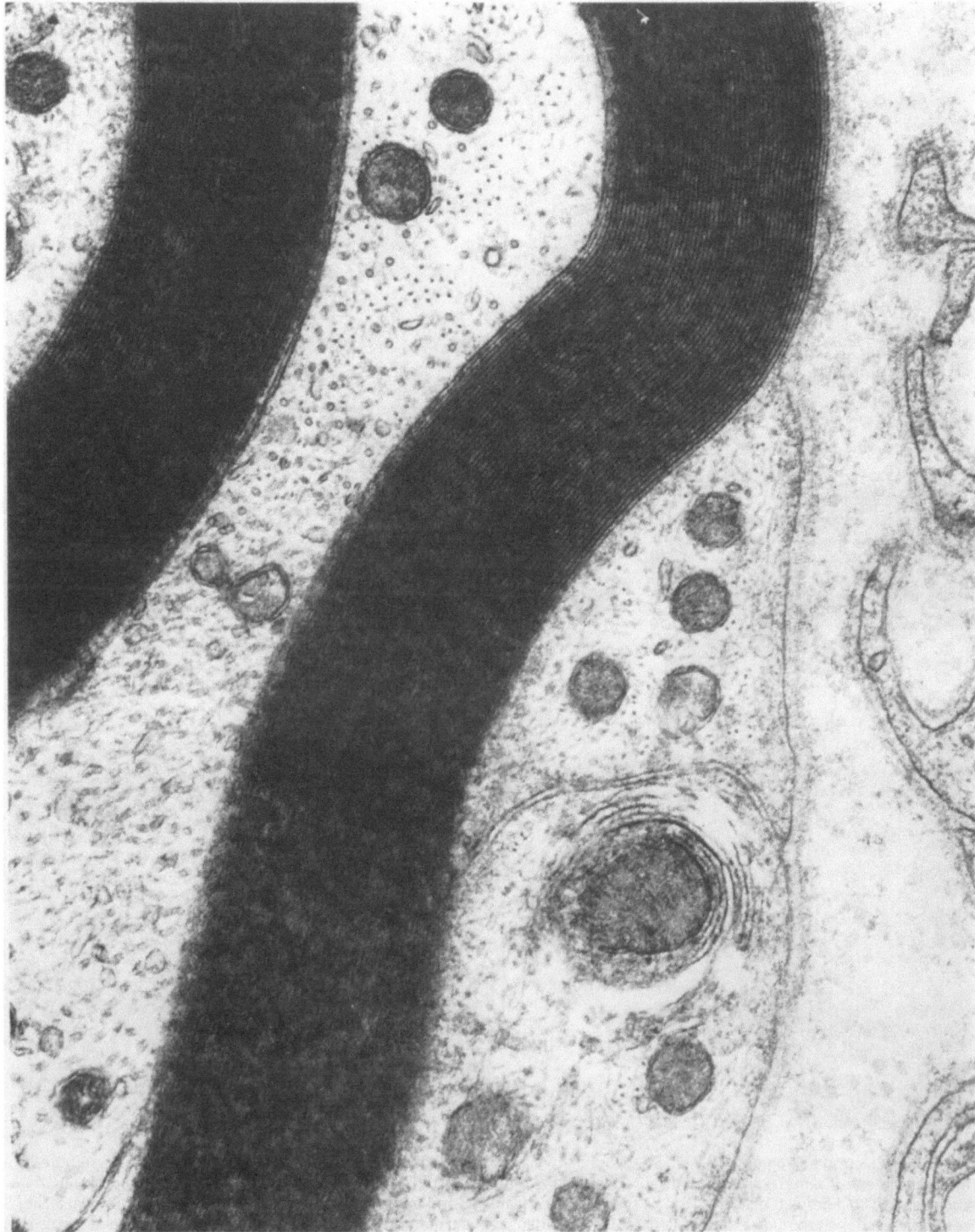

Fig. 3.35. Electron micrograph. TS. × 60 000. Normal myelinated nerve fibre. The axon contains neurofilaments and neurotubules, with small mitochondria. The myelin lamellae and the Schwann cell covering, surrounded by a layer of basement membrane, can be clearly seen.

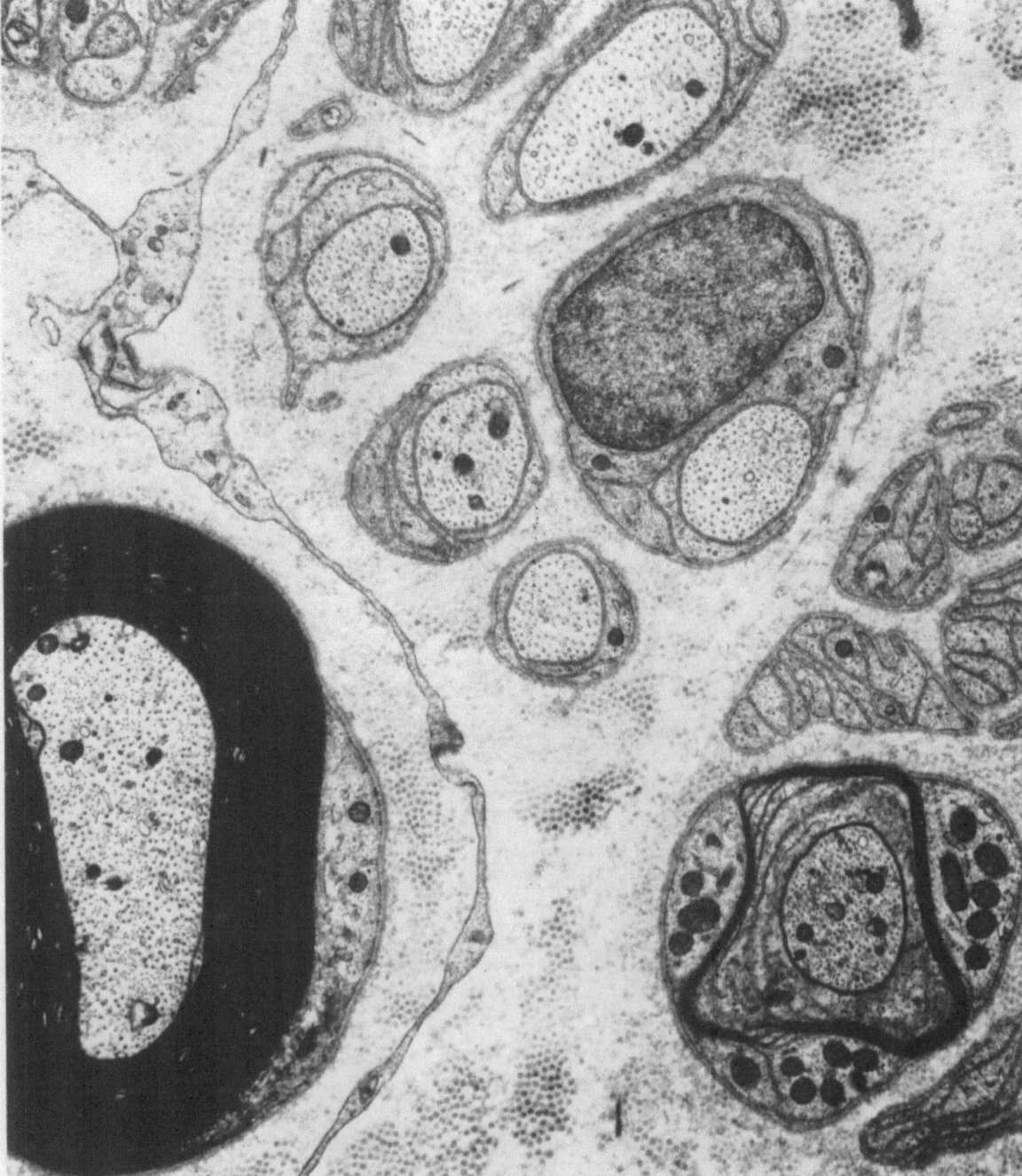

Fig. 3.36.   Electron micrograph. TS. × 22 500. Normal myelinated nerve fibre. There is a large, thickly myelinated nerve fibre. The internal and external mesaxon of its Schwann cell, and the dot-like neurofilaments and peripherally situated neurotubules, mitochondria and lipid droplets of its axon can be seen. Collagen filaments and part of a fibroblast separate this nerve fibre from an adjacent fibre, sectioned through a node of Ranvier. Note the dense axonal membrane. Unmyelinated nerve fibres, surrounded by thin layers of Schwann cell cytoplasm, occupy the remainder of the field.

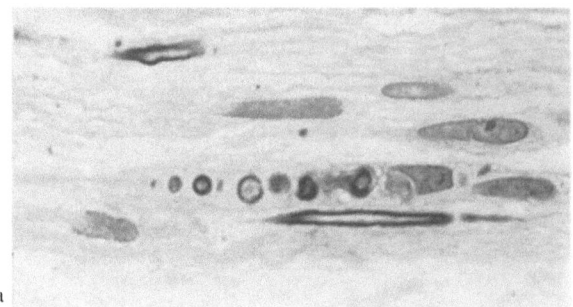

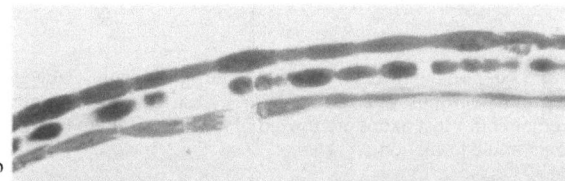

Fig. 3.37. a Toluidine blue. Plastic-embedded LS. Sural nerve biopsy. × 1600. Axonal neuropathy showing myelin ovoid formation during Wallerian degeneration. **b** Teased osmicated preparation. Sural nerve biopsy. × 1600. Three nerve fibres; in the lowermost fibre paranodal demyelination is seen and in the middle fibre there are myelin ovoids indicating Wallerian change. The upper fibre shows less marked abnormality.

nostic work. A full discussion of the technique of nerve biopsy with particular reference to the avoidance of artefact has been given by Dyck et al. (1984a) and Dyck and Thomas (1993).

Combined nerve and muscle biopsy is possible, when clinically appropriate. A useful method is to biopsy the posterior tibial muscle and the superficial peroneal nerve, using the same skin incision. The palmaris longus and its innervation – a motor nerve – may also be used, in the upper limb.

Indications for Nerve Biopsy

Nerve biopsy is limited in its application by three major factors. *First*, only sensory nerves are generally biopsied since biopsy of a motor or mixed nerve might cause persistent weakness. *Second*, biopsy of a sensory nerve, e.g. the sural nerve or the superficial branch of the radial nerve, causes some sensory loss and may occasionally lead to persistent dysaesthesia or painful neuroma formation in the proximal stump (Dyck et al. 1984a). Nerve biopsy should therefore only be considered when there is pre-existing sensory impairment in the distribution of the cutaneous innervation of the nerve to be biopsied. *Third*, the additional information gained by nerve biopsy is relatively restricted; it should be used only when full clinical, biochemical, immu-

nological and electrophysiological investigations are available. It is most valuable (Table 3.7) in the investigation of asymmetrical and multifocal neuropathies, when vasculitis is suspected, and in the presence of nerve enlargement. It is unlikely to yield useful clinical information in symmetrical polyneuropathies (Asbury and Gilliatt, 1984). Specific genetic DNA markers have increasingly obviated the role of nerve biopsy in Charcot–Marie–Tooth and related syndromes.

Table 3.7.   Indications for nerve biopsy

Severe progressive neuropathy of undetermined origin
Suspected inflammatory neuropathy
Suspected leprosy
Vasculitic neuropathies
Chronic painful sensory neuropathy
'Small-fibre' neuropathies
Suspected amyloid neuropathy
Asymmetrical and multifocal neuropathies
Some genetic and childhood-onset neuropathies when genetic markers are negative

Identification of Neuropathies by Nerve Biopsy

Peripheral neuropathies can be broadly grouped into *axonal degenerations* and *demyelinating neuropathies*.

Axonal degenerations occur when neuronal metabolism is disrupted so that axonal transport mechanisms fail. In the severest examples a motor or sensory neuron might die, resulting in degeneration of the whole length of the axon with consequent degeneration of the myelin sheath similar to the Wallerian changes which follow transection of a nerve fibre. Myelin ovoids may therefore be seen in longitudinal sections or in teased preparations (Fig. 3.37). Distal axonal degeneration (dying-back neuropathy) occurs when metabolism of the distal parts of the axon fails (Cavanagh 1964, 1979). This usually results from impaired axonal transport. Myelin breakdown occurs in the region of the distal axonal degeneration. This myelin breakdown appears as irregularities in axonal size and shape (Fig. 3.38). Recovery may be possible in some instances, for example by replacement of vitamin deficiencies, or cessation of exposure to neurotoxic chemicals or drugs. During regeneration after axonal injury axon sprouts grow from the proximal part of the damaged nerve and can be recognised in biopsies as clusters of tiny axons either free of Schwann cell covering and myelin, or surrounded only by a very thin layer of myelin (Fig. 3.39).

Segmental demyelination represents selective damage to Schwann cells causing disruption or loss

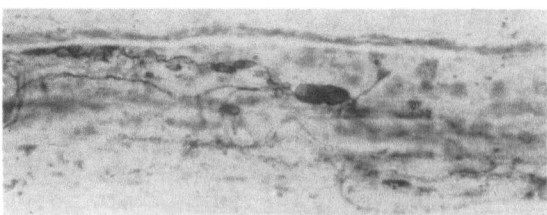

Fig. 3.38. Barker and Ip silver impregnation. Muscle spindle. Tabes dorsalis. The terminal sensory nerve fibre supplying the intrafusal muscle fibres shows axonal swellings and narrow bands typical of a distal axonopathy.

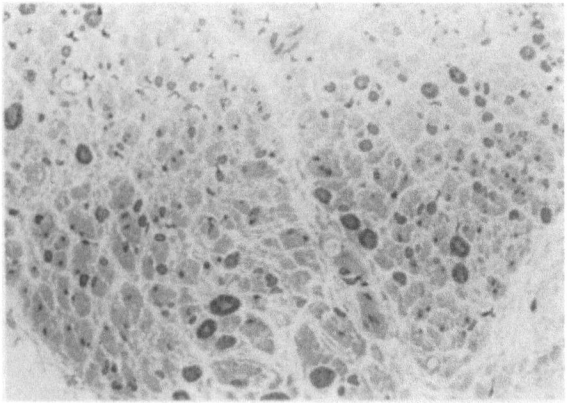

Fig. 3.40. Toluidine blue. TS. × 600. Sural nerve biopsy. Demyelinating neuropathy. A few enlarged, vesicular myelin rings remain but most axons are devoid of myelin and there is early onion bulb formation.

of myelin between two nodes of Ranvier. This process begins in the paranodal region. During the process of remyelination shortened "intercalated" nodes are formed. In demyelinating neuropathies a characteristic feature is the presence of large axons apparently devoid of myelin or surrounded by only a very thin layer of myelin (Fig. 3.40). After repeated episodes of demyelination and remyelination "onion bulbs" are formed (Fig. 3.41). These are circumferential leaflets of Schwann cell processes surrounding an axonal core. The outer leaflets are interspersed with collagen fibrils and fibroblasts. The proliferation of interstitial elements may result in palpable enlargement of affected nerves ("hypertrophic neuropathy"). Compression of a nerve, as in the carpal tunnel syndrome, causes localised segmental demyelination (Ochoa et al. 1971), but in severe or chronic nerve entrapment axonal damage also occurs.

In many neuropathies there is a combination of axonal degeneration and segmental demyelination.

It is uncertain, therefore, whether these two types of abnormality are independent processes. It has been suggested that increased intraneural pressure can itself lead to axonal or Schwann cell injury and this may be a factor in disorders such as the peripheral neuropathy associated with certain types of familial amyloidosis, in ischaemic nerve injury, and in the inflammatory polyradiculoneuropathies. Infiltration of a nerve with lymphocytes and macrophages is found in Guillain–Barré syndrome, and also in leprosy. In the latter disease, particularly in lepromatous leprosy, the characteristic acid-fast bacilli can sometimes be demonstrated in the Schwann cells. In diabetic neuropathy hypoxia of intraneural elements may be important in pathogenesis.

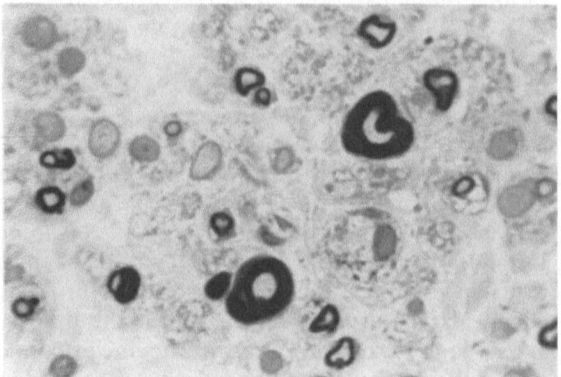

Fig. 3.39. Toluidine blue. TS. × 600. Sural nerve biopsy. Clusters of small axons devoid of myelin represent axonal sprouts. Several large axons are surrounded by unusually thin myelin rings indicating incomplete remyelination.

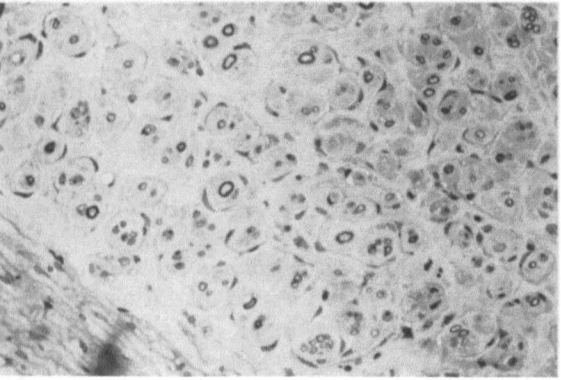

Fig. 3.41. Toluidine blue. TS. × 560. Median nerve biopsy. Onion bulb Schwann cell hypertrophy surrounding single or multiple thinly myelinated axons in a patient with burnt-out leprosy.

Chapter 4

Pathophysiological Correlations and Compensatory Mechanisms

Electromyography (EMG) is complementary to biopsy for a number of reasons. First, it can be used to examine several muscles and nerves in any individual patient. Secondly it can be used sequentially during the natural history and treatment of neuromuscular disorders, and thirdly it is a useful parameter for choosing a suitable muscle for biopsy or, indeed, in deciding whether biopsy should be undertaken. If the EMG is normal, muscle biopsy is unlikely to reveal abnormalities, although there are exceptions to this, as in some metabolic myopathies. The EMG may also provide information about neuromuscular transmission and early reinnervation: functional concepts which are beyond the scope of ordinary histological investigation.

Pathophysiological Correlations

The results of nerve conduction studies, EMG and muscle biopsy, and of nerve biopsy when indicated, are correlated with the clinical data and with the other investigations in the process of formulating a diagnosis. It is important to recognise that the abnormalities found in these tests are influenced by the stage of the disease process, and by the effects of treatment. The interpretation of these data in neurogenic disorders particularly illustrates the dynamic approach to understanding the disease process.

In general, nerve conduction studies show differing abnormalities in axonal and demyelinating neuropathies. In axonal neuropathies there is decreased amplitude of the compound muscle action potential (CMAP) and of the sensory action potential (SAP). In demyelinating neuropathies there is an increased distal motor latency and slowed motor conduction velocity. Increased distal motor latency and slowed conduction velocity can also occur in axonal neuropathies when there is

marked loss of large, fast-conducting nerve fibres. If the amplitude of the CMAP is more than 50% of the control value, and the conduction velocity is slowed more than 80% of control value, the neuropathy is likely to be demyelinating in type (Kimura 1989). In many clinical situations, such as Charcot–Marie–Tooth neuropathy Type 1, there is a close correlation between the physiological and pathological findings but, in other disorders, e.g. diabetic neuropathy, the correlation is less exact (Behse and Buchthal 1978).

Acute Neurogenic Disorders

In the EMG of neurogenic disorders fibrillation potentials are usually prominent in the acute stage although they do not appear for a week or more after the onset of denervation. Positive sharp waves may be found, but fasciculations do not occur. The interference pattern may be reduced; this is probably the earliest abnormality discernible during voluntary activation.

After a few weeks a number of polyphasic motor unit action potentials (MUAPs) may be recorded. They may resemble the MUAPs found in myopathies in that they may be of low amplitude and of normal or short duration. These features result from the presence of immature motor units consisting of only a few muscle fibres in the early phase of reinnervation of an acute neurogenic disorder. The potentials, when studied with a trigger-delay line and a low-frequency filter setting of 500 Hz or more, may show an increased neuromuscular jitter and impulse blocking (Fig. 4.1), indicating a decreased safety factor for neuromuscular transmission at motor end-plates. The motor unit firing rate may be normal or slightly reduced, especially in anterior horn cell disorders.

Motor nerve conduction velocity measurements are of great value at this stage of acute neurogenic disorders because they help to localise the lesion. In acute anterior horn cell disorders, e.g. in acute

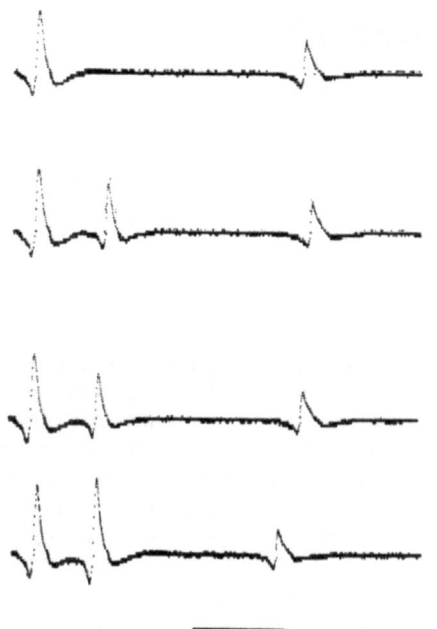

Fig. 4.1. Motor unit action potential, recorded with concentric needle EMG, and a trigger-delay line. Filters: 500 Hz and 10 kHz. The second component shows impulse blocking in the first of the four consecutive traces, and the third component shows a varying latency relative to the first, triggered component, indicating an increased neuromuscular jitter. Bar 4 ms.

poliomyelitis, the motor nerve conduction velocity is normal, but in radicular disease, e.g. in root compression syndromes, slowed proximal motor conduction can often be demonstrated with F wave studies. In some peripheral neuropathies, e.g. acute diabetic neuropathy, the conduction velocity may be slowed distally and in acute compressive neuropathies there is slowed conduction, localised to the damaged part of the nerve. Conduction block is characteristic of Guillain–Barré syndrome and of acute compressive neuropathies.

In the early stages of acute neurogenic disorders a muscle biopsy may show little abnormality. Since very little restructuring of the motor unit has occurred, fibre-type grouping is not usually found but scattered, small, pointed denervated fibres may be seen and there may be some general atrophy of muscle fibres.

Chronic Neurogenic Disorders

In chronic disorders, such as Charcot–Marie–Tooth disease and Kugelberg–Welander disease, the EMG abnormality is much more prominent. Fibrillation potentials can usually be recorded but are not as prominent as in the more acute neurogenic dis-

orders and may be found only after a diligent search. Fasciculations, on the other hand, may be very prominent, particularly in anterior horn cell disorders, especially motor neuron disease, and in some radiculopathies. Fasciculations are infrequent in distal symmetrical polyneuropathies, unless there is radicular involvement, as in Guillain–Barré syndrome; they may also be found in multifocal motor neuropathy and sometimes in chronic entrapment neuropathies.

The interference pattern is usually very abnormal in chronic neurogenic disorders. In severe cases only a few complex motor units may be recorded. The interference pattern is of higher amplitude than in normal subjects and is more variable in amplitude and density during maintained maximal isometric contraction than in normal subjects. This variation in interference pattern produces a characteristic wavering sound during the EMG recording.

During voluntary activation the first MUAPs recorded are similar in amplitude or larger than those of normal subjects. They are frequently polyphasic. These potentials are usually of normal duration. With increasing activation larger units are recorded and some of them may be of very high amplitude (>12 mV). The duration of these potentials is increased but, nevertheless, is often underestimated unless a trigger-delay line is used in the analysis of successive potentials. With the trigger-delay line, and the addition of a 500 Hz low-frequency filter setting, late components, some occurring more than 50 ms after the initial phase of the motor unit potential, can be recognised (Fig. 4.2). These late components represent activity in small muscle fibres with a slow propagation velocity (Stålberg et al. 1974). They may be mistaken for potentials originating from other motor units unless successive potentials are analysed in this way with the trigger-delay line. Indeed, when a motor unit is firing at 20 Hz or more, late components will appear on the oscilloscope screen synchronously with the reappearance of the first phase of the same motor unit potential. Since these late components are usually of lower amplitude than the earlier parts of the MUAP, and are often relatively isolated from the main part of the unit, they may resemble the low-amplitude, short-duration polyphasic units characteristic of myopathic disorders (Gath et al. 1969; Swash and Schwartz 1977). These potentials are found only in very longstanding neurogenic disorders.

In chronic neurogenic disorders due to anterior horn cell disease the firing frequency of individual motor units is often abnormal. MUAPs appear in irregular bursts; this is particularly well seen when the patient is asked to activate a single motor unit at

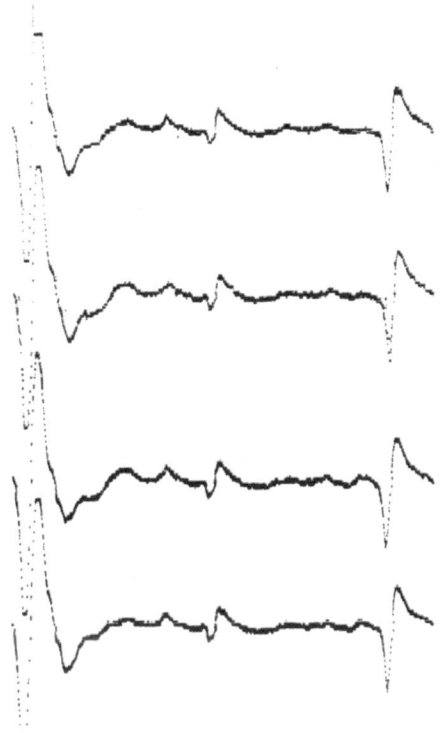

Fig. 4.2. Type 1 hereditary motor and sensory neuropathy. Single-fibre EMG recording. The consecutive traces show a complex unit with a duration of 18 ms, which shows a relatively stable configuration in the four recordings. Bar 4 ms.

a low firing rate (Stålberg et al. 1975a). Normal subjects can usually maintain a regular firing rate at about 8 Hz (Stålberg and Thiele 1973) but patients with anterior horn cell disorders have difficulty doing this, particularly when there is involvement of the corticospinal tracts. In general, upper motor neuron lesions lead to low firing rates, and lower motor neuron lesions to rapid firing rates. In both the interference pattern is decreased. Recruitment of motor units has been studied in motor neuron disease and ulnar entrapment neuropathy and found to be normal (Milner-Brown et al. 1974), but there is little information about the recruitment pattern in other neurogenic disorders. Disturbances of firing rate and instability of the interference pattern may result from defective central drive to the anterior horn cells, abnormalities of anterior horn cell firing capabilities, and disturbed recruitment pattern in a damaged motor neuron pool.

Single-fibre EMG has shown that the MUAPs in longstanding neurogenic disorders are more stable than those recorded in acute neurogenic disorders. Although many components of the MUAP in longstanding disorders may have an increased neuro-

muscular jitter, or show impulse blocking, these abnormalities are less prominent than in more acute neurogenic disorders.

In chronic neurogenic disorders motor nerve conduction is often abnormal. Very slowed conduction velocity (less than 10 m/s) is found only in demyelinating neuropathies. In general, in axonal neuropathies conduction velocity is only moderately slowed. In anterior horn cell disorders motor nerve conduction velocity is usually normal. However, in the late stages it may be somewhat slowed.

These EMG abnormalities in chronic neurogenic disorders are accompanied by characteristic findings in the muscle biopsy (Table 4.1). These consist of fibre-type grouping, suggesting effective reinnervation, with clusters of thin, pointed denervated fibres and, sometimes, with grouped atrophy. Collateral axonal sprouting, and reinnervation can be demonstrated by methylene blue or silver impregnation preparations. In longstanding neurogenic disorders Type 1 hypertrophy may occur and a few scattered necrotic fibres may be present. Other histological features of chronic neurogenic disorders are described later in this chapter.

Table 4.1. Histological features of neurogenic disorders

Denervation
Disseminated neurogenic atrophy
Target fibres
Grouped neurogenic atrophy
Changes in intramuscular nerve bundles

Reinnervation
Fibre-type grouping
Fibre-type predominance

Rapidly and Slowly Progressive Neurogenic Disorders

An objective assessment of the rate of progression of a neurogenic disorder can be made from the EMG and pathological findings. A disorder may pursue a rapidly or a slowly progressive course. Clearly, this varies from patient to patient. For example, some patients with motor neuron disease die in only a few months but as many as 20% of patients with this disease may survive for more than 5 years (Mulder and Howard 1976). It is important to consider the factor of rate of progression when assessing a patient since this has implications not only for investigation, but also for treatment and prognosis. When there is effective collateral reinnervation the rate of progression will be relatively slow. If collateral reinnervation is ineffective, and if active denervation is continuing, the rate of progression will be faster. These concepts can be evaluated both by EMG and by muscle biopsy. It is important to remember, nonetheless, that in a well-compensated disorder, apparently rapid deterioration may occur when the limits of functional compensation are reached or when other factors lead to further neuromuscular dysfunction. Wohlfart (1957) pointed out that even in motor neuron disease reinnervation may be so effective that as many as 30% of anterior horn cells may be lost without clinical weakness or wasting.

In a rapidly progressive disorder spontaneous activity, particularly fibrillation potentials, is prominent. Motor unit potential analysis shows potentials of varying amplitude. In motor neuron disease they may be very large (giant units). The duration of these MUAPs is moderately increased and polyphasic potentials are common. Macro EMG studies have shown that the motor unit potentials in rapidly progressive motor neuron disease are not as large as those in more slowly progressive cases (Stålberg et al. 1986). Single-fibre EMG studies show that rapidly progressive cases develop lower fibre densities, implying a reduced capacity for focal reinnervation compared to more slowly progressive cases (Swash and Schwartz 1982, 1984). Instability of MUAPs is probably the most important feature of rapidly progressive neurogenic disorders. Many MUAPs show a prominent neuromuscular jitter, with frequent impulse blocking. Stålberg et al. (1975a), using single-fibre EMG, found that 59% of the MUAPs in six patients with amyotrophic lateral sclerosis showed increased jitter.

In slowly progressive, well-compensated neurogenic disorders spontaneous activity is not a prominent feature. Motor unit potentials show a similar variability in amplitude to that found in more rapidly progressive (poorly compensated) cases but there is a larger proportion of polyphasic potentials in slowly progressive cases and these potentials may be of very long duration. Jitter determination shows that fewer potentials contain components with an increased jitter in patients with a slowly progressive course. Further, these potentials may contain only one or two components, usually the later components, with an increased jitter, whereas in more rapidly progressive neurogenic disorders, for example, motor neuron disease, many components within individual motor unit action potentials show increased jitter. Impulse blocking, likewise, tends to occur predominantly in late components in well-compensated disorders. Single-fibre EMG determination of fibre density in well-compensated neurogenic disorders is characteristically very increased and this is an important EMG indication of effective reinnervation.

The "giant" motor unit action potentials frequently recorded in the more rapidly progressive forms of motor neuron disease are less prominent in chronic neurogenic disorders, although there is a much greater fibre density in these disorders. Giant MUAPs are due to the summation of a large number of single muscle fibre action potentials, generated within a short time-period. In well-compensated, more chronic conditions these single muscle fibre action potentials are generated in a more extended period of time because of variations in fibre size and thus of propagation velocity in the muscle fibres, and variations in conduction time in axonal sprouts of varying length.

The biopsies of well-compensated neurogenic disorders are characterised by prominent fibre-type grouping. The muscle fibres are often of normal size but sometimes fibre hypertrophy, especially of Type 1 fibres, is prominent. Denervated fibres are uncommon in these biopsies. There may be some increased endomysial fibrosis and fibre splitting, scattered damaged fibres and, rarely, a few basophilic fibres may occur. These findings may lead to a mistaken diagnosis of myopathy unless careful attention is paid to the presence of fibre-type grouping (Schwartz et al. 1976a; Swash and Schwartz 1977, 1984). Lester et al. (1993) used a computer model to simulate the effect of progressive motor unit loss in neurogenic disorders. They found that about 60%–80% of motor units were lost (non-functional) before more than 10% of muscle fibres were denervated. In progressive disorders, e.g. motor neuron disease, 60% motor neuron loss, or even less, could result in easily detectable denervation pathologically, but in non-progressive disorders, e.g. old poliomyelitis or chronic spinal muscular atrophy, up to 80% motor unit loss could occur without detectable muscle fibre denervation, indicating the role of compensatory reinnervative processes. Fibre-type grouping was only noted when there was more than about 40% loss of functioning motor units, a figure that corresponds with Wohlfart's estimation of 30% loss without detectable change.

Late clinical deterioration in a well-compensated or slowly progressive neurogenic disorder may be accompanied, or preceded, by changes in the pattern of the EMG abnormality. In particular, a larger proportion of potentials may show increased jitter and blocking (Swash and Schwartz 1984).

Axonal and Demyelinating Neuropathies

Axonal neuropathies are accompanied by denervation of muscle, but in demyelinating neuropathies

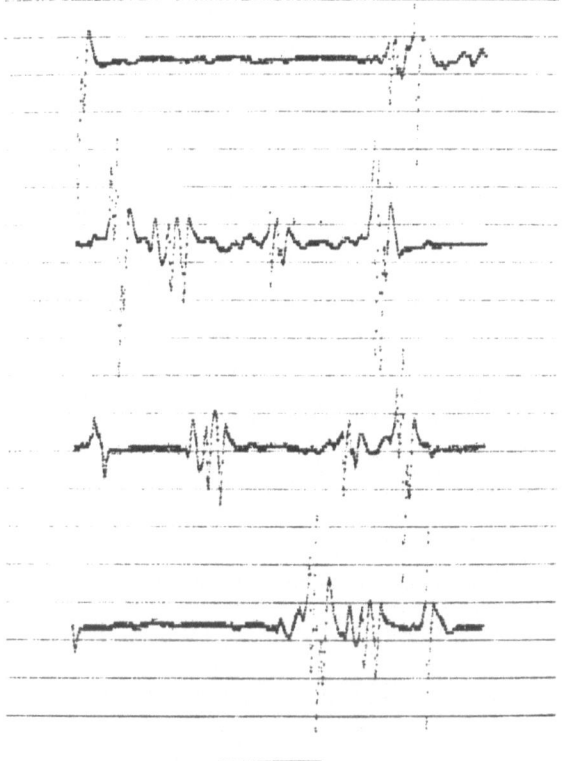

Fig. 4.3. Polyphasic, long-duration, high-amplitude/MUAP in a chronic axonal neuropathy (alcoholic neuropathy). Concentric needle EMG. Filters: 100 Hz and 10 kHz. Bar 20 ms.

axonal function is relatively preserved and EMG and pathological evidence of denervation is less prominent, or may be minimal. Fibrillation potentials and polyphasic, high-amplitude, long-duration, MUAPs are more prominent in axonal neuropathies (Fig. 4.3). In demyelinating neuropathies the MUAPs may be normal. Assessment of the interference pattern is not useful in differentiating axonal and demyelinating neuropathies, since it is moderately reduced in both types of neuropathy. In axonal neuropathies increased neuromuscular jitter is more prominent than in demyelinating neuropathies (Thiele and Stålberg 1975).

The major differentiating EMG feature between these two groups of neuropathies is the nerve conduction velocity measurement. Both sensory and motor nerve conduction velocity are markedly slowed in demyelinating neuropathies (Kimura 1993) but in axonal neuropathies conduction velocity is less affected (Gilliatt 1966). A median motor conduction velocity less than 30 m/s is indicative of a demyelinating neuropathy, e.g. Type 1 Charcot–Marie–Tooth syndrome (Buchthal and Behse 1977;

Bouché et al. 1983; Gherardi et al. 1983). Sensory nerve action potentials are delayed, or even unobtainable, in demyelinating neuropathies. When present, the sensory action potential (SAP) is more dispersed and of lower amplitude than normal (Gilliatt and Sears 1958; Buchthal and Rosenfalck 1966; Gilliatt 1966). In axonal neuropathies sensory nerve action potentials are smaller than normal and the sensory nerve conduction velocity is usually normal, or only slightly slowed. In severe axonal neuropathies no sensory nerve action potential can be obtained (Buchthal and Rosenfalck 1971).

Measurements of distal motor latency are important, particularly when considered in relation to conduction in the nerve itself. In demyelinating neuropathies the distal motor latency is prolonged and conduction in the myelinated part of the nerve is markedly slowed in demyelinating neuropathies. In severe axonal neuropathies the distal motor latency may also be increased, due to loss of fast-conducting fibres. The distinction between demyelinating and axonal neuropathies is often unclear (Behse and Buchthal 1978). Pathological investigation of nerves in peripheral neuropathies has shown that many neuropathies show features of both processes and the distinction is therefore less absolute than was previously thought.

The initial nerve conduction data may be useful in prognosis in Guillain–Barré syndrome. Small or absent compound motor action potentials indicative of the severe axonal form of the disease are associated with a poor prognosis (Feasby et al. 1986). Early fibrillation potentials may also imply a poor prognosis. Resolution of conduction abnormalities begins 6–10 weeks after onset of the disease (Albers et al. 1985).

Myopathic Disorders

The EMG abnormalities in myopathic disorders are less precise than those characteristic of neurogenic disorders. For example, there is no specific feature in myopathic disorders as unique as a slowed motor conduction velocity in a demyelinating peripheral neuropathy.

In some myopathic disorders fibrillation potentials can be recorded, but never to the degree found in acute denervation. The parameters of fibrillation potentials in myopathies are the same as those of the spontaneous potentials in neurogenic disorders. Positive sharp waves, however, are very unusual in myopathies. *Insertional activity* may be very prominent and prolonged, even lasting for several seconds, in patients with myopathies (Fig.

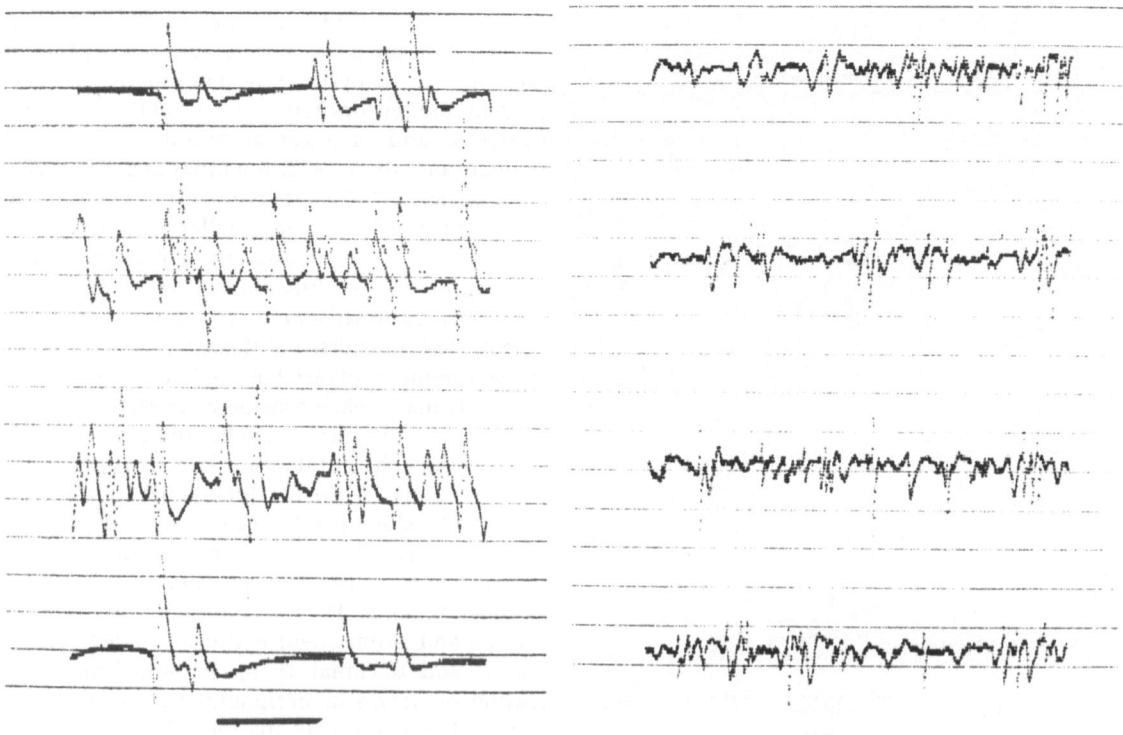

Fig. 4.4. Increased insertional activity in polymyositis. The motor unit activity continued for more than 200 ms. Concentric needle EMG. Filters: 100 Hz and 10 kHz. Bar 10 ms.

Fig. 4.5. Short-duration polyphasic motor unit action potentials of low amplitude in limb-girdle muscular dystrophy. Concentric needle EMG. Filters: 100 Hz and 10 kHz. Bar 20 ms.

4.4). In neurogenic disorders only a mild increase in insertional activity is found. Bizarre high-frequency potentials may be found, particularly in polymyositis and Duchenne muscular dystrophy.

The most striking feature of voluntary activity in the EMG of patients with myopathies is the finding of a full interference pattern during only slight force. In particular, even very weak muscles usually show a full interference pattern, a finding in contrast to that in neurogenic disorders in which the interference pattern is nearly always reduced in a weak muscle. Buchthal and Rosenfalck (1963) in a study of very weak muscles (MRC grade 0–2 only) in patients with myopathy or neuropathy found that a full interference pattern could be obtained in 81% of muscles in patients with myopathies but in only 2% of muscles in patients with neuropathy.

Motor unit potentials in myopathies (Daube 1978) are characteristically polyphasic potentials (more than four phases) of low amplitude (less than about 1 mV), even on maximal effort, and short duration (less than 9 ms in adults). These polyphasic units (Fig. 4.5) result from loss of functioning muscle fibres in the motor unit, giving a fractional appearance to the MUAP. Automatic

analysis shows an increased number of turns with an increased ratio of turns to mean amplitude (Stålberg et al. 1983; Liguari et al. 1992a,b).

The reduced amplitude of these potentials is largely due to the loss of functioning muscle fibres. Increased intramuscular fibrosis and the presence of atrophic muscle fibres also result in reduced action potential amplitude both by reducing volume conduction within the muscle, and because smaller action potentials are generated. The measurement of MUAP duration can be misleading. Because of the fractionation of the motor unit, from loss of individual functioning muscle fibres, the earliest and latest parts of the action potential may not be discerned (Buchthal and Rosenfalck 1963). In myopathies, myopathic potentials are often found in profusion in restricted parts of the muscle, but many normal MUAPs can usually be recorded in any individual muscle. A more complete assessment of MUAP parameters can be obtained by using the trigger-delay line. When successive MUAPs are studied in this manner, especially with a 500 Hz low-frequency filter setting, many potentials are seen to have an increased duration. This is particularly striking in Duchenne muscular dystrophy when the disease is at a stage of moderate disability (Stålberg et al. 1974; Desmedt and Borenstein 1976b). Macro EMG usually shows normal or small motor units in Duchenne dystrophy, but the fibre density is often increased reflecting local reorganisation of the motor units, and fibre splitting (Hilton-Brown and Stålberg 1986).

In the "benign" myopathies of childhood, myopathic potentials are often not very prominent. In these disorders there are only mild structural changes in the muscle although a number of characteristic abnormalities, for example rod bodies, may be present.

In polymyositis the motor unit potential parameters change during the course of the disease so that in the later stages of the disease the motor unit potentials become of larger amplitude and longer duration (Mechler 1974), resembling those seen in neurogenic disorders. In the earlier stages, however, typical myopathic motor unit potentials are prominent. The changing EMG features can be correlated, in chronic cases, with pathological features of restructuring of the motor unit, with fibre-type grouping (Swash and Schwartz 1977).

Single-fibre EMG reveals abnormalities in fibre density and, to a lesser extent, in the neuromuscular jitter, in most myopathies. The most striking changes are found in Duchenne muscular dystrophy, in which the fibre density increases until the disease is at a moderately advanced stage; in the later stages the fibre density decreases (Schwartz et al. 1977a). The individual single-fibre action potential components of the motor unit in myopathies are usually more dispersed than in neuropathies (Fig. 4.6), giving an increased inter-potential interval (Stålberg and Trontelj 1994). As in neurogenic disorders, the increased jitter found in some myopathies is most marked in the earlier stages of the disease.

In myopathies abnormalities in motor unit potentials can usually be demonstrated in weak muscles. In patients with little objective weakness, or in muscles apparently scarcely involved, a diligent EMG assessment may reveal the wide distribution of the disorder. EMG evidence of myopathic motor unit action potentials is also useful for carrier detection in Duchenne muscular dystrophy, in conjunction with blood CK measurement, and with muscle biopsy.

Nerve conduction in myopathies is normal except in myotonic dystrophy, in which the terminal motor latency is increased.

The *muscle biopsy* in patients with myopathy should be taken from a moderately involved muscle. The characteristic features of myopathies are degeneration and regeneration of single muscle fibres,

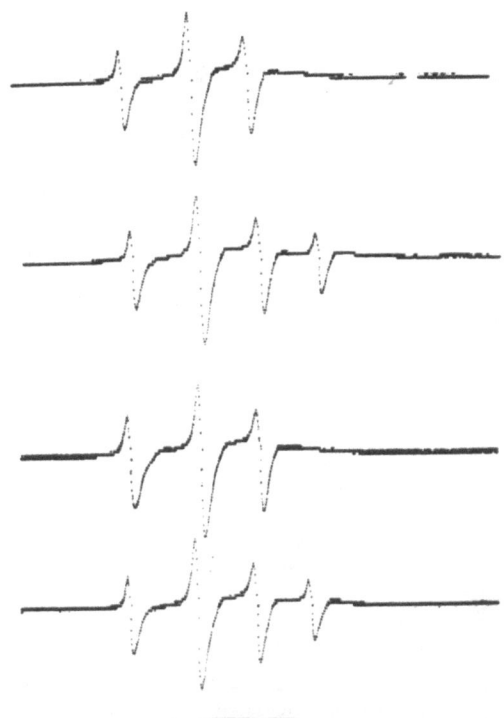

Fig. 4.6. Single-fibre EMG recording, showing dispersion of the four single-fibre action potentials of a motor unit in polymyositis. The last component shows impulse blocking. The dispersion of the individual action potentials is particularly characteristic of a myopathy, but may also be seen in secondary myopathic change in chronic neurogenic disorders. Bar 2 ms.

with increased variability in fibre size, increased central nucleation, and increased endomysial fibrosis. In addition, a number of more specific abnormalities in muscle fibres have been described in certain myopathies but these cannot be correlated with the EMG features. In metabolic and endocrine myopathies degeneration and regeneration of muscle fibres is not a feature and the typical myopathic EMG abnormality may be less evident.

End-Plate Disorders

Disorders of neuromuscular transmission are due to *presynaptic* dysfunction in which there is an abnormality of release of acetylcholine, as in the myasthenic syndrome and in botulism, or to *post-synaptic* abnormalities, as in myasthenia gravis. These two types of end-plate disorder can be differentiated by conventional and single-fibre EMG techniques (see Chap. 12).

The most important conventional EMG technique utilises repetitive motor nerve stimulation at

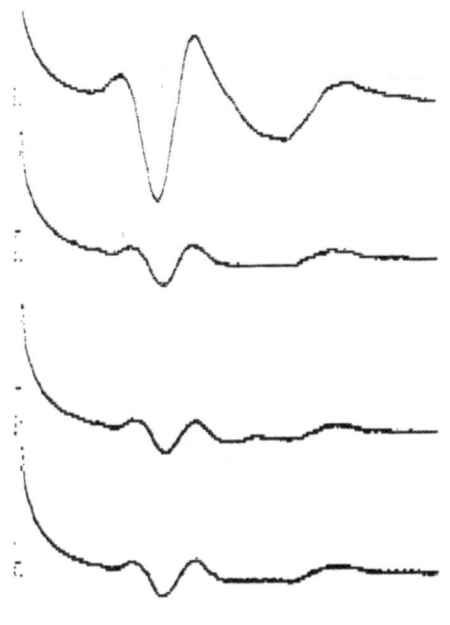

Fig. 4.7. Decremental response in abductor digiti minimi on stimulating the ulnar nerve at the wrist at frequency of 2 Hz, in a patient with myasthenia gravis. The first response shows an amplitude of 4 mV, but the fourth is only 0.4 mV, a decrement of 90%. Bar 4 ms.

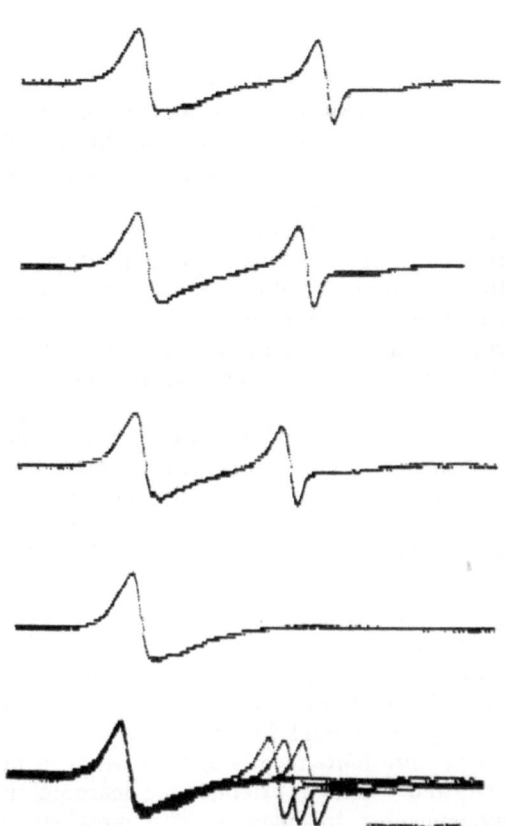

Fig. 4.8. Single-fibre EMG recording in the biceps muscle in myasthenia gravis. Four consecutive discharges are shown separately, and superimposed to illustrate the increased jitter of the second component in relation to the first, triggered component, and the blocking of this second component. The calculated jitter is greater than 150 μs. Bar 1 ms.

various rates, recording the evoked motor action potential from a suitable muscle. The three principal sites of stimulation for this study are the *ulnar* and *median* nerves at the wrist, recording from the abductor digiti minimi or abductor pollicis brevis respectively, and the *accessory* nerve, recording from the trapezius. Surface stimulating and recording electrodes are usually used and stimulation rates vary from 2 to 20 Hz. In presynaptic disorders the MUAP, initially of small amplitude, increases in size at rapid rates of stimulation, but in post-synaptic disorders, as in myasthenia gravis (Chap. 12), the characteristic feature is a reduction in size of the MUAP at low rates of stimulation (Fig. 4.7). The fourth potential evoked at 3 Hz shows a decrement of more than 10% of the amplitude of the first potential (Desmedt 1973; Desmedt and Borenstein 1976a). This decrement is less pronounced with faster rates of stimulation and at very fast rates a slight facilitation may be observed.

With single-fibre EMG the principal abnormality in both presynaptic and post-synaptic disorders is an increased neuromuscular jitter, with impulse blocking (Fig. 4.8). The fibre density may be mildly increased. Muscle biopsy gives little information in these disorders.

Compensatory Mechanisms

Compensatory factors are important in all neuromuscular disorders (Swash and Schwartz 1977). They are most easily recognised in slowly progressive disorders, when they are at their most effective. It is a striking clinical observation that patients with slowly progressive neuromuscular disorders retain their mobility even when their muscles are very weak and wasted, and that recovery from other disorders, such as polymyositis, may occur even in patients with extreme weakness, when the muscle biopsy may show marked and widespread muscle fibre necrosis. In neurogenic disorders, as in motor neuron disease or in Kugelberg–Welander disease, degeneration of motor neurons leads to denervation of muscle fibres and loss of function. This loss of innervation is partially compensated for by peripheral collateral sprouting from nearby functional motor nerve fibres (Edds 1950; Wohlfart 1957), leading to an increase in the number of muscle fibres within the surviving motor units. This process of compensatory collateral axonal sprouting is so effective that as many as 30% of anterior horn cells may be lost in motor neuron disease before weakness becomes clinically apparent. Later, however, with further loss of anterior horn cells this compensatory mechanism fails, collateral sprouting having reached its biological limitation, and weakness and muscular atrophy develop fairly rapidly (Lester et al. 1993).

In myopathic disorders, as in polymyositis, regeneration of damaged muscle fibres is important. Regeneration can continue during periods in which the disease is active and during quiescent phases, and if treatment is successful or the disorder ceases to be active, recovery may occur. Clinical recovery is then limited by the ability of muscle fibres to regenerate, and by the interposition of other factors, such as fibrosis. The latter interferes with muscular elasticity and contractility by its mechanical presence, and may impair reinnervation of regenerating muscle fibres by preventing regenerating axonal sprouts from making contact with the new muscle fibres. This is probably an important factor limiting recovery in Duchenne dystrophy, and it may account for the finding of fibrillation potentials in this disorder (Desmedt and Borenstein 1976b). Muscle fibre hypertrophy with training is perhaps the best-known example of a compensatory response in muscle. Muscular hypertrophy develops in response to increased loading during contraction; this phenomenon has been studied in some detail (Denny-Brown 1960). One maximal contraction held for as brief a period as six seconds, only once a day, will cause progressive hypertrophy to develop (Mueller and Hettinger 1953). Fibre hypertrophy is a common feature of many neuromuscular disorders, of both neurogenic and myopathic type, and occurs independently of special training. It probably represents the response of some fibres to the functional overloading found in muscles in which there has been loss or dysfunction of other fibres. The diameter of individual fibres may increase to two or three times the normal. The effects of increased functional loading on muscle have been studied experimentally. Denny-Brown (1960) reviewed the earlier literature. More recently, it has been found that exercise-induced fibre hypertrophy is often accompanied by longitudinal splitting of the hypertrophied fibres. Fissures, extending up to 100 μm along the length of individual fibres, develop at the periphery of hypertrophied fibres, presumably as a result of the increased functional stress during work-induced compensatory hypertrophy (Hall-Craggs 1970). Hall-Craggs and Lawrence (1970) observed that the longitudinal splits were accompanied or preceded by the appearance of centrally located nuclei, and that the separated peripheral segments of muscle fibres were often slightly basophilic. James (1973) found that longitudinal splits or fissures developed more frequently in Type 1 than in Type 2 fibres and that the separated fragments often contained several vesicular nuclei. He stressed that splitting induced by functional overload could not be regarded simply as a degenerative or traumatic response, since there was histological evidence that it was associated with a regenerative response in the separated fragments. Similar findings have been observed in human neuromuscular disorders.

Fibre Splitting in Disease

In neurogenic disorders splitting predominantly affects hypertrophied fibres and in most instances individual clefts or splits are associated with a centrally located sarcolemmal nucleus (Banker 1960; Schwartz et al. 1976a). Splitting may consist only of a single central or lateral fissure (Fig. 4.9), or it may lead to the formation of two or more apparently separate fibres, of identical histochemical type, each surrounded by a layer of basement membrane (Schwartz et al. 1976a). Splitting affects Type 1 fibres more commonly than Type 2 fibres (Schwartz et al. 1976a). In serial sections, some separate fibres may enlarge to attain a cross-sectional diameter similar to that of normal muscle fibres (Fig. 4.10). Others may fuse with each other, or insert onto adjacent interstitial connective tissue. It is likely that some split fibres become entirely separated from their parent fibres by this process but in such instances it is difficult to be certain that the separate smaller fibres were derived by splitting from their neighbouring fibres. Bell and Conen (1968) aptly termed these fibres "nesting fibres". Splitting also leads to the formation of very small separated fragments, some anuclear and non-viable, and others nucleate but probably too small to become functionally innervated (Schwartz et al. 1976a).

The ultrastructural features (Fig. 4.11) of this process of splitting in neurogenic disorders are similar to those shown experimentally in the rat (Hall-Craggs and Lawrence 1970). James (1973) found that fibre fragments of this type were often faintly basophilic, and there is histological evidence of active protein synthesis and of increase in size in such fragments of split fibres in chronic neurogenic disorders in man (Schwartz et al. 1976a; Swash et al. 1978a). The histological features of these split fibres,

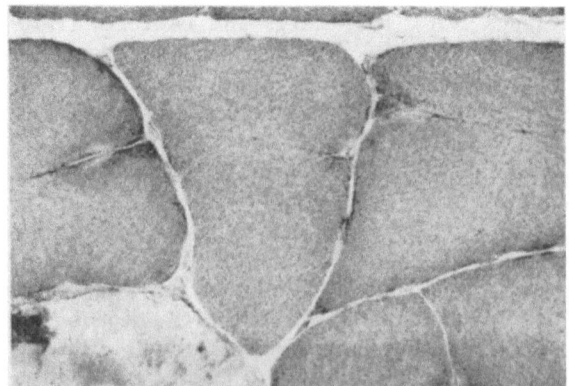

a

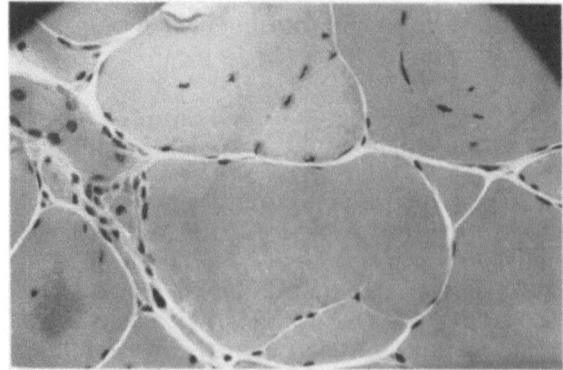

b

Fig. 4.9. Kugelberg–Welander disease. **a** NADH-tr. Three hypertrophied fibres showing longitudinal splitting. In each the split
commences at the periphery of the fibre. An NADH-tr dark zone
can be seen within the cleft in areas where separation of the
fibre fragments is incomplete. **b** H and E. Fibre splitting is usually
associated with centrally placed nuclei, and it often begins in
association with an endomysial nucleus at the edge of a fibre. To
the left of the field several pointed, denervated fibres, and a dark
central cored fibre can be seen. Both parts × 560.

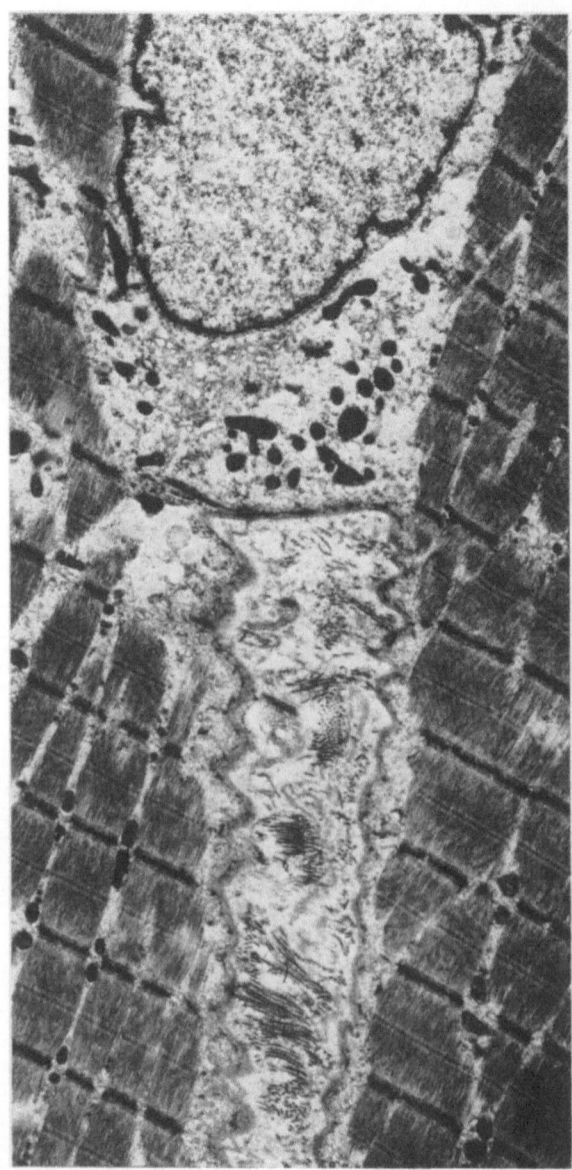

a

Fig. 4.11 *(continued on next page)* ▶

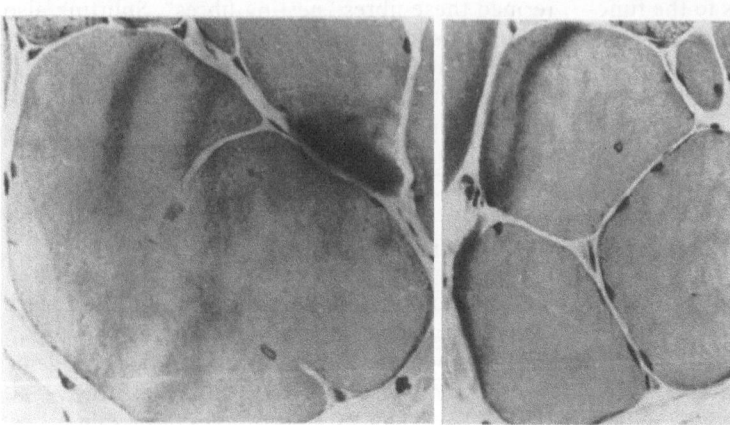

Fig. 4.10. H and E. × 560.
Kugelberg–Welander disease. Two
serial sections showing the process
of splitting of a single hypertrophied
fibre to form three apparently
separate fibres each about 50 μm in
diameter. Note the two enlarged
central nuclei near the splits.

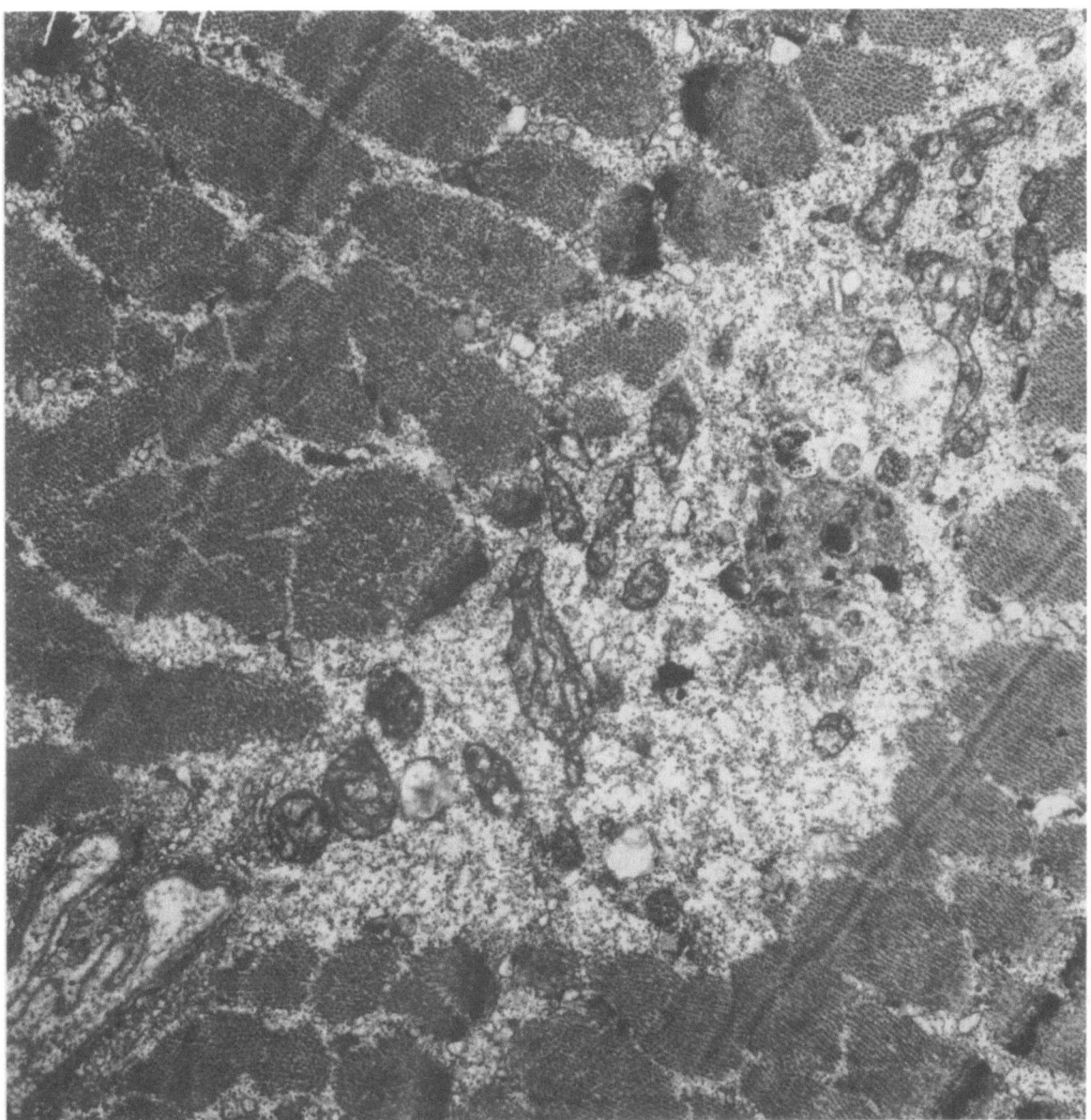

b

Fig. 4.11. Kugelberg–Welander disease. Electron microscope studies of affected fibres. **a** LS. × 15 000. A cleft, lined by plasma and basement membrane, invaginates the fibre. A centrally placed nucleus is situated at the end of the cleft, and the sarcoplasm in this region contains a number of mitochondria, and tubules of the Golgi apparatus. The Z bands are in register across the cleft, and at the end of the cleft Z band material is streamed across the advancing edge of the split itself. **b** TS. × 20 000. Beyond the cleft itself a zone of sarcoplasm containing enlarged mitochondria and some myofibrillar debris extends between the myofibrils, which are themselves of abnormal size at the margins of the zone of splitting. (*continued overleaf*)

however, are not those of active subendomysial regeneration (Fig. 4.12) of the type discussed by Schmalbruch (1976). Sulaiman and Kinder (1989) noted internal vascularisation in hypertrophic fibres, especially in distal muscles of chronic neurogenic disorders, and suggested this was related to splitting and induced by hypoxia in these enlarged fibres.

In the chronic form of polymyositis hypertrophied fibres sometimes show splitting similar to that found in hypertrophied fibres in neurogenic disorders. In other fibres "splitting" consists of extrusion of necrotic portions of damaged fibres, or is due to subendomysial regeneration from myoblasts formed after segmental necrosis, the sarcolemmal tube remaining intact (Schmalbruch 1976;

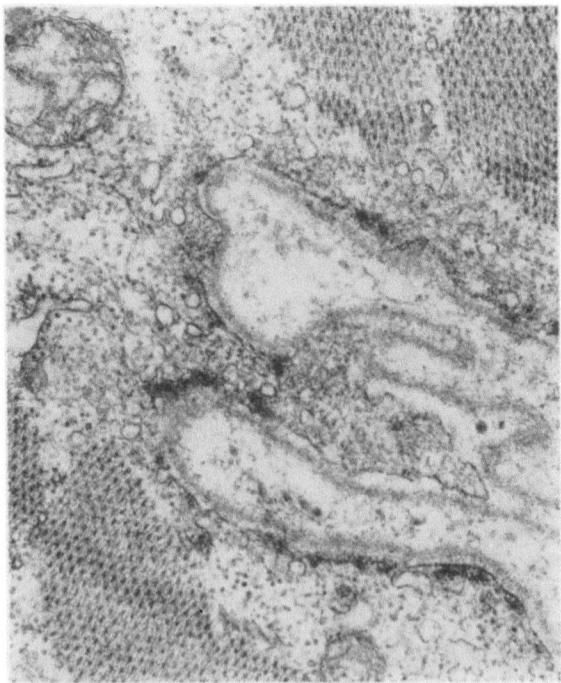

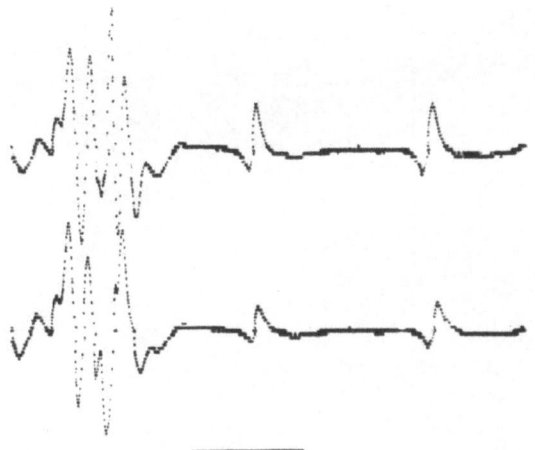

Fig. 4.13. Hereditary sensory and motor neuropathy Type 1 (Charcot–Marie–Tooth syndrome). Late potentials, occurring after the beginning of the triggering potential, are seen. Concentric needle EMG. Filters: 500 Hz and 10 kHz. Bar 4 ms.

Fig. 4.11c. Kugelberg–Welander disease. Electron microscope studies of affected fibres. c. TS. × 60 000. Enlargement of cleft shown in **b**. In this region pinocytotic vesicles can be seen free in the sarcoplasm and attached to the immature plasma membrane. This probably represents formation of the new plasma membrane.

myotubes having failed to undergo lateral fusion with one another beneath the basal lamina. The split fibres will be innervated by the same nerve fibre and will then be of the same histochemical type, forming small "myopathic groups" (Swash and Schwartz 1977).

Electromyographic Evidence

Swash et al. 1978a). Splitting associated with fibre hypertrophy is not a feature of acute polymyositis. In this disorder "splitting" is usually related to segmental fibre necrosis, or to regeneration. Splitting of hypertrophied fibres in Duchenne dystrophy and in limb-girdle dystrophy is well recognised (Erb 1891; Bell and Conen 1968). It probably results from regeneration after fibre necrosis, the regenerating

In EMG and single-fibre EMG investigations with a trigger-delay line, late components (Fig. 4.13) appearing more than about 10 ms after the initial action potential of a motor unit, have been found both in neurogenic disorders (Borenstein and Desmedt 1973; Stålberg et al. 1975b) and in muscular dystrophy (Borenstein and Desmedt 1973; Stålberg et al. 1974; Desmedt and Borenstein 1976b). Since the oscilloscope is triggered by the first part of the complex action potential of a single motor unit, the late components in these studies probably represent fibres innervated by collateral axon sprouts derived from the same motor unit. In neurogenic disorders the late components usually have a greatly reduced propagation velocity (Stålberg et al. 1975b) and similar late potentials with reduced propagation velocities have been found in Duchenne muscular dystrophy (Stålberg 1977). The slowed propagation velocity of the late components of these abnormally complex motor unit potentials implies that the action potentials arise in fibres of small diameter. Hilton-Brown et al. (1985), using an intramuscular nerve stimulation technique, found that split fibres were much more common than has been

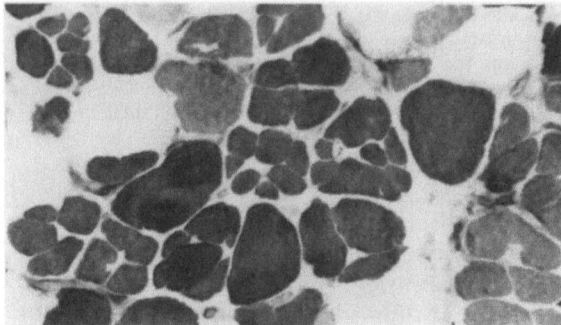

Fig. 4.12. Myosin ATPase, pH 4.3 × 350. Acute dermatomyositis. Subendomysial regeneration. Small rounded fibres can be seen contained within the subendomysial tube left by necrosis of muscle fibres.

concluded from conventional EMG and single-fibre EMG studies, as shown in muscle biopsies. In neurogenic disorders the neuromuscular jitter of the late components is usually increased, with intermittent impulse blocking, suggesting that reinnervation of the small-diameter fibres is functionally unstable (Stålberg et al. 1975b). In some moderately advanced cases of Duchenne dystrophy similar potentials with increased jitter and, rarely, with paired blocking, have been recorded (Stålberg et al. 1975b; Schwartz et al. 1977a), but the explanation of the phenomenon in this condition is uncertain.

Implications of Fibre Splitting

Splitting and Fibre-Type Grouping

Fibre-type grouping is regarded as a phenomenon found exclusively in neurogenic disorders (Dubowitz and Brooke 1973). In neurogenic disorders, increased fibre density found in single-fibre EMG recordings can be correlated with histochemical fibre-type grouping (Schwartz et al. 1977a). In addition, histological studies of the terminal motor innervation in these disorders, using the supravital methylene blue technique, have shown an increased terminal innervation ratio, and the presence of two or more motor end-plates on single muscle fibres (Coërs et al. 1973). Fibre-type grouping is thus usually taken as strong evidence of reinneration by axonal sprouting. However, small groups of fibres of similar histochemical type also occur in the myopathies (Ringel et al. 1976), including Duchenne muscular dystrophy (Schwartz et al. 1977a) and polymyositis (Ringel et al. 1976). The late motor unit components (Desmedt and Borenstein 1976b) and increased fibre density found in these myopathies with single-fibre EMG also indicate that enlargement of the motor unit has occurred (Schwartz et al. 1977a).

There are several possible mechanisms which might account for enlargement of motor units in the myopathies.

First, small clusters of regenerating fibres must receive innervation by axonal sprouting in order to become functional. This phenomenon has been studied in regenerating fibres after experimental crush injuries (Reznik and Engel 1970) and after ischaemic necrosis (Allbrook and Aitken 1951).

Second, segmental fibre necrosis may separate a viable part of a fibre from its innervation (Denny-Brown 1960). The denervated part of a fibre will then develop extrajunctional acetylcholine receptors (Katz and Miledi 1964; Ringel et al. 1976). Either denervation atrophy (Hall-Craggs 1971) or re-

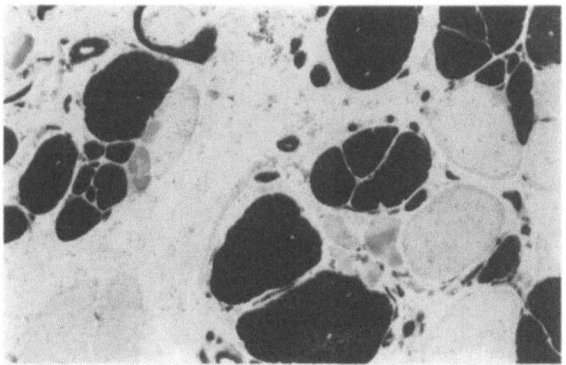

Fig. 4.14. Myosin ATPase, pH 4.3 × 140. Kugelberg–Welander disease. Two (dark) Type 1 fibres have become split into several separate fragments; these retain the histochemical type of their parent fibres and thus mimic fibre-type grouping. However, the difference in size between the fibre fragments and the adjacent unsplit fibres indicates that splitting has occurred.

innervation by axonal sprouting from a nearby motor unit will follow (Miledi 1962). Functional reinnervation of the denervated portion of a fibre can also occur if regenerating myotubes derived from the damaged segment re-establish continuity either between the denervated and reinnervated parts of the fibre (Reznik 1973) or with split or otherwise damaged, but innervated, nearby fibres. The continuity of the basement membrane scaffold of the damaged fibre (Vracko 1974) will determine which of these processes occurs.

Third, longitudinal fibre splitting can lead to forking of individual fibres. In serial sections the separated parts, which retain functional innervation through their connection with their parent fibre, often become larger in cross-sectional area, resulting in a compensatory increase in myofibrillar mass and in an apparent increase in the number of fibres in individual motor units. In random transverse sections this phenomenon may sometimes resemble fibre-type grouping (Fig. 4.14) and in single-fibre EMG recordings it is one factor leading to an increased fibre density, a phenomenon observed in both neurogenic (Stålberg et al. 1975b; Schwartz et al. 1976a) and myopathic disorders (Stålberg et al. 1974; Schwartz et al. 1977a). The forked branches themselves may insert in the perimysium of adjacent fibres, fuse with their parent fibres, or continue for variable distances through the muscle belly before ending blindly (Isaacs et al. 1973; Schwartz et al. 1976a). Ekstedt and Stålberg (1969) have suggested that forked fibres can be recognised with single-fibre EMG by the finding of an abnormally low neuromuscular jitter between two action potentials belonging to the same motor unit (Schwartz et al. 1976a).

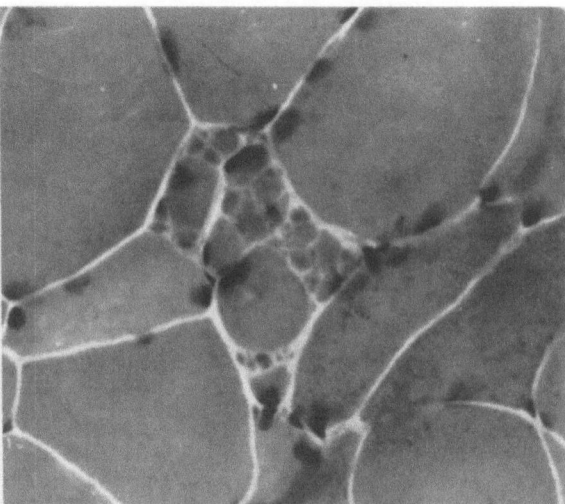

Fig. 4.15. H and E. × 350. Kugelberg–Welander disease. Fragmentation results in fibres of too small a size to attract innervation and become functional.

Fourthly, longitudinal fibre splitting may result in the formation of completely separate fibres. At first these fibres will lack innervation, but if axonal sprouting and new end-plate formation occur the split fibres will become functional components of an enlarged motor unit. The newly formed fibres will be of shorter length than normal fibres and will vary in cross-sectional area. They will probably arise and insert from the perimysium of adjacent fibres. In transverse sections this phenomenon can usually be recognised by the presence of clusters of fibres of similar histochemical type, but of varying size (Fig. 4.14). Split fibres may change their histochemical type in response to their new innervation but this will only very rarely be recognisable (Aloisi et al. 1974; Schwartz et al. 1976a).

Splitting as a Compensatory Process

In biopsies of longstanding neurogenic disorders secondary "myopathic" abnormalities are common (Drachman et al. 1967; Schwartz et al. 1976a). Fibre splitting is an important factor in the development of these abnormalities (Schwartz et al. 1976a). It may result in an increase in the number of fibres and thus of myofibrillar mass in the weakened muscle, or it may lead to the formation of small non-viable fragments and thus to failure of compensation. In Duchenne muscular dystrophy EMG evidence of late components (Desmedt and Borenstein 1975, 1976b) with a markedly increased fibre density, and histochemical fibre-type grouping, are all most prominent in the intermediate stages of the

disease (Schwartz et al. 1977a). In addition, Bell and Conen (1968) noticed that longitudinal fibre splitting was most common at this stage, when mobility is still possible. Later in the course of the disease compensation fails to keep pace with the progress of the disease, perhaps because regeneration fails, but also because continual fibre splitting results in the formation of fragments of insufficient size to become functional (Fig. 4.15). Reinnervation of fibre fragments, or of regenerating fibres, may also be less successful at this stage. Reinnervation could be impaired because increasing interstitial fibrosis acts as a physical barrier to axonal sprouts, because there is less muscle fibre regeneration, or because split or regenerating fibres may be unable to attain a sufficient size to provide a suitable stimulus to attract innervation, or to form end-plates. These factors are probably important in the rapid decompensation that occurs in the later stages of the disease.

In histological studies of the motor innervation in Duchenne muscular dystrophy, fine, beaded subterminal nerve fibres, forming small irregular endings on "atrophic" fibres, have been found, but the terminal innervation ratio is normal (Coërs et al. 1973). Further histological work is needed to resolve the apparent conflict between this observation and the other histological (Schwartz et al. 1977a) and physiological evidence (Borenstein and Desmedt 1973; Desmedt and Borenstein 1975, 1976b; Schwartz et al. 1977a), but it is possible that the late potentials found in EMG studies of this condition represent action potentials arising in small-diameter atrophic or regenerating fibres.

In healed, longstanding polymyositis large polyphasic potentials of increased duration are often recorded (Mechler 1974) and in such patients fibre-type grouping is seen (Ringel et al. 1976). In addition, we have noted that fibre splitting is present (Swash et al. 1978a) and this may thus also be a contributory factor leading to functional compensation in polymyositis.

In biopsies of chronic or slowly progressive neurogenic disorders fibre hypertrophy with fibre splitting and scattered regenerating fibres (Drachman et al. 1967; Schwartz et al. 1976a) are common features and lead to random variability in fibre size, giving a myopathic appearance. These features probably represent a *compensatory process* leading to an increase in myofibrillar mass of functionally innervated fibres within enlarged motor units. However, in very longstanding neurogenic disorders, for example in long survival after poliomyelitis, this secondary "myopathic" change may itself lead to functional decompensation, as suggested by Drachman et al. (1967).

Relation of Fibre Splitting to "Myopathic" Changes in Denervated Muscle

"Myopathic" features are commonly found in chronically denervated muscle; (Drachman et al. 1967; Mastaglia and Walton 1971a,b). These consist, in descending order of frequency, of central nucleation, longitudinal splitting of muscle fibres, muscle fibre hypertrophy, degenerative changes, random variation in fibre size and interstitial fibrosis (Cazzato 1970). Various suggestions have been made to explain the presence of these "myopathic" changes in denervated muscle. These include:

1. Coincidental myopathy and neuropathy
2. Reinnervation of denervated fibres (Adams et al. 1962)
3. Work-induced hypertrophy of innervated fibres, disappearance of denervated fibres and superimposed minor injury (Drachman et al. 1967)
4. Reduction of trophic factor due to "poor innervation" (Cazzato 1970)
5. Inadequate nutrition of hypertrophied fibres due to proliferation of collagenous tissue around small arteries (Mittelbach 1966)
6. Inadequate nutrition due to disproportion of muscle fibre mass attained during hypertrophy in relation to capillary blood supply (Cazzato 1970, Sulaiman and Kinder 1989).

In considering the pathogenesis of these "myopathic" changes in denervated muscle it must be realised that they are not identical to the typical histological abnormality found in the myopathies. In the myopathies, degeneration and phagocytosis of single fibres is common and small basophilic fibres, often found in small clusters, are frequently seen but both these abnormalities are less common in denervated muscle. Furthermore, areas of fat replacement and of marked interstitial fibrosis typically occur early in the natural history of some myopathies, but only much later in denervated muscle, while central nucleation, hypertrophy and splitting of muscle fibres occur in both neurogenic and myopathic disorders.

"Myopathic" features are most evident in those cases in which splitting is most prominent (Schwartz et al. 1976a) and it has been suggested that the following sequence of events occurs in chronic denervation. Functional overload of surviving, innervated or reinnervated muscle fibres leads to compensatory hypertrophy and this is accompanied by central migration of nuclei (Denny-Brown 1960). Splitting or fissure formation then occurs (Wohlfart and Wohlfart 1935), either affecting the hypertrophied

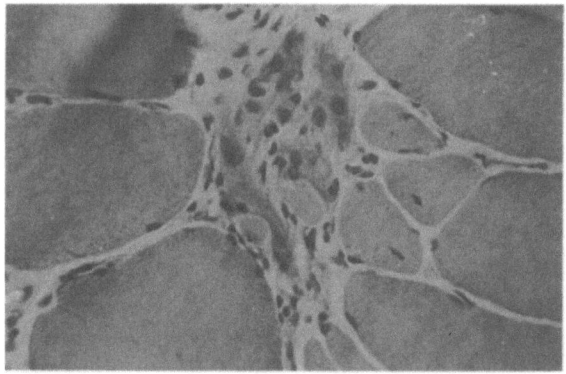

Fig. 4.16. H and E. × 400. Kugelberg–Welander disease. Regeneration is sometimes seen in cases in which secondary myopathic changes are prominent.

fibres themselves or adjacent, less hypertrophic fibres, perhaps less able to withstand the overloading force. Splitting is irregular in plane and length, and may be complete or incomplete, simple or complex, or may even lead to fragmentation of a fibre (Cazzato 1970). The latter phenomenon allows the possibility of regeneration from nucleated fragments, or degenerative change and phagocytosis of extruded fragments (Hall-Craggs 1970). A similar process has been observed in the intrafusal muscle fibres in myotonic dystrophy (Swash and Fox 1975a,b). Splitting of muscle fibres might thus account for the occurrence of isolated degenerating or regenerating fibres in denervated muscle in which "myopathic" changes are present (Fig. 4.16).

Isolated fragments derived from completed fibre splitting are functionally denervated. If collateral innervation by axonal sprouting becomes ineffective, as probably occurs in the later stages of chronic denervating disorders (Wohlfart 1958), the fibre fragments will undergo irreversible denervation atrophy. Other fragments will receive collateral innervation by axonal sprouts derived from the same or adjacent motor units, and this may be recognisable by a change in their histochemical type (see also Jennekens et al. 1974). The combination of hypertrophy, splitting and denervation atrophy will lead to pronounced variation in fibre size, becoming randomly distributed as the process advances. Further, it would be expected that interstitial fibrosis would become marked only late in the course of such a process, when destruction of individual fibres or fragments becomes a prominent feature.

Longitudinal fibre splitting thus represents an adaptive response to the increase in the load placed on remaining muscle fibres that accompanies a reduction in number of functioning muscle fibres. It is important in determining the histological and physiological features found in the muscle, and in the development of compensatory mechanisms in neuromuscular disease.

Compensatory mechanisms thus include:

1. Muscle fibre regeneration

2. Muscle fibre hypertrophy
3. Reinnervation
4. Remodelling of the motor unit, with fibre-type grouping
5. Fibre splitting, leading to increased muscle fibre mass

Chapter 5

Classification of Neuromuscular Diseases

A large number of different neuromuscular diseases are recognised. Classification is important for purposes of nomenclature and standardised diagnosis, but classification itself depends on knowledge of the underlying pathogenesis of the different diseases and, as new advances in knowledge develop, the classification of diseases alters. For example, the impact of molecular biology and genetics on neuromuscular diseases has had a particularly profound impact on classification of the genetically determined neuropathies. As the relationship between acquired and genetic syndromes in the progressive proximal neurogenic disorders becomes better understood there will probably also be profound changes in classification of these disorders. Even as this book has been in preparation, the limb-girdle dystrophy syndromes have begun to be unravelled. The World Federation of Neurology Committee on Neuromuscular Diseases modified its classification of Neuromuscular Diseases in 1994 in response to the changes necessary since its previous classifications of 1968 and 1988, and this internationally accepted classification of the neuromuscular diseases forms the basis of the organisation of chapters in this book.

We have adhered to the convention of classification according to a combination of topographic and pathogenetic criteria. For example, the neurogenic disorders are grouped according to the site of the lesion leading to neurogenic weakness. Thus the anterior horn cell disorders are classified separately from the neuropathies. Within each of these two categories, however, diseases are grouped according to whether they are acquired or congenital, and where their underlying basis is understood this information is also used in classification. In neurogenic disorders anterior horn cells, nerve roots, peripheral nerves with their myelin sheaths and the motor end-plates are vulnerable to different pathological processes by virtue not only of their different tissues, but also of their different anatomical locations. The myopathies are less easy to classify conveniently. We have used the compromise adopted by the World Federation of Neurology (WFN), namely to recognise the large number of genetic myopathies and dystrophies, and to then utilise a category of acquired myopathies due to external toxins, and further groupings of acquired inflammatory myopathies. The metabolic myopathies, however, comprise both acquired and hereditary diseases.

The classification given here is intended as an outline to enable the reader to understand the principles of the procedure used by the World Federation of Neurology in deriving this grouping of the neuromuscular disorders. In the detailed discussion of these groups of disorders in the following chapters of this book the reader will find more detailed classifications of the relevant subgroups.

Main Headings Used in the WFN Classification of Neuromuscular Diseases

1. Spinal muscular atrophy and other disorders of motor neurons
2. Disorders of motor nerve roots
3. Disorders of peripheral nerve
4. Disorders of neuromuscular transmission
5. Disorders of muscle

Classification of Neuromuscular Diseases

1. Spinal Muscular Atrophy (SMA) and Other Disorders of Motor Neurons

a] *Spinal muscular atrophies*
   Type 1 (Werdnig–Hoffmann disease)

Type 2 (intermediate SMA)
Type 3 (Kugelberg–Welander disease)
Type 4 (proximal SMA of adult onset)
Other types of SMA
  distal SMA
  scapuloperoneal SMA
  bulbospinal atrophy (Kennedy SMA)
  Vialetto–Van Laere syndrome
  arthrogryposis syndromes
  Fazio–Londe syndrome
  restricted forms of SMA (monomelic SMA)

b] *Motor neuron disease*
Sporadic amyotrophic lateral sclerosis
Familial amyotrophic lateral sclerosis

c] *Viral disorders*
Poliomyelitis and post-polio syndrome
Herpes zoster myelitis
HIV infection

d] *Creutzfeldt–Jakob disease*

e] *Motor neuron disorders with hyperactivity*
Stiff man syndrome
Myoclonic encephalomyelitis
Myokymia
Isaac's syndrome
Tetanus

2. Disorders of Motor Nerve Roots

a] *Physical compression of nerve roots*
Disc prolapse
Bony compression
Tumour
Trauma

b] *Radiation*

c] *Infective and post-infective*

d] *Immunologically mediated radiculopathies*

e] *Neoplastic infiltration*

3. Disorders of peripheral nerves

a] *Genetically determined polyneuropathies*
Charcot–Marie–Tooth (CMT) syndromes (also classified by specific mutations)
  CMT 1 (hypertrophic demyelinating)
  CMT 2 (neuronal)
  CMT 3 (infantile onset: Dejerine–Sottas)
  other CMT syndromes (including familial liability to pressure palsies)
Hereditary sensory and autonomic neuropathies

Hereditary neuropathies with known biochemical abnormalities
  Familial amyloid polyneuropathies
  Porphyria
  Metachromatic leukodystrophy
  Refsum's disease
  Lipoprotein deficiencies
  Others
Miscellaneous hereditary polyneuropathies
  Familial liability to pressure palsies (see CMT syndromes)
  Giant axonal neuropathy
  Friedreich's ataxia

b] *Acquired polyneuropathies*
Guillain-Barré syndrome and related disorders
  Acute demyelinating or axonal polyneuropathy
  Chronic relapsing demyelinating polyneuropathy
  Miller–Fisher syndrome
Polyneuropathy with paraproteinaemia or dysproteinaemia
  Multiple myeloma
  Benign monoclonal gammopathy
  Macroglobulinaemia and cryoglobulinaemia
Polyneuropathy with malignant disease
  Paraneoplastic neuropathies
  Infiltrative polyneuropathy
Polyneuropathy with connective tissue disease
Polyneuropathy with infection
  Leprosy
  Herpes zoster
  HIV
Metabolic polyneuropathies
  Nutritional neuropathy
  Alcoholic neuropathy
  Diabetic neuropathy
  Uraemic neuropathy
  Hepatic neuropathy
  Others
Polyneuropathy with other systemic diseases
  Critical care neuropathy
  Sarcoidosis
Toxic polyneuropathy
  Diphtheria
  Heavy metal poisoning
  Organic solvent toxicity
  Drug toxicity
Polyneuropathies of unknown cause

c] *Mononeuropathies*
Physical injury
  Trauma
  Compression

Radiation
Ischaemic and vasculitic
Haemorrhage
Tumours arising in nerves

4. Disorders of Neuromuscular Transmission

Myasthenia gravis
Lambert–Eaton myasthenic syndrome
Congenital myasthenic syndromes
Botulism and other toxins
Envenomation

5. Disorders of Muscle

a] *Genetically determined myopathies*

X-linked muscular dystrophies
Dystrophinopathies
Duchenne muscular dystrophy
Becker muscular dystrophy
McLeod syndrome
Scapulo-peroneal myopathy
Centronuclear myopathy
Emery–Dreifuss syndrome

Autosomal muscular dystrophies
Facio-scapulo-humeral muscular dystrophy
Scapulo-peroneal muscular dystrophy
Limb-girdle muscular dystrophy syndromes
Distal muscular dystrophy (Welander
disease)
Oculo-pharyngeal muscular dystrophy

Myotonic disorders
Myotonic dystrophy
Congenital myotonic disorders
Childhood myopathies
Central core disease
Nemaline myopathy
Myotubular myopathy
Myopathy with tubular aggregates
Congenital myopathies
Others

b] *Acquired myopathies*

Myopathies due to toxins or drugs
Drug-induced myopathies
Steroid myopathy
Alcoholic myopathy

Inflammatory myopathies
Polymyositis
Dermatomyositis
Inclusion body myositis
Paraneoplastic dermatomyositis
Others, e.g. sarcoidosis, granulomatous
myositis

c] *Metabolic myopathies*

Acquired endocrine myopathies
Dysthyroid myopathies
Osteomalacic myopathy
Cushing's syndrome

Hereditary metabolic myopathies
Glycogen storage diseases
Periodic paralysis
Mitochondrial and lipid storage diseases
Malignant hyperthermia
Rhabdomyolysis syndromes and
myoglobinurias

Chapter 6

Diseases of Anterior Horn Cells

Diseases affecting anterior horn cells may present at any age from infancy to the senium. Those diseases beginning in infancy, childhood or adolescence are usually limited to the anterior horn cells, but in adults other parts of the motor system, i.e. the upper motor neuron may be involved. The latter are classified as motor neuron disease, a disorder which is very rare in childhood. Certain viruses, particularly poliomyelitis, show a predilection to infect anterior horn cells but other viruses, for example Herpes zoster and Coxsackie virus, may also affect anterior horn cells. In most anterior horn cell disorders motor nuclei in the brainstem are also involved; the term spinal muscular atrophy does not, therefore, exclude bulbar involvement.

The cardinal features of neurogenic disorders are muscular weakness and wasting. In addition, anterior horn cell disorders in adults are often characterised by prominent fasciculation at rest. This is particularly evident in rapidly progressive disorders, such as motor neuron disease. In more slowly progressive disorders, such as Kugelberg–Welander disease, fasciculations are uncommon at rest, but partial voluntary contraction against resistance induces irregular contraction of large fascicles in affected muscles, a phenomenon which is uncommon in myopathic disorders. In neurogenic disorders anticholinesterase drugs, e.g. neostigmine, will induce fasciculation at rest at lower dosage than in normal subjects. When there is involvement only of the lower motor neuron the tendon reflexes may be reduced or absent but in motor neuron disease, in which lower and upper motor neuron lesions usually co-exist, the tendon reflexes are characteristically brisker than normal, even in wasted muscles. This finding of an increased tendon reflex in a wasted muscle occurs in other disorders in which upper and lower motor neuron lesions are present, particularly in the cervical myelopathy associated with cervical spondylosis. However, in the anterior horn cell disorders themselves sensory abnormalities are not present, although some patients with motor neuron disease complain of paraesthesiae.

The Spinal Muscular Atrophies

The term spinal muscular atrophy (SMA) was first used by Hoffmann in 1893 to distinguish progressive muscular weakness and atrophy in infancy, due to anterior horn cell degeneration, from muscular dystrophy (Werdnig 1891). Since then this designation has been used to include a group of related diseases, all characterised by anterior horn cell degeneration and muscle weakness and wasting, with differing ages of onset and progression. The sensory system is clinically normal. There have been many attempts at classification of these disorders (Dubowitz 1964; Emery 1971; Hausmanowa-Petrusewicz 1978; Pearn 1980, 1982; Harding 1984), all based on a combination of clinical features, especially on age of onset, outcome and pattern of inheritance. Thus the separation of different disorders within this group of diseases is still, to some extent, controversial. The classification used in this chapter (Table 6.1) takes account of the varying views expressed by previous workers (Dubowitz 1991).

The spinal muscular atrophies usually present as proximal weakness. In some rare varieties of these syndromes, however, the weakness is distally predominant, and asymmetrical. Scapulo-peroneal and bulbospinal forms have been described. Genetic factors are important; most are inherited as autosomal recessive traits (Pearn 1980). Within any individual family there is usually a high degree of concordance so that affected siblings or cousins tend to develop similar forms of the disease (Dubowitz 1995). In the adult forms many cases are inherited as

Table 6.1. Classification of spinal muscular atrophies (SMA) (major types)

SMA	Synonyms	Inheritance	Age of onset	Disability	Life expectancy	EMG	Muscle biopsy
Type I	Werdnig–Hoffmann disease Acute infantile SMA	Autosomal recessive 5q 11.2-13.3	0–6 months	Severe, generalised bulbar weakness common	Usually <2 years	Spontaneous motor unit activity at rest Neurogenic	Large group atrophy Rounded hypertrophic fibres
Type II	Intermediate SMA	Autosomal recessive 5q 11.2-13.3	<18 months	Never able to walk unaided, arms relatively strong, no bulbar involvement	>2 years	Neurogenic	Similar to SMA I but usually less severe
Type III	Kugelberg–Welander disease Mild SMA	Autosomal recessive 5q 11.2-13.3	>18 months	Variable. Slowly progressive weakness; may be mild or severe	Normal	Neurogenic with myopathic features	Fibre-type grouping Group atrophy Myopathic change
Type IV	Adult-onset SMA	Autosomal recessive	adult	Progressive weakness, unable to walk 20 years after diagnosis	Normal	Neurogenic with myopathic features	Similar to SMA III
	Adult-onset SMA	Autosomal dominant	adult	Slowly progressive proximal weakness Moderate disability	Normal?		

autosomal recessive disorders but autosomal dominant and sex-linked recessive forms also occur (Pearn et al. 1978). Diagnostic criteria for the common SMA syndromes were agreed at an International Consensus Conference (Munsat 1991a).

The separation of the different types of SMA is supported by the tendency for the clinical forms of the disease to appear consistently in different families. For example, SMA Type III never appears in families afflicted by SMA Type I more frequently than would be expected by chance (Pearn 1980, 1982). Bundey and Lovelace (1975a,b) found that chronic forms of SMA could be segregated by age of onset into two groups, those beginning before the age of two years and those manifesting after this age, and they noted that this division separated families into these two groups, suggesting that there are genetically distinct disorders. The classification, however, is unsatisfactory in other respects. In particular, the distinction between SMA Type I and SMA Type II is occasionally difficult since even in the same family cases of acute fatal and chronic forms of infantile onset have been reported (Hausmanowa-Petrusewicz 1978; Dubowitz 1995; Peran 1980, 1982). These problems have not been fully resolved, even with knowledge of the genetic loci for the common forms of childhood onset SMA (Munsat et al. 1990; Dubowitz 1991). Generally, autosomal recessive SMA is most severe in early onset cases, and least severe in late onset cases.

Types I, II and III are linked to a site on chromosome 5q at 5q 11.2-13.3. The locus has been mapped to a site between DNA marker D5 S4-35 and the microtubule associated protein MAP1b (Soares et al. 1993). The localisation of these three types of SMA to chromosome 5q 11.2-13.3 (Melki et al. 1990) led to the suggestion that the genetic locus is common to all three syndromes, the pheno-

typic difference resulting from other genetic or environmental influences (Muller et al. 1992). The genetic defect consists of a variable partial deletion near the NAIP gene (neuronal apoptosis inhibitory protein) at this site. The protein product of this gene, and its role in normal neuronal metabolism are of great interest (Roy et. al 1995) in understanding this group of disease.

Other SMA syndromes are not mapped to the SMA5q locus.

Clinical Presentation of Types I–IV SMA

Type I SMA (Werdnig–Hoffmann Disease)

This is virtually always a fatal disease, death occurring in 95% of cases by the age of 18 months (Pearn and Wilson 1973a), and in 100% by the age of 27 months (Pearn 1982). A few cases with a more chronic course have been described (Munsat et al. 1969b) but these may represent a different disorder.

The disease often begins in utero; in a third of cases the mother has noted unusually feeble fetal movements in pregnancy. In half of the affected children with SMA I the disease began before the age of one month, and all are affected by the age of five months (Pearn et al. 1978). The incidence of the disease is 1 in 20 000 live births and the two sexes are equally affected (Pearn 1973a). The carrier frequency is 1 : 60–80 and the gene frequency is 0.006.

The child is usually hypotonic at birth, with very weak limb and trunk movements. The child tends to lie with the arms abducted, flexed at the elbows, and with flexed knees and abducted legs (Fig. 6.1a). The child is never able to roll over and head control is poor. Movements of hands and feet may be relatively spared, although proximal weakness is severe.

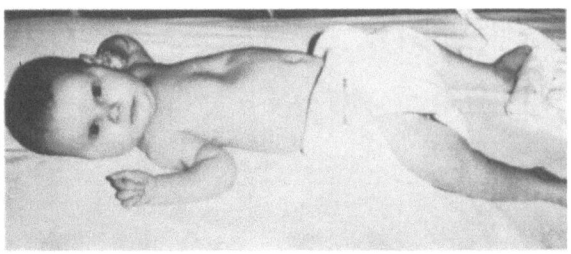

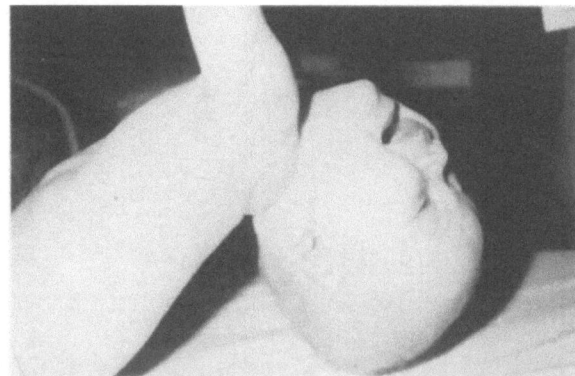

Fig. 6.1. Werdnig–Hoffmann disease. **a** The limbs are immobile and there is pectus excavatum. **b** Head posture cannot be maintained against gravity.

In some cases a tremor of the fingers is visible, probably representing fasciculation in the intrinsic or forearm musculature. There is poor swallowing and sucking and the tongue is often atrophic and fasciculating. Respirations are shallow, with paradoxical chest movements and the child cannot support its head (Fig. 6.1b). The normal startle and stepping reflexes are reduced or absent. The external ocular movements, however, are normal, and sphincter control is also normal. The facial musculature is also often spared at first so that the facial expression appears normal, but later facial weakness leads to a flat, expressionless face but with normal eye movements. The tendon reflexes are absent. On palpation the limb muscles are atrophic, but this is often obscured by subcutaneous fat. The clinical features are usually characteristic and the diagnosis can be made at birth or in the first few days of life in more than half the cases.

In most cases death occurs from pulmonary infection, often initiated by aspiration of food during feeding. Sometimes the diagnosis becomes evident after presentation in the first few months of life with pulmonary infection.

Very rarely diaphragmatic involvement may occur as a presenting feature (Schapira and Swash 1985), although this muscle is usually strikingly spared at all stages of the disease. This and other atypical features, such as arthrogryposis, eye muscle

weakness, visual and cardiac problems, marked facial weakness and evidence of CNS dysfunction, serve to exclude a diagnosis of Type I SMA. However, a number of other different disorders may also involve anterior horn cells, although these are not part of the SMA Type I phenotype (Dubowitz 1991).

Onset within the first few months of life is associated with early death, and onset after age 1 year with less severe disease and greater longevity (Munsat et al. 1990), resembling Type II intermediate SMA. With few exceptions, however, there is little intrafamilial variability (Munsat et al. 1990).

Type II SMA (Intermediate Type)

This form of SMA presents a little later than Type I SMA, usually before the first birthday, but after three months of age. Type II SMA is nearly as common as Type I SMA (Pearn 1978b). Development in infancy is normal but after six months of age the motor milestones become delayed and although the child may be able to sit, independent standing and walking are not achieved normally (Fig. 6.2). More than a third never walk, but 20%–40% can still walk, with assistance, at the age of ten years (Bundey 1985). The disease may sometimes seem to begin relatively acutely. In the majority of cases, in which the disease begins before the age of one year, weakness is generalised and severe, with a proximal emphasis. In cases with a later onset, in the second year of life, weakness is symmetrical and predominantly proximal, with prominent involvement of truncal and pelvic muscles.

The disease is often complicated by the development of scoliosis, although this can be partially prevented by appropriate management. Although the legs are often very weak, the arms are less affected and respiratory movement and bulbar muscles are also usually relatively spared. Fasciculation of the tongue and other muscles is present in more than 50% of cases. Facial muscles are affected in about a third of cases. The external ocular and urinary and anal sphincter muscles are normal. There may be a tremor of the outstretched fingers, similar to that found in SMA Type I. The tendon reflexes are depressed or absent.

This disorder may have a relatively non-progressive course, particularly in children with a later age of onset (>1 year). The disorder may undergo slow or episodic deterioration. In many cases little change occurs after the initial development of the weakness and wasting during a period of several months. In some patients weakness of intercostal muscles develops, leading to pulmonary complications, and the scoliosis itself sometimes pro-

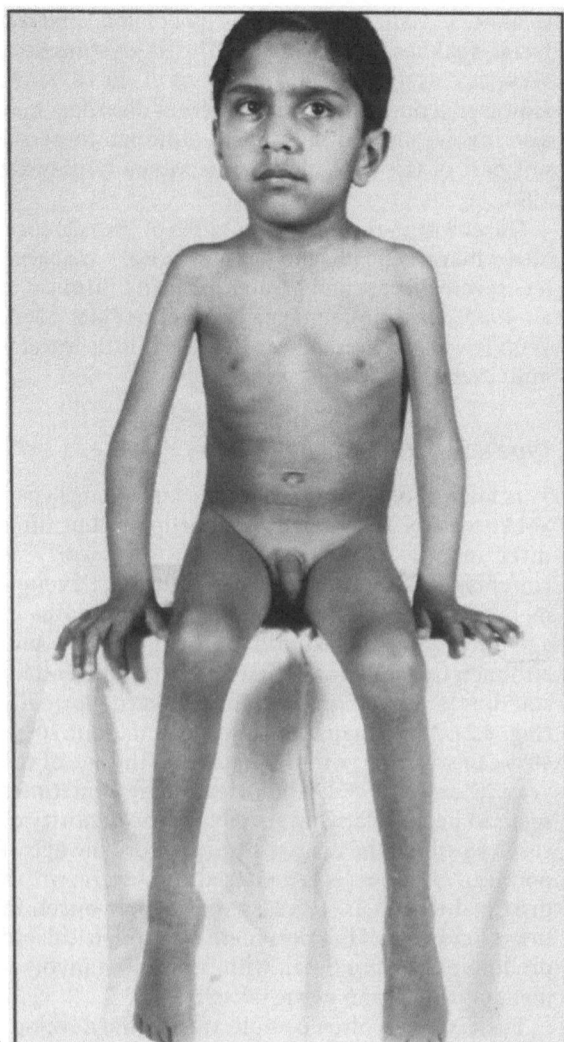

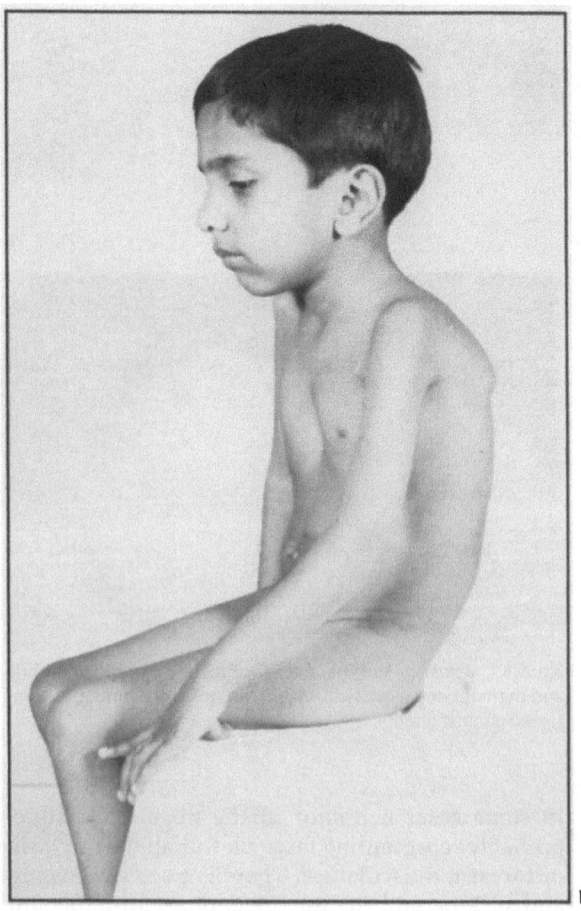

Fig. 6.2. Intermediate spinal muscular atrophy (Type II). There is prominent wasting, and the child never walked. Scoliosis has developed subsequently.

gresses, to the extent that it may interfere with respiration unless checked by orthopaedic correction.

Type III SMA (Kugelberg–Welander Disease)

The Type III variety of SMA presents in infancy or childhood (Wohlfart et al. 1955; Kugelberg and Welander 1956), with onset after the age of 18 months. The majority of cases begin before the age of 5 years. Many series show a male excess, but this is probably due to a relative excess of severe disease in males rather than a true sex difference (Hausmanowa-Petrusewicz et al. 1984; Bundey 1985). This form of spinal muscular atrophy is less common than the Type I form (Bundey 1985). After the initial descriptions of Type III SMA, investigation of patients with proximal weakness revealed that a proportion of patients previously thought to

be suffering from limb-girdle muscular dystrophy had this disorder, indicating the similarity of the clinical features (Tomlinson et al. 1974).

Distinction between typical cases beginning in childhood and those with onset somewhat later in life has been attempted but is blurred; generally cases beginning somewhat later have a more benign course. The disorder may begin abruptly, apparently in relation to a febrile illness, but most cases begin insidiously. The first symptom is usually related to weakness of muscles of the thighs and hips. The child has difficulty getting up from the ground and climbing stairs. The gait is often waddling and in children with onset early in life acquisition of walking may be delayed. Later, shoulder girdle weakness becomes evident, causing weakness of the arms and winging of the scapulae (Fig. 6.2). Paraspinal muscles may also be involved so that

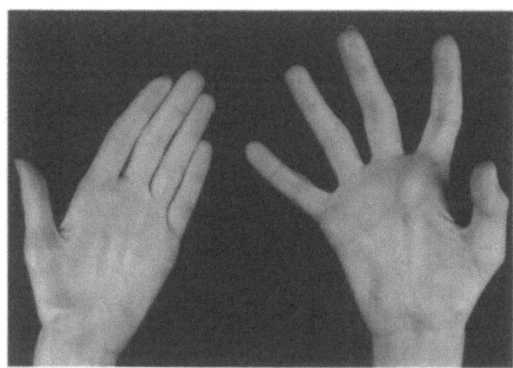

Fig. 6.3. Kugelberg–Welander disease. Wasting of the hands is a late feature.

neck extensors and flexors become weak and lordosis may develop. Scoliosis may also occur. Weakness is usually proximal and symmetrical and later may involve distal muscles (Fig. 6.3). Involvement of cranial musculature is less obvious, but facial weakness and palatal weakness may occur. The external ocular muscles are invariably spared, but ptosis has been reported. Selective involvement of brachioradialis, serratus anterior and deltoid muscles, with sparing of rhomboids and trapezius muscle was noted by Hausmanowa-Petrusewicz (1978).

Hypertrophy of the calves is a feature in about a quarter of all cases, but these are almost always males (Bouwsma and van Wijngaarden 1980). However, this finding should always raise the suspicion of an X-linked dystrophinopathy, e.g. Becker disease. Fasciculations can be found in limb muscles in about half the patients at some stage of the disease; they are detected most commonly in the relatively early stages. Fasciculation of the tongue is uncommon. The tendon reflexes are diminished or absent but sensory examination is normal. During slow active movements of affected muscles it is often possible to elicit "contraction fasciculations". These are fasciculation-like contractions of fascicles or groups of fascicles visible as irregular contraction of parts of a muscle during movement, and are a useful clinical sign of reinnervation demonstrable at the bedside.

Kugelberg–Welander disease is a relatively benign disorder. Survival into adult life is the rule and the life expectancy is normal. Walking may be possible for many years; Kugelberg and Welander (1956) described eight patients still able to walk 20–40 years after the onset of their disease. Intellect is normal and there are no associated abnormalities in other systems.

A number of variations of this clinical picture have been described in the older literature, but these probably mostly represent cases that would not be

acceptable according to current clinical and genetic diagnostic criteria (Munsat 1991a). Extensor plantar responses have occasionally been reported, without other clinical evidence of corticospinal tract involvement (Gardner-Medwin et al. 1967). This probably results from differential weakness in foot and calf muscles.

Autosomal dominant (Zellweger et al. 1972) and X-linked recessive forms have also been reported (Tsukagoshi et al. 1970). An autosomal dominant benign SMA not linked to chromosome 5q was described by Frijns et al. (1994).

Type IV SMA (Adult-Onset Type)

This form of SMA begins between the ages of 15 and 60 years, with a median age of onset of 35 years. The onset and progression is usually insidious, but periods of temporary arrest or progression of the disease may be noted. Pearn et al. (1978) noted that this disorder is relatively mild, ambulation being maintained throughout life. The incidence of the disease is less than 0.5/100 000 (Harding 1984). One-third of cases are dominantly inherited; these show a more rapid progression and may lose the ability to run after 5 years. The recessive form is more benign. This disease is rare and is difficult to distinguish from the proximal muscular atrophy type of motor neuron disease and from the axonal variety of Charcot–Marie–Tooth disease.

Other Types of SMA

Additional clinical forms of SMA have been described (Table 6.2) and some of these are relatively common. For example, the distal form of the disease represents about 10% of all cases of SMA (Pearn and Hudgson 1979). There are various schemes of classification but, currently, a classical clinical classification is most useful. For example, autosomal dominant SMA (non 5q) has juvenile and adult forms, the latter relatively benign (Rietschel et al. 1992).

Distal SMA. The distal form of SMA, which accounts for 10% of all cases of spinal muscular atrophy, is genetically heterogeneous. Cases with dominant inheritance begin before the age of 20 years whereas in the recessive form the disease may be very mild and of later onset. Most patients have distal weakness and wasting of the legs, especially affecting anterior tibial and peroneal compartments; and pes cavus and scoliosis are frequent (Pearn and Hudgson 1979). In other cases the hands may be predominantly involved (O'Sullivan and McLeod

Table 6.2.   Rare forms of spinal muscular atrophy (SMA)

SMA	Inheritance	Age of onset	Disability	Life expectancy	Sex
Distal	Dominant or recessive	2–20 years	Usually mild	Normal	M=F
Distal SMA upper limbs	?	15–30 years	Moderate	Normal	90% M
Chronic asymmetrical	?	16–45 years	Mild	Normal	M=F
Monomelic	?	Variable	Mild	Normal	90% M
Scapulo-peroneal	Autosomal recessive	3rd or 4th decade	Moderate	Normal or reduced	M=F
Bulbar SMA with deafness	?	1st or 2nd decade	Severe	Death less than 10 years from diagnosis	?
Bulbar SMA (Fazio–Londé)	Autosomal recessive	2–12 years	Severe	Death less than 8 years from onset	?
Kennedy SMA	X-linked	20–60 years	Moderate	Normal or slightly reduced	M
Oculo-pharyngeal	?Dominant	4th decade	Mild	Normal or slightly reduced	M=F
Facio-scapulo-humeral	Dominant	2nd decade	Mild	Normal or slightly reduced	M=F
Hexosaminidase A deficiency	?Recessive	Childhood or adult	Moderate or severe	Reduced	M=F

1978; Tan 1985). In some families vocal cord paralysis was a feature (Young and Harper 1980; Pridmore et al. 1992). It has been suggested that dominant distal SMA might be identical with the axonal form (CMT Type 2) of Charcot–Marie–Tooth disease (Dyck and Lambert 1968a). It has also been termed hereditary motor neuropathy (Harding and Thomas 1980c), a term that emphasises this concept. However, more recent studies suggest that dominantly inherited distal SMA is a discrete entity, although it is not inherited on chromosome 5q (Green et al. 1993). SNAPs are normal in distal SMA, but reduced or absent in CMT Type 2 (Harding and Thomas 1980).

Monomelic SMA. A few cases have been described in Japan and India, and perhaps also in Western countries (O'Sullivan and McLeod 1978), of wasting of an arm or leg apparently due to anterior horn cell disease (Singh and Jolly 1963; Sobue et al. 1978; Chopra et al. 1984). It has been noted that this disorder, which predominantly affects males, is often difficult to distinguish from poliomyelitis (Chopra et al. 1984). It seems to begin relatively rapidly and then to enter a non-progressive phase. EMG studies reveal that the abnormality is not limited to one limb, other muscles, including bulbar muscles, being affected (Virmani and Mohan 1985), particularly in the homologous muscles of the opposite limb (Kay et al. 1994). This syndrome has been aptly termed "the wasted leg syndrome" (Chopra et al. 1984). The affected extremity shows marked changes in selected muscle groups, e.g. soleus/gastrocnemius and posterior thigh muscles, with much less marked abnormalities in the opposite limb (Kay et al. 1994). De Visser et al. (1988) described EMG and CT findings in five patients with this disorder.

Distal SMA of Upper Limbs. This syndrome, also known as distal juvenile SMA, has mostly been reported in South Asia and the Far East, with rare cases in the West (O'Sullivan and McLeod 1978; Sobue et al. 1978; Singh et al. 1980). The C8-T1 myotomes are typically most affected. The illness progresses relatively rapidly during the first 1–2 years and then enters a stable phase. About 80% of cases are men, and the onset is between 15 and 30 years. The bulbar muscles are unaffected. Reflexes are depressed or absent in the affected limbs, and the plantar responses are flexor. The EMG shows a higher single-fibre EMG fibre density in the more affected arm, and mild abnormalities in the clinically unaffected lower limbs (Chan et al. 1991). The CSF is normal.

Chronic asymmetrical SMA syndromes. There are a number of patients with unclassifiable syndromes, often distal more than proximal, and asymmetrical, with involvement of two or more limbs either from the onset or later in the illness. There are no features of upper motor neuron involvement and the rate of progression is slow. Motor and sensory nerve conduction studies are normal. The natural history of these syndromes is long, even with a normal life expectancy, but the disease gradually becomes more widespread (Meadows et al. 1969b; Harding et al. 1983). In two of the 18 cases described by Harding et al. (1983) there was a family history of Werdnig–Hoffmann disease, but in most cases the disorder is sporadic and of uncertain genetic background.

Scapulo-peroneal SMA. This disorder affects the shoulder girdle and the distal musculature (Brossard 1886; Davidenkow 1939). Autosomal recessive inheritance predominates, and these cases are clinically more severe than dominant cases. In the recessive form pes cavus is frequent and involvement of the small hand muscles occurs in addition to severe weakness of the peri-scapular and shoulder muscles, and of the anterior compartment of the shin. Distal sensory loss is a feature of some cases (Davidenkow 1939; Schwartz and Swash 1975).

The presence of sensory involvement in these cases clearly distinguishes them from the myopathic form.

A myopathic disease with a similar scapulo-peroneal predilection shows sparing of the small foot muscles, including extensor digitorum brevis, but in this disorder (Chap. 14) there is more prominent involvement of facial muscles. The recessive form of scapulo-peroneal SMA presents earlier than the dominant form but there is great variability. Most cases present in the third or fourth decade (Kaeser 1965) but presentation in childhood is not unknown (Emery et al. 1968). The disorder may progress to cause moderately severe disability. One such recessively inherited case was described by Gharbi Ben Ayed et al. (1993).

Scapulo-humeral SMA. Spinal muscular atrophy in a facio-scapulo-humeral distribution presenting in the second decade was described by Fenichel et al. (1967). It is inherited as an autosomal dominant trait (Furukawa and Toyokura 1976).

Bulbar SMA with deafness (Vialetto-van Laere syndrome). This is a severe disorder, presenting in the first and second decades with facial weakness, dysphagia and dysarthria, usually preceded by bilateral deafness of variable severity. Later, more generalised weakness, either proximal or distal, develops, sometimes with respiratory muscle involvement including diaphragmatic paralysis (Vialetto 1936; van Laere 1966; Alberca et al. 1980; Gallai et al. 1981; Summers et al. 1987). The syndrome was probably first described by Brown in 1894.

Bulbar SMA of childhood (Fazio-Londé syndrome). This syndrome usually presents between the ages of two and 12 years with unilateral facial weakness, followed by dysarthria and difficulty chewing food (Fazio 1892). It is a progressive autosomal recessive disorder that leads to death within 1–8 years of the onset. Autopsy examination shows (in order of severity) loss of motor cells from the VIIth, XIth, Vth, IIIrd and VIth nerve nuclei (Gomez et al. 1962). The pyramidal tracts are not affected but anterior horn cells in the cervical spinal cord may also be affected, perhaps accounting for the later respiratory difficulties (Alexander et al. 1976). The Fazio-Londé syndrome is rare and less than 20 cases have been reported (Della Giustina et al. 1979; Gomez 1994).

Oculo-pharyngeal SMA. This is a very rare variant of adult onset SMA. Progressive ophthalmoplegia, dysarthria and dysphagia are the main features with distal weakness and wasting in the limbs (Matsunaga et al. 1973). The variant of distal SMA with vocal cord paralysis may be a related syndrome.

Clinical Investigation of Spinal Muscular Atrophies

The creatine kinase (CK) level is frequently moderately raised in the chronic, slowly progressive forms of SMA. In the severe infantile form (Type I SMA) the CK level is invariably normal, in the intermediate infantile onset form (Type II SMA) it is occasionally raised, and in the Type III Kugelberg–Welander form of SMA it is usually raised, sometimes to as much as ten times normal. The increase in CK level in slowly progressive SMA can be related to the development of secondary myopathic changes in the muscle (Schwartz et al. 1976a; Swash and Schwartz 1977). In Type I and Type II SMA the level of the MB isoenzyme of creatine kinase is often elevated, but in Type III SMA the CK consists mainly of the MM isoenzyme (Hausmanowa–Petrusewicz 1978). Later, with progression of the disorder, the CK gradually increases, but it begins to fall as the muscles become increasingly atrophic in the later stages of the disorder, e.g. in Type III SMA. This is in contrast to Duchenne muscular atrophy, in which the CK level reaches its peak in infancy, and gradually declines thereafter (see Hausmanowa–Petrusewicz 1978).

The ECG is usually normal. Cardiomyopathy is not associated with the SMA group of disorders. In Type III SMA heartblock has been reported (Tanaka et al. 1976), but this association has not been confirmed.

The differential diagnosis between spinal muscular atrophy and most forms of muscular dystrophy can be made by CT scanning of limb muscles (Bulcke and Baert 1982; de Visser and Verbeeten 1985). In SMA the muscles have a ragged outline and progressively develop diffuse low density lesions, reflecting loss of muscle tissue, and fatty replacement (Bulcke 1984). In muscular dystrophy larger low density lesions spread to involve the whole muscle. In SMA there is relatively generalised weakness of pelvic and thigh muscles, but in muscular dystrophy there is differential involvement of particular muscles at one cross-sectional level (see Chap. 14). Pseudohypertrophy is relatively uncommon in SMA. Horikawa et al. (1986) found that in patients with chronic SMA, aged 6–22 years, the quadriceps were more severely affected than the hamstring muscles, and that the abductor longus muscles were always less affected than other thigh muscles. Ultrasound has also been used to image muscles (Heckmatt et al. 1980). This technique involves no radiation and therefore has certain clinical advantages.

Electrophysiological Investigation

The electrophysiological findings in the four main types of SMA reflect the severity and rate of progression of the disease. The abnormalities found are similar in the four types, consisting of fibrillation potentials, fasciculations, complex motor unit action potentials (MUAP) often of increased amplitude and duration, and a reduced interference pattern. In the slowly progressive Type III and Type IV forms of SMA potentials of "myopathic" and "neurogenic" type may be recorded in the same muscle. Myopathic MUAPs are most prominent in patients in whom the CK level is raised (Gath et al. 1969; Mastaglia and Walton 1971b). In some cases the EMG may only show features of a myopathic disorder. In these cases neurogenic features evident in the muscle biopsy indicate a diagnosis of Kugelberg–Welander syndrome, and there is discordance between the electromyographic and clinical features (Black et al. 1974). The significance of this problem is discussed in Chap. 4.

Motor conduction velocity is slowed in Type I SMA (Moosa and Dubowitz 1976), but is normal in the other clinical types of SMA (Schwartz and Moosa 1977). Motor and sensory conduction velocity in normal children in the arm is >30 m/s by age 3 months, and >40 m/s by 1 year of age (Moosa and Dubowitz 1976). Sensory nerve conduction velocity is normal in children with Type I SMA (Schwartz and Moosa 1977), although involvement of sensory fibres has been reported in pathological studies (Marshall and Duchen 1975).

Needle electromyography shows fibrillations and positive sharp waves in all forms of SMA, but they are more prominent in SMA Type I than in the other forms of SMA. Fibrillations are widespread; they occurred in 100% of cases of Type I SMA studied by Hausmanowa-Petrusewicz (1978). In Type III SMA fibrillations are less widely distributed than in Werdnig–Hoffmann disease, occurring in about 60% of cases (Namba et al. 1970). Fasciculation potentials are uncommon in Type I SMA, occurring in about 20% of cases, but are more frequent, occurring in 50% of cases, in Type III SMA (Swift 1984). Complex repetitive discharges are relatively common in Type III SMA, but are rare in Type I SMA. A feature unique to Type I SMA is that MUAPs discharging spontaneously at 5–15 Hz can be recorded from limb muscles apparently at rest

(Hausmanova-Petrusewicz and Karwanska 1986). This activity may persist for hours, even during sleep and was found in 75% of cases irrespective of severity and duration of the disease by Buchthal and Olsen (1970).

During voluntary activity the interference pattern is reduced in all forms of SMA; this may be particularly prominent in Type I SMA in which only single motor units, firing at a rapid rate, may be activated (Kimura 1983). Reduction in the interference pattern is evidence of loss of motor units. The amplitude of surviving motor units may be increased in all forms of SMA but MUAPs of greater amplitude than 10 mV (giant units) are rare in Type I SMA, and are seen in a third of cases of Type III SMA (Swift 1984). The percentage of high-amplitude MUAPs, and of MUAPs of increased duration in Type III SMA, increases with increasing duration of the disease (Hausmanowa-Petrusewicz et al. 1981; Hausmanowa–Petrusewicz and Karwanska 1986). In the more advanced cases of Types III and IV SMA small polyphasic MUAPs, resembling myopathic potentials, are noted (Kugelberg 1949). They can be correlated with the development of secondary myopathic change in the muscle biopsy of these cases (Schwartz et al. 1976a). In Type I SMA small, polyphasic potentials may also be recorded, but these wave forms are of varying shape, representing intermittent impulse blocking within the motor units. This abnormality is sometimes consistent with the decremental responses noted in MUAPs evoked by nerve stimulation at both slow and fast rates in some cases of Type I SMA (Kimura 1983).

Single-fibre EMG recordings require controlled voluntary activation and the technique is thus difficult to apply to very young children. Single-fibre EMG shows prominent abnormalities in Type III SMA (Fig. 6.4). The fibre density, on average, is more than twice normal and it may reach a value of 9.0 (Stålberg et al. 1975b). It is most increased in chronic cases. The duration of individual MUAPs is variable; very late components (40 ms or more) may be seen but other potentials are of normal duration. Although many potentials show increased neuromuscular jitter and impulse blocking, generally only one or two of the components of an MUAP show this instability. The initial components of these potentials are usually stable; later components are more likely to show increased neuromuscular jitter or impulse blocking (Fig. 6.5). Stålberg et al. (1975b) found that the later components of the MUAP in a case of Kugelberg–Welander syndrome had a much slower propagation velocity of the wave of depolarisation of the muscle fibre membrane (the speed of conduction along the muscle fibre itself, measured with a multi-electrode) than the earlier components.

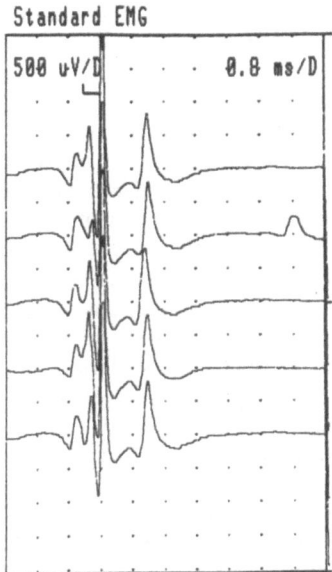

Fig. 6.4. Type III SMA. Concentric needle EMG. 500 Hz low-frequency filter. Complex stable potential of normal duration.

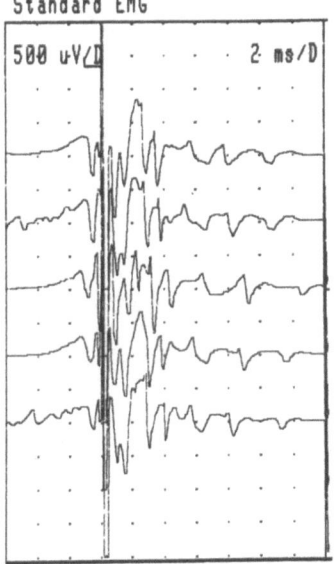

Fig. 6.5. Type III SMA. Concentric needle EMG. 500 Hz low-frequency filter. There is increased jitter and blocking of late components and the MUAP is of increased duration (about 10 ms).

This observation implies that the later components represent action potentials recorded from smaller muscle fibres, as propagation velocity is inversely related to fibre size (Håkanson 1956). In some MUAPs, recorded with single-fibre EMG, individual components are separated from each other by comparatively long intervals, a finding commonly associated with myopathic disorders. We have studied a number of children with the Type II form of SMA and have found similar abnormalities to those in Type III SMA.

Macro EMG recordings show an increased amplitude in 25% of the potentials studied in Type III SMA, indicating an increase in the number of fibres in the motor unit (Stålberg 1985).

Pathology

Muscle biopsy is often utilised to establish diagnosis in the spinal muscular atrophies. The hallmark of the muscle pathology is evidence of denervation and reinnervation. The appearances in Type II, III and IV SMA are generally similar, but Type I SMA shows unique features probably due both to the fact that biopsies of patients with this disorder are made in the first few months of life, and to the onset of the disease in most cases prior to birth, at a stage when muscle fibre development is still in progress.

In the muscle biopsy of Type I SMA the characteristic features are the presence of large groups of small atrophic fibres, often encompassing whole fascicles. Scattered hypertrophied fibres, often three to four times normal size, may be present in small clusters with these atrophic fibres, and inter-fascicular fibrosis is often present (Fig. 6.6a). The atrophic fibres are usually round rather than angular as in other neurogenic disorders and they usually show incomplete fibre-type grouping. Both fibre types show these changes but the hypertrophied fibres are more commonly Type I fibres (Dubowitz and Brooke 1973). The small fibres may be poorly Type II differentiated (Fig. 6.6b). The muscle spindles appear normal, but are unusually prominent, probably because the extensive fibre atrophy and loss of fibres occurring in the disease has allowed them to become more closely spaced than usual (Swash and Fox 1974).

The origin of the rounded atrophic fibres, which occur in sheets of fibres of slightly varying size and of mixed histochemical types, is uncertain. They show histological features similar to those of immature fibres and the phenomenon might therefore be due to maturational arrest during development. One explanation put forward is that it results from widespread loss of anterior horn cells which have previously contributed to reinnervation of denervated muscle fibres in utero. The reinnervation itself may have been maintained for too short a period to cause a complete change in histochemical fibre-type profile in the reinnervated fibres, or the neuron itself may have been unable to complete this trans-

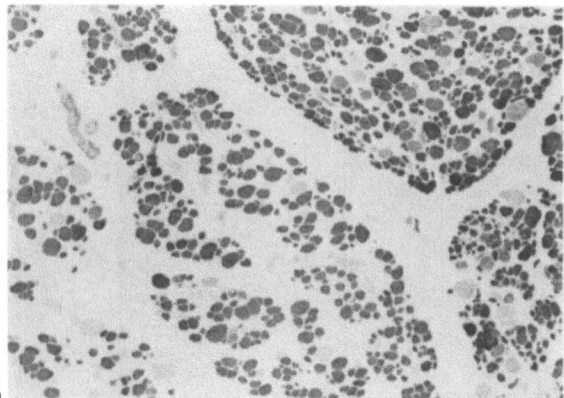

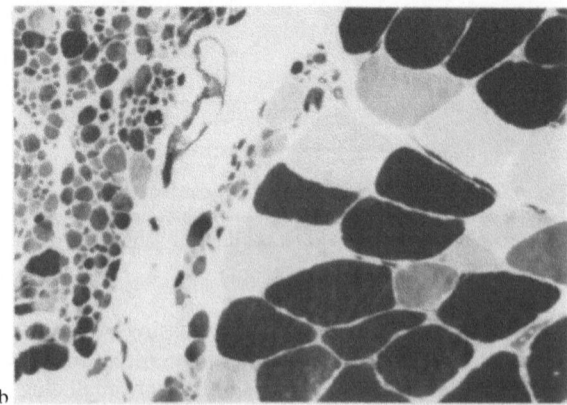

Fig. 6.6a. Type I SMA. ATPase pH 9.4 × 560. There is widespread fibre atrophy without fibre-type grouping. Larger Type I fibres are present. There is prominent thickening of the interfascicular connective tissue. **b** Type II SMA. ATPase pH 4.6 × 560. One fascicle is relatively preserved, but there are small rounded atrophic fibres in this fascicle and in the adjacent fascicle.

formation because it was already affected by the underlying disease process. Little is known about the time course of abnormality in the anterior horn cells in any of this group of neurogenic disorders. Hausmanowa-Petrusewicz et al. (1975, 1980) have suggested that the presence of immature fibres is due to arrest of their development occurring because of denervation, or even failure of innervation, in fetal life. The presence of persistent fetal fibres then interferes with the normal development of fibres within the muscle by preventing the orderly innervation and maturation of other muscle fibres. The ultrastructural features of the small, round fibres are very similar to those of fetal muscle at an early stage of development, and this hypothesis thus seems likely to be correct.

The atrophic fibres express fetal myosin heavy chain isoforms in Types II and III SMA, and these fibres tend also to express vimentin and desmin, whereas more mature, innervated fibres express either slow or fast myosin isoforms and do not show the characteristic features of undifferentiated muscle (Ben Hamida et al. 1994). The hypertrophied fibres show unusual histochemical features. Although usually Type I fibres according to the ATPase-based classification, they may react strongly or weakly for NADH and thus are not as clearly defined as normal Type I fibres. Fibre hypertrophy often occurs in weak muscles as a compensatory response to loss of muscle fibres, the remaining fibres being subject to increased load, and this is the probable cause of fibre hypertrophy in Werdnig–Hoffmann disease, as in other neurogenic and myopathic disorders. The predilection for Type I fibre hypertrophy in Werdnig–Hoffmann disease, however, is unexplained.

The pattern of innervation of muscle was studied by Woolf (1960) who found, in methylene blue preparations, that intramuscular motor axons terminated in a tangle of fine, beaded axons, with poorly formed motor end-plates. He interpreted this phenomenon as evidence of a severe "dying-back" disorder (Cavanagh 1964). In muscle biopsies intramuscular nerve twigs, if present, show almost complete absence of myelinated nerve fibres.

In the spinal cord there is widespread loss of anterior horn cells at all levels, with similar changes in the motor nuclei of the cranial nerves. The lumbar anterior horn cells are particularly severely affected (Marshall and Duchen 1975). Chou and Nonaka (1978) observed glial proliferation in the subpial zone of the ventral roots and suggested that this might account for degeneration in the lower motor neuron by compressing motor axons at this site. Malamud (1968) noted that the spinal cord appeared small and immature, with underdeveloped anterior horns, in two cases. The corticospinal tracts may also be relatively poorly myelinated for chronological age. In the sensory systems there may be degeneration of cells in the dorsal root ganglia with pallor of the posterior columns (Marshall and Duchen 1975). Fidzianska-Dolot and Hausmanowa-Petrusewicz (1984) have pointed out that the presence of anterior horn cells with immature features, and the presence of immature or "fetal" muscle fibres in the muscle in Type I SMA suggests that in this disease there is impairment of maturation of the lower motor neuron during development. Remaining anterior horn motor neurons do not contain ubiquitin deposits, unlike the pathognomonic features of amyotrophic lateral sclerosis.

The muscle biopsy in Type III SMA shows rather different features. In some cases the biopsy may show only mild changes, consisting of small groups of fibres of similar histochemical type, containing fibres of relatively normal size. Patients with the mildest form of the disease show fibre-type group-

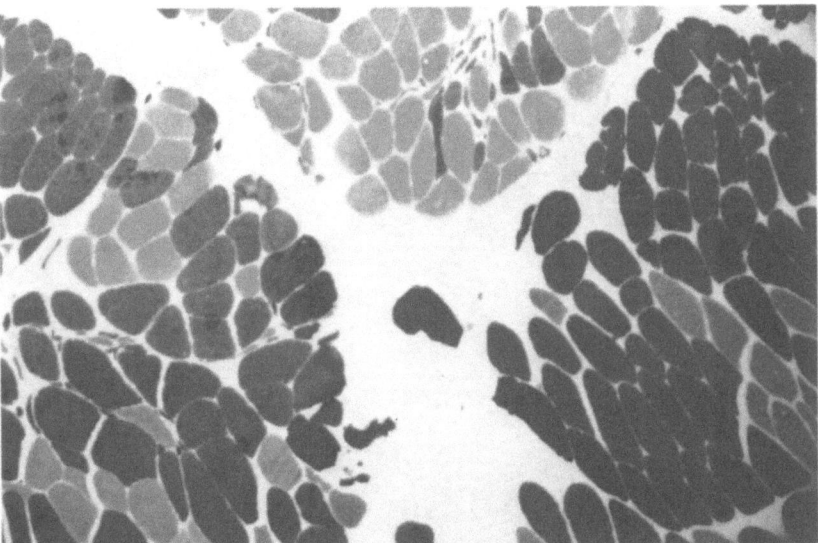

Fig. 6.7. Kugelberg–Welander disease. Fibre-type grouping: both Type I and Type II fibres are affected and there are scattered small pointed denervated fibres of both fibre types. Myosin ATPase, pH 4.3. × 140

ing in their biopsies, with few atrophic fibres. These features indicate only slight loss of motor neurons, with effective collateral reinnervation. In more severe cases, the biopsy appearance varies according to the duration of the illness. In children small fibres predominate with prominent fibre-type grouping. Later in the course of the disease well-marked fibre-type grouping is the major feature, with grouped atrophy or clusters of small, pointed atrophic fibres (Fig. 6.7). Individual fascicles may be composed entirely of hypertrophied fibres, others of atrophied fibres, and others mixed (Ben Hamida et al. 1994).

Hypertrophied fibres are often very prominent, reaching 100–150 μm in diameter. Hypertrophy probably represents work hypertrophy of the inner-vated muscle fibres, and it particularly affects Type I fibres (Swash and Schwartz 1977). These fibres often show fibre splitting, and central nucleation, espe-cially when they are examined in serial transverse sections. Even within areas of fibre-type grouping there may be some variation in fibre size and in some biopsies this feature is very prominent. In these biopsies other features suggestive of "myo-pathic" change may be found, consisting of in-creased numbers of central nuclei, longitudinal fibre splitting, particularly affecting Type I fibres, moth-eaten and whorled fibres (Fig. 6.8), seen best in NADH preparations, and in the later stages, fibrosis and fat replacement. Small basophilic regenerating

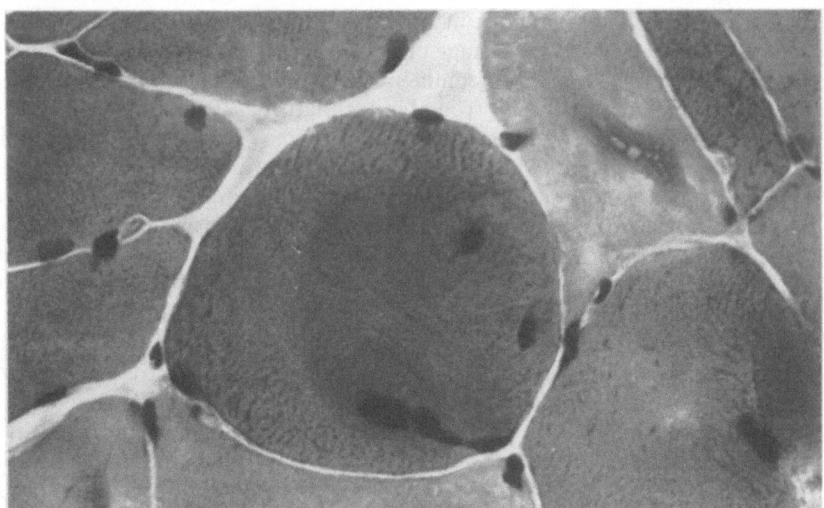

Fig. 6.8. Kugelberg–Welander disease. A whorled fibre, contain-ing several nuclei. H and E, × 560.

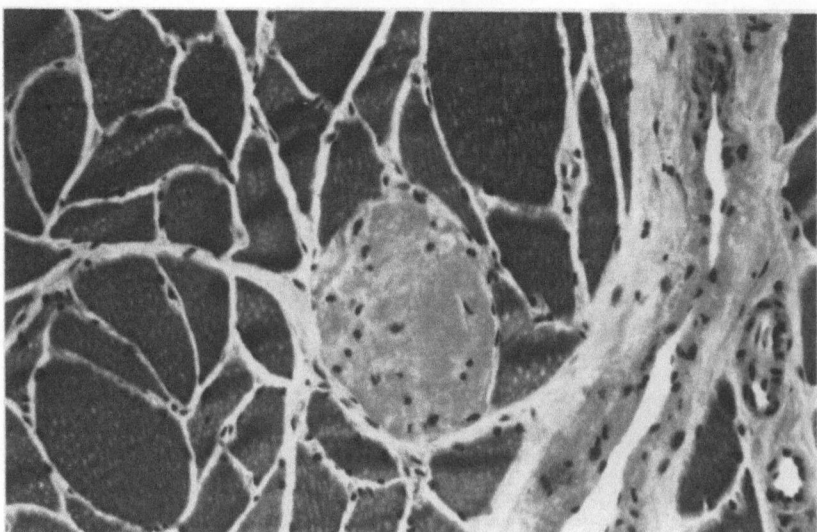

Fig. 6.9. Kugelberg–Welander disease. A necrotic fibre. H and E, × 350.

fibres, and pale necrotic fibres (Fig. 6.9) sometimes showing phagocytosis, may also be found. These features may be so prominent, in longstanding cases, that they suggest a diagnosis of myopathy, but the fibre-type grouping found in the ATPase preparations is the clue to the primary neurogenic disorder. The myopathic changes are thus secondary features (Schwartz et al. 1976a); their pathogenesis is discussed in Chap. 4. The myopathic features can be correlated with the myopathic potentials recorded with conventional EMG (Gath et al. 1969).

Small, rounded, poorly differentiated fibres, like those found in Werdnig–Hoffmann disease, are also a feature of Kugelberg–Welander disease (Type III SMA) and Hausmanowa-Petrusewicz et al. (1980) have suggested that this observation is evidence that the disorder also probably begins during development, in utero, but at a later stage of development than that at which Type I SMA commences. The relative proportions of small, rounded immature fibres, normal fibres and hypertrophied fibres, together with the extent of fibre-type grouping, may thus be a measure of severity of the disorder. In those cases with grouped atrophy, or scattered small pointed fibres, collateral reinnervation has proved ineffective, probably because of loss of large numbers of anterior horn cells. The development of secondary "myopathic" change probably reflects damage to individual muscle fibres in the later stages of the disease when reinnervation has developed to its maximal degree and effective movement is still possible.

The central nervous system in Type III SMA has been studied in only a few autopsies. There is loss of anterior horn cells, with degenerated, pyknotic cells adjacent to normal cells. This differs from Type I SMA in which all the anterior horn cells are abnormal. In Type III SMA the brain and brainstem are normal (Gardner-Medwin et al. 1967; Tomlinson et al. 1974). Remaining motor cells are nor ubiquitinated.

In Type II SMA the abnormalities in the muscle biopsy resemble those found in Werdnig–Hoffmann disease, but large groups of atrophic fibres are not commonly found (Fig. 6.4b). Rounded hypertrophied fibres, usually Type I fibres, occur and the smaller fibres also tend to be rounded, and not angulated as in other neurogenic disorders. In older patients, who have entered a stable phase of the disease, secondary "myopathic" changes, consisting of increased central nucleation and fibre splitting, may be found and it is in these patients that the higher CK levels are found. It is important to recognise that the changes found in the muscle biopsy in Type II SMA are not a reliable indicator of the prognosis (Dubowitz and Brooke 1973), as in this disorder the abnormality in the muscle biopsy may be indistinguishable from that found in the severe form of infantile muscular atrophy (Type I SMA).

In general the electrophysiological and pathological features of the less common varieties of SMA (Table 6.2) resemble those of the major types (Table 6.1). The abnormalities found in these investigations are often quite marked in clinically weak or wasted muscles, but may be much less prominent, or even normal, in clinically unaffected muscles. Further understanding of the spinal muscular atrophies may follow studies of the spontaneously occurring dominantly inherited disorder found in the Brittany spaniel (Sack et al. 1984), in which alterations in neurofilament in MRNA have been described (Muma and Cork 1993), and intense ubiquitination of of the peripheral neuronal cytoplasm has been found in surviving motor neurons (Hiraga et al. 1993). Schmalbruch et al. (1991) reported an autosomal mouse mutant.

Management and Treatment

In all SMA syndromes three disabilities require management. These are skeletal deformities, respiratory complications and contractures. All should be prevented by appropriate measures whenever possible.

In the severe infantile Type I SMA form no specific treatment is possible. Bulbar weakness may necessitate tube feeding, but this carries a risk of inhalational pneumonia. Respiratory assistance is rarely required before the extent of the disease and its severity is evident, and death usually results from ventilatory failure. Chest drainage and lying in bed in the prone posture may be useful in preventing pulmonary complications.

In the intermediate Type II form, the most important aspect is the prevention or treatment of skeletal deformities, especially scoliosis. Even when the spine is still straight the affected child should be fitted with an appropriate lightweight spinal support; the child should sit upright and not slumped to one side. If scoliosis does develop to beyond 50° surgical procedures will be required to straighten the spine, e.g. Milwaukee brace, Harrington rods or Luqué procedure. Scoliosis is more likely to develop in ambulatory children. Many affected children with Type II SMA can ambulate with long leg calipers from the age of about 5 years, with the aid of sticks, but others remain wheelchair-bound. Hip deformity may impair walking, but probably does not require treatment (Watt and Greenhill 1984). Contractures must be prevented by physiotherapy as necessary.

In Type III SMA no treatment may be required until weakness is relatively marked, since the growth phase is relatively normal. Contractures may develop later and if the patient becomes chairbound scoliosis may be a hazard. These can be prevented by appropriate splints, well-designed chairs, and by intermittent physiotherapy. For example, contractures of the ankles and feet can be prevented by lightweight plastic foot supports fitted while the foot is weak but not yet deformed (Watt and Greenhill 1984). The usual problems of immobilisation, including skin sores, osteoporosis, renal stones and joint and skeletal pain, may develop at this stage of the disease. Respiratory problems may dominate the clinical picture in the later stages of Type II and Type III SMA and it is important to avoid recurrent infections and bronchiectasis by careful physiotherapy and chest drainage as required.

Genetics and Genetic Counselling

The three major SMA syndromes of childhood onset, i.e. Type I SMA, Type II SMA and Type III SMA, are inherited as autosomal recessive disorders. The defective gene in each of these three syndromes is located on chromosome 5q at the 11.2–13.3 locus (Melki et al. 1990). Autosomal dominant proximal SMA syndromes are not linked to chromosome 5q (Kausch et al. 1991). A prenatal diagnosis is possible in the commonest forms of the disease, the autosomal recessive SMA syndromes, in informative families (Brzusnowicz et al. 1990), even though the putative gene product, and the DNA abnormality, or abnormalities, have not yet been identified.

Older studies have suggested a gene frequency for SMA Type I of 1 in 80 (Pearn 1982, 1983), allowing a calculated risk to children of unaffected siblings of 1 in 480 ($\frac{2}{3} \times \frac{1}{80} \times \frac{1}{4}$), assuming no parental consanguinity. SMA occurs with equal frequency (1 in 20 000 live births) in all races, and in all parts of the world, except where there is consanguinity, as in certain Moslem countries (Hausmanowa-Petrusewicz 1978; Pearn 1982; Hausmanowa-Petrusewicz et al. 1984). Hausmanowa-Petrusewicz et al. (1984) found that 63% of cases of SMA Type III were males in Poland but this effect has not been observed elsewhere. A few instances have been recorded of SMA of infantile and late childhood type in the same family; Gardner-Medwin et al. (1967) reported two brothers with onset at age 18 months and 15 years respectively, and another sibship with onset at birth and 4 years. Munsat et al. (1969) noted that four of their cases of typical Type I SMA had prolonged survival, but these would now be classified as Type II (intermediate) SMA. Clearly, these phenotypic variations will better be understood when the genetic locus for autosomal recessive SMA has been characterised.

X-linked Recessive, Bulbospinal SMA (Kennedy Syndrome)

This syndrome, consisting of progressive muscular weakness and wasting affecting bulbar and spinal musculature with gynaecomastia and reduced fertility, usually presents between the third and fifth decade (Kennedy et al. 1968). Proximal muscles are

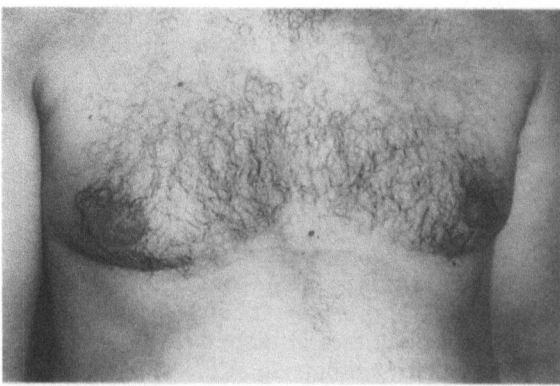

Fig. 6.10. Gynaecomastia in Kennedy syndrome; x-lined bulbospinal muscular atrophy.

often affected first, and lingual and facial fasciculations are prominent, so that a diagnosis of ALS may be suspected, but the tendon reflexes are reduced and the plantar responses are flexor. Resting or contraction fasciculations in the facial muscles are probably characteristic of the disease (Harding et al. 1982). Distal muscles are affected only later in the disease, but dysphagia and dysarthria may be prominent early features. Life expectancy is thought to be normal (Tsukagoshi et al. 1970; Arbiza et al. 1983; Schiffer et al. 1986). The CK is raised up to five times normal. The disease may progress only very slowly after a relatively rapid onset.

Gynaecomastia (Fig 6.10) is an evident feature of about half the cases, but oligospermia, testicular atrophy, impotence and elevated gonadotrophin levels are found (Warner et al. 1990). These endocrine anomalies are the result of androgen insensitivity. A high incidence of diabetes mellitus has been noted in Japanese cases (Sobue et al. 1989). The CSF is normal.

Electrophysiological Assessment

Motor nerve conduction studies are normal. The sural sensory nerve action potential is usually small or absent (Harding et al. 1982; Serratrice et al. 1988). EMG shows chronic partial denervation. EMG analysis of the facial muscles reveals repetitive discharges of groups of motor units resembling myokymia, or single motor unit discharges occurring repetitively (Olney et al. 1991); both these EMG abnormalities occur during volitional activity rather than spontaneously. True fasciculations are relatively uncommon in Kennedy syndrome, the clinical observation of spontaneous activity representing volitionally induced repetitive motor unit activity.

Distal muscle EMG studies are often nearly normal in the early phase of the disease.

Inheritance and Pathogenesis

The association with testicular dysfunction led to the recognition of an abnormality in androgen receptor function and to speculation on the role of androgen receptors in anterior horn cell survival and function. Genetic analysis has revealed a trinucleotide repeat sequence in the androgen gene on the proximal long arm of the X chromosome (Fischbeck et al. 1986) consisting of an expansion in the number of CAG repeats in a polymorphism in this location. The severity of the disease correlates with the degree of genetic abnormality, i.e. with the number of CAG repeats, as is the case in myotonic dystrophy in which a trinucleotide repeat occurs on a different chromosome (La Spada et al. 1991, 1992; Igorashi et al. 1992). How this genetic defect leads to the phenotypic expression of the disease is not yet understood.

Pathology

Several autopsies have been reported. Sobue et al. (1989) described three autopsies together with sural nerve pathology in a further six cases and reviewed the previous data. They found loss of neurons in the Vth, VIIth and XIIth nerve nuclei with relative sparing of the IIIrd, IVth and VIth cranial nerve nuclei. There was myelin pallor in the gracile columns but the corticospinal tracts were normal. The spinal roots showed loss of large myelinated fibres. Neurons were preserved in the nucleus of Clarke's column, in the intermedio-lateral cell columns and in Onuf's sacral nucleus. The latter nucleus innervates the pelvic floor striated sphincter muscles. Terai et al. (1994) studied the spinal cord at the L4 level in two cases in a comparative study of ALS, Kennedy syndrome and multiple system atrophy. They found that Kennedy syndrome was characterised by profound loss of large and medium-sized motor neurons in the medial zone, probably consistent with the paraspinal distribution of weakness found in the disease.

Management

No direct treatment is available. Diagnosis by DNA testing is important in establishing that the patient does not suffer from ALS, but clinical diagnosis is usually possible at the bedside. The prognosis is generally good, and bulbar failure does not usually occur (Kennedy et al. 1968). Genetic counselling can be given to family members on the basis of DNA testing of potential carriers or potential disease sufferers, based on family data.

Motor Neuron Disease

Motor neuron disease is a progressive disorder characterised by muscular wasting and weakness, with fasciculation, and by spasticity, hyperreflexia and extensor plantar responses. Bulbar involvement is frequently prominent, leading to dysphagia and dysarthria, but external ocular muscles are almost invariably spared. Sensory symptoms may occur but there are no objective sensory signs. The first case recognisable in the literature appears to be that of a French circus owner, Prosper Laconte, who died in 1853 (Veltana 1975), but the disease was first clearly described by Charcot (1869) who used the term *amyotrophic lateral sclerosis*. Motor neuron disease was formerly regarded as occurring in three forms; *progressive muscular atrophy, progressive bulbar palsy* and *amyotrophic lateral sclerosis*. These subdivisions reflect older concepts of nosology and they are now usually accepted as variations on a common theme, relatively severe muscular atrophy indicating predominant anterior horn cell disease and prominent spasticity and hyperreflexia being a sign of severe corticospinal tract involvement. *Primary lateral sclerosis*, a term reflecting the relatively isolated involvement of corticospinal tracts, is a rare related disorder.

Pathologically the whole motor system is involved, including the motor cortex, the posterior limb of the internal capsule, corticospinal pathways in brainstem and spinal cord, the motor neurons of the bulbar nuclei, usually with much less marked involvement of the IIIrd, IVth and VIth nerve nuclei, and degeneration of the anterior horn cells of the spinal cord. Secondary degeneration of the anterior spinal roots and motor nerve fibres occurs and there is widespread neurogenic atrophy in the skeletal muscles. In addition there may be involvement of spinocerebellar tracts and, in some cases, of the dorsal root ganglia and of axons in the posterior columns, but this does not result in clinically apparent sensory disturbance (see Oppenheimer 1976; Kawamura et al. 1981). In view of the similar pattern of pathological involvement of the motor system in these three forms an all-encompassing term such as motor neuron disease is probably justified. In some countries, particularly in the USA, the term amyotrophic lateral sclerosis (ALS) is used interchangeably with motor neuron disease (MND) in this general sense. Nonetheless recognition of the clinical subtypes of MND may be of value in prognosis, as will be discussed later.

Epidemiology

Motor neuron disease accounts for about 0.1% of adult deaths (Kondo 1978). It has an incidence of 0.4–2.0/100 000 (Juergens et al. 1980; Kurtzke 1982, 1985; Yoshida et al. 1986). The prevalence of the disease has been estimated at 2–6/100 000 although areas of increased prevalence, such as Guam, and the Kii peninsula of Japan, have been described in which a related disease is as much as 100 times more common (see reviews by Kondo 1978; Kurtzke 1985). Epidemiological surveillance of this Western Pacific form of ALS has shown a decrease in incidence from 50/100 000 in 1950 to 5/100 000 in 1990 (Kurland et al. 1994).

Motor neuron disease in Western countries is a disease of late middle life but the age-specific incidence and mortality rates increase with increasing age (Juergens et al. 1980; Li et al. 1985); the average age of onset in a survey of the disease in Finland was 58 years (Jokelainen 1977a). It is uncommon before the age of 40 years; 90% of cases begin between the ages of 40 and 70 years (Jokelainen 1977b). The median age of onset is 55 years (Juergens et al. 1980) and the mean age of death is 64 years (Neilson et al. 1994). There is a sharp decline in mortality after the age of 75 years. Most studies have shown that there is a slight predominance of cases in men; the male/female ratio is about 1.5 : 1.0 (Kondo 1978). There is a family history of motor neuron disease in 5%–10% of cases. The duration of the disease is generally 2–5 years, although some patients die in less than a year and others may survive for 12 years or more (Jokelainen 1977b). Mulder and Howard (1976) and Mortara et al. (1984) found that 20% of their patients were still alive 5 years after the onset of the disorder, and 10% were living 10 years after onset, but these figures probably reflect selection of material (Mulder and Howard 1976). Cases with onset after age 65 years have a mean survival of less than 2 years, but onset before 65 years is associated with survival greater than 3 years (Jokelainen 1977b; Kondo 1978; Juergens et al. 1980).

Jokelainen (1977b) found that patients with predominant bulbar involvement survived for a mean period of 2.2 years, whereas those with mainly spinal signs survived for a mean period of 3.3 years. Patients with mixed spinal and bulbar features had an intermediate prognosis. Patients with a much longer clinical course were not included in this assessment, since they were still alive; these patients probably had little or no bulbar involvement. Generally, the earlier the age of onset, the longer the survival (Jokelainen 1977b; Kondo 1978). The median survival of patients with the syndrome of progressive muscular atrophy was 10 years in the series described by Mortara et al. (1984). In amyotrophic lateral sclerosis the median survival was 4.3 years in one series (Caroscio et al. 1984).

Eisen et al. (1993) reported a prospective study of 246 patients of whom 138 died during the study. Disease duration in patients aged less than 40 years at presentation was 8.2 years; with onset in the seventh decade it was 2.6 years. Average duration was 4 years in men and 3.2 years in women, a difference that was not important. In people aged less than 40 years the sex ratio was 3.6 men to 1 woman. There was no difference in survival between men and women, or in bulbar versus non-bulbar onset cases.

A rising trend in both the incidence and mortality of the disease has been reported from several different countries (Durrleman and Alperovitch 1989; Flaten 1989; Lilienfeld et al. 1989). The cause of these trends has proved controversial. The suggestion that it might be due to an artefact of increased recognition of existing cases of the disease at diagnosis or death (Swash et al. 1989; Williams and Windebank 1991) has been challenged. Neilson et al. (1994), applying a Gompertzian model to the analysis of mortality data, concluded that the evolving mortality pattern of ALS is attributable to changing inter-disease competition resulting from the increased life expectancy of the population rather than to changing causative factors.

Clinical Features

The first symptom is normally weakness. This is usually first recognised as undue fatiguability, dragging of a leg during walking, or difficulty manipulating objects with the fingers (Fig. 6.11). This presentation occurred in 63% of 318 patients studied by Gubbay et al. (1985), and a similar frequency of this presenting symptom has been noted by others (Mulder and Espinoza 1969; Jokelainen 1977b; Rosati et al. 1977). In Jokelainen's series weakness of a leg was a slightly more common presenting feature than weakness of an arm. Monoparesis affected 23% and hemiparesis 4% of the series of Gubbay et al. (1985). Weakness of both legs was the presentation in 20%, and bulbar features were the presenting problem in 22% (Gubbay et al. 1985). Other presenting features include muscle atrophy (10%), muscle pains and cramps (9%), fasciculations (4%) and stiffness of gait (1%). Weight loss (2%) and paraesthesiae (3%) are

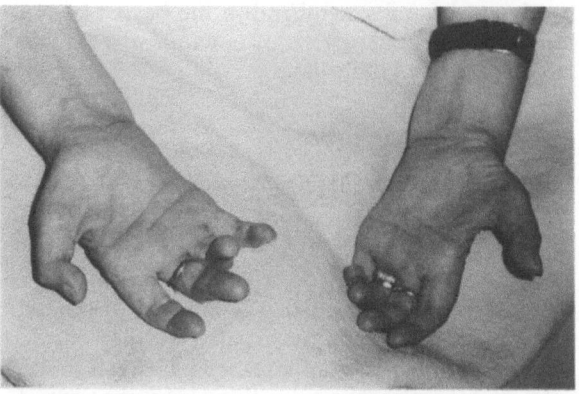

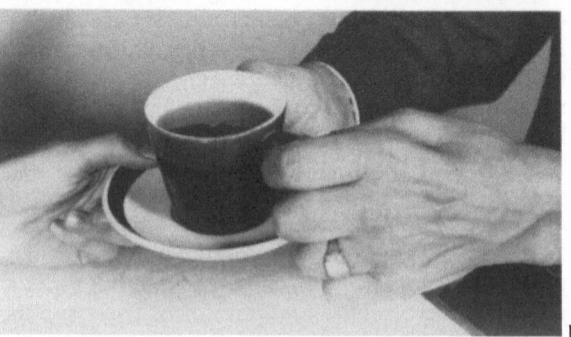

Fig. 6.11a, b. Wasting of the small hand muscles in motor neuron disease.

also occasionally presenting features of the disease (Gubbay et al. 1985). Sometimes a patient may notice ankle clonus as a first symptom, for example while driving. Exertional dyspnoea is a rare presentation (Sivak and Streib 1980). Belsh and Schiffman (1990) recorded similar initial symptoms in a study of misdiagnosis of ALS. The less common presentations tended to lead to misdiagnosis, or delay in diagnosis of 16 months or more.

Fasciculations, although uncommon as a presenting symptom, are frequently observed on examination. Nonetheless fasciculations are not themselves pathognomonic of motor neuron disease since they may occur in other myelopathies, e.g. cervical spondylosis, or in old poliomyelitis, and in some root or peripheral nerve disorders. Furthermore, fasciculations are quite common in normal subjects, especially after exercise. Reed and Kurland (1963) noted that 70% of a group of medically sophisticated people had experienced fasciculations, but only a quarter reported episodes of fasciculations more frequently than monthly. In motor neuron disease, fasciculations generally occur every 3 or 4 s, whereas benign fasciculations occur at a rate of about 1/s (Trojaborg and Buchthal 1965). When looking for fasciculations in motor neuron disease it is particularly important to examine the tongue carefully since fasciculations are easily detected in this muscle.

Although fasciculations, wasting and weakness may commence in a limited distribution, sooner or later the disease becomes generalised, especially in those patients with a longer survival. Spasticity, hyperreflexia and extensor plantar responses are characteristic features of almost all cases at some stage in the disease. However, severe lower motor neuron involvement may mask these upper motor neuron signs, and in some cases the degenerative process is largely limited to the lower motor neuron. Nonetheless the combination of atrophy and fasciculations of a limb muscle, with a very brisk tendon reflex, without sensory signs, is a rather characteristic feature of the disease. Only cervical spondylosis with myelopathy commonly mimics this finding. Cervical spondylosis is a common finding in patients with motor neuron disease because of the relative preponderance of both disorders in the age range affected and this may lead to problems in diagnosis. Brooks et al. (1994) noted that weakness developed faster in muscles in related spinal segments than more distally and involvement of other spinal segments is more likely than bulbar involvement, suggesting a proximity effect in spread of the disease process rather than a purely selective vulnerability model (Swash et al. 1986, 1988). Quantitative assessment of isometric force has shown a linear decline after the first year (Munsat et al. 1988; Ringel et al. 1994).

The urinary and anal sphincters are invariably spared. In an autopsy study Mannen et al. (1977) showed that a small group of anterior cells in the S3–4 segment, presumably innervating these voluntary sphincter muscles, were preserved. The autonomic nervous system is usually also spared, except in those patients with very prominent upper motor neuron signs. Extra-ocular movements are usually thought to be normal at the bedside, but abnormalities of pursuit movements consisting of a breakdown of smooth tracking into a series of saccadic interruptions, similar to those found in Parkinson's disease, have been reported (Jacobs et al. 1981). Rarely, partial or complete ophthalmoplegia has been described in advanced cases, with loss of motor cells from the cranial nerve nuclei subserving ocular muscles (Harvey et al. 1979).

Dementia is uncommon in patients with motor neuron disease, although Hudson (1981) noted that dementia of Alzheimer type occurred in the families of about 15% of patients with the sporadic form of motor neuron disease. David and Gillham (1986) found that patients with motor neuron disease were slightly impaired on tests of cognitive function, particularly picture recall, learning novel material and card sorting. These findings correlated with cerebral atrophy on CT scanning in these patients. Nearn et al. (1990) reported four patients in whom the clinical and pathological features of motor neuron disease were accompanied by a profound, rapidly progressive dementia with prominent frontal features, consisting of a bland, insight-less personality and disinhibition without specific neuropsychological deficits.

Although sensory symptoms, especially paraesthesiae, are frequent, sensory loss itself does not occur as a feature of the disease (Mulder 1982). Quantitative sensory testing in patients with motor neuron disease revealed an increased threshold to vibration in 14 of 80 patients (Mulder et al. 1983), but no change in other sensory modalities. Shahani and Russell (1969) found that ischaemic paraesthesiae are less likely to develop in patients with motor neuron disease than in controls. Heads et al. (1991) noted pathological changes in sural nerve biopsies consistent with a sensory neuronopathy.

Pressure sores are strikingly uncommon in ALS. Ono and colleagues have described decreased elasticity ("delayed return phenomenon" after skin pinch) associated with decreased collagen content, altered collagen cross-linkage and deposition of amorphous material which includes glycosaminoglycans in skin in the disease. It is uncertain, however, whether these changes are secondary to immobility and nutritional change, or have primary importance (Ono et al. 1994). The former seems more likely.

The majority of patients with motor neuron diseases show features of both upper and lower motor neuron disturbance in the limbs, hence the term *amyotrophic lateral sclerosis (ALS)*. The other clinical types of the disease are less common, and primary lateral sclerosis itself is rare (Table 6.3).

Table 6.3. Incidence and sex distribution of different clinical forms of motor neuron disease

	Sex ratio (M : F)	Incidence (% of all cases)
Amyotrophic lateral sclerosis	1.7	80
Progressive bulbar palsy	1.0	10
Progressive muscular atrophy	1.7	8
Primary lateral sclerosis	1.3	2

From Caroscio et al. (1984).

In *progressive bulbar palsy* the main presenting features are dysarthria and dysphagia, with difficulty in chewing. The tongue is weak and atrophic and fasciculations of the tongue may be prominent. Facial weakness is sometimes present. There is clinical evidence of combined upper and lower motor neuron involvement of the bulbar musculature, and similar abnormalities develop in the limbs during the course of the disease. The prognosis is determined by the severity of the bulbar abnormality.

In *progressive muscular atrophy* there is lower motor neuron involvement of limb muscles without definite evidence of upper motor neuron involvement. The tendon reflexes, however, are brisk even in the wasted muscles, a clinical feature that serves to differentiate this progressive disorder from adult-onset spinal muscular atrophy. The diagnosis of progressive muscular atrophy can only be considered in the absence of a family history of similar problems, and if the disorder begins after the age of 20 years (Mortara et al. 1984).

Primary lateral sclerosis is characterised both clinically and pathologically by degeneration restricted to the upper motor neuron. Pseudobulbar features may develop (Beal and Richardson 1981). Younger et al. (1988) described this syndrome, pointing out an onset after the age of 50 years, with symmetrical involvement of legs more than arms, predilection for men, and a progressive course in the absence of any identifiable cause.

Familial Motor Neuron Disease

About 5%–10% of cases of motor neuron disease are familial (Alter and Schaumann 1976). The majority of these cases show an autosomal dominant mode of inheritance, with adult onset. The clinical features resemble those of sporadic cases. Although several clinical differences have been reported, e.g. the mean age of onset is about a decade younger (45 years), the sex ratio is equal and the duration of the disease is slightly shorter (Emery and Holloway 1982), with a median survival of 2 years (Horton et al. 1976; Hawkes et al. 1984), subsequent descriptions have revealed few clinical differences between familial and sporadic cases (Li et al. 1988; Williams et al. 1988). Considerable phenotypic variation occurs in affected families, some patients showing pure lower motor neuron syndromes when probands developed the full amyotrophic lateral sclerosis syndrome (Siddique et al. 1989). Mulder et al. (1986) noted variability in age of onset, duration of disease and clinical features in affected families with the adult-onset syndrome.

Familial cases with prominent sensory features, including glove and stocking sensory loss, have also been reported but these cases fall outside the accepted definition of motor neuron disease (Horton et al. 1976). *Juvenile-onset* familial cases, with prolonged survival, of dominant or recessive inheritance and sometimes associated with demen-

tia, have been described (Myllyla et al. 1979; Emery and Holloway 1982). Ben Hamida and Hentati (1984) reported that a slowly progressive form of the disease, with onset before 30 years of age, is common in Tunisia. In southern India a sporadic, juvenile-onset form of amyotrophic lateral sclerosis is associated with deafness (Jagganathan 1973; Sayeed et al. 1975; Summers et al. 1987).

Differential Diagnosis

The typical clinical presentation of motor neuron disease is characteristic, with weakness, wasting and fasciculations (perhaps generalised) and with bulbar signs and evidence of bilateral corticospinal tract involvement with very brisk reflexes even in wasted muscles, in the absence of sensory signs (Table 6.4). It is uncommon for other disorders to produce this clinical picture. However, when motor neuron disease presents with disability limited to one limb, diagnosis may be more difficult.

Table 6.4. Diagnostic criteria (El Escorial criteria) for motor neuron disease (amyotrophic lateral sclerosis) proposed by the World Federation of Neurology Subcommittee on Motor Neuron Diseases

The diagnosis of ALS requires the presence of:
1. LMN signs (including EMG features in clinically normal muscles)
2. UMN signs
3. Progression of the disorder

The diagnosis of ALS requires the absence of the following clinical features:
1. Sensory signs
2. Sphincter disturbances
3. Visual disturbances
4. Autonomic dysfunction
5. Parkinson's disease
6. Alzheimer-type dementia
7. ALS "mimic" syndromes

The diagnosis of ALS is supported by the following features:
1. Fasciculation in one or more regions
2. Neurogenic change in EMG studies
3. Normal motor and sensory nerve conduction (distal motor latencies may be increased)
4. Absence of conduction block

Diagnostic categories:

Definite ALS	UMN plus LMN signs in 3 regions
Probable ALS	UMN plus LMN signs in 2 regions with UMN signs rostral to LMN signs
Possible ALS	UMN plus LMN signs in one region, or UMN signs in 2 or 3 regions, e.g. monomelic ALS, progressive bulbar palsy, and primary lateral sclerosis
Suspected ALS	LMN signs in 2 or 3 regions, e.g. progressive muscular atrophy, and other motor syndromes

Regions are defined as follows: brainstem, brachial, thorax and trunk, crural. UMN, upper motor neuron; LMN, lower motor neuron.
From Brooks (1994).

In the differential diagnosis, in particular, entrapment neuropathies, cervical or lumbar spondylosis, brachial neuritis, syringomyelia and multiple sclerosis must be considered. In most of these disorders, however, there will be absent reflexes or sensory signs and these should lead to appropriate investigation.

Motor neuropathies may also be mistaken for motor neuron disease (Chad et al. 1987) but in these cases the tendon reflexes are usually reduced or absent, an unusual finding in motor neuron disease, even in its late stages. Motor neuropathies involve legs more than arms. The syndrome of *multifocal motor neuropathy* (Krarup et al. 1990), however, may closely resemble motor neuron disease (Nobile-Orazio 1996). In 80% of cases weakness and wasting develops initially in the hands, is slowly progressive and asymmetrical and more frequent in men. Two-thirds of cases are younger than 45 years. Fasciculation may be present in weak muscles (Parry and Clarke 1988; Pestronk 1991). Conduction block in one or more nerves is an essential feature of this syndrome (Lewis et al. 1982b). Anti GM_1 antibodies are found in 30% (Lange and Trojaborg 1994) or more (Pestronk 1991) of these patients. In motor neuron disease conduction block is not a feature and anti GM_1 antibodies are found no more commonly than in control subjects (Willison et al. 1993). This syndrome is relatively uncommon in practice but is important since it is not a form of motor neuron disease, has a better prognosis and may respond to immunosuppressive treatment and immunoglobulin therapy (Van der Berg et al. 1995), (see chapter 11).

The most difficult differential clinical diagnosis is from *cervical and lumbar spondylosis with canal stenosis*, in which there may be upper and lower motor neuron signs in all four limbs, with fasciculations. However, sensory abnormalities usually occur in canal stenosis, although the sensory disorder may be subtle. In these patients the fasciculations are repeated at a faster rate than in motor neuron disease (Trojaborg and Buchthal 1965). The presence of bulbar involvement, particularly fasciculation of the tongue, in motor neuron disease is an especially important point in differential diagnosis and, of course, motor neuron disease and spondylosis may co-exist in patients in middle life. This problem may be difficult to resolve by any investigative technique, including EMG and neuroimaging.

Other neuromuscular disorders, such as polymyositis, should also be considered. Myasthenia gravis may also lead to diagnostic difficulties when there is bulbar involvement, but external ocular movements are characteristically spared in motor neuron disease. Hyperthyroid myopathy may present with systemic and bulbar involvement and fasciculation can occur in this disorder. Although the

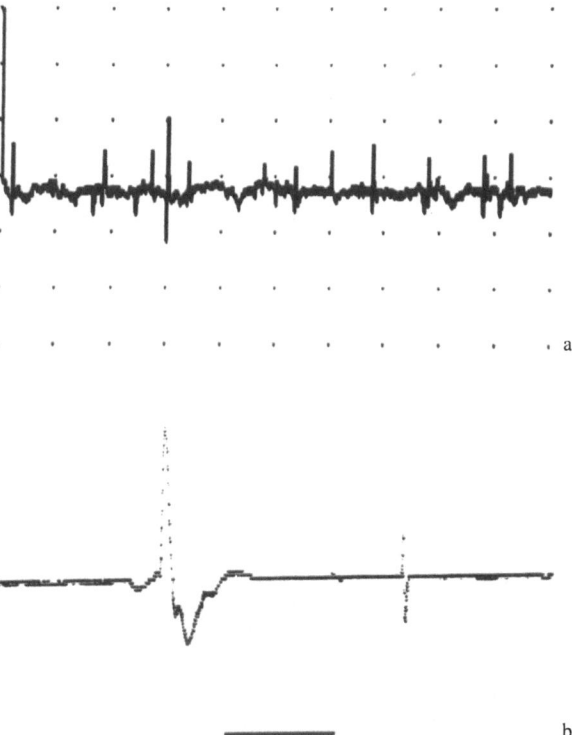

Fig. 6.12. Motor neuron disease: **a** Fibrillation potentials. **b** Polyphasic fasciculation potential, and fibrillation potential. Concentric needle EMG. Filters: 100 Hz and 100 kHz. Bar 20 ms.

reflexes are brisk in hyperthyroidism the signs of thyrotoxicosis itself usually give the clue to the underlying diagnosis. Hyperparathyroidism is also said to cause fasciculation. Adult onset spinal muscular atrophy differs in that there are no long tract signs at any stage of the illness and this feature, together with reduced reflexes, enables these two disorders to be distinguished even when the spinal form of motor neuron disease is only slowly progressive.

In *hexosaminidase deficiency* a motor neuron disorder may be associated with involvement of other neuronal systems, including cerebellum, cerebral cortex and peripheral nerve. The clinical manifestations and age of onset are variable (Mitsumoto et al. 1985).

Electrophysiological Assessment

With conventional, concentric needle EMG, fibrillation potentials (Fig. 6.12) and positive sharp waves, although not prominent, are almost invariably found, particularly in atrophic muscles. Fibrillations tend to become more prominent in the later stages of the disease (Goodgold and Eberstein 1983). Complex repetitive discharges are sometimes recorded.

Fasciculation potentials are often found. They may be very polyphasic (Fig. 6.12). They are more easily recorded when several surface electrodes, placed on different muscles, are used for simultaneous recording in a multi-channel recording system using several separate input amplifiers. This is a particularly convenient method for demonstrating involvement of upper and lower extremities in the disease. EMG sampling is much more sensitive than clinical observation in detecting fasciculations, revealing them to be widespread in motor neuron disease (Howard and Murray 1992). Howard and Murray (1992) found that in motor neuron disease fasciculations were recorded in more than five of eight muscle sites sampled. When fasciculations are less widespread another diagnosis should be suspected. In motor neuron disease fasciculations are usually repeated at a rate of about one per 3 or 4 s (Trojaborg and Buchthal 1965), but faster rates are occasionally found. Fasciculation at a slow rate was termed "malignant fasciculation" by Trojaborg and Buchthal (1965) to indicate its association with progressive motor neuron disease. These fasciculations usually appear to involve larger parts of a muscle than the benign fasciculations found in radiculopathies, or even in normal subjects. EMG studies demonstrate that in motor neuron disease fasciculations may occur repeatedly in the same motor unit. Although fasciculations are strongly associated, clinically, with anterior horn cell disease (Denny-Brown and Pennybacker 1938; Denny-Brown 1953), and have been thought to arise at or near the soma of motor neurons, Conradi et al. (1982), using a combination of collision techniques with single unit recordings and pharmacological experiments, have shown that fasciculations probably arise from distal sites of excitation within the motor axon arborisation (Roth 1984), or at the end-plate synaptic terminals themselves. About 10% of fasciculating motor units can be voluntarily activated (Guiloff and Modarres-Sadeghi 1992) and are mostly less complex low threshold units with conduction velocities between 30 and 45 m/s (Conradi et al. 1982). More complex fasciculations discharge at a lower rate than simpler fasciculations in motor neuron disease. The mean fibre density of fasciculations was increased (4.3) and the more complex the units the more unstable (Janko et al. 1989). The spike order of complex fasciculations varies suggesting that the generator site is multiple, perhaps rather distal in the case of units that cannot be voluntarily activated and more proximal in those that can be voluntarily activated. Axon reflexes may be involved when the generator site is distal (Janko et al. 1989).

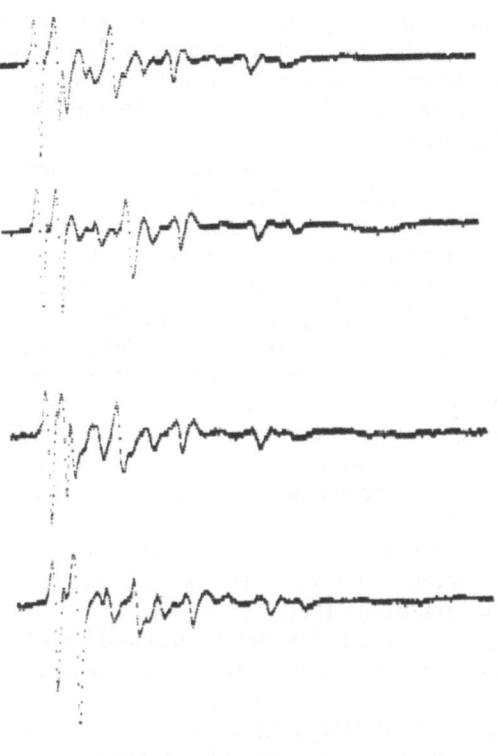

Fig. 6.13. Motor neuron disease: a triggered recording of a high-amplitude polyphasic motor unit action potential. Many components are seen and the potential is of increased duration (12 ms). Concentric needle EMG. Filters: 500 Hz and 10 kHz. Bar 4 ms.

On volition the MUAPs are typical of a neurogenic disorder. They are of increased amplitude, long duration and polyphasic (Fig. 6.13). The shape of the MUAPs may be highly unstable (Schwartz and Swash 1982). In atrophic muscles "giant" MUAPs (>12 mV) may be recorded; these are sometimes of very considerable amplitude (Erminio et al. 1959). The interference pattern in these atrophic muscles is usually greatly reduced and only single units may be recorded in any particular electrode position (Fig. 6.14).

Motor nerve conduction may be abnormal; in particular an increased distal motor latency (Lambert 1962) and a slightly slowed motor nerve conduction velocity may be found (Argyropoulos et al. 1978). This is more prominent in motor nerves supplying atrophic muscles and probably represents loss of the largest, fastest-conducting axons of large anterior horn cells; these are probably lost first in the disease. Sensory nerve conduction is normal, although occasionally small SNAPs may be found (Mondelli et al. 1993).

Repetitive nerve stimulation tests may show a decremental response at slow stimulation rates

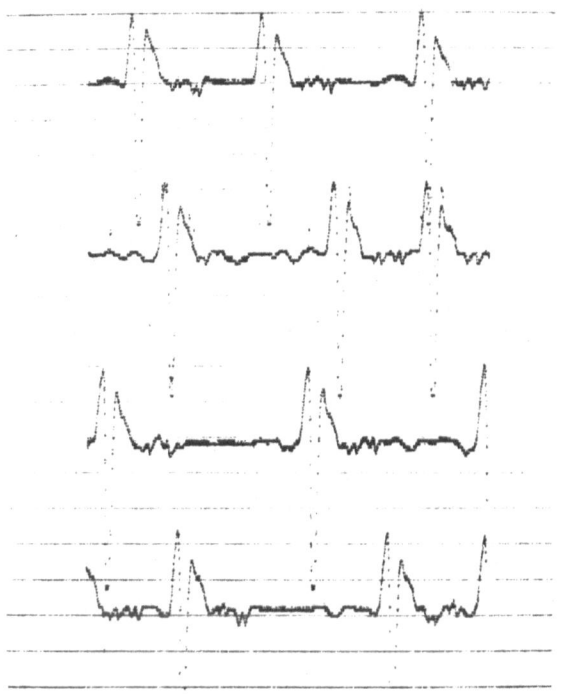

Fig. 6.14. Single unit activity during maximal volition. The unit is of high amplitude with a polyphasic following component of lower amplitude. Concentric needle EMG. Filters: 100 Hz and 10 kHz. Bar 20 ms.

(2 Hz), and potentiation at higher rates of stimulation (20 Hz) (Mulder et al. 1959). These abnormalities are found in about a third of patients, but neither of these abnormal responses to repetitive nerve stimulation is as prominent as that found in myasthenia gravis or in the myasthenic syndrome (Norris 1975). Killian et al. (1994) found a mean decrement of 10% in all patients tested, recording from trapezius, and noted abnormalities of greater severity in trapezius than in the hand. Bernstein and

Antel (1981) found that a decremental response to 2 Hz stimulation was associated with a rapidly progressive course, and atrophy of the muscle tested. Killian et al. (1994) found that the abnormality did not change in serial studies, and that it was not related to the duration of the disease. MEPP amplitudes are decreased in motor neuron disease (Maselli et al. 1993). This is due to reduced quantal content, quanta available for immediate release and quantal storage. These findings probably explain fatiguability and impaired neuromuscular transmission in the disease.

Single-fibre EMG provides further information. The fibre density is increased. It is most increased in weak muscles but is also increased in the limb muscles in patients with bulbar signs in whom there is no definite clinical evidence of the involvement of limb muscles (Stålberg et al. 1975a,b). Since the distribution of the neurogenic process is not uniform in different muscle groups, the EMG abnormalities may be strikingly different even in homologous muscles on the two sides of the body (Schwartz and Swash 1982; Swash and Schwartz 1982). These observations imply that the disease begins in certain motor neuron pools before it becomes generalised (Swash and Schwartz 1984). The neuromuscular jitter is increased in most potentials and usually several components of the MUAP complex show this increased jitter and impulse blocking (Fig. 6.15). The latter were observed in 20% of potentials by Stålberg et al. (1975b). The duration of the MUAPs recorded by single-fibre EMG is moderately increased but late units (units occurring >8ms after the first component of the motor unit action potential) are uncommon.

The different phases of the disorder can be staged on the basis of single-fibre EMG data as in Table 6.5.

In the first stage of the disease strength is normal and there is no detectable wasting of muscles, but the single-fibre EMG fibre density is slightly increased. This is the phase of early reinnervation. In the second stage, strength and muscle bulk remain normal but the fibre density has increased (>2.5). There may be some jitter and blocking. The latter is the first electrophysiological indication of impend-

Table 6.5. Stage of involvement of individual muscles in motor neuron disease

Stage	Strength	Wasting	Fibre density	Jitter and blocking	Interpretation
1	Normal	None	Normal or slightly increased (usually <2.5)	None or slightly increased	Phase of early reinnervation
2	Normal	None	Increased (>2.5)	Increased	Phase of well-compensated reinnervation
3	Weak and easily fatiguable	Often present	Markedly increased (>3.0)	Markedly increased	Phase of early decompensation: late reinnervation
4	Very weak	Prominent	Slightly increased: may not be recordable	Prominent if recordable	Late decompensated phase: reinnervation failure

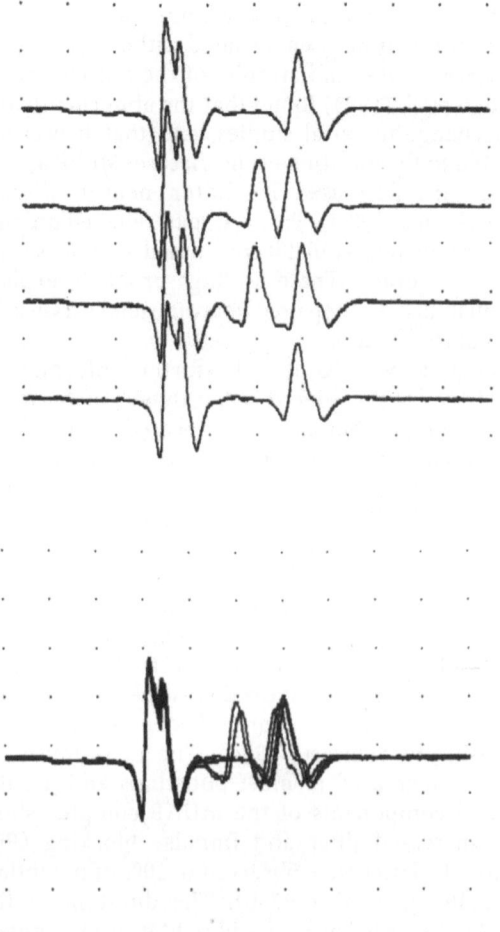

Fig. 6.15. Complex MUAP with two late units one showing jitter and blocking.

same patient at any particular time of observation. Further, it should be recognised that not only is there single-fibre EMG evidence of widespread involvement of anterior horn cells from the time of diagnosis, but the fibre density in this disorder does not increase to levels comparable with more chronic neurogenic conditions, particularly spinal muscular atrophy (Swash 1980), chronic neuropathies, syringomyelia, or poliomyelitis, indicating that the process of compensatory reinnervation is incomplete at all stages of the disease. This is consistent with the almost inevitably progressive course of the disease. The increased jitter in motor neuron disease probably results from a decreased safety factor for neuromuscular transmission at motor end-plates or in the terminal axonal tree. Impulse blockings in motor neuron disease are important in relation to the clinical phenomenon of fatiguability, and to the decremental response to repetitive nerve stimulation; these phenomena are similar to the findings in myasthenia gravis and myasthenic syndrome and probably reflect abnormalities in transmitter release.

The "giant" potentials recorded with concentric needle EMG represent the summation of single muscle fibre action potentials within an individual motor unit of increased size and compactness; this is probably evidence of fibre-type grouping. In Kugelberg–Welander disease, although the fibre density is even greater than in motor neuron disease, giant potentials do not occur. This is because the individual components of these potentials are distributed in a longer time period, the potentials being of longer duration, thus giving a lower amplitude. This probably represents variations in propagation velocity in fibres of varying size and the greater dispersion of the end-plate zone from axonal sprouting that occurs in Kugelberg–Welander disease.

With macro EMG the MUAP amplitude was increased in more than half the muscles studied, but was never abnormally small. The highest amplitudes were recorded in patients with slowly progressive disease (Stålberg 1982, 1983).

Estimation of the numbers of surviving motor units in weak muscles, usually the extensor digitorum brevis muscle, using the technique described by McComas and colleagues (see McComas 1977), in patients with motor neuron disease, has shown that reinnervation from surviving motor units can compensate for the loss of up to a half of the motor neuron pool, but that reinnervation apparently ceases when less than 5% of the motor units remain viable (Hansen and Ballantyne 1978). Bromberg et al. (1993) studied a group of 31 patients with motor neuron disease using motor unit number estimation, and EMG studies including turns/amplitude

ing failure of the process of functional reinnervation. This is the phase of relatively well-compensated reinnervation. In the third stage of the disease the muscle is weak and easily fatiguable. Wasting is often present. The fibre density remains markedly increased (>3.0), but impulse blocking is now a prominent feature. This is the phase of early decompensation of the process of reinnervation. Many anterior horn cells have been lost. In the fourth stage the muscle is very weak and wasting is prominent. The fibre density is not as high as in stages 2 and 3, but it is often difficult to calculate because only a small number of motor units may be detected. Jitter and blocking may be very prominent in the potentials recorded. In this phase reinnervation has failed and the muscle is irreversibly wasted.

It is important to recognise that individual muscles may be affected to varying degrees, i.e. they may show different phases of involvement in the ratios, SFEMG, macro EMG and isometric strength measurements, using the biceps and brachialis muscle groups. They concluded that collateral re-innervation was sufficient to prevent isometric strength and EMG measures, including fibre density, from accurately reflecting loss of functioning motor neurons. Only estimation of motor unit numbers is capable of analysing this loss of units. McComas (1995) has reviewed this technique.

Bosch et al. (1985) found abnormal somatosensory evoked potentials in 17 of 30 patients with motor neuron disease, with delay of the N32 and N60 peaks. These findings seem to indicate a disturbance of somatosensory pathways at cortical or subcortical levels.

Involvement of central motor pathways can be evaluated by transcranial cortical stimulation. Hugon et al. (1987) and Ingram and Swash (1987) used electrical stimulation and showed increased latencies to muscle of the upper limbs, and lower limbs (Ingram and Swash 1987), with increased conduction times in brain and spinal cord motor pathways. Magnetic stimulation (Ingram and Swash 1987; Eisen et al. 1990) revealed abnormal motor evoked responses, delayed, absent or reduced in amplitude in nearly all patients.

Laboratory Investigations and Imaging

The CK level is increased in more than half the patients. It may be increased to two or three times the normal range (Williams and Bruford 1970). The higher levels are found in patients whose muscle biopsies show secondary myopathic changes (Achari and Anderson 1974; Schwartz et al. 1976a), and is especially correlated with the presence of regenerating fibres (Tandon and Bradley 1985). The CSF protein may be slightly raised in some patients (Kjellin and Stibler 1976). In the series of Gubbay et al. (1985) 136 patients had CSF examinations. None showed a pleocytosis and the CSF protein was normal in two-thirds of those tested; in the remainder it was mildly raised. Reports of abnormalities of parotid and pancreatic function (Quick and Greer 1966; Charchaglie et al. 1974) led to treatment with pancreatic extract, but no benefit was observed (Quick 1969), and these abnormalities, including mild steatorrhoea, abnormal glucose tolerance with decreased insulin secretion and an abnormal response to secretin stimulation, are ascribed to the malnutrition which often accompanies the disease in its late stages. In a group of patients in whom motor neuron disease was associated with lymphoma (Younger et al. 1991) the CSF protein was increased and oligoclonal IgG bands were present in

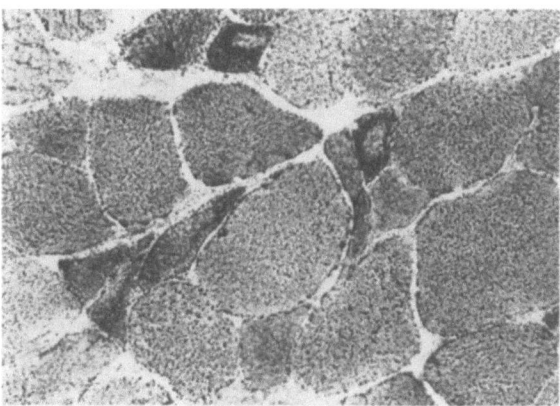

Fig. 6.16. Motor neuron disease. TS NADH × 560. There are clustered and isolated atrophic angulated fibres (disseminated neurogenic atrophy), and some show typical target-fibre formations, with dense enzyme reactivity surrounding the central target. These features suggest acute denervation.

three of nine patients. Monoclonal paraproteinaemia has been reported in 5%–10% of patients (Sanders et al. 1993), but this was not confirmed in a case control study (Willison et al. 1993). Anti GM_1 antiglycolipid antibodies are not increased in CSF in the disease (Willison et al. 1993). MRI of the brain shows high signal in the corticospinal pathways (Gooden et al. 1988; Friedman and Tartaglino 1993).

Haverkamp et al. (1995) reviewed 1200 cases, 831 of whom had typical sporadic disease. Of the latter group of 831 patients the CK level was normal in 45%, the CSF protein was raised in 40% with monoclonal IgG bands in 3%. In 2% AChR antibody levels were raised and 10% had IgM antibody to ganglioside GM_1. Rheumatoid factor titres were raised in 7%. Interpretation of these data is difficult without community-based age- and sex-matched control data. Haverkamp et al. (1995) present an analysis of prognostic variables and survival statistics in this untreated group of patients.

Muscle Biopsy

The most prominent finding is the presence of small angular fibres (Fig. 6.16), which are often found in small clusters of two or more fibres. These fibres stain darkly in NADH and non-specific esterase preparations and may be of either histochemical type. These are the typical features of disseminated neurogenic atrophy. In atrophic muscles, or in more advanced cases of the disease, fibre-type grouping is common (Fig. 6.17). Both fibre types are affected. Grouped fibre atrophy occurs in most patients, but these groups do not usually occupy whole fascicles.

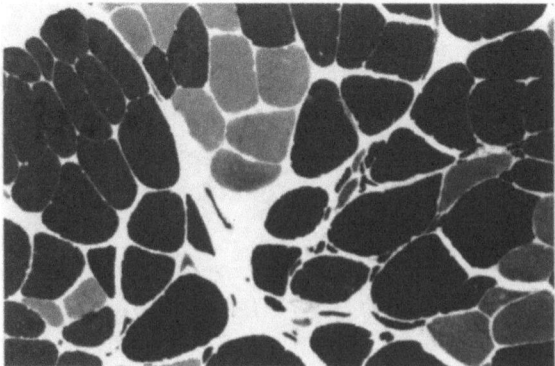

Fig. 6.17. Motor neuron disease. Fibre-type grouping and disseminated neurogenic atrophy. Myosin ATPase, pH 4.3.

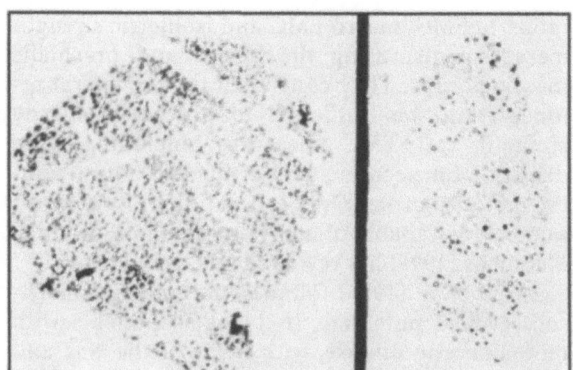

Fig. 6.18. Motor neuron disease. Atrophy of the ventral motor roots; normal and atrophic roots compared. Note the loss of axons in the atrophic roots.

Type 2C fibres may be present in increased numbers, and some fibres, nearly always Type 1 fibres, show target change (Fig. 3.21). These features indicate both denervation and reinnervation (Table 6.6).

Table 6.6. Muscle pathology in motor neuron disease

Denervation	Reinnervation	Other compensatory processes
Small angulated fibres	Fibre-type grouping (of normal-sized fibres)	Type 2 fibre hypertrophy
Small group atrophy		Fibre splitting (regenerating fibres)
Target fibres	Type 2C fibres present	

Coërs et al. (1973), using the intravital methylene blue impregnation technique, found that the terminal innervation ratio, the mean number of muscle fibres supplied by a terminal axon, was 1.8 (normal 1.26). They found that some end-plates and terminal axons showed degenerative changes consistent with a dying-back process (Cavanagh 1964) and that fine-beaded regenerating axonal sprouts were also present (Coërs and Woolf 1981). Wohlfart (1957) also demonstrated collateral axonal sprouting in this muscle by histological techniques. These direct observations of the pattern of innervation indicate that collateral sprouting is important in the process of reinnervation and fibre-type grouping in motor neuron disease; this process is part of the compensatory mechanism for loss of motor neurons which enables function to be retained in the muscle.

Patten et al. (1979) noted that the prognosis seemed to be better in patients in whom Type 1 fibre grouping was present, and worse in those with clusters of small atrophic fibres. Another such compensatory process is fibre hypertrophy. This is a feature of the earlier stages of the disease (Brooke and

Engel 1969b) and principally affects Type 2 fibres. In the late stages of motor neuron disease atrophy of both fibre types supervenes and secondary myopathic changes consisting of fibre splitting, variation in fibre size, fat replacement and fibrosis, and rare degenerating or regenerating fibres can be found (Schwartz et al. 1976a). Achari and Anderson (1974) found myopathic changes of this type in 67% of a series of 111 muscle biopsies from patients with motor neuron disease.

Other Pathological Aspects

At autopsy the striking macroscopic change is atrophy of the ventral roots (Fig. 6.18), and of the motor cranial nerves, and atrophy of the skeletal muscles. The peripheral nerves show Wallerian degeneration; the features of a dying-back axonopathy are not prominent, although it has been suggested that this is a basic pathological process in the disease (Greenfield et al. 1957). There is widespread loss of anterior horn cells (Fig. 6.19) (Lawyer and Netsky 1953). Some remaining motor cells show chromatolysis and accumulations of neurofilaments (Hirano et al. 1984). Loss of anterior horn cells in the disease may be strikingly asymmetrical in homologous segments (Brownell et al. 1970; Tsukagoshi et al. 1979; Swash et al. 1986). In addition, these cells show focal and patchy zones of loss and relative preservation within individual cervical segments (Swash et al. 1986). This focal loss does not extend, however, through individual cell columns as it does in poliomyelitis (Sharrard 1964). The gamma motor neurons are also involved (Swash and Fox 1974; Kawamura et al. 1977). The concept of selective vulnerability of motor neurons has received some attention. Tsukagoshi et al. (1979, 1980) noted more

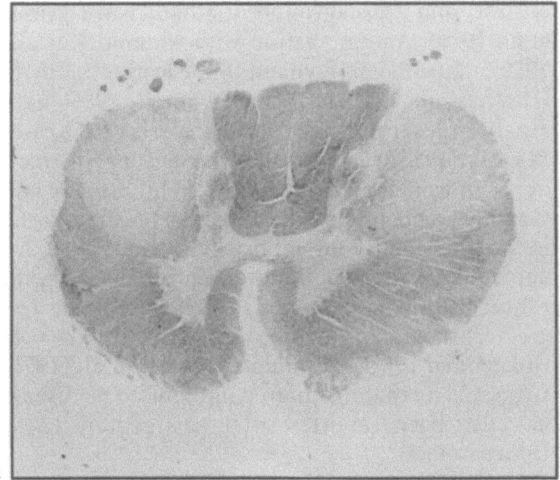

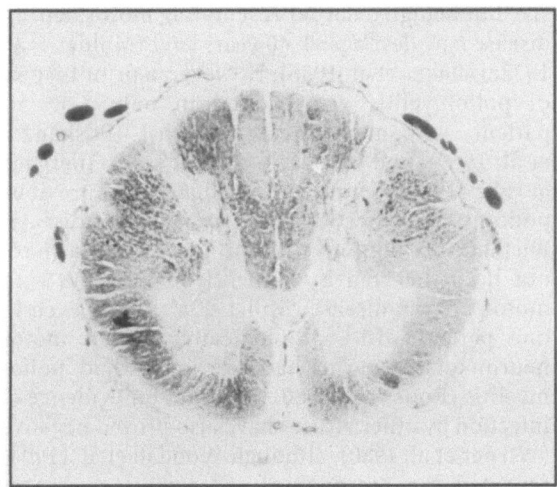

Fig. 6.19. Motor neuron disease. Loss of anterior horn cells and degeneration of the cortocospinal tracts. **a** In Werdnig–Hoffmann disease; **b** the corticospinal tracts are unaffected.

marked loss in the C8 than in the C6 segments, and the relative resistance of the neurons of Onuf's sacral nucleus, and of the cells of the oculo-motor nuclei is well recognised. Wohlfart (1958) suggested that motoneuronal death occurred sequentially as the disease progressed but there is little direct evidence supporting this assertion (Swash et al. 1986).

Bunina bodies – eosinophilic cytoplasmic inclusions – may be present in some anterior horn cells. Spheroidal axonal enlargements, containing 10 μm neurofilaments may occur in up to 60% of cases (Leigh and Swash 1991) and may be found in motor axons in sections of the spinal cord (Delisle and Carpenter 1984). The most characteristic feature of anterior horn cell and motor cortex involvement is the presence of ubiquitinated inclusion bodies consisting of skeins of thread-like structures possibly

related to Bunina bodies, and spherical, apparently solid inclusions (Leigh et al. 1988; Lowe et al. 1988). The latter are related to hyaline Lewy-like inclusions described by Hirano (1991). These inclusions have been reviewed by Lowe (1994).

The corticospinal tracts are degenerate (Fig. 6.19), with demyelination and gliosis, and this abnormality may be detectable even as far rostrally as the motor cortex in some cases. In some spinal cords there is reduction in myelin density in the whole of the anterior and lateral white matter, with normal myelin only in the posterior columns (Lawyer and Netsky 1953; Brownell et al. 1970). Senile plaques resembling those found in Alzheimer's disease, with intraneuronal neurofibrillary tangles may be found in increased number in the cortex in some cases (Oppenheimer 1976). In long-surviving cases there is widespread neuronal degeneration in subcortical structures, including basal ganglia, brain stem and cerebellum (Mizutani et al. 1992).

Aetiology

The cause of motor neuron disease is unknown (Swash and Schwartz 1992). Many possible causative factors have been considered.

Familial factors appear to be important in less than 10% of cases (Emery and Holloway 1982 and see above). The genetic locus reported in familial cases (FALS) maps to chromosome 21q 22.1–22.2, at the locus for the enzyme superoxide dismutase SOD-1 (Siddique et al. 1991; Rosen et al. 1993). Many different mutations in the SOD-1 gene have been reported but fewer than half the patients in the USA with FALS map to this locus, and this association is even less common in Europe. SOD-1 mutations in sporadic cases have been recognised (Jones et al. 1995). Decreased neuronal SOD activity can lead to cell death from peroxide toxicity (superoxide free radical damage) reinforcing an earlier concept that neuronal cell death in neurodegenerative diseases such as motor neuron disease can result from excitotoxic mechanisms.

The majority of these mutations are point mutations with single base substitutions leading to a single amino acid change without change in the size of the protein. Occasional mutations lead to the production of a premature stop codon, and have a truncated protein (see de Belleroche et al. 1995 for review). Mutations in exon 3 of the SOD-1 gene, important in the active pore region of the enzyme, appear fatal in utero, since none have been reported. Experiments in transgenic mice, carrying a human SOD-1 mutation have shown that the mice develop a progressive neurogenic disorder, with early vacuolation in the neuronal cytosol, neurofilamentous accumulations in the motor axon, and degeneration of motor cells in the spinal cord. It is believed likely that this transgenic form of motor neuron disease results from the gain of function related to the addition of the third, abnormal SOD-1 gene to the mouse genome (Dal Canto and Gurney 1995, et al. 1996). This has suggested that the motor neuron disease itself might be due to a gain of function disorder of the SOD-1 enzyme in the cytosol of the motor system, at least in FALS, if not in sporadic motor neuron disease. The sensitivity of the motor system to this mutation may be due to other mutations, or post-translational defects in glutamate transporter proteins, and in calcium binding protein activity in the motor cells in the spinal cord (Rothstein et al. 1995), and in the brain (Bristol and Rothstein 1996). The SOD-1 mutation may convert the enzyme from an anti-apoptotic to a pro-apoptotic protein.

Increased glutamate levels have been found in serum, CSF and brain in motor neuron disease (Rothstein et al. 1992; Camu et al. 1993). Glutamate is an excitotoxic neurotransmitter that facilitates calcium entry into the cell resulting in upregulation of calcium-activated proteases, and release of free radicals (Choi 1992). Rothstein et al. (1992) found a defect in high-affinity uptake of sodium-dependent glutamate in synaptosomes. Glutamate seems to have its excitotoxic action by activation of NMDA, AMPA and kainate receptors, all post-synaptic. Plaitakis et al. (1988) made early observations leading to the excitotoxic hypothesis (Shaw 1994).

Premature ageing or abiotrophy is suggested by the increasing incidence with advancing age (Calne et al. 1986) but this concept is, as yet, poorly formulated despite observation of loss of motor neurons with increasing age, and decreased capacity to form axonal sprouts, in normal ageing (McComas et al. 1973). Heavy metals, for example lead (Campbell et al. 1970; Conradi et al. 1978), mercury (Adams et al. 1983), manganese (Yase 1972) and selenium have all been suggested as playing a role in the disease but there appears to be no direct relationship between exposure to these substances, their levels in the tissues, and the disease (Conradi et al. 1982). Analogies between hyperparathyroidism and motor neuron disease perhaps associated with environmental calcium and magnesium deficiency (Yase 1984) have led to a hypothesis interrelating calcium and aluminium with degenerative neuronal disease and neurofibrillary tangle formation (Gajdusek 1985). Epidemiological searches for risk factors have implicated an excessive frequency of limb-bone fractures, a high milk consumption through-

out life, and a background of athleticism (Felmus et al. 1976). An association with trauma (Kurtzke 1982) and with employment in the leather industry (Hawkes and Fox 1981; Buckley et al. 1983) have also been recorded. In a cohort analysis of 356 cases Li et al. (1985) reported that the age-specific incidence in women declined in the eighth decade and that the incidence of the disease appeared to be increasing slightly for cohorts born since 1900. An apparent association of motor neuron disease with cancer (Brain and Norris 1965) is probably no greater than can be accounted for by chance (Jokelainen 1977a), although Younger et al. (1991) suggested a relationship to lymphoma. The disease has also been reported after gastrectomy (Ask-Upmark 1950).

In some patients with poliomyelitis, a progressive but benign disorder resembling motor neuron disease may develop 30–40 years later (Mulder et al. 1972; Dalakas et al. 1986). However, a prior history of poliomyelitis was elicited in only 2.5% of patients with motor neuron disease (Poskanzer et al. 1969), and in a case–control study Juergens et al. (1980) found no evidence of previous poliomyelitis infection in 35 cases of the disease. Furthermore poliomyelitis antigen or virions have not been detected in tissues from patients with motor neuron disease (Miller et al. 1980), even in one patient with pathologically verified motor neuron disease, who had previously had poliomyelitis (Roos et al. 1980). Searches for evidence of infection by other viruses have also proved negative (Wiener et al. 1980), although Woodall et al. (1994) reported the presence of enteroviral sequences related to Coxsackie B infection in spinal cord from eight of 11 cases of sporadic motor neuron disease and one of two familial cases. Armon et al. (1990) noted that only two patients in the USA rather than the seven expected had developed ALS following previous poliomyelitis in the 30-year period 1960–1990, suggesting that polio might have a protective rather than causative effect (see Martyn et al. 1988).

Immunological theories of causation have included the finding of immune complexes containing IgG and C_3 on the basement membrane and mesangium of the kidney in patients with the disease (Oldstone et al. 1976), and an increased frequency of HLA-A3 in rapidly progressive cases, and of HLA-B12 in slower cases (Antel et al. 1976). Other HLA studies have not confirmed these results (Zaiwalla et al. 1984). Gurney et al. (1984) reported that sera from patients with the disease inhibited sprouting induced in terminal motor axon of mouse gluteus muscle by prior treatment with botulinum toxin, and suggested that this inhibitory effect was due to an antibody in the serum of the patients. However the disease cannot be passively transferred to animals (Denys et al. 1984). Conradi and Ronnevi (1985) have reported that plasma from patients with motor neuron disease was cytotoxic to erythrocytes, and that this effect is retained in purified immunoglobulins from these patients (Ronnevi et al. 1984). Roisen et al. (1982) found that serum from patients with the disease was cytotoxic against cultured spinal cord neurons. Appel and colleagues found infiltration of lymphocytes and deposits of IgG around motor neurons in motor neuron disease at autopsy, and antibodies to L-type calcium channels in muscle of 38 of 48 patients with the disease, but not in familial cases (Smith et al. 1992). These observations require replication, and their possible significance in pathogenesis requires further work.

An association between motor neuron disease and monoclonal or polyclonal gammopathy (plasma cell dyscrasia) has been reported (Bauer et al. 1977; Patten 1984; Shy et al. 1986). Shy et al. (1986) found a gammopathy in 5% of 206 patients with motor neuron disease, but in only 1% of control subjects. Of the ten cases, four had IgM and six IgG paraproteins in their peripheral blood; all but one of these were kappa chain proteins. Cryoglobulins were detected in four patients. No clinically distinct features were recognised, although raised CSF protein values (780 mg/1) were detected in several of the patients in whom lumbar puncture was performed. Plasma exchange and chemotherapy have been used in patients with this association and improvement has been noted in a few cases. In assessing the clinical and theoretical importance of this association of motor neuron disease with plasma cell dyscrasia it is important to exclude the common and well-recognised motor neuropathy that may complicate benign or malignant paraproteinaemias (Kelly et al. 1981b) since this disorder may simulate motor neuron disease (Rowland et al. 1982; Parry et al. 1986). This distinction may be difficult since the finding of slowed motor conduction need not necessarily imply absence of anterior horn cell involvement. No specific immunocytopathological reaction between the paraprotein and anterior horn cells has yet been demonstrated (Doherty et al. 1986) and Donaghy and Duchen (1986) were unable to inhibit experimentally induced sprouting of motor nerve terminals with the serum of two patients with IgG kappa paraproteinaemia associated with motor neuron disease. Indeed, Willison et al. (1992) have disputed that any association with paraprotein exists (see above). The problems of the immunological theory have been succinctly reviewed by Rowland (1992).

Mann and Yates (1974) reported a reduction in neuronal RNA content in spinal motor neurons independent of disease duration or severity. This reduction of neuronal RNA may reflect aberrant transcription following unrepaired damage to neuronal DNA (Tandon and Bradley 1985).

Glycine tolerance is impaired in the disease (Lane et al. 1993), a finding that might be related to the excitotoxic hypothesis. In lathyrism and konzo, two forms of upper motor neuron degeneration related to ingestion of excitotoxins derived from the chickling pea (Spencer et al. 1987) and cassava respectively (Tylleskår et al. 1992), the toxin is believed to be a neuron-specific excitotoxin. Plasma cysteine levels were reported elevated in motor neuron disease by Steventon et al. (1988), a finding that Perry et al. (1991) could not confirm.

The epidemiologic evidence for genetic susceptibility in a cohort of the population has been reviewed above.

Management

There is no specific effective treatment available for motor neuron disease. Many potential therapies have been studied but all have been found ineffective, including immunosuppressive drugs such as cyclophosphamide (Smith et al. 1994), cyclophosphamide with steroids (Tan et al. 1994), bovine brain gangliosides (Bradley et al. 1984 Harrington et al. 1984), intravenous thyrotropin-releasing hormone (TRH) (Brooke et al. 1986; Coroscio et al. 1986; Mitsumoto et al. 1986), a long-chain alcohol octacosanol (Norris et al. 1986), vitamins, chelating agents, pancreatic exocrine replacement therapy, L-dopa, amantadine, isoprinosine, idoxuridine, lecithin, hormone therapy, naloxone, interferon and plasma exchange (see Tandon and Bradley 1985 for review). Other approaches, including antiglutamatergic drugs, anti-excitotoxic and anti-free radical therapies, and branched-chain amino acid supplements are also ineffective (see Swash and Schwartz 1992, and Leigh and Ray Chaudhuri 1994 for reviews). Certain neurotrophic factors, especially ciliary neurotrophic factor (CNTF), brain-derived neurotrophic factor (BDNF) and insulin-like growth factor (IgF) synthesised using recombinant DNA technology have been or are about to be tried (Mitsumoto et al. 1993, 1994; Longo 1994).

The advent of an era in which complex biological compounds, and new classes of drugs are coming forward for clinical trial has resulted in much discussion regarding trial methodology, particularly regarding appropriate methods of clinical measurement, e.g. strength measurements, clinical endpoints, disability scales and quality of life measures, and a code of practice has been agreed by the World Federation of Neurology Committee on Neuromuscular Disorders. An example of the difficulty was shown by a French trial of riluzole, a drug with anti-excitotoxic effects, that seemed to result in slowing of the rate of progression of the disease as shown by reduced mortality in a subgroup of patients with bulbar-onset motor neuron disease, although it was ineffective in patients with limb-onset disease (Bensimon et al. 1994). Rowland (1994) has pointed out that in this trial tracheostomy was set as an end-point equivalent to death, but criteria for tracheostomy in the different centres were not rigidly defined. In addition bulbar-onset could mean dysarthria, a relatively mild symptom, or dysphagia, a potentially fatal symptom. Nonetheless, a larger second trial showed a 7% reduction in mortality in all patients with ALS treated with Riluzole for 18 months (Lacomblez et al. 1996).

In patients with motor neuron disease syndromes associated with plasma cell dyscrasia, plasma exchange and chemotherapy was found by Shy et al. (1986) to be effective. However, these patients may well have had the syndrome of motor neuropathy with multifocal motor conduction block, rather than motor neuron disease itself, and plasma exchange is *not* helpful in idiopathic motor neuron disease (Kellerman et al. 1983). Tan et al. (1994) found that the presence of anti GM_1 antibodies in motor neuron disease did not serve as a marker for a response to steroid and cyclophosphamide therapy.

Bulbar Problems. These consist of excess salivation, dysphagia, choking, dysarthria and, in combination with proximal and respiratory muscle weakness, respiratory failure may develop.

Excess salivation can be reduced by anticholinergic drugs, and in severe cases, parotid irradiation and managed by proper head position, particularly preventing a "drooped head" position.

Dysphagia is a common problem, especially later in the disease, resulting in malnutrition and loss of weight, as well as choking episodes. Generally, semi-solid foods are easier to manage than liquids, but dry foods are also difficult to swallow. Newrick and Langton-Hewer (1984) found dysphagia was a major problem in up to 60% of patients. Dysphagia may improve with anti-spasticity therapy, such as baclofen or dantrium, and a palatal splint is sometimes helpful in controlling nasal escape of air or fluids during swallowing. Cricopharyngeal myotomy was formerly much used (Lebo et al. 1976; Loizou et al. 1980), although there is a treatment failure rate

of about 50% (Norris et al. 1985) and some centres experienced a significant post-operative mortality. The advent of percutaneous, endoscopic gastrostomy (PEG) has superseded myotomy, nasogastric tube feeding and open gastrostomy, since it is a quick procedure which is simple, safe and effective and cosmetically unobtrusive. The resultant improved nutrition results in weight gain, better general health and some improvement in strength (Norris et al. 1985).

Dysarthria is due to weakness and spasticity; 75% of patients develop major speech problems during the disease. Communication aids, employing a voice synthesizer are often well tolerated both by the patient and friends and family.

Respiratory Failure. Sometimes respiratory failure develops at a time when the patient is otherwise relatively mobile (Parhad et al. 1978; Sivak et al. 1982) and, in this situation, ventilatory support with a cuirass ventilator during sleep, or with intermittent positive pressure ventilation, may be used. A simple widely applied technique applicable to home use delivers oxygen under pressure via a tightly fitted face mask, or endotracheal tube (continuous positive airway pressure: CPAP). However, the cuirass respirator is technologically simple and can be managed with little help (Howard et al. 1989). Ventilator dependence in the terminal stage of motor neuron disease is not an option that should be lightly recommended, being costly, and posing problems for patient and family (Moss et al. 1993). This treatment results in an inevitable ethical dilemma concerning the end-point (see Carey 1986).

Pain. In a survey of the symptomatic problems disclosed by 42 patients with motor neuron disease nursed at home in the UK, Newrick and Langton-Hewer (1985) found that musculo-skeletal pain, falls, constipation and swelling of the legs were major problems. Many patients had difficulty sleeping, mainly because of inability to turn or position themselves comfortably (O'Brien et al. 1992). Sleep is frequently a problem. Diphenhydramine (50–100 mg) at bedtime is safe and has the additional benefit that it may be useful in suppressing muscle cramp and spasms. Respiratory depression with sedation must be avoided.

Cramps may sometimes be troublesome, and treatment with quinine sulphate (300 mg tds) or with phenytoin (100 mg tds) is sometimes effective.

Spasticity. Spasticity is not usually a major problem, since difficulty in walking more frequently results from lower motor neuron, rather than from upper motor neuron lesions. Tendon transfers may occasionally be useful in improving hand function in patients with relatively localised and slowly progressive disease (Sinaki et al. 1984).

Other Problems. Since the disease is progressive, rehabilitation plans must be adapted to the likelihood of increasing disability. Complex techniques or pieces of apparatus are often superseded by more severe disability. The most important principles are to prevent contractures and to retain mobility by range of motion, and isometric exercises (Janiszewski et al. 1983). A comfortable and properly fitted wheelchair is an important aid to social mobility, and electrically operated chairs with special controls adapted for people with weak arms are available. Emotional disturbances may be a major problem as bereavement reactions occur, and much help may be needed, both for patient and family.

Other Anterior Horn Cell Disorders

There are several disorders in which anterior horn cell disease occurs. In some of these, as in poliomyelitis, anterior horn cell degeneration is the major feature but in others, as in Creutzfeldt–Jakob disease, anterior horn cell involvement is only one aspect of a disorder involving other parts of the nervous system.

Degenerative Conditions

Three foci of motor neuron disease have been recognised in the Western Pacific: in Guam, the Kii peninsula of Japan and in Western New Guinea (Western Pacific ALS) (Garruto and Yase 1986). Motor neuron disease is ten times as common in Western New Guinea as in the Kii peninsula and Guam, and 100 times as common as in the West (Gajdusek 1984). In the Kii peninsula there is a strong family history, but the incidence of the disease has been declining in recent years in all three foci. Yase (1972) suggested that the disease might be related to dietary deficiency of calcium and magnesium. Clinically, the disease is similar to sporadic motor neuron disease, but neurofibrillary tangles are a characteristic feature at autopsy (Brody et al. 1971).

In the same areas in which Western Pacific ALS is found a syndrome of Parkinsonism-dementia with motor neuron disease has been reported (Brody et al. 1971), Hudson (1981) reviewed 42 sporadic

cases of motor neuron disease of which 26 also had dementia, eight had Parkinsonism and eight had both Parkinsonism and dementia. The clinical distinction of this syndrome from Creutzfeldt–Jakob disease may be difficult.

Western Pacific ALS has decreased in incidence since the 1990s. Chen (1994) noted that on Guam only one new case was recognised in the first 8 months of 1993, and in 1992 the incidence of the disease on Guam was about the same as that on the Kii peninsula of Japan. About 5% of the Guam cases developed Parkinsonism-dementia complex features, and about 35% of the latter developed features of ALS in the final stages of the illness (Veda 1993).

Amyotrophy, with fasciculation, may develop late in the natural history of a number of system degenerations (Table 6.7) (Rosenberg 1982).

Table 6.7. Other disorders associated with anterior horn cell degeneration

Degenerative conditions
Guam-type motor neuron disease (Western Pacific ALS)
Parkinsonism-dementia complex
System degenerations
Spino-cerebellar degeneration
Shy–Drager syndrome
Olivo-ponto-cerebellar degeneration
Joseph–Machado disease (Rosenberg et al. 1976)
Huntington's disease
Syringomyelia
Stiff man syndrome (see Chap. 21)
Viral and transmissible
Poliomyelitis
Herpes zoster
Post-encephalitic disease
Creutzfeldt–Jakob disease
Intoxications
Lead
Mercury and other heavy metals
Lathyrism
Metabolic and immunological
Hexosaminidase deficiency
Plasma cell dyscrasia
Post-irradiation syndromes

From Swash and Schwartz (1988).

Syringomyelia

This is a chronic degenerative disorder, in which a cavitating lesion develops in the cervical cord and lower brain-stem leading to dissociated sensory loss in affected segments, with lower motor neuron involvement in these segments, and corticospinal signs in the legs. There may be other signs of bulbar involvement including nystagmus and cerebellar signs, and Horner's syndrome. The disease is often asymmetrical and progression and pain in the affected segments is a feature of some cases. The pathogenesis of the disease is uncertain (see review by Barnett et al. 1973); a similar clinical syndrome can follow trauma to the cervical spine, or may occur with other diseases affecting the central part of the spinal cord, e.g. spinal cord tumours.

The EMG shows typical neurogenic features in the atrophic muscles. Double discharges may sometimes be recorded (Fig. 2.12). Motor and sensory nerve conduction studies are normal. Single-fibre EMG studies have shown a constant pattern of segmental involvement in the arms, the C8/T1 segment being most affected, the C7 segment less severely involved, and the C6 segment least affected. The MUAPs are very complex in the small hand muscles, with a very high fibre density (Stålberg et al. 1975b; Schwartz et al. 1980b). These complex potentials are usually stable (Fig. 6.20) but some show increased neuromuscular jitter with impulse blocking. It is very unusual for neurogenic changes to occur in the legs in syringomyelia, but in motor neuron disease the arms and legs are commonly both affected. Muscle biopsy studies of this disorder are not available, but at autopsy well-marked grouped atrophy is seen.

Poliomyelitis and the Post-Polio Syndrome

Poliomyelitis is an acute viral disorder in which anterior horn cells and motor nuclei in the brainstem undergo selective, rapid and irreversible degeneration leading to neurogenic atrophy and weakness of varying severity and distribution (Russell 1952). Some other enteroviruses may produce a similar syndrome.

In some patients deterioration occurs much later in life, with increasing weakness and fatiguability. This occurs in 25%–80% of cases of polio, a mean period of 29 years after the original attack (Windebank et al. 1987; Munsat 1991). It must be recognised that fasciculations and cramp in weak and wasted muscles in patients with residual disability are common and do not indicate that the disease has entered a progressive phase. Although it has been shown that late, progressive, neurogenic weakness resembling motor neuron disease occurs more frequently than would be expected in patients previously affected by poliomyelitis (Zilkha 1962; Poskanzer et al. 1969), the question arises as to whether this syndrome is really true motor neuron disease. The late progressive lower motor neuron involvement usually affects muscles on either side at the same segmental level as the major site of longstanding atrophy from poliomyelitis (Campbell et al. 1969). The anterior horn cell population at this spinal level has been depleted by the original infec-

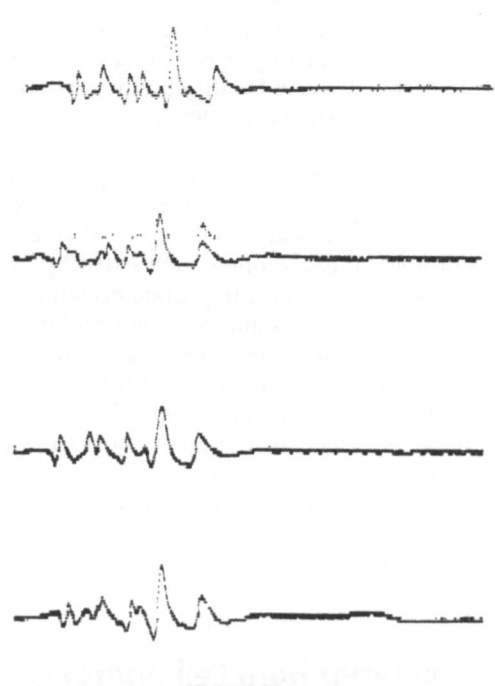

Fig. 6.20. Syringomyelia. Single-fibre EMG recording of a complex, stable motor unit action potential. Bar 4 ms.

tion and the surviving anterior horn cells have taken part in axonal sprouting to compensate for this loss, so minimising denervation atrophy in the affected muscles. These cells are further depleted as part of the normal ageing process after the age of about 60 years; further, these cells may not survive normally to this age because of damage sustained during the acute infection. These factors may thus lead to a progressive, localised neurogenic atrophy.

Post-polio syndrome has been defined as follows:

- History of documented acute paralytic polio
- Partial recovery and stability for at least 15 years
- Residual asymmetric muscle atrophy with weakness, areflexia, and normal sensation, in at least one limb
- Normal sphincteric function

In the post-polio syndrome new weakness and atrophy develops in previously affected muscles, but regions not thought to have been involved may be affected. Fatiguability, weakness, myalgia, loss of muscle bulk and fasciculation are the main features. There may be weakness of bulbar muscles, particularly swallowing, and sleep apnoea has been reported (Munsat 1991). The syndrome may progress with or without long periods of stability, during many years. Sharief et al. (1991) reported the presence of oligoclonal IgM antibodies to polio virus in the CSF of patients with post-polio syndrome together with increased amounts of interleukin-2, suggesting a persistent or reactivated low level polio virus infection.

The relationship, if any, of previous infection by poliomyelitis virus to the later development of classical motor neuron disease is doubtful. In a case-control study, in contrast to the data of Poskanzer et al. (1969), Juergens et al. (1980) found no evidence of previous infection with poliomyelitis in a group of 35 patients with motor neuron disease. In addition, Ahlskog and Mulder (see Alter et al. 1982) found no evidence of motor neuron disease in 47 patients who had poliomyelitis many years previously.

In acute poliomyelitis EMG evidence of denervation, i.e. fibrillation potentials, appears after about 3 weeks. Prior to this there is usually electrical silence in the paralysed muscles. Later, when recovery begins, polyphasic MUAPs of progressively larger amplitude can be recorded, indicating reinnervation. In the late stages, after many years, short-duration low-amplitude MUAPs similar to those recorded in myopathies, can be recorded among the other typically neurogenic potentials. Fibrillation potentials can be recorded, many decades after the onset and do not imply progression. Single-fibre EMG shows the typical features of a longstanding neurogenic disorder. The fibre density is increased and some potentials are of very long duration. In a group of 10 patients studied 22 years or more after poliomyelitis, in whom no progression of weakness had occurred, the neuromuscular jitter was more increased, with blocking, the longer the interval after poliomyelitis and the older the patient (Wiechers and Hubbell 1981; Ravits et al. 1990). These changes were thought to represent ageing of the motor unit superimposed on reinnervation following poliomyelitis (see Maselli et al. 1992).

Muscle Biopsy

In the acute stages severely affected muscles show generalised atrophy of muscle fibres, only a few islands of larger fibres remaining (Adams et al. 1962). This itself probably indicates a degree of re-innervation, and Coërs and Woolf (1959) showed collateral sprouting in one case 2 months after onset. In less severely affected muscles, fibre type grouping would be expected but biopsies of such patients have not been studied by enzyme histochemical techniques. In the chronic phase fat replacement and fibrosis are prominent features in some muscles. Remaining muscle fibres are arranged in groups of fibres of similar size; in some cases the muscle fibres show myopathic features, consisting of variability in fibre size, with hyper-

trophied rounded fibres, central nucleation, fibre splitting and some basophilic regenerating fibres (Drachman et al. 1967). These myopathic changes probably result from functional overload of weakened muscles, leading to muscle fibre hypertrophy and damage (see Schwartz et al. 1976a); it may be a factor in the deterioration observed in some patients many years after the onset of the disease. Pseudo-hypertrophy of weakened muscles, due to accumulation of adipose tissue together with marked hypertrophy of remaining muscle fibres has been reported (Bertorini and Igarashi 1985).

Herpes Zoster and Anterior Horn Cell Involvement

Herpes zoster virus is neurotropic. It usually invades the primary sensory neuron, in which it may lie dormant for many years, and the skin. In some patients there may be involvement of the lower motor neuron in the same spinal segment. Segmental paresis due to Herpes zoster infection occurs in about 5% of patients with cutaneous Herpes zoster (Thomas and Howard 1972). The segmental weakness follows the cutaneous manifestations of the disease, usually developing within 2–3 weeks. Half the patients have cranial nerve involvement, the facial muscles being most commonly affected, and in the remainder limb muscles are affected. The EMG shows typical neurogenic features. The prognosis is good; 85% of patients show complete or partial recovery (Thomas and Howard 1972). In some patients with Herpes zoster, involvement of sensory and motor roots may be accompanied by a transverse myelitis, leading to long tract signs in the legs. Similar involvement of the motor fibres in the facial nerve may occur in Ramsay–Hunt syndrome. The prognosis for recovery is poor. The reader is referred to texts of general neurology for reviews of Herpes zoster infection in the nervous system (see Kennedy 1987).

Creutzfeldt–Jakob Disease

Creutzfeldt–Jakob disease is a degenerative disease of the central nervous system leading to dementia, myoclonus and spasticity. In about 10% of cases there may be striking lower motor neuron involvement, with generalised fasciculation, weakness and muscular atrophy, most prominent in the distal upper limb muscles (Matthews 1975). The disease is fatal within a year of onset. There is evidence that it is due to a transmissible agent, i.e. a prion (Prusiner

1982, 1991). The infectious prion particle is a modified form of the normal host protein and infection depends on the host's prion-gene constitution, as well as exposure to prion particles (Palmer et al. 1991). Creutzfeldt–Jakob disease (CJD) is one of a group of diseases associated with prion accumulation in the nervous system. These are Gerstmann–Straussler–Scheinker syndrome, a fatal disease consisting of ataxia and dementia, Kuru, iatrogenic CJD, atypical prion disease, a disorder of long duration, and fatal familial insomnia. Motor neuron syndromes occurring with CJD and atypical prion diseases are not well characterised and may consist, it is believed, of an ALS syndrome, of an upper motor neuron syndrome or of a lower motor neuron syndrome. These all appear exceptionally rare in practice. The disease has been transmitted inadvertently by corneal transplantation from an affected donor (Duffy et al. 1974), and by means of intracerebral recording electrodes which had previously been used in a patient with the disease (Bernoulli et al. 1977).

The possibility of transmission by contaminated instruments limits investigation since adequate sterilisation is difficult. Gajdusek et al. (1977) suggested that needle electrodes should be autoclaved for 1 h at 121 °C and 20 lb/in^2 pressure, or incinerated and discarded. Simple boiling, or chemical or ionising radiation methods of sterilisation are not adequate. However, the epidemiological evidence does not suggest an unusual risk of Creutzfeldt–Jakob disease for medical and ancillary personnel; only direct contact, as in corneal transplantation from an infected donor, or by the use of brain electrodes formerly used in infected patients have been reported to transmit the disease from one person to another

(see Gajdusek et al. 1977 for full discussion). Salazar (1982) reported that 35 cases of Creutzfeldt–Jakob disease in which amyotrophy and fasciculation were prominent early features failed to show a transmissible spongiform encephalopathy, in contrast to the more typical form in which dementia is prominent and amyotrophy is slight or absent.

The EMG and single-fibre EMG features of the disease are very similar to those found in motor neuron disease (Schwartz, unpublished data). The muscle, at autopsy, shows typical neurogenic atrophy (Allen et al. 1971).

Intoxications

Heavy metals may cause motor axonopathy (see Chap. 11) with amyotrophy. *Lathyrism* is a self-limited upper motor neuron disorder characterised by loss of nerve fibres in the corticopinal tracts, especially in the lumber cord with pallor of the fasciculus gracilis (Román et al. 1985). The disease begins weeks or months after consumption of peas containing a neurotoxic glutamate agonist amino acid β-N-oxalylamino-L-alanine (BOAA) (Spencer et al. 1986). Amyotrophy is not a feature. Lathyrism is commonly associated with malnutrition (Cohn and Streifler 1981).

Post-Irradiation Syndromes

Amyotrophy due to denervation from loss of anterior horn cells can occur after irradiation therapy involving the spinal cord (Palmer 1972; Sadowsky et al. 1976).

Chapter 7　A Clinical Approach to the Neuropathies

Neuropathies are disorders of peripheral nerves. The peripheral nervous system consists of the peripheral and cranial nerves together with their nerve cells, i.e. the anterior horn cells and cranial motor nuclei, the dorsal root ganglia and cranial sensory nuclei, and the autonomic ganglia of the sympathetic and parasympathetic nervous systems. Disease may affect these structures proximally or peripherally, or even at their central cell body. The latter is sometimes termed *neuronopathy*, but the clinical expression of this pathological process consists of dysfunction in the peripheral nervous system and thus resembles that of primary disorders of the peripheral parts of the cell, i.e. the axon. Either motor cells and their axons, or sensory cells and their axons, or both, may be affected. Although autonomic disturbances rarely form a major aspect of the clinical features of peripheral neuropathy, autonomic neuropathy, e.g. in diabetes mellitus, can be a major source of disability.

Neuropathies fall into two main clinical groups. In *mononeuropathies* individual nerves, nerve roots or parts of a nerve plexus may be preferentially affected. The lesion is localised. A nerve may be injured or compressed or preferentially involved as part of a more generalised disorder, as in lead neuropathy. Nerves already abnormal by virtue of an occult or mild generalised neuropathy, as in diabetes mellitus, are peculiarly susceptible to pressure or entrapment. In these mononeuropathies motor and sensory symptoms and signs are limited to the distribution of the nerve affected. In some of these disorders a radiating tingling sensation is felt in the sensory distribution of a nerve when it is is percussed firmly at the point of damage or regeneration (Tinel 1917). The tendon reflexes are preserved unless the reflex tested depends on muscles supplied by a damaged nerve.

Mononeuritis multiplex is a syndrome in which several individual peripheral nerves are affected; it is usually due to vascular disease, e.g. polyarteritis nodosa, or diabetes. Multiple entrapment syndromes may present similarly and the term *multiple mononeuropathy* is often preferred to describe this syndrome.

In the second major group of neuropathies there is symmetrical, diffuse or generalised involvement of the peripheral nervous system. These syndromes are termed *peripheral neuropathies* or *polyneuropathies*. Clinically, polyneuropathies are characterised by distal, symmetrical sensory or motor abnormalities, or both. The distal tendon reflexes are usually absent, particularly the ankle jerks. There is weakness and, in established cases, wasting of the affected distal musculature, but fasciculations are uncommon. The sensory disturbance is distal and it becomes gradually less severe in more proximal parts of the limbs, thus assuming a "glove and stocking" distribution. There may be trophic and autonomic changes, including loss of hair, impaired sweating and shininess of the skin in these distal regions. Pure motor or sensory neuropathies occur, but in most instances there is a combination of motor and sensory involvement to varying degrees. In the early stages, or in very mild polyneuropathies the clinical features may be limited to tingling of the feet and fingertips, without objective findings on examination. In some predominantly motor polyneuropathies, weakness is mainly proximal, e.g. in Guillain–Barré syndrome. The peripheral nerves themselves are usually apparently normal to clinical examination (palpation) but in some *hypertrophic neuropathies* they are enlarged (Fig. 7.1). Focal nerve hypertrophy in which a localised swelling, that is often tender, can be palpated at pressure or entrapment points is a common feature.

Autonomic nerve fibres are usually involved as part of a generalised polyneuropathy; *autonomic neuropathy* occurring without sensory polyneuropathy is rare.

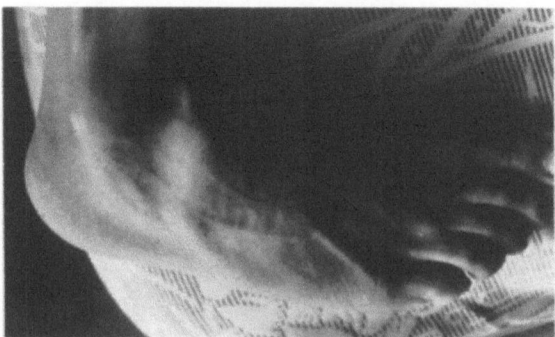

Fig. 7.1. Déjérine–Sottas disease. Hypertrophy of branches of the sural nerve on the lateral aspect of the foot.

Acquired symmetrical polyneuropathies are common and, despite the similar clinical features found in different cases, there are a large number of different causes for the syndrome (see Table 7.2 and Chapter 11).

Clinical Features of Neuropathies

The clinical features of peripheral nerve disorders are dependent on a number of inter-related variables. Careful assessment of these (Tables 7.1 and 7.2) enables diagnosis to be approached at the bedside, and appropriate investigation to be planned. The importance of syndrome analysis has been shown in a quantitative analysis based on a complete questionnaire consisting of several hundred questions (Dyck et al. 1986b). A series of simple questions should be posed by the clinician in assessing and planning management in a patient with neuropathy (Table 7.3).

Clinical Evaluation

The first consideration must always be to determine whether the disorder is a mononeuropathy, a syndrome of multiple involvement of single nerves as in mononeuritis multiplex, or a symmetrical polyneuropathy. Generally, difficulty arises only in patients with relatively slight sensory involvement in whom the motor signs can, perhaps, be interpreted in a number of different ways. As an example, the predominantly proximal weakness of Guillain–Barré syndrome may sometimes mistakenly be ascribed to an acute myopathy such as polymyositis. Corticospinal weakness must also be considered in this context since the tendon reflexes

Table 7.1. Factors influencing clinical features in peripheral nerve disease

Rate and mode of progression	
Acute	Onset in less than 4 weeks
Subacute	Onset in less than 1–3 months
Chronic	Onset in more than 3 months
Relapsing	Multiple episodes after acute or subacute onset

Subclinical
  e.g. chronic, or hereditary
  (without objective signs),
  drugs, uraemia, diabetes
  mellitus	

Table 7.2. Clinical patterns of neuropathies

Clinical pattern	
Mononeuropathy	Often due to entrapment or injury
Mononeuritis multiplex	Diabetes mellitus, polyarteritis nodosa
Symmetrical sensorimotor neuropathy	Many common neuropathies
Symmetrical sensory neuropathy	Diabetes mellitus, drugs
Motor neuropathy	Lead poisoning, porphyria
Radiculopathy	Cervical spondylosis
Autonomic neuropathy	Diabetes mellitus
Painful distal sensory neuropathy	Cancer, uraemia, diabetes mellitus

Table 7.3. Clinical analysis of a patient with suspected neuropathy

1. Does the patient have a neuropathy?
2. What is the clinical pattern of the symptoms and signs, e.g. mononeuropathy, mononeuritis multiplex etc? (Table 7.2)
3. Is the neuropathy acute, subacute, chronic or relapsing?
4. Is it predominantly motor, sensory or mixed?
5. Is there any evidence of autonomic involvement?
6. What are the positive or negative manifestations?
7. What investigations are appropriate?
8. What is the pathology?

After Thrush (1992).

may be depressed in acute cord lesions. The neuropathy of porphyria also presents with predominantly motor involvement and, in this condition, the ankle jerks are often preserved, although all the other reflexes may be absent. In proximal diabetic motor neuropathy weakness predominantly affects thigh extensor muscles and is often asymmetrical.

Neuropathies with severe sensory disturbance, but without prominent motor disability, include alcoholic neuropathy, which is frequently painful, and some drug-induced neuropathies. A number of hereditary neuropathies also preferentially involve the sensory system. In most neuropathies with sensory involvement all modalities of sensation are similarly affected but when there is associated posterior column disease (as in Friedreich's ataxia, subacute combined degeneration of the spinal cord and

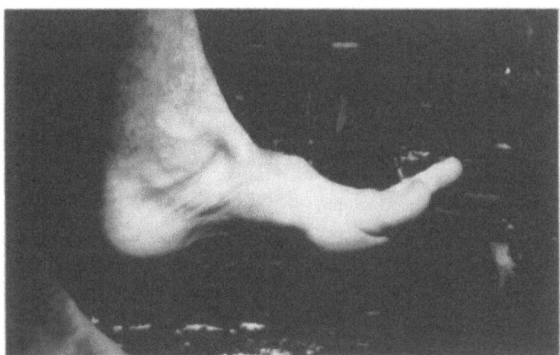

Fig. 7.2. Refsum's disease. Pes cavus. In this patient there is a sensorimotor neuropathy and the small muscles of the feet are atrophic.

carcinomatous sensory neuropathy) impairment of position sense, two-point discrimination and vibration sense outweigh alteration of pinprick and temperature. Touch sensation is also relatively little affected in these patients. In some other neuropathies, for example diabetic neuropathy, pinprick sensation may be more affected. Enlargement of the peripheral nerves is an important sign; it is found in leprosy, chronic or recurrent Guillain–Barré syndrome and in certain hereditary neuropathies, for example the hypertrophic form of Charcot–Marie–Tooth disease and Refsum's disease. These neuropathies are all predominantly demyelinating neuropathies.

Certain physical signs are of particular importance in patients with polyneuropathy. Pes cavus is a sign of a longstanding disorder (Fig. 7.2), beginning in infancy; most such cases are due to hereditary neuropathies such as Charcot–Marie–Tooth disease or Friedreich's ataxia. Sometimes pes cavus is found in asymptomatic relatives who may have no other obvious signs of neurological disorder. Retinitis pigmentosa, sensorineural deafness and cardiomyopathy are also often found in such patients, and signs of central nervous system involvement such as ataxia, nystagmus and extensor plantar responses may be present in those with spino-cerebellar degeneration.

Acquired polyneuropathies or mononeuropathies may be a manifestation of underlying systemic disease and this can often be recognised by clinical criteria. One of the commonest causes of sensorimotor polyneuropathy is drug-induced neuropathy. A careful history is necessary to discover the offending drug, which may be a medication that has been taken for a long time without apparent untoward effects. Similarly, a history of exposure to neurotoxic chemicals at work or in the environment, such as mercury, lead and industrial solvents, is often

very difficult to establish. Polyneuropathy is also a feature of some patients with advanced renal or hepatic disease, myxoedema, rheumatoid arthritis and other collagen-vascular diseases, and an occult neoplasm, particularly carcinoma of lung or ovary, and lymphoma, should also be considered. Mononeuropathies, particularly the carpal tunnel syndrome, are frequently associated with myxoedema, acromegaly and rheumatoid arthritis. Subclinical polyneuropathy may sometimes present with a mononeuropathy. For example amyloid neuropathy may present with a carpal tunnel syndrome, lead poisoning with a wrist drop and diabetes mellitus not uncommonly presents with a foot drop.

Clinical evidence of autonomic involvement in polyneuropathies is often neglected, but this is an important aspect of functional disability since it is associated with impaired sweating, impaired bladder and bowel control, impaired sexual performance and postural hypotension. Pupillary involvement is also often a feature in these patients. Autonomic failure is particularly a feature of the polyneuropathies associated with diabetes mellitus, carcinomatous sensory neuropathy and Guillain–Barré syndrome, but it may also occur as an isolated phenomenon following an infective illness (Thomashefsky et al. 1972).

Progression

Very *slowly progressive* polyneuropathies are most likely to be genetic in origin. However, diabetic and dysproteinaemic neuropathies may also be chronic. *Acute relapsing* polyneuropathy is commonly due to Guillain–Barré syndrome but certain metabolic neuropathies, e.g. porphyria and Refsum's disease, and repeated toxic exposures, may present acutely and develop a relapsing course. *Subacute* polyneuropathies, with a rate of progression involving a period of 1–3 months (Table 7.1) are frequent and include the major causes of acquired neuropathies, e.g. diabetes, alcohol and uraemia. Some acquired neuropathies pursue a more chronic course, e.g. leprosy. Entrapment and compressive mononeuropathies may have a very *acute* onset, often with local pain, or may develop gradually over many months. Acute polyneuropathies are less common; the most characteristic examples are Guillain–Barré syndrome, and toxic neuropathies.

Prevalence in Clinical Practice

The most common of the symmetrical polyneuropathies is diabetic neuropathy, but this is often mild. Of the mononeuropathies, entrapment of the median nerve in the carpal tunnel – *carpal tunnel syndrome* – is the most common. Leprosy is a common neuropathy in many countries, particularly in tropical climates. The hereditary neuropathies are relatively uncommon and of these Charcot–Marie–Tooth syndrome is the most frequent. Acquired neuropathies associated with drugs, malignant disease or metabolic disorders, although infrequent, are commonly seen in hospital populations. Some polyneuropathies, although uncommon, are important because they are life-threatening as in the Guillain–Barré syndrome. Similarly it is important to recognise neuropathies due to exposure to drugs, toxins, noxious chemicals, etc. since removal of the neurotoxic agent will result in recovery from the neuropathy.

Pathological Correlation in Peripheral Neuropathies

Classification of the polyneuropathies is complex (see Dyck et al. 1975b). Attempts have been made to classify these disorders according to the underlying pathology and particularly according to the predominance of axonal or demyelinating change. Such attempts are, in many respects, unsatisfactory; the main problem is that, in practice, the distinction has proven difficult to sustain on clinical or electrophysiological criteria. Most clinicians therefore prefer a mixed classification in which emphasis is placed on the causative factor, if known, and genetic factors rather than on the underlying pathology. In some disorders, for example the diabetic neuropathies, various clinical presentations occur in the different syndromes reflecting different aspects of the interaction of vascular and metabolic factors.

The main pathological and clinical interactions in the polyneuropathies are shown in Tables 7.4–7.8. This classification attempts to integrate clinical, electrophysiological and pathological data. Inevitably, there is overlap and some disorders, e.g. diabetes mellitus, can lead to several different neuropathic syndromes (Donofrio and Albers 1990). The pathology of the entrapment and compressive mononeuropathies is discussed in Chapter 8.

Axonal Transection

Wallerian degeneration follows transection of a nerve (Waller 1850); a series of well-known mor-

Table 7.4. Uniform (non-symmetrical) demyelination: sensorimotor polyneuropathy (these are hereditary disorders of myelin structure in some of which there is an abnormality of myelin metabolism)

Hereditary motor and sensory neuropathy
    Charcot–Marie–Tooth diseases Types I and IV
    Déjérine–Sottas disease (CMT Type III)
Metachromatic leucodystrophy
Krabbe's globoid leucodystrophy
Congenital hypomyelinating neuropathy
Tangier disease
Cockayne's syndrome
Cerebro-tendinous xanthomatosis

Table 7.5. Segmental demyelination: polyneuropathy with motor involvement more prominent than sensory involvement

Guillain–Barré syndrome: acute and chronic forms
Polyneuropathies with paraproteinaemia
Hereditary neuropathy with susceptibility to pressure palsies
Leprosy
AIDS
Paraneoplastic neuropathy
Amiodarone toxic neuropathy
Perhexilene toxic neuropathy

Table 7.6. Axon loss: sensorimotor polyneuropathy with predominant motor involvement

Porphyria
Charcot–Marie–Tooth Type II
Paraneoplastic polyneuropathy
Lead neuropathy
Dapsone neuropathy
Vincristine neuropathy

Table 7.7. Axon loss: sensory neuropathy or neuronopathy

Hereditary sensory neuropathy Types I–IV
Paraneoplastic sensory neuronopathy
Paraproteinaemic polyneuropathy
Friedreich's ataxia
Abetalipoproteinaemia (Bassen–Kornzweig disease)
cis-platinum toxicity

Table 7.8. Axon loss: sensorimotor polyneuropathy

Nutritional: vitamin B_{12} deficiency, thiamine deficiency
Alcoholism
Connective tissue disease: rheumatoid arthritis, SLE, PAN, etc.
Toxic neuropathies: acrylamide, hexacarbons, organophosphorus esters, etc.
Metal neuropathies: arsenic, mercury, thallium, gold
Drug-induced: metronidazole, chloroquine, phenytoid, colchicine
Paraneoplastic sensorimotor polyneuropathy
Giant axonal dystrophy
Critical care neuropathy
Lyme disease
AIDS
Multiple myeloma with polyneuropathy

phological events occurs distal to the transection and in the cell body of the neuron itself. These degenerative changes are followed by axonal sprouting from the proximal surface of the sectioned axon. Following nerve section there is an accumulation of organelles in both stumps of the transected axon and this is followed, in about 48 h, by discontinuities in the distal axolemma, swelling of the distal axon, and then by retraction of nodes of Ranvier and later by destruction of myelin lamellae, producing myelin ovoids. In acquired polyneuropathies Wallerian change is found only in distal parts of axons affected by *axonal degeneration* (see below). There is controversy concerning the role of increased pressure within nerves, resulting from amyloidosis, ischaemic swelling or inflammatory polyneuropathies, as a factor leading to axonal and Schwann cell injury. Such a mechanism would explain the axonal change that sometimes occurs in severe demyelinating neuropathies, for example in Guillain–Barré syndrome and in experimental diphtheritic neuropathy.

Neuronopathy

Axonal degeneration can occur from failure of the metabolic machinery of the neuron itself, an example of neuronopathy (proximal-distal axonopathy) (Spencer and Schaumburg 1980; Stenman et al. 1980); this results in impaired transport of metabolites and proteins along the axons to the periphery. If the neuronal cell body dies axonal degeneration occurs along the length of the axon, with resultant Wallerian change. Such a process will be selective, affecting only certain populations of neurons and their axons (Table 7.7).

Distal Axonopathy

Distal axonal degeneration ("dying back" neuropathy) occurs when metabolism of the distal parts of certain axons fails (Cavanagh 1964, 1979). It is usually thought that this results from impaired metabolism of the perikaryon of the nerve cell itself, but local abnormalities in distal axonal metabolism could also produce this change. Myelin breakdown, often segmental in character, occurs in the region of the axonal degeneration. The latter takes the form of irregularities in axonal size and shape and degeneration of axoplasmic constituents and the axonal terminations themselves, e.g. sensory receptors and motor endplates. Recovery from this process is possible if the metabolic abnormality can be corrected,

for example by replacement of vitamin deficiency or cessation of exposure to neurotoxic drugs or industrial chemicals. Distal axonal atrophy also occurs in inherited disorders such as spinocerebellar degeneration with neuropathy. In most distal axonopathies there is both a central and a peripheral component, with degeneration in large-diameter myelinated fibre tracts in the central nervous system as well as peripheral neuropathy (Spencer and Schaumburg 1977a,b). However, signs of corticospinal disease may be masked by the severity of peripheral nerve and posterior column involvement.

Cavanagh (1979, 1985) suggested a subclassification of acquired axonal degenerations (Tables 7.6 and 7.8) using a combination of morphological and biochemical criteria. This is summarised in Table 7.9.

Table 7.9. Cavanagh's (1979) classification of axonal neuropathies

Group 1   *Energy dependent axonal neuropathies* (? failure of oxidative metabolic pathways) – a limited distal axonopathy, restricted to peripheral nervous system
Thiamine deficiency
Alcoholic neuropathy
Arsenic and thallium poisoning
Tri-ortho-cresyl phosphate poisoning
Riboflavine deficiency
Friedreich's ataxia
Group 2   *Pyridoxine dependent axonal neuropathies*: distal, sensory greater than motor axonopathy, with more proximal nerve damage than Group 1 disorders
Isoniazid neuropathy
Acute intermittent, and variegate porphyria
Group 3   *Neuropathies with involvement of long spinal pathways and peripheral nerves*
a *With filamentous inclusions in axons*
n-Hexane
Methyl *n*-butyl ketone
2,5-Hexane dione
Acrylamide
Vincristine
b *With vacuolar or membranous changes in axons*
Organophosphorous insecticides
n-Bromophenylacetyl urea

Myelinopathy

Segmental demyelination (Gombault 1880–1881) occurs in neuropathies (Table 7.5), such as those caused by diphtheria toxin, experimental lead poisoning or Guillain–Barré syndrome, in which the Schwann cells are selectively damaged and myelin breakdown occurs. This may be restricted to individual Schwann cells so that degeneration is limited by the nodes of Ranvier. During the process of remyelination shortened, "intercalated" nodes are formed, a characteristic finding indicating that segmental demyelination has occurred. After repeated episodes of demyelination and remyelination *"onion bulbs"* are seen. This term refers to the presence of circumferential leaflets of Schwann cell processes surrounding an axonal core. The outer leaflets are interspersed with collagen fibrils and fibroblasts. This proliferation of interstitial elements may result in palpable enlargement of affected nerves (*hypertrophic neuropathy*).

Uniform demyelination (non-segmental demyelination) occurs in a group of hereditary neuropathies in which there is a genetic defect in myelin structure or metabolism. Segmental demyelination does not occur in these disorders and conduction block is not a feature.

Positive and Negative Symptoms in Neuropathies

Positive and negative phenomena are conspicuous in the sensory system (Table 7.10) and a similar classification of motor features of neuropathies is useful (Table 7.11).

Table 7.10. Sensory symptoms in neuropathies

	Positive	Negative
Paraesthesiae	Tingling, pins and needles	Numbness (hypoaesthesia and hypoalgesia)
Hyperpathia *Allodynia*	Painful or unpleasant sensations from non-noxious stimulation of skin	Loss of specific sensory modalities, e.g. pain, touch; and sensory ataxia, associated with loss of position sense, pseudo-athetosis
Dysaesthesiae	Spontaneous painful sensation	
Causalgia	Severe dysaesthetic pain, usually associated with autonomic disturbances, probably due to ephaptic transmission in damaged nerves	Loss of sensory discrimination. Replacement of sensation by pain
Neuralgia	Paroxysmal pain, e.g. trigeminal neuralgia or painful neuromas, sciatica, brachialgia	

Sensory Symptoms in Neuropathies

Damage to a peripheral nerve may cause negative or positive symptoms. Negative *sensory symptoms* consist of loss of sensation or reduced sensory acuity. They are often described as numbness or

Table 7.11. Motor symptoms in neuropathies

Positive	Negative
Fasciculations	Weakness
Myokymia	Wasting
"Spasms", e.g. hemifacial spasm	
Cramps	
Neuromyotonia and "continuous muscle fibre activity"	
Tremor	
Restless legs and moving toes	

dullness of sensation and may be modality-specific. Hypoaesthesia refers to reduced light touch and hypoalgesia to reduced pinprick (pain) sensitivity. Responses to cold, warm, vibration, position sense, tickle and itch may also be impaired. In polyneuropathies sensory impairment is typically distal with a gradual increase in acuity to more proximally located stimuli. In root lesions or mononeuropathies the sensory disturbance conforms to the sensory distribution of the affected nerve.

Positive symptoms may occur spontaneously, i.e. in the absence of cutaneous stimulation, e.g. paraesthesiae and spontaneous pain, or as an excessive response to cutaneous stimulation, e.g. hyperalgesia, dysaesthesia and allodynia (see Table 7.10). Positive sensory symptoms are largely due to abnormal generation of impulses in sensory axons.

Painful sensations in peripheral neuropathy are particularly associated with axonal neuropathies. Pain may be related to the type and size of fibre predominantly affected. When large, heavily myelinated, sensory A-fibres are stimulated no painful sensations are felt, but when smaller A-delta fibres are stimulated a burning feeling may be experienced, and C-fibre stimulation may cause intolerable pain (Collins et al. 1960; Ochoa and Torebjork 1989). These observations at first suggested that pain was perceived as a result of C-fibre activation. However, subsequent clinical studies have shown that loss of large fibres is not associated with pain, for example in Friedreich's ataxia and phenytoin neuropathy (Thomas 1974; Dyck et al. 1976; Nathan 1976), an observation not consistent with the gate control theory as initially set out by Melzack and Wall (1965). Patients with selective involvement of small fibres, e.g. in Fabry's disease (Ohnishi and Dyck 1974) and certain forms of diabetic neuropathy (Brown et al. 1976; Said et al. 1983), suffer severe pain. Said et al. (1983) noted that axonal sprouting was a prominent feature of painful, small-fibre, diabetic neuropathy (Archer et al. 1983), but both primary and secondary demyelination also occur in this disease and the cause of the pain in this and other painful neuropathies is thus complex. The pain in some cases of painful diabetic neuropathy may be reduced rapidly by normalisation of the blood sugar, and thus seems to be related to its level (Morley et al. 1984). Hyperglycaemia may lower the pain threshold and reduce the anti-nociceptive effects of morphine (Simon and Dewey 1981).

Chronic hereditary sensory neuropathy is associated with analgesia and with loss of small nerve fibres, but pain is not a feature (Schoene et al. 1970), illustrating the important role of rate of progression of the disorder in the generation of painful sensations in peripheral neuropathies. Pain is thus probably related to degeneration of unmyelinated and small myelinated nerve fibres, and to partial degeneration and regeneration of these fibres (Yiannikas and Shahani 1984). Studies of neuromas following experimental nerve injury support the concept that neuropathic pain arises when there is preferential regenerative sprouting of small diameter primary afferents. These regenerating axons are sensitive to sympathetic efferent activity, thus leading to the symptoms and signs of *causalgia* in man (Devor 1983; Asbury and Fields 1984; Wall 1985).

In nerve entrapment syndromes pain may be a major feature. The entrapped nerve is compressed and ischaemic, and acts as a source of spontaneous nerve fibre discharges (Ochoa and Torebjork 1980) and pain. Decompression thus provides relief of these symptoms (Yiannikas and Shahani 1984). Pain is a prominent early feature of brachial and lumbar plexus lesions; it may precede weakness and sensory disturbance in progressive lesions by days or weeks. The pain is deep, aching and exacerbated by movement of the limb. It may be due to swelling of the nerve causing stimulation of nociceptive afferents innervating the nerve sheaths (Asbury and Fields 1984).

Allodynia (hyperpathia) and *dysaesthesiae* are associated with immature regenerating axonal sprouts in a segment of damaged nerve. These sprouts are hyperexcitable and a source of ectopic or spontaneous impulse generation. They may also facilitate ephaptic transmission of electrical activity in the nerve, leading to inappropriate or painful sensations occurring after cutaneous stimulation, or even spontaneously (Torebjork et al. 1979; Ochoa 1982). Capsaicin, a pepper derivative, applied to the skin mimics spontaneous burning pain, such as occurs in erythralgia. This is generated in C-fibres (Culp et al. 1989). A clinical syndrome of spontaneous burning pain and mechanical hyperalgesia associated with fluctuations in skin temperature seems to be due to dysfunction in the C-fibre system. It has been colourfully termed the ABC syndrome (Angry Backfiring C nociceptor) (Ochoa 1986). This functional disorder is a feature of painful diabetic neuropathy.

Motor Symptoms in Neuropathies

Both negative and positive motor symptoms develop in patients with neuropathies (Table 7.11), but negative symptoms generally predominate and cause more disability.

Negative motor features consist of weakness and wasting of muscles. These features are usually most marked distally and are most prominent in axonal disorders. Focal weakness occurs in root lesions and mononeuropathies, usually as a result of compression syndromes, or trauma. In longstanding, slowly progressive neuropathies deformities of the digits or distal parts of the limbs may develop, e.g. Charcot–Marie–Tooth disease and leprosy.

Positive features are relatively unusual. Cramp may be a feature of chronic neuropathies, and fasciculations occur in affected segments in root lesions. Cramps are due to mass discharge of motor nerve fibres causing painful contraction of part of a muscle. This may be facilitated by ephaptic transmission in the damaged nerve. Fasciculations also most commonly arise in ectopic sites of impulse generation, usually in the distal axon or its branching points. Neuromyotonia consists of repetitive spontaneous activity of motor units, or groups of motor units, leading to stiffness and resting contraction of affected muscles. It arises in the damaged peripheral nerves. Restless legs and moving toes is a clinical description of a syndrome in which distal movements occur in the context of uncomfortable sensations in the lower legs, especially following a period of rest or sleep. In some patients with chronic polyneuropathy, especially in chronic demyelinating neuropathies, there may be an irregular distal tremor of the outstretched fingers. This is due to contraction of the reduced number of large, reinnervated motor units, with loss of the usual smooth recruitment pattern of normal motor units.

Clinico-Pathological Correlations

Axonal neuropathies tend to involve motor and sensory functions equally, and to produce disability distally at first, which gradually creeps more proximally as the disease progresses. The distal tendon reflexes are lost before the proximal reflexes are affected. Thus, weakness of foot muscles precedes weakness of intrinsic muscles of the hands. The symptoms and signs of progressive demyelinating neuropathies are not dissimilar, although the sensory abnormality is often less severe, and in some acquired demyelinating neuropathies proximal weakness is a major feature, as in Guillain–

Table 7.12.   General clinico-pathological correlations of neuropathies

Distal axonopathies	Demyelinating neuropathies
Insidious onset	Insidious or acute onset
Legs first affected	Both proximal and distal involvement of arms and legs
"Stocking and glove" sensory impairment	Sensory loss may be slight
Ankle jerks lost early; proximal tendon reflexes preserved	All reflexes lost early
CSF protein normal (nerve roots spared)	CSF protein raised (nerve roots involved)
Recovery may take months or years	Recovery may be rapid
Residual disability common	Residual disability slight
Toxic neuropathies often accompanied by central involvement, e.g. cord and optic nerves	Central involvement rare
Nerve conduction normal or only moderately slowed	Nerve conduction very slow
Needle EMG shows prominent neurogenic changes (denervation and reinnervation)	Needle EMG shows slight changes, unless disorder is chronic

Barré syndrome. Sometimes the degree of slowing of conduction velocity in demyelinating neuropathies is such that there is a recognisable delay in the recognition of a sudden cutaneous stimulus, e.g. a simple touch or pinprick, that is sufficiently characteristic to allow the underlying pathology to be recognised. In chronic demyelinating neuropathies nerve enlargement, especially of distal nerves, e.g. the cutaneous branch of the radial nerve at the wrist and the superficial branches of the sural nerves on the feet, may be a feature. In leprosy, nerve enlargement is also obvious, and this affects proximal as well as distal nerves, especially the posterior auricular nerves. Electrophysiological assessment, however, is by far the most reliable method of recognising axonal and demyelinating disorders (Behse et al. 1977) and especially of evaluating mononeuropathies. The latter are commonly associated with focal enlargement, tenderness and Tinel's phenomenon at the site of nerve enlargement or entrapment. The major clinical and electrophysiological features of axonal degenerations and myelinopathies of the peripheral nervous system are listed in Table 7.12.

Unfortunately the correlation between the clinical features and the pathology in the neuropathies is rarely as clear as might be expected. Longstanding demyelinating neuropathies may be accompanied by severe atrophy of muscles and in severe axonal neuropathies there may be dense sensory loss. The correlation of sensory findings with the pathology is particularly poor. This probably reflects varying patterns of damage to large and small, myelinated and unmyelinated fibres. In some very slowly progressive demyelinating neuropathies there may be severe damage to nerves, with palpable hypertrophy and greatly slowed nerve conduction velocity, but little or no motor or sensory deficit. Since the axonal neuropathies represent a disorder of neuronal function, there may be selective degeneration of certain populations of sensory and motor fibres,

and this will produce differing patterns of symptoms and signs in different polyneuropathies. Such differences are observed, particularly, in some hereditary neuropathies; for example, in porphyria the neuropathy is mainly a motor disorder, and distal movements and reflexes in the legs may be spared. Attempts have also been made to correlate the clinical features of the peripheral neuropathies with the size spectrum of nerve fibres involved (Table 7.13). Although this view of the clinical symptomatology of peripheral neuropathies has general relevance in the clinical assessment of patients it does not hold in absolute terms.

Table 7.13.   Relation of fibre involvement to clinical features in polyneuropathies

Small fibre neuropathy (Brown et al. 1976; Asbury and Gilliatt 1984)
      e.g. Diabetic polyneuropathy
Selective loss of pain and temperature sense
Burning painful dysaesthesiae
Tendon reflexes normal
Strength normal

Large fibre neuropathy (Nathan 1976)
      e.g. Charcot–Marie–Tooth Type 1
Sensory ataxia with impaired joint position sense and two point discrimination
Areflexia
Variable weakness
Minimal loss of sensation

Involvement of all fibres
All sensory modalities affected
Weakness and areflexia

Electrophysiological Correlations

The compound action potential recorded from a nerve consists of components conducting at various rates, depending on axonal diameter, myelination and internodal length. The fastest fibres, Aa fibres, about 11–12 μm in diameter, conduct at 60 m/s or more and the slowest, unmyelinated C fibres, 0.5–2.0 μm in diameter, conduct at about 20 m/s or less. In clinical studies of nerve conduction velocity only the fastest-conducting fibres are studied, because the shortest latency is used as the criterion for measurement. Slower-conducting fibres can be studied by measuring the dispersion of the averaged compound action potential, or by looking for peaks of varying latency within this potential. Such studies are difficult in situ but they have been carried out on sural nerve biopsies, recorded in vitro (see Lambert and Dyck 1975). Collision techniques can also be used for this purpose, but special equipment is required (Hopf 1962; Ingram et al. 1987a).

The important parameters in studies of motor nerve conduction in patients with suspected poly-neuropathies are the distal motor latency and the conduction velocity in the distal and proximal nerve trunks. Generally, in demyelinating neuropathies the distal motor latency is prolonged and conduction in the main trunk of the nerve is also slowed. The most proximal part of the nerve is usually also slowed, as demonstrated by F wave studies. Reduction in amplitude of the compound muscle action potential when stimulating proximally compared with distally, termed conduction block, is characteristic of acquired demyelinating neuro-pathies. In uniform demyelinating neuropathies, e.g. Charcot–Marie–Tooth disease, Type 1, marked reduction of motor conduction velocity occurs, but this is disproportionate to the relatively normal compound muscle action potential amplitude from distal stimulation (Dyck and Lambert 1968a). In axonal neuropathies, on the other hand, the distal latency is usually only slightly prolonged and there is only mild slowing in the distal trunk of the nerve, the most proximal part being less abnormal.

Sensory conduction studies may also differentiate between axonal and demyelinating polyneuro-pathies. In axonal neuropathies sensory potentials are usually smaller than normal, but the sensory conduction velocity is only slightly decreased. In demyelinating neuropathies the sensory conduction velocity is decreased, and in more severe cases the sensory nerve action potential becomes very small, or may be absent even when averaging techniques are used.

Generally, abnormalities in sensory nerve conduction can be recognised when motor nerve conduction studies are normal, and both motor and sensory nerve conduction studies are more likely to be abnormal in the legs than in the arms. In axonal neuropathies electromyographic (EMG) studies show prominent neurogenic changes in muscles sampled, with evidence of denervation and reinnervation. These changes are typically far less prominent in demyelinating neuropathies. In severe demyelinating neuropathies there may be a reduced interference pattern on voluntary activation due to conduction block.

Although this attempt to classify polyneuro-pathies into axonal and demyelinating disorders has the attraction of simplicity, in practice not only is it often difficult to decide by electrophysiological criteria whether in an individual case the disorder is axonal or demyelinating in type, but most neuropathies show pathological features of both axonal and demyelinating disorders. It has thus become increasingly apparent that a strict division along these lines is impracticable (Behse and Buchthal 1978). Nonetheless the finding of very slowed motor nerve conduction velocity (<25 m/s) is nearly always correlated with a severe demyelinating neuropathy. Gilliatt (1966) suggested that a motor nerve conduction velocity of less than 40% normal indicated the presence of segmental demyelination. These features are summarised in Table 7.12. Very mild neuropathies may be detected electrophysiologically by measuring motor and sensory nerve conduction in a number of different nerves. Wennberg (1984) evaluated 10 nerves, using a mean of the summed standard deviations as an index of function.

Assessment of autonomic disorders is difficult. Conventional neurophysiological investigations are not relevant, but the sympathetic skin response (SSR) may be reproducible. This consists of a potential recorded from skin following a cutaneous stimulus applied at a distant site. Variations in amplitude or morphology occur in patients with autonomic neuropathy but the latency of about 1 m/sec is unchanged (Shahani et al. 1984). Autonomic involvement is more a feature of axonal neuropathies than of demyelinating neuropathies, and correlates with loss of small unmyelinated nerve fibres in sural nerve biopsies. Other autonomic function tests, based on cardiological studies, bladder function, pupillary responses, sweat tests and gastro-intestinal motility disorders are used in clinical practice.

Clinical Investigation of Polyneuropathy

Careful clinical assessment of the motor and sensory signs is important not only for recognition and diagnosis, but also to provide a baseline for following progress of the disease, or improvement. Attempts have been made to develop quantitative and objective methods of sensory testing (Dyck

1975a; Conomy et al. 1979) but these are time-consuming and complex and are not generally employed. In some neuropathies there is relatively greater involvement of certain sensory modalities; for example, position and vibration sense are particularly affected in some sensory neuropathies. However, attempts to correlate these deficits with loss of particular groups of axons in pathological studies (Table 7.13) have not revealed consistent results, although it has for a long time been thought that fine tactile sensations are mediated by fast-conducting myelinated fibres and painful sensations by smaller myelinated fibres, and by a group of unmyelinated fibres (see Sinclair 1967; Burke et al. 1975).

Autonomic tests may occasionally be useful. These consist of tests of sweating in response to heat-induced rise in core temperature, pupillary assessment and tests of vasomotor function. In the latter orthostatic hypotension is a major manifestation. Changes in blood pressure and pulse rate following the Valsalva manoeuvre may also be tested, both at the bedside and by more accurate recording techniques. Bladder function can be assessed by cystometrography. These tests have been reviewed by Johnson and Spalding (1974), Bannister et al. (1979) and by Appenzeller and Atkinson (1984). Thermography, using a liquid crystal detection system or infra-red imaging to detect heat radiation from the skin, has been used to detect the distribution of abnormal autonomic innervation of skin in nerve root and nerve entrapment syndromes, e.g. carpal tunnel syndrome (So et al. 1989a,b).

Biochemical tests should include blood count and erythrocyte sedimentation rate since possible underlying causes such as malignant disease or autoimmune disorders may be implicated. Urinary- and blood-glucose tests are important in view of the common occurrence of diabetic neuropathy, which often presents in patients not known to be diabetic. Tests of liver and renal function are also important screening tests. The serum protein electrophoretic pattern is helpful in excluding dysgammaglobulin-aemic neuropathies. In severe, acute neuropathies porphyria should be excluded by testing for urinary porphyrins and urinary δ amino laevulinic acid. Measurement of the level of phytanic acid in the blood is the definitive investigation in Refsum's disease. The CK is slightly elevated in some patients with chronic motor neuropathies, but it is usually normal. The vitamin B_{12} level may be useful. Screening tests, using blood and urine samples, for toxins, chemical exposures and drugs may be helpful.

Examination of the CSF was formerly considered an essential part of the investigation of a patient with polyneuropathy. In subacute or chronic polyneuropathies the CSF protein level may be moderately raised. This is especially prominent in patients with demyelinating neuropathies, e.g. in diabetic neuropathy. In Guillain–Barré syndrome a raised CSF protein level is one of the criteria for diagnosis, particularly if it can be shown to increase during the first 6 weeks of the illness (Haymaker and Kernohan 1949). The CSF protein concentration is often normal in the first few days of the illness and, rarely, it may be normal throughout.

Genetic linkage and marker studies are proving increasingly valuable in the investigation of inherited neuropathies. Stereotyped clinical phenotypes, such as Charcot–Marie–Tooth disease, are revealed by genetic analysis to be associated with more than one possible genetic locus. Genetic studies on DNA isolated from circulating white blood cells can have a major role in the clinical investigation of peripheral neuropathies even, in some instances, when the disorder appears sporadic (Roa et al. 1993).

Electrophysiological Assessment

Studies of both sensory and motor nerve conduction are essential, and the upper and lower limbs should be evaluated. Because of the frequency of symptomatic or occult entrapment neuropathies, especially of the median, ulnar and common peroneal nerves, it is important to study nerves not commonly susceptible to entrapment or pressure injury when investigating patients with possible symmetrical polyneuropathies. A useful plan is to measure the velocity of motor conduction in the medial popliteal nerve and of sensory conduction in the sural and radial nerves. F responses are also important, particularly in the Guillain–Barré syndrome, in order to assess conduction in the proximal part of the nerve. The median and ulnar motor conduction velocities can also be studied but, if conduction in these nerves is slowed, entrapment neuropathy must be excluded. In generalised neuropathies such as diabetic neuropathy and Guillain–Barré syndrome, in which segmental demyelination occurs, slowing of nerve conduction may be particularly prominent in the median nerve at the carpal tunnel.

Sampling of weak distal muscles with concentric needle EMG is usually not necessary for diagnosis in demyelinating neuropathies when nerve conduction studies give clearly abnormal readings, but in axonal neuropathies when measurements of nerve conduction velocities are less clearly abnormal EMG may show evidence of denervation and reinnervation. Single-fibre EMG gives little additional diagnostic information in this context, but is useful in quantifying the extent of reinnervation.

Nerve Biopsy

Pathological studies of nerve biopsies rarely provide important diagnostic information. This is, in part, due to the limited sites available for biopsy; only the sural nerve, a pure sensory nerve, is commonly biopsied. Occasionally the superficial branch of the radial nerve, also a sensory nerve, is biopsied and in very severe chronic neuropathies it is sometimes appropriate to biopsy fascicles of mixed sensorimotor nerves. In a few conditions, such as hereditary amyloidosis, leprosy, metachromatic leukodystrophy and other metabolic or storage disorders of childhood, and in some cases of chronic or relapsing polyradiculoneuritis, diagnosis can be achieved by biopsy, but these conditions are rare. Biopsy can provide confirmation of axonal or demyelinating change and in chronic demyelinating neuropathies onion-bulb formation is characteristic and may be useful in suggesting a diagnosis. In chronic or relapsing Guillain-Barré syndrome the changes of longstanding demyelination and remyelination are associated with inflammatory cells.

No clinical difference in extent of sensory loss or dysaesthesiae has been observed in whole sural nerve or fascicular sural nerve biopsies, when patients were followed up five years later (Pollock et al. 1983b). Tactile-induced dysaesthesiae were the only long-term sequelae in this study. However, many clinicians do not recommend sural nerve biopsy unless there is sensory loss in the territory of the sural nerve. Some patients complain of pain from neuroma formation at the site of the biopsy. Solders (1988) noted discomfort in 11% of 67 patients followed up 6 months or more after fascicular sural nerve biopsy. These complications occurred to a similar extent in Dyck et al.'s (1993b) follow-up of the Mayo Clinic experience.

Outcome of Investigation of Polyneuropathies

It is common experience that in many patients with progressive or moderately severe polyneuropathy even intensive investigation fails to reveal a cause. Sometimes reinvestigation after an interval of about a year will provide an answer, and it is important to evaluate relatives in considerable depth, including electrophysiological assessment in order to exclude genetically determined neuropathy. Dyck et al.

(1981b) in a study of 205 patients with polyneuropathy found that 42% had inherited disorders, 21% inflammatory demyelinating polyradiculoneuropathy, 13% had miscellaneous disorders including diabetes mellitus, toxic exposures, leprosy and dysproteinaemias. Nonetheless, 24% of this series of patients remained undiagnosed.

Principles of Management of Polyneuropathies

Since neuropathies have many possible causes, accurate diagnosis is an essential prerequisite to management. Specific treatment is possible only in relatively few neuropathies, e.g. leprosy. Non-specific treatments, such as vitamins, thyroxine or gangliosides to promote axonal sprouting, are either unproven, toxic or still experimental (Hallett et al. 1981).

Trophic lesions of skin and joints are common in sensory neuropathies because of the vulnerability of these tissues to damage when they are not protected by normal sensation. The feet may thus be injured painlessly by poorly fitting shoes, and the fingers by thermal or physical injury. Prolonged pressure should be avoided; it is useful to soak the feet and to apply vaseline to them daily. The weakened, atrophic foot and hand is also more liable to injury because of the atrophy of muscle and subcutaneous tissues leading to prominence of bony structures and a propensity to skin ulceration and joint injury. When skin is denervated it tends to become more brittle and may split at skin flexures.

When there is autonomic involvement hyperhidrosis may be a feature leading to skin softening, and heat intolerance may occur. Postural hypotension may lead to syncope and thus to injury. This can be managed with mineralo-corticoids and elastic stockings. Metoclopramide may be helpful for gastric paresis (Snape et al. 1982).

In generalised neuropathies, particularly in hypertrophic neuropathies and in diabetic neuropathy, the nerves are susceptible to entrapment at the vulnerable sites, including cervical and lumbar intervertebral foramina. Entrapment should always be carefully considered because of the possibility of effective and relatively simple surgical treatment.

Physical therapy, including massage, manipulation and passive movement of muscles and joints to overcome venous and lymphatic stasis, to encourage use of affected limbs and to prevent joint contractures, is especially important in chronic neuropathies. Splintage with appropriate footwear is useful in the care of patients with severe weakness around the ankle or knee. Wrist splints may relieve pain and produce objective benefit in carpal tunnel syndrome. Cervical collars and lumbar corsets are useful in painful radiculopathies associated with degenerative disc and joint disease.

Neural pain in diabetic polyneuropathy can be partially alleviated by a number of drugs, but individual patients show varying responses to treatment and the results are often disappointing. Pain may subside within a few weeks of commencing therapy with insulin (Boulton et al. 1982). Generally, anticonvulsants, especially phenytoin and carbamazepine (Albert 1974), and analgesics, e.g.

paracetamol, aspirin and other anti-inflammatory drugs such as ibuprofen may be useful. Narcotics, e.g. dihydrocodeine, also have a place in treatment. Tricyclic antidepressants are frequently useful, perhaps because patients with chronic pain are often depressed. However, these drugs potentiate morphine analgesia by a direct action on the central nervous system (Botney and Fields 1983) and they are more effective if combined with a neuroleptic drug. Transcutaneous nerve stimulation, or stimulation of areas of painful skin is often beneficial. Dorsal column stimulation is of value in very severe pain. Sympathectomy has long been used in the treatment of causalgia and focal nerve blocks also have a place.

Chapter *8*   Nerve Entrapment and Compression Syndromes and Other Mononeuropathies

Mononeuropathies are perhaps the most common abnormality of the nervous system; indeed everyone has experienced transient paraesthesiae from minor injury to the ulnar nerve at the elbow, or to the common peroneal nerve at the lateral aspect of the knee. More severe injury, or more prolonged compression or entrapment of nerves will lead, however, to more pronounced and less transient sensory disturbance and weakness in the distribution of the affected nerve. The various causative factors are listed in Table 8.1. By far the most common causes of mononeuropathy are entrapment and compression syndromes.

Table 8.1.   Causes of mononeuropathies

Entrapment	Constriction or mechanical distortion of a nerve by a fibrous band, or within a fibro-osseous tunnel, e.g. carpal tunnel syndrome
Compression	Sustained pressure to a localised region of nerve, e.g. Saturday night palsy
Nerve injury	Blunt or sharp trauma
Stretch of nerves	Usually associated with trauma, may be a factor in certain entrapment and occupational palsies
Infarction of nerves	May affect multiple nerves, e.g. mononeuritis multiplex in polyarteritis nodosa
Tumours of nerves	Common only in neurofibromatosis
Infection of nerves	Leprosy
Predisposition to compressive or entrapment neuropathy	Underlying metabolic disturbances of peripheral nerve, e.g. diabetes, renal failure, alcoholism, Guillain–Barré syndrome, and hereditary predisposing factors

Injuries to Nerves

Acute nerve injury results from laceration, crush injuries (external pressure) and stretch injuries, e.g. in some brachial plexus lesions. Chronic compression

from fibrous bands, scars and narrow fibro-osseous tunnels causes nerve damage in entrapment neuropathies. Chronic stretch and angulation leads to nerve damage, for example when a nerve is stretched or rubbed over a bony promontory, or through a tight fibro-osseous tunnel during repetitive activity. Direct injury may result from inadvertent injection of foreign substances, infiltration or constriction by tumour or haemorrhage, by radiation injury and by laceration.

Direct injury to nerves by penetrating wounds is comparatively unusual in peacetime, but injuries sustained in road accidents are a common cause of peripheral nerve trauma. *Penetration wounds* from high-velocity missile injuries may directly sever a nerve or injure it in proximity by a shock-wave effect, which acutely disturbs or stretches the nerve. Some of these injuries may be recoverable, depending on the degree of disruption of endoneurial tissues.

Stretch or traction injuries can occur during birth; these usually affect the brachial plexus but the radial, posterior interosseous and sciatic nerves may also be damaged in this way. Most of these injuries are reversible, recovery occurring rapidly. Stretch injuries also occur in patients unconscious during anaesthesia. They usually result from unusual positioning of the patient on the operating table. Stretch injuries to nerves in the upper limb are more common than to those in the lower limb and often involve the brachial plexus; they are particularly associated with hyperabducted and extended arm postures (Kwaan and Rappaport 1970). Cervical root lesions may also occur in this situation. Compressive injuries may also occur during anaesthesia and are discussed below.

Peripheral nerves are resistant to stretch since there is a certain amount of slack in most limb positions, and they have innate elasticity (Sunderland 1978). Stretch injury results firstly in reversible conduction block, then in axonal fracture. With progressively increasing stretch, endoneurial rupture with disruption of fasciculi and even breakage of the whole nerve may occur. The latter occurs in the cervical roots in torsional injuries, particularly if the arm in pinned down and rotational force is applied to the rest of the body. Even with incomplete stretch injuries, vascular disruption may lead to swelling and increased intraneural pressure, causing secondary ischaemic infarction of the nerve.

Closed fractures and dislocations are also associated with nerve injuries. Goodall (1956) found that 95% of these involved nerves in the arm; the radial nerve accounted for more than half, the ulnar and median nerves being less commonly affected. In the leg the common peroneal nerve was most often affected. Nerves may be damaged at the time of fracture or afterwards from the effects of movement or of reduction of a dislocation. Delayed effects of trauma, such as entrapment of a nerve in scar tissue or callus may lead to nerve damage much later by a different mechanism.

Iatrogenic injuries occur from penetrating injury to nerves. These usually occur during intramuscular injection of drugs, for example, a sciatic nerve injury may occasionally follow drug injections into the buttock. The femoral nerve is also vulnerable in the thigh. Attempted cannulation of veins or arteries, especially in the antecubital fossa where the median nerve is vulnerable, may cause a severe nerve injury.

Functional Classification of Acute Nerve Injuries

Seddon introduced a three-part classification of acute peripheral nerve injuries in 1943. *Neuropraxia* is a temporary failure of nerve conduction without loss of axonal continuity between the neuron and its end organ. Functional recovery occurs in 1–6 months. Sunderland (1991) recognised three types of "conduction block injuries". In the mild, *transient* form symptoms persist for only a few minutes or hours, without pathological change. In *moderately severe lesion* the clinical disturbance persists for up to 4 weeks, with oedema, hyperaemia and cellular infiltration. The myelin at the site of injury is fissured and vacuolated and the axons may be thinned. In the *severe lesion* the conduction block may last for up to 6 months with similar pathological features, but with additional nodal dislocation, in which nodes are telescoped into the neighbouring paranode, away from the deforming force (Ochoa et al. 1972; Lundborg et al. 1983). *Axonotmesis* describes severance or damage to the axon with subsequent Wallerian degeneration distal to the axonal lesion, but with preservation of the basement membrane and the connective tissue of the nerve bundles. Axonal regeneration occurs after this lesion at a rate of 1–2 mm/day. In more severe injuries, termed *neurotmesis* by Seddon (1943), there is damage to the basement membrane and connective tissue and the perineurium may also be damaged. In the most severe instances the nerve may actually be severed. In these more severe injuries regeneration is less effective because of the damage to the basement membrane or to the connective tissue sheaths of the nerve, so that functional recovery is less complete (see Sunderland 1978; Lundborg 1987).

EMG evaluation is valuable in distinguishing these different types of acute nerve injury. In the first few days after injury the presence of voluntary activity in the territory of the injured nerve implies that the nerve is in continuity. In the absence of motor or sensory function in this territory in the first few days, stimulation of the nerve above the level of the lesion may evoke a response distally if the nerve is not completely severed. An absent response at this time is not informative as there could be severe neuropraxia or axonotmesis, or even neurotmesis. Two weeks after the injury a normal response from stimulation of the nerve *below* the lesion in the absence of EMG features of denervation indicates neuropraxia since Wallerian degeneration has not commenced. If the EMG shows denervation and the distal segment becomes electrically unresponsive 2 weeks after the injury, either neurotmesis or axonotmesis has occurred. The important clinical distinction between axonal damage and nerve section, requiring surgical repair for recovery to be possible, cannot be made by electrophysiological techniques. It may require surgical exploration.

Entrapment Neuropathies

Nerve entrapments are a common cause of mononeuropathy. In a review Nakano (1978) described 38 different syndromes, but many more have been described although only a few are common. The most common is entrapment of the median nerve at the wrist (carpal tunnel syndrome). The ulnar nerve may be entrapped at the elbow and the common peroneal nerve at the head of the fibula, but these two syndromes are more commonly due to compression injury rather than entrapment. The anterior interosseous branch of the median nerve may be damaged by entrapment at its origin from the median nerve as it passes between the two heads of pronator teres; the posterior interosseous branch of the radial nerve is vulnerable at the elbow. The lateral cutaneous nerve of the thigh may be damaged at the inguinal ligament and the posterior tibial nerve in the tarsal tunnel at the ankle. These and other entrapment syndromes are summarised in Table 8.2.

Table 8.2. Common sites of nerve entrapment

Nerve	Site	Motor (M) and/or sensory (S) involvement
Upper limbs		
Median nerve	Wrist (carpal tunnel)	SM
Anterior interosseous branch	Between heads of pronator teres	M
Digital nerves	Hand	S
Ulnar nerve	Elbow (cubital canal)	SM
	Wrist (Guyon's canal)	SM
Radial nerve		
Posterior interosseous branch	Elbow	M
Brachial plexus		
(Thoracic outlet syndrome)	Cervical rib	SM
Cervical roots	Scalenus anterior	SM
	Intervertebral foramen	SM
	Cervical spondylosis	SM
	Cervical disc disease	S or M
Lower limbs		
Sciatic nerve	Sciatic notch	SM
Common peroneal nerve	Fibular tunnel at head of fibula	SM
Posterior tibial nerve	Tarsal tunnel at ankle	SM
Lateral femoral cutaneous nerve of thigh	Inguinal ligament	S
Lumbo-sacral roots	Intervertebral foramen	
	Lumbar spondylosis	SM
	Lumbo-sacral disc disease	

Compression syndromes may also occur at many of these sites, particularly when a nerve is superficial or relatively unprotected.

Entrapment neuropathies present as subacute or slowly progressive disorders. Although there may be relatively sudden worsening of symptoms in patients with entrapment syndromes, such episodes represent the increased susceptibility of an entrapped nerve to compression injury and recovery usually occurs. In entrapment of mixed sensorimotor nerves pain or paraesthesiae are often early symptoms. Weakness is a somewhat later symptom; atrophy is not prominent until much later. Although the patient may be aware of altered sensation in the distribution of the nerve it is often difficult to confirm this by examination. However, in well-developed entrapment syndromes sensory loss and muscle atrophy may be present. In such cases treatment directed towards alleviation of the entrapment is unlikely to result in complete recovery. It is therefore important to be aware of the *early* symptoms and signs of entrapment syndromes.

Pathogenesis

There is controversy about the cause of entrapment mononeuropathies, partly because of a failure to distinguish between nerve compression, which is usually acute, and entrapment, which is usually chronic. Compression syndromes may also occur at many of these sites, particularly when a nerve is superficial or relatively unprotected. Entrapment lesions occur at sites at which nerves traverse narrow anatomical passageways and are therefore susceptible to constriction. That entrapment neuropathies do not result from nerve compression alone is shown by the worsening in symptoms which follows periods of activity of the affected limb and the improvement which is almost invariably produced by rest or splintage of the limb. Compressive neuropathies occur at any site in the course of a nerve, but are more frequent at sites of anatomical vulnerability, such as the radial nerve in the spiral groove of the humerus.

When explored, visible swelling is characteristically seen at the proximal edge of the trapped segment of nerve and sometimes a distal swelling is apparent at the distal edge also. The histological evidence suggests that proximal nerve swelling is largely due to folding and thickening of the perineurium and endoneurium with deposition of collagen, which causes enlargement of the individual fascicles of the nerve. Axonal degeneration may occur in severe entrapment neuropathies, but in early or "subclinical" entrapment perineurial swelling and fibrosis may be found in the absence of detectable axonal degeneration. In the naturally occurring entrapment neuropathy of the guinea-pig foot Ochoa and Marotte (1973) found a characteristic distortion of myelin sheaths. In each segment the myelin sheath was tapered at the end nearest the entrapment, while a bulbous swelling of folded myelin was produced at the far end of the segment. In segments close to the zone of entrapment telescoping of myelin internodes, similar to that later demonstrated in acute nerve compression syndromes (Rudge et al. 1974) was found. Ochoa and Marotte (1973) and Marotte (1974) observed segmental demyelination, Wallerian degeneration and regenerating axons in more severely affected nerves in their guinea-pigs. The nerve fascicles were smaller than normal, there was a loss of large-diameter fibres and the amount of intrafascicular collagen was increased. Neary and Eames (1975) and Neary et al. (1975) examined ulnar and median nerves in 14 subjects at autopsy. Half the nerves examined in their elderly subjects (ten were aged more than 60 years) showed abnormalities at potential sites of entrapment, viz; the elbow and the wrist. The abnormal nerves showed segmental demyelination and internodal myelin folds at the paranodal region away from the sites of entrapment, similar to those described by Ochoa and Marotte (1973) in the guinea-pig. Paranodal bulbous swellings were also present and clusters of regenerating axons were seen in the nerve distal to the site of entrapment (Neary and Eames 1975). Renaut bodies are seen in increased numbers in the endoneurium at sites of entrapment; these bodies, consisting of randomly oriented collagen fibrils, fibroblasts and acid mucopolysaccharide ground substance (Asbury 1973) are associated experimentally with recurrent trauma or sustained compression of a nerve (Jefferson et al. 1981; Ortmann et al. 1983). The role, if any, of vascular factors, either from the entrapment itself or from capillary closure caused by endoneurial thickening (Gelberman et al. 1981), is uncertain.

There are other clinical features, however, which cannot readily be explained simply by a compression theory in the entrapment neuropathies. In particular, sensory symptoms, especially paraesthesiae, may seem to arise proximal to the site of entrapment (Lishman and Russell 1961; Crymble 1968). Entrapment neuropathies are especially common in those who use their limbs for repetitive tasks over prolonged periods (Spaans 1970) and immediate relief from sensory symptoms, with rapid recovery of function, occurs after decompression of the entrapped nerve (see Sunderland 1978).

The occurrence of proximal sensory symptoms suggests that the nerve may be damaged proximal to the site of entrapment. Whether this results from a coincidental, second and more proximal entrapment, for example, at the intervertebral foramen ("*double-crush" syndrome*) as suggested by Lishman and Russell (1961) and by Upton and McComas (1973), or from stretch injury (McLellan and Swash 1976) is difficult to define, although Anderson et al. (1970) showed that in severe chronic carpal tunnel syndrome in the guinea-pig there was reduction in fibre diameter at the level of the intervertebral foramen. In longstanding entrapment lesions Wallerian change occurs distally, from axonal injury at the site of entrapment, and secondary atrophic changes develop in the axon proximally. The latter are followed by secondary demyelination and, ultimately, by loss of anterior horn cells which implies that irreversible changes have occurred (Dyck et al. 1981). Swenson (1993) noted that two insignificant entrapment lesions were not likely to impair function in a nerve, nor does a clinically insignificant lesion worsen symptoms from a pre-existing symptomatic lesion. However, two significant lesions along the course of a nerve might be additive.

The clinical effect of limb movement could be explained by frictional injury to nerves at potential sites of entrapment during the to-and-fro sliding movement of nerves that occurs with limb movement, as a necessary result of accommodation to changing lengths of the paths taken by nerves through a limb during flexion, extension and torsional movements (McLellan and Swash 1976). Nerves have some elastic capacity and the nerve fascicles within nerves are arranged in a zigzag course, the spiral bands of Fontana, that allows for some nerve stretch to occur during normal limb movement without causing axonal damage (Clarke and Bearn 1972). If a nerve is tethered by compression at points of entrapment, stretch-induced injuries may occur at these sites, or more proximally and distally because normal nerve movements are prevented during changes of limb posture (McLellan and Swash 1976). This hypothesis offers an explanation for the beneficial effect of rest in entrapment neuropathies.

The rapid recovery which often occurs after operative decompression (Hongell and Mattsson 1971) has suggested to Sunderland (1978) that vascular factors might be important, since recovery from a structural abnormality, such as the segmental demyelination and the internodal telescoping abnormality, could not occur so quickly. Recovery after compression neuropathies, for example, is much slower. Vascular effects on the nerve trunk induced by intrafascicular oedema – itself caused by venous and capillary stasis around the entrapment site – might be an important factor, and Sunderland (1978) has suggested that the paranodal bulbous swellings might be evidence in favour of this hypothesis. However, current evidence suggests that much of the rapid beneficial effect of surgical decompression is due to relief of conduction block in a relatively limited zone of abnormality (Gilliatt and Harrison 1984). In patients in whom recovery is less good it is likely that repair of myelination is incomplete, or that permanent axonal damage with Wallerian degeneration has occurred (Miller and Olney 1982).

It will be evident from this discussion that in entrapment neuropathies a number of factors are important (see Thomas and Holdorft 1993).

General Principles of Electrophysiological Assessment

Measurements of sensory and motor nerve conduction velocity are essential in the electrophysiological assessment of patients with entrapment of mixed nerves. The most important parameters are the amplitude, latency and duration (shape) of the sensory and motor action potentials, recorded across the site of suspected entrapment. In mixed nerves sensory symptoms are an early and often a prominent manifestation and the electrophysiological abnormalities are also most marked in sensory nerve fibres. Indeed, abnormalities of sensory conduction and of the evoked sensory action potential may occur with normal motor nerve conduction and normal sensory nerve action potentials. Only when nerve damage is severe are electromyographic (EMG) features of denervation found in muscles supplied by the affected nerve.

The most important feature of the abnormality of motor conduction is *conduction block*. Conduction block occurs in a nerve fibre when depolarisation of the axon membrane fails because of the increased capacitance caused by demyelination (Lafontaine et al. 1982). The definition of conduction block has proved controversial (see Chapter 12). Over short distances, e.g. less than 40 mm, phase cancellation and temporal dispersion are probably not major contributing factors in reduction of muscle action potential (MAP) area or amplitude, and a reduction in peak to peak amplitude of the compound muscle action potential (CMAP) by more than 20% is strong evidence for conduction block (Brown and Feasby 1984; Brown and Bolton 1993; Uncini et al. 1993). This reduction in peak to peak amplitude is associated with an increase in the duration of the negative component of the CMAP peak of less than 15% between the proximal and distal stimulating sites (Brown and Feasby 1984; Abu-Shakra et al. 1991). Conduction is especially likely to be blocked when there is paranodal demyelination; internodal demyelination produces less abnormality (see Rasminsky 1985). In practice, conduction block is recognised by the finding of a smaller amplitude MAP from stimulation proximal to the lesion, than from stimulation distally. In addition, proximal stimulation evokes a more dispersed MAP than distal stimulation. These features imply activation of fewer motor units from proximal compared with distal stimulation and they are usually associated, especially in more severe cases, with slowing of conduction velocity over the short, entrapped and compressed region of the nerve and its immediately adjacent regions (Denny-Brown and Brenner 1944; Rudge 1974; Harrison 1976).

Compression Neuropathies

Compression injuries occur when a nerve is compressed by an external force. Superficially placed nerves are vulnerable to this injury and include the common peroneal nerve at the head of the fibula, the radial nerve in the spiral groove of the humerus,

the ulnar nerve at the elbow and the lateral femoral cutaneous nerve of the thigh at the inguinal ligament. The brachial plexus may be compressed in the axilla by crutch injuries. Nerve roots are also vulnerable; prolapsed cervical, thoracic or lumbar disc material may compress nerve roots as they leave the spinal canal.

Compression injuries can occur in various situations. For example, common peroneal nerve injuries are common in ill or cachectic patients restricted to bed rest. This nerve is then vulnerable to injury from the weight of the leg resting on the mattress. Similarly, the common peroneal nerve may be injured in people who habitually sit with one leg crossed over another, or who habitually lean a leg against the hard wooden or metal edge of a desk or chair. The ulnar nerve can be compressed by the pressure of leaning an elbow on a chair, or by resting the point of the elbow on a ridged surface, for example the projecting edge of a car window. The deep branch of the ulnar nerve can be compressed or injured by the pressure of the palm of the hand against a hard object, as in changing gear. The radial nerve in the spiral groove is commonly injured by pressure as the arm is rested, when the patient is asleep, on the back of a hard chair or by trauma from elbow crutches. The lateral femoral cutaneous nerve of the thigh can be compressed during surgery, the leg being flexed on the abdominal wall in the lithotomy position.

Unconscious patients are particularly vulnerable to pressure injuries to nerves. The radial, common peroneal, median and ulnar nerves are most commonly affected, and in most instances the compression injury results from direct pressure applied to the nerve by strapping a limb against a hard object or by a tourniquet. Parks (1973) noted that in most cases pressure had been applied for 2 h or more. After overdoses of hypnotic drugs or in patients unconscious for several hours from other causes, e.g. stroke, diabetic coma and infections, compression injuries to these nerves also occur. Most of these patients have also been unconscious, lying on a hard surface, often with the limb at risk beneath the weight of the body, for several hours.

Some patients are more susceptible to the effect of compressive nerve injuries than others. Patients with diabetes mellitus are susceptible in this way (Gilliatt and Willison 1962), as are patients with alcoholism and Guillain–Barré syndrome (Lambert and Mulder 1964). Some families show a hereditary susceptibility to pressure palsies, a disorder inherited as an autosomal dominant trait (Earl et al. 1964). In these families recurrent mononeuropathies occur in response to pressure injury. The nerves show evidence of demyelination and remyelination, and the myelin sheaths show localised sausage-like swellings (tomaculi) or thickening, with increased numbers of myelin lamellae. Sensory conduction velocities are slowed and so, to a lesser extent, are motor conduction velocities, indicating the underlying neuropathy (Behse et al. 1972).

Compression injuries may lead to complete loss of function in a nerve, especially when the nerve is compressed while the patient is unconscious. Compression while a patient is conscious leads first to paraesthesiae in the distribution of the sensory supply of the nerve. This occurs in a few minutes, as everyone knows from common experience, but both its severity and the interval from application of the force before paraesthesiae occur depend on the compressive force and the time for which it is applied. With a slight compressive force, recovery from these paraesthesiae occurs in a few minutes once this force is relieved. Similarly, weakness resulting from such a mild injury, as when an arm "goes to sleep" or is found numb and weak after sleeping in an unusual posture, recovers in a few minutes or hours; "first-degree conduction block" (Sunderland 1978). In more severe compression injuries of this benign type recovery may be delayed for days or even longer. Paraesthesiae may persist for several weeks or even months. Sunderland (1978) has referred to this delayed recovery as indicating "second-degree conduction block". In some patients compression injury may be so severe that recovery is incomplete.

Acute compression syndromes mainly affect large, thickly myelinated fibres, the smaller myelinated and unmyelinated fibres being relatively spared. Thus motor function is affected early and paraesthesiae are prominent. Sparing of sensation on examination is often quite striking and is probably due to the relatively selective involvement of the larger fibres; there may be abnormalities of fine discriminative sensation, e.g. two-point discrimination. In more chronic compressive neuropathies weakness is associated with wasting, probably because of axonal injury in addition to conduction block. Generally, lesions of limited length recover more rapidly than lesions involving long segments of a nerve (Rudge et al. 1974).

Pathophysiology

Understanding of the pathophysiological basis of compression neuropathy has been complicated by controversy concerning the relative roles of the compressive force itself and of ischaemia of the nerve induced by the compression.

Caruso et al. (1973) suggested that nerve injury from a tourniquet is due both to the compression of the tourniquet and to ischaemia of the nerve below the level of the tourniquet. The sensory action potential in the distal nerve to the tourniquet was reduced in amplitude in normal human subjects 10 min after application of the tourniquet and, after 30 min, the sensory potential was reduced by more than 60% and the sensory conduction velocity was reduced by 25% (Caruso et al. 1973). The effect might therefore be due to ischaemia of the nerve distal to the tourniquet.

Gilliatt and his colleagues examined the effect of the pressure under the tourniquet itself in a series of experiments in which they measured the conduction velocity across the compressed segment of the nerve, and also studied the pathological changes in this part of the nerve. In the baboon they found that compression for 2 h at 500 mm Hg produced clinically evident nerve dysfunction which recovered in 24 h, although electrophysiological studies showed that motor nerve conduction was slowed across this segment for a longer period of time. A cuff pressure of 1000 mmHg produced a severe and longer-lasting paralysis of distal muscles, with slowed motor conduction velocity across the damaged segment. This disturbance of motor conduction velocity persisted for several months (Fowler et al. 1972). In patients with tourniquet paralysis, although nerve stimulation above the level of the compression injury may fail to elicit a twitch in the distal muscles, stimulation below the level of the injury will produce muscular contraction, indicating not only that there is conduction block at the site of the lesion, but that Wallerian degeneration, if it has occurred at all, is only slight (Moldaver 1954; Fowler et al. 1972). Moldaver (1954) was able to record a muscle twitch from proximal nerve stimulation after 7 weeks but recovery was not complete until 14 weeks after the compression injury. Recovery from conduction block due to compression injury to a nerve may thus be delayed for a long time.

In the compressed segment of nerve in these tournique experiments Ochoa and his colleagues found evidence of direct damage to myelin sheaths. There was dislocation and invagination of paranodal myelin with subsequent localised demyelination. The nodal displacement was maximal under the edges of the cuff, with relative or complete sparing under its centre. The direction of displacement was always away from the cuff, toward the uncompressed parts of the nerve, suggesting that the pressure gradient between the zone of pressure under the edge of the cuff and the nerve proximal and distal to the compressed segment was the factor responsible for nodal damage (Ochoa et al. 1971, 1972). That these changes, and the consequent localised conduction block, were due to the mechanical effects of nerve compression, and not to ischaemia, was shown by Rudge et al. (1974), who compressed the common peroneal nerve of the baboon against underlying bone with a suitably weighted nylon cord, so sparing the blood supply to the distal parts of the nerve and limb. They found similar nodal invagination on either side of the narrow band of compression induced by the cord, and a localised conduction block. Despite this elegant demonstration of the distortion induced by the compressive force itself, the blood supply to the segment of nerve compressed, however narrow, must be compromised during the period of compression (see Nobel et al. 1974; and discussion in Sunderland 1978). However, experiments in which this local nerve compression was combined with ischaemia of the whole limb of 3–4 h duration revealed no additional effect compared with the effect of local nerve compression itself (Williams et al. 1980).

Clinical Implications

It will be apparent from this discussion that tight, constricting bandages or plaster casts may cause acute dysfunction or even irreversible damage to peripheral nerves, even after comparatively short periods of compression. These causes of mononeuropathy are preventable.

Electrophysiological Assessment of Nerve Compression

EMG investigation of patients with compression injuries to nerves can provide diagnostic and prognostic information. The lesion can be localised by stimulation of the nerve above and below the level of compression injury, with evidence of conduction block. The distal limit of the lesion can be determined by finding the most proximal point from which a muscle action potential can be evoked in a distal muscle supplied by the injured nerve. It is more difficult to establish the proximal limit of the lesion. This can be attempted by recording an evoked *nerve action potential* from a more proximal segment of the nerve, following stimulation of the nerve above the lesion. The potential recorded will be the summated orthodromic sensory and antidromic motor potential.

During the first few weeks it is difficult to give a prognosis by electrophysiological investigation in a patient in whom clinical recovery has not begun. If there is return of sensory or motor function, however slight, in this time the prognosis is good even though the nerve may remain electrically inexcitable in the region of the lesion. Fibrillation potentials may be recorded in muscles distal to the lesion, supplied by the nerve, within about 2 weeks of the injury but this evidence of denervation is not necessarily a bad prognostic sign. Fibrillation potentials appear earlier the nearer the nerve lesion is to the muscle tested, indicating the shorter length of nerve degeneration necessary in this instance. The size of the muscle action potential evoked by stimulation distal to the lesion is more useful. The larger the evoked muscle action potential recorded 2 or 3 weeks after the injury, the better the prognosis (Smith and Trojaborg 1986). A large muscle action potential implies that little Wallerian degeneration has occurred in the distal part of the damaged nerve, and that the lesion is largely a neuropraxia. Another useful test is to study the nerve action potential evoked from distal nerve stimulation, recorded distal to the compression injury. The size of this nerve action potential can be related to the number and size of functioning axons. Even the presence of such potentials, although small, favours a return of useful functions (Kline and De Jonge 1968). These electrophysiological methods are also useful in assessing the effects of nerve injuries from other causes.

Upper Limb Syndromes

Median Nerve Syndromes

The median nerve is formed from branches of the lateral and medial cords of the brachial plexus, representing C5, C6, C7, C8 and T1 segments. It runs in the medial part of the upper arm, crosses the elbow anteriorly in the cubital fossa close to the brachial artery, and enters the flexor compartment of the forearm between the two heads of pronator teres, after innervating this muscle. It then divides distally into a purely motor anterior interosseous branch and a main trunk which enters the wrist, passes through the carpal tunnel and supplies motor and sensory branches to the hand. In the forearm the laterally placed flexors are all innervated by the anterior interosseous branch of the median nerve, including the flexor digitorum profundus I and II, flexor pollicis longus, and pronator quadratus muscles. The flexor carpi radialis, palmaris longus and flexor digitorum superficialis are all supplied by the main trunk of the median nerve. In the hand the abductor pollicis brevis, opponens pollicis and lumbricals I and II are supplied by the median nerve. The sensory branches of the median nerve innervate the skin of the lateral three-and-a-half digits on their ventral surfaces, and the palm of the hand, to a level just above the wrist together with the dorsal surfaces of the distal phalanges of the lateral digits.

The main sites of entrapment are in the carpal tunnel and at the point of entry between the two heads of pronator teres where the main trunk, or the anterior interosseous nerve may be compressed. The median nerve may be compressed at the shoulder by crutches or by unusual sleeping postures, and direct injuries may occur at this site or in the upper arm or antecubital fossa. Rarely, the latter injury occurs during attempted catheterisation of the brachial artery or vein as part of medical investigation.

Carpal Tunnel Syndrome

Entrapment of the median nerve in the carpal tunnel is by far the commonest of the entrapment mononeuropathies. The age-adjusted incidence is about 100/100 000 person years (Amadiro 1992). Women predominate in all series by about 3 : 1. Carpal tunnel syndrome is most common in the fifth and sixth decades. The nerve is compressed against the proximal edge of the flexor retinaculum (Brain et al. 1947; Phalen 1966) and this is accentuated by wrist flexion (Phalen 1972). During movement of the wrist or fingers the nerve normally slides proximally or distally beneath the retinaculum, but this is prevented if the nerve is trapped by the retinaculum, leading to stretch and frictional injuries to the nerve (McLellan and Swash 1976) and hence to the well-known deleterious clinical effects of movement, or of sleeping with the wrists flexed, and to the beneficial effects of splintage in a neutral position. In the normal wrist the pressure in the carpal tunnel is 7–8 mmHg. In carpal tunnel syndrome the pressure is increased to about 30 mmHg and with wrist flexion it may reach 90 mmHg; enough to cause nerve damage (Szabo et al. 1989).

The syndrome is associated with hypothyroidism, acromegaly, rheumatoid arthritis, amyloidosis, mucopolysaccharidosis (MacDougall et al. 1977), pregnancy, obesity, the menopause and local injuries to the wrist. O'Duffy et al. (1973) noted that 35 of a series of 100 patients with acromegaly had carpal tunnel syndrome. About 25% of patients with rheumatoid arthritis have carpal tunnel syndrome (Nakano 1978). Injuries to the wrist may cause acute damage to the median nerve, or the later development of median nerve compression, e.g. following Colles fracture (Lewis 1969). Voitk et al. (1983) found by questionnaire that 25% of 1000 women had symptoms of carpal tunnel syndrome during pregnancy, 75% of which were bilateral. Nearly all resolved spontaneously within a few days or weeks. Carpal tunnel syndrome has also been reported in uraemic patients treated with long-term haemodialysis. After 15 years 70% of patients have had carpal tunnel decompression, and the first patients require decompression after only about 8 years of dialysis (Chanard et al. 1989). The carpal tunnel syndrome in these patients has been associated with amyloid deposition in the transverse carpal ligament, probably derived from β_2 microglobulin (Chanard et al. 1989). Nerve ischaemia associated with vascular shunt surgery can also lead to median nerve palsy in haemodialysis patients (Halter et al. 1981). Further, patients with diabetes mellitus are unduly susceptible to mechanical nerve damage and Phalen (1972) noted that 14.5% of patients with carpal tunnel syndrome had diabetes. In other conditions in which the median nerve is enlarged or damaged, such as amyloid neuropathy, leprosy and Guillain–Barré syndrome symptomatic median nerve damage may occur from entrapment in the carpal tunnel. Inglis et al. (1972) found that in 53% of their 101 patients with carpal tunnel syndrome there was an underlying cause. Dekel et al. (1980) used computed axial tomography (CT) of the wrist to study the cross-sectional diameter of the carpal tunnel. They found that there was an association of a congenitally small carpal canal and symptoms of the carpal tunnel syndrome. The canal was particularly small in women, even in those in the control group, an observation which might explain the high incidence of the syndrome in women.

Bleecker et al. (1985) showed that a small carpal tunnel, assessed by measurement of the cross-sectional area by CT scanning, was associated with either clinical or subclinical features of carpal tunnel syndrome, whereas subjects engaged in the same occupation who were normal clinically and electrophysiologically had larger carpal tunnels. One diabetic patient had a normal canal and normal electrophysiological studies. These observations could be important in assessing the role of occupation in the initiation of carpal tunnel syndrome. Magnetic resonance imaging has been used to calculate the cross-sectional area of the carpal tunnel and to identify structures within it, including the nerve, tendons and vessels. Any areas of focal flattening of the nerve can be recognised. However, this technique does not have a clinical role in this disorder (Mesgarzadeh et al. 1989). In carpal tunnel syndrome there is a zone of increased pressure, particularly in the distal third of the carpal tunnel. This has been correlated with the clinical symptoms and with reduction in amplitude of the SNAP (Luchetti et al. 1990).

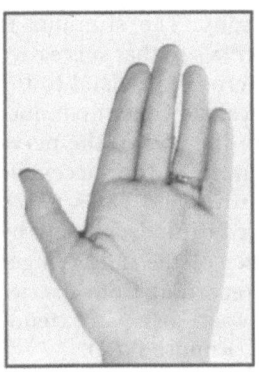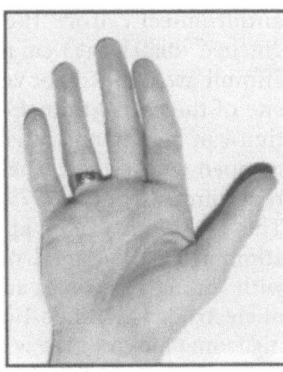

Fig. 8.1. Carpal tunnel syndrome. There is atrophy of the left thenar eminence; this is often a subtle sign.

Inglis et al. (1972) found numbness and pain the most prominent presenting symptoms of carpal tunnel syndrome. Only 3% of their patients presented with weakness. The sensory symptoms are prominent at night; 96% of Kendall's (1960) 327 patients experienced this symptom. Nocturnal discomfort is often felt in the flexor compartment of the forearm, as well as in the hand itself. The symptoms are often exaggerated by movement of the wrist or fingers, or by prolonged wrist flexion. As the disorder progresses weakness of thumb abduction and apposition develops so that the patient has difficulty buttoning clothes, winding a watch and tying shoelaces. Wasting of the thenar eminence develops at this time (Fig. 8.1). Rarely, the carpal tunnel may seem swollen at the wrist. Sensory abnormalities are found on examination in relatively advanced cases; the palmar surfaces of the thumb, index and part of the middle digits are affected, extending proximally to the wrist. On the dorsal surface of the hand sensory loss is found only in the terminal phalanx of these digits. The digits may feel swollen and provocative tests involving simulated grasping with the hand can induce an increase in hand volume of 20 mls or more, accompanied by discomfort and increased numbness (Braun et al. 1989). In such patients painless injuries to the median-innervated digits may occur.

In 43% of cases both hands are involved, but the dominant hand is usually the first and more severely affected (Reinstein 1981; Pryse-Phillips 1984). Pain in the median-innervated tissues of the hand, i.e. on the lateral side of the palm, may be conspicuous and may extend into the forearm or even to the shoulder.

A number of provocative signs have been advocated. The Tinel sign, evoked by tapping the nerve at the site of compression at the wrist, or slightly proximally is positive in some cases, but reports vary from 0–80% and it may even be positive in normal subjects (Bowles et al. 1982). Phalen's wrist flexion test (1966), in which full voluntary flexion of the wrist for more than 1 minute causes exacerbation of the sensory symptoms, especially in the middle finger, is positive in 48%–80% of patients. Pryse-Phillips (1984), in a study of 212 patients with carpal tunnel syndrome in a group of 505 patients with various upper limb mononeuropathies, noted that patients with carpal tunnel syndrome tended to relieve their sensory symptoms by flicking the wrist and hand "as though shaking down a clinical thermometer". This sign was present in 93% of patients with carpal tunnel syndrome, and was found only rarely (<10%) in patients with other brachial entrapment syndromes. It was not present in 32 patients with cervical spondylosis.

Because the median nerve divides into three branches in the carpal tunnel, one mixed branch to the muscles of the thenar eminence and the skin of the thumb, and sensory branches to the index and middle fingers, there may be variable involvement within the overall sensorimotor distribution of the nerve. Further, the clinical features, both motor and sensory, are not always typical because of anomalous innervation resulting from communications between the median and ulnar nerves in the forearm so that the ulnar nerve may innervate some of the usual sensory and motor innervation of the median nerve or vice versa. This anomaly occurs in about 15% of the population, an observation first made by Martin (1763) by dissection and confirmed by Gruber (1870). Electrophysiological studies have shown a similar incidence of the Martin-Gruber anastomosis (Iyer and Fenichel 1976). In two-thirds of cases the anomaly is bilateral; it may be dominantly inherited (Crutchfield and Gutmann 1980). Less commonly, an anastomosis may be present between the motor branches of the median nerve and the deep branch of the ulnar nerve in the hand (Riche–Cannieu anastomosis). In this anomaly the interossei and hypothenar muscles may be innervated by the median, rather than by the ulnar nerve (Riche 1897; Cannieu 1897).

Electrophysiological Assessment. The most sensitive parameter for diagnosis of the carpal tunnel syndrome is the sensory nerve action potential (SNAP). It is important to recognise that the amplitude and the conduction velocity of the SNAP decrease with age. For example, the lower limit of sensory conduction velocity in the median nerve from digit III (middle finger) to wrist is 55 m/s at age 20 and 45 m/s at age 80 years (Buchthal et al. 1974). There is a marked reduction in the amplitude of the SNAP in normal subjects over the age of 60 years, and the

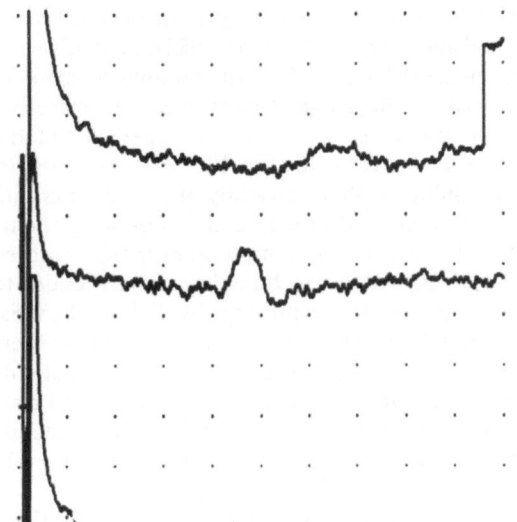

Fig. 8.2. Carpal tunnel syndrome. SNAPs recorded from middle finger (top) and index finger (lower). The response from the middle finger is delayed, and of reduced amplitude. Orthodromic technique recording from median nerve at wrist.

potential may be difficult to record with surface electrodes even in normal subjects of this age or more. However, with needle recordings a SNAP can be recorded (Buchthal et al. 1974), even in subjects with severe carpal tunnel syndrome.

Since not all of the branches of the median nerve in the carpal tunnel may be affected it may be important to record individually the SNAPs from the thumb, index and middle fingers (Buchthal et al. 1974). In a study of SNAP recordings from stimulation of digits I–IV MacDonell et al. (1990) found that stimulation of the index finger was least sensitive and stimulation of the middle finger was preferred in the diagnosis of carpal tunnel syndrome (Fig. 8.2). Sensory symptoms in carpal tunnel syndrome are often experienced, or provoked by the Phalen test, in the middle finger (digit III). Stimulation of digit IV produces a similar sensitive result (Lauritzen et al. 1991).

These three branches of the median nerve can also be studied in the short segment between the palm and the wrist, by stimulating the palm and recording the SNAP at the wrist in the usual manner. The patient experiences paraesthesiae with nerve stimulation in the digit supplied by the branch that is stimulated (Eklund 1975) and the latency of the response is delayed in the affected branch.

Precise localisation of the zone of entrapment can be achieved by using the "inching" technique. The stimulus is applied to the median nerve about 3 cm rostral to the wrist crease and SNAPs are recorded antidromically from the index. The stimulus is "inched" distally at 1 cm intervals so that successive stimuli are applied above, across and distal to the site of the carpal tunnel. Focal slowing of conduction can be demonstrated in the part of the nerve trapped within the carpal tunnel in the successive recordings (Kimura 1979; Brown and Yates 1982). This technique can be applied orthodromically by stimulating the digital nerves of the index finger with surface electrodes and recording from a series of electrodes mounted 1 cm apart on a pad extending from palm over the wrist (Kimura 1984).

Sedal et al. (1973) found that the ulnar nerve SNAPs were abnormally small in 39% of patients with carpal tunnel syndrome, and suggested that this indicated a subclinical neuropathy in such cases. Buchthal et al. (1974) argued that these small ulnar nerve SNAPs were probably due to coincidental traumatic lesions to the ulnar nerves at the elbow. Harrison (1978) studied the ulnar and radial SNAPs in patients with carpal tunnel syndrome and found no evidence of a generalised neuropathy. This controversy underlines the importance of studying nerves not usually susceptible to trauma when looking for evidence of a generalised neuropathy. In normal subjects the amplitude of the SNAPs recorded from the ulnar and median nerves after stimulation of digit V and digit III respectively should be greater from the median than the ulnar recording. In carpal tunnel syndrome the ulnar response is often larger.

The distal motor latency is an important parameter (Table 8.3), although it must be recognised that reliance on absolute values for the lower limit of this measurement may be misleading because of the variability in hand size between different subjects. In one study abnormalities of motor conduction were seen in 69% of subjects, but sensory conduction was abnormal in 93% (Kemble 1968). However, an abnormal distal motor latency can sometimes occur when sensory conduction is normal.

A difference in the distal motor latency of more than 0.5 ms between the two hands is abnormal, suggesting the presence of entrapment injury to the median nerve in the carpal tunnel even when the median motor latency is still within normal limits. Preston and Logigian (1992) described a technique utilising lumbrical and interossei recording with surface electrodes placed over the third metacarpal bone. A prolonged lumbrical (median stimulation) versus interosseous (ulnar stimulation) latency (>0.4 ms difference) was a sensitive indicator of carpal tunnel syndrome. Only 54% of their patients had an increased distal motor latency to APB, but 95% had an abnormal lumbrical-interosseous latency difference.

Table 8.3.   Normal values for motor and sensory conduction

Sensory			Motor Median nerve		
Digit I to wrist	CV[a] >42 m/s Amplitude >10.0 μV[b]		Wrist to APB Elbow to wrist	Latency CV	<4.2 ms >50 m/s
			Ulnar nerve		
Digit V to wrist	CV >41 m/s Amplitude >7.0 μV[b]		Wrist to ADM Below elbow to wrist Across elbow	Latency CV CV	<3.2 ms >52 m/s >50 m/s
			Common peroneal nerve		
Toe I to ankle	CV >32 m/s		Ankle to EDB Below knee to ankle Across head of fibula	Latency CV CV	<5.0 m/s >43 m/s >41 m/s

[a]CV, conduction velocity.
[b]After age 60 years the sensory potential amplitude decreases.
Modified from Rosenfalck (1975).

In addition, increase in the distal motor or sensory latency can occur after short periods of full voluntary wrist flexion, as in Phalen's manoeuvre. Schwartz et al. (1980a) found that wrist flexion for 2 min was sufficient to increase the distal motor latency in patients with carpal tunnel syndrome, so that the latency was abnormal only *after* wrist flexion in some patients (Fig. 8.3). This phenomenon has also been investigated by Marin et al. (1983), who found that wrist extension had a similar but less marked effect on motor and sensory conduction. Wilson-Macdonald et al. (1984) found a diurnal variation in motor conduction velocity in patients with positive Tinel and Phalen signs.

When the motor latency is markedly longer than normal there is often slowing of motor conduction velocity in the elbow to wrist segment of the median nerve (Fig. 8.4). Sampling the abductor pollicis brevis muscle with concentric EMG is usually not necessary for diagnosis, but the presence of EMG signs of denervation in this muscle is regarded by some as an indication for surgical decompression of the nerve. Stevens (1987) noted that needle EMG, in addition to being painful, was the least sensitive part of the EMG investigation of suspected carpal tunnel syndrome.

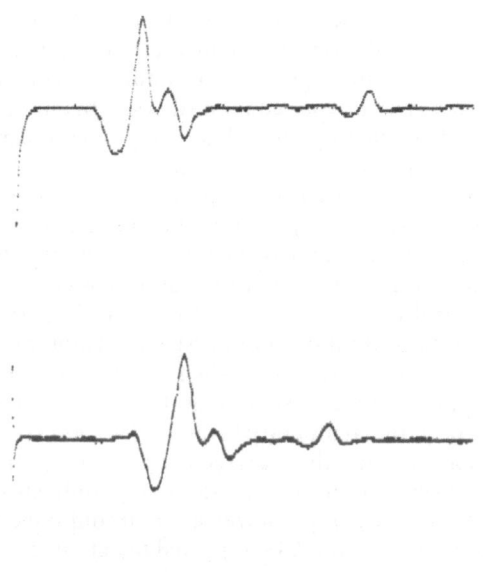

Fig. 8.4.   Carpal tunnel syndrome. Surface recording from abductor pollicis brevis following stimulation of median nerve at wrist and elbow. In the upper trace, recorded after stimulation at the wrist, the first (M) response shows a latency of 9.4 ms, and the second (F) response has a latency of 36 ms. In the second trace, recorded after stimulation at the elbow, the M wave latency is 13.8 ms and the F wave latency is 31 ms. The F response latency is shorter after stimulation at a more proximal site. The major abnormality is the increase in the distal motor latency. Bar 10 ms.

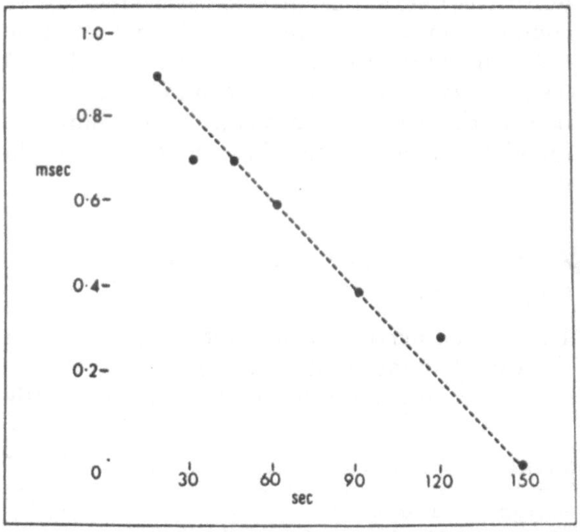

Fig. 8.3.   Electrophysiological changes following Phalen's test. The wrist was fully flexed for 2 min. Fifteen seconds after cessation of wrist flexion the distal motor latency was increased over the control value by 0.9 ms. It returned to the pretest value after 2 1/2 min. (From Schwartz et al. 1980a)

In patients with Martin–Gruber anastomosis (crossover) from the median to the ulnar nerve in the forearm, entrapment of the median nerve at the wrist may not be accompanied by typical symptoms or EMG features of carpal tunnel syndrome (Iyer and Fenichel 1976). In such cases there may be little evidence of denervation of small hand muscles since they are supplied by fibres travelling in the undamaged ulnar nerve. The crossover from median to ulnar nerves in the forearm may result in a normal motor latency from the median nerve at the elbow to abductor pollicis brevis in the face of a prolonged latency to this muscle from the wrist; sometimes the proximal latency may be shorter than the distal. Stimulation of the median nerve at the wrist evokes a compound muscle action potential (CMAP) in the thenar eminence of lower amplitude than stimulation of the median nerve at the elbow, because stimulation at the elbow excites both median and ulnar fibres through the crossover from median to ulnar in the forearm, so that the whole thenar eminence will be excited after median nerve stimulation at the elbow (Gutmann 1977).

Management. Rest is important and effective. Patients with carpal tunnel syndromes of mild severity without weakness or sensory loss often respond to splinting of the wrist in a slightly dorsiflexed position. Such splints are especially useful at night and in pregnancy since spontaneous improvement after delivery can be expected in most cases. In one series 21% of pregnant women had symptomatic carpal tunnel syndrome, usually commencing in the last trimester; only 3% had symptoms continuing for a month after delivery (Gould and Wissinger 1978). Treatment of causative factors such as hypothyroidism or recent weight gain may also be effective.

A local injection of steroid is useful in patients with intermittent or mild persistent symptoms, or in the elderly, particularly when pain is a prominent symptom (Phalen 1966). This treatment is often only of initial, temporary benefit; 127 of 497 treated patients eventually required surgery. Gelberman et al. (1980) found that at 18 months only 40% of patients were symptom free after steroid injection treatment. Green (1984) reported benefit in 81% of patients but symptoms recurred 2–4 months after the injection. Grannini et al. (1991) evaluated steroid injection using electrophysiological assessment. They found that at 6 months 35% were asymptomatic and 58% had partial improvement. Motor conduction improved in 65% and sensory nerve conduction in 73%. Many of their patients were only of mild severity.

Dawson et al. (1990) recommended 20 mg methylprednisolone mixed with 1–2 ml 1% xylo-caine. A fine gauge (25) needle is inserted proximal to the transverse wrist crease and medial (ulnar) to the palmaris longus tendon. Any paraesthesiae in a median nerve distribution indicate undue proximity to the median nerve and the needle should then be repositioned. Generally, repeated injections are not recommended, although the procedure may safely be repeated once or twice at intervals of several months. Steroid injection therapy is contra-indicated in the presence of sensory loss or motor deficit. In patients aged more than 50 years, or with symptoms for more than 10 months, or with constant paraesthesiae, conservative treatment is unlikely to succeed (Kaplan et al. 1990).

More than 90% of patients with carpal tunnel syndrome show a good response to surgical decompression and this outcome can be expected both in cases with short and long durations of symptoms (Harris et al. 1979). Clinical improvement usually precedes electrophysiological recovery. Motor symptomse have a more favourable prognosis than sensory symptoms (Harris et al. 1979). A longitudinal incision is preferred; a transverse incision gives a less good exposure of the transverse carpal ligament and carries with it the risk of section of the motor branch of the median nerve. An endoscopic technique for dividing the transverse carpal ligament has been developed. The most common cause of failure of surgical decompression is inadequate decompression; this can be recognised by repeated electrophysiological investigation which shows the continued abnormality expected when the nerve remains compressed. However, electrophysiological tests never return completely to normal if the nerve compression was severe. Hongell and Mattson (1971) noted improvement in electrophysiological tests of nerve conduction, using intraneural recordings, during surgery. Yates et al. (1981), however, found no change in the distal motor latency in intraoperative recordings.

Acute Compression of the Median Nerve in the Carpal Tunnel

The median nerve may be acutely compressed in the carpal tunnel (Table 8.4). In most of these syndromes the problem resolves spontaneously

Table 8.4. Causes of acute carpal tunnel syndrome

Wrist fractures and dislocations
Haematomas (haemophilia and anticoagulant medication)
Pyogenic infections of the hand and wrist
Rheumatoid arthritis
Vasculitis
Prolonged, unaccustomed manual work

From Stewart (1994).

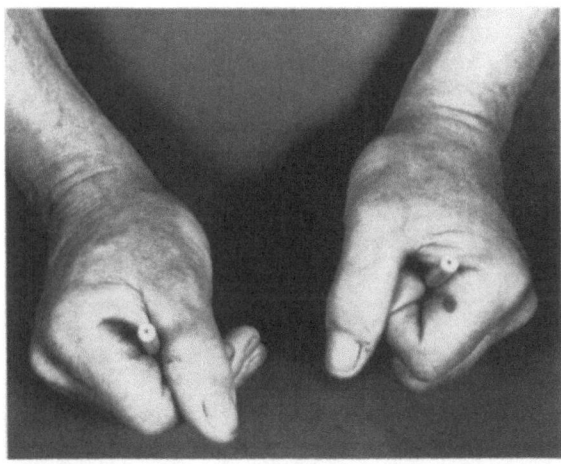

Fig. 8.5. Right anterior interosseous palsy. The patient is unable to flex fully the terminal parts of the thumb and index fingers around the pencil.

although a period of rest and analgesia may be required. In severe cases urgent decompression may be helpful, but in the presence of severe weakness and sensory loss the prognosis is guarded (Bauman et al. 1981).

Anterior Interosseous Syndrome

In this uncommon syndrome (Kiloh and Nevin 1952; Nigst and Dick 1979) the anterior interosseous branch of the median nerve in the forearm is trapped between the two heads of pronator teres under the tendinous arch of the flexor digitorum sublimis in the pronator tunnel (Geenen and Bunker 1985). There is weakness of the flexor pollicis longus, of the long flexors of the index and middle fingers (Fig. 8.5) and of the pronator quadratus. This results in a rather characteristic inability to "make an O" between the index and thumb due to loss of flexion of the tips of these two digits, so that a triangle rather than a circle is formed. There is no sensory loss, but pain in the forearm and wrist may be marked. The thenar muscles in the hand are strong but there is slight weakness of pronation. Bilateral cases have been recorded, and neuralgic amyotrophy can mimic this syndrome (Rennels and Ochoa 1980). Insidious onset cases are associated with fibrous bands arising from pronator teres or flexor digitorum sublimis, and compressing the anterior interosseous nerve in the pronator tunnel. The syndrome can occur acutely from direct trauma, e.g. stab wounds and fractures of the shaft of the radius (Warren 1963), and some cases have an inflammatory cause as a localised neuritis associated with a previous viral infection. Unaccustomed

vigorous supination/pronation exercise may also cause this nerve palsy (Hill et al. 1985).

Electrophysiological Assessment. There are EMG features of denervation in the long flexor muscles, but the SNAPs recorded at wrist and elbow are normal since the anterior interosseous nerve is a motor nerve (O'Brien and Upton 1972). The motor conduction velocity in the main part of the nerve is also normal, but the latency of the motor response from elbow to affected flexor muscles is prolonged when compared with similar stimulation in the unaffected limb (Nakano et al. 1977).

Management. Spontaneous recovery may occur, but is delayed and may take 6–18 months. Avoidance of forced or repeated pronation/supination activities, such as using a screwdriver, should be advised, and local steroid injections may be used. If recovery does not commence in 2 months surgical exploration of the pronator tunnel is advised (Stern 1984).

Pronator Teres Syndrome

The median nerve may be compressed proximal to the origin of the anterior interosseous branch. This rare syndrome is due to repetitive exercise involving pronation and supination, or in weightlifters, and may also occur from trauma. There is weakness in the hand as in carpal tunnel syndrome but, in addition or the long flexors of thumb, index and middle fingers, and the pronator quadratus, as in the anterior interosseous syndrome. There is sensory impairment in a median nerve distribution in the hand, together with involvement of the rostral portion of the palm. There is pain in the volar aspect of the forearm near the site of entrapment that can be reproduced by pressure over the pronator muscle during pronation with the elbow flexed (Hartz et al. 1981). Indeed, pain is often the major feature. In most patients conservative measures, especially avoidance of pronating movement, and steroid injection into the region of the pronator muscle, are helpful and surgery is rarely needed (Morris and Peters 1976).

There may be slowed motor conduction in the forearm, with a normal distal motor latency (Morris and Peters 1976). Needle EMG may demonstrate partial denervation in the long forearm flexors.

Other Median Nerve Syndromes

The median nerve may be injured by compression in the axilla, e.g. by the use of crutches. It may rarely be compressed beneath the ligament of Struthers which extends from a supracondylar bony spur to the medial epicondyle of the humerus (Sunderland 1978).

Ulnar Nerve

The ulnar nerve consists of branches from the C7, C8 and T1 roots. The nerve is infrequently damaged in the *axilla*, usually in association with trauma which often also involves median or radial nerves. This may occur from a hyperextended position of the arm during sleep in the prone position. The most common site of damage to the ulnar nerve is at the *elbow in the ulnar groove* behind the medial epicondyle of the humerus or in the cubital tunnel between the aponeurosis of the flexor carpi ulnaris muscle and the medial ligament of the elbow joint. The nerve may be entrapped in the cubital tunnel 1–3 cm distal to the epicondyle (Payan 1969, Miller 1979), or injured by pressure, trauma or deformities secondary to healed fractures in the ulnar groove. Injury at the latter site quite frequently occurs from direct pressure on the nerve after a period of unconsciousness or anaesthesia (Miller and Camp, 1979). The nerve is rarely entrapped in *Guyon's canal at the wrist* as it passes between the transverse carpal ligament and the volar carpal ligament bounded on either side by the bony margins of the pisiform bone and the hook of the hamate bone (Shea and McClain 1969). This canal also contains the ulnar artery and vein; in the canal the nerve bifurcates into motor and sensory branches and in the arm either branch can be separately damaged (Dawson et al. 1990). The deep, motor branch of the nerve is vulnerable to injury from *trauma in the palm*, especially from repeated trauma such as from power tools, manual labour etc. and from compression due to fractures of the hook of the hamate, ganglion formation or lipoma (Shea and McClain 1969). The ulnar nerve may be palpated only at and a little above the elbow. It is frequently more easily felt, thickened and sensitive to manipulation with a positive Tinel sign when injured at this site.

Ulnar Nerve Lesion at the Elbow

The elbow is the most common site of damage to the ulnar nerve. The clinical signs are variable. The most common presentation is with intermittent tingling on the ulnar border of the hand, extending into the little and ring fingers. This is often induced by movement or by minor trauma to the nerve at the elbow and it may be accompanied by local pain

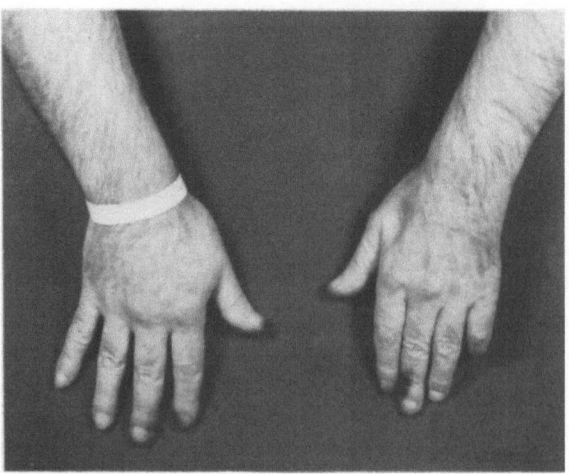

Fig. 8.6. Left ulnar palsy. There is wasting of the interossei, especially of the first dorsal interosseous muscle, with characteristic flexion of the little finger. There was osteoarthritis at the left elbow.

and tenderness at the site of the nerve in the ulnar groove or cubital tunnel, with a positive Tinel sign. Cubital tunnel syndrome occurs without evidence of joint deformity or trauma, is often bilateral, is associated with enlargement of the ulnar nerve in the ulnar groove, and symptoms are often induced by prolonged elbow flexion. The nerve is sensitive to percussion or slight external compression and Tinel's sign is localised to the cubital tunnel, rather than to the olecranon groove (Miller 1991).

In some patients sensory symptoms are minimal and presentation consists of a weak hand with atrophy of the hypothenar eminence, of the web of the thumb and of the interossei (Fig. 8.6). In these cases the lesion is of gradual onset and progressive ("tardy" ulnar nerve palsy). A characteristic posture develops, with flexion of the interphalangeal joints and hyperextension of the metacarpo-phalangeal joints of the ring and little fingers, due to weakness of the lumbricals, interossei and flexor digitorum profundus muscles, and unopposed action of the finger extensors and flexor digitorum superficialis. In other patients sensory symptoms predominate for many years without subjective weakness (van der Pool et al. 1968). Weakness of the hand causes difficulty with grip, writing and manipulative tasks involving the fingers; this can be a severe disability. In some patients the ulnar groove of the olecranon process is abnormally shallow, and this implies susceptibility to injury to the ulnar nerve from pressure at this site, even in everyday postures such as resting the elbow on a table or chair during work or rest.

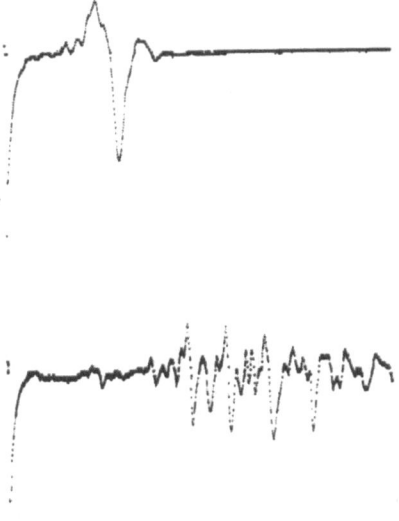

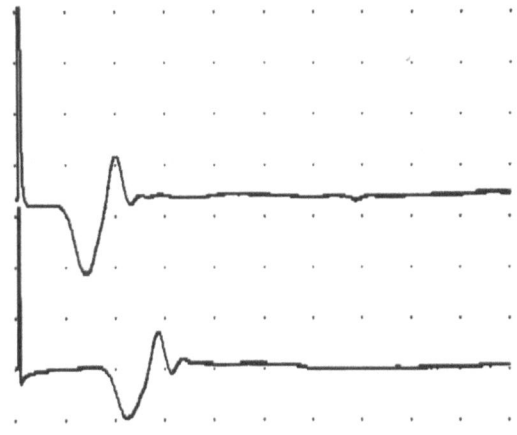

Fig. 8.8. A mild degree of conduction block.

Fig. 8.7. Ulnar nerve lesion at the elbow. Surface recording from the abductor digiti minimi following stimulation of the ulnar nerve at the wrist (upper trace), and elbow (lower trace). The conduction velocity from elbow to wrist was 10 m/s, and the evoked muscle action potential after proximal nerve stimulation is dispersed (lower trace). Bar 20 ms.

During flexion of the elbow the cubital tunnel becomes narrowed, causing compression of the ulnar nerve in susceptible people. In patients in whom motor conduction is slowed in this region, 1–3 mm distal to the epicondyle, surgical decompression of the appropriate segment of the nerve is effective (Miller 1979, 1991).

Electrophysiological Assessment. As in the case of the median nerve, the most useful parameters are the amplitude and latency of the SNAP. Payan (1969) found that, in lesions at the elbow, the SNAP recorded above the elbow was smaller than normal in 37 of 38 cases, and desynchronised in 35 of the cases, but only 23 showed slowing of sensory conduction velocity. In severe cases the SNAP will be absent and the nerve action potential (wrist to elbow) will be small (Payan 1969). The motor conduction velocity was slowed in 85% of his cases, the mean being 29% slower than normal. There may be marked dispersion of the evoked MAP (Fig. 8.7). Conduction block can be demonstrated at the level of the elbow by recording the MAP from abductor digiti minimi, stimulating the nerve above and below the elbow (Fig. 8.7). The amplitude of the CMAP in normal subjects stimulated at the elbow and the wrist, should be similar. When ulnar nerve compression causes conduction block the ampli-

tude of the CMAP stimulated at the elbow will be at least 20% less than after stimulation at the wrist (Miller and Olney 1982). A mild degree of conduction block is shown in Fig. 8.8

In evaluating possible ulnar nerve lesions at the elbow it is important to stimulate the nerve above and below the elbow, in order to assess conduction in this short segment of the nerve. The conduction velocity in the segment of the nerve across the elbow should not be slowed more than 12% compared with conduction in the below-elbow to wrist part of the nerve (Eisen 1974). Another useful test is to record the mixed nerve action potential at the elbow, stimulating the ulnar nerve at the wrist. The amplitude of this response should normally exceed 15 μV.

Concentric needle EMG may show chronic partial denervation in ulnar-innervated forearm and small hand muscles, but in patients with purely sensory symptoms EMG studies may be normal (Jabre and Wilbourn 1979).

Management. Surgical exploration with decompression or transposition of the ulnar nerve at the elbow is indicated only if there is weakness of the hand or forearm muscles, sensory loss and clear evidence of fibro-osseous abnormality at the elbow. Surgery is particularly indicated if the ulnar nerve palsy has developed insidiously. However, a long history, with marked weakness and atrophy, is a poor prognostic sign and recovery is unlikely even if the nerve is adequately decompressed (Payan 1969). When surgery is successful clinical improvement is accompanied by improvement of conduction velocity over the ulnar segment of the nerve (Lugnegard et al. 1977; Odusote and Eisen 1979). Several surgical techniques are used, including cubital tunnel decompression (Miller and Hummel 1980), anterior transposition of the nerve (Harrison and Nurick 1970), simple decompression (MacNicol 1979) and excision of the olecranon process. If the elbow joint is abnormal or the nerve dislocates when the elbow is flexed, transposition is the treatment of choice. However, this procedure can lead to worsening of symptoms, probably because of vascular factors (Payan 1969).

The majority of patients do not require surgical treatment, as the disturbance can be improved by preventing pressure on the elbow, and by limiting repetitive movement at the elbow, especially into full flexion. Appropriate soft protection of chairs and of table surfaces is helpful and a splint limiting elbow flexion may be used. Improvement should occur in the first 6–12 weeks. Ulnar nerve palsies following compression associated with unconsciousness or prolonged bed rest should always be treated expectantly in the first instance, since recovery usually occurs in 6–8 weeks. If there is no improvement in 3–4 months surgical exploration should be considered. In mild cubital tunnel syndrome without weakness 90% improve spontaneously (Eisen and Danon 1974).

Ulnar Nerve Lesions at Wrist and Hand

Four syndromes have been described (Eberling et al. 1960; Shea and McClain 1969; Urihurne et al. 1976).

1. Compression in, or proximal to, Guyon's canal. This produces weakness of all the ulnar-innervated muscles in the hand with sensory disturbance in the whole distribution except that supplied by the palmar cutaneous branch of the nerve, since the latter originates in the forearm. A small patch of skin on the palm near the wrist is therefore spared. The dorsal cutaneous branch originates in the forearm, so the dorsal surface of the hand is normal.
2. Damage to the motor branch. This occurs distal to Guyon's canal *before* the motor branch to abductor digiti minimi is given off. All the small muscles of the hand are weak, but there is no sensory loss.
3. Damage to the deep palmar branch of the nerve. This lesion usually occurs with recurrent trauma to the palm, e.g. cycling, the use of screwdrivers, catching heavy objects in the palm, or from ganglion formation (Shea and McClain 1969). Other causes, e.g. piso-hamate entrapment, lipomas etc., are rare, but fractures of the hamate bone are a well-known cause. There is weakness of the interossei, lumbricals and first dorsal interossei,

with sparing of the hypothenar eminence; there is no sensory loss.
4. Lesion of the superficial terminal branch that supplies sensation to the palmar surface of the distal part of the hand, and the ring and little fingers. There is no motor involvement.

Electrophysiological Assessment. There is normal conduction across the elbow, with normal nerve action potentials, and normal F responses. The lesion is thus localised distally. Damage to the motor branch or to the deep palmar branch (2 and 3 above) are the most common lesions. The SNAPs from the digital nerves of the little finger are normal and motor conduction studies show an increased distal motor latency to the first dorsal interosseous or abductor pollicis muscles. The distal motor latency to the first dorsal interosseous muscle should not normally exceed 4.5 ms (Eberling et al. 1960; Olney and Wilbourn 1985). The distal motor latency to the abductor digiti minimi is normally no longer than 3.4 ms, and in deep palmar branch lesions this will be normal. There is partial denervation of the affected muscles in needle EMG.

In the case of a lesion in Guyon's canal the SNAPs from the digital nerves of the little finger are small, of increased latency, or absent but sensory studies of the dorsal branch, recording from the dorsal surface of digit V and stimulating 8 cm above the wrist, are normal (Jabre 1980). The mean latency of the SNAP in this branch is $2.0 \pm 6 \ \mu V$.

Management. In occupational palsies, avoidance of recurrent trauma to the nerve in the palm or wrist is usually sufficient to result in improvement but if this fails, decompression with removal of a ganglion or of any other cause, e.g. lipoma or fractured hook of hamate, should be carried out. Entrapment in Guyon's canal should be treated by surgical decompression.

Ulnar nerve lesions proximal to the elbow are rare.

Radial Nerve

The radial nerve originates from the posterior trunk of the brachial plexus, comprising C5–T1 roots. In the upper arm it winds around the medial surface of the spiral groove of the humerus and passes through the heads of the triceps, which it innervates by two branches, to enter the superficial part of the upper arm before passing in front of the lateral epicondyle of the humerus. The posterior interosseous branch, a pure motor nerve, arises just distal to the elbow joint and enters the supinator muscle through the arcade of Frohse, a fibro-tendinous band representing the origin of this muscle. All the extensor muscles of the forearm except extensor carpi radialis longus and brevis muscles, which are supplied by the radial nerve itself through more proximal branches, are innervated by the posterior interosseous branch. The radial nerve innervates a small zone of skin, of variable extent, on the dorsal surface of the hand, especially in the web between thumb and index.

Compression Injuries in the Upper Arm

The radial nerve is vulnerable as it winds round the humerus in the spiral groove. The nerve is injured in 10–15% of patients with closed fractures of the humerus (Packer et al. 1972) and may be damaged in the axilla by crutches. The commonest cause of spontaneous radial nerve palsy is pressure during sleep when the arm hangs over a table or chair. There is wrist and finger drop due to paralysis of all the extensor muscles of the forearm. The clinical syndrome is often incomplete and recovery is complete and almost invariable (Berry 1993). Two-thirds of 114 cases in Berry's (1993) series were traumatic. Radial nerve palsy may also develop as a complication of arthroscopy of the elbow joint (Papilion et al. 1988). The triceps muscle and its reflex is spared since most of these injuries occur distal to the origin of the triceps branches. There may be sensory disturbance on the dorsum of the hand, but this is often difficult to detect. In radial nerve lesions above the level of the spiral groove the triceps and anconeus muscles are also paralysed, often incompletely.

Electrophysiological Assessment and Management. Electrophysiological measurements may be useful in predicting the outcome. If the SNAP in the radial nerve is reduced 6–14 days after injury and there is denervation on EMG examination of the radial-innervated muscles recovery will be prolonged or incomplete (Downie and Scott 1967). If the SNAP is present at this time and there is conduction block between the spiral groove and the lateral epicondyle of the humerus, recovery should occur within 6–8 weeks (Trojaborg 1970).

Management is conservative. A "cock-up" splint that provides extension of wrist and fingers is a useful orthotic aid, especially if provided with spring resistance against which the flexors may act. Fractures of the humerus should be treated according to orthopaedic principles. Displaced fractures

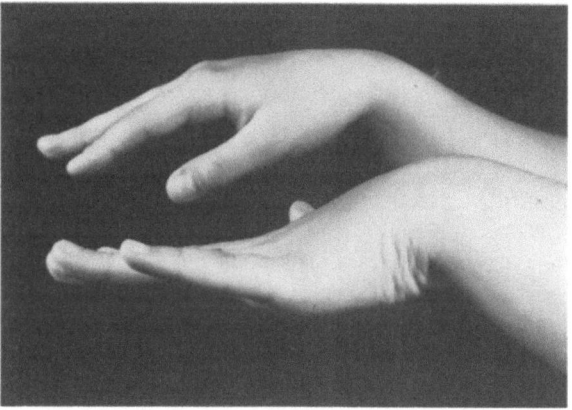

Fig. 8.9.   Right posterior interosseous palsy. There is weakness of finger and wrist extension, especially involving the radial digits.

will need operative fixation and the nerve should be explored at this time to ensure that it is free and not compressed or transected (Packer et al. 1972).

Posterior Interosseous Nerve Lesions

In lesions of the posterior interosseous nerve there is weakness of extension of the thumb and fingers, but less severe weakness of the wrist because the extensor radialis longus and brevis muscles, and the supinator muscles, are spared. This results in radial deviation of the wrist during attempted wrist extension. There is usually pain felt deeply in the forearm, often worsened by attempted extensor movements, especially of the middle finger, and by repeated pronation/supination. Pain often precedes weakness (Spinner 1968). Finger extension is therefore weak (Fig. 8.9) and painful. There is no sensory loss. In some patients weakness of extension of thumb and index is more marked than that of the other fingers because these branches are relatively more severely affected.

The nerve is compressed in the arcade of Frohse (Hagert et al. 1977) or by lipoma (Campbell and Wulf 1954) by synovial bulging in rheumatoid arthritis or by dislocation of the elbow. This is a site of predilection for damage in other neuropathies, e.g. chronic post-infectious polyneuropathies or diabetes, especially when the nerve is enlarged. Repeated unaccustomed extension/pronation movements may also cause posterior interosseous palsy. These causes of this syndrome have been reviewed by Carfi and Dong (1985). Kaplan (1984) followed 12 patients with posterior interosseous palsies, seven of which were due to blunt trauma, and noted

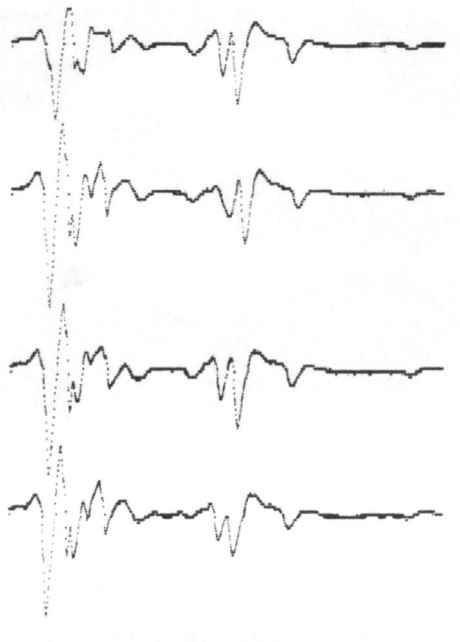

Fig. 8.10. Concentric needle EMG recording from extensor digitorum communis in posterior interosseous nerve entrapment. The motor unit action potential is complex and of increased duration, but it is stable, indicating effective reinnervation. Filters: 500 Hz and 10 kHz. Bar 4 ms.

that they all recovered spontaneously. Posterior interosseous nerve palsy represents only 25% of radial nerve lesions in clinical practice (Cravens and Kline 1990).

Tennis elbow may mimic this syndrome. In tennis elbow tenderness is mainly over the lateral epicondyle rather than over the supinator muscle, and elbow extension, wrist flexion and finger flexion all increase the pain. In about 5% of patients with tennis elbow, however, there may be a co-existent entrapment of the posterior interosseous nerve in the supinator canal (Werner 1979).

Electrophysiological Assessment and Management. There is increased motor latency from the radial nerve at the elbow to the extensor indicis proprius muscle (Carfi and Dong 1985). Rosen and Werner (1980) found that in some patients in whom the motor latency to extensor digitorum communis was normal, forced supination induced an increased latency. Needle EMG studies reveal partial denervation in the appropriate extensor muscles of the forearm (Fig. 8.10). Sensory potentials are normal. Falck and Hurme (1983) described a technique to measure motor conduction velocity across the arcade of Frohse in this nerve lesion.

Management should be conservative, with rest and restriction of supination/pronation movements of the arm. If recovery does not occur in two months surgical exploration should be advised. Lipoma can be recognised by soft tissue X-ray or MRI of the arm. A good result from surgical decompression can be expected in more than 80% of patients (Werner 1979).

Superficial Branch of the Radial Nerve

The superficial branch of the radial nerve, a sensory branch which may be palpated at the head of the radius near the wrist, is vulnerable to injury from pressure, for example by a tight wristband or handcuffs (Massey and Pleet 1978). Such a lesion to this nerve has been termed cheiralgia paraesthetica.

Musculocutaneous Nerve

The musculocutaneous nerve originates from the C5 and C6 roots. It supplies the biceps and brachialis muscles and innervates the skin of the radial side of the forearm. It may be injured by stretch, especially with hyperextension of the forearm (Trojaborg 1976; Spindler and Felsenthal 1978). The syndrome may be distinguished from root lesions affecting the C5 and C6 roots by sparing of spinati, deltoid and brachioradialis muscles. Sensory conduction studies in the lateral cutaneous nerve of the forearm may be useful in showing increased latency and reduced amplitude of the SNAP in lesions of the musculocutaneous nerve and of the lateral cutaneous nerve of the forearm, which may be damaged during vene puncture at the elbow (Spindler and Felsenthal 1978).

Notalgia Paraesthetica

Pleet and Massey (1978) suggested that a syndrome of burning, itching and paraesthesiae over the medial margin of the scapula might be due to damage to the dorsal roots of T_2–T_6 as they pass through the multifidus spinal muscles. There may be impairment of sensation in this distribution. Improvement occurs spontaneously.

Rectus Abdominis Syndrome

Pain in the abdominal wall, exaggerated by pressure over the rectus muscle, or by elevating a leg, may be due to entrapment of intercostal nerves T7–T12 within the rectus muscle (Komar and Varga 1975).

Lower Limb Syndromes

Nerves of the Pelvic Girdle

Several small nerves arising from the lumbar plexus innervate the muscles of the pelvic girdle and anterior thigh (Table 8.5). They are generally susceptible only to trauma. Although the lateral femoral cutaneous nerve of the thigh, femoral nerve, saphenous nerve and obturator nerve may be liable to entrapment, only entrapment of the lateral femoral cutaneous nerve of the thigh is a common syndrome.

Electrophysiological Assessment and Management. Generally, electrophysiological tests are not much used in the diagnosis of these pelvic neuropathies since the clinical features are usually characteristic. EMG studies are relatively difficult, and many of these nerves are inaccessible.

Management of these syndromes is generally conservative. When improvement does not occur spontaneously surgical exploration may be advised at the site of nerve compression or entrapment as revealed by the clinical and electrophysiological data.

Meralgia Paraesthetica

This syndrome is due to compression or entrapment of the lateral femoral cutaneous nerve of the thigh beneath the inguinal ligament (Jefferson and Eames 1979) or as it penetrates the deep fascia of the thigh to reach the skin. It is often initiated in the context of obesity or weight gain and weight control may often result in cure. The syndrome is characterised by burning pain and discomfort on the lateral surface of the thigh (Meros: thigh, and Algos: pain). Alternatively the nerve may be explored and freed by section of the ligamentous entrapment. Section of the nerve relieves the symptom but may be followed by neuroma formation with intractable pain. Injection with steroid is unlikely to result in lasting relief (Nakano 1978). Sigmund Freud in 1895 himself suffered from this condition, but believed initially that it might be of psychological origin, although he later recognised that it was organic (Dawson et al. 1983). The history of the condition was reviewed by Williams and Trzil (1991). Freud's

Table 8.5. Syndromes of nerves of the pelvic girdle

Nerve	Root innervation	Syndrome	Cause	Electrophysiological studies
Ilioinguinal	L1/2	Pain in groin and crura	Trauma, Surgery	–
Genitofemoral	L1/2	Inguinal pain Sensory loss in femoral triangle Loss of cremasteric reflex	Adhesions	–
Lateral femoral cutaneous	L2/3	Painful sensory loss antero lateral thigh ("meralgia paraesthetica")	Entrapment with obesity	Slowed sensory conduction in this nerve (Stevens & Rosselle 1970)
Femoral	L2/3/4	Quadriceps weakness	Compression beneath inguinal ligament	Slowed motor conduction in femoral nerve from inguinal ligament (Gassel 1963)
		Sensory loss anteromedial thigh and medial aspect lower leg	Stretch or pressure on psoas during pelvic surgery	Denervation of quadriceps muscle
		Absent knee jerk	Compression by tumour or abscess	
Obturator	L2/3/4	Weakness of hip adduction	Childbirth injuries	Denervation of adductor femoris and gracilis muscles
		Sensory loss upper medial thigh	Pelvic fractures	
Saphenous	L3/4	Pain medial aspect of knee and foot worsened by exercise	Entrapment in Hunter's canal	Sensory conduction may be useful
Superior gluteal	L4/5/S1	Weakness adduction and medial rotation of hip. Pain and tenderness at sciatic notch	Injections Trauma (fracture of femur)	Denervation of gluteus medius
Inferior gluteal	L5/S1/2	Weakness of gluteus maximus (extension, adduction and external rotation of thigh)	Injections Trauma (fracture of femur)	Denervation of gluteus maximus

illness may have been caused by wearing tight clothes.

Electrophysiological Tests. SNAP amplitude is reduced in the lateral femoral cutaneous nerve on the affected side, but there was no correlation with outcome (Lagueny et al. 1991).

Management. Most cases improve spontaneously. Williams and Trzil (1991) reviewed 277 patients. Of these only 24 required surgical section of the lateral femoral cutaneous nerve for pain relief. A local injection of 5–10 cc of local anaesthetic with corticosteroid is often effective.

Femoral Mononeuropathy

The femoral nerve arises from the L2, L3 and L4 nerve roots. It innervates the psoas muscle, passing through this muscle to lie adjacent to the iliacus muscle, which it also innervates. It leaves the pelvis beneath the inguinal ligament to enter the anterior thigh where it supplies motor branches to the quadriceps, sartorius and pectineus muscles, and sensory branches to the skin of the anterior thigh and, via the saphenous nerve, the medial surface of the leg below the knee. The femoral nerve can be injured in the pelvis during surgery by traction on the psoas muscle, by haematoma or malignancy. Beneath the inguinal ligament it is vulnerable to compression by prolonged hip flexion or malignancy, or to direct trauma (Al Hakim and Katirji 1993). The femoral nerve is vulnerable to ischaemic damage, e.g. as a complication of diabetes mellitus (Raff et al. 1968). However, in diabetics femoral nerve palsy is nearly always part of a more widespread lumbar plexopathy. The nerve can also be damaged by hyperextension injuries of the hip and during childbirth (Fox et al. 1990).

Femoral neuropathy causes weakness and atrophy of the muscles of the anterior compartment of the thigh, sensory loss over the lower anterior thigh and the medial aspect of the leg below the knee and reduced or absent knee jerk. Ilio-psoas involvement implies that the lesion is in the lumbar plexus or in the L2-3 roots, and obturator involvement, shown by weakness of hip abduction, indicates a proximal lesion, as in obstetric trauma or pelvic lesions.

Electrophysiological Assessment. Conduction studies, described by Gassel (1963) allow measurement of motor conduction in the femoral nerves, but EMG studies of the distribution of partial dener-

vation change are more useful in separating femoral from root or plexus lesions.

Obturator Mononeuropathy

The obturator nerve (L2–L4) supplies the adductor muscle of the thigh, the gracilis and small muscles in the deep upper thigh, e.g. pectineus, and the skin of the medial thigh. When this nerve is damaged the leg is circumducted because of the unopposed action of the abductors of the thigh. There may be pain in the medial thigh above the knee. The quadriceps muscles and the knee jerk are normal. Obturator nerve palsies occur with local lesions, e.g. malignancy, penetrating trauma, damage during hip arthroplasty, retroperitoneal haematoma or obstetric injury (Patterson and Morton 1973; Melamed and Satya-Murti 1983; Fox et al. 1990). Treatment depends on the cause.

Electrophysiological Assessment. The diagnosis can be confirmed by finding EMG evidence of chronic partial denervation in adductors, but not in quadriceps muscles. If no cause is evident MR or CT imaging of the pelvis should be undertaken.

Sciatic Nerve Syndromes

The sciatic nerve, the largest and longest nerve in the body, consists of two components, the common peroneal and tibial nerves. The sciatic nerve arises from the L4–S3 roots. These nerve roots pass through the cauda equina, where they are vulnerable to compression from herniated disc, canal stenosis or tumour before the two trunks of the sciatic nerve are formed in the lumbo-sacral plexus. The sciatic nerve leaves the pelvis through the sciatic notch below the piriformis muscle and passes between the ischial tuberosity and the greater trochanter, beneath the gluteus maximus muscle. In the posterior compartment of the thigh it lies deep to the hamstring muscles. The sciatic nerve supplies the hamstrings and, by branches from its two components, all the muscles below the knee. It also innervates the skin of the leg and posterior thigh.

Sciatic Neuropathies

In a series of 34 patients with sciatic nerve lesions (Stewart et al. 1983) ten patients, four of whom had bilateral sciatic neuropathies, had compressive lesions acquired during coma, anaesthesia or working with the buttock engaged against a hard object, ten had traumatic fracture-dislocation of the hip, six had hip surgery (Bonney 1986), four had sustained direct trauma to the nerve and four had miscellaneous disorders including endometriosis at the sciatic notch, haematoma, intramuscular injections and mononeuritis multiplex. The association of nerve lesion with hip surgery was reviewed by Weber et al. (1976) who noted sciatic obturator and femoral lesions in their patients, and observed subclinical EMG changes in other patients. Sciatic nerve palsy is now a rare complication of difficult childbirth or forceps delivery (Snooks et al. 1984). The nerve is well known to be vulnerable during therapeutic intramuscular injections given in the buttock.

The sciatic nerve is only rarely damaged by entrapment. It may be trapped beneath a band connecting the short head of the biceps femoris with the abductor magnus in the upper thigh, or by the piriformis muscle at the sciatic notch (Nakano 1978). The piriformis syndrome may present as buttock pain, with radiation down the back of the leg, resembling sciatica from lumbo-sacral disc protrusion (Robinson 1947). Mizoguchi (1976) reported improvement of sciatic pain in 12 of 14 patients in whom the piriformis muscle was divided; there was no radiological evidence of disc disease in these patients. In the piriformis syndrome there may be localised tenderness in the buttock. This syndrome, however, remains controversial.

In all these syndromes the common peroneal component of the sciatic nerve is more likely to be damaged than the tibial component, probably because it is located laterally (Sunderland 1953; Kimura 1983). When the nerve is damaged in the popliteal fossa, e.g. by pressure from a Baker's cyst, or by direct trauma, it is common for one or other component to be relatively selectively affected (Nakano 1978). Arthrography is a useful diagnostic technique in elucidating this problem. MR and CT imaging may be useful in demonstrating haematomas in the pelvis or along the course of the nerve (Pillary et al. 1988).

Electrophysiological Assessment. Conduction in the sciatic nerve can be assessed indirectly by F wave and H reflex studies from the distal part of the limb. Conduction velocity can be studied by stimulating the sciatic nerve directly with needle electrodes inserted at the gluteal fold (Gassel and Trojaborg 1964). Needle EMG studies will show abnormal potentials in the flexor muscles of the thigh and in the muscles below the knee, but normal motor unit potentials in the paraspinal and gluteal muscles. The latter muscles are innervated by the superior and inferior gluteal nerves, direct branches of the lumbo-sacral plexus. SNAPs recorded from peroneal or sural nerves are small in sciatic nerve lesions, but of normal amplitude in root lesions.

Common Peroneal Syndromes

The common peroneal nerve (L4–S1 roots) leaves the popliteal fossa laterally and winds around the neck of the fibula to enter the fibular tunnel. Here it divides into superficial peroneal (musculocutaneous) and deep peroneal (anterior tibial) branches. The superficial branch innervates the peroneus longus and brevis muscles and the skin of the lateral part of the leg and the dorsum of the foot. The deep peroneal branch supplies the tibialis anterior, extensor hallucis longus, extensor digitorum longus and brevis and the peroneus tertius muscles. It supplies the skin between the first and second digits of the foot. In 28% of people the extensor digitorum brevis muscle is also innervated by the accessory deep peroneal nerve, a branch of the superficial peroneal nerve (Gutmann 1970). The double innervation of the muscle is a source of difficulty in electrophysiological studies of common peroneal nerve function as a larger CMAP may be recorded from the extensor digitorum brevis when stimulating at the knee than at the ankle. In some patients, with the complete anomaly, the muscle may be innervated entirely by the accessory deep peroneal nerve. Clinically, it is important to recognise that a drop foot with sensory disturbance on the lateral aspect of the leg can also be due to L5 radiculopathy. In the latter syndrome, however, both the tibialis posterior (which inverts the ankle) and the hamstrings are also weak. In S1 lesions the ankle jerk is reduced or absent (Berry and Richardson 1976), but in common peroneal nerve lesions the ankle jerk is normal.

The common peroneal nerve may be damaged in the popliteal fossa but it is most vulnerable to compression injury as it winds round the head of the fibula near its division into deep and superficial branches (Garland and Moorhouse 1952). Persistent leg-crossing, and the common lesion sustained during bed rest, cause compression against the head of the fibula. Ganglia in this region may also damage this nerve (Cobb and Moiel 1974). Berry and Richardson (1976) found that the commonest causes were trauma to the knee, compression and underlying neuropathy, but they also noted that forced inversion of the ankle could produce a stretch injury of this nerve. Katirji and Wilbourn (1988) reviewed 116 common peroneal nerve lesions in 103 patients. The onset was acute in 57 patients, gradual in 35 and indeterminate in 11. Acute lesions were peri-operative in 29 patients and due to trauma in 24. Gradual lesions were associated with weight loss, prolonged hospitalisation and leg-crossing. In most patients there is equal involvement of all muscles innervated by the common peroneal nerve but in some the superficial peroneal branch may be relatively spared causing the peroneal muscles to be spared. Tinel's sign may be positive at the head of the fibula. Entrapment of the common peroneal nerve is rare, but may occur under the tendinous edge of the peroneus longus muscle at the head of the fibula. The terminal portion of the cutaneous branch of the deep peroneal nerve innervating the dorsum of the foot, especially the first dorsal web space, may be entrapped beneath the fascia of the dorsal surface of the ankle (Krause et al. 1977).

Electrophysiological Assessment and Management. Singh et al. (1974) found that motor nerve conduction velocity across the neck of the fibula, recording from the extensor digitorum brevis, or from other muscles, was slowed in only a third of patients with suspected common peroneal palsy. A reduction of motor conduction velocity of greater than 12% across the knee is significant. In severe cases, no response can be obtained from the extensor digitorum brevis muscle and in these patients functional recovery may be incomplete (Smith and Trojaborg 1986). Katirji and Wilbourn (1988) found that most lesions were at the fibular head. They confirmed the results of Singh et al. (1974), and found that recordings made from extensor digitorum brevis or anterior tibial muscles after stimulation at the fibular head were both useful. There was reduction in CMAP amplitude across the fibular segment suggesting that most lesions were accompanied by axonal loss rather than conduction block. Motor conduction velocity in the common peroneal nerve in the across-knee segment can be measured by recording from the peroneus brevis, innervated by the superficial branch of the nerve, and the tibialis anterior, innervated by the deep branch of the nerve (Devi et al. 1977). Sensory nerve conduction velocity was abnormal in two-thirds of these patients (Singh et al. 1974). EMG sampling of muscles innervated by this nerve is sometimes a useful test, but denervation is found only in more severe cases.

F response latencies are useful to differentiate common peroneal nerve lesions from more proximal lesions as slowed F wave responses will be found in root, plexus or sciatic nerve lesions. An underlying symmetrical peripheral neuropathy must be excluded by studying conduction velocity in the opposite limb or in the ipsilateral tibial nerve.

If the palsy is due to external compression, e.g. in the context of coma or anaesthesia, recovery can usually be expected within 2–15 months, but if the clinical deficit is severe the prognosis may be less good (see Smith and Trojaborg 1986). If the clinical disturbance is progressive, or recovery has not commenced by clinical or electrophysiological criteria during a 6-month period, surgical exploration may be useful. Splintage, with heel cup splints or orthotic shoes may provide functional benefit, and is important to prevent secondary genu recurvatum and arthrosis of the ankle.

Tibial Nerve Syndrome

The tibial nerve, a continuation of the medial trunk of the sciatic nerve, leaves the popliteal fossa through the two heads of gastrocnemius, passes through the posterior compartment of the lower leg, innervating gastrocnemius and tibialis posterior, and enters the foot through the tarsal tunnel having passed around the medial side of the ankle. In the foot it divides into medial and lateral plantar branches, innervating the small muscles of the foot and supplying sensation to the sole and to the medial side of the foot and ankle. The first branch, the sural nerve, innervates the skin of the posterior part of the leg.

The tibial nerve itself is rarely injured, but it may be compressed by Baker's cyst or by popliteal artery aneurysm in the popliteal fossa. The clinical features include pain, sensory loss and weakness in the distribution of the nerve.

Electrophysiological Assessment and Management. The motor conduction velocity in the tibial nerve can be measured from stimulation in the popliteal fossa, recording from the abductor hallucis muscle, but EMG studies of muscles innervated by this nerve are more useful in electrophysiological diagnosis (Thomas et al. 1959). Sural nerve sensory action potentials will be reduced in amplitude, or absent. If the disorder is progressive the nerve should be explored. Arthrography may aid preoperative diagnosis.

Tarsal Tunnel Syndrome

The tarsal tunnel syndrome is characterised by intermittent burning pain, tingling and numbness of the foot, usually aggravated by prolonged standing or by walking long distances (Edwards et al. 1969; DeLisa and Saeed 1983). Sensory symptoms invariably precede weakness. The distribution of symptoms depends on the pattern of differential involvement of the three branches of the posterior tibial nerve in the foot. The calcaneal branch supplies the skin of the heel; the medial plantar branch is a mixed nerve that supplies the abductor hallucis and the intrinsic foot muscles, and the skin of the medial side of the sole of the foot; and the lateral plantar branch supplies the abductor digiti quinti muscle and the skin of the lateral side of the foot. On examination there may be a positive Tinel sign on percussion just below the medial malleolus at the ankle, with diminished sensation to touch or pain on either the medial or lateral aspect of the sole of the foot, or on both. There may be atrophy of the abductor hallucis, but weakness of these muscles is difficult to detect. Pain is therefore the major feature of this syndrome, and may radiate proximally to the calf and leg, like carpal tunnel syndrome in the arm. Radiography of the foot may show evidence of arthritis or old fractures.

Tarsal tunnel syndrome may co-exist with peripheral neuropathy, and may be difficult to differentiate from an S1 root lesion by clinical criteria. The sensory disturbance is usually more medially distributed in tarsal tunnel syndrome, and the ankle jerk is diminished or lost in S1 root lesions. Further, in the latter, back pain and sciatica may be a feature.

Tarsal tunnel syndrome has been reported with post-traumatic fibrosis of the tarsal tunnel, hypertrophy of the abductor hallucis muscle, tenosynovitis, ganglion, rheumatoid arthritis, and with generalised disorders such as diabetes mellitus, leprosy and hypothyroidism (Linscheid et al. 1970; Bourel et al. 1976; Baylan et al. 1981; Schwartz et al. 1983).

Electrophysiological Assessment. The diagnosis is supported when the distal motor latency to the abductor hallucis from stimulation of the tibial nerve at the medial malleolus is increased (McGuigan et al. 1983); a value greater than 7.5 ms is abnormal in this medial plantar nerve. Similarly, recording from abductor digiti quinti enables a distal motor latency in the lateral plantar branch of the tibial nerve to be measured; a value greater than 6.6 ms is abnormal (Fu et al. 1980).

Measurement of sensory potential latency and amplitude in the medial plantar nerve after stimulation of the digital nerves in the toes increases diagnostic accuracy and yield (Guiloff and Sheratt 1977). Similar sensory studies are possible in the lateral plantar nerve (Oh et al. 1979). Ponsford (1988) described a method for stimulating the medial and lateral plantar nerves just lateral to the first metatarsal and between the fourth and fifth metatarsals, on the sole of the foot. SNAPs are recorded at the medial malleolus.

Management. Tarsal tunnel syndrome in many respects resembles carpal tunnel syndrome. Splinting with an arch support or plastic arthrosis may be helpful. Local steroid injection in the tarsal tunnel just distal to the medial malleolus has been tried. Operative decompression is helpful (Kaplan and Kernohan 1981). Oh et al. (1991a) documented recovery of sensory and motor potentials after surgical decompression of the tarsal tunnel. Anti-inflammatory drugs are indicated in patients with inflammatory arthropathy. The syndrome may often occur bilaterally by electrophysiological criteria, like carpal tunnel syndrome, but treatment should be restricted to the symptomatic limb. It is always important to exclude generalised sensorimotor neuropathy by appropriate investigation of other nerves in the leg and in the upper limbs.

Morton's Metatarsalgia

This syndrome consists of pain radiating into the fourth toe from the head of the metatarsal bone. It is worsened by standing and relieved by lying down. Pressure over the head of the fourth metacarpal bone induces the pain. The only neurological abnormality consists of loss of sensation on the medial side of the fourth toe (Kite 1966). Rarely the third toe may be affected. The condition was described by Morton (1876) but its cause, a mass of fibrinoid and fibrous degeneration in the soft tissue around the nerve, was recognised by Reed and Bliss (1973). It is caused by trauma from wearing high-heeled shoes, jogging or prolonged squatting.

Electrophysiological Assessment and Management. The sensory conduction velocity in the plantar interdigital branches of the medial or lateral plantar nerves, depending on the location of the symptom, may be slowed (Falck et al. 1984). Conservative management with a small pad under the affected metatarsal region may alleviate symptoms but surgical treatment may be necessary. The fibrous nodule should be excised, but release of the intermetatarsal ligament at the level of the deep plantar fascia may also be successful (Gauthier 1979).

Double-Crush Syndrome

There is sometimes an association between entrapment of a peripheral nerve, e.g. in carpal tunnel syndrome, and entrapment of a root in the course of this nerve at the neck (Lishman and Russell 1961; Upton and McComas 1973). Entrapment or compression of a nerve root seems to confer increased susceptibility to clinically significant entrapment of the same axons more distally. Upton and McComas (1973) suggested that this occurred because the more proximal lesion interfered with axoplasmic flow in the more distal segment, but another explanation is that tethering of the nerve at one point may lead to increased stretch and movement through other points of possible entrapment (McLellan and Swash 1976; Sunderland 1978).

Entrapment at two sites, the double-crush syndrome, can be demonstrated electrophysiologically. For example, in the carpal tunnel syndrome with a coincidental C8 root entrapment, the *motor double-crush syndrome*, the distal motor latency from wrist to abductor pollicis brevis will be increased and there will also be a delayed F response from stimulation of the medial nerve more proximally, e.g. at the elbow. It is important to look for electrophysiological evidence of both proximal and distal lesions in patients with distal nerve entrapment syndromes, particularly if their clinical presentation is somewhat unusual; not only may their symptoms result from a combination of proximal and distal entrapment but simple decompression of the distal entrapment, e.g. a mild carpal tunnel syndrome, will then probably fail to relieve all the patient's symptoms.

Confusion may arise electrophysiologically in patients referred for evaluation of presumed carpal tunnel syndrome if the examination is restricted to distal motor latency measurements in the median nerve. In a root lesion (C8) the distal motor latency may be increased, but the sensory potentials from the index will be of normal amplitude and latency, thus excluding compression of the median nerve in the carpal tunnel. Sensory symptoms affecting the index finger may arise either from carpal tunnel syndrome or from a C6 posterior root lesion, and both may co-exist in the same patient, the *sensory double-crush syndrome*.

Hurst et al. (1985) reported 1000 cases of carpal tunnel syndrome and noted an association with cervical arthritis and with diabetes mellitus. However, they did not report evidence of cervical radiculopathy. Swenson (1993) commented, in a critical review, that multiple symptomatic lesions of a nerve produced additive disabilities, but that multiple or single insignificant lesions, when added to a clinically symptomatic lesion, do not result in any added deficit.

Adequate Electrophysiological Studies in Entrapment Neuropathies

A certain minimum number of investigations are necessary in evaluating patients with entrapment neuropathies. Once an entrapment has been confirmed by clinical and electrophysiological assessment, sensory and motor nerve conduction in another nerve *in the same limb* should be studied to exclude a more widespread or generalised neuropathy. The opposite limb should also be studied, particularly in patients with carpal tunnel, ulnar nerve or common peroneal entrapment syndromes, since there is frequently subclinical entrapment of the homologous nerve which can be shown by changes in conduction velocity. F responses should probably also be performed.

It is important to remember that sensory nerve action potentials may be small, or even unobtainable, in older patients. Absence of a SNAP, recorded with surface electrodes, in the median nerve of an elderly subject is thus not necessarily evidence of carpal tunnel syndrome. Even in younger subjects the ulnar nerve SNAP is smaller than that recorded in the median nerve.

Other Mononeuropathies

Bell's Palsy

Sudden paralysis of one side of the face is a common event. The annual incidence in Rochester, Minnesota, was 22/100 000 (Hauser et al. 1971). The disorder often begins with pain in the mastoid region, poorly localised to the ear or the side of the jaw and this may precede weakness by a day or so. Weakness of the face, which is usually unilateral, may begin suddenly during the day, or come on overnight. It usually progresses to its maximal extent, which is often of complete hemifacial immobility, in a few hours but progression may continue for a few days in some cases. Eye closure is affected so that the patient complains of soreness and lacrimation and the eyelid remains open. The side of the mouth droops and speech may therefore be slurred. Taste on the anterior part of the tongue may be disturbed, especially in the more severe cases, and this is evidence that the nerve must be damaged proximal to the origin of the chorda tympani. In addition, some patients observe hyperacusis because of denervation of the stapedius muscle, which is also supplied by the facial nerve.

Rarely, Bell's palsy may be bilateral.

Recovery occurred completely in about half the cases in Taverner's (1955) series. In the remainder there was some degree of residual weakness and in about 20% this was severe, leading to contractures, conjunctival scarring in the unprotected, open eye, and sometimes to disfiguring hemifacial spasm. In some of these patients unusual movements of the face occur from aberrant regeneration so that, for example, attempted eye blinking is associated with movement of the side of the mouth, or vice versa. Similarly, lacrimation may occur on eating, from innervation of the lachrymal gland by parasympathetic fibres destined to supply salivary glands.

Recurrent idiopathic facial palsy is uncommon, occurring in less than 10% of cases (Park and Watkins 1949). In children the prognosis is better than in adults, about 80% of cases recovering completely in the 6 months after onset (Paine 1957). The prognosis in children, as in adults, is less good if recovery is delayed for more than 3 weeks, but recovery may continue for as long as 6 months (Manning and Adour 1972). If recovery from a complete or partial palsy begins in the first 10 days the prognosis is good. Overall, despite residual abnormalities, e.g. aberrant regeneration, only 10–15% of patients are dissatisfied with their recovery (Taverner 1955). Indicators of a poor recovery are complete palsy, reduced salivation and loss of taste. Electrophysiological studies (see below) are also useful. In the elderly recovery is often rather incomplete. Persistent pain is also a poor prognostic factor.

The disorder commonly follows an upper respiratory tract infection experienced a few days before. A seasonal incidence has been suspected, but was denied by Leibowitz (1969), who reported epidemiological evidence of an epidemic distribution of cases. Infection with Herpes zoster (Ramsay Hunt syndrome) or Herpes simplex may also be aetiological factors. About 10% of cases of idiopathic facial palsy are associated with H zoster infection (Robillard et al. 1986). There is an association with diabetes mellitus in the elderly (Korczyn 1971). A variety of other factors, including trauma, surgery, otitis media and other virus infections were described in earlier reports (Paine 1957; Manning and Adour 1972) but in many instances these are better regarded as causes of facial weakness *other* than idiopathic Bell's palsy. Hypertension may also be an associated and possibly predisposing or causative factor.

Leibowitz (1966) suggested that there might be two different aetiological factors, an infectious/inflammatory causation in young people and a vascular/ischaemic mechanism, including diabetes mellitus, in the older age group. In patients who develop bilateral facial palsy within a few days or weeks the diagnosis of idiopathic Bell's palsy should be questioned and, in particular, Guillain–Barré polyradiculoneuritis, leprosy, leukaemia, sarcoid, meningitis and syphilis should be considered. Multiple sclerosis should be borne in mind when other atypical clinical features, such as involvement of the abducens nerve, are present. Bell's palsy may also occur in patients with AIDS (Brown et al. 1988), occurring in 4% of a series reported by Schielker et al. (1989). Facial palsy is a frequent feature of Lyme disease.

Electrophysiological Assessment. In the first 4 days after the onset the only abnormality found with concentric needle EMG is a reduction in the number of MUAPs activated during voluntary contraction, causing a reduction in the interference pattern. At this stage fibrillation potentials are absent. The complete absence of voluntary activity during EMG at this stage is not necessarily a bad prognostic sign since it does not imply that the facial nerve has been transected. Reduction in the interference pattern in EMG recordings made in the second week, when compared with earlier studies, is also not helpful in prognosis. However, at the end of the second week fibrillation potentials may appear and there may be evidence of reinnervation; viz. polyphasic MUAPs. These two features indicate the presence of axonal damage but, unless the fibrillations are very profuse, they are not of prognostic value.

Conduction studies are useful in determining prognosis when performed at least 5 or 6 days after the onset (Zander Olsen 1975; Boongird and Vejjajiva 1978). In cases in which there is conduction block without destruction of the nerve (neurapraxia) the distal latency and the amplitude of the evoked motor response remain normal (>0.5 mV). The latency from the angle of the jaw to the orbicularis oris should be less than 4.0 ms, with a difference between the two sides of less than 0.5 ms. In these cases the prognosis for recovery is excellent regardless of the severity of weakness. Further, if the distal latency is increased but the amplitude of the evoked motor response is within the normal range the prognosis is good, since the lesion is incomplete with partial conduction block suggesting demyelination with axonal integrity. In the acute stage, using magnetic stimulation of the facial root, there is no response, although the M response is present from direct nerve stimulation (Roessler et al. 1989).

Zander Olsen (1975) found that the prognosis could be related to the amplitude of the evoked motor response 1 week after the onset regardless of the motor latency or the degree of paralysis, as shown in Table 8.6.

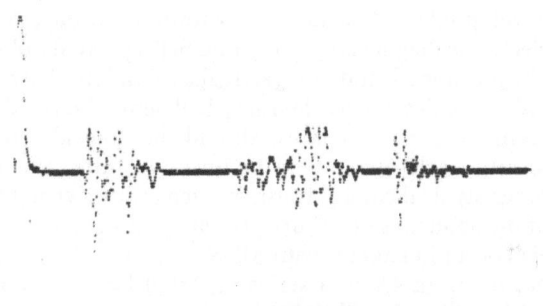

Fig. 8.11. Blink reflex in facial palsy. Three distinct components can be seen in this recording of orbicularis oculi with a facial EMG electrode after stimulation of the supraorbital nerve. The first component has an increased latency (16 ms). Bar 20 ms.

Table 8.6. Prognosis of facial palsy related to motor response amplitude 1 week after onset

Amplitude of motor response in relation to other side	Time of recovery	Extent of recovery
>30%	>2 months	Complete
10%–30%	2–8 months	Good to excellent
<10%	6–12 months	Incomplete or poor

Boongird and Vejjajiva (1978) suggested that these three groups of patients represented, respectively, those with segmental demyelination with only minimal terminal sprouting, those with a combination of axonal injury and regrowth with terminal collateral sprouting and, finally, a group with slow recovery in whom an almost total axonal injury necessitated regrowth before reinnervation could occur.

The blink reflex can be used to confirm the localisation of the lesion (Fig. 8.11). The latency of the first component of the blink reflex is increased within 2 days of the onset of a Bell's palsy and increases further during the first week (Kimura et al. 1976). The blink reflex latency, and the latency of the evoked motor response from facial nerve stimulation at the angle of the jaw, are increased similarly in idiopathic Bell's palsy, but in Guillain–Barré syndrome, in which facial weakness may be a feature, the distal latency may be normal but proximal conduction is slowed so that the blink reflex latency is increased. Further, in distal lesions, as in parotid tumours, distal slowing forms the major component of slowing both of the distal and the blink reflex latencies.

In the recovery phase, most patients develop aberrant reinnervation with synkinetic contraction of eyelid and perioral muscles. This may be accompanied by muscle spasm or contracture consisting of continuous EMG activity with myokymic discharges

at 12–26 Hz (Valls-Sole et al. 1992). Blink reflex studies will demonstrate reflex contraction of all the muscle groups of the face (Kimura et al. 1975).

Pathology. Little is known of the pathology of the condition; ischaemia, haemorrhage and oedematous swelling within the bony facial canal are probably all important factors. An immune pathogenesis in relation to the preceding infection has long been suspected but remains unproven (Abramsky et al. 1975). The presence of irreversible denervation atrophy in severe cases shows that severe axonal damage may occur.

Management. In 50% of patients recovery is complete, although it may be delayed in 20% of these. In the remainder there is a substantial recovery in most. In the majority of these patients recovery occurs without medical intervention. Steroid therapy seems to be useful in improving prognosis (Taverner et al. 1971) but since the weakness does not advance after the first few days there is little to be gained by treatment started more than 4 days after the onset. Usually prednisone 40–60 mg daily for 5 days is used, the dose being reduced decrementally after this. Acute surgical decompression has been advocated in the past but probably has little value. The exposed cornea must be protected and this may rarely require tarsorrhaphy in addition to hypromellose drops.

In patients in whom recovery fails and electrophysiological tests show no evidence of functionally useful nerve regeneration, a number of plastic surgical procedures are available, including free autogenous muscle transplants of the palmaris longus muscle (Hakelius and Stålberg 1974). Less than 5% of patients are sufficiently disabled to need surgical reconstruction, and this should not be recommended for at least a year after the palsy (Ludman 1981).

Hemifacial Spasm

The syndrome of hemifacial spasm consists of involuntary tonic or clonic activity in the facial muscle; bilateral involvement is rare. The disorder begins with infrequent twitches in the orbicularis oculi, but gradually becomes more severe and persistent, spreading to involve all the muscles of facial expression and even the platysma. Involvement of the frontalis muscle is less frequent. Paroxysms of muscular contraction develop, often initiated by voluntary contraction, and these may be accompanied by simultaneous (synkinetic) contraction of other components of the ipsilateral facial muscle.

Two-thirds of cases are women, and most are middle-aged. Spontaneous recovery has not been reported (Kielsen 1984a,b). The disorder is not associated with Bell's palsy (Auger 1979), but has been found to be due, in most cases, to vascular compression of the root exit zone of the facial nerve (Jannetta et al. 1977). This causes myelin abnormalities at this site leading to ectopic excitation and ephaptic transmission (cross-talk) in axons of the nerve (Nielsen, 1984a,b). Regular, writhing, rapid movements passing across one side of the face, not accompanied by synkinesis, may occur in nuclear facial lesions, e.g. from tumour or multiple sclerosis, and this facial myokymia must be distinguished from hemifacial spasm.

Electrophysiological Assessment. EMG recordings reveal episodes of continuous motor unit activity in all the parts of the facial muscle. Two patterns of EMG abnormality have been described. Willison (1982) described "blink burst" activity, consisting of contraction of muscle fibres in several facial muscles following a blink, the extent varying according to the force of the blink eye closure. In the second type spontaneous activity occurs, unrelated to blinks or voluntary activity, consisting of a long-lasting slow contraction. The blink burst consists of a high-frequency burst (200–400 Hz) of EMG activity and the slow contractions correspond to 20–50 Hz activity. These abnormalities represent activation of motor units by ephaptic transmission at the site of facial nerve compression. Synkinetic responses occur both in hemifacial spasm and in facial palsy, after reinnervation, although the pathophysiology is rather different. Blink reflex studies in hemifacial palsy (Esteban and Molina-Negro 1986) revealed evidence of central facial hyperexcitability together with impaired afferent conduction in the facial nerve. Stimulation of any single branch of the facial nerve induces synkinetic responses, with long periods of after-discharge, in all parts of the facial musculature innervated by the facial nerve. Hyperventilation may induce synchronous tonic/clonic activity (Nielsen 1984a) and blink reflexes also produce synkinetic responses widely distributed in the facial muscles. A similar abnormality in the blink reflex response is found in Bell's palsy in the recovering phase, but in facial myokymia or blepharospasm no such synkinetic response occurs (Auger 1979).

Management. Treatment with carbemazepine is generally not very successful. Surgical vascular decompression of the facial nerve in the posterior fossa, by the technique advocated by Gardner and Sava (1962) and Jannetta et al. (1977), produces excellent clinical results in 80% of patients. If untreated, the condition progresses and the twitching only ceases when degeneration of the nerve has progressed to the point that there is paralysis of the affected side of the face. Injections of botulinum toxin into the affected areas of the periorbital muscles have been used to cause neuromuscular blockade and partial weakness of the facial muscle, with relief of the symptom that is maintained for several weeks or months (Savino et al. 1985).

Facial Myokymia

Myokymia consists of undulating, wavelike movements across the muscle surface. Facial muscles are commonly affected (Gutmann 1991). It occurs in several disorders, especially multiple sclerosis, but also in brainstem tumours and Guillain–Barré syndrome. The movement occurs transiently, repeatedly or even continuously. As many as 15% of patients with Guillain–Barré syndrome show myokymia of the face by EMG studies (Mateer et al. 1983). Treatment is not usually required, since the disorder is self-limited in most patients, but phenytoin or carbamazepine may be effective.

Other Cranial Nerve Syndromes

Involvement of cranial nerves is a common feature of neurological disease. The *facial nerve* is often affected in neuromuscular disorders, e.g. in Guillain–Barré syndrome, leprosy, sarcoidosis, other peripheral neuropathies, and in anterior horn cell diseases. The *trigeminal nerve* may also be involved in some of these disorders and dysfunction in the trigeminal nerve can be assessed in its afferent limb by the use of blink reflex latency measurement. In trigeminal motor neuropathy, a disorder due to local infiltration or infection, or of sudden onset and a post-infectious aetiology, the blink reflex is normal but EMG shows neurogenic change in masseter and temporalis muscles (Chia 1988). The jaw-jerk latency can be used to assess the efferent side of this system. The *spinal accessory nerve* can be involved in neoplastic compression, or during surgical procedures in the posterior triangle of the neck, causing weakness of trapezius and sternomastoid muscles (Olarte and Adams 1977). The prognosis is better following blunt trauma, stretch, or in cases beginning spontaneously, e.g. in weightlifters. If EMG shows surviving motor units in trapezius the nerve is intact and the prognosis is good (Berry et al. 1991). *The external ocular nerves* may also be involved in some diseases that also affect other nerves, for example diabetes mellitus and polyarteritis nodosa. All the muscles involved in these cranial neuropathies can be studied by needle EMG, although special expertise is required in some instances.

Mononeuritis Multiplex and Multiple Mononeuropathies

Sometimes a patient may present with features of damage to more than one nerve (Table 8.7). This may take the form of isolated multiple mononeuropathies indicating local involvement of more than one nerve, or a more widespread disorder in which multiple mononeuropathies merge producing a clinical syndrome resembling polyneuropathy. In the latter instance asymmetry and variable severity of involvement in the territory of individual nerves is characteristic. In some instances, especially in patients with multiple mononeuropathy occurring in association with diabetes mellitus, or with acquired or hereditary liability to pressure palsies, there is clinical and electrophysiological evidence of plexus involvement. In vasculitis, on the other hand, distal nerves are more likely to be affected. Multiple mononeuropathies occur relatively frequently with multiple entrapments, other forms of external injury, infiltrative disorders or vascular disorders of

Table 8.7. Causes of multiple mononeuropathies (mononeuritis multiplex)

Vascular
Vasculitis
   Polyarteritis nodosa
   Churg–Strauss angiitis
   Other connective tissue disorders
   Rheumatoid arthritis
   Systemic lupus erythematosus
   Non-systemic vasculitis
   Wegener's granuloma and Sjogren's syndrome
Diabetes mellitus

Multiple entrapment or compressive neuropathies
Idiopathic and traumatic
Chronic inflammatory polyradiculoneuropathy and Guillain–Barré syndrome
Hereditary predisposition to pressure palsies
CMT Type 1 and other hereditary demyelinating neuropathies
Diabetes mellitus
Leprosy
Other focal presentations of generalised neuropathies, e.g. uraemia

Infiltrations and neoplasms
Lymphoma and leukaemia
Granuloma
Neurofibromatosis
Amyloidosis

Adapted from Parry (1985)

nerve (see Hellmann et al. 1988).

The term *mononeuritis multiplex* has often been used to denote inflammatory or vasculitic nerve lesions, particularly in relation to polyarteritis nodosa and related syndromes, but in the majority of patients with multiple peripheral nerve lesions the clinical syndrome is due either to multiple entrapments or to other diseases, e.g. Guillain–Barré syndrome, diabetes mellitus or uraemia, in which an underlying generalised neuropathy is associated with multiple mononeuropathies on the basis of susceptibility to entrapment, or to vascular or metabolic factors. The two terms mononeuritis multiplex and multiple mononeuropathy are thus interchangeable. In patients with vasculitis and multiple mononeuropathy the location of the nerve lesion is not necessarily related to potential sites of entrapment. Indeed, in many such patients clinical and electrophysiological assessment suggests that individual affected nerves are damaged at several sites.

The *vascular forms* of multiple mononeuropathies usually present acutely or subacutely, with poorly localised, aching pain. Lesions of plexus or proximal nerve trunks tend to be predominantly motor, and distal neuropathies show mixed sensorimotor features with marked involvement of pain and temperature sensation (Parry 1985). The tendon reflex in the territory of an affected nerve may be lost. Cranial nerves may be affected. The predominant pathological feature is nerve infarction with axonal degeneration. Electrophysiological assessment shows near-normal maximal motor conduction velocity with EMG features of partial denervation. The amplitude of the CMAP is reduced (Hopf 1963). The electrophysiological disturbance is multifocal and asymmetrical. Transient conduction may be a feature in nerves studied within a week of the onset of the illness, due to the fact that the distal portion of the nerve is still able to conduct before Wallerian degeneration sets in (Ropert and Metral 1990).

In *demyelinating neuropathies* presenting with multiple mononeuropathy there is slowed maximal motor conduction velocity, especially at sites of potential entrapment and also often in other segments of affected nerves. The underlying generalised neuropathy can be demonstrated by nerve conduction velocity studies in clinically unaffected nerves. In some such cases, e.g. in patients with leprosy or chronic Guillain–Barré syndrome, nerve enlargement may be evident on clinical examination (Lewis et al. 1982b). Treatment and management, including the indications for nerve biopsy, depend on the nature of the underlying disorder. These aspects are discussed elsewhere in this book.

Chapter 9

Nerve Root and Plexus Lesions

Lesions of the cervical and lumbar nerve roots are common. These proximal lesions may involve motor and sensory nerve fibres to varying degrees. The initial symptoms of root lesions are nearly always sensory, consisting of paraesthesias and dysaesthesias in a radicular distribution. These sensory symptoms are often related to particular postures or activities. Radicular pain may be a major feature. Motor disability develops later and consists of the typical features of a lower motor neuron lesion, with weakness, atrophy, cramp and fasciculation in the distribution of the lesion. The relevant tendon reflex, if any, is absent. In cervical root lesions Horner's syndrome may be present if the lesion is near the T1 root. The roots most commonly affected by entrapment are those leaving the spinal cord at points where spinal movement is greatest, especially at the C5, C6, C7 and C8 levels in the arm, and at the L4, L5 and S1 levels in the leg. The most commonly affected root in the cervical region is C7 (70% of cases), followed by C6, C8 and C5 (Yoss et al. 1957).

Cervical Root Lesions

The nerve roots that innervate the arms comprise the C3 to T1 motor and sensory roots. These nerve roots are especially vulnerable to traumatic or compressive injury in the intervertebral foramina, but they may also be damaged by primary or metastatic tumour and by infection (Table 9.1). However, degenerative zygoapophyseal joint disease and intervertebral disc prolapse are by far the most common causes of cervical root disease.

Cervical spondylosis is an almost universal phenomenon with increasing age, probably due to the wear and tear imposed by the frequent neck movements of daily life. Root lesions associated with spondylosis are commonest in the fifth and sixth decades (Lunsford et al. 1980) whereas acute disc prolapse tends to affect younger people. In *cervical spondylosis* nerve roots are commonly damaged by entrapment in the intervertebral foramina. These foramina may be narrowed by osteophyte formation from osteoarthritis of the apophyseal joints. The root is then compressed or repeatedly subject to injury during movement of the spine (Adams and Logue 1971) or of the limb (McLellan and Swash 1976), probably by stretching from the point of entrapment. A further factor is ischaemia, from interference with the radicular arterial circulation related to compression and to the co-existence of degenerative vascular disease. Nerve roots may also be compressed or entrapped by other abnormalities

Table 9.1. Causes of cervical root lesions

Degenerative and other bony disorders
Cervical spondylosis
Spinal canal stenosis
Rheumatoid spondylitis
Ankylosing spondylitis
Paget's disease

Trauma
Prolapsed cervical disc
Cervical hyper-extension injuries
Fracture/dislocation of cervical spine
Root avulsion from traction injuries to the arm

Neoplasms
Primary neoplasms of nerve roots
    Neurofibroma, Schwannoma
Meningioma
Metastatic neoplasms of cervical spine
    Carcinoma of bronchus and breast

Infections
Tuberculous osteomyelitis
Pyogenic osteomyelitis
Herpes zoster radiculitis
Post-infectious brachial neuritis

Vascular
Ischaemia
Dural arteriovenous malformation
Haemorrhage

near the intervertebral foramina. These include compression by enlargement of the ligamentum flavum, by prolapsed intervertebral disc, and by other lesions such as tumours of the spine.

Trauma is a particularly important cause of root lesions especially when there is stenosis of the spinal canal. The latter occurs as a congenital anomaly in about 5%–10% of the population, and is also a feature of cervical spondylosis and achondroplasia (Payne and Spillane 1957; Burrows 1963). There are often signs of a combination of cervical root and cord disease in such patients.

Clinical Features

The major clinical feature of cervical root lesions is pain. This pain is sharp, often with a shooting quality, and is associated with unpleasant tingling dysaesthesias in the sensory distribution relevant to the affected root (Table 9.2). These positive sensory symptoms are frequently exacerbated by movement of the spine, especially when the arm is elevated, stretching the affected root. Impaired sensation, particularly marked to pain and temperature rather than to discriminative touch and vibration sense, may be found in affected dermatomes. Tinel's sign may be positive in affected roots when evoked by tapping the neck in some cases, especially in traumatic lesions (Wynn-Parry 1984).

Table 9.2.   Distribution of pain and sensory loss in cervical root lesions

C5:	interscapular, deltoid areas
C6:	radial forearm, digits I and II
C7:	arm, forearm, digit III
C8:	arm, ulnar forearm, digits IV and V
T1:	axilla

The relevant tendon reflexes may be diminished; for example the biceps reflex is reduced in C6 lesions, the triceps jerk in C7 lesions. However, reduction of the amplitude of a mechanically elicited tendon reflex is often a difficult clinical sign to elicit. In cervical spondylosis accentuation of the finger and triceps reflexes, with loss or diminution of the amplitude of the biceps reflex, is an important and virtually diagnostic pattern of signs that indicates a root or root entry zone lesion at the C6 level, with an associated corticospinal tract lesion at the same level. There may be signs of corticospinal dysfunction in the legs, usually more marked on the side of the brachial root lesion. Weakness with signs of a lower motor neuron lesion is also a feature of root disease, although in most instances this is far

Table 9.3.   Distribution of weakness in brachial root lesions

C5:	deltoid
C6:	biceps, brachioradialis, wrist abduction and extension
C7:	triceps, wrist adduction, metacarpophalangeal extension
C8:	intrinsic hand muscles, interphalangeal extension
T1:	intrinsic hand muscles, especially lumbricals

less prominent than pain and other sensory features (Northfield 1973) (Table 9.3).

Electrophysiological Assessment of Root Lesions

The first step in electrophysiological diagnosis is localisation of the disturbance of function to root, plexus or nerve. Motor nerve conduction studies are useful in establishing whether or not there is a more generalised peripheral neuropathy, or a localised entrapment, such as a carpal tunnel syndrome. F-wave responses may be abnormal in radiculopathies but F waves recorded in hand muscles are relevant only to C8 or T1 root lesions, and these are uncommon. Sensory nerve action potential amplitude studies are normal in root lesions since the lesion is proximal to the dorsal root ganglia. H reflex studies in the upper limb are inconsistent. The monosynaptic tendon reflex amplitude, recorded electrically, is reduced in root lesions at C6 and C7 (Schott and Koenig 1991). EMG studies, somatosensory evoked potential responses, nerve root stimulation and magnetic stimulation techniques are all useful in assessing the localisation and extent of root lesions (Mills and Murray 1986; Wilbourn and Aminoff 1988; Evans et al. 1990).

EMG is useful in the diagnosis of root lesions since it can extend and confirm the results of clinical examination (Levin et al 1996). EMG evidence of denervation, especially fibrillation potentials, is present in the early stages (8–21 days from onset) of an acute root lesion, e.g. from trauma. However, EMG assessment is of relatively little value during the first week after a traumatic root lesion, except in deciding whether or not there has been complete section of the root. The presence of any volitional motor unit action potential (MUAP) activity in muscles innervated by the damaged root excludes a complete root section (Goodgold and Eberstein 1983) (Table 9.4). In this clinical situation further investigation is unnecessary and an expectant course should be pursued. Commonly, the information sought by EMG examination can be obtained equally reliably by meticulous attention to the history and physical examination.

Concentric or monopolar needle EMG studies can also be used to define the location of a root lesion in

Table 9.4. Electromyography in root lesions

Early
Reduced recruitment of motor units
Incomplete interference pattern
Fibrillations in paraspinal muscles after 7–10 days

Later
Fibrillation in distal muscles in root distribution
Positive sharp waves
Chronic partial denervation, with increased jitter and blocking in
  single-fibre EMG recordings

Chronic
Fibrillation less prominent
Polyphasic MAUPs of increased amplitude

Compound muscle action potential is of reduced amplitude at all stages
until recovery

Table 9.5. Differentiation of brachial root and plexus lesions

	Root lesions	Plexus lesions
Histamine skin response	+	0
SAP	+	0
EMG of posterior neck extensors	denervated	normal
SSEP	–	–

relation to the intervertebral foramen. The posterior primary rami of the ventral roots that innervate the erector spinae muscles arise within these exit foramina so that in root lesions in which there is no EMG evidence of denervation in these muscles the lesion must be distal to the foramen. In root lesions in which the erector spinae muscles show EMG features of denervation the lesion is located proximal to, or within, the foramen (Benecke and Conrad 1980). The latter is a feature of neurofibroma and meningioma, but traumatic lesions can fall into either category. EMG evidence of denervation may develop in the lumbar paraspinal muscles as early as 10 days after lumbo-sacral nerve root injury (Johnson and Melvin 1971). Generally, in acute or progressive nerve root lesions fibrillation potentials are prominent and the MUAPs are unstable, with increased neuromuscular jitter, and impulse blocking in single-fibre EMG recordings. In chronic, static lesions fibrillation potentials are less prominent, the MUAPs are of increased amplitude and more stable, and the interference pattern is reduced. Even at this stage, concentric needle EMG examination is a useful technique for assessment of the distribution of abnormality that can be used to localise the lesion to one or more motor roots (Hatt 1970). Generally, the EMG examination should be centred on muscles in the affected myotome and those overlapping this innervation. The finding of abnormalities in two or more muscles innervated by a single root, preferably from different peripheral nerves, is consistent with localisation of the lesion to this nerve root (Wilbourn and Aminoff 1988).

EMG evidence of denervation or of chronic partial denervation (reinnervation) in the rhomboid and serratus anterior muscles is also of potential localising value since the dorsal scapular and long thoracic nerves innervating these muscles arise proximal to the brachial plexus, but distal to the dorsal root ganglia (Table 9.5). For example, these muscles are usually affected in the "brachial neuri-

tis" syndrome, indicating that this disorder is not limited to the brachial plexus.

Somatosensory evoked potentials have been much used in recent years in the diagnosis of cervical root and brachial plexus lesions (Pratt et al. 1979a,b; Jones 1979). The stimulus is usually applied to the median or ulnar nerve at the wrist, since relatively few supramaximal stimuli are then needed for averaging (Jones 1979; Cohen et al. 1985; Yu and Jones 1985), but more exact discrimination in the diagnosis of post-ganglionic root lesions can be obtained by stimulating individual digital nerves with ring electrodes, e.g. digit I for the C6 root, digit II for the C7 root and digit V for the C8 root (Cohen et al. 1985). Direct stimulation of the skin to excite dermatomes directly is a relatively more painful and more prolonged procedure than nerve stimulation (Pratt and Starr 1981) and evokes smaller potentials that may be difficult to use for measurements of latency (Pratt et al. 1979a,b; Yu and Jones 1985).

The motor nerves can be examined by utilising F wave (Eisen et al. 1977; Fisher et al. 1979) and H reflex (Schimseiden et al. 1985) studies. In the former method the anterior horn cell pool is excited by antidromic stimulation of the nerve; in the presence of a root, or plexus, lesion the response may be delayed. However, normal F wave latencies do not preclude the diagnosis of root or plexus lesions, particularly when the symptoms are mainly sensory. H reflexes are difficult to obtain in the arms, but may provide useful information in the recognition of isolated lesions of the posterior roots (Schimseiden et al. 1985). Cortical latencies have also been recorded from tendon taps, and from other mechanical stimuli (Cohen et al. 1985). The combination of delayed F responses or H reflexes, with normal peripheral motor conduction velocity, is strongly suggestive of a proximal disturbance. Stimulation of the cervical roots at the level of the transverse processes of the C7, C8 and T1 vertebrae, using monopolar electrodes, may reveal abnormalities in motor latency and in the amplitude of the compound muscle action potential in some cases (Berger et al. 1985). The M response in nerves derived from an affected root, especially in C8 and T1 lesions, may be small, reflecting axonal loss (Goodgold and Eberstein 1983).

Imaging

Radiological investigations, especially straight X-rays of the cervical spine, CT scanning of the cervical spine and thoracic outlet and MR imaging of these regions, are important in providing full diagnostic information. These investigations are particularly useful in spondylosis, trauma and in suspected neoplastic lesions. However, the functional state of the affected roots can only be revealed by clinical and electrophysiological investigations. Davies et al. (1966) noted that clinical evidence of root avulsion, with the presence of two or more meningoceles, carried a poor prognosis for functional recovery. Root lesions of this type cannot be repaired surgically (Wynn-Parry 1984; Birch 1984). MRI is especially valuable in assessing clinical disc disease, and intrinsic lesions of the cord.

Brachial Plexus Lesions

The brachial plexus is formed by the exchange of motor and sensory nerve fascicles between the brachial roots to form the nerves innervating the arm and shoulder. It extends from the sensorimotor roots to the thoracic outlet. A detailed knowledge of the anatomy of the divisions of the brachial plexus into roots, cords, trunks and nerves is not necessary for everyday clinical practice, although a number of features are important. The first and second thoracic anterior primary rami contribute preganglionic sympathetic fibres to the stellate ganglion by a white ramus communicans. The stellate ganglion lies close to the C7 transverse process. Lesions of the lower part of the brachial plexus, situated close to the vertebral column, may thus result in injury to the cervical sympathetic nerve, causing ipsilateral Horner's syndrome with impaired sweating and vasomotor reactivity on the face and neck. This is an important sign of neoplastic invasion of the lower part of the plexus. It also occurs in some traumatic lesions of the plexus, and in patients with axillary artery aneurysms. The dorsal scapular and long thoracic nerves, innervating the rhomboid and serratus anterior muscles respectively, arise from nerve roots proximal to the brachial plexus and are spared in lesions limited to the brachial plexus. A classification of the common causes of brachial plexus lesions is given in Table 9.6.

The upper trunk of the brachial plexus is formed from the anterior rami of C5 and C6 roots; the middle trunk from the anterior ramus of C7 and the lower trunk from the anterior rami of C8 and T1.

Table 9.6. Classification of brachial plexus lesions

Trauma
Birth injury
    Upper cord: Klumpke's palsy
    Lower cord: Erb's palsy
Penetrating wounds
    Gunshot and stab wounds
Stretch injury
    Traction to arm in industrial and road traffic injuries
    Thoracotomy
Shoulder fractures and dislocations
    Lateral cord of plexus at risk more than medial cord
    Axillary nerve lesion rare: deltoid weakness
    Musculocutaneous nerve: biceps and brachialis paralysis

Crutch palsy
Medial cord at risk

Idiopathic and allergic brachial neuritis
(Parsonage–Turner syndrome: neuralgic amyotrophy)

Neoplasms
Metastatic carcinoma (breast and lungs)
Lymphoma

Radiation therapy (usually for carcinoma of breast)

Thoracic outlet syndrome and cervical rib compression syndromes

These three trunks undergo rearrangement to form the lateral, posterior and medial cords of the plexus. The nerves supplying the arm are derived from these cords, with branches from the trunks of the plexus.

Clinical Features

In lesions of the *upper trunk* of the brachial plexus muscles innervated by the C5 and C6 roots are affected. Thus there is weakness of deltoid and biceps brachii, and of the supraspinatus and infraspinatus muscles. The pectoralis and lower fibres of trapezius may also be involved. Sensory loss is usually evident in the C5 and C6 dermatomes, affecting both pain and light touch. The biceps reflex is reduced or absent. In patients with lesions of the *lower trunk* of the plexus similar motor and sensory abnormalities develop in the hand, but there is associated triceps weakness and atrophy. The weak, atrophic muscle may show fasciculation.

In plexus lesions muscular atrophy usually develops rapidly. Pain is not usually a conspicuous feature, but in traumatic or neoplastic plexus lesions it may be severe. In the weeks after plexus injury pain may intensify, so that the intense, continuous, stimulus-sensitive pain and discomfort of causalgia may develop. This causalgic pain may radiate beyond the anatomical limits of the cutaneous distribution of the affected trunks or cords of the plexus. Horner's syndrome is an important

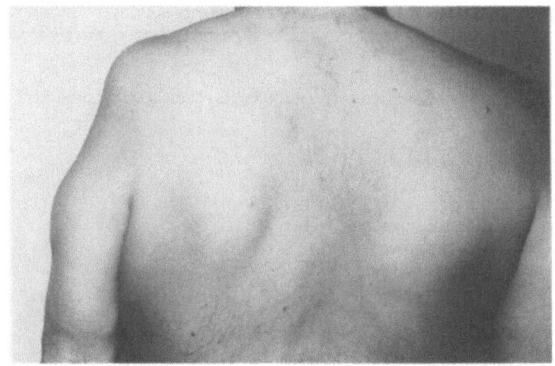

Fig. 9.1. Neuralgic amyotrophy (brachial neuritis). There is atrophy of the left deltoid muscle. The patient recovered over the following 18 months.

localising feature in such patients (Wynn-Parry 1980, 1984). When the plexus lesion follows a stretch injury, recovery ultimately may be satisfactory, although sometimes delayed for up to 2 years.

The *axillary nerve*, a branch of the posterior cord of the brachial plexus consisting of C5 and C6 root components, is vulnerable to injury in fractures and dislocations of the shoulder (Liveson 1984). There is weakness of the deltoid with sensory impairment on the lateral aspect of the upper arm. The supraspinatus is spared so that the initial few degrees of shoulder abduction are normal; clinical testing should be carried out with the arm held a little anterior to the coronal plane in order to exclude abduction by the supraspinatus.

Brachial Neuritis

Whether occurring without evident cause or following immunisation or viral infection, brachial neuritis (Wyburn-Mason 1941), also known as *neuralgic amyotrophy*, is a characteristic illness (Turner and Parsonage 1957; Tsairis et al. 1972). There is frequently shoulder pain of an aching and often severe character for 7 to 10 days before weakness, mainly of C5, C6 and C7 muscles, develops. Men are affected twice as often as women. Sensory loss is unusual and Horner's syndrome is uncommon. Individual branches of the plexus, especially the axillary, suprascapular and long thoracic nerves, may be selectively affected. Isolated involvement of more distal nerves, including the radial, anterior interosseous and phrenic nerves (Mumenthaler et al. 1984) may also occur. The rhomboids and serratus anterior muscles are almost invariably involved and it is thus likely that the lesion extends into the brachial roots. The disorder is bilateral in 25% of

cases, and the right side is more commonly affected than the left. Affected muscles develop wasting (Fig. 9.1) but the prognosis for recovery during the subsequent 1.5 to 3 years is good (Tsairis et al. 1972). However, 10% fail to recover useful function.

In about half the cases there is an antecedent event, e.g. immunisation, viral infections, trauma and vasculitis (Eisen 1993). Brachial neuritis may also occur in polyarteritis nodosa and in diabetes mellitus. A rare, dominantly inherited, familial form of brachial neuritis has been reported in which recurrent episodes occur, and paralysis of the vocal cord may develop (Taylor 1960; Geiger et al. 1974; Dunn et al. 1978). Some of these familial cases have tomaculous neuropathy (Bradley et al. 1975).

Brachial Plexus Lesions Due to Malignant Infiltration or Radiation Injury

The distinction between neoplastic invasion of the brachial plexus and radiation injury in patients with carcinoma of the breast and other metastases in the brachial plexus, especially lymphomas, is important in clinical practice, but is not always easy (Thomas and Colby 1972). Neoplastic invasion usually leads to signs of lower trunk dysfunction, with weakness of the hand and triceps muscles, and Horner's syndrome. Sensory impairment is relatively inconspicuous in the early stages. Pain in the shoulder and forearm is a major feature in 80% of cases. In radiation plexopathy pain is less frequent (20%) and less severe; weakness affects the upper trunk distribution causing weakness of deltoid and biceps, and sensory impairment is not a major feature. In carcinoma of the breast, invasion of the brachial plexus tends to develop within a year of surgery, but radiation plexopathy only rarely develops less than a year after treatment (Kori et al. 1981).

Electrophysiological Studies in Brachial Plexus Lesions

In plexus lesions the SNAP is reduced in amplitude and paraspinal muscle EMG is normal. Localisation of the plexus lesion can be surmised from SNAP studies in peripheral nerves in the arm. Responses from thumb stimulation are reduced in upper trunk lesions. Index and middle finger stimulation elicits SNAPs of reduced amplitude in middle trunk lesions, in recordings from the median nerve. The ulnar nerve response, recorded after stimulating the little finger, is of reduced amplitude in lesions of the lower trunk and medial cord of the plexus (Subrameny 1988).

In pressure palsies of the brachial plexus motor and sensory nerve action potentials are dispersed and of reduced amplitude, and conduction is slowed from stimulation at proximal sites, e.g. from Erb's point (Trojaborg 1977). In traumatic lesions of the plexus, as in trauma to the cervical roots, needle EMG studies are generally more valuable than conduction studies, since it is important to know whether there is denervation, and particularly whether or not motor units can be activated in the affected muscles. If continuity in the damaged plexus can be established by evidence of volitional EMG activity in affected muscles, then conservative management is indicated. Absence of volitional activation of motor units after trauma to the brachial plexus, on the other hand, indicates that surgical exploration and nerve grafting may be worthwhile (Stanwood and Kraft 1971). Other investigations, e.g. F wave studies and somatosensory evoked potential (SSEP) studies, do not add much useful information immediately after trauma. However, paralysis of the arm in a patient with normal SNAP amplitude, after severe trauma, with absent SSEP studies, is a typical EMG pattern associated with root avulsion proximal to the posterior root ganglion. The upper limit of normal for motor latency from Erb's point to deltoid, biceps and triceps muscles is 5.6 ms (Trojaborg 1977), and from nerve root stimulation it is 6.6 ms (Eisen 1993).

In very longstanding cases of brachial plexopathy aberrant regeneration of phrenic motor nerve fibres to biceps or triceps has been noted, causing rhythmic discharges of abnormal motor units in the latter muscles during inspiration; arm-diaphragm synkinesis (Swift et al. 1980).

In brachial neuritis, electrophysiological studies may be useful (Table 9.7) in demonstrating denervation and reinnervation in a distribution consistent with plexus or root disease, by showing slowed motor conduction in the plexus from stimulation at Erb's point (Trojaborg 1977), and in giving evidence of additional abnormalities, especially an increased F wave latency and slowed proximal motor conduction. They may sometimes reveal slowing of distal motor or sensory conduction, features suggestive of a relationship to Guillain–Barré syndrome (Weichers and Mattson 1969; Tsairis et al. 1972). Improvement can be monitored using these simple techniques, but SSEPs are also useful for this purpose (Jones 1979; Eisen 1988, 1993).

In plexopathies due to radiation therapy or to malignant invasion electrophysiological tests provide relevant information (Kori et al. 1981) (Table 9.8), but this is usually non-diagnostic. Probably the most reliable information is that obtained by clinical history and examination, and by CT or MRI

Table 9.7. Electrophysiological features of brachial neuritis

Motor conduction
Slowed latency from Erb's point
May be widespread abnormality resembling Guillain–Barré syndrome

F wave studies
Slowed proximal motor conduction

EMG
Fibrillations and positive sharp waves
Paraspinal muscles spared
Chronic partial denervation later

SAPs
Reduced amplitude in median and ulnar nerves

SSEPs
All components delayed.

Table 9.8. Cancer and radiation plexopathies, and thoracic outlet syndromes

Cancer plexopathy
Motor conduction slowed from Erb's point
SAP amplitude reduced

Radiation plexopathy
Motor conduction normal (not invariably)
SAP amplitude reduced

Thoracic outlet syndromes
Reduced or absent SAP ulnar nerve; normal in median nerve
SSEP: N13 delayed in ulnar, but not in median nerve
EMG: denervation intrinsic hand muscles
F wave latency increased

scans of the upper thorax and plexus region. Imaging also has a place in order to exclude invasion of the spinal canal and vertebrae.

Treatment of Brachial Plexus Lesions

The indications for surgical exploration in closed lesions are to establish diagnosis (and prognosis), e.g. in some patients with suspected malignant infiltration of the plexus, and in traumatic injuries. In the latter repair of associated vascular injury is imperative (Birch 1986). Repair of damaged nerve trunks or cords can also be attempted in selected cases, using cutaneous nerve grafts, and muscle or tendon transfers may be useful in improving function in a damaged limb, especially if sensation is relatively preserved (Narakas 1978, 1984).

Thoracic Outlet Syndrome

In thoracic outlet syndrome the brachial plexus or subclavian artery, or both are compressed in the root of the neck by cervical ribs, fibrous bands or muscles.

Peet et al. (1956) used the term thoracic outlet syndrome to encompass neurovascular compression syndromes within the region bounded by the first rib medially, the clavicle laterally and the scalene muscles. The history of the syndrome has been reviewed by Panegyres et al. (1993). Pain and paraesthesias are the most common features, but are often poorly localised, affecting upper arms and axillae more than the hands. Pain characteristically radiates toward the medial two digits, and may be worsened by certain postures or activities, e.g. carrying a heavy case. Tenderness and a positive Tinel sign may be elicited by palpation in the supraclavicular fossa. Sensory loss is uncommon. Sometimes the sensory symptoms may be elicited by particular manoeuvres, especially pulling down on the arm while the shoulders are thrown back with the patient standing in a "military position" (Young and Hardy 1983). In severe cases there is weakness and wasting of the intrinsic hand muscles, especially of the thenar eminence (Gilliatt et al. 1970; Gilliatt 1976; Lascelles et al. 1977), sometimes with ipsilateral Horner's syndrome (Gilliatt et al. 1970). The fully developed syndrome (Thorburn 1907) is rare.

The syndrome is due to compression or stretching of the medial cord of the brachial plexus against a fibrous band that extends from the transverse process of the seventh cervical vertebra to the scalene tubercle of the first rib, or by an accessory cervical rib. The subclavian artery may be involved in this compression, occasionally causing vascular complications, including arterial emboli, or venous thrombosis (Lascelles et al. 1977). There are thus two syndromes, a neurological disorder mainly affecting C8/T1 motor and sensory function, and a vascular syndrome that may have a rapid presentation leading to ischaemia of the hand, with ischaemic pain and a clinically evident circulatory disturbance (Panegyres et al. 1993). At least 90% of cases are neurological in type (Young and Hardy 1983).

Involvement of the subclavian vessels can sometimes be detected by obliteration of the radial pulse, or reduction of blood pressure when examined during rotation and elevation of the chin towards the palpated radial artery, coupled with hyperinflation of the chest (Adson's manoeuvre) or during hyperabduction and elevation of the upper limb (Wright's manoeuvre) (Panegyres et al. 1993).

Thoracic outlet syndrome is rare, occurring in about one per million people per year, but incomplete forms of the syndrome may be more frequent. Women are affected nine times more frequently than men (Gilliatt 1976). Cervical ribs occur in 1% of the population and the syndrome is often overdiagnosed in a patient presenting with pain in the arm.

Electrophysiological Assessment

Electrophysiological studies (Table 9.8) show that the SAP in the ulnar nerve is of reduced amplitude and the F wave latency in the ulnar nerve is increased (Gilliatt et al. 1970; Wulff and Gilliatt 1979). Somatosensory evoked potentials may be useful in diagnosis (Yiannikas and Walsh 1983). The ulnar N9 potential is reduced in amplitude and the N9–N13 latency (brachial plexus to cord segment) is increased. SSAPs probably yield the most reliable results in suspected cases. In the C8/T1 innervated muscles, especially the thenar eminence, there may be EMG features of chronic partial denervation. The study of Panegyres et al. (1993) suggested that no single electrophysiological test was preferred for diagnosis; SNAPs from digit V were abnormal in six of 13 patients and the F response was abnormal in six of nine patients in whom it was studied.

Imaging

MR imaging appears a sensitive investigation (Panegyres et al. 1993), revealing deviation of the brachial plexus in 79% of arms studied, with a false positive rate of 9.5% in asymptomatic arms. MRI was capable of demonstrating cervical ribs, and fibrous cervical bands, but also detected these features in three of 18 normal arms. Hypertrophy of the serratus anterior muscle was found in one patient. Of course, MRI will also demonstrate other pathologies, such as malignant invasion of the plexus.

Management

Surgical treatment, involving removal of cervical ribs or fibrous bands causing neurovascular compression is indicated in symptomatic arms. Adequate imaging should be a prerequisite of exploration. In patients with a vascular presentation angiography is useful in demonstrating the subclavian compression, and the presence of intra-arterial thrombus prior to endarterectomy and vascular repair.

Lumbo-Sacral Root and Plexus Lesions

Localisation of the site of lumbo-sacral lesions is more difficult than that of brachial root and plexus lesions. The lumbo-sacral roots are commonly damaged at their site of exit from the spinal canal, i.e. near the intervertebral foramina, but they may

Table 9.9. Causes of lumbar root and plexus lesions

Lumbar root disorders	Lumbo-sacral plexus disorders
	Degenerative and other bony disorders
Lumbo-sacral canal stenosis	
Ankylosing spondylitis	
Paget's disease	
	Trauma
Prolapsed lumbo-sacral disc	Penetrating wounds
Fracture/dislocation of spine	Traction injuries, e.g. during hip surgery
Root avulsion (rare)	Pelvic fractures
	Childbirth injuries
	Neoplasms
Neurofibroma and meningioma	Retroperitoneal neoplasms
Metastases and lymphomas	Intra-pelvic metastases, e.g. CA colon and cervix
Primary bone tumours	Intra-pelvic lymphoma
	Radiation plexopathy
	Congenital disorders
Sacral meningocele	
Spina bifida	
Lipoma	
Achondroplastic or idiopathic spinal stenosis	
	Infections and inflammatory disorders
Tuberculomas and pyogenic infections	Tuberculosis (of psoas)
Pott's disease	Autoimmune, e.g. Churg–Strauss syndrome
Arachnoiditis	Lumbo-sacral neuritis
	Vascular disorders
Infarction of conus medullaris	Aneurysm and haemorrhage
Arterio-venous malformations	Vasculitis
	Diabetic radiculoplexopathies lumbo-sacral neuritis (post-infectious)

also be damaged in the conus medullaris, in the cauda equina within the lumbo-sacral spinal canal, and in the lumbo-sacral plexus. Generally, the pattern of disorders that affect the lumbo-sacral roots and plexus is similar to that in the cervico-brachial region. Because the lumbo-sacral nerve roots traverse the lower lumbar and sacral spinal canal en route to their exit foramina, lesions of individual roots may occur from spinal canal disorders, e.g. spinal stenosis, or neurofibromata, as well as from disease within the exit foramina themselves.

The causes of lumbo-sacral root and plexus lesions are outlined in Table 9.9. The commonest of these are lumbo-sacral disc disease, and the lumbo-sacral lesions associated with lumbo-sacral spinal stenosis. Many of the latter patients also suffer from degenerative, hypertensive or diabetic vascular disease.

Lumbo-Sacral Disc Prolapse

This is a common cause of disability, causing pain, paraesthesiae, sensory disturbance and weakness in the distribution of the damaged nerve root. The prolapsed disc material compresses and distorts one or more lumbar or sacral nerve roots as they pass into the intervertebral foramen to leave the spinal canal. The disorder is associated with osteoarthritic change, and is especially common in men in the fourth decade. Its onset is often associated with spinal trauma, with unaccustomed heavy exertion, e.g. digging, or with an unusual posture. In 95% of cases disc prolapse occurs at the L4/L5 or L5/S1 disc interspace (Maurice-Williams 1981), so that the fifth lumbar or first sacral nerve roots respectively will be affected. In many patients the characteristic symptoms of low back pain, buttock pain and sciatica resolve during a short period of rest but in others the pain intensifies or becomes recurrent and, in some patients, signs of sensorimotor root lesion develop. The ankle jerk is diminished or absent, and clinical manoeuvres that stretch the nerve root, e.g. passive straight leg raising, cause intensification of the sciatic pain.

There are three clinical syndromes:

1. Posterolateral disc protrusion with compression of a single nerve root

2. Acute central disc protrusion with compression of the cauda equina

3. Lumbar canal stenosis causing chronic cauda equina compression and intermittent clinical symptoms.

Both lateral disc protrusions and canal stenosis may produce unilateral sciatica. The pattern of motor and sensory disturbance frequently enables recognition of involvement of the L4, L5 or S1 nerve roots. However, as many as 20% of patients with prolapsed lumbo-sacral disc lesions have no neurological abnormality other than sciatic pain. Between 60% and 80% of the population have had low back pain, and 14% have experienced back pain persisting for longer than 2 weeks. Sciatica has occurred in 2% of the population (Deyo and Tsui-Wu 1987).

Investigation

Plain X-rays often disclose osteoarthritic change with narrowing of the disc interspace at the site of disc prolapse, and slight lumbar scoliosis, concave to the affected side. Plain CT scanning of the spine (Fig. 9.2) is an effective method for imaging disc lesions (see Aminoff et al. 1985b). Magnetic resonance imaging is also helpful, since it can demonstrate abnormal discs by their increased proton density, and may also visualise the prolapsed portion of the disc. Radiculography, using water-soluble contrast, will reveal the disc prolapse, together with displacement and thickening of the affected root, and failure of filling of the root pouch, but this investigation is now virtually always carried out with transverse axial CT scanning, which is capable of differentiating disc prolapse from scar tissue, for example in the post-operative patient with recurrent pain. MRI with gadolinium enhancement can also provide this information (Ross et al. 1990). However, in some patients radiological studies reveal no abnormality.

Electrophysiological Assessment

Electrophysiological investigation is useful. EMG is the single most useful technique in diagnosis of lumbo-sacral root lesions (Wilbourn and Aminoff 1988). About 75% of patients with clinical features of lumbar radiculopathies show abnormalities with needle EMG (Knuttson 1961; Eisen et al. 1983b). EMG studies may be normal in the first week before denervation potentials develop, and after a year, when recovery has occurred (Wilbourne and Aminoff 1988). Needle EMG can be used to delineate the radicular basis of the syndrome by studying the distribution of neurogenic change in the affected, and in the contralateral unaffected leg. Bilateral involvement is much more common in lumbo-sacral disc prolapse than in cervical disc prolapse.

Fibrillations develop in an affected root distribution (myotome) in a proximal–distal progression, and show a similar pattern of disappearance during

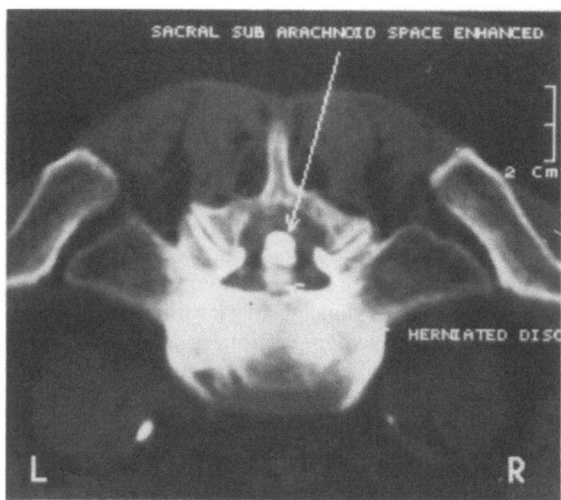

Fig. 9.2. CT myelogram (L5/S1) of central disc protrusion. The theca is displaced slightly dorsally by a free fragment of disc material.

recovery over the subsequent 12 to 18 months. Paraspinal muscle EMG is particularly useful in demonstrating fibrillation potentials in the acute phase and, during recovery, fibrillation potentials will be present in distal, but not in the proximal, paraspinal muscles (Wilbourn and Aminoff 1988).

F wave studies can be used to demonstrate the proximal lesion; they show increased latency in the damaged root, based on studies of distribution relative to the muscle sampled (Eisen et al. 1977; Tonzola et al. 1981; Tang et al. 1988). When abnormal, however, EMG studies are also abnormal and F wave studies are, in this sense, frequently redundant. H wave studies may also be useful in studies of the S1 root, in which gastrocnemius/soleus recordings can be made (Braddom and Johnson 1974). Abnormal F wave responses or H reflex latencies are found in 50% of patients with clinical features of L5 or S1 radiculopathies, a number of whom have normal myelograms (Tonzona et al. 1981). SSEP studies appear less reliable than other neurophysiological methods in diagnosis (Aminoff et al. 1985a; Cohen et al. 1985). SSEPs evoked from stimulation of relevant dermatomes may be helpful (Aminoff et al. 1985b). Magnetic stimulation (Banerjee et al. 1993) or electrical stimulation of motor roots (Swash and Snooks 1986) can be used to demonstrate an increased latency from stimulation at L1 or L4 to the muscles of the leg. This technique promises to be of practical value in the diagnosis of root lesions and cauda equina disease.

Electrophysiological investigation is particularly useful; *first* in establishing the diagnosis of lumbo-sacral root lesion in patients in whom there is doubt after clinical assessment either as to the extent of involvement or, particularly, whether the lesion is in the root, in the plexus, or in the common peroneal nerve. Thus paraspinal muscle EMG studies have a place in investigation of doubtful cases, and patients referred for electrophysiological assessment should always have motor and sensory conduction studies carried out to exclude neuropathy or distal entrapment. *Second*, electrophysiological assessment is useful in patients with recurrent symptoms whether or not they have previously had a laminectomy, since the finding of active denervation, especially prominent fibrillation and positive sharp wave potentials, implies ongoing damage to the motor root. *Third*, electrophysiological studies are useful if the clinical and imaging studies are in conflict. If EMG studies are normal the diagnosis is other than lumbo-sacral disc prolapse with nerve root compression.

Management

Bed rest is useful in the acute stages, but the back should be supported by a hard or firm bed and mattress. A lumbar brace is also useful, but sooner or later a period of active physiotherapy is required and the corset must be discarded. If there are definite neurological symptoms and signs in the acute stage of a disc prolapse laminectomy should be considered after appropriate investigation, but a period of conservative medical management may also be successful at this stage. Non-steroidal anti-inflammatory drugs are indicated for pain. Local injections of analgesic or steroid into facet joints or discs are not of proven benefit, and epidural analgesic is also of doubtful efficacy (Frank 1993). When pain is severe, or paralysis and sensory loss are marked, or if there are features suggestive of cauda equina involvement, investigation and consideration of surgical exploration should be advised. Surgery is indicated when pain is severe, there is an identifiable neurological syndrome, with disc prolapse visualised by imaging, and conservative treatment for 4–6 weeks has been ineffective. The main benefit of surgery is relief of sciatica (Deyo et al. 1990). Surgical treatment is less likely to be effective if low back pain, or sciatica, is the only symptom. After surgical treatment a programme of active physiotherapy to strengthen back muscles and improve spinal mobility is essential.

It is important to recognise the natural history of low back pain without sciatica. Most such patients do not have intervertebral disc prolapse. Most patients will recover, untreated, in less than 2 weeks, and even in patients with sciatica 90% do not require intervention (Deyo et al. 1990). In patients older than 55 years with back pain, 46% have an abnormality in the spine and 11% have malignant disease (Waddell 1982). Investigation is therefore particularly important in older age groups in planning management, especially when there are neurological signs on examination.

Lumbo-Sacral Canal Stenosis

Lumbo-sacral spinal stenosis may be congenital, occurring in people in whom the whole spinal canal is narrow, and the neck shorter and broader than normal, or in people with achondroplasia in whom spinal stenosis leads to both cervical cord compression and cauda equina root compression at a relatively early age (Verbiest 1955; Wackenheim and Babin 1980). Lumbo-sacral spinal stenosis may also develop in association with spondylotic degenerative disease of the lumbo-sacral discs, especially at the L3/4 and L5/S1 disc interspaces. In one series (Hall et al. 1985) the mean age of presentation was 63 years, and the mean duration of symptoms before diagnosis was 32 months. The posture of patients with symptomatic spinal canal stenosis is often rather characteristic. The hips, knees and lumbar spine are held in slight flexion, with absence of the normal lumbo-sacral lordosis, producing a "simian stance" (Simkin 1982).

The commonest presentation is discomfort occurring in the buttock, thigh or leg on standing or walking, that is relieved by rest, thus resembling claudication. This symptom may consist of pain, numbness or weakness, or commonly a combination of these. The pain and other symptoms may also be relieved by lying, sitting or by adopting a flexed posture at the waist. Pain may be caused by lying supine or by standing alone (94% in Hall et al. 1985). The association of these symptoms with spinal disease was first reported by Déjérine in 1911. Verbiest (1955) recognised that it was due to compression of the cauda equina and later descriptions were given by Bergmark (1950) and Blau and Logue (1961). Only 10%–25% of patients show abnormal restriction of straight leg raising (Hall et al. 1985; Editorial 1985). Examination may show little abnormality unless the patient is examined after postural or exercise stress tests. The ankle jerks are absent in fewer than half the patients and there is usually no weakness or sensory impairment at rest.

Investigation

Radiological investigation reveals degenerative disc disease, osteoarthritis of the facet joints, spondylolisthesis or, rarely, ankylosing spondylitis. CT scans usually show a narrowed lumbo-sacral spinal canal and myelography reveals partial or complete block to the flow of contrast at multiple levels, but especially at the level of L3 and L4 (Hall et al. 1985).

Electromyographic tests are usually abnormal, showing the features of multiple root involvement, often bilateral. The F waves may be delayed or absent depending on the degree of involvement of individual roots. F wave responses frequently show increased chrono-dispersion (Tang et al. 1988; London and England 1991).

Management

Patients with mild symptoms require no special treatment, but may derive subjective benefit from physiotherapy and lumbo-sacral support. If the symptoms are severe or progressive, decompressive laminectomy or foramenotomy may be indicated, depending on the nature of the radiological abnormality. The results of surgical treatment are generally good; Hall et al. (1985) reported that 62% of patients had good or excellent results, and that an additional 27% showed some improvement.

Cauda Equina Lesions

One of the commonest causes of cauda equina disease is lumbo-sacral spondylosis with canal stenosis as discussed above, but primary and secondary tumours (Mathew and Todd 1993), arachnoiditis, and congenital abnormalities, e.g. sacral meningocele, may cause this syndrome (Snooks and Swash 1985). There is pain, paraesthesiae and lumbo-sacral "saddle distribution" sensory impairment with weakness of pelvic floor and sphincter muscles. The ankle jerks may be absent and there may be weakness of the L5/S1 musculature, especially of dorsiflexion and eversion of the feet. These features are usually asymmetrical.

Electrophysiological investigations are useful. The CMAP is of reduced amplitude on the affected side and needle EMG shows chronic partial denervation in affected muscles. The F waves and H reflexes are delayed or absent, but SAPs are normal. The diagnosis is confirmed by radiological investigation, including CT scanning with contrast, and MRI.

EMG assessment of the external anal sphincter muscle and pubo-rectalis muscle can be useful if quantified (Henry and Swash 1985), and the motor conduction velocity across the motor roots of the cauda equina can be measured directly by using transcutaneous spinal stimulation at L1 and L4 spinal levels, and recording from sphincter muscles

(S3 and S4) or other, lower limb muscles representing the various lumbo-sacral motor roots (Snooks and Swash 1985; Maertens de Nordhout et al. 1988). In cauda equina lesions motor conduction in the affected cauda equina roots is slowed (Swash and Snooks 1986).

Treatment is surgical, with laminectomy, and radiotherapy if indicated. The prognosis depends on the nature and severity of the underlying disorder. Generally, in spondylotic cauda equina disease the prognosis is good provided that the disorder has not been very severe, or very longstanding prior to treatment.

Conus Medullaris Lesions

There is severe involvement of sphincters early in the clinical course, with impotence or incontinence, and with less marked involvement of the upper sacral and lumbar motor and sensory roots. Primary tumours, such as ependymoma, lipoma and dermoid cyst are the commonest cause of this rare syndrome. EMG examination shows denervation of pelvic floor and external anal sphincter muscles, with some abnormality in glutei and posterior thigh muscles symmetrically. The anterior thigh and upper limb muscles are normal. Radiological investigation, especially CT scanning with myelography, is necessary to delineate the diagnosis, and surgical treatment often alleviates disability.

Lumbo-Sacral Plexus Lesions

The lumbo-sacral plexus consists of two associated plexuses; the lumbar plexus comprises the L2, L3 and L4 roots, and the sacral plexus comprises the L5, S1, S2, S3 and S4 roots. Clinical distinction between lumbo-sacral root and lumbo-sacral plexus lesions may be difficult. In the latter the clinical features suggest involvement of more than one peripheral nerve or root, the weakness usually involves proximal muscles in lumbar plexus lesions (L2, L3, L4) and distal and peroneal muscles in sacral plexus lesions (S1, S2, S3, S4). In addition, pain in the buttock and leg in plexus lesions is usually not much affected by movement of the leg, e.g. by passive straight leg raising. In some disorders, e.g. trauma, malignancy, diabetes mellitus and radiation problems, a combination of root, plexus and peripheral nerve lesions may develop. Probably the most common cause of lumbo-sacral plexopathy is diabetes, but examination of the pelvis to exclude malignancy, especially vaginal and rectal examination, must not be omitted. The causes of lumbo-sacral plexopathy are listed in Table 9.9.

In diabetic polyradiculoplexopathy there is asymmetrical pain, and weakness in the proximal, anterior part of the thigh. Weakness affects hip girdle and quadriceps muscles but others, especially the thigh flexors, may be affected. This syndrome, formerly termed *diabetic amyotrophy, ischaemic monoeuropathy* or *femoral neuropathy* (Garland 1955) generally occurs in well-controlled Type 2 diabetes, but may be a presenting feature of the disease, and also occurs in young insulin-dependent Type 1 diabetics (Basron and Thomas 1981). Serious accidental injury to the lumbo-sacral plexus is uncommon because of the protected location of the plexus, but fractures of the pelvis are associated with damage to the lumbo-sacral plexus in about 10% of cases. Similarly, penetrating gunshot or knife wounds may damage the plexus.

Primary lumbo-sacral plexopathy, analogous to brachial neuritis in the upper limb, is an uncommon and poorly defined disorder. Only a few cases have been described (Sander and Sharp 1981; Evans et al. 1981). The onset is sudden with pain and weakness developing days or weeks later in an extended sciatic distribution, but sparing paraspinal muscles. Recovery may be partial or complete depending on the severity of the disorder, during a period of 1 or 2 years after the onset.

Retroperitoneal disease, for example metastatic tumour, lymphoma or leukaemic deposits, or haemorrhage, may also cause lumbo-sacral plexus damage and this may improve with appropriate treatment. Carcinomas of the prostate, cervix, uterus and rectum are particularly common causes of infiltration of this plexus. The plexus may also be injured in childbirth, especially in difficult forceps deliveries (Snooks et al. 1984). The plexus is damaged by the fetal head or by the forceps, and the deficit, which may be relatively localised to affect

sciatic or femoral nerve, is usually reversible (King 1950). Similar lesions of the plexus may develop during orthopaedic operations on the hip, particularly hip replacement, and these may also involve individual nerves, e.g. femoral, sciatic and obturator nerves. These also resolve spontaneously although recovery may be delayed.

Electrophysiological Assessment

Electrophysiological studies help to establish the location of the lesion in the plexus rather than in the lumbo-sacral roots. Needle EMG evaluation shows involvement of muscles in several root distributions, and paraspinal muscles are normal. SAPs may be small or absent. The F wave latencies are increased, or absent, in the L5/S1 segments from stimulation of the common peroneal and tibial nerves respectively, but these H reflex studies and SSEP studies do not allow differentiation of plexus lesions from radiculopathies. Near-nerve stimulation of individual roots, using needle electrodes insulated except at their tips placed adjacent to the nerve near the transverse process of the vertebral body, may reveal increased latencies across the affected parts of the plexus (McLean 1979).

Management

Lesions of the lumbo-sacral plexus are best managed conservatively. Radiation therapy is helpful in alleviating plexopathies due to malignant infiltration. Haemorrhages resolve spontaneously. Heparin and warfarin may be of value in radiation plexopathy (Glantz et al. 1994, Bowen et al. 1996). Steroids may be helpful in autoimmune disorders involving the lumbo-sacral plexus (Bradley et al. 1984a).

Chapter 10

Genetically Determined Neuropathies

The commonest form of the genetically determined neuropathies is a slowly progressive symmetrical disorder in which peripheral neuropathy, usually predominantly motor in type, is associated with deformities of the feet, particularly pes cavus. This group of disorders (Table 10.1) contains diseases inherited as an autosomal dominant or recessive trait. These disorders can often be recognised in apparently unaffected members of a family known to carry the trait by the foot deformity, which usually precedes the development of overt neuropathy by many years. None the less, the occurrence of pes cavus does not necessarily imply the presence of peripheral neuropathy and, conversely, in some patients with peroneal atrophy pes cavus may not be a feature. In some hereditary neuropathies an underlying metabolic defect has been characterised, e.g. Refsum's disease, amyloidosis, porphyria (see Table 10.4). Classification can thus be based firstly on an underlying metabolic derangement, to which the clinical features can be related. In those disorders known to be inherited but in which the underlying metabolic abnormality is unknown, on the other hand, clinical classification is more difficult. The genetic approach to these disorders has introduced a new approach to classification and to understanding of apparently intermediate phenotypes (see Tables 10.2–10.4). Inevitably classification of these latter syndromes is controversial and subject to change. Indeed, as new advances in understanding of the genetic and metabolic basis of these disorders are made, more precise criteria for recognition of disease entities can be established, leading to practical benefits in management and

Table 10.1. Classification of hereditary neuropathies

Charcot–Marie–Tooth (CMT)
Hereditary sensory neuropathies (HSN)
Hereditary neuropathies with specific metabolic defects

After Harding and Thomas (1984).

Table 10.2. Hereditary motor and sensory neuropathies (CMT)

Type 1 CMT (hypertrophic Charcot–Marie–Tooth disease)
  Autosomal dominant
    Type 1A (chromosome17p 11.2-12)
      duplication of PMP-22 gene
      point mutation of PMP-22 gene
    Hereditary liability to pressure palsies
      PMP-22 gene deletion or point mutations
    Type 1B (chromosome 1q 21-23)
      defects of Po
  Autosomal recessive

Type 2 CMT (neuronal form of Charcot–Marie–Tooth disease)
  Autosomal dominant
  Autosomal recessive
    adult type
    severe childhood type

Type 3 CMT (Déjérine–Sottas disease)
  Autosomal recessive in some cases
    congenital hypomyelinating neuropathy (PMP22 and Po defects described)

X-linked dominant CMT (chromosome xq 13)
  with or without connexin 32 defects

Complex syndromes
  with optic atrophy, deafness, spastic paraparesis (Xp26) or mental retardation (Xp22)

Table 10.3. Hereditary sensory neuropathies (HSN)

Autosomal dominant type (HSAN I)[a]

Autosomal recessive types
  congenital non-progressive sensory neuropathy (HSAN II)[a]
  progressive form
  familial dysautonomia (Riley–Day syndrome) (HSAN III)[a] (chromosome 9q 31-33)
  congenital sensory neuropathy with anhidrosis (HSAN IV)[a]
  HSN with spastic paraplegia
  HSN with predominant loss of small myelinated fibres (HSAN V)[a]
  other forms of HSN

X-linked recessive types

Sensory neuropathy in hereditary ataxias chromosome
  Friedreich's ataxia (9 cen-q21)
  autosomal dominant cerebellar ataxia
  others (see Table 10.8)

[a]Hereditary sensory and autonomic neuropathy, classified according to Dyck et al. 1983.

Table 10.4. Hereditary neuropathies with specific metabolic defects

A. Familial amyloid polyneuropathies (FAP)
    transthyretin-related FAP syndromes
        1. Portuguese, Swedish and Japanese syndromes
            (chromosome 18q 11.2-12.1)
            associated with methionine 30 (MET 30) substitution)
    Other transthyretin substitutions with various phenotypes
        2. Irish/Appalachian (ALA 10 mutation)
        3. Indiana (SER 84) and Maryland (HIS 58)
    Apolipoprotein A$_1$-related FAP syndrome
        4. Iowa type (chromosome 11q 23-qter)
            (associated with arginine substitution)
    gelsolin-related FAP syndrome
        5. Finnish type (chromosome 9q33)
            associated with asparagine substitution in the amyloid
            protein)

B. Porphyrias
    Acute intermittent prophyria
    Variegate porphyria
    Hereditary coproporphyria

C. Disturbances of lipid metabolism
    Phytanic acid storage (Refsum's disease)
    Leucodystrophies
        Metachromatic leukodystrophy
        Krabbe's globoid cell leukodystrophy
        Adreno-leuko-myeloneuropathy
    Lipoprotein deficiency
        Abetalipoproteinaemia (Bassen–Kornzweig disease)
        Alphalipoprotein deficiency (Tangier disease)
    Fabry's disease (alphagalactosidase deficiency)
    Cerebro-tendinous xanthomatosis (cholestanolosis)
    Sphingo-myelin lipidosis

D. Disorders with defective DNA repair
    Ataxia telangiectasia
    Cockayne syndrome
    Xeroderma pigmentosa

E. Neuropathies associated with mitochondrial disorders

genetic counselling. Most identifiable inherited neuropathies with a known metabolic basis are autosomal recessive traits. These represent a minority of patients with heritable neuropathies since dominantly inherited phenotypes predominate within individual families.

The Syndrome of Peroneal Muscular Atrophy

Classifications have been proposed by Dyck and Lambert (1968a,b) and Dyck (1984). The classification proposed by Dyck and Lambert (1968a,b) recognised that a pure motor form of peroneal muscular atrophy, without sensory abnormality clinically or by electrophysiological testing, is probably due to involvement of anterior horn cells alone, i.e. is a form of spinal muscular atrophy (Harding and Thomas 1980a). Those forms of peroneal muscular

atrophy with both motor and sensory involvement, whether recognised clinically or by electrophysiological testing, are also termed the hereditary motor and sensory neuropathies (HMSN) (Dyck 1984). The terms Peroneal Muscular Atrophy, Charcot–Marie–Tooth (CMT) syndrome and hereditary motor and sensory neuropathies (HMSN) are interchangeable.

Peroneal muscular atrophy can be classified into major types on the basis of clinical, electrophysiological and pathological data: CMT Type 1 and CMT Type 2 (Harding and Thomas 1984; World Federation of Neurology Research Committee 1994). CMT Type 1 is characterised by marked slowing of motor conduction, with segmental demyelination and onion bulb formation in peripheral nerves. CMT Type 2 is characterised by mild slowing of motor conduction and by axonal degeneration in peripheral nerves. There are few clinical differences between these two syndromes, but genetic studies have demonstrated the existence of several different types. Most cases of Charcot–Marie–Tooth syndrome are dominantly inherited, reflecting the predominance of the dominantly inherited CMT Type 1 syndrome. X-linked and autosomal recessive families have been described. A severe infantile form (CMT Type 3) was first described by Déjérine and Sottas (1893). The major features of CMT Types 1 and 2 are shown in Table 10.5. In Sweden CMT Type 1 was found to affect 1 in 20 000 schoolchildren (Hagberg and Westerberg 1983) but Harding and Thomas (1980a) estimated prevalence in the UK as 1 in 5000.

CMT Type 1 (Hypertrophic Form of Peroneal Muscular Atrophy)

CMT Type 1 is the most common form of peroneal muscular atrophy. In two-thirds of patients symptoms begin in the first decade and in almost all cases the disorder begins before the age of 20 years. CMT Type 1 is two to three times more common than CMT Type 2 (Harding and Thomas 1980a). The disease usually presents with foot deformity, or with difficulty walking, and with foot drop due to weakness of the peroneal and anterior tibial muscles (Fig. 10.1). Dyck et al. (1984a) noted that only a quarter of affected persons, ascertained clinically or on the basis of slowed motor conduction velocity in the first decade, had high arches, but in later decades about two-thirds had high arches (Harding and Thomas 1980a). Pes cavus (Fig. 7.2) implies muscular imbalance between the intrinsic muscles of the foot and the long flexors and extensors acting across the foot, resulting in progressive deformity during development.

Table 10.5. Comparison of features of Type 1 and Type 2 CMT

	Hypertrophic (Type 1)	Neuronal(Type 2)
Age of onset	Usually <10 years	Usually second decade
Reflexes	All lost	Absent ankle jerks
Distal sensory signs		
Hands	+	±
Feet	++	++
Weakness		
Hands	+	±
Feet	++	+++
Nerve enlargement	Present	Absent
CSF protein	Raised	?Normal
Sensory nerve conduction	Slowed	Normal or slightly slowed
Motor nerve conduction	Very slowed	Slightly slowed
Sural nerve biopsy	Onion bulbs, Segmental demyelination	Mild axonal degeneration
Course	Progressive	Variable

Weakness predominantly affects distal leg muscles at first, but later more proximal muscles in legs and small hand muscles are involved. In severe cases complete atrophy and paralysis of small foot muscles and of the anterior compartment of the leg develops. Fasciculations and cramps may occur in affected muscles. The ankle jerks are always depressed or absent, and in more than half the cases all the tendon reflexes are absent.

Symptomatic sensory involvement is uncommon but there is usually distal impairment of vibration

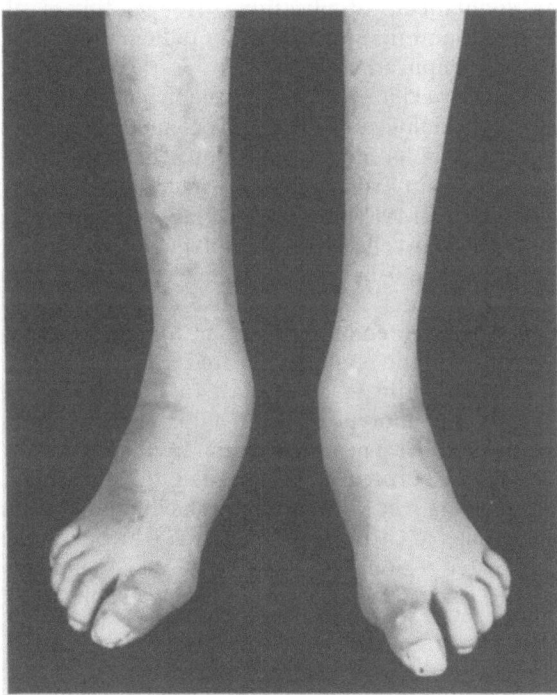

Fig. 10.1. HMSN Type 1 (Charcot–Marie–Tooth syndrome). There is atrophy of the calf and small foot muscles with atrophy of the skin of the toes and collapse of the dorsal arch of the feet. The Achilles tendons are shortened resulting in secondary impairment of gait.

and position sense. Cutaneous sensation is less markedly affected but a characteristic feature is marked delay in the appreciation of a touch or pin-prick applied to the foot, representing a clinical assessment of slowed conduction in the peripheral nervous system. Enlargement of peripheral nerves (Fig. 7.1) is present in about 25% of cases (Dyck and Lambert 1968a).

Scoliosis occurs in 14% of patients (Harding and Thomas 1984) but other skeletal deformities are uncommon. All of these clinical features may lead to presentation; Brust et al. (1978) found that 37% of their patients presented with abnormal gait, 26% with weak feet or legs, 16% with foot deformity and the remainder with delayed walking in infancy, weakness of the hands or sensory symptoms in the feet. The disease usually progresses slowly, but in some cases disability may remain static for many years, but then rapidly progress (Brust et al. 1978). The disorder is more severe in males than females.

Various other clinical manifestations have been described. Of these, tremor is the most frequent. This resembles intention tremor, and occurs in about 30% of cases of CMT Type 1. This association has been characterised as the Roussy–Levy syndrome (Roussy and Levy 1926), but probably represents an association of CMT Type 1 and essential tremor (Lapresle and Salisachs 1973). Ataxia may occur, but this is due to the motor and sensory disorder in the legs. Optic atrophy, pupillary abnormalities, deafness and pigmentary retinal degeneration have been reported but these features are not concordant within families and thus probably represent chance associations (Harding and Thomas 1980b). These complex clinical features have led to confusion between Charcot–Marie–Tooth syndrome and Friedreich's ataxia, but these disorders are not related (see Salisachs et al. 1982). Cardiomyopathy is not associated with CMT Type 1.

Pupillary constriction has been noted, but not consistently, but autonomic involvement does occur, consisting of impairment of sweating that may be generalised and is due to a defect in sympathetic innervation. Vasomotor control is normal, however (Ingall and McLeod 1991).

Early infantile onset forms are often autosomal recessive, and more severe than the more frequent autosomal dominant disorder (Vital et al. 1987).

Genetics of CMT Type 1 Phenotypes

Several patterns of inheritance have been identified. The most common pattern is an autosomal dominant inheritance, but X-linked dominant and X-linked recessive families have also been identified (see Dyck et al. 1993a). Autosomal recessive inheritance has also been reported in a few cases (Gabreëls-Festen et al. 1992a,b 1993). Autosomal dominant families show linkage either to chromosome 17p (CMT Type 1A) to chromosome 1q (CMT Type 1B) or to neither of these loci (CMT Type 1C), indicating additional loci for this syndrome (Chance et al. 1992; Chance and Pleasure 1993). Ionanescu et al. (1993) studied 730 members of 63 families, of whom 356 were affected with Charcot–Marie–Tooth disease. They found that 60% had CMT Type 1A (chromosome 17) and only 2% had CMT Type 1B. The remainder were CMT Type 2 or X-linked dominant pedigrees.

The phenotypic expression varies considerably even within individual families, but there is no clinically evident difference in phenotype between the Type 1A and Type 1B disorders. Families with Type 1A CMT may contain probands with severe disease, and others with minimal or even subclinical CMT syndrome.

CMT (HMSN) Type 1A and the Peripheral Myelin Protein 22 (PMP 22 gene)

In CMT1A the disorder is linked to band p11.2-12 on chromosome 17. In these patients the most common abnormality is duplication of a segment of this band spanning approximately 1.5 million bases. Thus affected patients have 3 copies of this segment, one on their normal chromosome 17 and two on the other chromosome 17, that bears the duplication

(Hallam et al. 1992). Patients with trisomies involving larger segments of this region of chromosome 17 may have mental retardation, micrognathia and hypoplastic, low set ears in addition to the CMT1A phenotype (Chance et al. 1992). Children who are homozygous for the duplication, i.e. with a tetrasomy (four copies), have a severe demyelinating neuropathy (Lupski et al. 1992). Some patients with CMT1A are sporadic cases of the disease, and have a de novo duplication (Hoogendijk et al. 1992). Taken together, these observations suggest that there is a dose effect in the expression of the genetic disorder.

The duplication of 17p11.2-12 that is associated with CMT1A is thought to arise from unequal crossing over of genetic material during meiosis, resulting in reciprocal duplication of the gene. These duplications appear to have arisen independently in different families because different and heterozygous alleles occur in different families, and fresh mutations are recognised (Hoogendijk et al. 1992; Harding 1995). The duplicated material is flanked by a repeated sequence 17–29 kilobases in length; this is present in three copies in the duplicated region. The recognition of de novo gene duplication at 17p11.2-12 suggests that many cases without a family history, in whom recessive inheritance might formerly have been suspected, should be reassigned as spontaneous duplications. Hoogendijk et al. (1992) found that nine of 10 sporadic patients had de novo duplications.

Further evidence for the genetic location and pathophysiology of CMT1A has come from studies of the Trembler mouse. This mouse has an autosomal dominant hypomyelinating neuropathy (Henry and Siddman 1988). In transplantation experiments the Schwann cells of the Trembler mouse cannot remyelinate normal axons (Aguayo et al. 1977). This mouse disorder maps to mouse chromosome 11 which has syntenic homology to human chromosome 17p in the region associated with the CMT1A locus (Valentijn et al. 1992a). In the mouse the Trembler phenotype is due to a missense mutation in the peripheral myelin protein -22 (PMP 22) gene. The PMP 22 protein is expressed on the transmembrane domain of Schwann cells. The human PMP 22 gene maps to chromosome 17p11.2, which is in the duplicated region associated with CMT1A, and may be the critical gene in this disorder (Table 10.6).

Table 10.6. Relation of PMP-22 abnormalities to clinical phenotype in hereditary motor and sensory neuropathy syndromes

Summary	Genotype	Phenotype
Minus 1 syndrome	Deletion of PMP-22 locus from one Ch17	Hereditary neuropathy with liability to pressure palsies
+2	One PMP-22 locus on each Ch17	Normal subjects
+3	One PMP-22 locus on one Ch17. duplication of PMP-22 on other Ch17	CMT 1A syndrome
+4	Duplication of PMP-22 loci on each Ch17	Severe form of CMT 1A

Further support for this hypothesis has been provided by the observation in a family described by Valentijn et al. (1992b) in Holland in which affected members had a missense mutation of PMP 22 identical to that in the Trembler mouse.

A deletion of the PMP 22 gene, leading to underexpression of the PMP 22 protein in peripheral nerve myelin, is associated with the phenotype of the autosomal dominant disorder, hereditary neuropathy with liability to pressure palsies (Chance et al. 1993). This finding suggests that duplication, point (missense) mutation, and deletion of PMP 22 gene result in different phenotypes, largely as a result of disturbances in expression of the PMP 22 protein. The normal function of the PMP 22 protein is, as yet, unknown although an effect on myelin stability has been suggested, perhaps implying a defect of cell adhesion (CAM).

CMT Type 1B

The CMT1B phenotype is identical to CMT1A. The disorder is linked to the Duffy blood group locus on chromosome 1 (Guiloff et al. 1982) at Ch1q21.2-23, the Fcγ receptor gene region (Lebo et al. 1991). In this syndrome it has been shown that there are deletions or point mutations in the myelin protein zero (Po) gene (Hiyasaka et al. 1993).

X-linked CMT Phenotypes

Families with X-linked inheritance usually show a dominant pattern of transmission. The phenotype usually resembles CMT Type 1, but is more severe in males in the few families in which males and females have been affected (Ionanescu et al. 1995). The gene has been mapped to the proximal long arm of the X chromosome at Xq13 (Hahn et al. 1990; Hiyasaka et al. 1993). This locus includes the gene for connexin 32 but not all families show defects in connexin 32 protein. Connexin 32 is a gap junction protein that forms intercellular channels for diffusion of small molecules and charged ions. It may be detected at nodes of Ranvier and Schmidt-Lanterman incisures (Bergoffen et al. 1993; Harding 1995).

Investigations

The ECG may rarely show conduction abnormalities (Brust et al. 1978). However, cardiomyopathy is not a feature of the disorder. The CSF protein is often moderately raised, an abnormality providing strong evidence of proximal involvement of the peripheral nervous system. The CK may be mildly or moderately raised, especially in patients with longstanding, severe weakness.

Electrophysiological Assessment

Diagnosis depends on slowed nerve conduction velocity, an abnormality which may be found even in apparently unaffected first-degree relatives. The motor conduction velocity in the median, ulnar and peroneal nerves is, on average, half the normal value (Dyck 1975b). Buchthal and Behse (1977) similarly found that the motor conduction velocity in the peroneal nerve was less than half normal in all their patients with clinical signs of the disease. The motor conduction velocity in the median and ulnar nerves is usually in the range of 15–35 m/s (Gutmann et al. 1983). In almost all cases the median nerve motor conduction velocity is less than 38 m/s (Harding and Thomas 1980a,b). The motor nerve conduction velocity in this disorder may be slower than that found in any other neuropathy; values as low as 2 m/s may be recorded in the legs. The severity of the abnormality of conduction, however, cannot be directly related to the severity of the clinical disorder. The distal motor latencies are often prolonged by a factor of two or three times normal. F wave conduction studies have shown that the proximal conduction is also slowed, the whole nerve thus being affected (Panayiotopoulos 1978; Lachman et al. 1980). Generally, motor conduction velocity is relatively slower than sensory conduction velocity. Because of the uniform distribution of the myelin abnormality temporal dispersion is not usually a feature. In addition, conduction block is not a feature. These two features clearly distinguish CMT1A and CMT1B from acquired demyelinating neuropathies (Lewis and Sumner 1982; Donofrio and Albers 1990). The amplitude of the motor evoked potential is reduced, and this abnormality is related to the disability more closely than is slowing of motor conduction, which does not change during the course of the disease (Dyck et al. 1989).

Sensory conduction is also abnormal. In the sural nerve the conduction velocity is usually about half the normal value (13–32 m/s) and the amplitude of the sensory action potential was less than 10% of normal in Buchthal and Behse's (1977) series of cases, in which recordings were made with needle electrodes. Using surface electrode recording techniques, SAPs can only rarely be recorded in the sural nerve, and median nerve SAPs are absent in 93% of cases (Harding and Thomas 1980b). Buchthal and Behse (1977) found a similar degree of slowing of sensory conduction and of reduction of the amplitude of the SAP in the median and

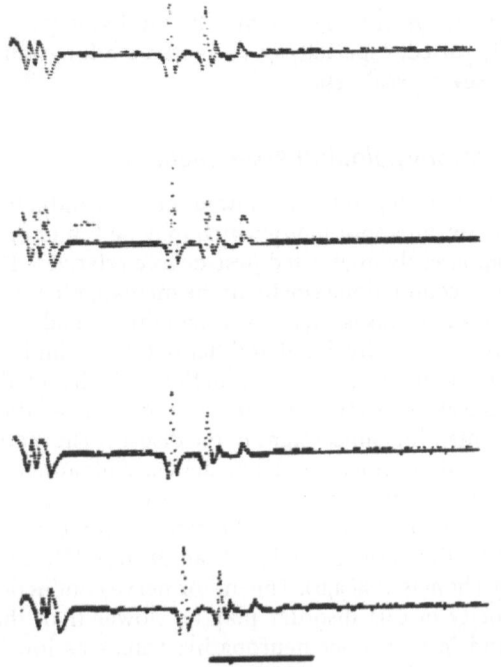

Fig. 10.2. CMT Type 1. Motor unit action potential of long duration (28 ms) and stable configuration. This is characteristic of a chronic neurogenic disorder. Concentric needle EMG. Filters: 500 Hz and 10 kHz. Bar 10 ms.

superficial peroneal nerves as in the sural nerve, indicating that conduction in the fastest conducting fibres is affected similarly in upper and lower limbs.

It is a characteristic finding that the hypertrophied nerves show an abnormally high threshold to electrical stimulation so that higher voltages are required to stimulate the nerve. Furthermore, nerve stimulation is unusually painful as compared with other neuropathies. This may be due to the relatively severe loss of large myelinated fibres in the disease.

Concentric needle EMG shows more abnormality in distal than in proximal muscles. The legs are characteristically more affected than the arms. Fibrillation potentials and positive sharp waves were recorded in a third of Buchthal and Behse's (1977) cases. With voluntary activation the MUAPs are polyphasic, of long duration and of increased amplitude. The interference pattern is usually reduced. With the trigger-delay line late components of these polyphasic MUAPs are often very prominent (Fig. 10.2) even as long as 50 ms after the triggering potential.

In older patients short-duration, low-amplitude, polyphasic MUAPs may be recorded, particularly in proximal muscles. These potentials are similar to those found in myopathic disorders and can be correlated with secondary myopathic changes found in the muscle biopsy (Swash and Schwartz 1977).

Single-fibre EMG also shows abnormalities. The motor unit fibre density is markedly increased. In a multi-electrode study Schwartz et al. (1976b) found large numbers of single-fibre action potentials within the uptake areas of the electrode. The fibre density in this form of neuropathy is as high as recorded in any other disorder, implying prominent reinnervation. The neuromuscular jitter may be increased and some potentials show intermittent blocking, but these abnormalities are not prominent.

Electrophysiological tests, particularly measurement of the motor nerve conduction velocity and distal latency, are useful in screening relatives of affected patients to establish inheritance and to identify possible carriers for genetic counselling. Many of these affected relatives will have abnormalities of their feet, such as pes cavus, or abnormalities of the toes, but some will show no clinical stigmata of the disease although their nerve conduction may be markedly slow. Abnormalities of motor nerve conduction can be detected in infancy, even when the child is asymptomatic and clinical signs are trivial or difficult to elicit (Combarros et al. 1983). Gutmann et al. (1983) showed that the slowing of motor conduction was similar in infants and adults over the age range 3 to 70 years. The slowing of motor conduction evolves over the first 3 to 5 years of life. Similarly the distal motor latency becomes abnormal during this time.

Muscle Biopsy

In early cases, or in relatively uninvolved muscles, fibre-type grouping may be the only abnormality. In clinically affected muscles more marked abnormalities are found. These consist of the typical features of denervation and reinnervation in a chronic, slowly progressive, neurogenic process. Small angulated atrophic fibres are prominent and may be found in groups; grouped denervation atrophy. Fibre-type grouping itself is also very prominent and is often as marked as in the chronic spinal muscular atrophies; all the fibres in a fascicle may be of one fibre type in advanced cases. Type 1 fibres are often hypertrophied and these may show fibre splitting (Swash and Schwartz 1977). Type 2 fibres, on the other hand, tend to be somewhat atrophic, even when reinnervated and grouped. Fibrosis is not a major feature but there is usually some increase in interfascicular and endomysial connective tissue. Hypertrophied fibres often contain centrally placed nuclei, and a number of other morphological changes may be found in individual muscle fibres. These, consisting of target, targetoid and whorled fibres, are particularly prominent in this disorder. Other architectural changes, including moth-eaten fibres and occasional scattered necrotic and regenerating fibres, occur and there are features of secondary myopathic change (Haase and Shy 1960; Drachman et al. 1967; Schwartz et al. 1976a).

The pathological changes in muscle in the hypertrophic form (Type I) have not been differentiated from those of the neuronal form (Type II). Buchthal and Behse (1977) found no difference between the two groups.

Motor end-plates also show abnormalities. The terminal innervation ratio is increased. In some instances the end-plates themselves show beaded degenerate terminal clumps but, in others, a collateral ramification consisting of branching axons and motor end-plates of normal appearance indicates the presence of well-developed collateral sprouting (Coërs et al. 1973).

Peripheral Nerve Biopsy

The pathological appearances are dominated by segmental demyelination and remyelination with the formation of classic onion bulbs consisting of concentric Schwann cell lamellae. There is a loss of both large and small myelinated nerve fibres to a variable degree. In transverse sections onion-bulb formations consisting of whorls of Schwann cell processes are the major feature and these may be very large, reaching 20–30 μm in diameter. Some onion-bulb formations surround large myelinated axons, but in others the central axon is demyelinated or only thinly myelinated. Some onion-bulb whorls are devoid of a central axon (collagen pockets). Onion bulbs are far more prominent distally than proximally (Dyck 1984). In young children demyelination is prominent, but onion bulbs are infrequent (Gabreëls-Festen et al. 1992b). Axonal loss occurs as the disease progresses. Behse and Buchtahl (1977b) noted that there was selective loss of nerve fibres greater than 7 mm and less than 5 mm in diameter resulting in a unimodal fibre diameter spectrum with a peak of 5–6 μm in affected nerves; normal nerves show a bimodal distribution of fibre diameter. The endoneurial space is enlarged and contains excess collagen fibrils. The perineurium is thickened, due to extra layers of perineurial cell cytoplasm, and to fibrosis. Unmyelinated fibres are probably also present in reduced numbers but this has not been quantified. Clusters of small myelinated fibres representing regenerating axon clusters are uncommon.

In teased-fibre studies segmental demyelination is found (Dyck et al. 1968). The evidence that the pathological changes are more prominent distally in a nerve than proximally suggested to Dyck et al. (1974) that the disease is due to a primary neuronal disorder with progressive atrophy of the distal ends of nerves, the segmental demyelination and remyelination occurring as secondary features. This concept is supported by distal axonal attenuation in relation to myelin thickness, and decreased axon calibre and neurofilament content. However, the genetic evidence, implicating abnormalities of the PMP-22 gene, strongly implies a primary abnormality in Schwann cells. Axonal loss is therefore likely to be a secondary process (Gabreëls-Festen et al. 1993). The primary pathological deficit may consist of unravelling of the inner layer of myelin on the axon and therefore might be associated with an abnormality of cell adhesion molecule (CAM) function.

In autosomal recessive Type 1 CMT two variations in the pathology have been noted. In one form onion bulbs of classical type, and onion bulbs involving unmyelinated fibres, inserting into basal lamina, have been reported (Gabreëls-Festen et al. 1992a). In the second type onion bulbs are frequent and tomaculous swellings are prominent on nearly all myelinated fibres, suggesting an abnormal axon–Schwann cell interaction. This syndrome is of infantile onset (Vital et al. 1987; Gabreëls-Festen et al. 1993).

Other Pathological Features

At autopsy there is degeneration of the posterior columns. Some loss of anterior horn cells in the lumbar cord has been reported. Separate studies of hypertrophic and neuronal forms of the disease are lacking (Hughes and Brownell 1972). Abnormal distributions of fatty acids in serum and peripheral nerve myelin have been reported (Yao et al. 1976; Williams et al. 1986) but the relation of this finding to the rate of progression of HMSN Type 1 has not been determined.

Prognosis

The course of the disease is progressive but disability remains moderate and the ability to walk is rarely lost, even in old age (Dyck 1975b; Buchthal and Behse 1977), although bracing of the ankle is usually required. Life expectancy is normal.

CMT Type 2 (Neuronal Type of Peroneal Muscular Atrophy)

This form of Charcot–Marie–Tooth disorder is recognised by the near-normal nerve conduction velocity which characterises it. It is usually autosomal dominantly inherited, but some recessive cases have been described (Harding and Thomas 1980a, c). CMT Type 2 is about a third as common as the Type 1 disorder (Harding and Thomas 1980a). This form of peroneal muscular atrophy usually begins in the second decade (Harding and Thomas 1980c). Two-thirds of Buchthal and Behse's (1977) cases began under the age of 10 years. This observation itself suggests that there may be two variants of the neuronal form of the disease, one beginning in childhood and one in middle life. Weakness of small hand muscles in CMT Type 2 is less severe than in CMT Type 1 and the disease is generally milder. A further point of difference is that the peripheral nerves are not enlarged in this form. Generally, the prognosis is better in CMT Type 2 than in the Type 1 disorder. Distal sensory loss is less prominent and is uncommon in the hands in the Type 2 disease. Position sense is the most affected modality and patients may appear restless, shifting their legs to maintain balance (Dyck and Lambert 1968a,b). The proximal tendon reflexes are often preserved, especially in the upper limbs. Kyphoscoliosis is an uncommon feature, and pes cavus occurs less frequently and is less severe in CMT Type 2. Progression is slow and disability less severe. Tremor and ataxia are uncommon features (Harding and Thomas 1980b).

The dominant gene for CMT Type 2 is not allelic to that for CMT Type 1; the two disorders are thus separate genetic entities (Guiloff et al. 1982). The genetic locus of Type 2 CMT is at Ch 1p 35-36 and a second locus, for a Type 2B disorder has been identified at Ch 3q 13-22.

Generally the autosomal recessive form shows more severe weakness of distal arm and leg muscles than the more common autosomal dominant form. An X-linked dominant mode of inheritance is more common than autosomal recessive inheritance (Hahn et al. 1990). The prevalence in Sweden was 1 in 9000 in Hagberg and Westerberg's (1983) series of Swedish children.

Investigations

There are few differences between the Type 1 and Type 2 forms. The CSF protein might be expected to be normal or only slightly increased in the Type 2 form . The ECG is normal.

Electrophysiological Assessment

The nerve conduction velocity in the sural nerve was normal in half Buchthal and Behse's (1977) cases, but in the remainder it was only mildly slowed: the slowest was 39 m/s. The amplitudes of

the sensory nerve action potentials in the sural nerves in these patients were all smaller than normal, ranging from 1% to 59% of the control values. However, the amplitudes of the SNAPs in this neuronal form of the disease are generally higher than the very low values recorded in the hypertrophic form (Buchthal and Behse 1977). Sensory conduction was similarly slowed in the median nerve but the amplitudes of the sensory potentials in the median nerve were normal in half the patients studied. Harding and Thomas (1980b) found that SNAPs were absent in 73% of cases and reduced in amplitude in the remainder of their patients. Unlike Buchtahl and Behse (1977) these observations were made with surface recording electrodes.

The distal motor latency is usually increased in the legs (Christie 1961), even when the motor nerve conduction velocity is normal (Buchthal and Behse 1977). The motor nerve conduction velocity may be difficult to study in patients with very wasted distal leg muscles, but motor conduction is usually slower than in normal subjects, although not nearly as slowed as in Type 1 disease. Buchthal and Behse (1977) found that the slowest motor conduction velocity in the peroneal nerve was 60% of normal. Median nerve motor conduction may be mildly slowed (Dyck 1975b). Harding and Thomas (1980b) confirmed Buchthal and Behse's (1977) finding that motor nerve conduction in the median nerve was always faster than 38 m/s in the Type 2 form of CMT. In some patients motor nerve conduction can be normal in arms and legs, and this observation illustrates the importance of sensory conduction studies in this disorder, when differentiating it from spinal muscular atrophy.

Conventional concentric needle EMG studies reveal evidence of denervation in the legs, with fibrillation potentials and positive sharp waves in distal, atrophic muscles. Fasciculations can be recorded in the legs in about 25% of cases (Buchthal and Behse 1977). Continuous motor unit activity (neuromyotonia) may be recorded, and this has been associated with calf enlargement (Vasilescu et al. 1984; Hahn et al. 1991). Neuromyotonia has not been reported in the hypertrophic (Type 1) form (Buchthal and Behse 1977). Single-fibre EMG shows an increased motor unit fibre density. Somatosensory evoked response latencies in patients with CMT (type unspecified) are normal (Noël and Desmedt 1980).

Muscle Biopsy

The changes found in the muscle biopsy are similar to those found in the Type 1 form of the disease (Behse and Buchthal 1977b).

Nerve Biopsy

Biopsies of the sural nerve, a sensory nerve, show slight loss of large myelinated nerve fibres; smaller fibres are normal (Behse and Buchthal 1977b). Fibre loss is due to axonal degeneration. Segmental demyelination with onion-bulb formation is not a feature (Dyck 1984). The endoneurial space is not enlarged. No information on changes at autopsy is available.

Prognosis

Progression is inconspicuous in some patients. Half of Buchthal and Behse's (1977) cases showed no progression during a period of five or more years, and in the others deterioration was more obvious in the legs than in the hands.

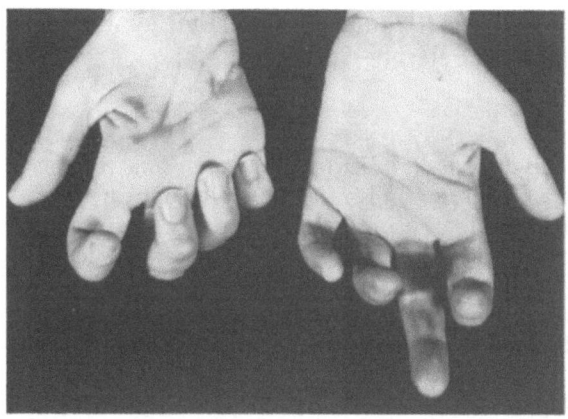

Fig. 10.3. Chronic progressive CIDP (steroid responsive). "Claw hand" deformity from longstanding weakness and wasting of forearm and small hand muscles.

Management of Charcot–Marie–Tooth Syndrome (CMT Types 1 and 2)

No specific treatment is available. Management is thus directed toward methods of preventing deformity and secondary disability. Skeletal deformity, especially kyphoscoliosis, can be prevented by appropriate bracing in some cases, but some otherwise require surgical correction to improve pulmonary function (Siegel 1977). Pes cavus can also be corrected surgically and, if a plantigrade gait can be restored, there may be considerable improvement in gait (Shapiro and Bresnan 1982). Orthotic correction of foot drop may be useful in less advanced cases, and lengthening of the Achilles tendon with triple arthrodesis may prevent progressive foot deformity at this stage of the disease. Periods of bed rest should be avoided, since these may cause permanent regression of function, even with subsequent intensive physiotherapy. Physiotherapy itself has little to offer in the management of the disorder on a day-to-day basis, but is useful when given intermittently, particularly if a new disability has arisen, e.g. after an accidental fall. When mobility is compromised weight gain becomes a hazard leading to further difficulty in movement, and regular exercise, for example swimming, is beneficial.

Dyck et al. (1982) reported seven patients with chronic progressive CMT with raised CSF protein, in whom prednisone therapy produced improvement. These patients showed features consistent both with CMT and with chronic inflammatory demyelinating polyradiculopathy and thus were not entirely typical of CMT Types 1 and 2 (Fig. 10.3).

Dyck et al. (1982) suggested, however, that occasional patients with CMT syndrome, especially when there is rapid worsening of disability with both proximal and distal limb involvement, and increased levels of CSF protein, may benefit from a trial of steroid therapy. Treatment with vitamin E supplements (81.6 IU/day) and essential fatty acids (3 g daily) produced some improvement in a placebo-controlled trial of one year's duration (Williams et al. 1986); this effect was probably largely related to the membrane effects of vitamin E.

Diagnosis of CMT Types 1 and 2

These syndromes have characteristic clinical features but the clinical differentiation of Type 1 and Type 2 CMT may sometimes be difficult. Since these two disorders are genetically distinct they do not occur in the same kinship (Dyck and Lambert 1968b; Harding and Thomas 1980a; Guiloff et al. 1982). The main technique for distinguishing these two disorders is based on nerve conduction velocity measurements.

Distal spinal muscular atrophy is a form of the peroneal muscular atrophy syndrome. However, it differs from CMT Type 1 and 2; there is less upper limb weakness, the tendon reflexes are usually present and the sensory examination is normal. Motor nerve conduction velocity and sensory nerve action potentials in upper and lower limbs are normal. Although this disorder is often classified among the hereditary motor neuropathies because of its clinical resemblance to the CMT syndromes (Dyck and Lambert 1968b), it is better classified with the spinal muscular atrophies (see Chapter 6).

CMT Type 3 (Hypomyelination Neuropathy of Infancy: Déjérine–Sottas Disease)

This disorder is inherited as an autosomal recessive trait (Déjérine and Sottas 1893; Davidenkow 1927). It consists of a progressive disorder beginning in childhood with bilateral foot deformity and delayed and difficult walking. There is a severe mixed sensorimotor neuropathy with distal wasting of all four limbs and small stature. Light touch and position and vibration sense are particularly affected. Lightning pains in the legs may be a feature of the disorder. The peripheral nerves may be palpably enlarged, although this is uncommon in this syndrome. Other features include miosis, and poor pupillary reaction to light, nystagmus and clumsiness of fine movements with sensory ataxia. The facial features may be coarse. The tendon reflexes are absent. These clinical features may not represent a single entity.

Guzetta et al. (1982) divided cases of Type 3 CMT into three subgroups; a *congenital* form with complete absence of myelin with severe disability and motor nerve conduction less than 5 m/s (Charnas et al. 1988), an *infantile* form with delayed motor development, eventually able to walk, also with extremely slowed motor conduction (less than 5 m/s), and a *juvenile* form with onset between the ages of 6 and 12 years in whom motor conduction velocity was less than 14 m/s.

In the *severe congenital form* death may occur in a few days or months and there may be complete absence of myelin in the peripheral nervous system, without onion bulbs (Charnas et al. 1988). In the *infantile form* of congenital onset with absence of myelin, first reported by Lyon (1969), hypotonia is present from early infancy, with absent tendon reflexes, distal wasting and delayed motor mulestones. Death usually occurs in infancy. The peripheral nerves are not enlarged in this form of the disorder. Biopsy of the sural nerve reveals preservation of axons, but absence of myelin sheaths. There is a mild endoneurial fibrosis and electron microscopy revealed concentric whorls of reduplicated basal laminae with scanty Schwann cell processes resembling onion bulbs (Lyon 1969). Similar findings have been described in an autopsied case (Karch and Urich 1975). In the *juvenile form*, the child is normal at birth, but fails to develop normally. There is motor and sensory loss with pes cavus, scoliosis and sensory ataxia. Nerve biopsy shows large classical onion bulbs, and the CSF protein is raised (Dyck et al. 1993). The pathological features of the juvenile form are more prominent than the similar abnormality found in the hypertrophic nerves of Type 1 CMT atrophy. In addition there is discontinuous, peri-axial absence of myelin more extensively than can be accounted for by segmental demyelination and the remaining myelin is thinner than normal when compared with axonal diameter. Further, myelin thickness is less than that found in other hypertrophic neuropathies, suggesting that there is a true "hypomyelination" representing an abnormality specific to Schwann cell formation (Dyck et al. 1971).

The autosomal dominant forms of CMT Type 3 are located at the CMT Type 1 loci, and the autosomal recessive form on Ch 8q.

Investigations

The CSF protein is raised (Dyck and Lambert 1968a). The motor nerve conduction velocity is very slow, even in the arms. In three or four patients studied the ulnar motor conduction velocity was less than 5 m/s (Dyck and Lambert 1968a). Sensory nerve action potentials are difficult or impossible to obtain with surface recording techniques. Nerve stimulation is often painful. Concentric needle EMG studies show prominent neurogenic changes similar to those found in peroneal musuclar atrophy. The parents show no electrophysiological abnormality (Dyck 1975b).

Other Forms of CMT

CMT Type 5 (Dyck 1984) is a term that has been used to describe an autosomal dominant disorder resembling CMT Type 2 in which corticospinal features, especially spasticity of gait, are found. The characteristic presentation is with difficulty running or walking in the second or later decades. The ankle jerks are absent, but the plantar responses are extensor (Harding and Thomas 1984). Life expectancy is normal. The motor nerve conduction velocity is usually normal in the arms, but slightly slowed in the legs and the sural sensory nerve action potential is usually small or absent (Dyck 1984). However, Harding and Thomas (1984) found normal sensory conduction in 20% of their cases, and slowed motor conduction in the arms. In some respects CMT Type 5 resembles atypical forms of hereditary spastic paraplegia with distal amyotrophy.

Other types of CMT have been described. In *CMT Type 6* peroneal muscular atrophy is associated with optic atrophy and deafness and lancinating pains. A variety of families with peroneal muscular atrophy syndrome associated with optic atrophy, deafness and pigmentary retinal degeneration (*CMT Type 7*) have been reported, with either autosomal dominant or recessive inheritance (see Dyck 1984; Harding and Thomas 1984). These syndromes cannot all yet be satisfactorily classified. Three X-linked forms have been described: CMTX-1 with peripheral neuropathy, CMTX-2 with peripheral neuropathy and mental retardation and CMTX-3 with peripheral neuropathy and spastic paraparesis (Ionasescu 1995).

Hereditary Neuropathy with Liability to Pressure Palsies

This term was introduced to describe a syndrome (De Jong 1947) in which pressure or traction on a nerve, caused, for example, by sleeping on a limb or with the arms elevated, may result in a mononeuropathy (Earl et al. 1964). The peroneal and ulnar nerves are most frequently affected. Verhagen et al. (1993) found that the peroneal nerve was the commonest affected nerve; 43 of their 99 patients had peroneal neuropathy. Occasionally several nerves, the brachial plexus and even cranial nerves, may be involved. In most cases nerves are involved at the usual sites of susceptibility to compression. The neuropathy may lead to transient or longer-lasting paraesthesiae with or without motor involvement. In normal subjects stress on a nerve would produce symptoms only for a few minutes but in patients affected by the syndrome recovery may occur only during several days or weeks. Sometimes recovery may be incomplete with residual mild weakness and wasting but little sensory impairment. In some older patients there may be signs of peripheral sensorimotor neuropathy and in some families some affected persons have developed a generalised sensorimotor neuropathy without focal attacks of weakness or sensory disturbance. The disorder usually presents in the third decade. The peripheral nerves are not usually thickened clinically, but pes cavus and hammer toes may be a feature. Most reported families have been of German or Dutch extraction. Clinically asymptomatic family members may be discovered when affected families are studied by electrophysiological or genetic testing; 31 of Verhagen et al. (1993) 99 cases were asymptomatic. In 11% of patients there is involvement of the brachial plexus; this is painless (Verhagen et al. 1993).

The disorder is inherited as an autosomal dominant condition, with a large interstitial deletion which includes the gene for PMP 22 on chromosome 17p11.2 (see Table 10.6) (Chance et al. 1993). A family with a frame shift mutation has also been recognized (Nicholson et al. 1994). The clinical phenotype is therefore associated with underexpression of PMP 22.

Laboratory Assessment

There are features typical of a demyelinating neuropathy. Even in unaffected limbs the nerve conduction velocity is mildly or moderately slowed and sensory and motor nerve action potentials are small and dispersed. Distal muscles show EMG features of denervation and reinnervation, but these are not marked. Conduction in proximal segments of affected nerves is usually normal (Behse et al. 1977). Behse et al. (1977) noted that slowing of conduction velocity was as pronounced in younger as in older patients, even in the same family. Sites of entrapment and pressure points, especially at the ulnar head and the olecranon groove, are particularly likely to be zones showing slowed nerve conduction, or even conduction block; the latter may persist for months or years and may improve if the nerve is decompressed (Magistris and Roth 1985).

Sural nerve biopsies have shown a relative shift to smaller diameter fibres with segmental demyelination and remyelination. In addition, thickened segments of myelin occur frequently on individual fibres, the number of myelin lamellae being increased as much as tenfold (sausage-shaped swellings or tomacula). The CSF is normal.

Hereditary Brachial Plexus Palsies

A similar liability to focal neuropathy in which susceptibility is limited to the brachial plexus has been reported in several families (Bradley et al. 1975). Isolated cranial nerve palsies causing hoarseness and difficulty swallowing, facial palsy and unilateral deafness and Horner's syndrome may occur. However, in this syndrome pain and weakness are major features (hereditary neuralgic amyotrophy) and recovery may be incomplete with persistent weakness and muscular atrophy (Davies 1954; Arts et al. 1983). The literature on this syndrome is difficult to review because many authors failed to recognise that brachial plexus palsy is common in patients with hereditary neuropathy with liability to pressure palsies. For example, the series of Bradley et al. (1975) probably consisted largely of patients with the latter condition. Arts et al. (1983) showed that motor and sensory conduction was normal and in an autopsy study found no evidence of tomaculous or demyelinating neuropathy (van Wensen 1991).

Treatment and Prognosis

Individual pressure palsies should be treated by splinting and physiotherapy to avoid joint contractures. The prognosis for recovery is excellent. The patient should be encouraged to avoid future pressure palsies, especially by avoiding sleeping in unusual positions or places, for example in a chair or a car, or on the ground. No other specific measures are necessary and life expectancy is normal. Occasionally foot ulcers may develop in areas of anaesthetic skin and these should be treated by rest, debridement and avoidance of ill-fitting footwear. Steroid therapy is not effective (Arts et al. 1983).

Migrant Sensory Neuritis of Wartenberg

This syndrome consists of recurrent episodes of pain with subsequent loss of sensation induced by movement of a limb causing stretching of a peripheral nerve (Wartenberg 1958). Inconclusive electrophysiological abnormalities were noted in three of the six cases reported by Matthews and Esiri (1983) and sural nerve biopsy in one case showed minor abnormalities including occlusion of a perineurial blood vessel. This syndrome thus remains ill-defined.

Hereditary Sensory and Autonomic Neuropathies (HSAN)

These rare syndromes were reviewed, with an autopsy of a single case, by Denny-Brown (1951) and, later, by Schoene et al. (1970). For many years these cases, in which distal sensory impairment with painless ulceration, spontaneous lancinating pain and various trophic changes in affected distal skin occur, were thought to be due to spinal dysraphism (see Dyck and Ohta 1975, for review of historical aspects).

Five types of hereditary sensory neuropathy have been described, in all of which autonomic symp-

toms occur (Dyck 1984). All these syndromes are rare (Table 10.7). Type I HSAN is dominantly inherited; all the other types are congenital and probably recessively inherited disorders.

Type I HSAN

This dominantly inherited disorder (Denny-Brown 1951; Nair 1976, 1978) is the commonest of these rare syndromes. There is slowly progressive distal sensory impairment which may initially be limited to loss of pain and temperature sensation distally in the legs. Later the upper limbs are also affected. Other sensory modalities are often relatively or even completely spared in the early stages of the disease (dissociated sensory loss) but later all modalities are affected. The distal tendon reflexes are reduced or absent. There may be slight distal muscle atrophy and weakness, with pes cavus, resembling peroneal muscular atrophy. Spontaneous, lightning-like pains are frequent and involve both lower and upper limbs. Painless, progressive, persistent and penetrating foot ulceration is a typical but not invariable feature. These ulcers usually occur after minor injury or infection of the feet and can be avoided by scrupulous care of the feet (Spillane and Wells 1969). Neuropathic arthropathy (Charcot joints) is a frequent feature in the feet and ankles. The disorder is slowly progressive over many years. Autonomic disturbances, despite the designation of this condition as HSAN Type I, are not a feature of this disorder. Progressive deafness was a feature of the kinship reported by Denny-Brown (1951) and Hicks (1972). The peripheral nerves are not enlarged. Nair (1978) noted optic nerve involvement and pupillary changes in some cases in India.

Electrophysiological Assessment

Sensory nerve action potentials are absent in upper and lower limbs (Ludin et al. 1977; Dyck et al.

Table 10.7. Major clinical features of HSAN syndromes

	HSAN I	HSAN II	HSAN III	HSAN IV	HSAN V
Age of onset	2nd decade	Infancy	Infancy	Infancy	Infancy
Inheritance	AD	AR	AR	AR	?AR
Sensory disturbance to pain	Distal loss	Absent	Decreased	Absent	Absent
Tendon reflexes	Usually normal	Decreased or absent	Decreased	?Decreased	Normal
Corneal reflex	?	Decreased	Decreased	Decreased	?
Fungiform papillae on tongue	?	Absent	Absent	Present	?
Autonomic features postural hypotension	–	–	Yes	–	–
Sweating	±	Normal	Increased	Decreased or absent	Normal
GI motility	?	Abnormal	Abnormal	Normal	?
Key references	Denny-Brown (1951)	Ohta et al. (1973)	Riley and Moore (1966)	Swanson et al. (1965)	Low et al. (1978) Landrieu et al. (1990)
Genetic locus			9q 31-33		

1984b). However, somatosensory evoked potentials can be recorded from cortex after stimulation of the index finger (Ludin et al. 1977). Motor nerve conduction is normal or slightly slowed. Concentric needle EMG may reveal polyphasic MUAPs and denervation. *In vitro* recordings of sural nerve removed at biopsy have shown a decreased amplitude of the compound nerve action potential, particularly of the C-fibre potential (Dyck et al. 1971).

Pathology

In the peripheral nervous system there is a marked loss of unmyelinated fibres, and of small myelinated fibres. The latter changes are more marked at the ankle, compared to the mid-calf level (Dyck 1984). These features are consistent with a slowly progressive axonopathy beginning at the periphery (Denny-Brown 1951). In the CNS there is loss of myelinated fibres, with gliosis, of the gracile tracts and loss of nerve fibres in the dorsal roots. These features are consistent with the loss of dorsal root ganglion cells, especially L4–S2, noted by Denny-Brown (1951) (Horoupian 1989).

Type II HSAN

In this disorder recessively inherited or sporadic sensory neuropathy becomes evident in infancy or childhood although it is probably present from birth. There is distal sensory neuropathy particularly affecting touch, but also involving pain and temperature sensation. Position sense and vibration sense are severely affected and Romberg's sign is usually positive. There is a prominent tendency for ulceration to occur on the tips of the fingers and toes, leading to a painless mutilating acropathy with loss of digits, sometimes associated with Charcot joints and with unrecognised stress fractures of hands and feet. There is no motor weakness. The disease is probably non-progressive but some reports have described very slow progression (Nukada et al. 1982). Scoliosis occurs in some patients. Lancinating pains are less common and less severe than in HSAN Type I. Autonomic involvement may develop; Nukada et al. (1982) reported defective sweating in one of 13 cases and incontinence in two of these patients. The tendon reflexes are often absent, but the nerves are not enlarged.

Electrophysiological Assessment

Electrophysiological assessment resembles the features of HMSN Type 1. Sensory nerve action potentials cannot be recorded and motor conduction is normal or slightly slowed. EMG may reveal fibrillation potentials in distal foot muscles. In *in vitro* recordings of sural nerves, only the C-fibre component of the compound nerve action potential can be recorded (Ohta et al. 1973; Nukada et al. 1982).

Pathology

There is striking loss of myelinated nerve fibres in sural nerve biopsies, with relative preservation of unmyelinated fibres. The clinical distinction between HSAN Types I and II is difficult and nerve biopsy has been recommended for genetic counselling.

Type III HSAN, Riley–Day Syndrome (Familial Dysautonomia)

This disorder is rare; most cases have been recognised in Ashkenazi Jews. Familial dysautonomia affects one in 10 000 births to Austrian Jews. It is inherited as an autosomal recessive trait, and consanguinity is common in the families of affected patients (Riley et al. 1949). The disease usually presents at birth, or in the first weeks of life, with features of involvement of the peripheral motor, sensory and autonomic nervous system. There is marked loss of neurons, up to 90% depletion, in the dorsal root ganglia and in the Gasserian ganglia, and cervical and thoracic sympathetic ganglia are similarly affected (Pearson and Pytel 1978). The clinical features and severity of the disease vary. Many affected children die in infancy from aspiration pneumonia. A quarter die before the age of 10 years and 50% before age 22 years (McKusick et al. 1967). The diagnosis is suggested by a history of severe feeding problems with poor sucking, dysphagia, recurrent pneumonia and failure to thrive. Severe episodic vomiting, which affects half the children, is not usually a problem before the age of 3 years. The major abnormalities on examination are lack of overflow tears (alacrima), corneal hypoaesthesia, postural hypotension, erythematous blotching of the skin, and absence of the tendon reflexes. The most distinctive feature, however, is absence of the fungiform papillae of the tongue. This is virtually pathognomonic of familial dysautonomia. During development additional features become evident. The gait is awkward and clumsy, the sense of taste is defective, there is growth retardation with scoliosis, which may be severe, and recurrent corneal ulceration may be a problem. Vomiting crises, lasting 1–3 days or more, are a serious and potentially fatal manifestation. They consist of attacks of sweating, erythema, hypertension, gastric distention and urinary retention, often associated with pulmonary infection and electrolyte imbalance. Incontinence is not a feature of the disorder. In the peripheral nervous system there is a disturbance of pain and temperature sensation, but other modalities are spared, or only slightly abnormal. Riley and Moore (1966) reviewed the clinical features.

The diagnosis can be substantiated by demonstration of suprasensitivity to methacholine, and by absence of a dermal histamine flare response. Instillation of methacholine (2.5%) or pilocarpine (0.0625%) into the conjunctival sac produces pupillary miosis, similar to that found in Holmes–Adie syndrome, because of parasympathetic denervation of the iris sphincter; in normal subjects the pupil size does not change. In the histamine skin test an injection of 1 : 1000 histamine phosphate intradermally normally produces a central weal surrounded by an axon flare. In familial dysautonomia the flare is replaced by a narrow violaceous areola, but the weal is formed normally. These two tests, together with the absence of fungiform papillae on the tongue, represent a diagnostic triad for familial dysautonomia.

Laboratory Assessment

Nerve conduction studies do not reveal marked abnormalities. There may be decreased amplitude of sensory nerve action potentials with normal conduction velocity (Aguayo et al. 1971), but sensory and motor conduction velocities are always in the low normal range (Brown and Johns 1967). The mixed nerve action potential may show two peaks representing two nerve fibre populations with different conduction velocities (Brown and Johns 1967).

Pathology

The pathological features are incompletely described. There is a marked decrease in the number of neurons in the cervical and sympathetic ganglia, and probably also in the Gasserian and posterior root ganglia (Pearson et al. 1971). In the sural nerve there is a marked decrease in the number of unmyelinated nerve fibres (Aguayo et al. 1971). Pearson and Pytel (1978) have reviewed the changes in sympathetic and parasympathetic ganglia. In the CNS abnormalities in the reticular substance and atrophy of neurons in the Xth and XIth cranial nerves have been reported (Cohen and Soloman 1955).

The level of dopamine beta hydroxylase in serum is decreased (Weinshilbourn and Axelrod 1971) and there are abnormalities in catecholamine metabolism. Abnormalities in nerve growth factor, leading to decreased activity in familial dysautonomia, have also been reported (Schwartz and Breakfield 1980).

Type IV HSAN

Type IV HSAN is distinguished by insensitivity to pain and anhydrosis. Mild mental retardation is also a feature. Very few cases have been reported (Goebel et al. 1980). Temperature regulation is abnormal and survival beyond childhood is unlikely. The failure to respond normally to painful stimuli leads to susceptibility to multiple, recurrent fractures, superficial injuries and mutilation of the limbs. On sensory testing sharp stimuli can be differentiated from dull stimuli and corneal testing is uncomfortable, so that the sensation of pain is not clinically absent. However, temperature sensation is much more severely affected. Sweating is virtually absent even in very hot conditions. Sural nerve biopsy shows a selective loss of small myelinated fibres, absence of unmyelinated nerve fibres but a normal population of larger myelinated fibres. About 20 cases have been reported (Ito et al. 1986). Axelrod and Pearson (1984) showed mild slowing of motor conduction in peroneal nerves, but Lee et al. (1976) found normal motor and sensory conduction.

Type V HSAN

Some five cases of a milder disorder than Type IV HSAN, with impaired pain sensibility in a distal distribution without major sweating abnormality, have been described (Dyck et al. 1983), in which there was selective loss of small myelinated fibres but preservation of large myelinated and unmyelinated fibres (Landrieu et al. 1990). Muscle strength and reflexes are normal.

Other cases have been described of hereditary sensory neuropathy associated with spastic paraparesis (Cavanagh et al. 1979a), but these are difficult to classify at present. A relation with the spino-cerebellar degenerations has been implied. Cases associated with skeletal dysplasia, neurotrophic keratitis (Donaghy et al. 1989) and tonic pupils have been described.

Congenital Universal Insensitivity to Pain

The HSAN syndromes are associated with relatively selective impairment of pain sensitivity and in some of these syndromes, particularly HSAN Type III, this abnormality is not limited to the distal parts of the limbs. The relative specificity of involvement of different modalities of sensation in peripheral nerve disorders can be associated with the particular myelinated and unmyelinated axons or nerves that are damaged. Selective involvement of large diameter fibres is associated with loss of low threshold mechanoreceptors leading to sensory ataxia, and to impairment of discriminatory cutaneous sensation, e.g. shape and texture, but superficial pain and temperature sensation is normal and spontaneous dysaesthesiae do not occur. Friedreich's ataxia and other spino-cerebellar degenerations are examples of this type of disorder. Selective loss of small afferent fibres is associated with raised thresholds to nociceptive and thermal stimuli, and with acral mutilation and distal perforating ulcers. Spontaneous painful sensations may occur in these disorders, e.g. in HSAN Type I, but are much more common in acquired neuropathies, e.g. alcoholic neuropathy, diabetic neuropathy, Guillain–Barré syndrome, in which ectopic impulse generation and ephaptic transmission are common (Ochoa and Torebjork 1980).

Indifference to pain consists of a failure to react in the expected defensive manner to painful stimuli, and the absence of autonomic effects usually associated with pain, e.g. increased pulse, respiration and blood pressure, in the presence of a normal threshold to the stimulus. Patients usually have normal tendon reflexes, normal sensory thresholds on examination and normal motor and sensory conduction (Dyck et al. 1983). The syndrome is a feature of several different disorders, especially HSAN Types II, III, IV and V, Fabry's disease, and in some cases of inherited amyloidosis. Dyck et al. (1983) have shown reduced levels of acetylcholinesterase and of dopamine beta hydroxylase in the sural nerve in HSAN Types II and V. In these patients there was a selective, virtually complete absence of small myelinated (A delta) afferent fibres. Dorsal root fibres, i.e. unmyelinated nociceptive fibres, were probably also involved (Dyck et al. 1983).

Indifference to painful stimuli may also occur in severe endogeneous depression (Ben-Tovim and Schwartz 1981) and in schizophrenia.

Management of HSAN Syndromes

Specific treatment for these disorders is not available. The special measures recommended for management of Riley–Day syndrome are discussed below. In HSAN Type I and II prevention of ulcers is of major importance since in severe cases digits may

be lost, leading to severe disability. Footwear should be properly fitted and daily foot washing is important to maintain skin pliability and to prevent minor infection. If ulcers develop, treatment by cleaning, debridement and rest afe essential. Walking barefoot should be discouraged because of the risk of painless injury.

Genetic counselling should take account of the pattern of inheritance; in HSAN Type I, children of an affected parent have a 50% chance of developing the disorder. The risk in HSAN Types II, III and IV is difficult to assess since these are autosomal recessive disorders. In one study of Type II HSAN 83% of affected persons were born of consanguineous parents (Kondo and Horikawa 1974).

Treatment and Management of HSAN Type III (Riley–Day Syndrome)

The disease is only slowly progressive but death occurs from the dysautonomia, particularly during the vomiting crises. Only about a third of patients reach the age of 20 years and sudden unexplained death is not unusual. The vomiting crises can be treated with diazepam or with chlorpromazine. The febrile response to infection is reduced so that serious infection may be accompanied by only moderate fever. The impairment of pain sensation may be sufficient to prevent recognition of serious injury, for example fractured bones. There is sometimes a propensity to develop electrolyte disturbances and symptomless hypercapnia and hypoxia so that the severity of pneumonia may be unrecognised. Careful assessment and treatment of these complications is thus necessary.

Sensory Neuropathy in Hereditary Ataxias

Peripheral nerve involvement is a feature particularly associated with the clinical manifestations of Friedreich's ataxia, and it is also found in a number of other spino-cerebellar degenerations (Table 10.8).

In one important group of patients with a hereditary ataxia syndrome associated with peripheral neuropathy there is a severe and prolonged deficiency of vitamin E. This may either occur secondary to chronic fat malabsorption (Muller et al.

Table 10.8. Hereditary ataxias associated with sensory neuropathy

Freidreich's ataxia (McLeod 1971)
Behr's syndrome (Thomas et al. 1984)
Olivo-ponto-cerebellar atrophy (McLeod and Evans 1981)
Marinesco–Sjögren syndrome (Serratrice et al. 1973)
Ramsay–Hunt syndrome (ataxia and myoclonus (Bird and Shaw 1978)
Spastic paraparesis

1983) or it may occur as a selective abnormality of vitamin E absorption (Harding et al. 1985). Ben Hamida et al. (1993) have described a syndrome resembling Friedreich's ataxia, with vitamin E deficiency, in which genetic mapping to chromosome 8q was found (Ben Hamida et al. 1994a). Early vitamin E replacement may arrest or improve the neurological disorder.

Friedreich's Ataxia

Friedreich's ataxia (Friedreich 1976) is an autosomal recessive disorder, beginning in the first or second decade (Harding 1981), in which progressive sensory and cerebellar ataxia and dysarthria is associated with severe impairment of position sense in the legs and with pes cavus. Spasticity in the legs is also a feature, and both plantar responses are extensor, although the ankle jerks may be absent. Cardiomyopathy is a frequent feature and retinal degeneration and deafness may also occur. The first symptoms are usually apparent in the legs, especially high foot arches and unsteady gait. Romberg's sign is positive. Later in the disease ataxia of the arms develops and speech may also become affected by the cerebellar disorder. Nystagmus is invariably present. Deterioration of handwriting may be an early symptom. Disability becomes severe, requiring a wheelchair by the age of 45 years. Later onset cases are less severely affected, and have a slower course. A few patients present in the third decade. Survival is variable; the mean age of death is 35 years (Hewer 1968; Harding 1981) but some patients, particularly the later onset cases, live longer.

The biochemical basis of Friedreich's ataxia is unknown. A genetic locus for the disease has been assigned to the proximal region of the long arm of chromosome 9 at 9q13-21.1 (Hanauer et al. 1990; Chamberlain et al. 1993). The gene product has been termed Frataxin, and is due to a trinucleotide GAA intronic repeat at the 9q13 locus (Campuzano et al. 1996). An identical clinical syndrome, but associated with vitamin E deficiency, has been described in Tunisia and mapped to chromosome 8q (Ben Hamida et al. 1993). Ouahchi et al. (1995) found that this disorder was due to a mutation in the α-tocopherol transfer protein raising the possibility of a vitamin E related defect in Friedreich's ataxia itself. Neither disorder improves with vitamin E supplementation.

Electrophysiological Assessment

The motor nerve conduction velocity is normal or mildly reduced, but the sensory nerve action poten-

tials are reduced in amplitude, or absent (McLeod 1971; Ackroyd et al. 1984). Concentric needle EMG may show mild neurogenic changes, particularly in the distal muscles. The blink reflex is normal (Shahani 1970). The latency of the P100 component of the pattern-evoked response (visual evoked response) is delayed. The ECG shows low voltage QRS complexes with deep Q waves, conduction defects and left ventricular hypertrophy. The echocardiogram shows a symmetrical, concentric hypertrophic cardiomyopathy (Ackroyd et al. 1984).

Pathology

Sural nerve biopsies show evidence of axonal degeneration especially affecting large myelinated fibres. Axonal atrophy is a feature. The brunt of the abnormality in the nervous system is found in the posterior and lateral columns of the spinal cord, and lesions elsewhere in the central nervous system are less marked. Cell loss is found in the deep cerebellar nuclei and fibres are lost from the optic tracts (see Greenfield 1976).

MRI scanning may show moderate atrophy of the medulla and, less commonly, of the cerebellum. The cerebrum appears normal (Ormerod et al. 1994).

Management

The neuropathy in this condition is insignificant in relation to the central manifestations. It has been suggested that oral choline or lecithin supplements might improve ataxia but the results of trials with these compounds have produced conflicting and disappointing results (Chamberlain et al. 1980). Most patients are bedridden by the third decade and die before their fourth decade, usually from the effects of the cardiomyopathy. Physiotherapy is useful in alleviating symptoms in the early stages.

Other Neuropathies Associated with Genetic Diseases

Peripheral neuropathy is a feature of other rare inherited syndromes of unknown metabolic cause (Table 10.8).

A mild neuropathy with sensory and motor features may accompany olivo-ponto-cerebellar atrophy. This neuropathy is of axonal type. In Behr's syndrome, an autosomal recessive disorder of infantile onset, there is mental retardation, visual failure, pyramidal signs and sensory neuropathy with loss of large myelinated fibres. Marinesco-

Sjögren syndrome is an autosomal recessive disorder with mental retardation, cerebellar ataxia and cataracts in which sensory neuropathy may occur. In hereditary spastic paraplegia sensory neuropathy with distal mutilation has been reported in a few families (Cavanagh et al. 1979a).

Chediak–Higashi Disease

In this disorder, inherited as an autosomal recessive trait, there is defective hair pigmentation (oculocutaneous albinism), mental retardation and pancytopenia. Lympho-reticular malignancy is an associated complication. Seizures, cerebellar ataxia and peripheral neuropathy may occur, associated with giant lysosomes in Schwann cells (Lockman et al. 1967). Nerve biopsy shows loss of large myelinated fibres and motor conduction is normal with reduced or absent SNAPs and delayed central motor conduction (Misra et al. 1991).

Chorea-Acanthocytosis Syndromes

Two major subdivisions of the acanthocytic neuromuscular syndromes occur, abetalipoproteinaemic and normo-betalipoproteinaemic (Estes et al. 1967). Normo-betalipoproteinaemic neuroacanthocytic syndromes are much the more frequent.

These disorders are sporadic, or inherited as autosomal recessive or dominant traits. The clinical features include dementia, sensori-motor neuropathy, mental retardation, seizures, cerebellar signs, tremor, choreoathetosis that often also involves the mouth and face, retinitis pigmentosa, corticospinal signs, pes cavus and torticollis. Malabsorption may also be a feature of those patients with abetalipoproteinaemia (Schwartz et al. 1963). Muscle biopsies and EMG studies have shown neurogenic muscle atrophy although myopathic features, with raised blood CK levels, probably secondary in type (Schwartz et al. 1976a; Swash and Schwartz 1977), have also been noted. Motor nerve conduction is normal, but SNAPs are reduced in amplitude or absent. Nerve biopsies may show an axonal neuropathy (Hardie et al. 1991). A pure myopathic form of acanthocytosis, inherited as an X-linked trait (McLeod's syndrome) has also been described (Swash et al. 1983).

Giant Axonal Neuropathy

This is a syndrome characterised by a slowly progressive sensorimotor neuropathy with clumsy gait, and often associated with optic atrophy and abnormal eye movement or nystagmus. A characteristic facies has been reported and in many cases the hair has been tightly curled and is of abnormal appearance (Asbury et al. 1972). The peripheral nerves show large focal axonal swellings (spheroids) which contain an excess of neurofilaments, and a similar histological change has been noted in the central nervous system (Asbury et al. 1972). The disorder is inherited as an autosomal recessive characteristic and parental consanguinity is common in reported cases. Carpenter et al. (1974) noted that the abnormal hair had a decrease in disulphides and an increase in thiol groups. In the central nervous system neurofilamentous axonal swellings also occur, and there may be changes resembling a spino-cerebellar degeneration (Mizuno et al. 1979). SNAP amplitudes are reduced but motor conduction is normal (Berg et al. 1972).

Infantile and Juvenile Neuro-axonal Dystrophy

In this disorder there is psychomotor regression leading to retardation and death. The disorder begins in the second or third year of life, and death occurs within the first decade, in a demented, spastic stage with peripheral neuropathy. Pathologically there are stacked membranes, tubular and vesicular profiles and abnormal mitochondria in peripheral nerves, and spheroids in grey and white matter that are PAS positive and argyrophilic (Cowen and Olmstead 1963; Duncan et al. 1970). More than 100 cases have been described (Aicardi and Castelein 1979).

Electrophysiological Assessment

Motor conduction is normal but the EMG shows chronic partial denervation; later motor conduction may become slowed. Visual evoked potentials are often abnormal (Aicardi and Castelein 1979). The EEG may show an excess of diffuse high voltage fast activity.

Hereditary Neuropathies with Specific Metabolic Defects

Familial Amyloid Polyneuropathy (FAP)

The familial amyloid polyneuropathies (FAP) are rare disorders. Several clinical types (Table 10.4) have been described, named by their place of discovery as Portuguese, Indiana, Irish/Appalachian and Iowa. A fifth type was described by Meretoja and Teppo (1971) in Finland. The Portuguese variety is the most common. All the familial amyloid polyneuropathies are dominantly inherited, all are progressive and all usually present in the third decade, but earlier and later presentations have been recorded. An isolated, progressive form of trigeminal neuropathy is associated with amyloid deposition in a trigemino-spinal distribution (Spillane and Urich 1976). Peripheral neuropathy also occurs in primary systemic amyloidosis, an acquired disease without a genetic basis (Kelly et al. 1979; Abarbanel et al. 1986).

Transthyritin-related FAP: Portuguese (MET 30) Amyloid Polyneuropathy (Type I FAP)

This is the most common form of FAP. It presents with the insidious development of impairment of pain and temperature sensation in the lower extremities, often associated with spontaneous shooting pain and paraesthesiae in the legs (Andrade 1952; Andrade et al. 1970). Sensory abnormalities develop later in the hands. Position sense is affected only in the later stages of the disorder, when distal weakness and wasting and loss of tendon reflexes become apparent. Carpal tunnel syndrome is a rare presenting feature. Autonomic disturbances, with impotence, diarrhoea, urinary and faecal incontinence, postural hypotension and abnormal pupils (particularly a scalloped edge to the pupil, which occurs in 30% of patients) are early and major clinical manifestations which may themselves be disabling. Ulcers may develop on the feet. Fasciculation may be a feature in the advanced stages of the disease. The disorder is steadily progressive leading to death 5 to 15 years after onset (Saraiva et al. 1993). Families with a later age of onset (Libbey et al. 1984) are particularly characteristic of Swedish kindreds (Dwulet and Benson (1984; Saraiva et al. 1993). Vitreous opacities are also frequent in Swedish compared to Portuguese families. This disease also occurs in Japan, where it has been suggested that the genetic defect was introduced by Portuguese sailors during the first European contacts with Japan in the sixteenth century, since the clinical and biochemical features are identical in Portugal and Japan (Ikeda et al. 1987). The disorder is also recognised in Greece, Italy, Brazil and Majorca, observations suggesting a Portuguese nautical origin.

Electrophysiological Studies. Sural nerve SNAPs may be normal in the early stages of the disease, but become smaller, and often undetectable, as the disease progresses. Sensory conduction velocity is normal. In most cases motor conduction is normal or only slightly slowed but, occasionally, may be severely slowed (Anderson and Blom 1972; Sobue et al. 1990). The EMG shows prominent neurogenic changes in tibialis anterior and extensor digitorum brevis, but less commonly in the thenar eminence. Carpal tunnel syndrome is not a feature of this form of familial amyloid polyneuropathy. Dyck and Lambert (1969), in in vitro studies of nerve biopsies, showed selective loss of A and C potentials. Autonomic function tests, e.g. R-R variation on deep breathing, are usually abnormal. The plasma catecholamine levels are normal (Ducla-Soares et al. 1991).

Pathology. Sural nerve biopsy shows large deposits of amyloid in the endoneurium and around blood vessels both in the endoneurium and epineurium; they can be identified by their birefringence in Congo red preparations viewed under polarised light. The amyloid filaments can be identified by electron microscopy (Coimbra and Andrade 1971); they consist of non-branching fibrils 7–10 nm thick, with a characteristic striated appearance. The fibril protein contains prealbumin (Libbey et al. 1984). Dyck and Lambert (1969) showed loss of unmyelinated nerve fibres, with axonal degeneration of myelinated nerve fibres. However, myelinated fibres near amyloid deposits show distortion of the myelin sheath, segmental demyelination and Wallerian degeneration (Coimbra and Andrade 1971; Sobue et al. 1990). Amyloid is formed to a minor extent in the basal foramina of Schwann cells.

Amyloid is deposited not only in peripheral nerves, but also in the vitreous of the eye, in the kidneys, heart, blood vessels and spleen and in the rectal mucosa and skin. The diagnosis can thus be established by rectal or skin biopsy, or sometimes by ophthalmoscopic examination, which shows vitreous opacities and perivascular amyloid deposition in retinal vessels. The CSF protein is raised. The peripheral nerves are not enlarged. The central nervous system is not involved.

Treatment. The basic, genetically determined biochemical disorder is not reversible. Plasma exchange has been tried to reduce the levels of circulating amyloid precursor protein, but was not effective. However, liver transplantation may improve autonomic disturbances, especially gastro-intestinal function, and has been reported to improve the neuropathy (see Reilly and King 1993).

Other Transthyretin Substitutions (Type II FAP)

The SER 84 syndrome was first described in an Indiana family (Rukavina et al. 1956) but a similar disorder has been recognised in a family of German ancestry in Maryland (Mahloudji et al. 1969), now known to be due to a mutation in the 58 position (HIS 58) of the transthyretin molecule. The disorder presents with pain and numbness in a carpal tunnel distribution followed some years later by thenar atrophy and weakness. Some patients develop discomfort and polyneuropathy in the feet many years later. Corneal and vitreous opacities cause visual symptoms, especially specks and floaters in the visual fields. The skin of the hand is smooth and shiny, and the wrist thickened. At carpal tunnel decompression, which is usually curative, amyloid is often found in the transverse carpal ligament (Andrade et al. 1970). Diagnosis can usually be made by rectal or gingival biopsy. Cardiac arrythmias and heart failure may occur as a late feature from cardiac amyloidosis, and other organs are also involved, especially kidneys, tongue, liver, spleen and larynx. Cardiomyopathy is more severe in the Rukavina (Type II FAP) syndrome and neuropathy is more severe in the Maryland type (HIS 58).

Laboratory Assessment. The major laboratory finding with Type II (Rukavina) FAP is the presence of the typical features of carpal tunnel syndrome. Motor nerve conduction velocity is otherwise normal, or only slightly slowed, but the terminal motor and sensory latencies are increased, suggesting an axonal "dying-back" process.

Pathology. There is widespread deposition of amyloid in blood vessel walls. Amyloid may also be demonstrated in the flexor retinaculum when carpal tunnel decompression is performed. Nerve biopsies also show amyloid deposition (Mahloudji et al. 1969).

Management. Carpal tunnel decompression usually leads to improvement in the initial symptoms. Treatment of vitreous opacities is also possible.

Apoprotein A₁-related FAP Syndrome (Type III, Iowa Type)

This syndrome is due to an arginine for glycine substitution at position 26 (Nichols et al. 1990). It is a painful distal symmetrical sensorimotor polyneuropathy beginning in the legs in the fourth decade, resembling Type I (MET 30) FAP. There is neither carpal tunnel nor autonomic involvement. The main feature is progressive renal failure from amyloid nephropathy; peptic ulceration is also a feature. The CSF protein is invariably increased. Death occurs less than 20 years after the onset. The dorsal root ganglia are characteristically involved, and many other organs show amyloid deposition.

Gelsolin-related FAP (Type IV Finnish FAP)

Ten cases of Type IV FAP in three Finnish families were reported initially but since then more than 200 families have been recognised in Finland, with some in Holland, Denmark and Japan (Meretoja and Teppo 1971; Reilly and King 1993). The disorder is associated with an abnormal fragment of plasma protein, gelsolin, in which there is a substitution of asparagine for aspartic acid at position 15 of the amyloid protein (Levy et al. 1990). The characteristic feature is paresis of the upper branch of the facial nerve beginning in the third decade. Other bulbar signs occur in some cases later in life and a mild sensorimotor neuropathy may also develop. Corneal opacities, due to corneal lattice dystrophy, consisting of opaque corneal specks containing amyloid, are a feature. Renal amyloid deposition and atrophy of facial skin are also prominent features. At post-mortem, amyloid is found deposited in most organs, especially around blood vessels. The meninges are involved but the CNS is spared. In the peripheral nervous system amyloid is deposited around blood vessels and in the endoneurium and perineurium.

Electrophysiological Studies. Motor conduction is normal. SNAPs are reduced in amplitude (Boysen et al. 1979). Denervation may be found in the tongue in EMG studies.

Other Forms of Hereditary Amyloidosis

A number of other mutations in transthyretin have been described and in all a sensorimotor neuropathy, often mild and of late onset, is a feature. In some variants a severe cardiomyopathy occurs, for example in the Irish/Appalachian type (transthyretin ALA 60 mutation) (Staunton et al. 1987, 1991). In others polyneuropathy occurs without autonomic involvement (Yasuda et al. 1994).

A Welsh family in which isolated progressive trigeminal neuropathy with destructive ulceration of the face occurred, associated with amyloid deposition in a trigemino-spinal distribution, was described by Spillane and Urich (1976). The disorder progressed during several decades. In the central nervous system amyloidosis as a familial disorder has been associated with seizures and dementia in a kinship from Ohio in which there was a mild peripheral neuropathy (Goren et al. 1980).

Cause of the Neuropathy in Amyloidoses

Three major categories of amyloidosis are recognised (Case Report 1986). In all types of amyloidosis there is deposition of a fibrillar protein that shows apple-green birefringence under polarised light with Congo red staining, due to the organisation of the fibrils in twisted, betapleated sheets. The amyloid fibrils are composed of normal serum proteins, but the precise composition of the amyloid varies in the different forms.

In *familial amyloidosis*, including the familial amyloid polyneuropathies (FAP), the amyloid protein fibrils (AF amyloid) are composed of monomeric units of pre-albumin (transthyretin) which is the transport molecule for thyroxine and retinol. AF amyloid is also found in the senile plaques of Alzheimer's disease (Glenner 1983).

Neuropathy in hereditary amyloidoses has several possible causes. Firstly, it is associated with deposition of amyloid fibrils in the endoneurium, perineurium, blood vessels, and in the basal lamina of Schwann cells and satellite cells. The amyloid fibrils themselves may cause distortion of the endoneurial space with misalignment of Schwann cells, basal lamina and collagen fibrils. This could induce disturbance of the Schwann cell–axon relationship. leading to axonal degeneration (Bunge and Bunge 1978). It has also been suggested that amyloid deposition in the nerve might cause ischaemia in the nerve by altering the functional capacity of endoneurial vessels (Hanya et al. 1989). Direct compression of nerve fibres, inducing axonal degeneration, by amyloid deposits, may also be a factor (Said et al. 1984). In Type II FAP amyloid is deposited particularly in nerve roots or dorsal root ganglia causing specific localised effects.

Secondary amyloidosis (AA amyloid) is associated with chronic diseases, especially rheumatoid arthritis, chronic inflammatory diseases such as tuberculosis and osteomyelitis, familial Mediterranean fever and in medullary cell carcinoma of the thyroid. AA amyloid protein has a molecular weight of about 8500 daltons, and represents a fragment of the much larger protein, serum amyloid-associated protein. AA amyloid is associated with a mild, acquired polyneuropathy.

In non-familial *primary amyloidosis* (myeloma-associated amyloid, AL amyloid) the amyloid protein consists of an immunoglobulin light chain (A kappa or A lambda) of 5000–23 000 daltons molecular weight. This AL amyloid protein is synthesised

by a clone of plasma cells; 20% of patients have multiple myeloma and 90% have monoclonal protein in serum or urine (Kyle and Greipp 1983). Neuropathy may complicate this acquired amyloidosis.

Porphyric Neuropathies

The porphyrias are a group of inherited disorders characterised by abnormalities in haem biosynthesis (Fig. 10.4). Excessive excretion of porphyrins or their precursors is a feature. Clinically, features of involvement of the skin, the liver and the peripheral and central nervous systems may be present. The term porphyria is derived from the reddish colour of urine containing excess porphyrins. Waldenström (1939) categorised the neurological symptoms caused by acute intermittent porphyria, and his work led to speculation concerning the possible relation of the episodic insanity of George III to the porphyria that has been traced in the Hanoverian line and the Prussian royal family as far back as Mary, Queen of Scots (Macalpine and Hunter 1967, 1969; Case Records 1984). Of the six recognised forms of porphyria (Table 10.9) only three – acute intermittent porphyria, variegate porphyria and hereditary coproporphyria – cause neuropathy. Mental disturbance may be a feature of each of these three varieties of porphyria.

Table 10.9. Classification of porphyrias

	Chromosomal locus
Hepatic types	
Acute intermittent porphyria	Ch11q24
Variegate porphyria	Ch14q32
Hereditary coproporphyria	
Porphyria cutanea tarda (symptomatic porphyria)	Ch1p34
Erythropoietic types	
Congenital porphyria (Gunther disease)	Ch10q35
Erythropoietic coproporphyria	

All forms of porphyria except congenital erythropoietic porphyria are inherited as autosomal dominant traits; the latter is autosomal recessive. A type of porphyria described in Chester, England (Chester porphyria) is due to inheritance of both variegate and cutaneous hepatic porphyria (Quadiri et al. 1986). This is associated with a genetic locus on chromosome 11q.

Peripheral neuropathy occurs in porphyria as an acute phenomenon. The clinical features are identical in all three hepatic porphyrias in which neurological involvement occurs, presumably on the basis of a common biochemical disturbance in them. The neuropathy usually occurs in the context of an acute

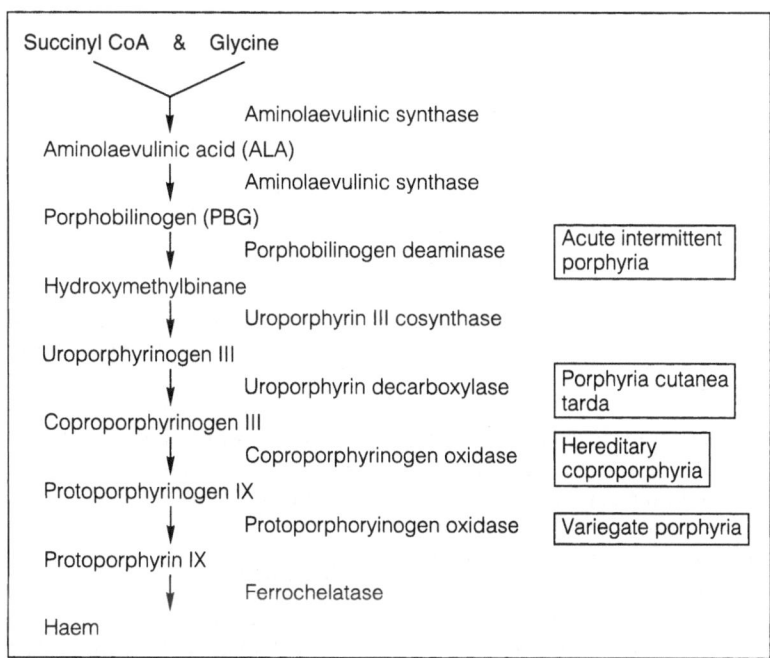

Fig. 10.4. Metabolic pathway for haem synthesis in the liver. The clinical syndromes associated with specific enzyme defects are indicated. Porphyria cutanea tarda is not associated with neurological disease and may be induced by alcoholism, or other liver disorders in susceptible people. Modified from Windebank and Bankovsky 1993.)

exacerbation of the porphyria, with abdominal pain, vomiting, tachycardia and sometimes also with central nervous system manifestations including anxiety and agitation, psychosis or seizures. Porphyric attacks, with or without neuropathy, are often precipitated by drugs, especially barbiturates, oral contraceptives, rifampicin, sulphonamides, chloramphenicol, phenytoin and alcohol. They may also be initiated by infection, and are particularly common in adolescence and premenstrually. Neuropathy may accompany or precede other manifestations of the porphyria; attacks in which neuropathy occurs are almost invariably drug-induced (Ridley 1969, 1975).

In acute intermittent porphyria, variegate porphyria and hereditary coproporphyria, affected subjects show few manifestations between attacks, although in variegate porphyria hyperpigmentation of face and hands with photo-sensitivity and susceptibility to abrasions often brings the disorder to notice in the first or second decades. This form of porphyria is particularly common amongst Afrikaaners in South Africa. In acute intermittent porphyria, a neuropathy is associated with about 30% of acute attacks of the disease.

The neuropathy may begin acutely or it may progress more slowly, even over a period of weeks or months. The arms are usually affected first and the presenting weakness may be symmetrical or asymmetrical. Paraesthesiae or an action tremor may occur at the onset but sensory loss is not a major feature, the neuropathy being almost entirely motor. Facial weakness is often seen. The legs are usually less affected than the arms and there is usually a proximal predilection. Distal weakness is less common. Ridley and Cavanagh (1972) suggested that the variable features might be explained by the pattern of exercise before the onset of the neuropathy. Sensory symptoms or sensory loss when present are usually proximal, producing a "bathing trunk" distribution of sensory loss in the buttocks and shoulders. Porphyric neuropathy thus seems to affect short fibres, perhaps by retrograde axonal transport of a toxic material (Case Records 1984). Autonomic features are common.

There may be retention of urine and alteration of bowel habit. Bladder sensation may be lost and the anal sphincter may be weak. The tendon reflexes are diminished or absent, but the ankle jerks are characteristically preserved, even when the neuropathy is clinically very severe, a point of considerable diagnostic importance. Hypertension may accompany tachycardia. Behavioural disturbances, consisting of irritability, confusion, mania or depression occur in about 30% of cases and seizures develop in 25%.

A third of patients with acute neuropathy associated with acute intermittent porphyria died in Ridley's (1969) series of 29 cases, usually from cardiac involvement and, of those who survived, recovery began within 2–3 weeks of the peak of the disability and continued for many months. Proximal muscles recovered first. Relapses can occur during the first part of this recovery, and may prove fatal. Recurrent attacks may occur at any time, and patients must be warned to avoid drugs known to precipitate acute attacks. There are many such drugs (see Windebank and Barkovsky 1993), including barbiturates, hydantoins, sulphonamides, oestrogens, ethanol, various antibiotics and hypnotics.

Laboratory Investigations

During acute attacks the porphyrin precursors delta amino-laevulinic acid (ALA) and porphobilinogen appear in the urine. The latter may be detected by the red colour that develops when it is converted to uroporphyrin either spontaneously or by the action of ultraviolet radiation in sunlight. This forms the basis of a simple bedside test. Two millilitres freshly prepared Erlich's aldehyde solution is added to an equal volume of urine. A pink/red colour indicates the presence of either urobilinogen or porphobilinogen. If the colour remains in the upper aqueous layer after the addition of 4 ml chloroform the urinary pigment consists of porphobilinogen, confirming the diagnosis of acute intermittent porphyria.

The faecal pigment coproporphyrin is present in increased amounts of the faeces in acute intermittent porphyria, porphyria variegata and in hereditary coproporphyria during attacks of neuropathy. The enzyme abnormalities in these different porphyrias have been reviewed by Brodie et al. (1977), but the biochemical pathology of the porphyrias is still incompletely understood (Case Records 1984).

Inappropriate antidiuretic hormone (ADH) secretion, with a low serum sodium and low osmolality can occur (Hellman et al. 1962); this electrolyte disturbance could also be due to a renal lesion caused by the excretion of delta ALA (Eales et al. 1971).

The CSF protein is often mildly raised in acute attacks and the ECG may show tachycardia and ischaemic changes. Increased urinary excretion of catecholamines may occur, suggesting sympathetic overactivity, a phenomenon which might explain both the tachycardia and the risk of sudden death.

Electrophysiological Assessment

The motor and sensory nerve conduction velocity may be mildly slowed (Wochnik-Dyjas et al. 1978), but is usually normal even in acute attacks (Gilliatt 1966; Zimmerman and Lovelace 1968), although the compound motor action potentials evoked by nerve stimulation are of reduced amplitude. Mustasoki (1980) found slowed conduction in some populations of motor fibres in patients between attacks of acute neuropathy, suggesting a possible subclinical selective neuropathy. Concentric needle EMG studies show profuse fibrillation potentials in the early stages (Nagler 1971). After several weeks polyphasic units are noted which subsequently increase in amplitude. The interference pattern gradually normalises as the patient improves. Sensory conduction velocity is normal. SNAPs may be reduced in amplitude, or normal. Sympathetic skin responses reveal normal function in these unmyelinated small fibres. It is believed that the disturbance of haem metabolism leads to abnormalities in oxygen transport causing axonal degeneration and cell death.

Nerve Biopsy

Few descriptions of the abnormality in peripheral nerve are available. Thomas (1971) noted axonal degeneration with some associated segmental demyelination and Cavanagh and Mellick (1965) thought that the disorder was a "dying-back" neuropathy, but more recent evidence suggests that this axonal neuropathy shows unique selective involvement of certain, short groups of motor nerve fibres that implies a unique causative process, perhaps due to retrograde axonal transport of toxic metabolites (Sweeney et al. 1970). Hierons (1957) noted changes in sensory nerve fibres at the root entry zone as well as in anterior horn cells.

Course and Management

In Ridley's (1969) series complete or almost complete recovery occurred in those patients who survived the acute stage of the neuropathy but Sorensen and With (1971) found that half the survivors of an acute attack had residual paralysis 3 years later, and recovery was not as good in men as it was in women. No specific treatment is available; drugs likely to have induced the attack must be withdrawn. Chlorpromazine can be used safely for pain and to manage the psychosis. Respiratory failure may occur if respiratory muscles are involved and weakening of the voice may be an early symptom of this complication. Tracheostomy and assisted ventilation may be necessary in these cases. The tachycardia can be controlled with propranolol.

Both glucose administration and vitamin B$_6$ (pyridoxine) 100 mg b.d. have been used to try to lessen the severity of the attack, but the effectiveness of these treatments is uncertain (Ridley 1969, 1975). Acute infection should be treated immediately, and hyponatraemia corrected gradually by fluid restriction.

Intravenous haematin, in a dose of 4 mg/kg I/V over 30 minutes twice daily lessens the duration and severity of acute attacks of neuropathy. It should be given during a 3–14 day period from the earliest phase of an acute attack. If relapse occurs when haematin therapy is discontinued, this therapy may be repeated (Pierach 1982).

Hypertrophic Neuropathy with Phytanic Acid Storage: Refsum's Disease

Refsum's disease is an autosomal recessive inherited disorder characterised by a mixed sensorimotor polyneuropathy in which the nerves may be palpably enlarged, and by ataxia and retinitis pigmentosa (Refsum 1946). Progressive deafness, due to cochlear involvement, is seen in most cases and cardiomyopathy, ichthyosis, night blindness and skeletal malformation with epiphyseal dysplasia, pes cavus and shortened metacarpal bones are all frequent manifestations. The age of onset varies from early childhood to the second decade. The first symptom is usually night blindness with atypical tapeto-retinal pigmentary degeneration of the retina. Later, optic atrophy and blindness may develop. Retinitis pigmentosa is a feature in all patients with the disease. Although the major manifestation in the fully developed disorder is the peripheral neuropathy, clinical diagnosis depends on the presence of night blindness, deafness and cerebellar ataxia; both arms and legs are ataxic. The peripheral neuropathy is progressive and symmetrical. Tendon reflexes are gradually lost during the course of the disease. The sensory manifestations include distal sensory impairment, especially of position sense and vibration sense, and both paraesthesiae and spontaneous pain may occur. The sensory features thus resemble those of Déjérine–Sottas disease. Cardiomyopathy may be clinically important in the later stages of the disease and death may occur from left ventricular failure, or from arrhythmia (Refsum 1981, 1984). A diagnostic tetrad of neuropathy, retinitis pigmentosa, cerebellar signs and increased CSF protein particularly suggests the diagnosis. However, the syndrome is heterogenous and cerebellar features are often absent (Skjeldal et al. 1987). In a study of 917 Norwegian patients Skjeldal et al. (1987) found that all the patients had retinopathy, night blindness and restricted visual fields, together with reduced tendon reflexes and increased serum phytanic acid levels. All but one had sensory disturbances, 14 had

deafness and 12 had anosmia. Only seven had ichthyosis and only five had ataxia.

Although the neuropathy is slowly progressive periods of remission occur in which the disease shows no progression, and sudden exacerbations of the neuropathy, in which the patient becomes much weaker, sometimes with both distal and proximal involvement, may occur. Complete recovery from the exacerbation of the disease may occur and such episodes often closely resemble Guillain–Barré polyradiculoneuropathy (Veltana and Verjaal 1961).

Laboratory Investigations

The CSF protein is markedly raised, sometimes being as high as 700 mg/100 ml or more, and the cell count is normal. The CSF protein is lower during periods of remission, and rises in exacerbations, a further source of potential confusion with Guillain–Barré syndrome. The ECG is usually abnormal, showing tachycardia, conduction disturbances and abnormalities of P waves and QRS complexes. The electro-retinogram may be reduced or absent. The skeletal anomalies, particularly the epiphyseal dysplasia, can be recognised by X-rays of the knees, feet and hands.

The diagnosis can be confirmed by measurement of the serum phytanic acid (3,7,11,15-tetramethyl hexadecanoic acid). In normal subjects phytanic acid is present in virtually undetectable quantities in blood (<0.2 mg/100 ml), but in patients with Refsum's disease phytanic acid is present in blood, urine, CSF and liver (Kahlke and Richterich 1965; Billimoria et al. 1982). A raised phytanic acid level in the serum is an essential criterion for diagnosis since patients with many of the clinical features of Refsum's disease are not infrequently seen, in particular, acute intermittent porphyria. Tangier disease, Déjérine–Sottas disease and Friedreich's ataxia may be mistaken for Refsum's disease. Phytanic acid is a phytic derivative which is found principally in plants and in animal fat, which is derived exclusively from the diet, and is not synthesised endogenously in man. Patients with Refsum's disease are unable to break the terminal carbon atom from the fatty acid chain, a process dependent on α-oxidation. Phytanic acid cannot therefore be metabolised by the usual process of β-oxidation and accumulates in the tissues, especially in fat and in the nervous system (Steinberg et al. 1966). In some patients ω-oxidation at the carbon atom furthest from the carboxyl end of the fatty acid chain on the phytanic acid molecule occurs as a partial adaptive response to the biological problem of deficient α-oxidation (Billimoria et al. 1982).

An infantile form of Refsum's disease has been described (Bolthauser et al. 1982), with dysmorphic features, mental retardation, retinopathy, deafness, hepatomegaly and, usually, peripheral neuropathy. Unlike classical Refsum's disease, peroxisomes are absent or abnormal in this syndrome, suggesting that it is a separate disorder (Stokke et al. 1984).

Electrophysiological Assessment

Both motor and sensory nerve conduction velocities are very slowed in the upper and lower limbs and there is EMG evidence of denervation. Nerve conduction velocity improves in parallel with clinical recovery and reductions in phytanic acid levels during treatment (Gibberd et al. 1979).

Nerve and Muscle Biopsy

Sural nerve biopsy has been systematically studied by Fardeau (1975) and by Fardeau and Engel (1969) who noted that the nerve was irregularly swollen and that the swollen areas contained a greyish mucoid matrix. Transverse sections revealed reduced numbers of myelinated nerve fibres with onion bulb formations. Many onion bulbs contain unmyelinated as well as myelinated nerve fibres. In longitudinal section the Schwann cells contain small sudanophilic and metachromatic droplets (Cammermeyer 1956); by electron microscopy these droplets have been shown to be osmiophilic and to be found within Schwann cell cytoplasm (Fardeau 1975). The droplets probably represent phytanic acid deposition, since increased phytanic acid levels have been demonstrated in the nerve biopsy itself (Fardeau et al. 1976). Teased nerve fibre studies show segmental demyelination (Fardeau 1984).

Other Pathological Aspects

At autopsy widespread changes in spinal cord and brain have been reported. Sudanophilic lipid droplets have been found in leptomeninges, choroid plexus, ependyma, and in glial cells of globus pallidus. Axonal reaction is found in anterior horn cells and degeneration of posterior root ganglion cells and of posterior columns occurs secondary to the peripheral nerve changes. The peripheral nerves are generally enlarged but the most severe enlargement occurs in their more proximal parts, for example in the brachial and lumbar plexuses. Cerebellar lesions are inconspicuous, but tract degeneration occurs in the cerebellar connections and in the medial lemniscus (Refsum 1946, 1984; Cammermeyer 1956; Alexander 1966). The myocardium shows fibrosis and the heart is enlarged (Alexander 1966).

Treatment and Outcome

Untreated cases pursue an unpredictable course; some cases may not be severely disabled but others have a series of exacerbations, or pursue a steadily progressive course, leading to death. Death may also occur suddenly from cardiac causes. Dietary management was introduced by Eldjorn et al. (1966). The diet excludes all dairy products, all vegetables except potatoes, and also fatty meats and fish, chocolate and nuts. Potatoes, fruit juice, bread, rice, eggs and lean meat thus form the basis of the diet. Vitamin supplementation is thus necessary. Such a diet has been shown to result in improvement in muscular strength with slow but progressive reduction in blood phytanic acid content and in CSF protein, together with improvement in nerve conduction velocity. In a severe life-threatening exacerbation plasma exchange has been employed with success (Lundberg et al. 1972; Gibberd et al. 1979). Dietary management improves the prognosis, reducing the risk of blindness and cardiomyopathy substantially (Skjeldaal et al. 1992). Generally, the risk of neurological complications is correlated with phytanic acid levels.

Screening for Susceptibility

Relatives of affected patients can be screened by blood phytanic acid assay (Kahlke and Richterich 1965), although it is unusual to find other affected relatives without clinical signs. Asymptomatic mothers of patients with the disease have been found to have raised phytanic acid levels, a finding suggesting that these women were heterozygous carriers of the disease with moderately reduced α-oxidative capacity, but without clinical expression of the disease. Fibroblast cultures can be used to check α-oxidation in suspected cases (Poulos et al. 1984). Heterozygotes show half the normal rate of α-oxidation of fatty acids in their fibroblasts, but are asymptomatic (Refsum 1984). Goldman et al. (1985) screened all patients presenting with retinitis pigmentosa by phytanic acid assay and found one case of Refsum's disease in 52 cases. Sixteen other patients in this group had signs of neurological disorder. The genetic locus is, as yet, unknown.

Other Genetically Determined Neuropathies with Metabolic Defects

There are a number of uncommon inherited neuropathies in which a metabolic defect is present, in addition to Refsum's disease and the porphyrias (see Table 10.4). The clinical and biochemical features of these rare disorders will be briefly discussed here (Table 10.10). Reviews are available (see Dyck and Thomas 1993; Menkes 1985).

Table 10.10 Genetic neuropathies with metabolic defects

	Genetic locus
Metachromatic leukodystrophy (sulphatide lipidosis)	Ch 22q 13.31
Globoid cell leukodystrophy (Krabbe's disease)	14q 21-q31
Angiokeratoma corporis diffusum (Fabry's disease)	xq 22
Tangier disease (alpha lipoprotein deficiency)	–
Bassen–Kornzweig's disease (abetalipoprotein deficiency)	–
Chediak–Higashi syndrome	–
Cockayne's syndrome	10q 21
Adrenoleukodystrophy	xq 28
Cerebro-tendinous xanthomatosis	2q 33
Xeroderma pigmentosa	various loci
Ataxia telangiectasia	11q 22

Neuropathies in Leukodystrophies (Table 10.4)

The leukodystrophies are a group of inherited disorders with abnormal metabolism of myelin, leading to progressive demyelination. The clinical syndrome consists of progressive dementia, with spasticity, cerebellar features and abnormalities of vision and of spinal afferent pathways. Cerebral imaging demonstrates prominent abnormalities in central myelin. The commonest of these disorders is metachromatic leukodystrophy, which occurs with an incidence of about one in 4000 births. Neuropathy is a feature of this disorder, and of Krabbe's disease, Fabry's disease and adrenoleucomyeloneuropathy (adrenoleukodystrophy).

Metachromatic Leukodystrophy (Sulphatide Lipidosis)

This disorder occurs in two forms, arylsulphatase A deficiency and multiple sulphatase deficiency (mucosulphatidosis), a disorder in which there are clinical features of both metachromatic leukodystrophy (MLD) and mucopolysaccharidosis.

MLD is due to abnormalities in the enzyme arylsulphatase A. The gene for this enzyme, which converts sulphatide, a major component of myelin, to cerebroside, is located on chromosome 22 at the q13.31-q ter region. The gene contains eight exons coding for 507 amino acids and a number of different mutations in these exons have been recognised. These mutations are responsible for different, but not for specific clinical syndromes. MLD presents as late infantile, juvenile and adult forms.

The *late infantile form of MLD* is the most common syndrome, presenting between 15 and 18 months of age with progressively difficult walking, weakness of the feet with hypotonia of the legs and with retardation of mental development. Between 2 and 3 years of age the child becomes unable to sit, there is truncal titubation, speech is slow and indistinct, optic atrophy develops and muscle tone increases in the legs, although the tendon reflexes are absent. Sensitivity to touch develops. In the later stages, 1 to 7 years after the onset, quadriparesis, seizures, blindness and dementia develop, before death occurs.

The *juvenile form* is of intermediate severity between the infantile and adult syndromes.

The *adult form of MLD* begins in late adolescence or early adult life, although an onset in the third decade is typical (Percy et al. 1977). The usual presentation of the adult-onset syndrome is with deteriorating memory, speech and thought processes with a schizophrenia like psychosis. The gait becomes wide-based and ataxic, muscle tone is increased, and the tendon reflexes brisk, and incontinence and optic atrophy are evident. Peripheral neuropathy may develop. Death occurs many years later after a phase of dementia, quadriparesis and spasticity (Austin et al. 1968). Rarely pes cavus may be a feature (Baquis et al. 1991).

Pathology. In the CNS there is loss of myelin with reduced numbers of oligodendroglia and deposits of metachromatic granules in macrophages, oligodendrocytes and free in the neuropil. The cerebellum is atrophic. The brain stem and spinal cord are atrophic in early-onset cases. In the peripheral nerves the myelin is thinner than normal and extensive segmental demyelination occurs, with metachromatic granules in macrophages and Schwann cells, and lying between nerve cells (Scholz 1925; Dayan 1967; Thomas et al. 1977). The granules are about 1 μm in diameter.

The CSF protein is raised, perhaps associated with the segmental demyelination, and increases during the course of the disease to 100–200 mg/ml. Urinalysis is important in diagnosis. The urinary sediment contains metachromatic granules and the urine contains increased amounts of sulphatide. Blood leukocytes, serum and cultured skin fibroblasts contain reduced activity of arylsulphatase A (Austin et al. 1968). Arylsulphatase A assays in leukocytes have been used to determine carrier status in potential heterozygotes (Beratis et al. 1975). Brain imaging by CT and MRI is important in diagnosis since it reveals evidence of central demyelination and cerebral atrophy, with ventricular enlargement.

Nerve biopsy is rarely necessary in establishing the diagnosis since assay of enzyme activity in leucocytes is informative.

Electrophysiological Assessment. Visual and somatosensory evoked potentials show delay. Brain stem auditary-evoked potentials show increased interpeak latencies and loss of some late components in the late infantile and juvenile forms but not in the adult-onset forms. The EEG often shows high voltage slow waves and spikes.

Nerve conduction studies in the late infantile and juvenile forms usually show slowed motor conduction, which may be very prominent (<10 m/s) (Thomas et al. 1977). Sensory potentials may be reduced in amplitude, or absent (Clark et al. 1979). In the adult form less abnormality is evident, and nerve conduction may be normal, even in advanced cases.

Other Forms of MLD

There are two other syndromes (Kolodny 1993). In *multiple sulphatase deficiency* several related enzymes are abnormal. The clinical features resemble those of late infantile MLD but there are dysmorphic, coarsened facial features, skeletal abnormalities (e.g. deformities of acetabuli) and hepatomegaly. Corneal clouding and hydrocephalus further resemble mucopolysaccharidosis. In *sulphatide activator protein deficiency*, an extremely rare syndrome, there is delayed development and progression of the core syndrome of MLD.

Treatment. Bone marrow transplantation is effective if carried out before signs of nervous system involvement develop, in the juvenile and adult forms of MLD (Krivit et al. 1990; Krivit et al. 1992). Arylsulphatase A in donor macrophages is sufficient to help correct the metabolic error in the host tissues and thus to prevent full expression of the disease.

Other Leukodystrophies with Neuropathy (Table 10.11)

Segmental demyelination is also a feature of the peripheral nerve abnormality (Bischoff 1975) found in *Krabbe's globoid cell leukodystrophy* (β-galactosidase deficiency). Irritability, sound-induced seizures, mutism, dementia and quadriplegia develop in childhood. The Schwann cell cytoplasm contains crystalline deposits and increased acid phosphatase activity (Dunn et al. 1969) and posterior root ganglia may show degenerative changes (Sourander and Olsson 1968). Globoid cells do not occur in the peripheral nervous system. Motor nerve conduction is slowed in 50% of cases (Dunn et al. 1969). Krabbe's disease is inherited as an autosomal recessive trait at Ch 14q21-q31.

In *Fabry's disease* (angiokeratoma corporis diffusum) sural nerve biopsy may show reduction of

Table 10.11 Major biochemical and electrophysiological features of some inherited disorders

Disease	Enzyme defect	Substance accumulated	CSF protein	Nerve conduction studies	Nerve pathology
Metachromatic leukodystrophy[a]					
infantile	Arylsulphatase A	Sulphatide	Raised	Very slow	Segmental demyelination
Adult	Multiple sulphatases	Mucosulphatide	Raised	Mild slowing	Loss of large fibres Lipid storage
Krabbe's disease	Cerebroside sulphotransferase and β galactosidase	Ceramide and dihexoside	Raised	Slow[a]	Segmental demyelination
Fabry's disease	α Galactosidase	Ceramide and trihexoside	Raised	Slowed[b]	Segmental demyelination Lipid deposition Loss of large myelinated nerve fibres
Tangier disease	α Lipoprotein deficiency, low level of high density lipoprotein		Normal or slightly raised	Normal or slightly slowed[c, d]	Mild axonal loss
Bassen–Kornzweig disease	β Lipoprotein deficiency Low cholesterol and other blood lipids Acanthocytes in blood		Normal or slightly raised	Normal[d, e]	Axonal loss
Tay–Sachs' disease (and variants)	Hexosaminidase	GM$_2$ ganglioside	Raised	?Slowed	Segmental demyelination Lipid storage[f]

[a]Dunn et al. (1969)
[b]Kocen and Thomas (1970)
[c]Kocen et al. (1973)
[d]Pleasure (1975)
[e]Mars et al. (1969)
[f]Kristensson et al. (1967)

myelinated nerve fibres with lamellated glycolipid (ceramide trihexoside) deposits in the perineurium (Kocen and Thomas 1970). However, the diagnosis is more easily made by skin biopsy. Intense pain in the legs and feet with tenderness and burning feelings is characteristic, with distal hypohidrosis. There is a red maculo-papular rash in flexures and nail beds. The disorder is inherited as an X-linked recessive trait at Xq22. Small neurons in dorsal root ganglia are selectively lost. Phenytoin may relieve pain (Lockman et al. 1971) and renal dialysis and transplantation may be needed to relieve renal failure from renal involvement (Desnick et al. 1972). The latter may partially correct the systemic disorder by replacing the missing enzyme. Sheth and Swick (1980) found that motor conduction was slowed, but Kocen and Thomas (1970) reported normal motor and sensory conduction.

Adrenoleukodystrophy is a progressive X-linked (Xq28) recessive disorder affecting adrenal cortex and central and peripheral nervous system (Moser et al. 1987). In one form, *adrenomyeloneuropathy*, peripheral neuropathy develops (Weiss et al. 1980), with primary Schwann cell abnormalities consisting of lamellar inclusions, comprised of long chain fatty acids. Fibroblasts of carriers demonstrate this biochemical abnormality (Moser et al. 1980; Goto et al. 1986). A diet low in very long chain fatty acids may decrease long chain fatty acid levels in the tissues and could be beneficial (Suzuki et al. 1986). A dietary lipid, glyceryl trioleate with glycerylerucate, has been advocated as a therapy and has even been the subject of a blockbuster film "Lorenzo's Oil". However, this remedy appears not to be effective (Moser 1993). Some patients with the disease show mild slowing of motor conduction with EMG evidence of denervation (Vercruyssen et al. 1982).

Gangliosidosis

Late infantile and *juvenile variants of amaurotic idiocy*, including Batten–Bielschowsky syndrome, some cases of Niemann–Pick disease and Spielmeyer–Vogt syndrome, may be diagnosed by a combination of biochemical and ultrastructural studies of sural nerve biopsies. Diagnosis is usually made more easily by biochemical examination of blood and other tissues.

Disorders of Lipid Metabolism

In *cerebro-tendinous xanthomatosis* (cholestanolosis), dementia, cerebellar ataxia, spasticity and peripheral neuropathy develop with cutaneous xanthomas located over tendons, e.g. Achilles region, and with cataracts. The disorder appears in late childhood or adolescence, and is associated with high circulating levels of cholestanol, a 5α dihydro derivative of cholesterol, and deposition of cholestanol in the tissues. It is inherited as an autosomal recessive disorder (Ch 2q33). There is a mild neuropathy, with predominantly sensory features (Ohnishi et al. 1979; Donaghy et al. 1990). In the peripheral nerves cholestanol is deposited in endoneurial tissue, and a demyelinating neuropathy develops with some lipid inclusions in Schwann cells (Donaghy et al. 1990). Motor conduction is slightly slowed and SNAPs are reduced in amplitude (Argov et al. 1986; Dohaghy et al. 1990).

Treatment with oral chenodeoxycholic acid, which supplements the intrahepatic pool of cholesterol metabolism, can result in improvement in the neuropathy and in the other clinical features, including the nerve conduction studies (Donaghy et al. 1990).

Two inherited lipoprotein disorders are associated with neuropathy. *Tangier disease*, an autosomal recessive disorder due to absence of high-density α-lipoproteins in the blood, with low blood cholesterol levels, presents in childhood with tonsillar enlargement due to accumulations of cholesterol ester. The viscera may also be enlarged and a progressive sensorimotor neuropathy with moderately slowed nerve conduction velocities develops. Histologically the neuropathy, which develops in one-third of affected patients, is characterised by loss of myelinated and unmyelinated nerve fibres without segmental demyelination, but with accumulations of cholesterol esters in Schwann cells (Kocen et al. 1973). Transient mononeuropathies or generalised neuropathy with weakness of facial and small hand muscles, and dissociated loss of pain and temperature sensation proximally, suggestive of small fibre disease, may develop (Pollock et al. 1983a; Gibbels et al. 1985). Congenital muscle fibre-type disproportion has been reported in muscle biopsies (Dehkarghani et al. 1981).

In abetalipoproteinaemia (*Bassen–Kornzweig's disease*) a variety of other clinical manifestations occur beside peripheral neuropathy, including acanthocytosis, retinitis pigmentosa, progressive posterior column degeneration, loss of anterior horn cells, mental retardation, steatorrhoea and hypocholesterolaemia (Mars et al. 1969). The disorder, an autosomal recessive trait (Ch 2p24) affects males more than females. Peripheral neuropathy in this disorder probably results from axonal damage secondary to the axonal disorder and partly from segmental demyelination. EMG studies may be normal or show partial denervation and slightly decreased conduction velocity. This disorder is characterised by profoundly low levels of vitamin E from birth. With vitamin E and A supplementation the neurological disorder may be prevented or partially reversed (Muller and Lloyd 1982; Harding et al. 1985).

Neuropathies Associated with Defective DNA Repair

In two disorders associated with abnormalities of DNA repair, *ataxia telangiectasia* (Ch 11q22) and *xeroderma pigmentosum* (several chromosomal locations identified), very mild peripheral neuropathy may occur (Thrush et al. 1974).

Cockayne's syndrome, another disorder of DNA repair, is a recessively inherited disorder with mental and physical retardation, with dwarfism, deafness, retinitis pigmentosa and other defects. It is inherited on Ch 10q21.1. It may be complicated by peripheral neuropathy (Moosa and Dubowitz 1970), with slowed conduction and loss of myelinated fibres (Lewis et al. 1982b). In the brain there

are features suggesting a leukodystrophy with marked white matter degeneration.

Other Metabolic Disorders

In *Chediak–Higashi syndrome*, a disorder characterised by partial albinism, hepatosplenomegaly and peroxidase-positive granules in polymorphonuclear leucocytes, cranial and peripheral neuropathy may be associated with spino-cerebellar degeneration and mental retardation. Intra-cytoplasmic inclusions are found in neurons and axons and perivascular infiltrates may be found both in the central and peripheral nervous system (Sheramata et al. 1971). The disorder is inherited as an autosomal recessive trait. The peripheral neuropathy is an axonopathy, with normal motor conduction velocity and small or absent sensory potentials. Central motor conduction is slowed (Misra et al. 1991).

Neuropathy occurs in mitochondrial cytopathies. In most of these cases there are abnormal mitochondria in the peripheral nerves, particularly in Schwann cells (Schroder 1993).

11 **Acquired Polyneuropathies**

Diabetic Neuropathy

Diabetes mellitus is one of the commonest causes of neuropathy. The neuropathy may present in a number of different forms but mixed syndromes are frequent. About half of all insulin-dependent diabetics have symptomatic neuropathy, representing about 0.5% of the population of developed countries (Brown and Green 1984; Brown and Asbury 1984) (Table 11.1)

Table 11.1. Classification of diabetic neuropathy

Symmetrical polyneuropathy
  Predominantly sensory neuropathy
  Predominantly motor neuropathy
  Predominantly autonomic neuropathy
Focal and multifocal neuropathies
  Asymmetrical proximal motor neuropathy (diabetic amyotrophy)
  Entrapment neuropathy
  Mononeuropathy and mononeuritis multiplex (including intercostal and cranial neuropathies)

Symmetrical Polyneuropathy

The commonest form of neuropathy in diabetes, symmetrical polyneuropathy, occurs in about 7.5% of diabetic patients at the time of diagnosis, but in as many as 50% after 25 years of the disease (Pirart 1978). It is most severe in patients with diabetes of long duration (Rundles 1945), and in those with poor control of blood sugar levels (Greenbaum et al. 1964). It may occur as a complication of established diabetes or it may precede other features of the disease, especially in patients presenting with diabetes after 40 years of age. It is relatively uncommon in children. Diabetes may thus be discovered by investigation in a patient presenting with polyneuropathy, particularly a predominantly sensory polyneuropathy. In other patients the neuropathy arises following an episode of severe ketosis, or after

starting treatment (Lawrence and Locke 1963). Neuropathy complicates both Type 1, insulin-dependent diabetes mellitus and Type 2, non-insulin-dependent diabetes. Autonomic dysfunction develops in about a quarter of patients 5 years after diagnosis of diabetes (Canal et al. 1978).

Objective distal sensory loss is often mild, but paraesthesiae or burning sensations may be prominent. Weakness is not a conspicuous finding in most cases. The distal reflexes, especially the ankle jerks, are usually lost and there may be impaired vasomotor control in the distal extremities, leading to coldness and loss of postural control of small blood vessels in the feet. In severe cases there may be marked impairment of position sense and of other sensory modalities, and neuropathic ulcers and Charcot joints may occur. When the latter are combined with pupillary abnormalities from associated diabetic autonomic neuropathy the clinical picture resembles tabes dorsalis. The "diabetic foot", consisting of chronic ulceration, is associated with neuropathy, and is a frequent cause for hospitalisation and amputation in diabetes.

These clinical features are relatively consistent and have led to the suggestion that four major clinical forms of distal symmetrical polyneuropathy can be recognised in diabetes.

Large Fibre Neuropathy. In this syndrome paraesthesiae in the feet and hands are prominent, associated with distal loss of position sense, vibration or light touch, mainly affecting the legs. There may be slight distal weakness. This is the commonest clinical syndrome.

Small Fibre Neuropathy. This is a rather less common syndrome. Aching pain in the legs with burning feelings in the feet is a major presenting feature. Distal pain and temperature sensation may be impaired and autonomic features may be present. The tendon reflexes and strength are preserved. There is electrophysiological and morphological evidence to support the concept that this syndrome is due to an axonal disorder mainly affecting small myelinated fibres (Brown et al. 1976). *Pseudo-tabetic neuropathy* is a severe form of diabetic neuropathy, associated with prominent autonomic dysfunction, Charcot joints and pressure sores.

Chronic Distal Motor Neuropathy. This is an unusual form of diabetic neuropathy. Some patients with this syndrome have had an acute onset and therefore have suffered from related Guillain–Barré syndrome (Brown and Greene 1984), but in most the disorder is progressive and metabolic control is adequate (Timperley et al. 1985). A distal motor neuropathy has also been reported in patients with hypoglycaemia due to insulinoma, but not in patients with hypoglycaemia associated with diabetes (Jaspan et al. 1982). This may be due to pressure palsies in some patients and the nosological status of the syndrome is uncertain (Editorial 1982b). However, there is evidence of specific involvement of motor axons, with EMG features of partial denervation in the presence of normal motor conduction velocity (Harrison 1976). This concept is supported by the poor prognosis for recovery. Timperley et al. (1985) reported microvascular occlusions in the vasa nervorum due to intimal hyperplasia and thrombi in nerve biopsies in this syndrome.

Autonomic Neuropathy. This syndrome, without marked sensory or motor features, is a common complication of diabetes. Most affected patients are young, and have Type 1 diabetes. Gastro-intestinal features include diarrhoea, vomiting, incontinence and gastric and colonic dilatation. Cardiovascular abnormalities, with postural hypotension and cardiac denervation, are important. Sudden death may occur. Impaired urinary continence, impotence, sweating disorders, and pupillary abnormalities may also develop. This syndrome varies greatly in severity, may be refractory to treatment and has been associated with iritis (Guy et al. 1984). Mild symptomatic autonomic neuropathy is frequent in patients with diabetes. For example, erectile impotence is a problem in 30%–60% of diabetics (Kolodny et al. 1974). Peripheral oedema, often found in diabetics with autonomic neuropathy, may be due to arteriovenous shunting (Ward et al. 1983) from autonomic denervation (Rayman et al. 1986). Autonomic neuropathy is associated with a poor prognosis for survival (Ewing et al. 1980). In 10 years 27% of symptomatic, and 10% of asymptomatic patients have died (Watkins 1991).

Focal and Multifocal Neuropathies

Mononeuropathies in diabetic patients are frequently due to the special susceptibility of the peripheral nerves in diabetes to the effects of compression or entrapment (Mulder et al. 1961; Gilliatt and Willison 1962); in some patients these lesions may be multiple. Other mononeuropathies in diabetic patients have been attributed to microvascular disease, e.g. third nerve and other cranial nerve palsies. The asymmetrical proximal motor neuropathy of diabetes has come to be recognised as a distinct clinical syndrome.

Proximal Motor Neuropathy (Diabetic Amyotrophy). This syndrome was probably first described by Bruns in 1890. It consists of asymmetrical or, less commonly, symmetrical weakness and wasting of the hip and thigh muscles, especially iliopsoas, quadriceps and adductor muscles. It thus tends to spare the hip extensors and hamstring muscles. Rarely proximal upper limb muscles and the muscles of the anterior compartment of the leg below the knee may be affected (Casey and Harrison 1972). It usually coexists with a mild sensory polyneuropathy. The onset is acute or subacute, associated with pain in the affected muscles, weight loss and often with the clinical onset of the diabetes itself. Most patients are older than 50 years, and have Type 2 diabetes (Garland 1955; Casey and Harrison 1972). A similar syndrome can occur rarely with other diseases, especially polyarteritis nodosa (Goodman 1954). When the weakness is asymmetrical the clinical pattern closely resembles that of mononeuritis multiplex (see Brown and Greene 1984). In diabetic proximal motor neuropathy, sensory impairment is unusual in dermatomes associated with the weak muscles, although there is often slight distal sensory loss associated with the coincidental distal symmetrical sensory polyneuropathy (Chokroverty et al. 1977). The knee jerk is typically absent, and the CSF protein is almost always increased (Garland 1955; Casey and Harrison 1972). Relapses after several weeks are uncommon.

This disorder is probably due to metabolic factors related to the diabetes and to weight loss, or to vascular disturbance leading to infarction. The clinical and electrophysiological features suggest involvement of motor roots, lumbo-sacral roots and femoral nerve in varying combinations (Raff and Asbury 1968; Asbury 1977). Some improvement occurs during the 6–12 months following beginning treatment in most newly diagnosed diabetic patients and with improved control of the diabetes in the remainder (Casey and Harrison 1972). Recovery continues over a period of several years and permanent disability is rare. The knee jerk remains absent in 40% of cases.

When the motor disturbance is strikingly asymmetrical it has been suggested that the term *mononeuritis multiplex* should be used, the designation proximal motor neuropathy being reserved, in this classification, for those cases in which proximal involvement is symmetrical and virtually exclusively motor (Brown and Asbury 1984). Although cases with asymmetrical involvement of proximal muscles are more likely to show sensory abnormalities in a proximal distribution, indicating involvement of sensory fibres in sensory roots or in the lumbo-sacral plexus, a rigid distinction between them along these lines seems unproductive and artificial, and does not imply a different view either on pathogenesis or on management and treatment. Other causes of mononeuritis multiplex, such as collagen vascular disease, sarcoidosis, leprosy and amyloidosis, must be excluded.

Cranial Mononeuropathies. Isolated palsies of cranial nerves are more common in diabetics than in the general population. Most instances occur in patients older than 50 years (Zorilla and Kozak 1967). Nerves to the external ocular muscles are most commonly affected, particularly the oculomotor nerves. The sixth and fourth nerves are less commonly involved; the fourth nerve is rarely affected in isolation. The third nerve palsy of diabetes is characteristic, being of sudden onset, accompanied by orbital and retroorbital pain; although often associated with complete involvement of external ocular muscles innervated by the nerve, the pupil is almost invariably spared. Recovery occurs spontaneously to a variable degree. In a small proportion of cases recurrent third nerve palsies may occur.

Differential diagnosis includes third nerve palsy from compression of the nerve by aneurysm of the posterior communicating or internal carotid arteries, but in these patients the pupil is usually affected early and the third nerve palsy is progressive over several days. Other causes include idiopathic third nerve palsies, and an association with dysglobulinaemias, sarcoidosis, chronic or subacute meningitis and Tolosa–Hunt syndrome. Rarely orbital granulomas associated with polyarteritis nodosa may affect the third nerve, and central causes, as in brain stem infarction, must always be considered.

The pathology of oculomotor palsy in diabetes has been studied by Dreyfus et al. (1957), Raff and Asbury (1968) and by Asbury et al. (1970). Their studies have shown focal lesions in affected nerves, with demyelination and axonal damage. Raff and Asbury (1968) demonstrated an occluded intraneural artery which seemed to account for some of the infarcts in the nerve. Thickening and hyalinisation of capillary and arteriolar walls, with narrowing of the lumina of these vessels, was also found and the studies suggest that isolated cranial nerve palsies are probably vascular in origin. A similar pathogenesis has been advanced for diabetic amyotrophy (Raff and Asbury 1968). Hopf and Gutmann (1990) found evidence of mesencephalic infarction as a cause of pupil-sparing diabetic third nerve palsy; MRI abnormalities and abnormal masseter reflexes were found.

Intercostal Mononeuropathies. The intercostal nerves may also be involved (Ellenberg 1978). The patient complains of abdominal pain or paraesthesiae in the distribution of individual dermatomes. It may be acute, unilateral and severe, but the prognosis for recovery is excellent (Kikta et al. 1982). It often co-exists with peripheral and autonomic neuropathies. There are abnormalities in thermoregulatory sweating on the trunk in this syndrome (Fealey et al. 1989).

Entrapment Neuropathies. Diabetics are prone to entrapment neuropathy, or to pressure palsies, e.g. of median nerve at the wrist and ulnar nerve at the elbow. The onset is often abrupt and painful (Fraser et al. 1979).

Laboratory Investigations

The most important laboratory test in diagnosis is a urinary analysis for glucose and ketone bodies, and a random blood glucose estimation. In some patients the underlying diabetes, especially Type 2 diabetes, may be recognised only when a formal glucose tolerance test, or perhaps a 2-hour post-prandial glucose level, is carried out. In patients with proximal motor neuropathy, or mononeuritis multiplex, mild diabetes mellitus may not be a sufficient explanation for the clinical disorder and other causes of the syndromes should also be considered.

Levels of sugar in urine during the period of stabilisation of diabetes may be only poorly correlated with blood sugar levels. The level of blood sugar itself can be self-monitored using appropriate portable colorimetric equipment, and the overall diabetic control can be checked by using the levels of glycosylated haemoglobin (HbA_{1c}). When there is hyperglycaemia for prolonged periods the level of HbA_{1c} rises above the normal upper limit of about 6% (Bunn 1981).

The CSF protein is raised in about two-thirds of patients with diabetes, but this is not pathognomic of symptomatic diabetic neuropathy, or of its severity, and a raised CSF protein level is often found in patients without clinical features of neuropathy (Bischoff 1966). Abnormalities of polyol metabolism in the peripheral nervous system are accompanied by changes in the ratio of sorbitol and myoinositol concentrations in the CSF. The sorbitol level tends to be increased, and the myoinositol level decreased (Servo et al. 1977). These changes correlate with the hyperglycaemia, rather than with the severity of the neuropathy.

Tests of autonomic dysfunction are sometimes useful in assessing the physiological defect prior to treatment, especially in patients with postural hypotension, diarrhoea or incontinence (McLeod 1992).

Electrophysiological Assessment

The most prominent abnormality is slowing of sensory conduction velocity (Gilliatt and Willison 1962). Studies of the sural nerve are more likely to reveal abnormalities than studies of nerves in the arm (Burke et al. 1974a). Behse and Buchthal (1978) found that reduction in the amplitude of the sural nerve sensory action potential was a more sensitive indication of abnormality than was slowing of the sensory conduction velocity in this nerve. Sensory nerve conduction was abnormal in the legs in 76% of patients studied by Behse et al. (1977) but in the median nerves of the same patients there was slowing in only 30%. When there was both sensory and motor involvement on clinical examination, the slowing of sensory nerve conduction velocity was more prominent (Behse et al. 1977), but when motor conduction is abnormal it is more closely correlated with clinical status than the abnormality in sensory conduction. Indeed, 40% of diabetic patients without clinical evidence of neuropathy may have abnormal sensory action potentials, with slowed conduction, in the upper limbs (Noel 1973).

Motor nerve conduction velocity is less abnormal than sensory conduction. Slowing of motor conduction velocity is more prominent in the legs than in the arms. Motor and sensory conduction is usually somewhat slower in distal than in proximal segments of a nerve, and slowing around zones of potential entrapment is very common in diabetic patients, even when asymptomatic (Kaeser 1970). Kuribayashi et al. (1982) found slowing of the N9–N13 interwave latency in diabetics with polyneuropathy, suggesting an important proximal component in the nerve roots. Troni et al. (1984) found abnormal H reflexes. Redmond et al. (1992) compared sensory and motor conduction velocities in asymptomatic diabetics, in patients with mild sensory symptoms and in severe diabetic sensory and autonomic neuropathy. Stud-

ies of the sural nerve sensory conduction were more sensitive than median nerve studies, and than motor studies, in the asymptomatic and mild groups. Peroneal conduction was also more sensitive than median conduction. In the severely affected upper and lower limb sensory studies were always abnormal. Quantitative sensory testing, using vibrational and thermal stimuli (Dyck et al. 1987), was less sensitive than electrophysiological tests.

In a study of patients with untreated maturity-onset diabetes Graf et al. (1979) found a negative correlation between the level of fasting plasma glucose and the motor nerve conduction velocity. None of these patients had symptomatic neuropathy. Lawrence and Locke (1963) showed that diabetic patients had a slower mean motor nerve conduction velocity than non-diabetic patients, and that in those with neuropathy the mean motor nerve conduction velocity was even slower. It has been suggested from studies of this kind that some degree of subclinical neuropathy is an almost universal accompaniment of diabetes mellitus, and subtle sensory abnormalities can often be found in such patients on careful sensory testing.

In sensory polyneuropathy concentric needle EMG shows only mild denervation changes but in patients with motor and sensory signs prominent denervation and reinnervation with polyphasic MUAPs of increased duration are found (Behse et al. 1977). EMG features of chronic partial denervation usually precede slowing of motor conduction velocity. In a single-fibre EMG study (Thiele and Stålberg 1975) the fibre density in the extensor digitorum communis muscle was normal in diabetic patients. However, the predominant involvement of the legs in diabetic sensorimotor neuropathy is associated with an increased fibre density in the tibialis anterior muscle in most patients (Martinez 1986).

In proximal motor neuropathy associated with diabetes there may be electrophysiological evidence of a mild symmetrical sensory neuropathy and at sites of potential entrapment or compression injury slowing of conduction may be demonstrated. In diabetic mononeuritis multiplex slowed conduction velocity is found in affected nerves in segments away from potential sites of entrapment or compression, and concentric needle EMG shows prominent denervation in severe cases. The F wave response is often slowed bilaterally in the legs in patients with proximal motor neuropathy syndromes, and there may also be slowing of conduction in the femoral nerves (Gassel 1963). When stimulating the femoral nerve below the inguinal ligament, the distal motor latency to the quadriceps muscle should not exceed 7.5 ms, with stimulating and recording electrodes 30 cm apart. The proximal location of the abnormality is shown, in some patients, by the presence of fibrillations and some long-duration polyphasic motor unit potentials in the paraspinal muscles, suggesting root involvement (Chokroverty et al. 1977). Other muscles outside the distribution of the femoral nerves are almost invariably involved. The disorder is radicular and plexus in location (Chokroverty 1989), although involvement of anterior horn cells has also been suspected.

Pathological Correlations

From the slowed nerve conduction velocity found in diabetic patients, especially with neuropathy, it would be expected that the nerve pathology should include segmental demyelination (Gilliatt 1966). Greenbaum et al. (1964) found that the main abnormality was loss of myelinated fibres. In teased preparations, Thomas and Lascelles (1965, 1966) found segmental demyelination in mild and severe cases, whereas axonal loss was also noted in severe, chronic cases. Since demyelination, but not axonal loss, was found by Chopra et al. (1969) in diabetic patients without clinical evidence of neuropathy, the earliest change was thought to be segmental demyelination, a view consistent with Bischoff's (1968) suggestion that a metabolic defect in Schwann cells is the primary abnormality. However, Bischoff (1973) later showed axonal degeneration early in the natural history of diabetic neuropathy and the independence of segmental demyelination and axonal degeneration in diabetic neuropathy has therefore been challenged (Thomas and Eliasson 1975). Loss of dorsal root ganglion cells and of anterior horn cells has been found in some autopsied cases (Greenbaum et al. 1964) and there is evidence of loss of myelinated and unmyelinated fibres of all sizes in sural nerve biopsies in diabetic neuropathy (Behse et al. 1977). It therefore seems likely that both axonal degeneration and segmental demyelination occur in this neuropathy. Further, remyelination is often found in sural nerve biopsies (Behse et al. 1977) and Ballin and Thomas (1968) found onion-bulb formation in 7 of 10 nerves examined at biopsy. Degenerative changes, with lipid inclusions, in Schwann cells are an early feature of symmetrical sensorimotor neuropathy and a characteristic change is thickening and reduplication of basement membranes, around both Schwann cells and capillaries.

Behse et al. (1977) concluded from their correlative studies of sural nerve conduction and pathology in diabetic neuropathy that slowing of conduction velocity, when severe, was related to loss of the large, myelinated fibres. However, mild slowing of conduction by up to 30% could not be explained by changes in myelin thickness, or loss of myelinated fibres, but must be due to a metabolic abnormality in the axons or Schwann cells associated with the diabetes itself. In patients with painful "small-fibre" diabetic neuropathy, with pseudosyringomyelic dissociation of sensation, spontaneous pain and autonomic features, sural nerve biopsies showed loss of unmyelinated and of small myelinated axons, with axonal sprouting suggesting a severe axonal neuropathy. However, there was also some evidence of primary and secondary demyelination in these biopsies (Said et al. 1983).

Studies of skeletal muscle have shown grouped denervation atrophy in severe cases of polyneuropathy (Greenbaum et al. 1964). Coërs and Hildenbrand (1965) have correlated the nerve conduction velocity, the terminal innervation ratio in methylene blue preparations of motor endplates, and neurogenic changes in the muscle. Patients with slowed nerve conduction velocity but without clinical evidence of neuropathy showed changes in the terminal innervation with swelling of the terminal expansion of the motor end-plates. In cases with areflexia, but without muscle weakness, there was collateral axonal sprouting in the terminal motor innervation with scattered small muscle fibres. In patients with a moderate degree of weakness fibre-type grouping was noted, with more prominent changes in the terminal innervation; these patients showed with EMG long-duration polyphasic MUAPs with fibrillation potentials. In less affected patients no denervation potentials were recorded.

The pathology of the proximal motor neuropathies may be somewhat different. In an autopsy of a 72-year old man who died 6 weeks after the onset of diabetic mononeuritis, multiplex numerous small infarcts were seen in the affected nerves (Raff et al. 1968). Although striking endothelial and perithelial proliferation was found in arterioles and capillaries in these nerves no focal arterial occlusion was recognised in this patient. Nonetheless, the presence of infarcts in the affected nerves is in keeping with a vascular basis for this neuropathy. Similar changes have been found in the third cranial nerve in a case of diabetic third nerve palsy (Asbury et al. 1970). Eames and Lange (1967) found that the first morphological effect of ischaemia in peripheral nerves is segmental demyelination, and this change has been found in the ischaemic cranial mononeuropathy associated with diabetes. Timperley et al. (1985) noted microvascular occlusions in peripheral nerve biopsies in patients with progressive neuropathies associated with good diabetic control.

Neurogenic changes may be found on muscle biopsy (Chokroverty et al. 1977). Chokroverty et al.

(1977) found clusters of small, grouped Type 1 and Type 2 fibres, with target formation in Type 1 fibres. These small fibres stained darkly with NADH-tr, but were negative in the phosphorylase reaction. In one patient 5% of Type 2 fibres showed tubular aggregates and intramuscular nerves showed patchy demyelination, axonal degeneration and fibrosis. Electron microscopy showed various other nonspecific abnormalities. The motor endplates showed degenerative changes, sometimes quite marked, without attempts at axonal regeneration. Chokroverty et al. (1977) concluded that diabetic amyotrophy was secondary to a metabolic derangement in the affected femoral and other nerves, rather than to diabetic microangiopathy but this conclusion must be regarded as speculative. In autonomic neuropathy there is severe loss of myelinated axons in the vagus nerve and in the sympathetic trunk (Low et al. 1975; Duchen et al. 1980).

Pathogenesis

Diabetes is a metabolic disorder and it has therefore been assumed that diabetic neuropathy has a metabolic cause. A number of different metabolic disturbances have been recognised, and these all have possible relevance to the development of neuropathy. Indeed, Thomas and Lascelles (1966) thought the primary abnormality might reside in Schwann cell metabolism. However, the pathological evidence of both axonal and Schwann cell involvement and, especially, the evidence for ischaemia of affected nerves must be considered. The following metabolic abnormalities have been documented:

- Reduced nerve Na/K ATPase activity (Das et al. 1976)
- Reduced nerve conduction velocity in diabetic rats does not correlate with structural change, but with hyperglycaemia (Sharma and Thomas 1974)
- Sorbitol accumulation in nerve (Kjeldsen et al. 1987)
- Myoinositol depletion in nerve (Gillon and Hawthorn 1983)
- Glycogen accumulation
- Reduced synthesis and transport of axonal proteins
- Impaired myelin metabolism (see Low 1987).

Rapid changes in blood glucose levels, including hyperglycaemia (Yasaki and Dyck 1991) are not factors leading to diabetic neuropathy (Andersen et al. 1994). Experimental studies on streptozotocin induced diabetes in the rat have been important in elucidating causative mechanisms of diabetic neu-

ropathy. Accumulation of sugar alcohols, such as sorbitol (Gabbay et al. 1966; Thomas and Ward 1975) or reduced nerve myoinositol levels (Greene et al. 1975; Clements and Reynertson 1977) may be important. Dietary myoinositol supplementation seemed to improve conduction in experimental diabetes (Greene et al. 1975). Dyck et al. (1980), however, found no correlation between myoinositol levels in nerve biopsies and the presence of neuropathy in human diabetes. The link between sorbitol metabolism, which involves aldose reductase metabolism, and myoinositol levels in nerves in diabetes is not yet understood. Brown and Asbury (1984) and Low (1987) reviewed the concept that the metabolic abnormality may be related to deficient energy metabolism in peripheral nerves. Disturbances of fatty acid metabolism in nerves have also been found in diabetes but these do not appear to account for the abnormality of nerve conduction (Thomas and Eliasson 1975).

Studies of peripheral nerves in rats made diabetic by treatment with alloxan or streptozocin have yielded controversial results. Slowing of conduction has been found in the largest myelinated fibres in these animals without segmental demyelination but with structural axonal changes similar to those found in humans. The abnormality in conduction in the fibres is partially reversed by insulin treatment. These findings have been discussed extensively (Sharma and Thomas 1974; Thomas and Sharma 1976 and Jakobsen 1979).

There is a relationship between the degree of hyperglycaemia and the occurrence of neuropathy (Pirart 1978) and between neuropathy and glycosylated haemoglobin levels (Drury et al. 1982), but current understanding of the metabolic abnormality in the diabetic neuropathies is incomplete, and the data from experimental studies of diabetes in the rat are often difficult to correlate with the findings in human diabetes.

Disease of the small intraneural vessels, due to diabetes, has also been proposed as a mechanism for neuropathy in the disease (Woltmann and Wilder 1929; Fagerberg 1959). In patients with severe polyneuropathy sural nerve biopsies have shown prominent small vessel disease, with capillary closure and endothelial hyperplasia (Dyck et al. 1985a; Timperley et al. 1985). In a study of 11 patients with diabetic polyneuropathy Newrick et al. (1986) found that intraneural oxygen tension, measured with an *in vivo* technique in the sural nerve, was reduced, and that the nerve/vein oxygen gradient was also reduced.

This work in human diabetic neuropathy is corroborated by similar observations in the diabetic rat (Tuck et al. 1984).

Management of the Diabetic Neuropathies

In general, the course of symmetrical polyneuropathy is improved by careful control of diabetes. Glycosylated haemoglobin levels (HbA_{1c}) are useful in checking long-term control and the patient should check the blood sugar level randomly during the day. Gregerson (1968) and Ward et al. (1971) observed improvement in motor nerve conduction within a few weeks of beginning treatment in patients with newly diagnosed diabetes with or without clinical evidence of neuropathy. Treatment with continuous subcutaneous insulin infusion ("insulin pump") may result in even more rapid, but incomplete, clinical and electrophysiological improvement (Boulton et al. 1982). Fraser et al. (1977) found that patients treated with insulin showed improvement in motor nerve conduction, but that those treated with sulphonylurea drugs showed no such improvement. In painful diabetic neuropathies there is some evidence that hyperglycaemia is a factor initiating pain (Morley et al. 1984) and insulin treatment may alleviate pain in most patients (Young et al. 1985). This improvement may occur within a few days of achieving diurnal euglycaemia (Samanta and Burden 1985). Sorbinil, an inhibitor of aldose reductase, prevents accumulation of sorbitol in the nerve, and has been found to reduce pain and improve nerve conduction in diabetic polyneuropathy (Jaspan et al. 1983), but the degree of clinical improvement was minimal in long-term administration (Sima et al. 1988). Progression of diabetic neuropathy may be halted, and clinical improvement induced, by euglycaemia following successful pancreatic islet cell transplantation (Kennedy et al. 1990). The place of this treatment in management is uncertain at present, however, since the degree of improvement was mild.

Cranial and other mononeuropathies usually improve spontaneously, independently of diabetic control, unlike symmetrical distal sensory polyneuropathy. Severe diabetic neuropathy has been treated by stringent dietary and insulin therapy for many years with beneficial results (Greenbaum et al. 1964). Both symmetrical polyneuropathy and the vascular single or multiple neuropathies respond in the same way. Diabetic amyotrophy improves similarly, if incompletely, with control of diabetes. Autonomic neuropathy is reversible only in the early stages (Hilton et al. 1983); in advanced cases nerve conduction may improve but autonomic symptoms persist (Campbell et al. 1976).

Gregerson (1967) showed that careful control of diabetes reduced the risk of development of severe neuropathy and suggested that there was a critical period in the first few years of the disease so that if there was only a mild or moderate neuropathy during this time later deterioration was unlikely.

In patients with chronic neuropathy resistant to treatment, care of the skin and of the feet is important. The major persistent problems following effective control of diabetes are symptomatic of autonomic involvement. Orthostatic hypotension and impotence are particularly resistant to therapy, but the former may respond to treatment with 9α-fludrocortisone, or sometimes to indomethacin. Elastic stockings and the maintenance of an erect or partially erect posture are important even in sleep. A somatostatin analogue (SMS 201–995) can improve blood pressure and may lead to effective treatment (Hoeldtke et al. 1986). The diarrhoea of autonomic gastro-intestinal involvement may improve with tetracycline or neomycin.

Because of the susceptibility to entrapment or compression injuries it is important to advise patients with occult or slight neuropathies to avoid postures likely to induce pressure palsies. Furthermore, such pressure palsies in diabetic patients usually improve with conservative management and decompression should be delayed until after a period of effective management of the diabetes. Patients with diabetic polyneuropathy are particularly susceptible to develop pressure sores and cutaneous infections in the feet, and careful surveillance is helpful in preventing these complications. About 10% of patients with diabetic neuropathy experience burning and unremitting pain (Pavy 1887; Max et al. 1991). Amitriptyline and desipramine may be useful (Max et al. 1991). Non-steroidal analgesics and carbamazepine are also used but are not very effective. Locally applied capsaicin cream may be of value (Ross and Varipapa 1989).

Uraemic Neuropathy

A neuropathy may occur with chronic renal failure. It was probably first described by Osler in 1892 but the first complete description was by Hegstrom et al. in 1961. Hegstrom et al. (1961) recorded the development of a moderately severe neuropathy during intermittent haemodialysis. Asbury et al. (1963) recorded the clinical and pathological findings in four uraemic patients who had not been treated by dialysis and Thomas (1978) found clinical evidence of peripheral neuropathy in 25% of patients referred prior to haemodialysis. This relatively low incidence, compared with the 65% reported by Robson (1968) 10 years earlier, probably reflects referral practice and the earlier treatment of uraemia. Savazzi et al. (1980) found that neuropathy was not present unless the glomerular filtration rate was less than 20 ml/min and the creatinine level was greater than 6 mg/dl. Nielsen (1973) showed a relationship between slowing of nerve conduction and the degree of abnormality in creatinine clearance. Asbury (1984) has emphasised that the diagnosis of uraemic polyneuropathy rests on the association of neuropathy with longstanding severe renal failure, and the exclusion of other causes. The CSF protein is usually normal, but may be slightly elevated. Polyneuropathy is not a complication of acute renal failure.

The neuropathy is usually distal, symmetrical and mixed sensory and motor in type. It varies considerably in severity and rate of cramps and restless legs (Callaghan 1966), but distal dysaesthesiae and numbness with absent ankle jerks are early signs. Nielsen (1971a,b) noted that two-thirds of 109 patients with renal failure had cramps and restless legs. Bolton and Young (1990) considered that water-soluble vitamin depletion might be a factor in the sensory component of the neuropathy. Most patients with neuropathy improve or become stable with dialysis; those with mild neuropathy usually improve but those with severe neuropathy show little benefit with this treatment. In a few patients neuropathy may worsen rapidly when dialysis is begun, but improvement usually occurs if the dialysis time is increased (Konotey-Ahulu et al. 1965). Rapid deterioration during haemodialysis may be associated with sepsis; the resulting axonal neuropathy resembles critical core neuropathy (Bolton and Young 1990). Nielsen (1974) found that a decrease in vibratory perception threshold was an indication of clinical deterioration in the neuropathy even when there was no rapid change in conduction velocity.

Carpal tunnel syndrome has been recognised as a complication of long-term dialysis. It is related to the duration of treatment and is probably not related to the pressure of the arteriovenous shunt in the forearm used for access to the circulation (Halter et al. 1981). However, Harding and Le Fanu (1977) have suggested that the shunt may cause local ischaemia of the median nerve and oedema in the carpal canal. Carpal tunnel decompression relieved the symptoms in the cases described by Halter et al. (1981). Amyloidosis secondary to renal failure may also cause carpal tunnel compression (Bolton and Young 1990). The amyloid is derived from β_2 microglobulin.

Electrophysiologial Assessment

Motor nerve conduction velocity is reduced in uraemic neuropathy. Further, slowing of motor nerve conduction is related to the severity of the uraemia, as assessed by serum creatinine levels (Jebsen et al. 1967). Jebsen et al. (1967) found clinical neuropathy only in patients with slow conduction velocity and severe impairment of renal function. The sensory nerve action potentials are usually reduced in amplitude, but there is only mild slowing of sensory conduction, except in very severe cases (Nielsen 1973). Nerve conduction velocity improves only slightly with dialysis but rapid improvement occurs after successful renal transplantation (Nielsen 1974). Concentric needle EMG usually shows features of denervation in distal muscles, as a consistent finding, early in the course of the disease. F responses may show proximal nerve involvement in uraemic neuropathy, especially in subclinical cases (Ackil et al. 1981; Asbury 1984).

Thermal thresholds were abnormal in six of 20 patients studied by Angus-Leppan and Burke (1992), but nerve conduction studies were abnormal in 16 of those patients. These findings are consistent with relative susceptibility of large fibres in this neuropathy.

Pathological Correlations

Asbury et al. (1963), in four autopsied cases, found striking loss of nerve fibres with maximal effect distally, and sparing of proximal portions of nerves, nerve roots and sympathetic ganglia. There was active Wallerian degeneration distally, but myelin sheaths appeared to be affected out of proportion to the axonal change. Dayan et al. (1970) found segmental demyelination alone in sural nerve biopsies in acute uraemia and segmental demyelination and axonal degeneration in chronic cases. Thomas et al. (1971) agreed with Asbury et al. (1963) that the main abnormality was secondary to axonal damage rather than a direct effect of uraemia on Schwann cells. Appenzeller et al. (1971) found features suggestive both of axonal damage and segmental demyelination. Thomas et al. (1971) concluded that demyelination in uraemic neuropathy was secondary to axonal loss and axonal thinning.

There is agreement that uraemic neuropathy is not due to vitamin deficiency (see Asbury 1984) and is multifactorial in relation to the uraemia.

Management

Renal dialysis stabilises or results in slow improvement in uraemic polyneuropathy (Bazzi et al. 1991). Renal transplantation produces more complete and more rapid improvement in the clinical features of polyneuropathy than does haemodialysis (Nielsen

1974; Asbury 1984). Following successful renal transplantation, the clinical features and neurophysiological abnormalities gradually improve; there may be resolution of sensory symptoms within a few days but motor function improves more slowly (Nielsen 1974; Bolton 1976). Diabetics with renal failure show no improvement in neuropathy after renal transplantation, or even after combined renal and pancreatic transplants (Van der Vliet et al. 1988).

Hepatic Neuropathy

A mild symmetrical sensorimotor neuropathy is occasionally seen in patients with chronic liver disease. Pathological studies of sural nerve biopsies have shown that this is mainly a demyelinating neuropathy (Dayan and Williams 1967; Knill-Jones et al. 1972). Nerve conduction is slowed (Vasilescu et al. 1978b). The relation of this neuropathy to the hepatic failure is controversial, however, since in many patients alcoholism, diabetes and drug therapy could equally be responsible. Guillain-Barré polyneuropathy has been reported in association with the recovery phase of hepatitis A (Johnston et al. 1981) and perhaps also earlier in the disease. In a few cases circulating hepatitis B antigen was present (Berger et al. 1981). A chronic relapsing demyelinating polyneuropathy associated with hepatitis B infection was described by Inoue (1987). Immune complex deposition was noted by electron microscopy. In hepatitis A many patients develop abnormal sensory conduction (Chari et al. 1977). In chronic primary biliary cirrhosis a mild sensory neuropathy may develop with xanthomatous deposits in the nerves (Thomas and Walker 1965). In childhood biliary atresia vitamin E depletion neuropathy may develop (Sokol et al. 1985).

Neuropathies Associated with Alcoholism, Malnutrition, Hypovitaminosis and Malabsorption

Alcoholic Neuropathy

Neuropathy is one of a number of neurological complications of alcoholism. It was one of the commonest neuropathies in the USA. Victor and Adams (1953) found clinical evidence of peripheral neuro-

pathy in 9% of patients admitted to the Boston City Hospital because of alcoholism. Some patients with alcoholic peripheral neuropathy also have other neurological complications of alcoholism, such as cerebellar degeneration, Wernicke–Korsakoff syndrome, delirium tremens or withdrawal seizures (Mawdsley and Mayer 1965). Peripheral neuropathy was found in over 80% of a series of 245 cases with Wernicke–Korsakoff syndrome (Victor et al. 1971).

The neuropathy itself may be asymptomatic, being evident on examination by thinness of the extremities, absent ankle jerks and decreased sensibility to all modalities in the feet and shins (Victor and Adams 1953). The symptomatic neuropathy is usually insidiously progressive but sudden worsening may occur. The legs are always more severely involved than the arms. Motor and sensory symptoms occur concomitantly and pain and paraesthesiae in the distal parts of the legs, particularly the soles of the feet, are characteristic symptoms. Pain may be very severe, and affected distal muscles are tender to pressure. Sensory loss may be severe distally and sensory ataxia may be a feature in such patients. The tendon reflexes are absent distally, and later more proximal reflexes also become unobtainable. The skin of the extremities is often sweaty and reddened but other manifestations of autonomic involvement, e.g. postural hypotension, are uncommon (McLeod 1992). Contractures may develop in severe cases and muscular atrophy may be very pronounced. Trophic changes may develop in the feet, with perforating ulcers, oedema and foot deformity in chronic cases. The sphincters are usually unaffected. The CSF protein is usually normal (Victor and Adams 1953).

Electrophysiological Assessment

Motor and sensory nerve conduction velocity may be slightly slowed even in the absence of motor and sensory symptoms, a finding consistent with the common occurrence of asymptomatic or subclinical neuropathy in alcoholic patients, as discussed above. In these patients, and in those with symptomatic neuropathy, sensory conduction is most abnormal in the distal segments (Mawdsley and Mayer 1965). Casey and Le Quesne (1972) found that sensory nerve conduction was slowed in the digits but not in the more proximal segments of the median nerve even in alcoholic patients *without* clinical evidence of peripheral neuropathy. Walsh and McLeod (1970) found that motor conduction velocity was slightly slowed in alcoholic neuropathy and Behse and Buchthal (1977a) reported mild slowing of sensory conduction with diminished amplitude of the SNAP in the sural nerve.

Reduction in the amplitude of the SAP in the sural nerve is probably the earliest change. Behse and Buchthal (1977a) found that the sensory potential in the sural nerve was small in 70% of patients and sensory conduction was slowed in this nerve in 60% of patients but in all of these patients slowing was to no more than 70% of normal. The distal motor latency in the peroneal nerve was increased in half the patients but in only a third was the common peroneal motor conduction velocity abnormal.

Concentric needle EMG shows evidence of chronic partial denervation (Fig. 11.1) in nearly all patients with overt alcoholic neuropathy. This is more prominent in the legs than in the arms (Behse and Buchthal 1977a). Single-fibre EMG studies have shown that the motor unit fibre density is increased (Thiele and Stålberg 1975).

Sympathetic skin responses were absent on the sole of the foot in 16 of 30 patients studied by Navarro et al. (1993).

Pathological Correlations

Both the clinical and electrophysiological features suggest that alcoholic neuropathy is due to axonal degeneration of distal type and the pathological studies of Walsh and McLeod (1970) and Behse and Buchthal (1977a) confirm this. Both sectioned and teased nerve fibres have been examined in sural nerve biopsies. In addition there is degeneration of dorsal root ganglion cells and of some fibres in the posterior columns. Evidence of remyelination has been found in the sural nerve biopsies (Walsh and McLeod 1970) and Behse and Buchthal (1977a) noted some slight evidence of segmental demyelination, but this is probably secondary to the primary axonopathy.

Experimental alcoholic feeding in the rat produces mild distal axonopathy without segmental demyelination (Bosch et al. 1979). Meyer et al. (1981) suggested that alcoholic neuropathy might be due to alcohol rather than to thiamine deficiency in patients with the disease. However, animals developing neuropathy when given alcohol are also nutritionally deprived, and thiamine depletion seems to be the major factor (Bosch et al. 1979).

Management

Alcoholic neuropathy resembles clinically that of thiamine deficiency and there is evidence that thiamine deficiency associated with alcoholism may be a causative factor. Nonetheless the response to treatment with parenteral thiamine is poor, an

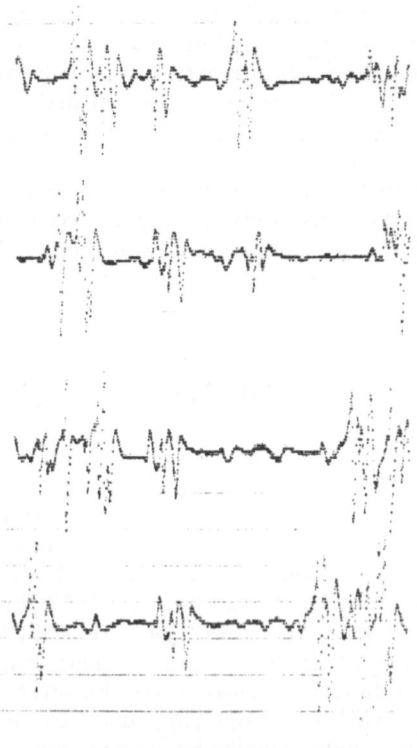

Fig. 11.1. Alcoholic neuropathy. Voluntary activity showing highly polyphasic units and a markedly reduced interference pattern. Concentric needle EMG. Filters: 100 Hz and 10 kHz. Bar 20 ms.

observation also made in beri-beri neuropathy. Novak and Victor (1974), in particular, have argued that alcoholic neuropathy is due to thiamine deficiency. It is probable that alcohol alone is not toxic to the peripheral nervous system in humans (Mayer 1966). The nutritional status of alcoholic patients is generally poor and the neuropathy may well be the result of several deficiencies (Strauss 1935). If a normal diet is resumed there is a slow and incomplete recovery over many months, and dysaesthesiae and pain remain prominent and disabling symptoms. Multi-vitamin supplementation should always be used in the initial stages. In mild cases the prognosis is good provided the patient's nutritional status is improved and there is abstinence from alcohol.

Malnutrition

Malnutrition is a complex metabolic disorder in which multiple deficiencies of protein, lipid, carbohydrates, vitamins and trace metals may develop. In starvation muscle wasting occurs, with atrophy of muscle fibres. Type 2 fibres are affected before Type 1 fibres. In infants and children with marasmus, although there is severe growth retardation, muscular weakness and wasting and loss of subcutaneous fat, motor conduction velocity is normal (Singh et al. 1976). In kwashiorkor, on the other hand, a disorder in which there is relatively selective protein malnutrition, together with variable degrees of vitamin deficiency, there is hyporeflexia, proximal muscle wasting and weakness with a waddling gait. In this condition motor conduction velocity is markedly slowed, often to about half normal, and the sensory nerve action potentials may be absent (Sachdev et al. 1971; Engsner and Woldemoriam 1974). Muscle biopsies in kwashiorkor show grouped atrophy and the EMG shows prominent fibrillation potentials (Sachdev et al. 1971). Motor conduction velocity returns to normal within 5 weeks of restoration of an adequate diet (Osuntokun 1971; Engsner and Woldemoriam 1974). Scott and Weir (1981) have suggested that the neuropathy of kwashiorkor is due to methionine deficiency, and that it is therefore biochemically related to the neurological effects of vitamin B_{12} and folate deficiency.

Gibberd and Simmonds (1980) reviewed the medical histories of 679 patients with neurological disease, from a group of 4684 ex-Far East prisoners of war released in 1945. In 89 neurological disease developed many years later. Peripheral neuropathy that commenced during captivity in 593 of 679 patients with neurological disease improved, but optic atrophy and cord lesions acquired during the period of captivity showed little improvement and, in some cases, progressed in later years. Spillane (1947) described the clinical syndromes in British soldiers released at the end of the second world war. Nutritional neuropathies with optic atrophy and sensory deafness are common in Southern India, and respond only partially to dietary and vitamin treatment.

Neuropathies Associated with Hypovitaminosis

Thiamine Deficiency

In clinical practice it is rare for thiamine deficiency to occur in isolation. In most patients in Western countries there is associated malnutrition induced by gastro-intestinal disease or by drug or alcohol addiction. The clinical features in these patients are therefore complex. Pure thiamine deficiency has been studied in special situations of dietary deprivation, as in prisoners of war kept on restricted diets

(Spillane 1947) or in alcoholic patients (Victor and Adams 1953).

The neuropathy of thiamine deficiency (dry beri-beri) is usually a mixed sensory and motor disorder but predominantly sensory or motor forms may occur. Foot drop is the commonest motor presentation. Wrist drop may also be a feature. There is usually distal sensory loss and dysaesthesiae and burning sensations are common, especially in the feet. Distal reflexes are lost. In nutritional, non-alcoholic thiamine deficiency cranial nerve involvement may occur, with tongue, face and laryngeal weakness (Daniels 1906).

Following treatment with thiamine or diet, motor symptoms and signs improve within 6 months, and sensory disturbances in about a year.

Electrophysiological Assessment. Motor nerve conduction velocity is slowed in rats with dietary thiamine deficiency by as much as 50% (Erbslöh and Abel 1970). In man it is not clear whether the nerve conduction velocity is slowed or not, but in alcoholics blood thiamine levels are always low in those with neuropathy, and in half of those without neuropathy, and the nerve conduction velocity is slowed in alcoholic neuropathy (see Mawdsley and Mayer 1965).

Pathological Correlations. Axonal degeneration predominates (Collins et al. 1964; Prineas 1970), mainly affecting large myelinated fibres (Takahashi and Nakamora 1976), but the earliest changes affect the myelin (Erbslöh and Abel 1970). Thiamine is required for decarboxylation of α ketoacids and as a cofactor for transketolase, an enzyme involved in the pentose phosphate shunt. This may be important in neurons which are metabolically active.

Vitamin B_{12} Deficiency

In patients with neurological manifestations of vitamin B_{12} deficiency the possibility that a peripheral neuropathy co-exists with the changes in the posterior and lateral columns of the spinal cord has for long been a controversial issue. Woltmann, in 1919, thought that five of his 100 patients with pernicious anaemia had an associated peripheral neuropathy, but others have ascribed the clinical features of distal sensory impairment and absent distal reflexes wholly to involvement of posterior columns and nerve roots (Buzzard and Greenfield 1921). Glove and stocking sensory loss is unusual in subacute combined degeneration with pernicious anaemia but some of these patients show abnormalities of nerve conduction (Gilliatt et al. 1961; Mayer 1965), suggesting primary involvement of peripheral nerves (Fine and Hallett 1980). Mayer (1965) found that there was distal slowing of sensory conduction. The pathology of the peripheral nervous system in pernicious anaemia has not been systematically studied. It has been suggested that peripheral nerve involvement is part of an axonal degeneration (Foster 1945) but it is not clear that this is more than would be expected in relation to the extensive cord and posterior root ganglion lesions found in these severe cases. McLeod et al. (1969) provided histological evidence of axonal degeneration in the peripheral nervous system in B_{12} deficiency with clinical evidence of neuropathy. Whatever the pathogenesis of the glove and stocking sensory disturbance, improvement with vitamin B_{12} (hydroxocobalamin) treatment is usually substantial. It has been suggested that the underlying defect in the central and peripheral nervous system is an inability to resynthesise methionine by methylation from homocysteine (Scott et al. 1981). Folate administration in the presence of B_{12} deficiency exacerbates the neurological disorder because folic acid, by stimulating cell division, uses methionine for protein synthesis thus diverting it from methylation in myelin (Scott and Weir 1981).

Electrophysiological studies (Fine et al. 1990) show reduction in amplitude of sural SNAPs. Motor conduction velocities were normal or minimally slowed but the evoked motor responses were of reduced amplitude. EMG showed distal denervation. F responses showed increased chronodispersion in 7 of 10 patients, indicating loss of some large, fast-conducting fibres. Somatosensory evoked responses were abnormal from peroneal nerve stimulation. VERs were normal or mildly abnormal. BSAERs were normal (Fine et al. 1990). Tomado et al. (1988) found that central and peripheral sensory conduction improved with treatment with hydroxocobalamin. These features suggest that the lesion in the peripheral nervous system is a distal-proximal axonopathy.

Other B Group Vitamin Deficiencies

Other B group vitamin deficiencies may also be associated with clinical syndromes in which peripheral neuropathy occurs but these syndromes, for example nutritional burning feet syndrome, may not be due to single vitamin deficiencies but to a combination of vitamin deficiency and malnutrition. *Pellagra* itself, however, is probably the result of nicotinamide deficiency and a peripheral neuropathy may be a prominent manifestation. However, the neuropathy that accompanies the cutaneous lesions, and the encephalopathy in this syndrome are probably due to coincidental deficiency of other B group vitamins (see Victor 1984). Nutritional *pyridoxine deficiency* is unknown in man but inhibition of pyridoxine metabolism by isoniazid, a drug used in the treatment of tuberculosis, is a well-known cause of peripheral neuropathy (see below). In addition the ingestion of large quantities of pyridoxine (2 g or more daily) may cause degeneration of neurons in the dorsal root ganglia, and a disabling toxic sensory neuronopathy (Schaumberg et al. 1983a). Other B group vitamin deficiencies have not been associated with damage to the peripheral nervous system and vitamin A, vitamin C and vitamin D deficiencies similarly do not cause peripheral neuropathy.

Vitamin E Deficiency

This vitamin (α-tocopherol) is an important cofactor in the metabolism of the human nervous system, but symptomatic deficiency syndromes are rare (Muller 1986). Lloyd and colleagues (Muller et al. 1983) have summarised the evidence for the role of vitamin E deficiency in human neurological disorders. First, in abetalipoproteinaemia early treatment with vitamin E delays and may prevent the development of neurological complications, especially sensorimotor neuropathy and ataxia. Secondly, in other chronic disorders of fat absorption, e.g. steatorrhoea, cholestatic liver disease and cystic fibrosis (Guggenheim et al. 1982; Harding et al. 1982), neurological dysfunction can be improved by oral or parenteral administration of vitamin E (Elia et al. 1981; Guggenheim et al. 1982). Thirdly, the neuropathological changes reported in vitamin E-deficient humans are similar to those reported in vitamin E-deficient animals (Muller et al. 1983).

In acquired vitamin E deficiency, associated with malabsorption, extensive intestinal resection, steatorrhoea and cholestatic liver disease, there is a sensory ataxia, with loss of vibration sense and disturbed position sense, absent distal reflexes and sparing of pain and temperature sensation. Paraesthesiae may be prominent (Traber et al. 1987). In advanced cases muscular weakness and atrophy, either proximal or distal, may develop. Tomasi (1979) described a case of vitamin E deficiency with myopathy that resolved with treatment. In about half of the cases progressive external ophthalmoplegia is a feature. The clinical features resemble those of spino-cerebellar degeneration and in patients with Bassen–Kornzweig syndrome, associated with abetalipoproteinaemia, cerebellar ataxia, dysarthria and pigmentary retinal degeneration are prominent. Autopsy studies of these patients have shown myelin abnormalities in the spino-cerebellar pathways and in the cerebellum (Sobrevilla et al. 1964).

These changes are reversible with vitamin E therapy if treatment is initiated early in life (Muller 1986).

Familial isolated vitamin E deficiency, due to a transport defect, may present with peripheral neuropathy or a spino-cerebellar syndrome (Harding et al. 1985). A familial syndrome resembling Friedreich's ataxia, with vitamin E deficiency has been recognised in Tunisia. It is linked to chromosome 8 (Ben Hamida et al. 1994a). Harding et al.'s (1985) patient had normal nerve conduction velocity and EMG studies but abnormal somatosensory evoked responses. In Traber et al. (1987) two of five patients had mild abnormalities of sensory conduction, but the nerves contained reduced amounts of α-tocopherol.

Investigations. Serum vitamin E levels are so low as to be undetectable, and vitamin E levels in CSF, adipose tissue and peripheral nerves are similarly very low (Traber et al. 1987). Motor nerve conduction velocity is slightly slowed, or normal, and sensory nerve action potentials are of reduced amplitude, or absent. There may be EMG features of denervation in distal muscles (Schwartz et al. 1963; Miller et al. 1980). In those cases associated with abetalipoproteinaemia, the ECG may show ectopic beats and ventricular hypertrophy (Harding 1984), and the electroretinogram is abnormal in some patients. The CK may be slightly increased and peripheral blood films may show acanthocytes. Muscle biopsies reveal neurogenic changes with fibre atrophy, grouped reinnervation and sometimes target fibres. Myopathic changes are not prominent. The CSF is normal.

In animal studies selective loss of large myelinated fibres in sensory tracts in the spinal cord and peripheral nerves have been reported, and similar abnormalities have been reported in sural nerve biopsies in patients with vitamin E deficient neuropathy (Miller et al. 1980). Axonal spheroids and dystrophy have been noted in the gracile columns (Sung et al. 1980; Rosenblum et al. 1981).

Treatment. Vitamin E supplementation is essential. This may be given orally, but parenteral therapy is usually necessary because of the problem of malabsorption with which this syndrome is so frequently associated. Harding et al. (1985) reported a case in which selective vitamin E malabsorption seemed to lead to a spino-cerebellar syndrome with neuropathy that was reversed with vitamin E treatment. Doses of the order of 100 mg/kg per day have been recommended (Muller et al. 1983). In some patients coincidental deficiency of vitamin A, another fat-soluble vitamin, has been suspected and this should probably also be supplemented.

Tropical Ataxic Neuropathy

In Africa and the Caribbean, methionine deficiency with associated chronic intoxication with cyanogenetic glycosides derived from dietary sources, e.g. cassava, may lead to ataxic neuropathy (Osuntokun 1981). This syndrome is believed to differ from tropical spastic paraplegia (TSP), a disorder associated with HTLV-1 infection. Tropical ataxic neuropathy (TAN) is a syndrome of burning feet with normal strength, severe distal sensory loss, absent ankle and knee jerks and sensory ataxia. Sural nerves show severe axonal loss with few signs of regeneration (Vallat et al. 1987a). This syndrome has been recognised in tropical Africa, e.g. in the Ivory Coast. It is assumed to be due to malnutrition.

Hypothyroid Neuropathy

Symptomatic polyneuropathy is rare in hypothyroidism, although 80% of patients have paraesthesiae in the hands, due to carpal tunnel syndrome associated with thickening of the transverse carpal ligament. A tarsal tunnel syndrome may also occur from ligamentous thickening (Schwartz et al. 1983). Although distal sensory thresholds are reduced in many patients, the ankle reflexes are present. The reflex may show a characteristic slowed contraction and relaxation phase, due to abnormal excitation/ contraction relationships in the muscle fibres. Deafness is a frequent feature, and some patients show cerebellar ataxia, and a mild dementia with personality change. Studies of the peripheral nerves have shown mild slowing of sensory and motor conduction (Martin et al. 1983). Dyck and Lambert (1970) found mild axonal degeneration with secondary demyelination in nerve biopsies (Pollard et al. 1982). Muscle is also involved, with cramps and fatigue. Severe neuropathy is very rare in hypothyroidism, mainly causing sensory deficits and ataxia (Dyck and Lambert 1970).

Acromegalic Neuropathy

A mild sensorimotor neuropathy, often associated with carpal tunnel syndrome, is a feature of acromegaly. Thirty-five of 100 patients reviewed by O'Duffy et al. (1973) had carpal tunnel syndrome.

Dinn and Dinn (1985) found segmental demyelination and onion-bulb formation in sural nerve biopsies from nine patients. Low et al. (1974) reported mild sensorimotor neuropathy in five of 11 acromegalic patients. Ulnar and peroneal nerves were enlarged. Sural biopsies showed increased perineurial tissue, reduced numbers of myelinated and unmyelinated fibres, segmental demyelination and single onion bulb formation. There is a mild reduction in motor conduction velocity.

Neuropathies Associated with Malignant Disease and Dysproteinaemias

Involvement of peripheral nerves in patients with cancer may be due to extrinsic compression or infiltration by tumour, metabolic disturbances, chemotherapy or remote effects. Peripheral neuropathies occurring as a remote non-metastatic complication of malignant disease have been reported in association with a number of different carcinomas, and with the lymphomas and other reticuloses. The concept was first clearly delineated by Denny-Brown (1948) and examined in detail in a large series of cases, reported from the London Hospital, by Brain and colleagues (Henson and Urich 1970). Carcinoma of the lung in men, carcinomas of the breast and ovary in women and lymphomas in both sexes are particularly commonly associated with neuropathy. Neuropathies in patients with lymphomas, however, may sometimes be due not to a non-metastatic complication of the disease, but to widespread invasion of nerves or nerve roots by the lymphoma itself. This can also occur with other lymphomas or carcinomas, and it is an important consideration because of the possibility of effective treatment by radiotherapy or by cytotoxic drugs. These drugs may themselves cause peripheral neuropathy in patients with cancer and in some patients cachexia and malnutrition may lead to neuropathy; these different causes of neuropathy have led to some controversy as to the frequency of peripheral neuropathy as a non-metastatic complication of malignant disease in different surveys (Croft and Wilkinson 1965; Brain and Norris 1965; Currie et al. 1970; McLeod 1984).

A number of other non-metastatic complications of malignant disease are recognised including central disorders such as carcinomatous cerebellar degeneration, carcinomatous myelopathy and carci-

nomatous encephalitis but peripheral neuropathy is far commoner than these. Further, polymyositis associated with carcinoma is a relatively common non-metastatic complication of malignant disease. The combination of proximal weakness with muscular wasting and decreased or absent tendon reflexes that occurs in some patients with cancer led to the use of the all-embracing term "carcinomatous neuromyopathy" (Henson and Urich 1970), but this confusing terminology has now been abandoned.

The clinical syndromes, their association with cancer, and recognised circulating antibodies are listed in Table 11.2.

Paraneoplastic Sensory Neuropathy

In this syndrome (Denny-Brown 1948) the major clinical feature is usually a profound sensory ataxia with pseudo-athetoid distal movements of the hands. The onset is usually subacute but may occur within a few days. The syndrome is sometimes asymmetrical. There is marked sensory loss to all modalities, including position and vibration sense and to two-point discrimination in all four limbs and this may be demonstrable in proximal as well as in distal joints. The arms are often more affected than the legs. Light touch is disturbed in a glove and stocking distribution, but pinprick and temperature sense is less affected. There may be distal paraesthesiae and this can be severe, disabling and painful in some cases. Weakness and atrophy of muscles occurs in the late stages of the syndrome. The tendon reflexes are all absent. In some cases there are associated features of carcinomatous brain-stem encephalitis, with nystagmus, and signs of autonomic neuropathy, including orthostatic hypotension, and pupillary paralysis may also occur. Symptoms of sensory neuropathy usually precede discovery of the underlying carcinoma by 5–16 months but this interval may be several years (Henson and Urich 1970). The carcinoma is almost invariably a smoking-related small cell carcinoma of the lung. Croft and Wilkinson (1969) noted that nine of their 11 cases were women. The mean survival of their patients was 14 months. There is little evidence that treatment of the carcinoma influences the course of the neuropathy (Croft et al. 1965), although some patients with sensory neuropathy in whom regression of the lung tumour occurred have been reported (Darnell and De Angelis 1993). It is characteristic that after an initial period of progression the disorder often enters a period of relative stability.

Henson and Urich (1970) have stressed the association of the clinical features of carcinomatous encephalomyelitis, with inflammatory lesions in

Table 11.2. Paraneoplastic syndromes affecting nerve and muscles

Syndrome	Neoplasm	Antibody
Neuropathies		
Subacute sensory neuropathy	Small cell lung cancer Other cancers	Type IIa pan-neuronal anti-Hu 34-42 kD proteins
Sensorimotor neuropathy	Carcinoma, lymphoma and myeloma	No single factor recognised
Guillain–Barré syndrome	Hodgkin's disease	Unknown
Mononeuritis multiplex	Small cell lung cancer, lymphoma	Unknown
Intestinal pseudo-obstruction (autonomic neuropathy)	Small cell lung cancer	IgG antibody to neurons of myenteric and sub-mucosal plexi
Neopathies associated with paraproteinaemia	Myeloma B cell lymphoma Benign paraproteinaemia	IgM/IgG/IgE antibodies
Acquired amyloid polyneuropathy	Myeloma Dysproteinaemias	
Disorders of Neuromuscular Junction		
Myasthenia gravis	Thymoma	Unknown
Lambert–Eaton myasthenic syndrome	Small cell lung cancer	IgG antibody to voltage-dependent calcium channel at neuromuscular junction
Muscle Disorders		
Polymyositis-dermatomyositis	Small cell lung cancer, breast and ovary cancer, lymphoma	See text
Subacute necrotising myopathy	Carcinoma, lymphoma	Unknown

brain stem and cervical spinal cord with this syndrome and regard them as part of the same nosological entity. Thus, most patients with sensory neuropathy show nystagmus and ataxia of the cerebellar type in the limbs and many develop mental changes, including memory impairment, during the course of their illness. Other common features include extensor plantar responses and vertigo. Chalk et al. (1992) reported 26 cases, of whom half had associated neurological syndromes, particularly autonomic, cerebellar and cerebral features, that were also paraneoplastic. Twenty of their cases were women. They suggested that prominent pain is a particular feature of this syndrome.

Paraneoplastic Mixed Sensorimotor Neuropathy

This is the most common neuropathy associated with malignant disease.

There are three main syndromes. In the *subacute* or chronic form the disorder is mild and of insidious onset, usually becoming evident months or years after diagnosis of the carcinoma itself. Indeed, it often occurs in the terminal stages of the illness. The legs are affected more than the arms and there is mild distal sensory impairment and weakness with diminished tendon reflexes. There is often mild proximal muscular weakness (Croft et al. 1967). Trigeminal sensory loss may be a feature.

An *acute* form also occurs. This may present before or after the carcinoma has become apparent. The typical features of distal sensorimotor neuropathy are present but respiratory and bulbar signs may be present. The mean survival was 27 months in Croft and Wilkinson's (1969) series and during this time there may be little progression of the neuropathy. This syndrome resembles Guillain–Barré syndrome (Lisak et al. 1977).

In a third form a *remitting and relapsing* course is characteristic (Croft and Wilkinson 1969). In this group mean survival was only 16 months after the onset. The relapsing form of sensorimotor neuropathy may precede diagnosis of the tumour. This form of the neuropathy seems to be more strongly associated with carcinoma of the lung than the other two subgroups of sensorimotor neuropathy but it may occur with other tumours, e.g. seminoma of the testis, and carcinomas of breast, uterus, thymus, stomach and cervix (Henson and Urich 1970). Improvement has been noted after steroid therapy, or after removal or other treatment of the primary neoplasm (Littler 1970a; McLeod 1984).

Paraneoplastic Autonomic Neuropathy

This rare complication, most frequently associated with small cell carcinoma of the lung, presents as recurrent or chronic intestinal pseudo-obstruction caused by intestinal dysmotility. Lennon et al.

(1991) found circulating autoantibodies to enteric neurons in this syndrome.

Paraneoplastic Vasculitic Neuropathy

A few cases of subacute, asymmetrical sensorimotor neuropathy, usually in men, associated with lymphoma or small cell lung cancer have been described (Oh et al. 1991b). The CSF protein and ESR are raised and there may be a few lymphocytes in the CSF. Nerve biopsy shows vasculitis with axonal neuropathy, and there is mild slowing of motor and sensory conduction. The syndrome responds slowly to immunosuppressive therapy and steroids (Oh et al. 1991b).

Types of Neoplasm

Neuropathy may be associated with a variety of different neoplasms (Henson and Urich 1970).

There are differences in the relative frequency of the association of the different types of neuropathy with different carcinomas. Sensory neuropathy is almost invariably associated with oat cell carcinoma of the lung (Dayan et al. 1965) but it has also been reported with carcinoma of the oesophagus or caecum (McLeod 1984). The mild form of mixed sensorimotor neuropathy, which usually occurs in the terminal stages of the cancer, is associated principally with carcinomas of lung, breast or stomach (Croft et al. 1967). The subacute variety of mixed sensorimotor neuropathy occurs with many different cancers but the majority are found in patients with carcinoma of the lung. The remitting relapsing form, however, is mainly found with cancers of the breast, cervix, uterus, bladder, testis and thymus, and is relatively uncommon with carcinoma of the lung (Croft and Wilkinson 1969).

Incidence

The incidence of neuropathies associated with malignant disease is a controversial topic because there are differences in ascertainment of cases in different surveys (Henson and Urich 1982). Furthermore, clinical examination alone leads to recognition of abnormalities in a smaller percentage of patients than clinical examination combined with electrophysiological assessment. In carcinoma of the lung clinical signs of peripheral neuropathy are found in about 5% of patients (Croft and Wilkinson 1965; Trojaborg et al. 1969). Electromyographic evi-

dence of a subclinical neuropathy, however, was found in 36% of such patients (Trojaborg et al. 1969; Donofrio et al. 1989). The next most common associated neoplasms are carcinoma of the stomach and breast. In reticuloses, sensory neuropathy is exceptionally rare (Currie et al. 1970) and mixed sensorimotor neuropathy is also uncommon, occurring in less than 1% of patients studied by Currie et al. (1970) when myeloma (see below) was excluded. Teravainen and Larsen (1977) found an overall incidence of clinical or electrophysiological evidence of peripheral neuropathy in 48% of their 33 patients with lung cancer. Hawley et al. (1980) noted that the incidence of neuropathy in patients with oat cell carcinoma was not increased in the early stages of the disease, but all their 71 patients showed features of neuropathy when their body weight had decreased by 15% or more. These incidence figures exclude the development of neuropathy in these patients during the course of treatment with cytotoxic drugs (see *Drug-Induced Neuropathies*).

An acute or relapsing polyneuropathy resembling Guillain-Barré syndrome occurs in patients with Hodgkin's disease and other lymphomas (Lisak et al. 1977; McLeod 1984), and in seminoma of the testis (McLeod 1984). This neuropathy may develop when the lymphoma is active, or in remission. The acquired amyloid neuropathies, associated with dysgammaglobulinaemias, are discussed under the latter heading. Peripheral nerve involvement is common in patients with cancer treated with chemotherapy. Indeed, this is a far commoner cause of neuropathy than remote complications of the tumour itself. Vinca alkaloids are particularly important in causing such toxic neuropathies (Weiss et al. 1974; Correale et al. 1991).

Pathogenesis

Wilkinson (1964) and Wilkinson and Zeromski (1965) found serum anti-nerve antibodies by an immunofluorescent technique in four cases of sensory neuropathy but not in patients with mixed sensorimotor neuropathy (Wilkinson 1964). Paty et al. (1974) found increased macrophage sensitivity to peripheral nerve antigen in patients with lung cancer and neuropathy. The significance of these findings was uncertain until the more recent demonstration that neuron-specific antineuronal antibodies could be detected in serum and CSF of patients with paraneoplastic syndromes involving both peripheral and central nervous systems, including peripheral nerve, retina and cerebellum. The presence of antineuronal antibodies represents an immunological response by the host immune system to the tumour. Three patterns of anti-neuronal antibodies have been recognised (Schiller and Jones 1993).

Type 1 antibodies react against Purkinje cell cytoplasm; these antibodies recognise the 34 and 62 kDa antigens of Purkinje cells (anti-Yo antibodies) (Petersen et al. 1992). Type IIa antibodies (anti-Hu) recognise 34–42 kDa proteins found in the cotyplasm of all neurons (Delman et al. 1992). Type IIb antibodies (anti-Ri) also recognise nuclear and cytoplasmic antigens found in all neurons, of 53–61 kDa and 79–84 kDa. Type IIb antibodies are often related to breast cancer and their presence is associated with the opsoclonus-ataxia syndrome. Type IIa antibodies are associated with sensory ataxia and encephalomyelitis-ataxia, and occur especially in patients in whom this paraneoplastic syndrome is linked to the presence of small cell carcinoma of the lung (Delman et al. 1992). Rarely these antibodies, and this syndrome, may develop in patients with cancer of the breast. Retinal degeneration is associated with anti-retinal antibodies that recognise a 23–25 kDa protein, and occurs in patients with small cell cancer of the lung (Polans et al. 1991). Kiers et al. (1991) have suggested that small cell lung cancer is particularly antigenic because of its propensity to undergo necrosis in the centre of tumour masses, leading to the release of antigen and inducing an IgG antibody response.

Sensory neuropathy may be a particularly common feature of paraneoplastic syndromes because the dorsal root ganglion cells are outside the blood-brain barrier. The prognosis and outcome, however, seem not to be related to antibody levels in the blood. Jean et al. (1994) explored the lymphocyte subclasses present in inflammatory cell exudates in patients with anti-Hu positive paraneoplastic encephalomyelitis. They suggest that anti-Hu IgG may be internalised by neurons and inhibit a protein essential for maintaining neuronal phenotype.

Laboratory Investigations

Apart from investigations appropriate to the diagnosis and management of the underlying carcinoma, the CSF examination is useful. The CSF protein is usually raised in all types of neuropathy apart from the mild "terminal" sensorimotor neuropathy. The CSF is usually acellular, but in those patients in whom an encephalitic illness is associated with sensory neuropathy the CSF may show a lymphocytosis, with a normal blood/CSF glucose ratio. Assay of neuron-specific antibodies in the blood (above) is useful in determining the immune basis of these paraneoplastic syndromes.

When a sensory or acute sensorimotor neuropathy occurs in a patient aged 60 years or more (Croft et al. 1965) it is reasonable to consider the possibility that there may be an underlying carcinoma, if other causes of neuropathy, such as diabetes, have been excluded. In these patients the chest X-ray and cytological examination of the sputum are most likely to lead to discovery of the causative lesion. Endoscopic bronchoscopy is also useful. Clinical and radiographic examination of the breasts should also be undertaken in women and the cervix should be examined. Routine haematological and biochemical studies may also be useful but more complex procedures are not only unlikely to reveal a causative neoplasm but will almost certainly not lead to treatment. If no tumour is discovered the chest X-ray should be repeated at intervals of several months.

Electrophysiological Assessment

The motor conduction velocity is usually normal in both sensory and sensorimotor neuropathies but in some patients it may be mildly slowed (Moody 1965; Croft et al. 1967; Trojaborg et al. 1969), particularly in advanced cases (Donofrio et al. 1989). Sensory conduction, on the other hand, is usually abnormal and the sensory nerve action potentials may be unobtainable with surface electrode recordings (Croft et al. 1967; Trojaborg et al. 1969). Motor conduction is normal in patients with typical sensory neuropathy, but may be mildly slowed in advanced cases (Donofrio et al. 1989; Chalk et al. 1992).

Campbell and Paty (1974) found slowing of motor and sensory conduction in some of their patients with sensorimotor neuropathy. Concentric needle EMG shows evidence of denervation, most marked in distal muscles, and fibrillation potentials and fasciculations may be recorded in distal muscles in patients with sensorimotor neuropathy (Trojaborg et al. 1969; Campbell and Paty 1974). These features suggest an axonal disorder. In the proximal muscles of these patients short-duration, low-amplitude polyphasic units are often found (Moody 1965; Campbell and Paty 1974), a feature that may be taken to lend support to the concept that the proximal weakness often found in these patients is due to an associated myopathy (see Croft et al. 1967), the so-called "neuromyopathy". Repetitive nerve stimulation should always be assessed in these patients in order to test for the presence of the myasthenic syndrome (Lambert–Eaton syndrome: see Chapter 12).

In patients with Guillain–Barré syndrome associated with Hodgkin's disease and in patients with the relapsing/remitting type of sensorimotor neuropathy motor and sensory conduction velocities may be markedly slowed, features suggestive of a demyelinating neuropathy.

Pathological Features

The muscle biopsy shows scattered small atrophic fibres (Hildebrand and Coërs 1967). Grouped denervation may be found in distal muscles, for example in small hand muscles studied at autopsy (Henson and Urich 1970). In the proximal muscles mild myopathic changes may occur, but these have not been well characterised. Hildebrand and Coërs (1967) found evidence of collateral ramification of the terminal innervation in some of their cases. The peripheral nerves have been studied at autopsy, but reports of sural nerve or other nerve biopsies taken at earlier stages of the disease are not available. Henson and Urich (1970) have emphasised the occurrence of segmental demyelination as being more prominent than axonal degeneration. There is increased cellularity in the nerves, probably from Schwann cell proliferation, and there may be a sparse lymphocytic infiltration in a perivascular distribution in the endoneurium and epineurium. The extent of axonal damage varies from case to case and when this is severe there may be fibrosis of the nerve. In sensory neuropathy the peripheral nerves show marked loss of myelinated nerve fibres, especially evident in sensory nerves. There is severe loss of nerve cells in the posterior root ganglia, loss of fibres in the posterior nerve roots, particularly in the cervical and lumbar regions, and Wallerian degeneration in the posterior columns (Croft et al. 1965; Henson and Urich 1970, 1982). These pathological features are characteristic of the terminal stages of the neuropathy and it is difficult to compare them with the electrophysiological abnormalities which are more consistent with a primary axonal disorder, rather than a demyelinating process.

Other pathological features, found in some cases, especially in patients with sensory neuropathy, include patchy lymphocytic infiltration of the temporal lobe, brain stem and spinal cord with destruction of nerve cells. The motor nuclei of the brain stem and cervical cord may be particularly involved (see Henson and Urich 1970). No malignant cells are found in the CSF or root pouches.

Management

In the relapsing form of mixed sensorimotor neuropathy steroid therapy may be useful, but in the other neuropathies no treatment is effective. Treatment of the underlying cancer is not usually helpful, although there are instances in the literature of remission of mixed sensorimotor neuropathy after removal of seminomas of the testis (Littler 1970a; Evans and Kaufman 1971) and of renal carcinoma (Swan and Wharton 1963). Dalmau et al. (1992) noted that none of their 71 patients with paraneoplastic encephalomyelitis and sensory neuropathy associated with anti-Hu antibodies responded to any treatment, including surgery, chemotherapy, radiotherapy, steroids, plasma exchange or immunosuppressive therapy. Although some patients become stable, a phase of lack of progression frequently occurs without treatment (Henson and Urich 1970).

Infiltration of Nerve Roots and Nerves

Direct infiltration of nerves and nerve roots is relatively common in lymphomas and in multiple myeloma but is a less common complication of carcinomas, except in breast carcinoma which may frequently invade the brachial plexus. Of 989 patients with lymphoma only 4% had compression of nerve roots or spinal cord (Correale et al. 1991). In most instances of direct invasion of the peripheral nervous system there is an asymmetrical multiple mononeuropathy. The clinical syndrome depends on the pattern of involvement of the peripheral nervous system (Urich 1974). In some of these cases there is an associated carcinomatous or lymphomatous meningitis (Henson and Urich 1982). The CSF shows a cellular response in many cases, with a raised protein and a low glucose level, and cytological examination of the CSF may reveal neoplastic cells. Intradural tumour deposits can be demonstrated by myelography, or by X-ray, CT or MRI. Occasionally a nerve lesion may occur from haemorrhage into a nerve in acute leukaemia, or other bleeding diatheses.

Neuropathies Associated with Monoclonal Gammopathies

Monoclonal gammopathies are a group of abnormal plasma proteins, secreted by a clone of plasma cells, consisting of homogeneous IgG fractions. Monoclonal gammopathies may be associated with a malignant clone of plasma cells, as in multiple myeloma or solitary plasmacytoma or, more commonly, may occur as a benign disorder. Peripheral neuropathy may be a feature of both malignant and benign gammopathies (Kissel and Mendell 1996). Monoclonal gammopathy is found in about 10% of patients with peripheral neuropathy of unknown cause (Kelly et al. 1981b). In a normal population the prevalence of monoclonal gammopathy is 0.1% in the third decade and 3% in the eighth decade (Kyle et al. 1972). The incidence of polyneuropathy associated with monoclonal gammopathy increases with increasing age; as many as 2/1000 people older than 50 years have this syndrome (Kelly et al. 1981b). The disorders associated with monoclonal gammopathy are listed in Table 11.3.

Table 11.3. Disorders associated with monoclonal gammopathy

Monoclonal gammopathy of undetermined significance (MGUS)
(Benign gammopathy)

Malignant plasma cell dyscrasia
Multiple myeloma
Plasmacytoma
Waldenström's macroglobulinaemia
Heavy chain disease (HCD)
Primary amyloidosis (light chain type)
Lymphoma
Cryoglobulinaemia

Each monoclonal protein is secreted by a clone of plasma cells in the bone marrow, and consists of two heavy polypeptide chains of the same class and two light chains of the same type. There are five types of heavy chain – γ in IgG, α in IgA, μ in IgM, δ in IgD and ϵ in IgE. IgG protein exists in four subclasses; IgG1, IgG2, IgG3 and IgG4, and there are two subclasses of IgA; IgA1 and IgA2. Light chains exist in two forms, the kappa (κ) and lambda (λ) chains.

Neuropathy Associated with MGUS (Table 11.3)

This is the most common of the neuropathies associated with monoclonal gammopathy. The syndrome is clinically heterogeneous, presenting with distal weakness, sensory loss and sometimes with autonomic disturbance. The disorder is chronic and slowly progressive. The CSF protein is raised. The clinical syndrome may be mild or severe. In some patients there is proximal weakness, a feature often associated with demyelination (Gosselin et al. 1991). Remission is unusual and there may be marked disability. The MGUS may be IgM, IgA or IgG in type. There is no relation between the level of abnormal circulating protein and the development of neuropathy or its severity. The neuropathy may be present even when the total IgG, IgM and IgA levels are normal. Sensory ataxia is more frequent in patients with IgM-associated neuropathies (Kyle

and Dyck 1993). This syndrome is similar to that found in patients with chronic inflammatory demyelinating peripheral neuropathy (CIDP), particularly in patients with MGUS IgG and IgA associated neuropathies. Extended follow-up of patients with MGUS associated neuropathy reveals that there is an increasing incidence of multiple myeloma, amyloidosis, macroglobulinaemia or other lymphoproliferative disorders, reaching 33% at 20 years follow-up (Kyle and Dyck 1993). Two-thirds of these patients developed multiple myeloma, with a median interval of 10 years from presentation.

Electrophysiological Assessment

The electrophysiological findings are variable, reflecting the range of pathology. Conduction velocity may be slowed (Fitting et al. 1979; Swash et al. 1979a), with conduction block (Smith et al. 1983) in patients with demyelinating neuropathy; in patients with axonal neuropathy conduction is only mildly slowed (Kelly 1983).

Pathology

Half the patients with IgM monoclonal gammopathy associated with peripheral neuropathy have circulating IgM κ antibody directed against an epitope shared by peripheral nerve glycolipid, the myelin-associated glycoprotein (MAG) and neuronal surface antigens (O'Shaunessy et al. 1986). The peripheral nerves show segmental demyelination and axonal loss, with preservation of small unmyelinated fibres (Swash et al. 1979a; Smith et al. 1983). IgM has been found in the myelin of the peripheral nerves (Propp et al. 1975; Chazot et al. 1976) as has amyloid (Bigner et al. 1971).

The deposition of IgM in peripheral nerve myelin in these neuropathies is of uncertain significance (see Swash et al. 1979a; Smith et al. 1983). While it is possible that IgM deposition is part of an immune process causing myelin destruction and axonal loss (Latov et al. 1981) studies with other normal and damaged peripheral nerves in in vitro experiments in which nerve sections were incubated with paraprotein taken from a patient with neuropathy suggest that IgM deposition simply reflects blood–nerve permeability (Swash et al. 1979a). An immunological specificity of circulating antibody to MAG in these neuropathies has been reported in a proportion of patients with dysproteinaemias (Braun et al. 1982); Freddo et al. 1985), but it may be a secondary immunological epiphenomenon rather than a primary process (Kelly 1985).

Haffler et al. (1986) noted that anti-MAG activity was associated with a slowly progressive, predominantly sensory neuropathy, and that these patients did not respond to treatment with plasma exchange or chemotherapy. This syndrome has been further delineated by Latov et al. (1988) and Kelly et al. (1988) who noted a slowly progressive syndrome with numbness and ataxia, areflexia and mild distal weakness, without pain. The peripheral nerves may be thickened. These features are consistent with the pathological features, which consist of demyelination with axonal loss. The outer lamellae of myelin may be split and widened and IgM is demonstrable in these lamellae. It is rare for IgA or IgG to be deposited on peripheral nerve myelin, even in the presence of Iga or IgG gammopathies. This syndrome is often an axonal neuropathy and Nemmi et al. (1990) reported that the IgG κ protein in their case bound to a neurofilament protein. However, demyelinating and axonal syndromes occur with IgG and IgA monoclonal proteins (Bailey et al. 1986).

Management

A number of different treatments have been tried with variable results. Although Dyck et al. (1991) reported that patients with IgG and IgA associated neuropathies responded better than those with IgM proteins, in a double-blind trial of plasma exchange, others have found little or no difference. Indeed, other treatments, such as prednisone, chlorambucil, cyclophosphamide and intravenous gammaglobulin, have all been reported to be effective in a varying proportion of patients, regardless of the monoclonal gammopathy (Simmonds et al. 1993a). Differences in response between demyelinating and axonal syndromes might be expected but the literature is unclear on this point. The neuropathy may be present with modest or marked quantities of monoclonal circulating protein and there is no precise relation between the change in level of abnormal protein and clinical recovery, when it occurs (Kelly et al. 1988).

Neuropathy Associated with Myeloma

Peripheral neuropathy in patients with myeloma is of variable severity and clinical type. The neuropathy is usually associated with a monoclonal IgM protein in the blood. Overall, as many as 13% of patients with myeloma develop neuropathy, but electrophysiological abnormalities are found in as many as 39% (Walsh 1971). In a retrospective survey, however, Currie et al. (1970) found an incidence of neuropathy of only 3%, and Kelly (1981b) reported an incidence of 5%.

The neuropathies found in patients with myeloma can be related to the two main types of the disease, i.e. to multiple myeloma with osteolytic lesions, and to osteosclerotic or solitary myeloma. In addition, amyloidosis (AL amyloid) may complicate myeloma and this may result in an acquired amyloid neuropathy.

In *osteolytic myeloma* three types of neuropathy have been recognised. *Symmetrical sensorimotor neuropathy* is the most common (Davis and Drachman 1972; Kelly et al. 1981a,b; Kelly 1983, 1985). This is usually a mild disorder, frequently beginning in the feet with an ascending course. Pain or dysaesthesiae may be prominent and the distal reflexes are absent. The neuropathy tends to parallel the clinical state of the patient, becoming worse when the disease progresses, or when there is weight loss. It must be distinguished from neuropathies associated coincidentally with cytotoxic chemotherapy. A *pure sensory neuropathy* also occurs, resembling that found associated with small cell carcinoma of the lung. A predominantly *motor form* that is progressive and that may resemble Guillain–Barré syndrome may develop during the course of osteolytic myeloma (Kelly et al. 1981a). In some cases cranial nerve palsies may develop, even involving the tongue.

The *osteosclerotic* form of myeloma is less common than the osteolytic variety, occurring in only 3% of patients with myeloma (Reitan et al. 1980). However, neuropathy may be a complicating factor in half of these patients (Iwashita et al. 1977; Kelly et al. 1983). They are predominantly male and the mean age of onset of neuropathy is lower than in the paraneoplastic neuropathies complicating osteolytic myeloma. The neuropathy was present for a mean duration of 20 months before myeloma was recognised in the patients described by Kelly et al. (1983). The diagnostic feature in these patients was the presence of solitary or multiple osteosclerotic lesions on X-ray (Driedger and Pruzanski 1980). Read and Warlow (1978) noted that more than 90% of patients in whom neuropathy was associated with *solitary plasmacytoma* were men. The neuropathy is sensorimotor with prominent motor features. It is usually slowly progressive but a more rapidly progressive form with severe disability within a year of onset is recognised. The CSF protein is usually raised and immunoelectrophoresis of plasma reveals monoclonal protein in low concentration. The bone marrow, however, may reveal little or no abnormality. In a subgroup of patients, pigmentation, endocrine disturbances (including gynaeco-mastia, impotence, hypothyroidism and diabetes mellitus), peripheral oedema, pleural effusion, hepatosplenomegaly, lymphadenopathy, hirsuitism and excessive sweating have been described. The syndrome was first clearly recognised in Japan (Iwashita et al. 1977; Bardwick et al. 1980; Nakanishi et al. 1984). It has been termed POEMS, an acronym for peripheral neuropathy, organomegaly, endo-crinopathy, monoclonal gammopathy and skin changes (Bardwick et al. 1980). Miralles et al. (1992) concluded that there was no clinical value in attempting to distinguish POEMS from osteoscle-rotic myeloma with peripheral neuropathy. They also noted that the survival of patients with multiple myeloma was 20% at 5 years, but that of patients with plasma cell dyscrasia was 60% at 5 years follow-up.

About 20% of patients have *amyloidosis* of light chain type (Kelly et al. 1979, 1981b). In these patients the neuropathy is of sensorimotor type, but autonomic features, especially impotence and pos-tural hypotension, are often present. Pain is also a particular feature of this syndrome, with relatively selective loss of pain and temperature sensation. Kyle and Bayard (1975) noted that of 61 patients with amyloidosis secondary to myelomatosis, 33% had peripheral neuropathy. Carpal tunnel syndrome was a presenting feature in 32%.

Laboratory Investigations

The CSF protein is raised in many cases, especially those with severe neuropathies associated with osteosclerotic myeloma (Kelly 1985). The CSF cell count is normal. In the blood there is almost invari-ably an abnormality in the serum proteins in patients with multiple myelomatosis. With immu-noelectrophoretic studies a raised IgM, with a mono-clonal distribution, is found in about 80% of patients with neuropathy; 40% of such patients have Bence Jones protein in their urine (Davis and Drachman 1972). The diagnosis of myelomatosis can often be suspected, therefore, from these studies. In about 10% of the patients with myeloma and neuropathy reviewed by Davis and Drachman (1972), however, no abnormal protein was found in blood or urine. A raised ESR with anaemia, multiple lytic or sclerotic lesions in bone X-rays, and the finding of plasma cell infiltration of the bone marrow are useful points in diagnosis. The diagno-sis of osteosclerotic myeloma or solitary plasmacy-toma is more difficult unless the tumour is biopsied, or it secretes monoclonal IgM or IgG. In Read and Warlow's (1978) review of neuropathy associated

with solitary plasmacytoma the ESR was normal in all cases and only two of 15 patients showed a para-protein; however, the CSF protein was raised in all of these cases.

Electrophysiological Assessment

In patients with myelomatosis, but without clinical signs of neuropathy, Walsh (1971) found that there was mild slowing of motor and sensory nerve con-duction velocity in all the nerves studied in 39% of patients. In several other patients there was localised slowing at sites of potential nerve entrap-ment, e.g. in the median nerve at the wrist and in the common peroneal nerve at the head of the fibula.

Motor conduction velocity is markedly slowed in the predominantly motor polyneuropathy associ-ated with osteosclerotic myeloma (Davis and Drachman 1972; Kelly et al. 1981a). The sensory nerve action potentials are usually absent. In the neuropathy associated with amyloidosis in patients with myeloma the main abnormality is carpal tunnel syndrome, with electrophysiological features of mild sensorimotor neuropathy.

Concentric needle EMG studies show evidence of partial denervation in distal muscles, with fibrilla-tion potentials at rest and polyphasic MUAPs of long duration with a reduced interference pattern during voluntary contraction.

Nerve Biopsy

Sural nerve biopsies have been studied by Hesselvik (1969) and by Walsh (1971). The major finding in these studies was axonal degeneration. Nerve fibres not undergoing degeneration were usually normal but some fibres with short internodal lengths, suggesting regeneration, were seen. Segmental demyelination was less marked except in the neuropathy associated with osteosclerotic myeloma (Dayan et al. 1971). In other studies of necropsy material axonal degeneration was found to be more prominent distally than proximally and segmental demyelination of varying severity has been recorded (McLeod and Walsh 1975). Lymphocytic infiltration and small plasma cell infiltrates have been recorded in relation to endoneurial blood vessels, but these are not prominent changes (Victor et al. 1958; Hesselvik 1969). Amyloid may be found in the peripheral nerves in myelomatosis (Davies-Jones and Esiri 1971). Dayan et al. (1971) noted that amyloid deposition in the transverse carpal liga-ment occurred in one of their patients.

Course and Prognosis

Improvement in the neuropathy may follow radiotherapy in patients with localised lesions. Davis and Drachman (1972) found that in 27% of their patients the neuropathy improved with treatment, but none improved spontaneously. In one patient there was a marked improvement in motor nerve conduction velocity during a phase of clinical improvement which continued for 18 months. We have observed a man in whom a solitary plasmacytoma was associated with neuropathy. Improvement followed radiotherapy and a subsequent deterioration in his neuropathy a year later led to further investigation. A second plasmacytoma was found and, after this was irradiated, his neuropathy again improved. In one of Davis and Drachman's (1972) patients no recurrence of neuropathy or myeloma occurred 10 years after irradiation of a plasmacytoma. Treatment of patients with generalised myelomatosis is more difficult, however, even with cytotoxic drug therapy (Driedger and Pruzanski 1980). The osteosclerotic form of myeloma responds to treatment with radiotherapy, and with melphalan and prednisolone, with improvement also in the neuropathy (Driedger and Pruzanski 1980; Reitan et al. 1980). Plasma exchange appears not to be helpful (Kelly 1985). The prognosis reflects the severity and extent of the underlying myeloma.

Other Neuropathies Associated with Paraproteinaemia

Peripheral neuropathy may also occur in other diseases in which paraproteins circulate in the blood (Table 11.3), such as Waldenström's macroglobulinaemia, lymphoma, leukaemia, cryoglobulinaemia (Vallat et al. 1980) and Castleman's disease (Frizzera et al. 1983).

Waldenström's Macroglobulinaemia

This is a disorder of men older than 60 years, presenting with weakness, fatigue, anaemia and nasal haemorrhage. There is often blurred vision with retinal haemorrhages, cutaneous haemorrhages, renal impairment, deafness and congestive heart failure. A sensorimotor neuropathy is common in this disease. There is a monoclonal IgM protein in the blood, of high molecular weight consisting of a kappa light chain in most instances. The neuropathy is usually demyelinating in type. A demyelinat-

ing syndrome resembling CIDP has been reported, and a spinal muscular atrophy-like motor disorder may occur (Latov et al. 1988)

Cryoglobulinaemias

These are immunoglobulins that precipitate in cooled blood. There is purpura of distal extremities. The neuropathy is a painful, axonal disorder. Cryoglobulins occur in plasma cell dyscrasias, lymphoproliferative disorders, and collagen vascular diseases (Chad et al. 1982).

Castleman's Disease

This is a syndrome characterised by abnormal lymphoid proliferation of unknown cause. There are whorls of lymphoid cells in abnormal lymph nodes. In some cases a monoclonal gammopathy has been reported, rarely associated with plasma cell dyscrasia and sensorimotor neuropathy. The disorder may be associated with functional immunosuppression, and with Kaposi's syndrome, in this respect resembling AIDS (Frizzera et al. 1983).

Neuropathies Associated with Collagen Vascular Disease

A neuropathy can occur in all the collagen vascular disorders, but is most common in rheumatoid arthritis and in polyarteritis nodosa (Moore and Cupps 1983). Peripheral nerve involvement is clinically evident in about 25% of patients with polyarteritis nodosa (PAN) (Bleehan et al. 1959), in 10% of patients with rheumatoid arthritis (Johnson et al. 1959) and in 5% of patients with systemic lupus erythematosus (Johnson and Richardson 1968). Neuropathy may also be associated with giant cell arteritis (Warrel et al. 1968), Wegener's granulomatosis (Stern et al. 1965) and scleroderma (Richter 1954). In these disorders involvement of a single nerve, multiple involvement of single nerves – mononeuritis multiplex – or symmetrical sensory or sensorimotor polyneuropathy may occur (Table 11.4). Guillain–Barré syndrome may occur in systemic lupus erythematosus (Feinglass et al. 1976).

Polyarteritis Nodosa

There is widespread inflammation and necrosis of medium-sized arteries which may also involve the

Table 11.4. Neuropathy syndromes with collagen vascular disease

Mononeuritis multiplex and peripheral neuropathy	Common:	PAN
		Churg–Strauss syndrome
		Hypereosinophilic syndrome
	Rare:	Giant cell arteritis
		Sarcoidosis
		Sjögren's syndrome
		Behçet's disease
		Non-systemic vasculitis limited to peripheral nerve
Dorsal root ganglionopathy		Behçet's disease

blood vessels supplying peripheral nerves, causing single or multiple ischaemic nerve lesions. These usually present with pain and paraesthesiae within the sensory distribution of the affected nerve, followed in a few hours by weakness and sensory loss in the same territory. A symmetrical polyneuropathy may develop during the course of the disease but both mononeuritis multiplex and symmetrical polyneuropathy may be presenting features (Bleehan et al. 1959), occurring in up to 50% of cases of PAN (Kissel et al. 1985; Bouche et al. 1986). The neuropathy is almost always associated with several other manifestations of polyarteritis nodosa, such as arthritis, hypertension, signs of renal, liver or pulmonary involvement, skin lesions or Raynaud's phenomenon. The ESR is raised, and there is a polyclonal increase in immunoglobulins (IgG). The pattern of involvement of the peripheral nerves resembles that found in rheumatoid arthritis. Cranial nerve involvement is uncommon but sixth and third nerve palsies sometimes occur. Generally mononeuritis multiplex occurs early, often before involvement of other organs, particularly of the CNS, develops.

Other Forms of Polyarteritis

Polyneuropathy may occur in other forms of polyarteritis, including drug-induced varieties, Churg–Strauss syndrome (Churg and Strauss 1951) asthma, eosinophilia and polyneuropathy, Sjögren's syndrome (Kaltreider and Talal 1969), serum sickness and narcotic abuse. In Sjögren's syndrome a pure sensory neuropathy (ganglionopathy) may also occur (Kennett and Harding 1986).

Rheumatoid Arthritis

Neuropathies associated with rheumatoid arthritis (Chamberlain and Bruckner 1970) have been classified into four types (see Pallis and Scott 1965).

Clinically evident neuropathy is uncommon in rheumatoid disease, affecting only about 1% of patients (Chalk et al. 1993).

Distal Symmetrical Sensory Neuropathy. This is an insidious, slowly progressive sensory neuropathy with little or no motor involvement. There is distal loss of all sensory modalities with absence of the ankle jerks. In severe cases motor involvement may develop, and even in mild cases evidence of chronic partial denervation and a reduced interference pattern in distal muscles are found with concentric needle EMG. The sensory nerve conduction velocity is often very slow. This neuropathy usually occurs in patients with longstanding nodular rheumatoid arthritis and marked joint deformities.

Mononeuritis Multiplex. Involvement of several nerves either simultaneously or sequentially occurs in rheumatoid arthritis as in polyarteritis nodosa, but is uncommon. Entrapment neuropathies are common in rheumatoid arthritis and it may be difficult to distinguish the rapidly progressive carpal tunnel syndrome of a patient with severe rheumatoid arthritis from a vasculitis involving the median nerve. However, in mononeuritis multiplex there may be focal slowing of conduction in segments of nerve at a distance from sites of potential nerve entrapment.

Digital Neuropathy. This is a mild neuropathy in the distribution of individual digital nerves in the hands. There is sensory loss in the distribution of the affected digital nerves. It can be assessed electrophysiologically by stimulating on one or other side of a finger, recording from median or ulnar nerves at a more proximal site.

Severe Mixed Sensorimotor Neuropathy. This may present as a mononeuritis multiplex, but progression is rapid and the symmetrical signs of a severe neuropathy supervene. In most patients this neuropathy is part of a more generalised vasculitis and the prognosis is poor (Chamberlain and Bruckner 1970). Indeed, death often occurs within a few years. The neuropathy is usually accompanied by moderately severe painful proximal weakness, probably due to an associated polymyositis. The EMG shows marked denervation in distal muscles and a mixed neurogenic and myopathic abnormality in proximal muscles. Pathologically there is both Wallerian degeneration and axonal loss, with segmental demyelination. Nerve infarction is rare (Beckett and Dinn 1972).

Systemic Lupus Erythematosus

Symmetrical sensorimotor neuropathy may develop in systemic lupus erythematosus (SLE) in 5%–7% of patients (Grigor et al. 1978). Root involvement, or mononeuritis multiplex may occur, and cranial neuropathy may also develop (Ashworth and Tait 1971), especially trigeminal involvement. Involvement of the peripheral nervous system is a manifestation of vasculitis and is a poor prognostic sign which usually develops in the later stages of the disease. An acute neuropathy resembling Guillain-Barré syndrome may occur (Feinglass et al. 1976). In systemic lupus erythematosus a severe neuropathy, sparing respiratory, trunk and cranial muscles, develops subacutely but may assume a chronic relapsing course. The CSF protein may be very raised, and papilloedema may occur. Nerve conduction velocity is greatly slowed.

Wegener's Granulomatosis

The clinical features of nerve involvement in this syndrome are those of mononeuritis multiplex. As in polyarteritis nodosa orbital involvement, sometimes presenting as pseudotumour of the orbit, may occur. The neuropathy in Wegener's granulomatosis is thus indistinguishable from that of polyarteritis nodosa (Stern et al. 1965).

Scleroderma

Isolated trigeminal sensory neuropathy may be a manifestation of scleroderma (Beighton et al. 1968). A mild generalised mixed sensorimotor polyneuropathy may also occur (Gordon and Silverstein 1970). Neuropathy in this syndrome is rare.

Cranial Arteritis

Mononeuritis multiplex or symmetrical polyneuropathy may occur in giant cell arteritis (Warrel et al. 1968). Peripheral neuropathy has been reported in 26% of cases in one series (Wilshe and Healey 1971) and improvement occurs with steroid treatment (Caseli et al. 1988).

Mixed Connective Disease

Trigeminal sensory neuropathy (Ashworth and Tait 1971), distal polyneuropathy and carpal tunnel syndrome may develop in this disorder, and these features may be a presenting problem.

Sjögren's Syndrome

Trigeminal neuropathy of sensory type, mononeuritis multiplex, distal sensory neuropathy and pure sensory neuronopathy have all been described in Sjögren's syndrome (Kaplan et al. 1990). Peripheral nervous system involvement occurs in about 10% of patients. Very rarely a CIDP-like syndrome may develop. The ESR is raised in about half the cases, and there may be positive tests for rheumatoid factor or anti-nuclear antibody, with anti-SSA or anti-SSB circulating antibodies. A nerve biopsy may reveal vasculitis with axonal loss (Mellgrew et al. 1989).

Hypersensitivity Vasculitis

This includes Henoch–Schonlein purpura and serum sickness. Mononeuropathies have been reported with Henoch–Schonlein disease, in which a circulating cryoglobulin is present. Brachial plexus neuropathy and radial neuropathy may occur in acute serum sickness, but the cause of this complication is uncertain.

Behçet's Disease

In this syndrome orogenital ulcers, ocular inflammation and stroke may occur. The disorder is a chronic inflammatory process and rare cases of peripheral neuropathy have been reported, including mononeuritis multiplex (Takeuchi et al. 1989).

Sarcoidosis

Neuropathy is a rare feature of sarcoidosis, occurring in only about 5% of patients with the disease (Delaney 1977). It is due to non-caseating granulomas in the endoneurium or perineurium of affected nerves, and thus represents a multiple, focal mononeuropathy (Challenor et al. 1984). Arteriolar involvement within affected nerves may be a feature. The *cranial nerves*, particularly the facial nerve and the auditory nerve, are especially vulnerable. Facial weakness is usually complete and sudden, and recovery is incomplete. Both sides of the face may be involved in sequence, and parotitis usually accompanies this complication (Matthews 1965, 1984). *Spinal mononeuropathies* also occur, affecting thoracic and other ventral roots, and may resemble Guillain–Barré syndrome (Strickland and Moser 1967) or mononeuritis multiplex (Stern et al. 1985). *Distal symmetrical sarcoid polyneuropathy* is a rare progressive disorder (Nemmi et al. 1981). In sarcoid neuropathy steroids are usually useful, although spontaneous remission may also occur (Matthews 1965, 1984).

Assessment, Pathology and Management of Neuropathies Associated with Collagen Vascular Disease

Laboratory Assessment

Apart from laboratory investigation of the underlying collagen vascular disease, only the CSF examination is useful. The CSF protein is usually raised in these symmetrical polyneuropathies but may be normal in mononeuritis multiplex.

Electrophysiological Assessment

There is moderate slowing of sensory and motor nerve conduction in most of these neuropathies (Bouche et al. 1986). Even in cases presenting with mononeuritis multiplex there is usually EMG evidence of a generalised neuropathy. In all generalised neuropathies, including collagen vascular diseases, there is usually localised slowing of conduction at potential sites of entrapment, particularly in the median nerve at the wrist, and the ulnar nerve at the elbow. A carpal tunnel syndrome may be the first indication of the disorder, especially in polyarteritis nodosa and rheumatoid arthritis and this can be differentiated from mononeuritis multiplex by the onset, in the latter condition, of severe pain and the involvement of more than one nerve. Nerve conduction across affected segments of nerve in mononeuritis multiplex is slowed sometimes with conduction block (Ropert and Metral 1990) and if this is not at a site of potential entrapment it is useful in diagnosis. EMG evidence of denervation cannot be found until about 2–3 weeks after the onset of the nerve lesion.

Pathology

In severe cases of all the neuropathies associated with collagen vascular disease there is evidence of obliterative arteritis of the vasa nervorum (Pallis and Scott 1965). Bywaters (1957) described a bland intimal proliferation leading to obliteration of the vascular lumen, but with preservation of the internal elastic lamina. Mild inflammatory cell infiltration may also be found and in some cases, especially in polyarteritis nodosa, there are acute necrotising lesions with nerve infarction. In the severe polyneuropathy of rheumatoid arthritis vascular changes and nerve fibre damage are found most prominently in the ulnar, median and sciatic nerves in the upper arm and thigh respectively. At these sites myelinated and unmyelinated fibres were absent and distal segments showed Wallerian degeneration and segmental demyelination (Dyck et al. 1972). Dyck et al. (1972) have suggested that these necrotic zones represent the watershed zone of the blood supply of these nerves.

Haslock et al. (1970) and Beckett and Dinn (1972) found segmental demyelination without arteritic lesions in the sural nerve biopsies from patients with mild sensory neuropathy associated with rheumatoid neuropathy, but in more severe cases there was axonal loss with arterial occlusion. Segmental demyelination thus occurs in these milder, slowly progressive cases.

Management

The mild neuropathies associated with collagen vascular disease do not themselves require treatment, although they probably improve with steroids when these are used to treat the causative disorder. Severe neuropathies, on the other hand, are themselves an indication of an active vasculitis and vigorous steroid or immunosuppressive therapy or plasma exchange is indicated. In rheumatoid arthritis nerve entrapment should be treated by surgical decompression. Plasma exchange has been used with benefit in polyarteritis and rheumatoid arthritis complicated by neuropathy (Brubaker and Winkelstein 1981). Intravenous immunoglobulin has also been used in the treatment of systemic lupus erythematosus, Sjögren's syndrome and rheumatoid arthritis, with benefit (Dwyer 1992). Specific use of this therapy in neuropathies complicating these disorders has not been objectively assessed.

Inflammatory Polyradiculoneuropathy

Guillain–Barré syndrome (Guillain et al. 1916) is an acute, symmetrical neuropathy with characteristic features. It is the most common cause of acute generalised paralysis with an annual incidence of 1 or 2 cases/100 000 (Langmuir et al. 1984; Hankey 1987). Kaplan et al. (1985) reported an incidence of 4/100 000 in Colorado and suggested that this was a high prevalence area for the disease. The major epi-

demiological studies do not reveal a seasonal incidence (Asbury et al. 1969), but Wiederholt et al.
(1964) and Dowling et al. (1977) reported data
showing seasonal clustering in the autumn and
winter months.

All clinical studies have shown a male predominance, generally about 1.5 : 1 (Hughes 1990; Ropper
et al. 1991). The disease occurs at any age, with a
peak between ages 45 and 75 years. The mean age of
onset is in the fifth decade (Ropper et al. 1991).
Older patients tend to have a slightly more severe
form of the disease. In addition, an explosive onset
of paralysis is associated with severe weakness and a
poorer prognosis for recovery (Winer et al. 1988).

The disease was first described by Landry in 1859,
as a severe ascending paralysis with respiratory
involvement. Guillain, Barré and Strohl (1916)
described two cases with a benign clinical course,
and noted that the CSF protein was elevated, and
the CSF cell count normal; the "albumino-cytologi-
cal dissociation" that formed part of the diagnostic
criteria for the disease. These two patients had a
benign course. Subsequently, there was controversy
concerning the clinical definition of the disorder,
and particularly as to whether severe cases with respiratory involvement represented severe forms of
the same disease, or a different disorder (Guillain
1938, 1953). The holistic view, expressed by Haymaker and Kernohan (1949), of an acute neuropathy of varying severity, and occasionally including
cases with a cellular response in the CSF, has subsequently prevailed. Nonetheless, the modern
approach includes a classification that allows a
number of variant clinical syndromes under the
eponymous title of Guillain–Barré syndrome (Table
11.5). The history of the syndrome has been well

Table 11.5. Classification of Guillain–Barré Syndrome (GBS) and its
variants

Acute typical Guillain–Barré syndrome (GBS)

Chronic inflammatory demyelinating polyradiculoneuropathy (CIDP)
    Relapsing syndrome
    Progressive syndrome

Clinical variants of Guillain–Barré syndrome
    Fisher syndrome
    Pure motor Guillain–Barré syndrome
    Pharyngo-cervico-brachial weakness
    Paraparetic form
    Ataxic form without ophthalmoplegia
    Acute axonal Guillain–Barré syndrome
    Acute paralytic disease of northern China
    Acute pandysautonomia

GBS associated with systemic disease
    Hodgkin's disease
    SLE
    Sarcoidosis
    HIV infection

Toxic causes, e.g. exogeneous gangliosides, jellyfish sting

described by Ropper et al. (1991) in their monograph on the disease.

Clinical variants of the basic syndrome are frequent, accounting for 15% of all cases of acute GBS
(Ropper 1992). The inclusion of these syndromes as
variants of GBS has gradually become accepted
since recognition of the similar CSF and electrophysiological findings in these syndromes and in
acute GBS, and the similar, resolving clinical course
that usually results. The axonal form of GBS differs,
however, in its pathology, course and clinical neurophysiology, and also in its lack of response to conventional treatment.

Acute Inflammatory Polyradiculoneuropathy (Guillain–Barré syndrome)

The typical illness (Asbury et al. 1978; Asbury and
Cornblath 1990) presents as a predominantly motor
disorder, with weakness of all four limbs, although
often affecting the legs before the arms and so having
an ascending course. Weakness is often quite strikingly proximal so that while the patient can move his
feet and grip his hands tightly, at the same time he
may be unable to stand and may show signs of
involvement of respiratory muscles. Respiratory
muscle weakness occurs in about 30% of cases admitted to hospital (Ropper and Shahani 1984). Bulbar
involvement may also occur and facial palsy is especially common. The external ocular muscles are
usually unaffected. Sensory symptoms may be inconspicuous although distal paraesthesiae may occur in
the early stages and distal sensory loss is demonstrable in about 50% of cases on examination. The initial
examination reveals that in half the patients legs are
more severely involved than arms, and in a third
there is a similar degree of weakness in arms and
legs. Although weakness is usually described as symmetrical there are almost always subtle differences
between the two sides. Striking asymmetry, however,
is so rare that another diagnosis should be considered if this is a feature. Muscle pain is a feature in
about a quarter of cases, often associated with
paraesthesiae. Although facial weakness is common,
major facial paralysis is less frequent. The illness is
often heralded by muscular pain. Weakness rapidly
worsens from the onset and is at its worst within a
week in 40%, and within two weeks in 77% of cases
(Ropper and Shahani 1984). After a short interval
recovery begins; this may be rapid or slow and some
patients, especially the elderly, make only a partial
recovery. Generally those patients most severely
affected show the slowest and least complete recovery. The reflexes are absent in most cases. Complete

areflexia has been reported in about 80% of patients (Winer et al. 1988a,b), but the biceps jerks were preserved in 50% of cases on admission in the series described by Ropper et al. (1991). Autonomic neuropathy may sometimes occur as part of the syndrome (Lichtenfield 1971). This autonomic disturbance may involve the heart, with vagal paresis, and cardiac dysrhythmia may cause sudden death. A finding of a fixed heart rate at >100 beats/min should raise suspicion of this risk (Oakley 1984).

As the disease progresses during the first few days, sensory symptoms develop in 70%, ataxia in 20%, sphincter dysfunction, usually urinary retention, in 18% and bulbar features in 40% (Ropper et al. 1991). Ventilatory weakness is present in 10% of cases on admission, but develops in 30% of cases in the fully developed syndrome.

Diagnostic criteria have been agreed for typical GBS (Asbury and Cornblath 1990; Ropper 1992). These are set out in Table 11.6.

Table 11.6. Diagnostic features of typical Guillain–Barré syndrome

Features required for diagnosis of GBS
  Progressive weakness in both arms and both legs
  Areflexia

Features strongly supportive of diagnosis of GBS
  Progression in days or first month after onset
  Relative symmetry
  Mild sensory symptoms or signs
  Cranial nerve involvement, especially facial diplegia
  Recovery beginning 2 to 4 weeks after progressive phase ceases
  Autonomic dysfunction
  Absence of fever at onset
  Increased CSF protein, with <10 cells/mm³ in CSF
  Typical electrodiagnostic features

Features casting doubt on diagnosis of GBS
  Sensory level
  Marked, persistent asymmetry of symptoms or signs
  Severe and persistent bowel/bladder dysfunction
  More than 90 cells/mm³ in CSF
  Presence of another cause for neuropathy or weakness

From Ropper (1992)

The CSF protein is raised in most cases after an interval of several days, and gradually returns to normal levels during the period of recovery (Haymaker and Kernohan 1949). The peak level is reached 2–4 weeks after the onset of the disease. In some patients the CSF protein level is not conspicuously raised (Prineas and McLeod 1976) and in others a slight lymphocytic response occurs, but this is rare. Papilloedema is a rare complication of GBS, associated with a CSF albumin level >200 mg/100 ml. The syndrome resembles benign intracranial hypertension (Ropper and Marmaron 1984), and is probably due to failure of absorption of CSF across the arachnoid villi (Davidson and Jellinek 1977).

Not all patients with GBS present the typical syndrome of an acute disorder with progression in

days, or in the first month after the onset. These patients with a longer phase of progression have been classified as *subacute GBS*, with progression continuing during the first 3 months and *chronic progressive CIDP* (chronic inflammatory demyelinating peripheral neuropathy), with progression continuing for more than 2 months (Hughes 1990, Cornblath et al. 1991a). *Recurrent acute GBS* consists of two or more attacks, with each phase lasting less than 4 weeks. In *chronic relapsing CIDP* at least two attacks occur, in one of which the progressive phase is of more than 4 weeks duration. The term AIDP (acute inflammatory demyelinating polyneuropathy) is a synonym for acute, typical GBS.

Antecedent Events

From the earliest descriptions of typical GBS an association with antecedent infection has been recognised. The infection generally occurs 1 to 3 weeks before the development of weakness, but some cases with a shorter interval have been recognised, the shortest being 2 days (Ropper et al. 1991). In cases beginning more than 6 weeks after an infection the relationship is uncertain. Half the cases of typical GBS follow an upper respiratory infection and 10% follow an episode of diarrhoea. In 27% of the series of Ropper et al. (1991) there was no prior illness. The symptoms develop somewhat more quickly after a gastro-intestinal infection than after an upper respiratory tract infection (Winer et al. 1988b). The mean interval between infection and the development of symptoms was 11 days in the Ropper et al. (1991) series of 120 patients from the Massachussetts General Hospital, studied prospectively.

Infections with certain viruses, bacteria and mycoplasma have been incriminated as leading to the development of acute GBS (Table 11.7). In many of these, e.g. hepatitis A, rubella and influenza A and B infections, the association is uncommon and, perhaps, doubtful but in others, e.g. cytomegalovirus (CMV), Epstein–Barr virus (EBV), HIV and *Campylobacter* infections the association is clearly documented. The clinical syndrome itself is similar in all these instances, except that GBS following *Campylobacter jejuni* infection (Rhodes and Tattersfield 1982) is often associated with severe or variant forms of the disease, e.g. acute axonal GBS, and with marked and persistent residual disability (Yuki et al. 1990; Arnason and Soliven 1993). Winer et al. (1988a,b) noted *C. jejuni* antibodies in 15% of their prospective series. Kaldor and Speed (1984) in a retrospective series, found antibodies to *C. jejuni* in 38% of a consecutive series of cases, many of whom had a poor outcome, Although this experi-

Table 11.7. Antecedent events in typical Guillain–Barré syndrome

Viral infection
 Cytomegalovirus
 Epstein–Barr virus
 HIV
 Others, less well documented

Bacterial infection
 Campylobacter jejuni
 Mycoplasma pneumoniae

Immunisation
 Rabies vaccine
 Influenza vaccine
 Poliomyelitis vaccine
 (Smallpox vaccine)

Systemic disorders (with immune dysfunction)
 Sarcoidosis
 SLE
 Hodgkin's disease
 Lymphoma

Pregnancy

Surgery

Spinal epidural anaesthesia

ence was not replicated elsewhere (Ropper et al. 1991; Enders et al. 1993; Vriesendorp et al. 1993), Rees et al. (1995) have confirmed the association, and Ho et al. (1995) noted it also in China.

Peripheral neuropathy occurs in about 20% of patients with AIDS, usually presenting as a persistent, distal, painful sensory neuropathy (De la Monte et al. 1988). Typical GBS is an infrequent complication of HIV infection (Cornblath et al. 1987). A CIDP syndrome may also occur in patients with HIV infection (Cornblath et al. 1987). In both these clinical syndromes there is a pleocytosis of up to 40 cells/mm^3 in the CSF, a feature that would be unusual in idiopathic GBS syndromes. Ropper et al. (1991) suggests that tests for HIV infection or for Lyme disease should be carried out if there are more than 10 cells/mm^3 in the CSF. The neuropathy responds to conventional treatment, suggesting it is a true GBS despite the cellular response in the CSF.

Many of the associations noted in Table 11.7 are apparently uncommon. For example, pregnancy has been associated with GBS in a number of cases but epidemiological evidence in support of an association is lacking. The question obviously arises as to whether pregnancy was a relevant factor in these cases (Hughes 1990). Two of Ropper et al. (1991) cases occurred post partum. The association with surgery is difficult to document. Six patients with GBS following surgery were reported by Arnason and Asbury (1968) and in retrospective series GBS occurs after surgery in 5%–10% of cases (Arnason and Soliven 1993). However, prospective studies reveal that this association is extremely rare (Ropper et al. 1991) and it has been suggested that

infection complicating the surgery is the causative factor. The suggested association with spinal epidural anaesthesia, reported in two cases (Steiner et al. 1985), is not supported by a prospective review of 10 440 patients given epidural anaesthesia (Phillips et al. 1969), of whom 38 had transient motor and sensory symptoms that followed the anaesthesia immediately and disappeared after 5 days.

The association with Hodgkin's disease has been reported in both the acute and chronic forms of this disease. The neuropathy follows the usual course of rapid onset followed by improvement, and recovery is usually complete (Lisak et al. 1977; Julien et al. 1980). Currie et al. (1970) reported the occurrence of peripheral neuropathy in 1.4% of 210 cases of Hodgkin's disease. The association was reviewed in 10 cases (Clinico-pathological conference 1990). All had disseminated Hodgkin's disease. Nine were male, and the neuropathy was severe in six cases. The outcome was favourable in five. Cases of GBS have been associated with autoimmune disease (see Hughes 1990) and with vasculitis (Hughes 1990), and diabetes mellitus.

Ganglioside therapy was used in Italy as a non-specific remedy for neurological disorders. Landi et al. (1993) reported 25 patients in whom typical acute Guillain–Barré syndrome developed 4–14 days after parenteral administration of gangliosides. In this series there were two deaths and most patients had severe residual disability, and many showed an antibody response to gangliosides. Only 12% had an antecedent infection. Pang and Schwartz (1993) reported a patient who developed GBS a week after being stung by the jellyfish *Pelagia noctiluca*.

Chronic Relapsing CIDP

One or more relapses occur in about 2% of patients (Guillain–Barré Syndrome Study Group 1985). Most relapses occur during the first 6 months after the onset (Arnason 1975) but some may occur months or even years later (Ashworth and Smyth 1969; Wijdicks and Ropper 1990). Relapses are usually preceded by another antecedent infection, and recovery is often less complete than after the first illness. The CSF protein level rises in a relapse as in the original illness, but it may not return to normal (Janeway and Kelly 1966) and it has been suggested that in these patients recovery never really occurs, the disease entering a quiescent phase of minimal activity which can be provoked into an active relapse by the appropriate antigenic stimulus (Asbury et al. 1969). Sometimes, after repeated relapses (Austin 1958), palpable nerve enlargement may occur (Bosches and Sherman 1953).

Chronic Progressive CIDP

This chronic form of Guillain–Barré disease may develop after several relapses or more commonly begin as a slowly progressive disorder. The patients enter a slowly progressive phase with marked proximal and distal "glove and stocking" sensory impairment. The peripheral nerves are usually enlarged and the CSF protein is moderately raised. Investigation reveals no systemic abnormality. An antecedent event is recognised in about 30% of cases (Simmonds et al. 1993a), including pregnancy and infection (McCombe et al. 1987). Men are more likely to enter a chronic phase of the disease than women and in children a chronic course without a typical subacute or acute onset, and without relapse, is rather common and may be mistaken for spinal muscular atrophy or even for a myopathic process (Tasker and Chutorian 1969). Thus CIDP may occur at any age. The clinical diagnostic features are summarised in Table 11.8. Idiopathic CIDP is associated with A1 and B8, DRW3 haplotypes.

Table 11.8. Clinical diagnosis of CIDP

Required features
  Progressive or relapsing course during at least 2 months
  Motor, sensory or sensorimotor syndrome
  Reduced or absent reflexes
  Increased CSF protein
  CSF cell count <10/mm³ (except HIV positive cases)
  Slowed motor nerve conduction
  Increased distal motor latency in at least two limbs
  Partial conduction block may be present

Features that exclude the diagnosis
  Sensory level
  Major sphincter disturbance
  Evidence of another cause, e.g. familial neuropathy

From Cornblath et al. (1991a).

In 80% of cases there is a gradual onset of symptoms. McCombe et al. (1987) noted that 65% had a relapsing course and 35% had a progressive or monophasic course. Patients with a progressive course have a later age of onset than those with a relapsing course. In that series of 92 patients, 76 were followed up for 10 years; 73% of these were living independently and had made a good recovery and only 2% were unable to walk. The mortality was 6% during this period. Although most patients had severe motor involvement with sensory involvement, 22% had a predominantly motor disorder, and 6% a predominantly sensory neuropathy. In the chronic stage of CIDP, distal weakness and wasting, with absent tendon reflexes in the distal extremities, and distal sensory impairment are found. The peripheral nerves may be enlarged and there may be an action tremor, with a distal postural tremor

(Dyck et al. 1975b). The CSF protein is usually raised, often to greater than 1 g/1.

Thomas et al. (1987) reported several patients in whom CIDP was associated with multifocal demyelination in the central nervous system. This association was recognised by clinical features suggestive of multiple sclerosis (de la Monte et al. 1986) and the MRI appearances were consistent with this diagnosis, but this association is rare and its aetiology is unknown. SLE was excluded in these cases.

CIDP may be associated with a number of other disorders (Table 11.9). Patients in whom CIDP is associated with MGUS tend to be older, male, more slowly progressive, less severely affected, and with less weakness and more marked distal sensory impairment (Simmonds et al. 1993a).

Table 11.9. Disorders associated with CIDP

Systemic lupus erythematosus

Monoclonal gammopathy
  Monoclonal gammopathy of uncertain significance (MGUS)
  Waldenstrom's macroglobulinaemia
  POEM syndrome
  Osteosclerotic myeloma

Castleman's disease

CNS demyelinating disease

HIV infection

Diabetes mellitus

Fisher Syndrome

Miller Fisher (1956) described an acute, self-limited disorder characterised by ophthalmoplegia, ataxia, areflexia and mild facial and bulbar weakness, and suggested that the syndrome was an unusual form of GBS. The CSF protein is usually raised. Presentation is usually with diplopia, ataxia developing a few days later. The first manifestation is usually bilateral abductor paralysis. The pupils may be fixed and dilated when there is oculomotor nerve involvement. The ataxia resembles cerebellar ataxia and has excited controversy. It is thought to be due to a mismatch of information from muscle spindles and other proprioceptors due to involvement of large Ia fibre input to the cerebellum (Ropper and Shahani 1983). There is no associated dysarthria or nystagmus. Fisher syndrome follows viral and other infections. Recurrent cases have been described, but typical GBS has not been a feature (Schapira and Thomas 1986). No evidence of brain stem lesion is present in these cases, as shown by the CT and MRI appearances (Ropper et al. 1991). However, an alternative view of the cause of this syndrome is that it is the result of a CNS lesion, perhaps a primary brain stem encephalitis (Bickerstaff 1978). This controversy probably reflects difficulties in clinical diagnosis (Petty et al. 1993; Al-Din et al. 1994) of brainstem encephalitis and Fisher syndrome. Fisher's variant of GBS accounts for 6% of cases (Ropper et al. 1991).

The electrophysiological studies may show evidence of peripheral neuropathy (Fross and Daube 1987). In 10 patients, 6 had mild slowing of motor nerve conduction with abnormal late responses. The major abnormality was small SNAPs, implying an axonal sensory neuropathy or predominantly proximal damage to the peripheral myelin. These features are an important component of the evidence that this disorder is due to a peripheral rather than a central nervous system disorder. However, F responses are reported to be normal (Sauron et al. 1984). Phillips et al. (1984) found no abnormalities in the brain stem nuclei but the extra-axial oculomotor nerves were demyelinated.

Roberts et al. (1994) have reported that serum IgG autoantibodies to GQlb ganglioside (Chiba et al. 1992) increased, and then rapidly increased the frequency of miniature end-plate potentials in a mouse phrenic nerve-diaphragm preparation, suggesting that this antibody could lead to failure of acetylcholine release from motor nerve terminals in this syndrome. The electrophysiological evidence for axonal neuropathy is not explained by the observation, and proximal demyelination is a better explanation.

Plasma exchange, used in patients with severe ataxia, is effective (Irvine and Tibbles 1981).

Pure Motor Guillain–Barré Syndrome

This syndrome accounts for 3% of cases of GBS. The disorder presents as progressive, symmetrical limb weakness with mild facial weakness, areflexia and a raised CSF protein (Haymaker and Kernohan 1949). There are no sensory disturbances, or abnormalities of sensory nerve conduction. Motor conduction shows proximal conduction block early in the clinical course (Spaans 1985). A severe form of this clinical syndrome shows axonal pathology (see below).

Pharyngo-cervico-brachial weakness is a localised pure motor form of GBS involving head and neck, shoulder and, later, leg muscles. It is often associated with ptosis and ophthalmoplegia. Recovery may be delayed and tracheostomy may be required (Ropper 1986).

The *paraparetic form* is rare, and also involves the motor system without sensory involvement. This syndrome was described by Guillain (1938).

A *painless multiple cranial neuropathy* variant of GBS was described by Munsat and Barnes (1965).

Acute Axonal Guillain–Barré Syndrome

Axonal degeneration occurs in almost all cases of acute GBS, but is often minor in degree and inconsequential (Feasby et al. 1993). In severe typical cases of GBS, in which recovery is poor, axonal degeneration is probably the cause of the persistent weakness and wasting. Axonal demyelination can occur as a consequence of severe acute inflammatory demyelination, or as a primary phenomenon without inflammation or demyelination.

The latter syndrome has been characterised as a disorder of rapid onset and progression, with peak deficit at 6 days. In six of eight cases reported by Feasby et al. (1993) ventilatory support was necessary within 2 days of the onset of symptoms. Thus an "explosive" onset implies severe disease, and this may be associated with primary or secondary axonal damage. In most cases complete or partial external ophthalmoplegia has been a feature. Respiratory or gastrointestinal symptoms may precede the onset of the neuropathy (Brown et al. 1993). The CSF protein may be normal or raised (Feasby et al. 1986). Yuki et al. (1992) reported IgG anti-GDIA antibodies in this disorder.

Cases of this axonal type have been recognised in the past, associated with relatively normal motor conduction, but the correlation of these features with pathological evidence of primary, noninflammatory axonal loss has been appreciated only more recently (Feasby et al. 1993). The motor nerves are inexcitable, although sensory potentials can usually be recorded but may be of reduced amplitude (Feasby et al. 1986). There is prominent denervation on needle sampling of muscles by EMG after about 3 weeks.

Recovery is slow, commencing in the facial and extraocular muscles. The outcome is often poor, with severe residual weakness and wasting (Feasby et al. 1986) in survivors.

Acute Paralytic Disease of Northern China

An acute paralysis, resembling GBS, called acute motor axonal neuropathy (Ho et al. 1995), has been described in children and young adults in China. The median age of onset was 7 years. More than 1000 cases have been recorded, occurring in annual epidemics, almost all in rural areas, with a peak incidence in August and September. The recurrence rate is 5%. The CSF protein is increased. The mortality is about 5%. A third of cases had an antecedent viral illness, two-thirds of whom had respiratory symptoms. The disorder begins with leg weakness, which rapidly ascends over a week to involve respiratory and bulbar muscles. External ocular muscle weakness is very rare (Zhao et al. 1981; McKhann et al. 1991). Classical acute Guillain–Barré syndrome of demyelinating type is less frequent than this motor neuropathy, and the seasonal variation is less marked in the former syndrome (Ho et al. 1995).

Electrophysiological studies of this syndrome have shown normal motor nerve conduction velocities, normal distal motor latencies, normal SNAP amplitudes, but low CMAP amplitudes (<80% normal), and denervation potentials on needle sampling of muscles (Ho et al. 1995). The latter are noted early in the natural history of the disease. These features are consistent with a pure motor neuropathy of axonal type. Serological studies excluded a diagnosis of poliomyelitis but there were raised titres to *C. jejuni* in 76% of patients (Ho et al. 1995).

This disorder may differ from the pure axonal form of GBS in that in the latter condition the motor nerves are inexcitable and SNAPs may be of reduced amplitude. McKhann et al. (1991, 1993) have therefore suggested that this acute axonal motor neuropathy of children in China may have a different aetiology. Most patients recover at least partly, but the outcome and the effect of attempted treatment is not well documented.

Acute Pandysautonomia

An acute or subacute autonomic neuropathy, occurring without motor or sensory involvement, or with sensory loss, decreased reflexes and an increased CSF protein, was first reported by Young et al. (1969, 1975), and was described also by Thomashefsky et al. (1972). Most cases have occurred in children. The disorder may progress over several weeks with abdominal pain, vomiting, constipation, urinary retention, pupillary abnormalities, diminished sweating and postural hypotension. Recovery is complete in about 50% of cases and disabling residual symptoms are rare. Nerve conduction studies are occasionally abnormal (Ropper et al. 1991).

Electrophysiological Assessment in Guillain–Barré Syndrome

Abnormalities in nerve conduction are both the most sensitive and the most specific laboratory findings in acute GBS. They occur earlier and more frequently than elevation in the level of the CSF protein and are therefore particularly important in the initial diagnostic evaluation. The most characteristic finding, implying demyelination in the peripheral motor system, is conduction block. Conduction block is a feature indicating failure of conduction in a major proportion of motor nerve fibres, and therefore correlates with weakness. The sensory nervous system is less markedly abnormal, but spontaneous discharges in partially demyelinated internodes probably account for dysaesthesiae and pain in this syndrome.

Proximal conduction block, with prolonged, dispersed or absent F waves, in the presence of normal distal conduction, is an early feature demonstrated by stimulation of cervical roots, Erb's point or axilla (Brown and Feasby 1984). Mills and Murray (1985a) used percutaneous electrical stimulation over the cervical vertebrae to demonstrate proximal conduction block between the cervical roots and axillae even when peripheral motor conduction was normal, during the first 3 weeks of the disease. Ropper et al. (1990), in a study of 113 patients with GBS, found generalised slowing of motor conduction in only 22% of adult patients, although this seems more common in children, in whom 61% showed generalised slowing if motor conduction (Bradshaw and Jones 1992). McQuillen (1971) also noted more marked slowing of motor conduction in children than in adults. In adults slowing of motor nerve conduction is often most prominent in sites of potential nerve entrapment, particularly in the median nerve at the wrist. Conduction block may also be a feature at sites of entrapment (Brown and Feasby 1984). Albers et al. (1985) reported that abnormal F wave studies were most prominent 3 to 5 weeks after onset of GBS, occurring in 68% of patients in the early stages of the disorder (Ropper et al. 1990).

The compound muscle potential amplitude is a more sensitive indicator of abnormality than conduction velocity. In the first 2 weeks the major abnormalities are small CMAP amplitudes and increased F response latencies. The maximum abnormality occurred in the third week for motor studies and in the fourth week for sensory studies (Donofrio and Albers 1990). Kimura (1978) found F wave abnormalities were more likely to be abnormal in the median and ulnar nerves than in the peroneal nerves, findings quite unlike a symmetrical sensorimotor neuropathy of other causation. In addition, the distal motor latency is usually more abnormal in the median than in the ulnar nerve (Rudnicki et al. 1992); the increase in the median nerve was 182%, and in the ulnar nerve 49%.

Sensory conduction is characteristically less abnormal than motor conduction in GBS. Sural conduction is normal in about half the patients in the first week, although median and ulnar sensory conduction is abnormal (Murray and Wade 1980; Albers et al. 1985).

In patients with the acute axonal form of GBS almost all motor nerves are inexcitable, and the responses when obtained are of extremely low amplitude (Feasby et al. 1986), 1993). Sensory nerves are also relatively inexcitable, although conduction velocity is normal.

Concentric needle EMG studies reveal abnormal spontaneous activity after about 2 weeks and abnormalities of motor unit organisation, with increasing polyphasia and increasing amplitude, appear between the fourth and fifth week (Donofrio and Albers 1990). With single fibre EMG, increased fibre density can be detected first in proximal muscles in the first three weeks, and later in more distal muscles (Gantayet et al. 1992). The prognosis seems to be related more to the presence or absence of denervation potentials than to the degree of slowing of motor conduction velocity (Eisen and Humphreys 1974). Denervation indicates that there has been axonal damage. Miller et al. (1988) demonstrated that a marked reduction in CMAP amplitude was a reliable indicator of a poor outcome, since it presumably correlated with secondary axonal damage. Ten of their patients had CMAP amplitudes less than 10% of normal, and only one of these patients could walk without assistance at 6 months. Conduction block, increased distal motor latency or slowing of motor conduction were not related to prognosis, and they found no relation to the presence of fibrillation potentials.

Electrophysiological Assessment in CIDP

In CIDP motor conduction is usually markedly slowed, usually to less than 60% of normal values, and this feature in two or more nerves is a diagnostic feature when associated with the clinical picture of CIDP. The distal motor latencies are increased. These features are often asymmetrical and usually affect upper and lower limbs. The compound muscle action potential shows dispersion and conduction block is frequently present, and multifocal in distribution. Conduction block is sometimes demonstrable only when nerves are stimulated proximally, and is not necessarily restricted to sites of entrapment. Conduction block and asymmetrical slowing of motor conduction velocity are useful features in differentiating CIDP from hereditary demyelinating polyneuropathy (CMT Type 1) (Lewis

and Sumner 1982; Uncini et al. 1993). Sensory conduction is also usually abnormal; SNAPs are often absent.

Electrophysiological investigations in chronic and relapsing forms of CIDP show no distinguishing features. CIDP differs from GBS in that in the latter it is uncommon for motor conduction velocities to be very slowed, as in CIDP (McCombe et al. 1987; Cornblath et al. 1991b). These features are summarised in the electrophysiological criteria for the diagnosis of CIDP which include:

- Prominent slowing of motor conduction in two or more nerves
- Increased F wave latencies
- Marked temporal dispersion of the CMAP
- Conduction block.

Pathological Correlations

Although in acute inflammatory polyradiculoneuropathy the abnormality is principally due to segmental demyelination, axonal degeneration occurs in severe cases (Haymaker and Kernohan 1949; Asbury et al. 1969). The demyelinating process is widely distributed in the peripheral nerve, involving both proximal and distal parts. Segmental demyelination is accompanied by a mononuclear cellular infiltration, with the lesions scattered randomly through the nerve. Myelin breakdown usually begins at the nodes of Ranvier or in the Schmidt–Lanterman incisures. In a case with oculomotor involvement coming to autopsy 38 days after the onset of the illness Dehaene et al. (1986) found demyelination and inflammation in the third and sixth cranial nerves, resembling the changes in other nerves, but no abnormality in the CNS. In the acute, early phase endoneurial oedema, macrophage-associated demyelination and axonal degeneration are found. Macrophages invade the myelin sheath by displacing the Schwann cell from the axon, thus effectively stripping myelin from axons (Brechenmacher et al. 1987). Macrophages also disrupt superficial myelin lamellae in this process. Most sural nerve biopsies contain lymphocytic infiltration, even with light microscopy.

After several days Schwann cell proliferation and, in recovering cases, remyelination occurs, but this process is delayed if axonal degeneration has occurred. New internodes are often shorter than normal, accounting for the permanently slowed conduction velocity often found even when clinical recovery has been complete. If recovery is delayed, or the disease enters a chronic or relapsing phase,

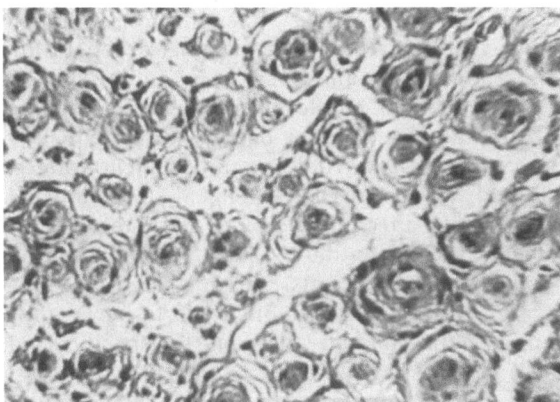

Fig. 11.2. Chronic Guillain–Barré syndrome. Toluidine blue. TS. × 350. Onion-bulb formations, and features of a demyelinating neuropathy are present.

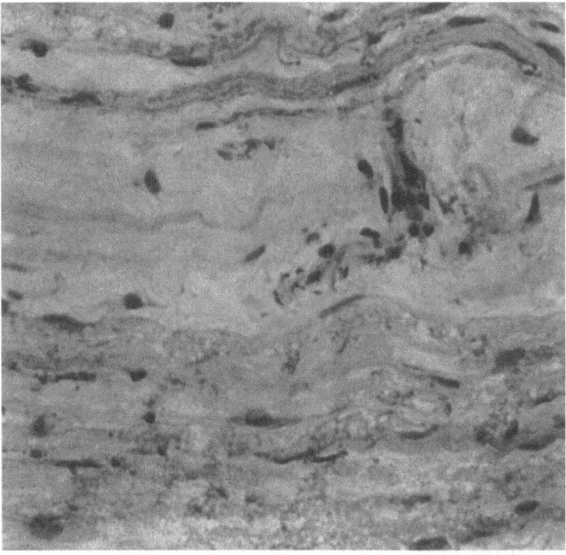

Fig. 11.3. Relapsing Guillain–Barré syndrome. Toluidine blue. TS. × 560. Demyelinated and remyelinating nerve fibres.

nerve hypertrophy may occur. This is due to the formation of onion bulbs, onion-like whorls or reduplicated Schwann cell cytoplasm (Fig. 11.2), and endoneurial fibrosis.

Inflammatory cell exudates (Fig. 11.3) may remain in the nerve fascicles in these chronic cases. In the less common acute axonal form of GBS, nerve biopsy shows severe axonal degeneration, without inflammation or demyelination (Feasby et al. 1993).

Oppenheimer and Spalding (1973) showed that grouped denervation atrophy was prominent in the muscles of fatal cases and they also noted that there was an abnormal proliferation of the terminal nerve tree so that some muscle fibres received multiple innervation. In addition, they noted inflammatory cell exudates in some of the muscles studied. Muscle biopsies in the earlier stages of the disease show mild neurogenic changes, consisting of scattered atrophic pointed fibres and small groups of fibres of similar histochemical type.

Pathogenesis

GBS is a demyelinating disorder in which peripheral nerve myelin is attacked by an externally triggered autoimmune process in which active T lymphocytes are involved. During the acute illness, activated T cells expressing several surface receptors are present in the circulation, and serum levels of interleukin-2 and its soluble receptor are increased (Hartung et al. 1990). Some of these lymphocytes are sensitized to PMP 22, a major peripheral nerve myelin antigen. In the peripheral nerve itself, there is loss of the myelin proteins P-0, MBP (myelin basic protein), PMP 22 and MAG (myelin-associated glycoprotein). Antineural antibodies have also been demonstrated in serum. The early antibody attack on myelin is followed by a lymphocytic response that leads to macrophage infiltration and destruction of myelin (Ropper 1992). The rise and fall of circulating antibody levels to peripheral nerve antigen correlates with the onset and recovery from the clinical syndrome, and with the development of the neurophysiological changes (Rudnicki et al. 1992).

Immunoglobulin appears not to be deposited on myelinated axons during the course of the disease (Brechenmacher et al. 1987), but several groups have reported finding membrane attack complement C3 and IgG in the endoneurium in some cases (Nyland et al. 1981). Acute phase serum from patients with GBS causes demyelination when injected intraneurally into rat sciatic nerve (Harrison et al. 1984) and Koski (1990) has demonstrated complement-fixing antibodies to peripheral nerve myelin in the serum of GBS patients which correlate with disease activity. The degree of demyelination in the rat sciatic nerve model correlates with the clinical severity of the GBS syndrome (Saida et al. 1982).

The target antigens for the process of immune-mediated demyelination in GBS are unknown but GM_1 ganglioside, LM_1 (a myelin glycoprotein) and β tubulin have all been incriminated, and perhaps all are involved since none is universally associated with GBS (Ilyas et al. 1992; Connolly et al. 1993). Anti-GM_1 antibody has been found in GBS, multifocal motor neuropathy and Chinese paralysis syndrome (Kornberg et al. 1994). In GBS these antibodies are particularly associated with the axonal form that follows infection with *C. jejuni* (Yuki et al. 1992). This antibody response has also been found in GBS, not of axonal type, associated with ganglioside therapy in Italy (Nobile-Orazio et al. 1992).

Anti-MAG antibodies and antibodies to the P_0 peripheral nerve glycoprotein are also possibly important in causing demyelination. The former lead to a characteristic widening of the intra-period line, due to failure of compaction of the external Schwann cell cytoplasmic surfaces.

The major physiological changes in nerve conduction in GBS occur early in the course of the syndrome, at sites where the blood-nerve barrier is defective, proximally in motor and sensory roots, distally in muscle, and in entrapped nerves (Sumner 1981). At sites of entrapment vesiculation of myelin and nerve oedema is particularly prominent (Prineas 1981).

In CIDP, the clinical syndrome is associated with a serum IgM protein in 30% of patients (Simmonds et al. 1993a). Selective high-titre IgG and IgM binding to β tubulin is more specific for CIDP than it is for GBS, occurring in about half all CIDP cases (Connolly et al. 1993).

The process of segmental demyelination and its association with immunologically competent cells and macrophages, and then remyelination, has been studied in experimental allergic neuritis, a disorder produced by immunisation with peripheral nerve in Freund's adjuvant (Waksman and Adams 1956). In this experimental model the CSF protein is raised, without a cellular response. This disorder is thought to be analogous to the naturally occurring acute inflammatory polyradiculoneuropathy (Astrom et al. 1968; Asbury et al. 1969; Arnason 1975).

Experimental allergic neuritis can be passively transferred to another animal by injecting extracts of lymphoid cells suggesting that it is due to delayed hypersensitivity to nerve antigens; it can be prevented by prior immunosuppression (Arnason and Chelmica-Szare 1972). The disorder has an acute phase, but may show relapses and exacerbations. It is associated with a cellular immune response to the PMP 22 and Po myelin antigens, leading to acute myelin breakdown. The disorder can be passively transferred lymphocyte transfusions from sensitised animals (Brosnan et al. 1984). This model thus differs in many respects from the naturally occurring GBS.

There appears to be no unitary basis for the pathogenesis of GBS. Even the relationship between GBS and CIDP is controversial; they may be considered as components of a single disorder, or separate disorders (Feasby 1992). In GBS demyelination is usually a primary process, axonal degeneration occurring as a secondary phenomenon, although rarely there may be primary axonal degeneration (see above). Immune complexes, and a slightly increased serum IgG level, may be found in the serum, and the disorder occurs more frequently than expected in partial immunodeficiency states. Antibody targets are GM_1, MAG, LM_1, β tubulin and Hu antigen, all components of peripheral nerve myelin. In CIDP antibody to β tubulin is found in about half the patients. Cell-mediated immune responses have been demonstrated to nerve antigens in both GBS and CIDP, but the specificity of these responses has varied from series to series. Schwann cells may express MHC Class 2 molecules in GBS, suggesting a role as antigen-presenting cells for the T cell response. The inter-relations of the humoral and T cell responses in pathogenesis in this disease are controversial, but clearly important (Hartung and Toyka 1990).

Management of GBS

Only two treatments, plasma exchange and intravenous immunoglobulin therapy (IVIG), alter the course of GBS. Other treatments are supportive. Steroid therapy, either in conventional doses for 2 weeks or in large intravenous "pulsed therapy" doses for 5 days, given at the onset of the disease is ineffective (Hughes; et al. 1978; Hughes 1991) and may even increase morbidity and mortality as a consequence of steroid-related effects (Hughes et al. 1978). In Hughes et al. (1978) study the clinical outcome of the untreated group was better than that of the treated group. This result was particularly important since it demonstrated the value of the controlled clinical trial in assessing an empirical therapy that was, at the time, believed by many neurologists to be effective.

Plasma Exchange. This treatment is of value in severe GBS. Even the early experience of this therapy demonstrated that some patients responded, while others did not (Brettle et al. 1978; Kennard et al. 1982). Rail et al. (1980) noted rapid improvement in motor conduction during plasma exchange. Patients in whom GBS is sufficiently severe that walking is impossible should respond well to plasma exchange (Guillain–Barré Study Group 1985). All the clinical evidence suggests that treatment is most effective when given in the first week of the illness, but may still be useful in the second week. After this, unless the patient is continuing to deteriorate, it is less likely to be effective. The Guillain–Barré Study Group (1985) concluded that the times required for recovery of unassisted walking, and the duration of the period of mechanical ventilation were halved. At 6 months the outcome was better than in untreated patients. In the French study (French Cooperative Group 1987) 44% of 111 control patients, and 67% of 109 exchanged patients had improved 4 weeks after the onset of GBS ($P < 0.001$). There was no difference in outcome after treatment with 5% albumin replacement compared to fresh frozen plasma replacement, and the precise number and volumes of plasma exchanges seems unimportant. In the French Cooperative Group (1992) study 71% of treated patients had recovered normal strength 1 year later, compared with 52% of controls. However, the frequency of severe residual disability (11%) was not affected by plasma exchange, and 21% of patients receiving plasma exchange progressed, despite the treatment, to require mechanical ventilation (French Cooperative Group 1987). In addition, relapses occurred in the first month in about 10% of patients (Ropper et al. 1988).

Plasma exchange is not free of other potentially serious side effects. Septicaemia occurred in 12.8% of treated and 4.5% of control patients in the French study, and was also a major problem in the American and other studies. Local discomfort from vascular access lines, hypotension, allergic reactions, haemorrhage and viral infection may also occur. It is difficult to use in children.

Intravenous Immunoglobulin (IVIg) Therapy. IVIg consists of pooled human IgG obtained from cold alcohol fractionation of plasma from 10 000 or more donors. A dose of 0.4 g/kg is given by an infusion pump daily for 5 days (Thornton and Griggs 1994). This treatment is easy to use compared with plasma exchange and appears to be as effective. Van der Meche et al. (1992) compared IVIg with plasma exchange in 150 patients and found that the IVIg-treated patients had a slightly better functional outcome, and fewer complications at 4 weeks. However, relapses occurred in 10% of cases, a similar proportion to that in patients treated with plasma exchange. Castro and Ropper (1993) and Irani et al. (1993) found that relapses were more frequent in patients treated with IVIg. Whether these differences between the Dutch and American experience are related to the immuno-modulatory effect of the IVIg used, or to other factors, is unknown.

The indications for IVIG, or plasma exchange, are currently uncertain. There are grounds for suggesting that these two treatments could act synergistically, IVIg inactivating immune complexes and plasma exchange removing immunoglobulins, but only further experience will resolve these issues (Dwyer 1992).

General Measures. The illness varies greatly in severity and special measures may be unnecessary in most cases. However, in more severe cases there is a risk of ventilatory failure from involvement of respiratory muscles and it is important, therefore, to monitor ventilation in all patients admitted to hospital with Guillain–Barré syndrome, especially during the initial week or two, during the phase of progression and before improvement has commenced. This can be done by measuring forced expiratory volume (FEV_1), peak flow or tidal volume. Elective mechanical ventilation should be undertaken with an endotracheal tube, when these tests show that the patient's ventilatory capacity is failing, since ventilatory collapse may occur suddenly and unexpectedly, for example during sleep or fatigue. Cardiac function should be monitored by ECG in these patients since elective atrial pacing is sometimes required (Oakley 1984).

Nursing procedures are necessary to prevent pressure on vulnerable nerves because these patients are especially liable to develop pressure palsies. Catheterisation may be necessary but loss of bladder and bowel control is relatively uncommon since autonomic involvement is usually relatively slight. Physiotherapy is important in management both in the acute stage and during rehabilitation.

Calorie intake should be maintained as far as possible by nasogastric and intravenous feeding, since a good nutritional state is important in preventing decubitus ulcers and in maintaining resistance to infection. Ventilatory muscle weakness and immobility lead to pulmonary infection. This must be recognised early and treated with antibiotics immediately. Frequent, even daily, chest X-rays are important.

Management of CIDP

Four treatments, steroids, oral immunosuppressant drugs, plasma exchange and IVIG, may be effective in CIDP. In many patients a combination of steroids and immunosuppressant drugs is necessary and plasma exchange is often also used as an early treatment in severe cases. The value of IVIG has been demonstrated.

Various *steroid regimes* have been tried and there are no comparative trials of, for example, oral versus intravenous steroids. Dyck et al. (1982) compared high dose alternate day steroids with placebo in an open design and noted more marked improvement in the treated group. The beneficial effect of steroids was first noted by Austin (1958) in a single case responsive to ACTH, a clinical observation later supported by Thomas et al. (1969) and Dyck et al. (1975). McCombe et al. (1987) reported that 65% of 76 patients improved with steroid treatment. Dyck et al. (1985b) found that steroids with azathioprine were no more effective than prednisolone used alone. A recommended regime is 60–100 mg/day for 2 months, or a shorter time if there is marked clinical improvement. The dose is then reduced over several months while improvement continues. If the patient relapses the dose is often increased. If improvement reaches a plateau immunosuppressive drugs should be considered.

Plasma exchange is useful in progressive or relapsing cases, especially in the first 2 years of the disease. It has particularly been used in initial therapy, in conjunction with steroid therapy, in securing a remission (Gross and Thomas 1981), although Feasby et al. (1983) have used it in long-term treatment. The latter is expensive and technically demanding. Dyck et al. (1986) conducted a 3-week controlled trial of plasma exchange in CIDP and reported improvement. Not all patients respond, however, (Gross and Thomas 1981) and the extent of improvement is often comparatively slight (Dyck et al. 1986a).

Immunosuppressant drugs are usually introduced after a course of high-dose prednisolone has proved inefficacious or only partially effective. Azathioprine is the drug most often used, but proof of its effectiveness in a controlled trial is lacking. Dyck et al. (1985) failed to show any effect when azathioprine was added to prednisolone therapy. Any beneficial effect noted may be delayed for 4–6 months. Cyclophosphamide and cyclosporin A have also been tried in uncontrolled studies (Hodgkinson et al. 1990) with apparently beneficial results.

IVIg treatment has been noted to cause rapid improvement that was initially encouraging. However, controlled studies have not confirmed this early enthusiasm, except for a transient response in some patients (van Doorn et al. 1990). Recent studies have showed the same efficacy as plasma exchange (Briani et al. 1996).

Management of Miller Fisher Syndrome

Plasma exchange has been widely used since the report of Littlewood and Bajada (1981) describing beneficial effects, and this is probably the treatment of choice for patients who are severely ataxic or unable to stand. Steroids are probably not effective.

Outcome

About 75% of patients recover almost completely but about 10% are left with a severe residual disabil-ity (Wiederholt et al. 1964; McLeod et al. 1976; Winer et al. 1988b). The remaining 15% have mild to moderate weakness. However, quantitative testing reveals that only 15% of patients are completely normal (Ropper 1992). About 10% of patients enter a relapsing course (Briscoe et al. 1987). The mortality of the disease is less than 5% in hospitalised series (Arnason 1975). Many cases are benign and are never admitted to hospital so that these figures refer only to those patients with sufficient initial disability to warrant admission to hospital. In the Massachussetts General Hospital series three of 120 patients remained wheelchair-bound 3 years later; these patients had an acute onset over 2 to 5 days (Ropper 1992).

Negative prognostic factors include age greater than 40 years, compound motor action potential at abductor pollicis brevis (APB) muscle less than 1 mV at the initial study (<120% normal), rapid onset of weakness and severe disease requiring ventilation (Winer et al. 1985). Winer et al. (1985) defined rapid onset as "bedbound within 4 days from the first symptom". These investigators also noted that a period of longer than 4 weeks before improvement commences, and a "plateau time" after peak deficit greater than 10 days were adverse factors (de Jager and Minderhoud 1991). Conduction velocity itself is not of prognostic importance in spontaneous recovery, although in chronic Guillain–Barré syndrome the motor conduction velocity tends to improve in parallel with improvement, or response to treatment (Gross and Thomas 1981). Conduction block and the CSF abnormalities, similarly, do not have prognostic significance.

A good outcome, conversely, is associated with slower onset over a 2-week period, retention of some tendon reflexes, no requirement for ventilation, younger age and a relatively large CMAP at the APB muscle. However, improvement generally ceases after 18–24 months. Children recover better than adults (Ropper 1992).

Multifocal Motor Neuropathy

This disorder (see Chap. 6) is a progressive, asymmetric disorder usually affecting distal muscles, particularly the arms. About 80% of patients are men. The age of onset is between 20 and 50 years but older cases are recognised. Weakness is progressive, but may show a stepwise course (Nobile-Orazio 1996). Fasciculation and cramps are a feature in two-thirds of patients; it is this feature which has led to confusion with motor neuron disease (Chad et al. 1986). Multifocal motor neuropathy, unlike CIDP, is distal, asymmetric and rarely accompanied by sensory impairment.

Electrophysiology

The hallmark of the syndrome is persistent, multifocal motor conduction block outside sites commonly associated with nerve compression or entrapment (Lewis et al. 1982). Motor conduction velocity is usually normal, or only slightly reduced, away from these abnormal sites. Sensory potentials are normal. EMG shows fibrillation and fasciculation potentials, with features of chronic partial denervation in abnormal muscles, whereas clinically normal muscles show no abnormality. In motor neuron disease the neurogenic disorder is always generalised in EMG studies, even of clinically normal muscles (Nobile-Orazio 1996).

The EMG examination should evaluate nerves supplying clinically involved muscles. The most commonly involved nerves are the median and ulnar nerves in the forearm (Chaudry et al. 1994). The crucial test to exclude this disease is adequate examination of portions of nerve not usually susceptible to compression or entrapment.

Laboratory Studies

The CSF protein is usually normal (Van den Berg et al. 1995). IgM antibodies to GM_1 ganglioside are found in some patients, but the specificity of this finding is limited and these antibodies are also found in motor neuron disease and CIDP (Pestronk et al. 1990).

Pathogenesis

A study revealed an inflammatory demyelinated polyradiculoneuropathy with segmental demyelination (Oh et al. 1995). It seems likely that the antibody response is in some way associated with the conduction block and demyelination in this disease (Kaji et al. 1993). The neurophysiological abnormality can be replicated in mice by passive transfer (Roberts et al. 1995), and may be due to an abnormality located at the nodes of Ranvier.

Management

Intravenous IgG is effective in 90% of patients, producing improvement within a week. Improvement is most marked in the most recently affected limbs and correlates, at least weakly, with resolution of conduction block (Van den Berg et al. 1995; Kaji

et al. 1992). Cyclophosphamide therapy, given orally in low dosage, may reduce subsequent dependence on frequent intravenous IgG infusions (Nobile-Orazio et al. 1993). The mechanism of action of intravenous IgG is not understood.

Steroid therapy and plasma exchange are generally not effective in treating this disorder.

Neuropathies Due to Infection

With the exception of leprosy, primary infections of peripheral nerves are an uncommon cause of peripheral neuropathy. Several syndromes develop in the aftermath of an infection, for example, Guillain–Barré syndrome, brachial neuritis and Bell's palsy, but these are usually classified separately as immunogenetic or other forms of neuropathy and are therefore discussed elsewhere in this book. The main syndromes are listed in Table 11.10.

Table 11.10. Neuropathies due to infection

Viral disorders
HIV
Herpes zoster
Herpes simplex
Rabies
Bacterial disorders
Leprosy (Hansen's disease)
Lyme disease
Diphtheria
Tetanus
Parasitic disorders
Tropical infestations

HIV-related Neuropathies

Peripheral neuropathy is the most common neurological complication of HIV-1 infection, occurring in 30% of patients with AIDS. There are several syndromes (Table 11.11). At autopsy, there is evidence of peripheral neuropathy in almost all patients (de la Monte et al. 1988). In some patients peripheral neuropathy is related to lymphoma, or its treatment.

Table 11.11. HIV-related neuropathies

Distal symmetrical sensory neuropathy
Inflammatory demyelinating polyneuropathy
Acute and chronic forms
Mononeuritis multiplex
Opportunistic radiculopathies
Cytomegalovirus
Herpes virus infections

Distal Sensory Neuropathy

This disorder presents in patients with AIDS as dysaesthesiae, confined at first to the soles of the feet, followed by hyperpathia and distal pain. The latter is so severe that the patient may not walk. The upper limbs are not usually so severely involved. The ankle jerks are absent, but the knee jerks may be increased. The thresholds for all sensory modalities are increased in the feet, but there is little or no motor involvement. The CSF protein may be slightly increased (Cornblath and McArthur 1988; Leger et al. 1989).

Electrophysiological studies show absent sural sensory nerve action potentials, with mild slowing of motor conduction velocity. F wave potentials may be delayed. There are distal chronic neurogenic features, mainly confined to foot and calf muscles, on EMG (So et al. 1988). Pathological studies have shown that there is loss of axons, involving both myelinated and unmyelinated fibres (de la Monte et al. 1988).

Fuller et al. (1990) noted axonal atrophy in addition to Wallerian degeneration. Most cases do not show inflammation in nerve biopsies, although this has been reported.

Treatment consists of pain relief, using carbamazepine, amitriptyline or simple analgesics (de la Monte et al. 1988). Steroids and plasma exchange are not effective.

Inflammatory Demyelinating Neuropathy

This syndrome resembles idiopathic Guillain–Barré syndrome in its clinical features, the CSF and EMG findings, and in the response to treatment and outcome. The patient presents with weakness as the most prominent symptom, usually involving all four limbs, with distal paraesthesiae and sometimes sensory loss and with reduced tendon reflexes. Although it may have an acute onset, subacute and chronic cases are more common. This neuropathy may develop at any stage of the course of HIV-related illness, including seroconversion and AIDS-related complex (Parry 1988; Leger et al. 1989). As in Guillain–Barré syndrome spontaneous recovery may occur (Cornblath et al. 1987). Nerve biopsy shows inflammation and demyelination. Treatment with IVIg or with plasma exchange may be effective.

Mononeuritis Multiplex

Abrupt-onset mononeuropathies occur in many nerves, involving face, trunk or limbs, often associated with AIDS-related conditions (ARC) Lipkin et al. 1985). Vasculitis has been demonstrated in some cases (Gherhardi et al. 1989), but in other patients this presentation leads to a chronic inflammatory demyelinating peripheral neuropathy (Parry 1988).

Opportunistic Radiculopathies

Cytomegalovirus (CMV) infection in patients with AIDS may present with a rapidly progressive cauda equina syndrome. The CSF shows a raised protein, a polymorphonuclear pleocytosis and sometimes a reduced glucose level (Miller et al. 1990). The infection may respond to treatment with ganciclovir (Miller et al. 1990), but the prognosis is poor if treatment is delayed. Herpes virus infection, syphilis, tuberculosis and lymphoma may cause a similar syndrome (Guiloff and Fuller 1992).

Neuropathies Associated with Critical Care

The development of muscle weakness in critically ill patients, especially in patients treated in intensive care units, has increasingly been recognised. This problem becomes evident when weakness and muscular atrophy, or difficulty weaning the patient off a ventilator are recognised after a period of severe illness, itself often involving multi-organ failure (Bolton et al. 1984). Sometimes there is a previously unrecognised neuromuscular disease, e.g. myasthenia gravis, motor neuron disease or porphyria, that is unmasked by the illness, but the commonest cause is a polyneuropathy of axonal type developing in the setting of multi-organ failure or sepsis (Witt et al. 1991). This disorder develops in about 70% of such patients and should be suspected when there is unexplained difficulty weaning the patient from mechanical ventilation.

Critical Care Neuropathy

The clinical features consist of flaccid weakness of the limbs, with shallow, rapid respirations. Sensory examination is often difficult because of the patient's general illness, but it may be possible to demonstrate distal sensory loss. Fasciculations are not present and facial weakness is not usually a feature, although respiratory muscle weakness is a problem (Bolton et al. 1993). Most affected patients have required mechanical ventilation for at least a week before the neuropathy develops.

Electrophysiological Assessment

Nerve conduction studies show normal or slightly slowed motor and sensory conduction velocities.

Sensory NAPs and CMAPs are reduced in amplitude and there is prominent evidence of denervation, with positive sharp waves and fibrillations. Motor unit action potentials may be difficult to study in these very sick patients, but complex potentials are not a feature of the early, acute phase of the illness. There is no abnormality of neuromuscular transmission, an important aspect of the diagnosis at the first EMG evaluation.

Nerve biopsy has shown prominent axonal degeneration without inflammation, and the muscle biopsy, if carried out, shows acute denervation with disseminated neurogenic atrophy (Chad and Lacomis 1994).

Prognosis and Treatment

Recovery occurs over a period of several weeks, except in very severe cases in which some weakness persists (Bolton et al. 1984; Witt et al. 1991). In many patients the disorder is mild and often unrecognised. No specific treatment is available, and the underlying cause of this neuropathy is unknown. Sepsis has been suggested as a factor by Bolton et al. (1993).

Differential Diagnosis of Critical Care Neuropathy

Several disorders must be considered in the diagnosis of this neuropathy. Guillain–Barré syndrome is generally a cause of weakness leading to the need for critical care, rather than a complication of critical care itself. Typical Guillain–Barré syndrome is a demyelinating neuropathy, with slowed nerve conduction and conduction block, but in the less common axonal form of this syndrome electrophysiological studies are similar to those of critical care neuropathy, itself an axonal disease. The main differences between axonal-type Guillain–Barré disease and critical care neuropathy are that in the former the onset is rapid, often during 24 hours, the disease is severe, the nerves are often inexcitable and the prognosis for functional recovery is poor.

Disorders of neuromuscular transmission, especially underlying myasthenia gravis, and treatment with neuromuscular blocking agents also need to be considered. In critical care neuropathy there is no abnormality of neuromuscular transmission, e.g. with "train of four" decrement tests at 3 Hz, and denervation potentials are present. Muscle wasting may occur in the intensive care unit as a consequence of prolonged, severe systemic illness and cachexia, and sometimes due to steroid myopathy.

A rapidly evolving myopathy has been recognised, developing over 1–2 weeks, in patients treated with high-dose steroids in intensive care units, who are also given neuromuscular blocking agents to aid mechanical ventilation, e.g. vencuronium (Danon and Carpenter 1991; Al-Lozi et al. 1994). These patients were not septic. There have been several case reports of this syndrome in patients with a myopathy of varying severity (see Sher et al. 1979; Al-Lozi et al. 1994). Recovery from this myopathy, which is characterised by selective loss of myosin fibrils in atrophic Type 2 fibres, is gradual over a period of 3–4 months (Barohn et al. 1994).

Diphtheria

Diphtheritic neuropathy results not from direct infection of the peripheral nervous system, but from the effects of a neurotoxin produced by the causative organism. Nonetheless it is best considered in this context. This disorder is now uncommon in developed countries, although sporadic cases occur in populations in which the level of immunity is low. The development of the neuropathy is related to the severity of the diphtheritic illness. Neuropathy occurred in about 20% of cases in Rolleston's review of an extensive experience when the disease was common. In patients with nasal diphtheria almost half developed neuropathy, but in those with laryngeal diphtheria no cases of neuropathy developed (Rolleston 1925). Neuropathy may also follow cutaneous infection, and the relation of site of infection to the development of the neuropathy has subsequently been disputed.

The neurological symptoms usually begin in the third or fourth week of the illness with palatal paralysis, producing nasal speech and regurgitation of fluid through the nose on swallowing. Weakness of arms or legs may also be a presenting feature of the neuropathy. Sensory symptoms are unusual, the motor involvement always predominating, but distal paraesthesiae with impaired position and vibration sense may be noted. The motor neuropathy tends to develop between the sixth and twelfth weeks of the illness, but may be delayed until the twentieth week. Asymmetrical weakness may be a feature. Ataxia, bulbar paralysis and proximal muscular weakness may occur and impaired pupillary reactions to accommodation have been noted (Kurdi and Abdul-Kader 1979). Solders et al. (1989) reported a recent case with autonomic involvement, affecting parasympathetic reflexes, e.g. vagal functions, but not involving the sympathetic nervous system. Cardiomyopathy and renal involvement may also develop; these are serious complications. Sphincters are involved only in severe cases.

Laboratory Investigations

Diphtheria toxin is thought to inhibit the synthesis of myelin basic protein and proteolipid (Pleasure et al. 1973), but there is no readily available assay for the toxin, although the organism can be grown in culture and is relatively easily recognised by Gram staining. The CSF protein is usually increased and may exceed 300 mg/dl (Gaskell and Korb 1946). There may be a mild lymphocytosis in the CSF. The ECG shows conduction abnormalities in many patients.

Electrophysiological Assessment

Early in the course of the neuropathy the motor nerve conduction velocity may be normal but it usually falls to about half normal values during the natural history of the neuropathy. Recovery of motor conduction occurs 4–8 months after the onset of the neuropathy. Strength usually improves at a stage when motor conduction velocity is still abnormal. Sensory nerve action potentials and conduction velocities are similarly affected. Concentric needle EMG shows fibrillation potentials, positive sharp waves and a reduced interference pattern at the height of the neuropathy. These are probably signs of axonal damage, superimposed upon the segmental demyelination responsible for the slowed conduction.

Pathology

The main feature of the changes in the peripheral nerves is segmental demyelination, with preservation of axonal continuity. The abnormality is most pronounced in the dorsal root ganglia and in the spinal nerve roots (Fisher and Adams 1956) but is less marked in the periphery. This selective involvement may reflect variations in the blood/nerve permeability of the toxin. Demyelination begins in the paranodal regions, affecting small fibres more severely than large (Cavanagh and Jacobs 1964). Involvement of nerves is patchy, adjacent paranodes being spared or severely involved. These changes have been studied experimentally (McDonald 1963). The toxin is thought to have a specific inhibitory effect on the synthesis of myelin proteolipid and basic protein (Pleasure et al. 1973).

Course

No specific treatment is available for the neuropathy associated with diphtheria, but it can be avoided by treatment with specific diphtheria antitoxin within 48 h of the infection. Recovery occurs gradually during several weeks in most patients, and the prognosis is good, the tendon reflexes reappearing when the patient has fully recovered some 2–4 months after the onset. Death may occur in the acute stages of the illness, or later from cardiac involvement. Myocardial involvement occurs in about 65% of cases, leading to death in about 10% of all cases. There is often a striking lack of correlation between the clinical features and the nerve conduction velocities during the phase of recovery (Kurdi and Abdul-Kader 1979), which may reflect the patchy distribution of involvement of the peripheral nervous system and consequent variation in the rate of recovery in individual nerves. During the recovery phase there is marked susceptibility to pressure palsies (Hopkins and Morgan-Hughes 1969) and care should be taken to avoid this complication, and to avoid contractures by the early use of physiotherapy and mobilisation.

Tetanus

A mild neuropathy, with distal weakness and sensory loss, occurs in some patients with severe tetanus (Shahani et al. 1979). This neuropathy is often asymmetrical and individual nerves may be particularly involved. Autonomic involvement is frequent and may cause sudden death (Sun et al. 1994). It is uncertain whether this autonomic disorder is of central or peripheral origin, but the former is more likely. Motor and sensory conduction velocity may be mildly slowed and concentric needle EMG shows evidence of denervation, with polyphasic motor unit action potentials. The abnormalities of nerve conduction are most obvious 3–6 weeks after the onset of trismus. The CSF is normal, but CK may be raised and myoglobinuria may occur in severe cases. Muscle biopsies late in the illness show fibre-type grouping consistent with reinnervation (Risk et al. 1981). The features are consistent with the principal pathological findings in the peripheral nervous system of axonal degeneration, often affecting motor end-plates first, in the typical distal distribution characteristic of a dying-back phenomenon.

Continuous EMG recordings show that muscle fibre activity in proximal muscles, especially in masseter muscles, is unceasing, with normal motor units. The silent period after reflexly generated muscle contraction is absent in tetanus, but is retained in patients with voluntary contraction, or with stiff man syndrome (Risk et al. 1981). This is presumed to indicate absence of Renshaw inhibition in tetanus with trismus.

Neuropathy is not the cause of the muscle spasms and weakness in tetanus; the disorder is characterised by involuntary muscle spasm caused by the action of a toxin, tetanospasmin, formed by *Clostridium tetani* infection. The toxin prevents the presynaptic release of acetylchorline (ACh) at the neuromuscular junction, and of the γ-aminobutyric acid (GABA), glycine and other inhibitory neurotransmitters in the spinal cord, thus resulting in reflex, released muscle spasms that are stimulus-sensitive.

Herpes Zoster

The most common syndrome of herpes zoster infection is the typical painful vesicular eruption limited to the distribution of one or more dermatomes, which may be accompanied by signs of motor involvement in the same root distribution, for example with facial palsy in geniculate herpes zoster infections. Motor involvement is more common in the elderly and in patients with malignant disease. The interval between the skin eruption and the development of muscular weakness is usually less than 2 weeks; facial weakness may appear as soon as 3–5 days after the first sign of sensory involvement. Motor weakness usually develops rapidly, in hours or days, and recovery is slow (Thomas and Howard 1972). In some patients there are clinical signs of cord involvement and the CSF may show a raised protein content and a mild lymphocytosis.

Rarely a symmetrical polyneuropathy resembling Guillain-Barré syndrome may occur 1–3 weeks after herpes zoster infection (Dayan et al. 1972; Sanders et al. 1987).

Electrophysiological Assessment

EMG studies may be useful in the assessment of the pattern of motor involvement. Fibrillation potentials can be found in affected muscles and, on activation, motor units are reduced in number but of normal amplitude (Thomas and Howard 1972). In the rare cases of symmetrical polyneuropathy following herpes zoster infection, the nerve conduction velocities are usually slowed.

Nerve Biopsy

The peripheral nerves show segmental demyelination, but there is also evidence of axonal degeneration and in autopsy studies loss of anterior horn cells and of neurons in the dorsal root ganglia may be prominent (Dayan et al. 1972).

Management

The basis of treatment is antiviral chemotherapy with acyclovir. Other antiviral agents, e.g. vidarabine, are less effective. Acyclovir has usually been given parenterally by intravenous infusion and treatment is most likely to be effective, especially in preventing post-herpetic neuralgia, when given in the acute stage of the illness, as soon after the onset as possible.

Recovery occurs in about half the cases of radicular involvement and partial recovery in a further third (Thomas and Howard 1972; Gardner-Thorpe et al. 1976). In patients with polyneuropathy the disease may be serious or mild (Dayan et al. 1972). In cases of radiculopathy in which there is evidence of cord involvement residual disability is common. Persistent pain is a problem in many patients, especially in the elderly in whom it may be unremitting, leading to depression and disability. Over the age of 70 years, 75% of patients develop post-herpetic neuralgia. This post-herpetic neuralgia is difficult to alleviate by medical or surgical means, including steroids, carbamazepine, opiates, tricyclic antidepressants, phenothiazines and transcutaneous or thalamic electrical stimulation.

Herpes Simplex

Herpes simplex virus invades the central nervous system through the peripheral nerves. It may rarely produce sensory impairment or pain in a root distribution. Guillain–Barré syndrome may follow the infection, but a causal link has not been established in the isolated cases reported (Hughes 1990).

Rabies

Rabies virus infection (Fishbein and Robinson 1993) is associated with a progressive, almost invariably fatal encephalomyelopathy. Paralytic or "dumb" rabies (rage tranquille) is a less familiar form of the disease that accounts for about 20% of cases (Editorial 1978). This clinical syndrome resembles Guillain–Barré syndrome both clinically and pathologically (Chopra et al. 1980). The incubation period was about 7 weeks in the 11 cases reported by Chopra and colleagues.

Rabies vaccination with duck embryo vaccine is effective and virtually free of neuritic complications (Rubin et al. 1973). The older vaccines (Semple vaccine) were prepared from brain and spinal cord and Guillain–Barré syndrome was a frequent com-

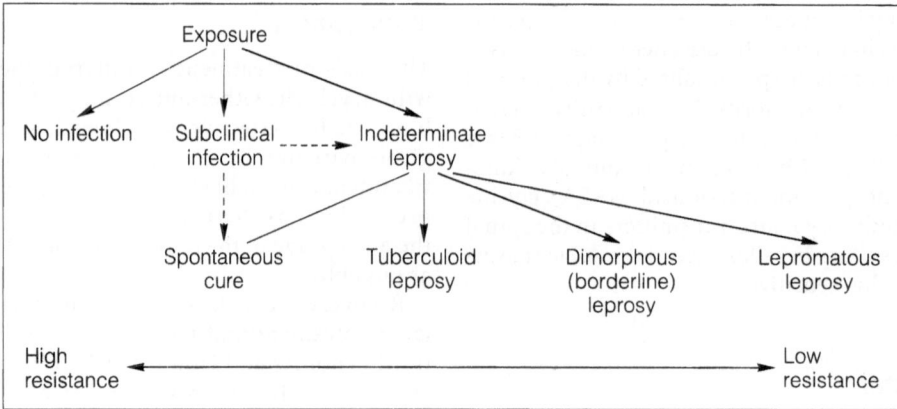

Fig. 11.4. Possible outcomes of leprosy.

plication of their use, with a mortality of up to 30% (Remlinger 1928; Lopez-Adaros and Held 1971). Chopra et al. (1980) found segmental demyelination with secondary Wallerian change in the peripheral nervous system in these patients. Concentric needle EMG shows prominent fibrillation after 2 weeks' illness, and the nerves may then be inexcitable to electrical stimulation (Prier et al. 1979).

Leprosy

Leprosy is widespread in tropical and subtropical zones, and cases occur in temperate zones among immigrant populations. Worldwide, it is one of the commonest of all neuropathies, affecting 6/1000 in South and East India, but even in these high prevalence zones diabetic neuropathy is commoner (Wadia 1984). In 1987 it was estimated that there were about 10 million people with leprosy in the world (World Health Organization 1988), but since the advent of drug therapy programmes sponsored by WHO this number has dropped to about 3 million known cases, of whom 80% live in India (2 million cases), Brazil (250 000 cases), Nigeria (150 000 cases), Myanmar (100 000 cases) and Indonesia (100 000 cases). These numbers probably represent only half the actual cases, indicating the extent of non-availability of diagnosis and treatment as to about 3 million people. The disease is due to infection by *Mycobacterium leprae*. It is acquired only after prolonged contact in overcrowded conditions. Many people appear not to be susceptible to the disease, perhaps because of previous exposure to *Mycobacterium tuberculosis*. The factors leading to susceptibility are complex, and largely determine the course and clinical type of the disease in individual patients. Nutritional and immunological factors are particularly important, but children are generally more susceptible than adults. Infection may occur through the skin or upper respiratory tract. Clinical manifestations of leprosy vary (Cochrane and Davey 1964; Sabin and Swift 1975) and several different types of the disease are recognised (Fig. 11.4).

After infection the response of the host is determined by immunological factors. In lepromatous leprosy blood-borne dissemination occurs before localised infection in superficial nerves develops (see below) (Sabin et al. 1974). Bloodstream spread is less important in tuberculoid leprosy in which the disease may be relatively localised (Dastur et al. 1973). In tuberculoid leprosy the patient produces a relatively effective response to infection, but in lepromatous leprosy the immune response is ineffective and the infection disseminates. During the course of the disease intercurrent infections and other factors may swing the disease from one extreme to the other.

Indeterminate Leprosy

This early lesion is most commonly found in children. There is an indolent, hypopigmented skin lesion, which may be anaesthetic. Biopsy of this lesion shows a few inflammatory cells near neurovascular bundles and *M. leprae* may be present in small cutaneous nerves. The lesion occurs after an incubation period of 3–5 years and may resolve or progress to the lepromatous or tuberculoid phase (Fig. 11.4) (Troutman 1984). In this form of the disease there is little immunological check to bacterial proliferation and skin and peripheral nervous system are extensively involved. It frequently represents the end-stage of the disease. The skin lesions may be macules, nodules or plaques, which are especially prominent in cool areas of skin (Fig. 11.5)

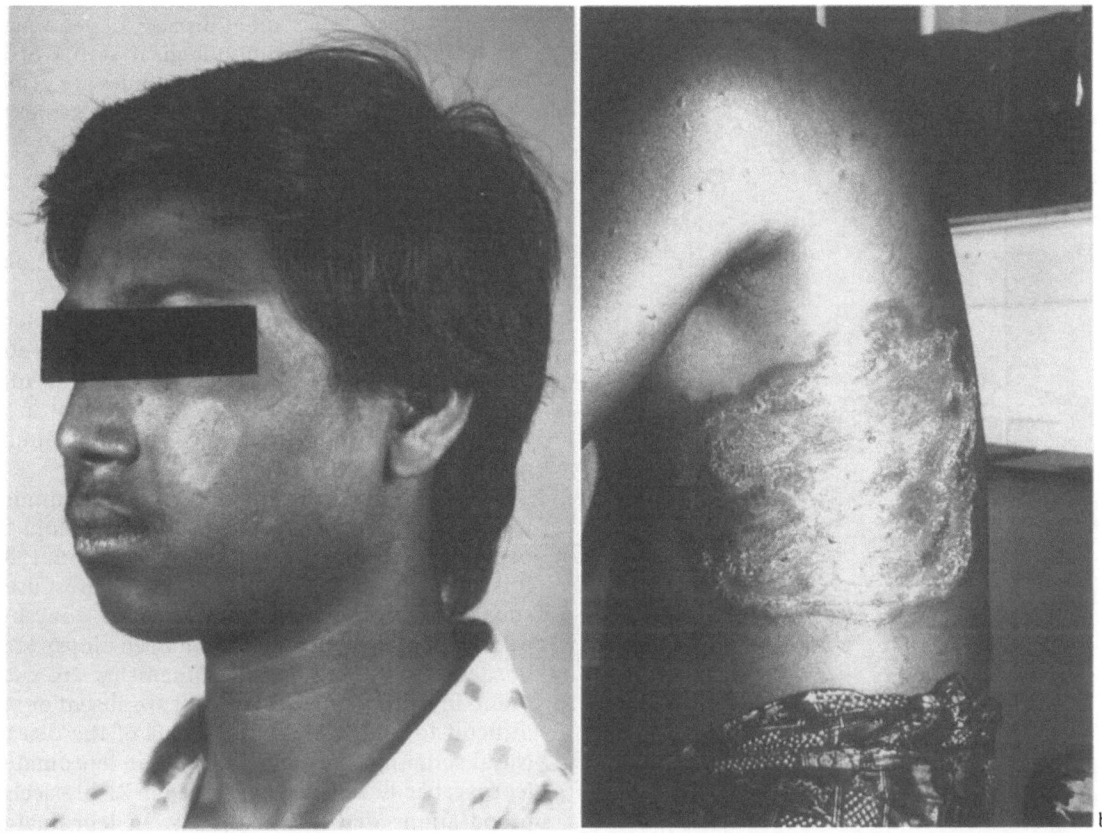

Fig. 11.5. **a** Lepromatous leprosy. The depigmented patch on the cheek has an irregular, well-marked edge. This patch was hypoaesthetic, and *Mycobacterium leprae* was isolated from nasal scrapings. **b** A large lepromatous lesion on the thoracic wall.

such as nose, chin, cheeks, fingertips, anterior chest wall and ears (Sabin et al. 1974). These lesions are usually numerous and symmetrical but they may be solitary. In advanced cases, infiltrated skin lesions lead to a characteristic leonine facies. These lesions are *not* always hypoaesthetic. Despite these lesions, which may contain large numbers of acid-fast bacilli, there is little evidence of systemic involvement or illness. Later, complications such as Charcot joints, loss of digits and facial structures, and osteomyelitis may develop. In lepromatous leprosy it is thought that there may be continuous leakage and dissemination of bacilli into the circulation from a primary intraneural focus, in association with suppression of cell-mediated immunity (Stoner 1979).

The main symptom is sensory loss, particularly affecting the hands and feet. It may be patchy at first, principally affecting shins, forearms, cheeks and ears; the coolest areas of the body. The palms and soles are spared. The peripheral nerve trunks are grossly enlarged by fusiform rather than nodular swellings, and small cutaneous nerves are usually similarly palpably enlarged. Affected nerves are often tender. Nerve abscesses, consisting of enlarged, tender inflamed lesions, laden with *M. leprae* may occur in affected nerves.

In more advanced cases a typical glove and stocking sensory disturbance to pain and touch is found, but position sense and vibration sense may be much less affected. Motor involvement occurs in a distribution consistent with involvement of individual nerves, the greater auricular, ulnar, median and common peroneal being particularly affected. These nerves become damaged both because they are superficial (cooler) and therefore involved by the disease and because, when enlarged, they are particularly susceptible to pressure and entrapment neuropathy. The tendon reflexes may be preserved, even when the neuropathy is established, but loss of sweating from autonomic involvement is a common feature leading to coolness of the extremities.

Tuberculoid Leprosy

Cutaneous lesions are less evident in this form (Jopling and Morgan-Hughes 1965) but the skin

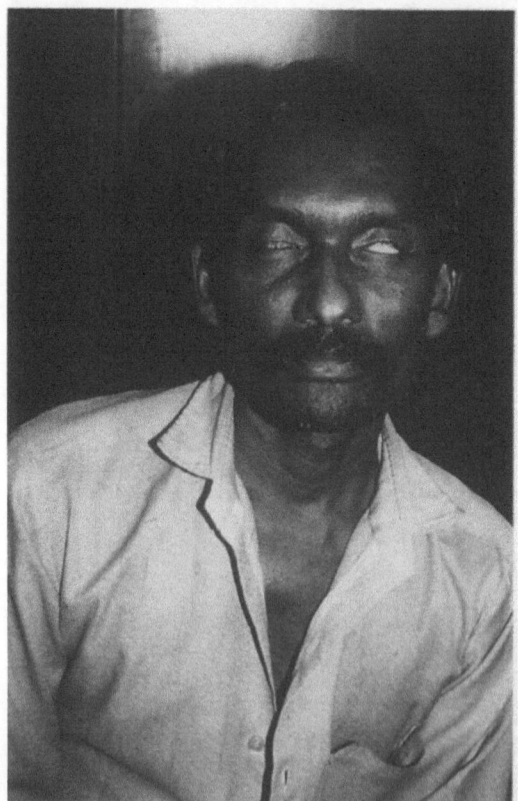

Fig. 11.6. Tuberculoid leprosy. Partial bilateral facial palsy is a frequent clinical finding that may be very subtle.

lesions show a characteristic sharply demarcated border, often erythematous and elevated, with anaesthesia, especially to pain and temperature sense, within the lesions. The skin lesions usually involve the face, the extensor surfaces of the limbs and the buttocks, and are hypopigmented in their central parts. The peripheral nerves show a peculiar nodular enlargement; both large nerves and small cutaneous branches may be affected. Glove and stocking neuropathy is not a feature of this form of the disease, the clinical features of nerve involvement being that of a mononeuritis multiplex. Ulnar, median, common peroneal and facial nerve involvement (Fig. 11.6) is particularly characteristic and radial, posterior auricular and sural nerve involvement is also a typical feature recognised by nerve enlargement and sometimes by sensory loss.

Dimorphous Leprosy

This form of the disease represents an intermediate disorder between the lepromatous and tuberculoid forms. Clinically, dimorphous (borderline) leprosy is unstable. The disease may evolve either towards

lepromatous or tuberculoid disease, depending on the nutritional and immunological status of the patient. Violaceous plaques and nodules are present on the skin and peripheral nerve enlargement is persistent.

Laboratory Assessment of Leprosy

The diagnosis is usually apparent clinically, although the skin lesions are easily missed by inexperienced observers since they may mimic the cutaneous manifestations of other diseases. The CSF protein may be raised but is often normal. The ESR is often raised in lepromatous leprosy; it is normal in the tuberculoid form. Circulating immunoglobulins may be raised.

The lepromin test is useful in assessing immunological reactivity; it is positive in tuberculoid but negative in lepromatous leprosy (see Melsom 1983). It is not, however, a diagnostic test. The most useful such test is skin biopsy which may be done by a punch-biopsy technique or by an open biopsy at the border of a suspect lesion. Organisms are easily found in lepromatous leprosy but are absent or very difficult to find in the other forms of the disease. Nasal scrapings may also be useful in lepromatous leprosy; bacilli can usually be seen in Ziehl–Neelsen preparations of these scrapings. In lepromatous leprosy bacilli are also prominent in affected nerves, and nerve biopsy may be useful in some cases.

Biopsies of skin lesions have been used to assess the presence of viable bacilli utilising a polymerase chain reaction (PCR) method to test for bacterial DNA as an index of bacterial viability. This test may have value in assessing the need for further antimicrobial therapy (Jamil et al. 1993).

Electrophysiological Assessment

In lepromatous leprosy sensory and motor nerve conduction velocity is slowed (Sohi et al. 1971) but in tuberculoid leprosy it may be normal, except in affected nerves (Jopling and Morgan-Hughes 1965). In lepromatous leprosy slowing occurs to the greatest degree in segments of nerves particularly involved, or affected by the combination of lepromatous enlargement and entrapment (Swift et al. 1973). The ulnar, median and common peroneal nerves are particularly affected (Magora et al. 1971). In both lepromatous and tuberculoid leprosy abnormalities of nerve conduction are found in those parts of nerves which are particularly affected, a pattern of abnormality similar to that found in other disorders in which mononeuritis multiplex occurs (Rosenberg and Lovelace 1968). In both forms of the disease there is a close relation between slowing of conduction and the presence of nerve enlargement and weakness (Verghese et al. 1970). Nerve conduction velocity improves with treatment and may prove useful not only in assessing the effect of treatment, but also in recognising deterioration during the prolonged clinical management necessary in severe forms of the disease (Jopling and Morgan-Hughes 1965; Rosenberg and Lovelace 1968).

Concentric needle EMG shows signs of partial denervation in the weak muscles (Sebille and Gray 1979).

Pathology

In nerve biopsies of patients with lepromatous leprosy there is a marked reduction in the number of unmyelinated axons, even in the early stages of the disease (Yoshizumi and Asbury 1974), and a loss of large myelinated fibres (Dastur et al. 1973). Affected nerves are oedematous, with relative preservation of their fascicular architecture. The perineurium is infiltrated by large numbers of foamy histiocytes and bacilli, especially near blood vessels. Bacilli are also found in Schwann cells, arranged longitudinal to the long axis of the nerve and Schwann cells are destroyed in this form of the disease. The nerve often contains large numbers of elongated macrophages.

In tuberculoid leprosy nerve biopsies are characterised by granulomatous nodular lesions, which destroy the normal architecture of the nerve. Langhans and foreign body giant cells are often found. Bacilli are usually absent. Segmental demyelination and remyelination are found in the involved nerves (Job 1973). In some fascicles there may be almost complete loss of axons. The most severe nodular lesions are often situated in parts of a nerve adjacent to overlying skin lesions.

Muscle biopsies may also show abnormalities, consisting of inflammatory cell infiltrates containing mononuclear cells and lymphocytes. Sometimes fragmented bacilli may be found in the macrophages but intact bacilli are rarely found (Sebille and Gray 1979).

Diagnosis

Certain clinical features are of major importance in diagnosis. The disease has a long asymptomatic precursor phase in which skin lesions may be the dominant feature. These features are listed in Table 11.12.

Management of Leprosy

Several anti-lepromatous drugs are available. Dapsone remains a mainstay of treatment (Jacobson

Table 11.12.   Diagnostic features of leprosy

Symptoms
Patchy change in skin colour
Shooting pain
Peripheral sensory loss
Deformities of digits
Nodules in skin/nerves
Chronic foot ulceration: usually painless
Shooting pains

Signs
Red or hypopigmented macules or papules
(these lesions are not dark and do not itch)
Painless injuries or burns to extremities
Deformities
   Asymmetrical ptosis or facial palsy
   Foot and/or wrist drop
   Claw hand
   Trophic ulcers
   Absorption of digits
   Loss of eyebrow hair laterally
   Loss of nasal septum
   Loss of incisor teeth from upper jaw
Induration of skin
Enlargement of peripheral nerves
Loss of sensation and sweating in skin patches

Bacteriological examination
Nasal scrapings
Skin scrapings
Nerve biopsy
PCR

and Trantman 1971). In lepromatous leprosy it is important to introduce anti-lepromatous drugs slowly to avoid a lepra reaction, a phenomenon in which death of large numbers of bacteria leads to an allergic reaction, requiring steroid therapy. Other newer drugs such as thiambutosine and clofazimine are also used. Oxfloxacin, a new antimicrobial with anti-leprosy activity may also be clinically useful. Rifampicin (600 mg monthly) and dapsone (100 mg daily) for 6 months has been recommended for paucibacillary borderline/tuberculoid and tuberculoid leprosy (WHO 1982). In multibacillary lepromatous and borderline/lepromatous disease rifampicin (600 mg monthly) and dapsone (100 mg daily) combined with clofazimine (300 mg monthly and 50 mg daily) is recommended for at least 2 years (Editorial 1982a; WHO 1982). Smaller doses may be used in children.

In all kinds of leprosy, especially in lepromatous leprosy, *acute exacerbations* (Type 2 ENL: erythema nodosum leprosy reaction) may occur with fever, erythema nodosum, deterioration of neuropathy and evidence of involvement of other structures, e.g. uveitis, suggestive of a sensitivity reaction. This phenomenon occurs during treatment. Anti-lepromatous therapy should be stopped and steroids begun. Clofazimine 200–300 mg daily is also effective and should be used with steroid therapy to control Type 2 reactions. The treatment of choice is thalidomide 300–400 mg/day, which controls the reaction in 1–3 days. A dose of 100 mg daily is continued for 2–6 weeks. Chloroquine may be helpful in such cases. *Reversal reactions* (Type 1 reactions), in which skin lesions suddenly become erythematous and swollen following initiation of chemotherapy, signify increased immunity and are usually followed by eradication of bacilli and healing (Ridley 1969). Steroids may be indicated (Joliffe 1977). Decreased immunity leads to *downgrading reactions* in patients with tuberculoid and dimorphous disease in whom a shift to lepromatous disease occurs with a failure of host immunity. Antimicrobial therapy is indicated.

Surgical treatment in patients with established neuropathy in whom the peripheral nerves are grossly enlarged is sometimes indicated, not only to relieve entrapment syndromes but, sometimes, to release intraneural pressure at sites of nodular or oedematous swelling (Selby 1974). Nerve grafting in patients with localised disease can improve sensory function (McLeod et al. 1975).

Physiotherapy is important, particularly in its educational role to teach patients to avoid trauma to anaesthetic extremities. The prognosis in tuberculoid leprosy is good, especially if it is diagnosed and treated early, but lepromatous leprosy can be difficult to manage, particularly if it is widespread before treatment is begun. It is particularly important to avoid injuries to the feet from ill-fitting footwear and to the fingers during cooking in patients with anaesthetic extremities. The typical absorption of digits that occurs in the disease appears to be due to poverty, and painless attacks by vermin, such as rats. Recurrent infection in anaesthetic digits is also important (Brand 1964).

Lyme Disease (Borreliosis)

Lyme borreliosis is a zoonosis transmitted by ticks and caused by the spirochaete *Borrelia burgdorferi*. The disease affects skin, nervous system, heart and joints. The ticks that transmit the disease are subspecies of *Ixodes*, a species that is restricted to temperate climates and which lives in relation to small mammals, deer and birds, depending on the subspecies and the stage in the life cycle of the tick. Rarely, the parasite may be transmitted by haematophagous insects, e.g. horseflies.

Humans are most likely to be infected between June and October. About 1500 cases a year are recognised in the USA, and in Europe the disorder is common in Austria and Southern Germany but has been recognised in most other European countries, including Britain, and also in Asia. There are three clinical stages of disease. In the *first stage* there is erythema chronica migrans, which appears at the location of the tick bite in the 2 weeks after the bite. Headache is common in this stage. Cutaneous lesions may be hypoaesthetic, resembling one of the features of leprosy. The *second stage* develops weeks or months later with neurological, cardiac and musculoskeletal symptoms. The neurological features consist of radiculoneuritis, cranial neuritis and meningitis. The *third stage* begins with arthritis, CNS manifestations develop, with encephalo-myelitis, ataxia, amnesia, irritability and depression. There may be a chronic peripheral neuropathy that may persist, with encephalopathy for many years (Logigian et al. 1990; Pfister et al. 1994).

Several types of neuropathy have been noted (Table 11.13).

Table 11.13.   Neuropathies in Lyme borreliosis

Radiculoneuritis
Facial and other cranial nerve palsies
Peripheral neuropathy

Cranial Neuropathies in Lyme Borreliosis

Facial palsy is the most common, often associated with headache and meningitis, occurring in about 10% of all cases, and being bilateral in half of affected patients (Clark et al. 1985). Involvement of all other cranial nerves, except the olfactory nerves, has been reported. The CSF shows a pleocytosis, a feature distinguishing facial involvement in Lyme disease from idiopathic Bell's palsy. The CSF may contain atypical plasmacytoid cells that may resemble those seen in lymphoma. The CSF protein is usually raised and the sugar normal. The outcome is usually favourable, but in about 10% of cases recovery is incomplete.

Radiculoneuritis

This develops in 40% of patients, with radicular pain, hyperaesthesia and with pain in the spine. Weakness develops focally and then multifocally, seeming to involve each limb in turn, gradually progressing over days or weeks, and leading to atrophy. The common clinical patterns include brachial or lumbosacral plexitis, mononeuritis or peripheral neuropathy. The tendon reflexes are usually depressed and a tetraparesis or Guillain–Barré-like syndrome may develop. Meningeal symptoms are prominent in about 25% of patients and facial palsy is present in about half. The CSF shows a pleocytosis with a raised protein level. Sensory loss is relatively infrequent, usually in a dermatomal distribution.

Peripheral Neuropathy

Mild, chronic polyneuropathy develops in about half the patients with stage 2 or 3 disease. In these patients there are distal paraesthesiae with glove and stocking sensory loss and mild asymmetrical distal weakness. Focal involvement, with carpal tunnel syndrome, may also be a feature. CNS manifestations are often also present in these patients. In patients with peripheral neuropathy alone the CSF is normal, but if there are associated CNS manifestations there may be an increased CSF protein and, less commonly, a CSF pleocytosis.

Electrophysiological Assessment

In the majority of patients with Lyme disease there is electrophysiological evidence of peripheral neuropathy of axonal type. Motor and sensory conduction is slightly slowed and SNAPs and CMAPs are of reduced amplitude (Hopf 1975; Kristoferitsch et al. 1988; Logigian et al. 1990). About 10% of asymptomatic patients with borreliosis, e.g. with cutaneous manifestations alone, have abnormal electrophysiological tests. The electrophysiological abnormalities improve in parallel with the clinical response to treatment. In a few patients with a Guillain–Barré-like presentation there are features consistent with a demyelinating peripheral neuropathy; in these patients the CSF shows a pleocytosis consistent with Lyme borreliosis.

In patients with the radiculoneuritis syndrome associated with Stage 2 borreliosis, there are features both of axonal and demyelinating peripheral nerve disease. About 5% of patients with Stage 2 disease have delayed F response latencies (Vallat et al. 1987b).

Laboratory Diagnosis

Diagnosis by isolation and culture of *Borrelia burgdorferi* is difficult and serological tests are therefore preferred. Occasionally the spirochaete can be recognised in silver stains of biopsied tissue, e.g. from skin lesions. The most commonly used serological tests are enzyme-linked immuno-absorbent assays (ELISA tests), indirect immunofluorescence assays (IFA) and Western blot. In Stage 1 disease only half the patients have detectable antibodies in blood, mainly consisting of IgM antibodies. In Stage 2 90% are positive and the antibodies are predominantly IgG, and in chronic Stage 3 cases IgG titres are high, even after treatment (Pfister et al. 1994).

In the diagnosis of Lyme disease with neurological involvement ("neuroborreliosis") both CSF and serum antibodies should be tested. Intrathecal production of IgG antibodies does not necessarily represent evidence of disease activity. False-positive IgM antibodies may be found in rheumatoid disease or after Epstein–Barr virus infections, and about 14% of forestry workers in endemic areas show IgG antibodies (Münchhoff et al. 1986).

Treatment and Outcome

Stage 2 Borreliosis with meningo-radiculoneuritis usually recovers spontaneously without sequelae (Pfister et al. 1993), and the value of antibiotic treatment in these cases is therefore uncertain. Ceftriaxone 2 g daily for 14 days intramuscularly, with or without penicillin G 1 g tds, may accelerate recovery and is useful in painful radiculitis.

Stage 3 disease, with peripheral neuropathy, improves with ceftriaxone 2 or 4 g daily, or cefotaxime 6 g daily. This treatment is effective in about 90% of cases. Patients with peripheral neuropathy without associated CNS manifestations may respond to cloxacillin 200 mg daily for 14 days or amoxycillin 1.5 g daily for 14 days (Weber and Pfister 1994).

If signs and symptoms persist or recur, or if IgM antibodies persist, treatment should be repeated. Treatment failure occurs in as many as 30% of patients (Logigian et al. 1990). A Jarisch–Herxheimer type reaction occurs in the first few days of treatment, with fever, chills and worsening symptoms. This is a mild response not necessitating steroid or other treatment, that resolves in a few days.

Drug-Induced and Toxic Neuropathies

A large number of drugs and toxic industrial or environmental substances have been found to cause damage to the peripheral nervous system. However, drugs that cause significant peripheral neuropathy at all frequently are usually withdrawn from clinical use except in the relatively unusual circumstances that their clinical value outweighs the severity of this complication, as in the case of vincristine. In the case of many other widely used drugs peripheral neuropathy occurs so uncommonly, or is so mild, that the neuropathic risk is acceptable to patients. Many drugs now recognised as causing peripheral neuropathy in humans have no known effect on the peripheral nervous system of other species, so that this relatively common toxic effect may escape detection during statutory drug-testing procedures.

In clinical practice it is relatively uncommon for a drug-induced neuropathy to present as an entirely

Table 11.14. Types of toxic neuropathies

Susceptible organ	Pathology	Clinical syndrome	Examples	Frequency
Neuron cell body (usually dorsal root ganglion)	Nerve cell death (toxic neuronopathy)	Rapid onset Usually purely sensory	Organic substances Mercury Procarbazine	Rare
Schwann cell myelin	Segmental demyelination (toxic myelinopathy)	Rapid onset Predominantly motor	Perhexilene Amiodarone Adriamycin	Rare
Axon	Distal axonal degeneration (distal axonopathy or "dying back")	Gradual onset Stocking and glove sensory disturbance	Most drugs and toxic compounds	Common
With central involvement	Central–distal axonopathy	Gradual or subacute onset	Heavy metals Tri-o-cresyl phosphate (TOCP)	–

After Schaumburg and Spencer (1979).

unexpected phenomenon in a patient with peripheral neuropathy as the only clinical problem. Most drug-induced neuropathies develop in the context of treatment for some other condition. In many instances drug-induced neuropathy will be subclinical, since its manifestations may be relatively insignificant and only detected by careful clinical examination. Drug-induced neuropathies are far more common than industrial or environmental causes of peripheral neuropathy. However, large clusters of cases appear when toxic exposure occurs in the community, as in the several well-documented outbreaks of organophosphorus poisoning, or in workers in certain industries exposed to organic solvents or heavy metals, and thus industrially and environmentally caused neuropathies have considerable social impact. Continuing low-level exposure to many compounds may cause a subclinical neuropathy that can be detected by screening examinations. Virtually all of these drug-induced and toxic neuropathies are axonal in type (Table 11.14).

Clinical Features

The toxic axonal neuropathies present with clinical features that are sufficiently constant to suggest the diagnosis. The onset is usually insidious, occurring in the context of chronic exposure to the drug or toxic substance at a relatively low level. Only the distal parts of axons in the peripheral nervous system are affected and the symptoms and signs reflect this distribution of abnormality. Since the longest axons are to be found in the legs sensory disturbance and sometimes weakness becomes evident first in the toes and feet and only later affects the hands. Dapsone and vincristine neuropathies, however, may predominantly affect the hands. The ankle jerks are often absent at the time

of presentation reflecting susceptibility of the heavily myelinated Group 1A spindle primary afferent axons, but the other tendon reflexes are usually present. Although distal sensory impairment is a common feature, the patient may complain not of numbness but of painful pins and needles, or of shooting pain in the distal parts of the extremities. In some cases, as in thalidomide neuropathy, this may be a persistent feature. Motor and sensory conduction velocities may be normal or only slightly slowed, although the sensory nerve action potentials in the sural nerves are usually small or even absent. The CSF protein is normal.

When the drug or toxic exposure is removed slow recovery commences. In some neuropathies, e.g. hexacarbon neuropathy, however, progression of disability may continue for several months after exposure to the toxic substance has ceased (Schaumburg and Spencer 1984). Recovery may continue during several months or even years but the extent of final recovery is dependent both on the severity of neuropathy at the time of diagnosis, and on the amount and duration of exposure to the toxic substance. In some patients evidence of involvement of pathways in the central nervous system becomes evident during recovery as improvement in distal sensation and strength occurs, especially in patients exposed to mercury salts.

In organic mercury poisoning the brunt of the pathological change is found in the dorsal root ganglia neurons (Hunter et al. 1940). The initial symptoms may consist of distal paraesthesiae that gradually progress centrally, even involving the tongue. Sensory ataxia may develop. In addition, features of central involvement with mental impairment and loss of central vision may develop, as in Minamata disease (Hunter et al. 1940; Takeuchi et al. 1962).

Management of toxic exposures consists of removing exposure and trying to promote excretion of the toxic substance and its metabolites. Generally, however, the prognosis is dependent on the dose ingested or absorbed and treatment is thus simply expectant. In the treatment of Paraquat-organophosphorus poisoning haemodialysis has been tried but without success and death occurs from multiple organ failure in a dose-dependent relationship.

Selective Schwann cell damage is a rare consequence of drug or toxic exposure. Although lead neuropathy has been considered a major example of segmental demyelination, pathological evidence suggests that there is a mixed axonal and demyelinating pathology (Cavanagh 1985). In perhexilene and amiodorone neuropathy, acute paraesthesiae and muscle weakness develop; the latter may be strikingly proximal, and autonomic features may be present. Nerve conduction studies show marked slowing of motor and sensory conduction (Said 1978). Recovery occurs rapidly following withdrawal of the drug.

Mechanisms of Neurotoxic Effects of Drugs and Other Substances

In most cases of drug-induced neuropathy the mode of action of the drug or toxic substance is unknown, although the end result is almost invariably distal axonal degeneration. The various known modes of action of these substances have recently been reviewed by Cavanagh (1985) and by Schaumburg and Spencer (1984).

Role of the Liver

Most drugs and chemicals are detoxified in the liver by microsomal enzyme systems. If this capacity for hepatic detoxification is decreased by metabolic disease or by concomitant therapy with other hepatotoxic drugs, toxic effects will result after apparently slight drug exposure. In addition, the microsomal enzyme systems can produce toxic metabolic substances from certain ingested chemicals, which are themselves not neurotoxic. For example, in arylphosphate organophosphate intoxication, a highly toxic active derivative is produced in the liver, and in n-hexane and methyl n-butyl ketone poisoning, a highly neurotoxic substance, 2, 5 hexanedione, is produced in the liver.

Role of the Vascular Bed

The vascular bed in the peripheral and central nervous system, especially in sensory and autonomic

ganglion, is also important. Drugs and chemicals show greater permeability across the blood-nervous system barrier at these sites, whereas motor nerve fibres appear to be less permeable, thus accounting for the preponderance of sensory symptoms. In metronidazole, misonidazole and nitrofurantoin toxicity, the vascular bed in the sensory and autonomic ganglia may be selectively affected.

Dying Back Change

The concept of "dying back" distal axonopathies includes a large number of disorders, including many examples of neuropathies due to drugs and toxic chemical exposures (Table 11.14). It represents the final expression of numerous "weak points" between the cell body and the end organ (see Cavanagh 1985). In these disorders the metabolic mechanism for expression of the neuropathy is as yet unknown.

Effects of Energy Metabolism

Interference with energy metabolism may produce a peripheral sensory neuropathy. In arsenic poisoning the clinical syndrome of painful sensory neuropathy resembles that of thiamine deficiency (beri beri), although the specific skin changes of arsenic poisoning are diagnostic. In thallium poisoning motor involvement develops after sensory symptoms (Cavanagh et al. 1974) and it has been suggested that the clinical features are the result of interference with flavoprotein metabolism. Misonidazole and its related compounds probably also cause neuropathy by interfering with energy metabolism, an effect that cannot be prevented by vitamin loading. Isoniazid interferes with pyridoxine metabolism, an effect that is likely to be more pronounced, at lower dosages, in people who acetylate the drug slowly, causing a severe, distal, painful sensorimotor neuropathy with sensory ataxia (Ochoa 1970). This neuropathy can be prevented by treatment with pyridoxine, and improves with this substance. However, pyridoxine overdosage may itself cause neuropathy (Schaumburg et al. 1983a). Hydralazine also causes pyridoxine deficiency neuropathy (Raskin and Fishman 1969).

Effects on Cell Constituents

Drugs and toxic chemicals may interfere with the functions of various cell constituents in axons or nerve cell bodies, thus causing neuropathy. Doxorubicin interferes with RNA transcription in cell nuclei, but this seems not to be important in human toxic neuropathies (see Cavanagh 1985, and Table 11.14). RNA and ribosomal structure and function are impaired by mercury, especially in the sensory cells of the posterior root ganglia (Cavanagh 1979). Microtubules are important in axons for the transport of metabolic materials. Vincristine depolymerises microtubular protein, producing peripheral neuropathy, with paraesthesiae, numbness and loss of distal reflexes, as a dose-related effect (Shalanski and Wisniewski 1969). Hexacarbon intoxication (Allen et al. 1975) affects neurofilaments, resulting in accumulations of neurofilamentous material in the central and peripheral nervous system. In the peripheral nervous system these neurofilamentous accumulations are found particularly in paranodal parts of axons, especially proximally (Chou and Hartmann 1965). The smooth endoplasmic reticulum is damaged in acrylamide neuropathy in experimental animals (Cavanagh and Gysbers 1983), a neuropathy that affects large fibres, and causes numbness, sweatiness and ataxia. The tendon reflexes are all diminished although the weakness and sensory loss are predominantly distal, perhaps from early involvement of spindle afferent fibres (Le Quesne 1984). Perhexilene maleate damages Schwann cells, cells that are normally relatively insensitive to toxins (Said 1978). Lead poisoning seems to produce neuropathy by inducing endoneurial oedema, leading to disorganisation of nodes of Ranvier, with myelin loss and also axonal degeneration (Ohnishi et al. 1977).

Drug-Induced Peripheral Neuropathies

In clinical practice a classification based on pathology and biochemical mechanisms is inappropriate. In addition, the clinical features of the neuropathies show considerable overlap, dependent on the individual drug effect, the length and amount of drug exposure and the presence of idiosyncratic factors affecting susceptibility, especially the presence of other latent or subclinical neuropathy due, for example, to hepatic or renal disease, or to diabetes mellitus. Thus the clinical features themselves are usually not very useful in the diagnosis of particular syndromes. Argov and Mastaglia (1979) avoided these problems by evolving a classification based on the therapeutic uses of the drugs concerned (see Table 11.15).

Antineoplastic Drugs

Peripheral neuropathy is particularly common with antineoplastic drugs. Vinca alkaloids are associated with peripheral neuropathy of some degree in all patients receiving antineoplastic drugs. Vincristine neuropathy produces a mixed sensorimotor neuropathy with dysaesthesiae. Position sense is usually spared. Weakness of the hands, especially of wrist extensors, and of distal muscles in the legs is a particularly prominent feature. The distal reflexes are

Table 11.15. Clinical syndromes of drug-induced neuropathy and drugs implicated

Clinical presentation	Antimicrobial drugs	Antineoplastic drugs	Cardiovascular drugs	Hypnotics and psychotropics	Antirheumatic drugs	Other drugs
Sensory neuropathy	Ethionamide Chloramphenicol Diamines	Procarbazine Nitrofurazone Cisplatin Taxol				Calcium carbimide Sulfoxone Ergotamine Propylthiouracil
Paraesthesiae only	Colistin Streptomycin Nalidixic acid	Cytarabine	Propranolol	Phenelzine		Sulthiame Chlorpropamide Methysergide
Sensorimotor neuropathy	Isoniazid Ethambutol Streptomycin Nitrofurantoin Clioquinol Metronidazone	Vincristine Podophyllum Chlorambucil	Perhexilene Hydrallazine Amiodarone Disopyramide Clofibrate	Thalidomide Methaqualone Glutethimide Amitriptyline	Gold Indomethacin Colchicine Chloroquine Phenylbutazone	Phenytoin Disulfiram Carbutamide Tolbutamide Chlorpropamide Methimazone
Predominantly motor	Sulphonamides Amphotericin			Imipramine		Dapsone
Localised neuropathies	Amphotericin Penicillin	Mustine Ethoglucid				Anticoagulants Paraldehyde

Modified from Argov and Mastaglia (1979).

absent in all patients taking effective doses of vincristine, and the effect of the drug can be monitored by measuring sensory nerve action potentials from the digital nerves; the responses are always diminished in amplitude with 2–4 weeks of beginning vincristine therapy, and the H reflex response is also reduced in size (Casey et al. 1973; Guiheneuc et al. 1980). Autonomic features may occur, including impaired bladder dysfunction and hypomobility of the gut. Laryngeal palsies may also develop and optic atrophy has been reported (Shurin et al. 1982). Vincristine neuropathy is said to be commoner in patients with lymphoma than in other patients (Watkins and Griffin 1978). Improvement occurs when the drug is stopped, but may be incomplete, especially if there is severe weakness. Vincristine is a microtubule polymerising agent. Acute neurotoxicity has been described in patients receiving other hepatotoxic drugs (Davies et al. 1985).

Treatment of solid tumours with cisplatin causes a progressive distal sensory neuropathy when high doses are used (Reinstein et al. 1980) and ototoxicity and optic neuropathy may also occur. The neuropathy begins with distal tingling and numbness, with preservation of pain and temperature sensation. The reflexes are reduced and Lhermitte's sign may be present. This toxic neuropathy is dose-dependent, beginning after doses of 300–600 mg/sq m. The sural nerve potentials are absent and motor nerve function is unaffected. Vincristine neuropathy affects large and small motor and sensory axons, but cisplatin specifically affects large sensory fibres (Gastaut and Pellissier 1985). The mechanism of this effect is unknown (Roelofs et al. 1984; Mollman 1990). The neuropathy can be partially prevented with ethiofos, a phosphorylated sulphhydryl compound (Mollman et al. 1988), and more effectively prevented or delayed by an ACTH analogue (Org 2766) (Gevritsen van der Hoop et al. 1990). After cessation of cisplatin therapy the sensory neuropathy slowly resolves during a year or more.

Taxol, a cytotoxic drug derived from the bark of the Pacific yew tree, is a tubulin polymerising agent that causes a rapid onset, ataxic, sensory neuropathy.

Antimicrobial Drugs

Many antimicrobial drugs, especially those used in the treatment of tuberculosis, may cause peripheral neuropathy (Table 11.15). Most of them, for example isoniazid neuropathy, are reversible on withdrawal of the drug, especially after pyridoxine therapy (see above). The incidence of isoniazid neuropathy is determined by several factors. The neuropathy is commoner in patients treated with more than 10 mg/kg. Other factors include the acetylator phenotype which determines the rate of metabolism of the drug, and the quantity of pyridoxine ingested in food or as supplemental therapy. Deficiency of pyridoxine itself produces a neuropathy and isoniazid administration results in the formation of a hydrazone of pyridoxine, thus causing a deficiency of pyridoxine. It has also been suggested that pyridoxine excretion is increased by isoniazid therapy. Both idiopathic pyridoxine deficiency and isoniazid therapy increase xanthenuric acid excretion in the urine, an indication of an abnormality in tryptophan metabolism (Bartolome et al. 1974). The neuropathy can be prevented by pyridoxine supplements. In patients with isoniazid neuropathy large daily doses (250 mg or more) should be used. Ethambutol may induce sensory or sensorimotor neuropathy, with optic nerve involvement occurring rather more frequently (Tugwell and James 1972). Neuropathy may also complicate treatment with ethionamide, a drug resembling isoniazid, but this does not respond to pyridoxine supplements.

Metronidazole causes peripheral neuropathy after treatment for several months, and in higher doses causes encephalopathy and cerebellar ataxia (Coxon and Pallis 1976; Kusumi et al. 1980). Dapsone, used in the treatment of leprosy, causes a motor neuropathy when used at high doses in the treatment of cystic acne and other skin disorders. It is less likely to cause neuropathy in the treatment of leprosy.

Nitrofurantoin may cause a distal neuropathy in which numbness is followed by severe weakness and profound sensory loss. Lindholm (1967) found that 62% of patients with normal renal function treated with nitrofurantoin developed electrophysiological evidence of denervation. The neuropathy may sometimes develop rapidly and is more likely to occur in patients with uraemia. The subacute form may clinically resemble Guillain–Barré syndrome, but the electrophysiological findings are those of an axonal neuropathy. If severe changes occur, recovery is slow and incomplete (Lindholm 1967).

Antirheumatic Drugs

Peripheral neuropathy is a rare complication of gold therapy for arthritis. The neuropathy is a typical sensorimotor disturbance, but it may be associated with severe cramps and a curious rippling, myokymia-like movement in the calf and foot muscles, probably representing neuromyotonia (Katrak et al. 1980). The incidence of neuropathy with gold treatment is 0.5% (Hatfall et al. 1937). The neuropathy associated with gold therapy, like that with nitrofurantoin, is not dose-related and may occur at any time during therapy, even after a single dose (Layzer 1985a). Penicillamine may also cause neuropathy during the treatment of rheumatoid arthritis but the association is poorly documented. The commonest cause of neuropathy in rheumatoid disease is the disease itself.

Anti-convulsant Drugs

The incidence of peripheral neuropathy, with stocking distribution sensory disturbance and diminished ankle jerks, in 186 epileptic patients was 11% (Swift et al. 1981). These patients had slightly slowed motor and sensory conduction velocity and abnormal H reflexes. Although this mild neuropathy in patients with epilepsy has been attributed to phenytoin (Lovelace and Horwitz 1968), it occurs also in patients taking several other anti-convulsant drugs, and in patients whose anti-convulsant drug regime does not include phenytoin (Swift et al. 1981). The frequency of peripheral neuropathy seems not to increase with increasing duration of phenytoin therapy, so that the role of phenytoin in this mild, clinically unimportant neuropathy is not proven.

Cardiovascular Drugs

Perhexilene maleate, a drug used in the treatment of angina, may cause painful distal paraesthesiae and, later, weakness that may be strikingly proximal. There may be bilateral papilloedema and the CSF protein is usually raised. Nerve conduction studies show marked slowing of motor conduction in the arms (less than 20 m/s). The slowing usually develops after several months' treatment, and the ESR may be raised. When the drug is stopped recovery occurs slowly (Said 1978). Hydralazine causes neuropathy, but only when high doses are used (Burley and Stein 1979). Neurological side effects, including tremor, gait instability, dizziness and peripheral neuropathy (6%) develop in about half of all patients treated with amiodorone for ventricular tachyarrhythmias. In 7% of patients these effects were so severe that treatment with this drug was stopped (Charness et al. 1984).

Other Drugs

Disulfiram, used in the treatment of alcoholism, may cause neuropathy. This neuropathy probably results from a metabolite of the drug, perhaps carbon disulphide (Casier and Merlevedi 1962), and is usually reversible when the drug is withdrawn (Mokri et al. 1981). Rothrock et al. (1984) reported severe neuropathy with only partial recovery after disulfiram and ethanol overdosage. Drowsiness and optic neuropathy may be associated clinical features. Other drugs causing neuropathy are listed in Table 11.15.

Peripheral Neuropathy Due to Toxic Chemicals and Metals

Peripheral neuropathy resulting from exposure to toxic chemical substances is a feature of the industrialised world; the exposure may occur in the home, at work or in the environment. When the neuropathy is due to exposure to a toxic substance on a single occasion the cause is usually obvious, and when exposure occurs at work, or even in the environment, there are often several other cases so that a toxic cause is suspected at once. Long-continued exposure at a lower dose level is much more difficult to detect, however, even after a careful history and assessment of possible risk factors. Le Quesne (1984) has summarised this clinical approach (Table 11.16). Only a limited number of these toxic neuropathies have proved reproducible in species other than man.

Neuropathies Due to Industrial Agents

Acrylamide

Acrylamide is used as a grouting agent in soil during mining and engineering operations, and in industrial chemical applications. Exposure to high concentrations produces a subacute encephalopathy whereas long-term but low-level exposure leads to a distal axonopathy with exfoliative dermatitis, especially of hands and feet. Exposure results from skin contact. Numbness and sweating of the hands and feet and ataxia are prominent features. The latter probably results from degeneration of muscle spindles but there is evidence of cerebellar involvement also. All sensory modalities are affected, and all tendon reflexes are diminished. Weight loss also occurs, and micturition may be affected (Le Quesne 1984).

Electrophysiological studies show reduction in sensory nerve action potential amplitude even in the

Table 11.16. Clinical features of toxic neuropathies (after Le Quesne 1984)

	Acrylamide	Arsenic	Carbon disulphide	Hexacarbons	Lead	Organophosphates	Thallium
Motor	++	++	+	+	++	++	++
Sensory	++	++	++	+	–	+	++
Pain	+	+	+	–	–	+	++
Reflexes	Absent	Ankle jerk absent	Absent	Ankle jerk absent	?	Ankle jerk absent	Ankle jerk absent
CNS involvement	Ataxia Encephalopathy	–	Optic atrophy Psychosis Parkinsonism	Spasticity	Encephalopathy in children	Spastic paraparesis	Optic atrophy Involuntary movements Confusion
Other systems	Weight loss Red, peeling hands & feet	GI disturbance Pigmentation Mee's lines	–		Anaemia Colic Lead line in gums	Acute GI disturbance	Acute GI disturbance Alopecia
Treatment	–	BAL	–	–	Penicillamine	Atropine Cholinesterase reactivator drugs (pralidoxime)	Potassium salts Prussian blue

GI, gastro-intestinal; BAL, British anti-Lewisite
After Le Quesne (1984).

early stages (Fullerton 1969). Improvement occurs when exposure ceases. Residual ataxia may be a problem after severe neurological complications.

Gold et al (1988) found that a single large dose in rodents caused proximal axonal swelling in dorsal roots with impairment of transport of all slow component axonal proteins and interference with axonal sprouting.

Hexacarbons

Both *n*-hexane and methyl *n*-butyl ketone are metabolised in the liver to 2,5-hexane dione, a neurotoxic substance. Hexacarbons are used in industrial solvents and in glue, and outbreaks of neuropathy have been reported among Italian shoemakers (Cianchetti et al. 1976) and in "gluesniffers" (Korobkin et al. 1975). The neuropathy is particularly severe in the latter group. It begins with sensory disturbance but severe weakness develops. Severe autonomic disturbance has been noted, with distal hyperhidrosis, sometimes followed by anhidrosis, and impotence (Altenkirch et al. 1977). Motor conduction velocity is markedly decreased, suggesting that there is segmental demyelination. However, only the distal reflexes are lost, even in severe cases. Pathological studies show a giant axonal neuropathy with neurofilamentous inclusions at nodes of Ranvier, with secondary paranodal myelin breakdown (Spencer et al. 1975). Progression continues for up to 4 months after expo-

sure and recovery is delayed during a year or more and may be incomplete. Clinically, this form of neurotoxicity may be confused with Guillain–Barré syndrome. Both industrial and "glue-sniffer" outbreaks have been studied (Allen et al. 1975; Korobkin et al. 1975).

Carbon Disulphide

This chemical is used in the rubber and textile industries. Low-level exposure causes distal paraesthesiae, weakness and painful muscles; optic neuropathy may be an associated feature. Recovery is slow. Exposure to high doses may produce an acute psychosis, and Parkinsonism has also been reported (Vigliani 1954).

Ethylene Oxide

Used in hospitals for sterilisation, ethylene oxide may cause sensorimotor neuropathy after repeated low level exposure (Kuzuhara et al. 1983).

Trichlorethylene

This substance, used in dry cleaning, may cause trigeminal neuropathy of relatively sudden onset, only rarely with involvement of other cranial nerves, e.g. facial, oculomotor and optic nerves, and never with limb involvement. Recovery occurs gradually over several months. The cause of this neurotoxic response is uncertain (Cavanagh and Buxton 1989) and it has been suggested the syndrome may be due to activation of latent herpes virus infection.

Organophosphates

Organophosphorus compounds are used as insecticides and as plasticisers in lubricating oils. Neuropathy occurs from attempted self-poisoning, from adulteration of food and cooking oil, and from contamination by insecticides. Organophosphates are long-acting cholinesterase inhibitors. Intoxication may follow a single dose, causing initial gastro-intestinal symptoms with paraesthesiae and rapidly progressive distal weakness developing 1–3 weeks later. Spasticity and incontinence occur with TOCP poisoning, evidence of both CNS and PNS involvement. Motor conduction velocity is normal but sensory nerve action potentials are small or absent (Hierons and Johnson 1978). The prognosis for recovery is poor. The neuropathy is due to formation of a neurotoxic esterase. Assay of this esterase in lymphocytes after acute exposure may predict the development of the neuropathy (Lotti et al. 1984). Treatment with atropine and cholinesterase reactors in the acute stages may control the anticholinesterase inhibition, but does not prevent the neuropathy. Outbreaks affecting thousands of people have occurred (Senanayake and Johnson 1982). The diagnosis depends on the history of toxic exposure and, without this information, there are no specific diagnostic features.

Electrophysiological studies may indicate early evidence of the severity of the impending neuropathy, with spontaneous repetitive activity and a decrement of the 2nd potential during repetitive stimulation (Wadia et al. 1989).

Toxic Oil Syndrome

Toxic oil syndrome consists of a multisystem disorder presenting with fever, skin rash, dyspnoea, myalgia, eosinophilia and chronic pneumonitis. A few months after the initial outbreak in 1981, about 10% of patients developed a sensorimotor peripheral neuropathy. The syndrome was linked with the ingestion of adulterated cooking oil, but its precise cause has not been determined. Pathological investigation revealed epineurial inflammation, perineurial fibrosis and intrafascicular necrosis, perhaps representing nerve infarction. An immune-mediated pathogenesis has been suggested (Tabuenca 1981). No fresh cases have been reported

after the initial outbreak, suggesting a toxic exposure from adulterated cooking oil.

Metal Neuropathies

Lead

Although formerly common, lead neuropathy is now a rare disorder. It is predominantly motor and usually asymmetrical, with wrist drop, proximal shoulder girdle weakness, peroneal muscle weakness and laryngeal paralysis as the five principal patterns of presentation in decreasing order of frequency (Schaumburg et al. 1983b). Distal weakness with absent distal reflexes is perhaps now a more frequent presentation. The possibility that minor clinical and electrophysiological changes occur in workers exposed to slightly raised environmental lead levels has received increasing support (Seppalainen et al. 1979) from the finding of slightly slowed motor nerve conduction velocity in these workers. The nerves show axonal degeneration (Buchthal and Behse 1979; see above).

Arsenic

Arsenic poisoning remains a problem, whether induced deliberately or from accidental ingestion of poisons intended for rats. After a single large dose a gastro-intestinal illness is followed about two weeks later by burning painful paraesthesiae in the hands and feet. Distal weakness develops and may progress for as long as 5 weeks (Le Quesne and McLeod 1977). In mild cases neurological abnormalities may be restricted to glove and stocking sensory loss with loss of distal reflexes. Recovery is very slow, taking place during months or years. In severe cases ventilatory failure and drowsiness may develop. The transverse white line or stria on the nails is a diagnostic feature, and arsenic can be detected in the hair and urine, even several months after a single dose. Basophilic stippling of red blood cells may be noticed and aplastic anaemia may complicate the clinical course. Chronic ingestion results in mild sensorimotor neuropathy that evolves slowly during many months. Le Quesne (1984) has stressed the use of pubic hair for analysis – cranial hair may contain arsenic from cosmetic applications. The normal level of arsenic in hair is less than 1 mg/kg, and in blood less than 30 μg/1. Treatment of the established neuropathy is disappointing but chelation therapy with British anti-lewisite (BAL) is important in increasing the rate of urinary excretion of arsenic, so hastening recovery. BAL treatment is particularly important in preventing neuropathy if given within a few hours of exposure to arsenic.

Thallium

Thallium poisoning causes a characteristic clinical syndrome, with a severe sensory neuropathy that is often painful, with a less marked motor component, confusion, behavioural changes, convulsions and even coma. Tremor may develop. There is a sensory ataxia in the early stages with distal limb weakness, limb pain and ptosis. Proximal tendon reflexes are preserved. Alopecia develops 2–3 weeks after acute intoxication. Recovery occurs over many months once thallium exposure ceases.

Thallium inhibits Na-K ATPase, thus interfering with cell metabolism. Pathologically there is axonal degeneration in peripheral nerves, with a "dying back" distribution. However, the pathophysiological basis for the acutely developing clinical syndrome is probably biochemical rather than degenerative, the axonal degeneration developing after the clinical features have become established (Cavanagh et al. 1974; Yokoyama et al. 1990).

Electrophysiological studies show small CMAPs, and small or absent SNAPs. These tend to normalise as the patient improves. EMG shows chronic partial denervation, with fibrillation potentials, in distal muscles (Yokoyama et al. 1990).

Mercury

Organic mercurials cause damage to the CNS, with visual field constriction, ataxia, dysarthria and tremors. Inorganic mercury leads to gastro-intestinal symptoms and nephrotic syndrome. A few cases of sensory neuropathy have been described. The best-known example of mercurial poisoning in modern times occurred from exposure of the local population to organic mercurials discharged into the sea at Minamata Bay in Japan. The mercurials entered the food chain after ingestion by fish (Kurland et al. 1960).

Electrophysiological and Laboratory Assessment

In all the toxic axonal neuropathies similar abnormalities are found. In patients with mild clinical abnormalities motor nerve conduction velocity is normal but the compound muscle action potential may be of reduced amplitude. The sensory nerve action potentials are often small and this may be the most sensitive indicator of abnormality, e.g. in acrylamide neuropathy (Takahashi et al. 1971). EMG shows evidence of denervation, with fibrillation potentials, and single-fibre EMG shows increased jitter, and blocking in distal muscles. In more advanced cases motor conduction is slightly slowed and the sensory potentials may be absent. EMG reveals polyphasic MUAPs and with single-fibre EMG the fibre density is increased. In perhexilene neuropathy, associated with Schwann cell involvement, motor conduction is slowed, often to less than 20 m/s, and the CSF protein is greatly increased. The CSF protein level in axonal toxic neuropathies is normal, or only slightly raised.

Screening for Low Level Toxic Effects

People potentially exposed to neurotoxic chemicals at work or in a domestic environment pose a public health problem in that, if subclinical toxic effects can be demonstrated, then clearly exposure to the substance should cease. However, this concept has proved difficult to introduce in practice because the methods available, particularly electrophysiological tests and quantitative sensory testing, have generally not been shown to be useful in recognising a predictable abnormality. When the neurotoxic effect is directed towards myelinated axons, as in lead exposure, nerve conduction velocity may be slowed (Seppalainen et al. 1979). However, most toxic substances affect the axons and in these instances nerve conduction may be normal, the first abnormality being reduction in size and slight dispersion of the sensory potential in sural nerve conduction studies (Rosen et al. 1978; Rosen 1984). In some cases, e.g. in organic solvent exposure, there may be an associated psycho-asthenic syndrome consisting of fatigue, instability and subjective memory problems. In some of these patients EEG abnormalities may be present (Seppalainen et al. 1980).

Chapter *12* Myasthenia Gravis and Other Myasthenic Syndromes

In this group of disorders transmission at the motor end-plates is abnormal. There are a number of possible abnormalities in motor endings which might result in inadequate neuromuscular transmission. These include abnormal synthesis of acetylcholine (ACh), defective release of ACh quanta, abnormalities in the neuromuscular cleft itself, abnormal post-synaptic ACh receptors and abnormal breakdown of ACh because of defective cholinesterase. In a number of congenital myasthenic syndromes discrete abnormalities in various components of the post-synaptic ACh receptor have been found, and in the Lambert–Eaton myasthenic syndrome release of ACh vesicles is abnormal (Table 12.1).

Table 12.1. Classification of disorders of the neuromuscular junction

Myasthenia gravis
Myasthenic syndrome (Lambert-Eaton syndrome)
Congenital myasthenic syndromes
    Pre-synaptic defects
    Pre- and post-synaptic defects
    Post-synaptic defects
    Partially characterised syndromes
Botulism
Tick paralysis and other toxins

Myasthenia Gravis

Myasthenia gravis is an acquired autoimmune disorder of neuromuscular transmission in which there is destruction of acetylcholine receptors at the neuromuscular junction. Most patients have circulating antibodies to the nicotinic acetylcholine receptor (AChR). Immune deposits of IgG and complement are present on the post-synaptic membrane of the neuromuscular junction in all cases. Both the clinical and electrophysiological features are explained by the reduction in number of available acetylcholine receptors at the neuromuscular junction.

The disorder is characterised by fluctuating weakness, consisting principally of abnormal fatiguability, with improvement after rest. Remissions and relapses are common. The muscular symptoms may be restricted to certain muscle groups, especially the eyelids and external ocular muscles, the bulbar musculature, and proximal limb muscles, but in many cases weakness and fatiguability become generalised. Permanent muscular weakness and wasting may develop in the later stages in more severely affected patients.

The disease seems to have been described first by Willis (1672), who gave a succinct description of a patient with prominent bulbar weakness and fatiguability. The aetiology was obscure for many years. Early studies of the pathology failed to reveal any abnormality in the central nervous system or marked changes in the muscles (Campbell and Bramwell 1900) and the diagnosis from hysteria was, for a long time, difficult. The observation that anticholinesterase drugs produced rapid but transient improvement in strength in the disease (Remen 1932; Walker 1934) led to the realisation that the disease was due to abnormal neuromuscular transmission and our present understanding of the disease stems from the morphological, electrophysiological and immunological studies of motor end-plates begun as a result of Walker's (1934) observation. Myasthenia gravis shows several clinical subgroups (Table 12.2). The clinical subgroups of adult-onset myasthenia gravis were defined by Compston et al. (1980).

The category of adult-onset myasthenia gravis in the classification given in Table 12.2 includes both ocular and generalised myasthenia. Although myasthenia may be restricted to involvement of the external ocular muscles in 40% of cases at presenta-

Table 12.2. Classification of myasthenia gravis

Acquired, adult-onset myasthenia gravis
1. Without thymoma
   (a) Onset before age 40 years
   (b) Onset after age 40 years
2. With thymoma
Drug-induced myasthenia gravis
Transient neonatal myasthenia gravis

tion it remains confined to these muscles in only 16%, and most cases show electrophysiological changes in other muscles (Grob et al. 1981; Bever et al. 1983). Osserman (1958) and Osserman and Genkins (1971) utilised a classification that is used more as an index of severity than a classification of different syndromes (Table 12.3). Drachman et al. (1982) modified the Osserman scale to relate it to antibody levels (Table 12.3).

Table 12.3. The Osserman clinical severity classification of myasthenia gravis

	Osserman and Genkins (1971)		Drachman et al. (1982)	
20%	Grade 1	Ocular	Focal	Grade 1
30%	Grade 2A	Mild generalised	Mild generalised	Grade 2
20%	Grade 2B	Severe generalised	Severe generalised	Grade 3
11%	Grade 3	Acute fulminating	Myasthenic crisis	Grade 4
9%	Grade 4	Late severe		

Neonatal myasthenia is a transient disorder which occurs in about one in seven babies born to myasthenic mothers. Juvenile-onset myasthenia does not differ from adult-onset myasthenia with onset before age 40 years in this classification (Table 12.2) (Bundey 1972). The term congenital myasthenia has been superseded by the recognition of a number of discrete, congenital myasthenic syndromes (see Table 12.1) (Engel 1984).

The modal age of onset is lower in women than in men (Simpson 1981). Grob et al. (1981) found a mean age of onset in women at 28 years and in men at 42 years. The overall female to male preponderance is 6 : 4 (Osserman and Genkin 1971). Simpson (1978) noted a prevalence of about 1 in 25 000. In Denmark Somnier et al. (1991) found a point prevalence of 1 in 10 000 for women and 0.6 per 10 000 for men. The annual incidence of the disease was 4.4 per million, with an early-onset peak for women in the third decade and a late-onset peak for both sexes in the eighth decade. Schwab and Leland (1953) noted a male predilection in the elderly. The disease occurs in all races, all over the world. In Chinese people it is more common in children (40% of cases) than in Western races (20%) (Wang et al.

1992). The adult-onset form shows a rare familial occurrence (Namba et al. 1971).

Adult-Onset Myasthenia Gravis

The cardinal feature of the disorder is fatiguability. In 10% generalised fatigue is the presenting feature (Grob et al. 1987). Since this symptom is subjective the diagnosis is very difficult in the early stages. A number of other diseases, especially nervous tension and depression, may present with this complaint. The onset of myasthenia gravis is usually gradual and symptoms are often most evident in the evening when the patient is tired, or following a period of unusual exertion. Acute infections also frequently exacerbate underlying and perhaps undiagnosed or latent myasthenia.

Weakness and Course

Weakness is usually first evident in the external ocular muscles, producing unilateral or bilateral ptosis, and diplopia (Fig. 12.1). This is the presenting symptom in about half the cases. In patients with clinical features limited to external ocular muscles 1 month after the onset, two-thirds develop generalised disease (Grob et al. 1987). In a third, difficulty in swallowing or chewing, indicative of weakness of bulbar muscles, is the presenting symptom and in the remainder weakness of the limbs, which may be proximal or distal, unilateral or bilateral, is the major feature (Perlo et al. 1966; Grob et al. 1981). The symptoms become more generalised in the first few months after the onset in most patients, and reach their maximum intensity in 65% of patients within a year of the onset. The symptoms vary from day to day, and in longer cycles, in relation to remissions and exacerbations. In some patients spontaneous remission may continue for many years but in others the disease tends to pursue a downhill course, although variable from month to month. In the more severely affected patients permanent relatively unvarying weakness may develop (Fig. 12.2a), especially in proximal muscles, and this is often accompanied by wasting.

Ocular Myasthenia

Patients with involvement of external ocular muscles alone, in whom no marked change has occurred for 2 years or more, seem to show little or no progression or involvement of other muscles (Osserman 1958). Grob et al. (1981) noted an 88% likelihood that the disease would remain localised

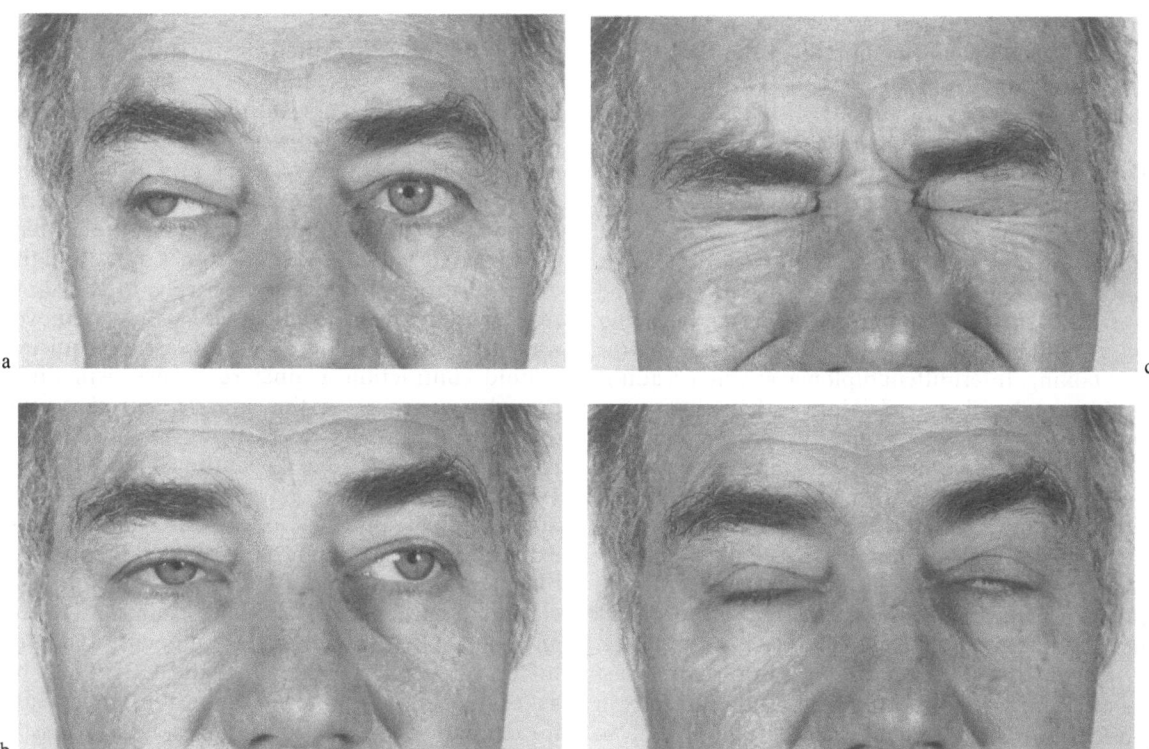

Fig. 12.1. Myasthenia gravis. **a** Gaze to the right. There is partial ophthalmoplegia with predominantly right-sided ptosis, and a corrugated brow from frontalis muscle overaction. **b** Gaze to the left. There is partial ophthalmoplegia with similar associated features. **c** Maximal forced eye closure. **d** After eye closure there is marked bilateral ptosis ("fatigue").

after this time. In patients with external ocular weakness alone, 3 years after the onset, there is only a 5% chance of the development of generalised disease (Grob et al. 1987). Nonetheless, we have seen a patient in whom limb muscle weakness developed 50 years after presentation with myasthenia gravis limited to the external ocular muscles. Only 16% of 168 patients with myasthenia gravis followed by Grob et al. (1981) for a mean period of 12 years showed myasthenia gravis clinically localised to the external ocular muscles.

Generalised Myasthenia

The facial muscles are involved in most patients, even in those who present complaining only of diplopia or ptosis. In patients with predominant bulbar involvement, weakness of the respiratory musculature is particularly likely to occur and this may be a life-threatening complication. It may develop relatively rapidly in such patients either shortly after the disease begins, or during an exacerbation.

Exacerbation of myasthenic weakness (*myasthenic crisis*) may occur spontaneously, or in response to a number of extraneous factors. The latter particularly include intercurrent infection, whether a trivial viral upper respiratory ailment or a more serious bacterial infection. Patients with predominantly bulbar myasthenia are particularly at risk of developing respiratory infections, and ventilatory failure may occur in relation to such infections. Other common factors leading to exacerbations of myasthenic weakness are emotional stress, pregnancy, fever, exposure to a warm environment such as a hot bath or sunbathing (Borenstein and Desmedt 1974), and overmedication with anticholinesterase drugs. The latter, representing *cholinergic crisis*, may occur because of fluctuations in the safety factor for neuromuscular transmission, or because of incorrect medication. Other drugs, such as phenytoin, muscular relaxant drugs used in anaesthesia, and certain antibiotics, such as neomycin, may also lead to an exacerbation of myasthenic weakness, which may sometimes be clinically important. Prior to the use of modern immunosuppressant drugs 50% of patients with generalised myasthenia developed an episode of severe weakness within 8 months (Grob et al. 1987) to 21 months (Cohen and Younger 1981) of the onset. Myasthenic crises occurred in 16% of 447 patients reviewed by Cohen and Younger (1981). The first crisis occurred at a mean age of 38 years in women, and 62 years in men. The mortality from myasthenic crisis improved from 42% in 1960–1964 to only 6% in 1975–1979 (Cohen and Younger 1981).

Some symptoms are particularly characteristic. Patients with bulbar myasthenia often notice that their voice becomes quieter, or may disappear altogether, during continued conversation. Similarly, they find that they are unable to chew strongly towards the end of a meal. Many such patients tend to sit with their jaw supported in one hand in order to prevent it hanging open, and to facilitate chewing and talking. Intermittent diplopia, as when reading, watching television, or driving is a frequent symptom in patients with ocular myasthenia. Fatiguability of the limbs, or of a hand, may be noticed as a feature of repetitive tasks in patients whose myasthenia mainly affects the limb musculature. Involvement of respiratory muscles is usually relatively asymptomatic, the patient presenting with flaccid proximal and bulbar weakness, and with drowsiness, but not with shortness of breath or dyspnoea. The functional effectiveness of the respiratory musculature must thus always be evaluated carefully in patients with myasthenia gravis presenting in an exacerbation.

Physical Examination

On examination there may be few pathognomic features. A triple-furrowed tongue, an appearance in which the tongue has three long longitudinal furrows, is a useful feature when present, but is found only in relatively longstanding cases (Buzzard 1905). In addition to weakness of the lower jaw, bilateral facial weakness and ptosis (Fig. 12.1) there may be a tendency for the head to fall forward, from weakness of the neck extensors, a sign found otherwise only in polymyositis, very advanced myotonic dystrophy or in dropped head syndrome. External ocular muscle weakness is found in as many as 90% of cases. Variable squint is thus a frequent manifestation and a nystagmus-like inability to sustain gaze, especially laterally, is a common feature. This may mimic internuclear ophthalmoplegia and lead to diagnostic confusion in early cases (Glaser 1966). Proximal weakness is prominent only in severe cases, and distal weakness may also be found, often strikingly asymmetrical in distribution. In severe cases, particularly of long duration, muscle atrophy may develop.

Since, in milder cases, clinical diagnosis rests on the demonstration of fatiguability, a symptom which is both subjective and difficult to quantitate because of variations in exercise tolerance, a

number of clinical tests for the disease have been devised and these are often very useful. It is particularly important to test muscles commonly affected by the disease, such as external ocular, bulbar and proximal, e.g. deltoid, muscles. The extensors of the neck can also be readily tested. A prolonged conversation, as in history-taking, is often sufficient to demonstrate myasthenic fatigue in the bulbar muscles. The patient's voice becomes quiet, and the lower jaw begins to close ineffectively. After a short rest, strength is restored. Repeated abduction movements of the shoulders, a movement requiring deltoid contraction against resistance, will often provoke weakness of this muscle, but since the deltoid is ordinarily very strong repeated rapid movements may need to be continued for as long as 1–2 min, and this test may be stressful to patient and examiner alike. Simple maintenance of arm extension or abduction is often difficult to interpret but may also demonstrate fatiguability. Repeated clenching movements of the hand against the resistance of a sphygmomanometer bulb, or a dynamometer, can similarly be used, or the patient may be asked to get up from the sitting position repeatedly for a minute or so. Fatigue and weakness are easily recognised. It will be apparent that these tests may not always be appropriate, and suitable tests must be selected in each patient in order to demonstrate myasthenic weakness.

In patients with very mild myasthenia, especially when symptoms are limited to external ocular muscles and are only transient in nature, tests of maintained elevation or lateral gaze may be useful. With sustained gaze, squint may develop, or nystagmoid movements of the eyes may become apparent. Cogan has described a lid-twitch sign, in which rapid redirection of gaze from the downward to the primary position results in a quick twitch of the lid upward, followed by a gradual return of the lid to the ptotic position in the next fraction of a second (Cogan 1965). This sign is particularly useful because not only is it practically invariably present in patients with myasthenia, even in those with minimal disease affecting only external ocular muscles, but it does not occur in other disorders.

An interesting observation in some patients with myasthenia, originally noted by Mary Walker (Walker 1938) is that fatigue of the forearm muscles by repetitive clenching and unclenching of the hand induces increased ptosis. The test is best carried out under ischaemic conditions, the ptosis developing a few seconds after release of the cuff. This response may be due to the release of lactate from the exercised forearm muscles into the circulation. Lactate binds calcium and may thus interfere indirectly with release of ACh at motor end-plates (Patten

1975). The phenomenon does not therefore indicate that a "toxic" myasthenia-producing substance is released from the muscle.

Special Features

The different types of myasthenia gravis (Table 12.2) show a number of special features.

Neonatal Myasthenia

In the *neonatal period* myasthenia is usually a transient phenomenon, often presenting on the first day of life, which resolves within the first month (Stern et al. 1964; Namba et al. 1970). It occurs in 12% of the newborn children of myasthenic mothers (Namba et al. 1970). Although often mild it may be severe and life-threatening during the first 2 weeks after birth. In all cases the infant's mother has myasthenia.

Affected infants usually present with feeding difficulties, generalised weakness and floppiness, respiratory difficulty, a feeble cry and bilateral facial weakness after birth. Ptosis is comparatively uncommon (Namba et al. 1970). Treatment with neostigmine is effective, when indicated, but most cases are not sufficiently severe to require treatment. The risk of another child being similarly affected is about 70% (Namba et al. 1970). Neonatal myasthenia is associated with increased levels of circulating acetylcholine receptor (AChR) antibody found not only in infants born to myasthenic mothers with and without clinical evidence of myasthenia, but also in the affected mother herself. The severity of neonatal myasthenia correlates not with the clinical severity of the mother's disease, but with her antibody level (Ymard et al. 1989).

The half-life of AChR antibody in 15 unaffected children was 3 to 11 days but in two children with neonatal myasthenia it was 42 and 91 days respectively (Lefvert and Osterman 1983). It has been suggested that neonatal myasthenia may be transferred by IgG antibodies absorbed from the maternal milk (Brenner et al. 1992). Tzartos et al. (1990) showed that maternal and fetal AChR antibodies showed similar antigenic specificities. A fetal factor interfering with the action of passively transferred maternal AChR antibody has been described, and amniotic fluid itself will inhibit AChR antibody binding. This may explain the absence of neonatal myasthenia in most infants of myasthenic mothers (Abramsky et al. 1979).

Rarely, arthrogryposis is seen in an infant born to a myasthenic mother. This has been associated with circulating antibodies directed to fetal rather than to adult AChR protein (Vincent et al. 1995).

Myasthenia with Thymoma

Patients with myasthenia associated with thymoma are generally older, and have a shorter history of muscle weakness, with a more severe and progressive course. In other respects there are no clinical differences in the syndrome (Teoh et al. 1989).

Associated Disorders

Myasthenia gravis, principally the adult form, is associated with an increased incidence of other disorders known to have an immunological basis. The link between myasthenia and these disorders is probably genetic and forms the cornerstone of the evidence that myasthenia itself is due to a genetically determined disturbance of immune tolerance (Simpson 1960, 1978). Disorders of the thyroid gland, including Hashimoto's thyroiditis, goitre, or frank myxoedema or thyrotoxicosis, occur in about 9% of men and 18% of women with myasthenia at some time during their lives (Simpson 1978). Rheumatoid arthritis, pernicious anaemia, pemphigus, Sjögren's syndrome and systemic lupus erythematosus also occur more frequently than expected in patients with myasthenia gravis, and in their relatives (Namba and Grob 1970; Simpson 1960, 1978). Epilepsy may also occur in a slightly increased prevalence than in the general population (Hoefer et al. 1958). Johns et al. (1971) noted an association between myasthenia gravis and polymyositis in 14 patients. There was a tendency for exacerbation of the two diseases to occur at different times. An association between myasthenia and multiple sclerosis has also been reported (Patten et al. 1972; Aita et al. 1974). In chronic graft versus host disease associated with bone marrow transplantation about 0.5% of patients develop myasthenia gravis (Bolger et al. 1986). The myasthenia develops 2 to 3 years after bone marrow transplantation, usually after reduction or discontinuation of immunosuppressant treatment (Bolger et al. 1986).

The Autoimmune Causation of Myasthenia Gravis

There are five criteria for accepting an autoimmune basis for a disease (Table 12.4).

Table 12.4. Criteria for autoimmune pathogenesis

1. Antibody is present in patients with the disease
2. Antibody interacts with the target antigen
3. Passive transfer of the antibody reproduces the main features of the disease
4. Immunisation with antigen produces a model of the disease
5. Reduction in antibody titre ameliorates the disease

From Drachman and Kuncl (1994)

Myasthenia gravis satisfies these criteria.

Enlargement of the thymus gland, or a thymoma, is often found in adult-onset myasthenia gravis. Rather than simply an associated feature of the disease this thymic abnormality is important in pathogenesis, and will be discussed later. An association of myasthenia gravis, giant cell polymyositis and myocarditis has been reported with thymoma (Pasuzzi et al. 1986).

Pathophysiology

Electrophysiological recordings from intercostal muscle biopsies of myasthenic patients, in vitro, have shown that the miniature end-plate potentials spontaneously occurring at the motor end-plates are smaller than normal, although their frequency is normal (Elmqvist et al. 1964). The amount of ACh released is normal (Albuquerque et al. 1976), but the responsiveness of the post-synaptic membrane is decreased (Grob and Namba 1976). These studies indicate that the defect of neuromuscular transmission in myasthenia is post-synaptic.

This conclusion is supported by studies of the ACh sensitivity of motor end-plates in the disease. The sensitivity of motor end-plates to ACh, studied by micro-iontophoretic techniques, is decreased, even in those fibres in which neuromuscular transmission can be observed (Albuquerque et al. 1976). This finding correlates fairly well with the observation that the number of ACh receptors in the end-plate region of myasthenic muscle fibres is reduced by up to 30% (Famborough et al. 1973; Pestronk et al. 1985).

Ultrastructural studies of motor end-plates in myasthenia gravis have shown that the post-synaptic region is smaller than normal, with simplification and loss of the post-synaptic folds. The mean nerve terminal area is smaller than normal but the numbers of synaptic vesicles are normal (Santa et al. 1972). The area of post-synaptic membrane capable of binding α-bungarotoxin, a snake venom with specific affinity for ACh receptors at motor end-plates, is reduced (Engel et al. 1977d). In more abnormal end-plates the synaptic clefts may be greatly and irregu-larly widened. Albuquerque et al. (1976) noted that the number of ACh receptors is particularly reduced on the tops of the post-synaptic folds, where they are most exposed to the extracellular environment, and at the point where they should be closest to the pre-synaptic nerve terminal apparatus.

The pre-terminal apparatus has been studied extensively by light microscopy with the methylene blue technique. Two main types of abnormality have been found; expanded endings, sometimes formed by several motor arborisations with marked irregularity of axoplasmic expansions, and elongated endings with lack of side branches. In addition, increased collateral ramification of motor axons, resulting in an increased terminal innervation ratio, may occur (Coërs et al. 1973). Coërs (1975) noted that an increased terminal innervation ratio was found only in patients older than 50 years. Some of these changes might be due to anti-cholinesterase drug therapy since neostigmine induced similar changes in rat end-plates, at similar dose levels to those used in man (Schwartz et al. 1977b). These pre-terminal abnormalities are probably secondary responses occurring in relation to the destruction of post-synaptic folds and ACh receptors.

Engel et al. (1977c) have shown that IgG and C_3 are deposited in the post-synaptic membrane and in degenerate material seen in the junctional synaptic space. These immune complexes occurred in greater abundance in less severely affected patients than in more severely affected patients in a distribution similar to that of post-synaptic ACh receptors (Engel et al. 1977d), an observation consistent with the assumption that an antibody in the circulating IgG of myasthenic patients is directed against an antigenic component of the ACh receptor protein. Less severely affected patients show more affinity for circulating antibody because they have larger numbers of functional ACh receptors in their end-plates than more severely affected patients; destruction of the ACh receptors is the primary reason for absence or reduction in numbers of miniature end-plate potentials (MEPPs) (Engel et al. 1977d). The presence of C_3 and C_9 (Engel et al. 1981b) on the post-synaptic membrane indicates that IgG binding to the receptor protein leads to activation of the complement-dependent system required for lytic destruction of the post-synaptic membrane (Kolb et al. 1972). The lytic "membrane-attack" complex of the complement cascade thus accounts for the strikingly atrophic appearance of the post-synaptic membrane in severe cases of myasthenia gravis (Engel 1981b). IgG and C_3 deposition on the receptor sites does not necessarily directly interfere with receptor function.

Circulating ACh Receptor Antibody

A circulating antibody to nicotinic ACh receptor protein is found in the IgG fraction of the plasma proteins in 74–90% of patients with generalised myasthenia gravis (Lindstrom et al. 1976; Mittag et al. 1976; Oh et al. 1992), but only in 70% of those with symptoms restricted to eye muscles for more than 2 years. There is an inexact correlation between the level of ACh receptor antibody titre in the blood and the severity of the myasthenia (Lindstrom et al. 1976; Drachman et al. 1982), indicating that the antibody is heterogenous (Vincent and Newsom-Davis 1980). Procedures leading to a reduction in the level of this antibody in the blood, such as thymectomy (Newsom-Davis 1979b), treatment with immunosuppressive drugs (Reuther et al. 1979), plasmapheresis (Pinching et al. 1976) and thoracic duct drainage (Bergström et al. 1973) are associated with clinical improvement. Transfer of immunoglobulin from the serum of myasthenic patients to mice produces weakness, a decremental response to repetitive nerve stimulation, a reduction in MEPP amplitude, and a reduced number of ACh receptor sites (Toyka et al. 1977; Lerrick et al. 1982). This effect could not be produced by transfer only of the IgG fraction, although it was enhanced by the presence of the C_3 component of complement (Lerrick et al. 1982).

Patients with myasthenia gravis possess a heterogenous population of antibodies to different components of the acetylcholine receptor, mainly against the extracellular domain. Most antibodies bind to the α subunit (Vincent et al. 1987; Marx et al. 1990). One region of the α subunit seems to represent the main immunogenic region, but even to this region there are heterogenous antibodies. Thus, the titre of AChR antibodies in the disease correlates poorly with disease severity (Krolick et al. 1993). Since the antigenic specificity of the extraocular muscle AChRs differs from that of limb muscles, titres that use limb muscle AChRs as an assay inevitably show poor correlation with extraocular muscle weakness and fatigue (Oda 1993).

Although it was initially thought that the ACh receptor antibody induced myasthenia by a blocking action at the ACh receptor sites, this has been found not to be the case since the antibody binds the protein subunit at the ACh site, rather than at the ACh-sensitive part of the receptor, and the disease is produced by the acceleration of the ACh receptor degradation consequent to cross-binding of this protein component of the ACh receptor with ACh receptor antibody (Drachman et al. 1977).

The antibody itself is probably produced by lymphocytes as it can be detected in thymic lymphocyte cultures (Vincent et al. 1978b). This finding, in tissue culture, was particularly noted in hyperplastic thymus glands; antibody production was not detected in thymic lymphocytes cultured from thymomas (Vincent et al. 1979; Newsom-Davis et al. 1982). Kao and Drachman (1976) reported that muscle cells can be cultured from adult human thymus and that these cells bear ACh receptors. Engel et al. (1977) confirmed the latter observation but Nicholson and Appel (1977) were unable to demonstrate ACh receptors by α-bungarotoxin binding, or by antibody labelling in both normal and myasthenic thymus tissue. In experimental autoimmune myasthenia gravis, however, a disorder induced by immunisation with an exogenous nicotinic ACh receptor, antibody to ACh receptors is produced at sites other than thymus gland (Lennon et al. 1975).

There is a relative increase in the number of B cells in thymus gland in patients with myasthenia gravis (Lisak et al. 1976). It is likely that the B lymphocytes produce the ACh receptor antibody since this antibody was found in 75% of thymus glands of patients with myasthenia (Mittag et al. 1976). It has been confirmed in cultures of cells from myasthenic thymus that the thymus is a site of anti-AChR antibody production (Scadding et al. 1981) to which plasma cells, as well as lymphocytes, may contribute (Newsom-Davis et al. 1982). T lymphocytes bearing thymosin a_1 on their surfaces are found in increased number in the blood of the majority of patients with myasthenia gravis. Thymosin α_1 specifically recruits helper T cells and may be important in the disturbed immunoregulatory mechanisms that initiate the disease (Dalakas et al. 1983). An increased number of T helper lymphocytes is also found in the thymus in the disease, and may be important in triggering the antibody response to AChR protein on myoid cells that seems an early feature of the disease (Hohlfeld et al. 1986).

ACh receptor antibodies from different patients seem to show similar binding potencies against ACh receptors in test preparations (Appel and Elias 1979). This observation, together with the inexact relation between clinical status and antibody levels, suggests that host factors are important in determining the effect of ACh receptor antibody in individual patients (Vincent and Newsom-Davis 1980). However, the ACh receptor antibody titre in patients with mild localised myasthenia is usually low or undetectable. Reduction of antibody levels with treatment is associated with clinical improvement (Oosterhuis et al. 1983; Vincent et al. 1983).

On the basis of comparison of clinical, pathological and HLA features, and of the levels of circulating ACh receptor antibody Compston et al. (1980) proposed that adult-onset myasthenia gravis is a disorder of heterogenous causation. However, as in other autoimmune diseases, the causative factors leading to the characteristic autoimmune response are unknown. There is evidence from thymomas that the autoimmune response is directed initially against the α subunit of the ACh receptor (Marx et al. 1990) before becoming generalised and self-replicating. It has been suggested that this could be initiated by molecular mimicry after exposure to Herpes simplex virus (HSV), since HSV has some homology with the amino acid sequence of the α subunit (Schwimmbeck et al. 1989). In the thymus, myoid cells are probably the source of ACh receptor protein and mRNA for the α subunit of the receptor found in thymic extracts (Wheatley et al. 1992).

Experimental Autoimmune Myasthenia Gravis

Muscular weakness resembling myasthenia gravis was produced in rabbits by immunising them with ACh receptor derived from the electric organ of electric eels by Patrick and Lindstrom (1973). In this model of the human disease there is a similar disturbance of neuromuscular transmission (Toyka et al. 1975), and the number of ACh receptor sites at motor end-plates, measured by α-bungarotoxin binding, is reduced (Engel et al. 1976; Engel et al. 1977d). The acute phase of the experimental disorder is characterised by phagocytic invasion of the neuromuscular junction (Engel et al. 1976), a phenomenon not seen in the naturally occurring disease in man, or in the naturally occurring variety found in the dog (Zacks et al. 1966). A similar model in the rat more closely resembles the human disorder and has enabled detailed study of the immunopathogenesis of receptor breakdown at the motor end-plate (see Lindstrom 1980). Experimental myasthenia can be induced in the mouse by passive transfer of human IgG from myasthenic patients (Toyka et al. 1977). Spontaneous myasthenia has been reported in the dog (Lennon et al. 1981).

Other Immunological Features of Myasthenia Gravis

The striking clinical response to thymectomy, and the association of other autoimmune disorders with myasthenia gravis led to the development of the immune hypothesis of its causation. A variety of autoantibodies have been found in the sera of patients with myasthenia. A 7S gammaglobulin,

binding specifically to the A band of striated muscle, is found in nearly all cases with thymoma, but in only 10% of other patients with myasthenia (van der Geld et al. 1964). Patients with thymoma show anti-titin circulating antibodies in 97% of cases (Gantel et al. 1993). This antibody is not found in autoimmune myasthenia associated with thymic hyperplasia. Anti-muscle antibodies may be found in low titre in control subjects but there the antibody binds to I band (Vetters 1965). The A band antibody cross-reacts with thymic myoid cells (Feltkamp-Vroom 1966). However, there is no correlation between the severity of myasthenia and the titre of this antibody. Other antibodies commonly found include thyroid antibodies, anti-nuclear factor, gastric parietal cell antibodies and rheumatoid factor (Simpson 1966). Other abnormalities, such as positive Coombs factor, are rare.

One of the factors determining initiation of the disease must be the susceptibility of the host; indeed 7% of cases of myasthenia gravis are familial (Pirskanen 1977). In young patients with myasthenia without thymoma, particularly in women, there is an increased occurrence of HLA-A1 and B8 antigens (Pirkanen et al. 1972) and of B12 in Japanese myasthenic patients (Yoshida et al. 1977). This association was found in 79% of patients, mostly women, under the age of 40 years and in 59% of all patients, compared with 19% in the general population, in the 100 patients studied by Feltkamp et al. (1984). In myasthenic patients with thymoma there is no association with HLA-A1 or B8 (Sachs 1979) but an increased occurrence of HLA-A2 has been reported (Feltkamp et al. 1984). The association of myasthenia with HLA-B8 probably represents the association of the disease with autoimmune factors (Dausset et al. 1974). No association has been found between HLA status and the presence or titre of ACh receptor antibody (Christiansen et al. 1978).

The immunological abnormalities found in myasthenia gravis have suggested a classification (Table 12.5).

Table 12.5. Subgroups of myasthenia gravis

	Generalised			Ocular
Age of onset (years)	<40	30–50	>40	Wide range
Sex ratio M : F	1 : 3	1 : 1	3 : 1	3 : 1
Serum anti AChR titre	+++	++	+	±
Anti-striated muscle antibody	20%	90%	60%	30%
HLA associations (caucasoids)	A1, B8, DRw3	None	A3, B7, DRw2	Variable
Thymus pathology	Hyperplasia	Thymoma	Atrophy	None

From Newsom–Davis and Murray (1984)

Pathogenesis of Myasthenia Gravis

The following processes can be envisaged in the pathogenesis of the disease:

1. Induction of acetylcholine receptor (AChR) expression on thymic myoid cells
2. (a) Release of AChR from myoid cells
   (b) Uptake of AChR by thymic antigen-presenting cells
   (c) AChR antigen epitope presentation by HLA class II cells
3. Recognition of AChR fragments by specific CD4+ T cells
4. Stimulation of B cells by AChR-specific T cells in thymus and in the periphery to produce AChR antibody
5. Antibody-mediated destruction of AChR protein at motor end-plates. This process involves complement T cells and macrophages.

CD4+ T cells are helper T cells that respond to antigen that has been processed by antigen-presenting cells. This is associated with major histocompatibility complex (MHC) class II molecules. These MHC class II molecules contain a groove that accomodates linear peptides 15–20 amino acids in length, and thus can select those peptides which can be bound and presented. The T cell receptor recognises peptides only in association with the MHC class II molecule; thus indicating the importance of HLA phenotypes in the pathogenesis of this, and other, autoimmune diseases.

Antibody-Negative Myasthenia Gravis

About 15% of patients with generalised myasthenia have no detectable circulating AChR antibodies. Nonetheless these patients respond in a similar fashion to immunosuppressant medication, as do patients with increased AChR antibody titres (Newsom–Davis et al. 1987), and they have a reduced number of ACh receptors at motor end-plates, again, as in those patients with circulating antibody (Drachman et al. 1987). Burges et al. (1994) found that passive transfer of plasma or purified IgG from patients with antibody-negative myasthenia to mice caused a reduction in MEPP amplitudes or reduced end-plate potential quantal content, but without changes in ACh-induced depolarisation. These observations suggested that antibody-negative myasthenia is heterogenous, with several physiological defects, implying a number of different antigenic targets. In the human sero-negative form of myasthenia gravis the neurophysiological features resemble those of antibody-positive myasthenia

gravis (Oh et al. 1992). Clinically, the disorder is usually relatively mild, or relatively restricted to ocular muscles. The latter is perhaps dependent on the assay procedure which uses AChR derived from limb muscles, rather than ocular muscles (Oda 1993).

Pathology of the Thymus in Myasthenia Gravis

Thymomas occur in about 10% of patients with myasthenia gravis (Schwab and Leland 1953); in patients with thymoma, myasthenia gravis occurs in 30% (Namba et al. 1978). About 60% of myasthenic patients with thymomas are male (Simpson 1958). Other pathological changes, excluding thymoma, occur in about 60% of patients with myasthenia gravis, but in the remainder the thymus gland appears histologically normal. The hyperplastic changes found in this group of patients consist of the presence of germinal centres in the thymic medulla. However, there is no correlation between the number of germinal centres observed and the severity of the myasthenia. Hyperplasia consists predominantly of lymphoid follicle prominence with increased numbers of lymphocytes and plasma cells, but without epithelial cell hyperplasia. Despite the histological appearance of hyperplasia the thymus gland is usually of normal weight (Castleman and Norris 1949). The density of Hassal's corpuscles, and the pattern of involution of the cortex and medulla of the thymus gland with increasing age is normal (Goldstein and Mackay 1966). With fluorescence techniques the striations of myoid thymic cells show A band autoantibody affinity in many patients (Goldstein and Mackay 1966).

Thymomas are classified broadly into lymphoblastic and epithelial cell tumours but this division is, to some extent, artificial and most such tumours are described as lymphoephtheliomatous (Henson et al. 1965; Castleman 1966). The epithelial cell component of these tumours is derived from Hassal's corpuscles. Thymomas, although locally invasive, rarely metastasize beyond the pleural cavity. Rarely, myasthenia gravis may develop some time after removal of a thymoma (Castleman 1966). Namba et al. (1978) found that this occurred in 10% of patients with thymoma, within 18 months of the removal of the tumour. In myasthenia gravis, thymomas are found by routine radiographic or CT (Fig. 12.2b) investigation of the anterior mediastinum or during surgical exploration; they do not present with mediastinal compression or other intrathoracic complications. There is, however, a very rare association of thymoma with pure red cell aplasia and peripheral neuropathy. Thymoma in

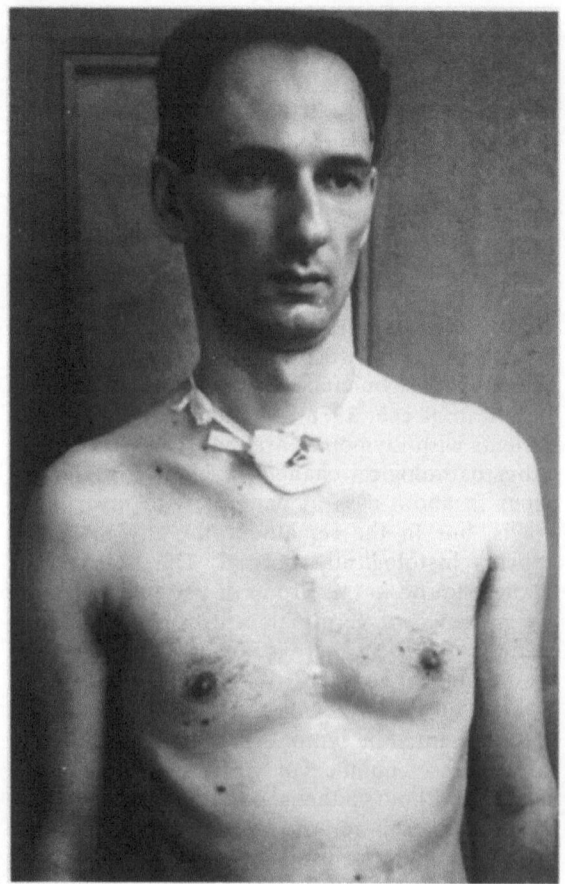
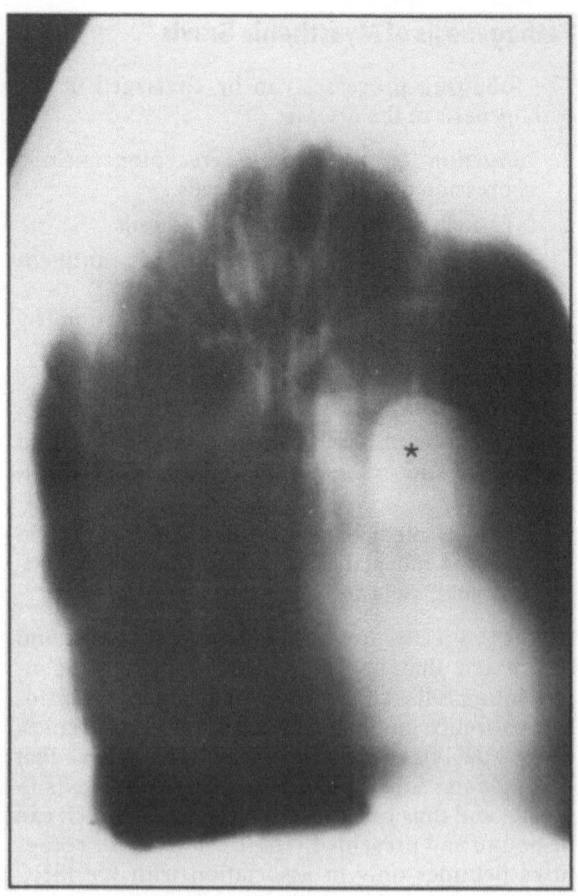

Fig. 12.2. Myasthenia gravis. **a** There is a myopathic facies with slight atrophy of limb muscles. This patient has had a thymectomy, but required tracheotomy post-operatively. **b** Lateral tomogram of chest in a patient with myasthenia gravis. There is a thymic tumour superior and anterior to the cardiac shadow (star).

infants and children is very rare (Namba et al. 1978).

Muscle Pathology

There may be little or no abnormality in some biopsies. In most, however, abnormalities are seen and these are most prominent in patients with marked weakness. Dubowitz and Brooke (1973) noted that Type 2 atrophy was often not uniformly distributed, even appearing focally within the biopsy, suggesting that it was not necessarily a non-specific phenomenon related to disease. Lymphorrhages, focal aggregations of lymphocytes, usually unrelated to blood vessels, are common (Russell 1953). However, lymphorrhages are not unique to myasthenia gravis since they also occur in neurogenic disorders and in polymyositis. Engel and McFarlin (1966) found Type 2 atrophy in about half of their patients, and

lymphorrhages in a quarter. Scattered small fibres of either histochemical type and some isolated necrotic fibres may also be found (Engel and McFarlin 1966). Clusters of small, pointed fibres, or even fibre-type grouping, have also been reported, suggesting that denervation and reinnervation occurs during the course of the disease (Fenichel and Shy 1963; Brownell et al. 1972). Denervation has usually been attributed to myasthenic damage to motor end-plates (see Schwartz et al. 1977b). The abnormalities found in motor end-plates have been described above. Similar changes have been described in the motor innervation of muscle spindles in the disease (Swash and Fox 1975c).

Diagnosis

Although the diagnosis of myasthenia can often be made with confidence from the clinical features of

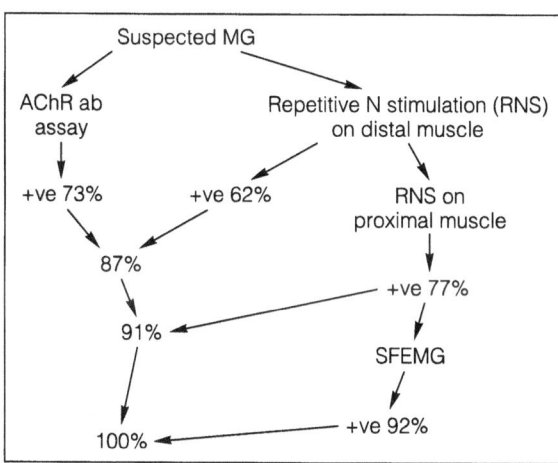

Fig. 12.3. Sensitivity of clinical tests for myasthenia (Oh et al. 1992)

the disease, in mild cases and in patients with restricted ocular or bulbar involvement there is a wide differential diagnosis. A number of pharmacological and electrophysiological tests are available for diagnosis and, ultimately, diagnosis is confirmed by the response to treatment with anticholinesterase drugs. Measurement of levels of ACh receptor antibody is also useful in diagnosis, although there is no clear relation between level of antibody and severity of myasthenia, and in 15% of patients the test is negative (see above).

The role of the various diagnostic tests is shown in Fig. 12.3. Note that both biological assessment by AChR assay, and physiological testing by EMG are important. Pharmacological tests assess the response to cholinergic (anticholinesterase) drugs and are still commonly used in diagnosis and in assessing the response to treatment.

Pharmacological Tests

The first pharmacological methods for establishing the diagnosis of myasthenia consisted of the administration of 1.5 mg neostigmine IM, or 15 mg orally (Viets and Schwab 1935). With intramuscular neostigmine, improvement in strength begins in 10–20 min, with a peak effect at about 30 min. Because of muscarinic effects on the gastro-intestinal tract and the heart it is a wise precaution to give 0.6 mg atropine IM just before neostigmine is given. Because neostigmine has an effect for an hour or more careful clinical evaluation of many different muscle groups can be carried out, and patients can make their own assessments of the effectiveness of the drug during exertion. Lessening of fatiguability is a subjective, but impressive, result in typical cases.

The effect of neostigmine is gradual and it is not always easy to be sure of improvement, particularly in patients with minor degrees of weakness, with limited ocular involvement, or with fatiguability as the only symptom (Eaton 1943). A shorter-acting drug, edrophonium hydrochloride (Tensilon) is useful in diagnosis of such patients because it can be given intravenously (Osserman and Kaplan 1952), its effect becoming obvious very rapidly and disappearing within 5–10 min (Osserman and Genkins 1966). An initial dose of 2 mg is given intravenously and if no reaction occurs within about 45 s an additional 8 mg can be injected slowly, through the same needle. Since the duration of action of the drug is short it is important to select a moderately weak muscle in which to assess strength or fatiguability; examination of ptosis is often useful. Because the drug is given intravenously it is usually convenient for an observer to assess the response.

There is a small risk of cholinergic crisis, manifested by extreme bradycardia or even transient severe weakness requiring brief ventilatory support, and the test should never be performed without facilities for resuscitation being immediately available. This risk is very small when the drug is used for diagnosis, but is more appreciable when it is being used to assess the effectiveness of anticholinesterase therapy in the management of patients in whom the diagnosis is well established (see below). If the response to edrophonium is uncertain the test can be repeated using a placebo normal saline injection and the two clinical responses compared directly. Normal subjects and patients with myasthenia often develop sweating, bradycardia and abdominal cramps with edrophonium, but the fasciculations frequently observed about the face, and sometimes in other muscles, in normal subjects after edrophonium are rarely observed in myasthenic patients, unless cholinergic crisis is imminent (see below). It is a curious phenomenon that patients with myasthenia frequently show a rather prolonged beneficial response, even for longer than 30 min, after their first injection of edrophonium, a response in excess of anything observed subsequently.

The edrophonium test is positive in 90%–95% of all cases of myasthenia. False-positive results may occur in Lambert–Eaton syndrome, botulism, Guillain–Barré syndrome and motor neuron disease (Oh and Cho 1990).

Patients with myasthenia show an increased sensitivity to curare, a phenomenon that formed the basis of a curare test for myasthenia, in which a small dose of curare (2% of the normal curarising dose) was given intravenously and the development of weakness, which would not occur in a normal individual, was observed (Bennett and Cash 1943). This test and its modification, a regional curare test, (Brown et al. 1975) is dangerous, unpredictable and no longer used in clinical practice. One interesting feature of the response of myasthenic patients to curare was the sensitivity of muscles clinically uninvolved by the disease, a feature well known to anaesthetists, and indicating the generalised nature of the disease even in patients with apparently restricted ocular myasthenia (Horowitz et al. 1975).

Electrophysiological Tests

All electrophysiological tests for myasthenia test neuromuscular transmission. Since this is variable and the abnormality is always worsened by repetitive or continuous activity, the tests themselves depend on assessing the effects of activity on the defect of neuromuscular transmission. The most important of these electrophysiological tests is repetitive supramaximal nerve stimulation with recording of the evoked MUAPs.

Repetitive Nerve Stimulation. When supramaximal stimuli are applied in a train a decrement in the amplitude of the evoked response is observed in many patients with myasthenia (Harvey and Masland 1941a; Desmedt 1973). Jolly (1895) described a decremental response to repeated faradic stimulation of the belly of affected muscles; this technique probably stimulated the terminal innervation rather than the muscle fibres themselves.

The repetitive nerve stimulation test is usually carried out on the median or ulnar nerve at the wrist, recording from small hand muscles with surface electrodes, but proximal muscles may also be studied. It is important that the limb tested should be warm, especially when small hand muscles are tested since skin temperatures less than 34 °C may lead to false-negative results (Ricker et al. 1977). Recordings made from the deltoid are particularly useful, the stimulus being applied at Erb's point. In addition, the facial nerve can be stimulated, recording from the orbicularis oculi muscles. A supramaximal stimulus, at least 150% of the stimulus required to give a maximal evoked muscle action potential, is applied to the nerve. The response to the first stimulus is normal, or slightly small, in myasthenia (Harvey and Masland 1941b). When the nerve is stimulated at 2–3 Hz in normal subjects the amplitude of the fourth or fifth response does not decrease by more than 8% of the amplitude of the first response. In patients with myasthenia, however, the amplitude of the fourth or fifth response to stimuli applied at 3 Hz often shows a decrement of 10% or more (Fig. 12.4). Ozdemir

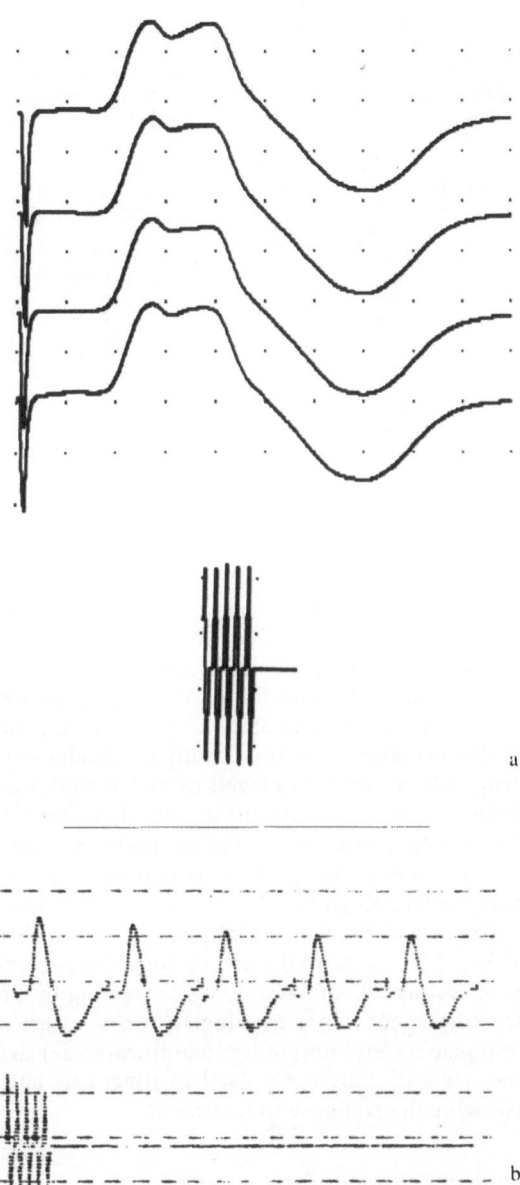

Fig. 12.4. **a** Decremental response in a normal individual, there is no decrement to 3 Hz stimulation. **b** Decremental response of 25% in myasthenia gravis, with ulnar nerve stimulation at a frequency of 3 Hz, recorded from abductor digiti minimi.

and Young (1976) found an abnormal decremental response in 52% of patients when recordings were made from the abductor digiti minimi after ulnar nerve stimulation at the wrist. Recordings made from the deltoid muscle, after stimulation at Erb's point, increased the yield of abnormal responses to 89%, and facial studies yielded 62% of such myasthenic responses.

Stimulation of the spinal accessory nerve in the neck, recording from the trapezius muscle, has also been recommended and is less uncomfortable than the deltoid technique (Dong et al. 1980; Schumm and Stöhr 1984); 87% of patients showed decremental responses.

The radial nerve–anconeus muscle system can also be used (Kennett and Fawcett 1993), although only 10% of ocular myasthenics and 53% of generalised myasthenics show an abnormal response. Exercise prior to testing increased the proportion of abnormal responses in the small hand muscles by a further 15%. Desmedt (1973) and Desmedt and Borenstein (1977) have suggested that the repetitive nerve stimulation test can be made more sensitive. They found that the yield of positive results was increased when the four repeated supramaximal stimuli were applied 30 s after repetitive stimulation at 3 Hz for 4 min. When the test is performed in this manner after repetitive stimulation at 3 Hz for 4 min, *with the limb made ischaemic by a cuff*, myasthenic patients show a more marked decrement, but some patients with ocular myasthenia still show a normal response (Ozdemir and Young 1976; Desmedt and Borenstein 1977).

At higher rates of stimulation than 3 Hz a paradoxical potentiation of the size of the evoked MUAP may be observed (Mayer and Williams 1974). This may represent recruitment of blocked neuromuscular junctions, or a transient facilitation of neuromuscular transmission occurring with higher rates of stimulation (20–50 Hz). The latter could occur from release of stored quanta of ACh neurotransmitter at presynaptic sites. After a brief period of facilitation neuromuscular block increases again with further tetanic stimulation, or exercise; the phenomenon called post-facilitation (post-exercise) exhaustion. This results from decreased safety factor for transmission, depletion of ACh quantal stores and changes in the post-junctional part of the neuromuscular junctions.

Electromyography. In most patients conventional concentric needle EMG is normal but in some, particularly those with persistent weakness unresponsive to anticholinesterase drugs, short-duration polyphasic MUAPs of low amplitude suggesting myopathy may be found (Pinelli et al. 1975); evidence of myopathy associated with myasthenia is found in about 10% of patients with longstanding myasthenia. Some of the patients may have a coexistent polymyositis (Johns et al. 1971). Conversely, there may be a reduced interference pattern with polyphasic MUAPs of normal amplitude, suggesting a neurogenic component, in some patients. Short-duration polyphasic units of low amplitude in myasthenia could occur because of intermittent loss of functioning muscle fibres within motor units,

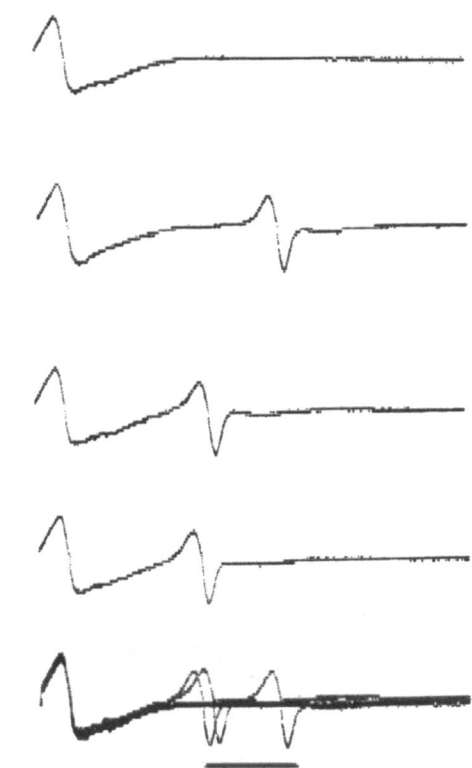

Fig. 12.5. A potential pair showing increased jitter and impulse blocking. Single-fibre EMG. Bar 1 ms.

consequent on the neuromuscular block itself. There is a characteristic variability in the configuration of a given MUAP in successive recordings, for example using a trigger-delay line. The initial few MUAPs show a progressive decrease in amplitude and duration (Kimura 1983).

Single-Fibre EMG. Single-fibre EMG has proved a useful tool in the diagnosis of myasthenia gravis. All other clinical and neurophysiological tests for myasthenia depend on the demonstration of intermittent failure of transmission at a proportion of motor end-plates in a muscle (neuromuscular blocking). With single-fibre EMG this feature can be easily recognised by intermittent blocking of single muscle fibre action potentials (Fig. 12.5) in recordings in which two or more muscle fibre action potentials belonging to the same motor unit can be seen (see Chaps 2 and 3). However, the earliest recognisable abnormality with single-fibre EMG is the presence of an increased neuromuscular jitter (Fig. 12.6) (Stålberg et al. 1974), representing a decreased safety factor for neuromuscular transmission at the end-plates and muscle fibres studied (Stålberg et al. 1975a). In patients with myasthenia gravis there is considerable variation in the degree

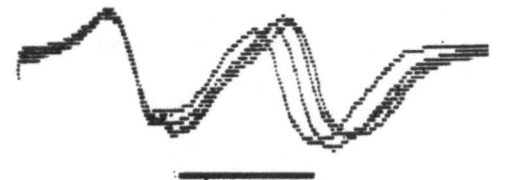

Fig. 12.6. A potential pair showing increased jitter (65 μs) but without impulse blocking. Single-fibre EMG. Bar 0.4 ms.

of abnormality found in different muscles, and within the same muscle. Even within the same motor unit increased neuromuscular jitter and impulse blocking may affect different single neuromuscular junctions, yet others may be normal (Stålberg et al. 1976b). It is important to recognise this variation in the degree of involvement of individual end-plates in a motor unit; at least 20 potential pairs must be studied before it can be accepted that the neuromuscular jitter is normal. Even in patients with severe myasthenia one or more of the potential pairs recorded usually shows a normal jitter, but in ocular myasthenia recordings from the forearm extensors may reveal an abnormal neuromuscular jitter in only one or two of the 20 potential pairs. Single-fibre EMG nearly always reveals increased jitter, and usually impulse blocking in patients with generalised myasthenia (Stålberg et al. 1974).

It is interesting to note that an increased neuromuscular jitter was found in seven of 21 close relatives of myasthenic patients (Stålberg et al. 1976b), although myasthenia is clinically evident in only 5% of close relatives of such patients (Namba et al. 1971).

In ocular myasthenia about 20% of patients show a normal jitter in limb muscles, but the jitter seems more frequently (88%) abnormal in the frontalis muscle (Sanders and Howard 1986). In generalised myasthenia, abnormalities are often more prominent in deltoid than in extensor digitorum communis. During a single-fibre EMG examination in a patient with myasthenia gravis it is common to find that jitter and blocking become more prominent as the examination proceeds, and the muscle often becomes weak at this time. Even motor units with a jitter in the normal range may show abnormal jitter and blocking after several minutes spontaneous activity at low firing rates (8–12 Hz) (Ingram et al. 1985). This corresponds to the clinical fatiguability of myasthenia and to the effects of repetitive nerve stimulation on the evoked MUAP. Increased jitter and blocking correlate with neuromusclar transmission failure occurring during exercise, or nerve stimulation.

Schwartz and Stålberg (1975a) showed that there was a progressive decline in the numbers of muscle fibres activated within individual motor units during repetitive nerve stimulation, although other muscle fibres were sometimes recruited as some became blocked. With rest, jitter and blocking decrease. During repetitive nerve stimulation, using the technique of single axon stimulation at the motor point (Trontelj and Stålberg 1991), or stimulating the nerve, and recording by SFEMG from the same muscle used for standard single-fibre EMG of voluntarily activated units, a relationship between decremental responses and neuromuscular blocking was confirmed (Gilchrist et al. 1994).

Intravenous edrophonium decreased neuromuscular jitter and impulse blocking in myasthenic muscles (Stålberg et al. 1976b) and regional curare increased the blocking. The motor unit fibre density is slightly increased, especially in older patients (Stålberg and Trontelj 1994). In patients treated with anticholinesterase drugs there is usually an improvement in the single-fibre EMG abnormality. Impulse blocking is less frequent and the neuromuscular jitter is less abnormal. In nearly all patients, however, even those with little or no weakness or fatigue, an abnormal jitter can be demonstrated. Rarely, in patients who have entered a clinical remission, the single-fibre EMG studies become normal (Sanders et al. 1979). Sanders and Howard (1986) reported that 32% of patients in remission have normal single-fibre EMG studies in limb muscles.

In assessing patients for the diagnosis of myasthenia by single-fibre EMG a number of points must be remembered. *First*, one of 20 potential pairs (5%) may show increased jitter in normal subjects (Stålberg and Thiele 1975). *Second*, an increased neuromuscular jitter is found in many different disorders other than myasthenia; it is not a specific feature of myasthenic weakness ("all that jitters is not myasthenia"). A transient increase in neuromuscular jitter may be found, for example, after non-specific influenza-like viral infections (Friman et al. 1977). *Third*, if the muscle examined by single-fibre EMG shows a normal jitter, yet is weak, the diagnosis is other than myasthenia gravis (Stålberg et al. 1976b).

Other Electrophysiological Tests

Another non-invasive test in patients with bulbar myasthenia depends on fatigue in the stapedius muscle of the middle ear, shown by decay of the acoustic impedance measured during application of a continuous tone to the opposite ear (Blom and Zakrisson 1974; Kramer et al. 1981). However, the results of this test appear variable (Oosterhuis et al. 1985). Electronystagmography and tomography have also been used in diagnosis. Saccadic velocity increases, and intraocular pressure also increases, after edrophonium chloride in myasthenic patients. In normal subjects intraocular pressure decreases after edrophonium chloride (Campbell et al. 1970).

AChR Antibody Level

The AChR antibody level is raised in about 85% of patients with generalised myasthenia gravis (Oh et al. (1992) reported only 73%), and only about 50% of patients with ocular myasthenia (see Drachman and Kuncl 1994). False-positive results are rare. The level of antibody correlates poorly with the severity of the disorder (see above). Patients with myasthenia gravis associated with thymoma invariably have increased AChR antibody levels (Vincent et al. 1993). Most patients whose myasthenia is associated with thymic involution are sero-negative (Vincent et al. 1993). The AChR antibody test is the only biological test for myasthenia which shows specificity and, although of slightly limited sensitivity, is recommended as an initial test in all patients in whom the diagnosis is suspected.

Other Clinical Investigations

It is important to consider the possibility of thymoma. CT of the anterior mediastinum is probably the most reliable method for detecting thymic enlargement, but it does not reliably distinguish benign enlargement from tumour (Janssen et al. 1983). Ordinary lateral X-ray tomography (Fig. 12.2b) is notoriously unreliable. Radio-isotope scanning is particularly valuable for demonstrating recurrence of thymomas in patients who have relapsed after thymectomy, or in indicating the presence of ectopic thymic tissue (Testa and Angelini 1979). Striated muscle antibodies are present in 84% of patients with thymoma; in non-thymoma patients these antibodies are found in 5% of those under 40 years and 47% of those older than 40 years (Limburg et al. 1983). Thymomas are exceptionally rare in childhood.

Management

The objectives of treatment are to improve neuro-muscular transmission and to prevent further destruction of ACh receptors by interfering with the autoimmune lytic process in the motor endings, and by preventing or slowing down synthesis of ACh receptor antibody. Neuromuscular transmission can be improved by using anticholinesterase drugs, and

the other objectives are partially achieved by thymectomy and by immunosuppressive therapy. Plasma exchange has a role in severe, relatively acute cases or relapses, and in preparation for thymectomy.

Anticholinesterase Drugs

The two commonly used drugs are neostigmine and pyridostigmine (Mestinon). These drugs inhibit the enzyme cholinesterase which hydrolyses acetylcholine to choline and acetyl CoA in the synaptic cleft. Cholinesterase is produced in the post-synaptic junctional folds of the motor end-plate but is also present presynaptically in the subterminal apparatus itself. Anticholinesterase drugs improve neuromuscular transmission by increasing the concentration of ACh in the synaptic cleft but their mode of action is probably much more complex than this.

Neostigmine is relatively short-acting; most of its clinical effect wanes after 2–3 h and it has a rapid onset of action, with a peak effect in rather less than an hour after oral ingestion. Pyridostigmine has a slower effect and a longer duration of action, remaining effective for some 3–5 h after ingestion. Neostigmine is thus useful intermittently, especially to provide a short boost of increased strength before exertion, or before a meal, and pyridostigmine is used to provide more longlasting benefit throughout the day when given in divided doses. Patients vary in their requirement for these drugs. A few mildly affected patients may need only neostigmine before meals, or pyridostigmine 60 mg three or four times daily, but severely affected patients require frequent dosage with pyridostigmine, even 3-hourly, throughout the day and, sometimes, even nocturnal medication. In severely affected patients the mortality of myasthenia treated with cholinergic drugs alone was 25% (Rowland et al. 1956; Glaser 1966), but the use of the other methods of treatment including thymectomy, immunosuppressant therapy and plasma exchange, has greatly improved the outlook. Other, longer-acting cholinergic drugs such as ambenonium hydrochloride (Mytelase) and distigmine are little used because their effects are cumulative and difficult to predict. As a rule of thumb, it is generally unwise to allow a myasthenic patient to take more than 18 anticholinesterase tablets, of whatever type, in 24 h. If a patient needs approximately this number of tablets daily one of the other forms of treatment is probably indicated, especially since high doses of the drugs can themselves damage the motor end-plates (Schwartz et al. 1977b).

In patients with severe myasthenia, already taking anticholinesterase drugs, muscular weakness may be due either to an exacerbation of the myasthenia, or to *cholinergic crisis* – weakness due to competitive depolarisation block of ACh receptors by these drugs. Cholinergic crisis can sometimes be recognised by fasciculations, small pupils, salivation, sweating, pallor, bradycardia, diarrhoea and abdominal cramps but if the patient is also taking atropine and probanthine to prevent the unwanted muscarinic effects of anticholinesterase drugs it may be extremely difficult to recognise on clinical criteria. The diagnosis can be made by using the short-acting intravenous anticholinesterase drug edrophonium chloride. If the patient shows no improvement, or is made weaker by 2–10 mg edrophonium iv, cholinergic crisis is present. This test must *never* be performed in this situation without the immediate availability of full respiratory support. Further, it must be recognised that the respiratory muscles may be in incipient cholinergic block while other muscles may still be responsive to cholinergic medication so that assessment is doubly difficult. A practical course to follow is to stop all anticholinesterase drugs, ventilate the patient electively if necessary and, after a period of 2–3 days, gradually reintroduce anticholinesterase drugs in small increments (Osserman and Genkins 1966). Elective withdrawal of anticholinesterase drugs was formerly in vogue as a way of "resting the endplates" since it seemed sometimes to induce substantial remission but this relatively hazardous plan of management is used now rather less because of the availability of other forms of treatment, especially plasma exchange.

In the long term, treatment with high doses of anticholinesterase drug may itself affect neuromuscular transmission (Engel et al. 1973) and cause morphological changes in motor end-plates (Schwartz et al. 1977b). Stålberg (1980) found that the fibre density in single-fibre EMG recordings of patients with myasthenia treated with anticholinesterase drugs was 2.2 standard deviations greater than normal subjects, but that in untreated patients it was only 1.2 times greater, suggesting that the deleterious effect of the drugs might have functional significance. Further, since neurogenic atrophy occurs in such patients (Brownell et al. 1972) it is probably wise to avoid such treatment by advising thymectomy or immunosuppressive drug treatment.

Thymectomy

Thymectomy was first performed in myasthenia gravis by Sauerbruch in 1911. Several large series have been reported (Simpson 1958; Ferguson 1962;

Henson et al. 1965; Papatestas et al. 1976) and there is agreement that thymectomy is beneficial. Remission occurs in about 10% of cases in the first year after operation but seems to occur in more patients later, e.g. in 30% at 5 years (Papatestas et al. 1976; Oosterhuis 1981). Remission occurs in 8% of patients treated medically and in 30% of those treated by thymectomy (Buckingham et al. 1976). A good result is most common in patients with a short history of myasthenia, irrespective of age; it was concluded from the earlier studies that young women (under 30 years of age) with a history of less than 2 years (Henson et al. 1965) or 5 years (Simpson 1958), had the best chance of remission after thymectomy but this conclusion is probably unduly restrictive since older people of either sex may have an excellent result. Overall, improvement can be expected in 65%–85% of patients after thymectomy if no thymoma is found (Rowland 1980). No controlled studies of the effect of thymectomy are available (Genkins et al. 1993); in general patients having the operation are often those with the more severe disease. Remission and improvement are least likely to occur in patients with thymoma (Simpson 1958). In a review of 261 surgically treated patients, 75 had thymomas of which 26 were locally invasive. The prognosis in these patients, who tended to be older, was poorer than in those with non-invasive thymoma. In this series post-operative irradiation seemed to cause a transient deterioration in myasthenic symptoms. Nonetheless 17 of 19 patients with invasive thymomas treated by thymectomy and irradiation were alive 6.5 years after surgery (Monden et al. 1984). The finding of large numbers of germinal centres in a thymus showing thymic hyperplasia has also been associated with a less good prognosis (Papatestas et al. 1976). However, improvement sometimes occurs within a few days of operation. After thymectomy the AChR antibody may fall rapidly or slowly during many months. There is a significant correlation between the AChR antibody titre and the clinical state in patients re-evaluated 1.5–3 years after thymectomy (Vincent et al. 1983).

Few of these studies of the effect of thymectomy have included control observations in a parallel group of patients treated medically, so that it is difficult to draw firm conclusions about the effectiveness of this operation. Simpson (1958) attempted to do this in his review of Keynes's surgical material and Rowland et al. (1956) have also given an account of the severity of the disease before thymectomy and adequate anticholinesterase drugs were available. Recent studies (Genkins et al. 1993) of the effectiveness of thymectomy in myasthenia gravis suggest that:

1. Progression to severe disease is made less likely
2. A high proportion of total remissions is induced
3. The older patient (>45 years) is likely to have the best result; this differs from earlier experience
4. The incidence of thymomas is reduced
5. Pre-pubertal children should not be operated on unless symptoms are life-threatening or very severe; thymectomy in children carries a small risk of late malignancy
6. All thymomas should be removed.

It is our policy to recommend thymectomy in adult patients with generalised myasthenia soon after diagnosis, since this seems to improve the long-term prognosis, and to make subsequent medical management easier. In addition, it is never possible to be absolutely certain by clinical and radiographic investigation whether or not a thymic tumour is present pre-operatively.

Patients with myasthenia restricted to ocular muscles do not usually require thymectomy, but such patients also improve if operated on and intervention may be indicated in those in whom ocular palsies are intractable to anticholinesterase medication. Schumm et al. (1985), in a study of 18 patients with ocular myasthenia treated by thymectomy, found that 80% improved and none developed generalised myasthenia during a mean follow-up period of 26 months. The operation carries a very low morbidity and mortality in experienced centres.

Post-operative management requires nursing in an Intensive Therapy Unit, with reduction of anticholinesterase drugs to about half pre-operative levels during the first few days. Neostigmine is particularly useful during this period because it can be given parenterally. If rapid improvement occurs during the first few weeks the dosage of these drugs must be reduced accordingly, and this can be done empirically, or with edrophonium tolerance testing. Patients with thymomas should be treated with irradiation to the anterior mediastinum post-operatively.

In some very weak patients plasma exchange may be valuable in preparing the patient for surgery, since it may cause a temporary remission. A few patients require intermittent plasma exchange for several months before and after thymectomy (Perlo et al. 1981).

Immunosuppressant Therapy

Steroids are useful in inducing remission, but steroid therapy, because of its well-known adverse effects, should be reserved for severe cases. Thymectomy is best carried out before steroids are considered in the management of severe cases both because of the adverse effects of steroids and because steroid therapy makes operation and wound-healing more difficult.

Steroids were first given as ACTH (Torda and Wolff 1951) but oral prednisolone or prednisone is now usually used. Dexamethasone has also been used. Torda and Wolff (1951) noted a high incidence of increased weakness with ACTH treatment. The weakness is very severe, even requiring ventilatory support in some patients, and also occurs, although to a lesser extent, with high doses of prednisone. An incremental regimen during the first two weeks was introduced by Seybold and Drachman (1974) to obviate this steroid-induced weakness, and alternate-day regimes also seem less likely to induce it (Warmolts and Engel 1972b; Sghirlanzoni et al. 1984). However, with the alternate-day regime some patients observe weakness either on the steroid, or later on the non-steroid day, and a once-daily schedule is probably preferable during the first month, followed by an alternate-day regime (Brunner et al. 1976). Pascuzzi et al. (1983) found that 48% of patients begun on high-dose prednisone worsened initially but with slowly increasing doses Sghirlanzoni et al. (1984) noted that only 19% deteriorated at the start of treatment. None of the latter developed respiratory crisis but 8% of cases treated with high-dose steroids developed this problem (Pascuzzi et al. 1983). Doses of 50–100 mg prednisolone orally are usually used for the first month, and then the dose is gradually reduced. Treatment with antacids and potassium supplements, and with an anti-tuberculous drug for prophylaxis (isoniazid), may be given if indicated. Improvement occurs in 80% of patients in the first month or so but fewer than 50% remain improved when assessed at 3 months. In addition, maximum improvement did not develop until treatment had been continued for 9 months (Pascuzzi et al. 1983). A few patients seem to remain improved only while steroids are continued and this can be a problem in long-term management because of the increasing risk of adverse effects of steroids. Drachman and Kuncl (1994) recommended daily steroids for 3 months followed by alternate-day treatment.

Previous thymectomy, and the thymic pathology bear no relation to the expectation of improvement with steroid therapy. Levels of ACh receptor antibody usually decrease during steroid therapy (Seybold and Lindstrom 1979). Serious side effects greatly limit the application of steroid therapy; Pascuzzi et al. (1983) reported that 67% of their patients developed vertebral collapse. Thymectomy is therefore a much safer primary treatment.

Other immunosuppressant drugs have been used and of these azathioprine is the most effective (Witte et al. 1984), at a dose of 150–200 mg daily calculated according to body weight (Mertens et al. 1969, 1981). This drug, when given with prednisolone, allows the dose of the latter to be reduced more rapidly than when steroids are given alone (a "steroid-sparing" effect) and seems to have a long-term effect in reducing production of ACh receptor antibody in the lymphoid system. A clinical effect of azathioprine is not apparent before 6–12 weeks and reaches a maximum more than a year after starting (Mattell et al. 1976; 1981). As the patient improves dosage of anticholinesterase drugs must be slowly reduced.

Azathioprine therapy is indicated in many patients with generalised myaesthenia, and should be started at diagnosis. The thymic pathology is irrelevant to the clinical response observed; the level of ACh receptor antibody gradually falls during treatment (Reuther et al. 1979). Some patients have been treated with azathioprine for more than 10 years; it is only possible to stop the drug without relapse in very few patients (Mertens et al. 1981). About 40% of cases achieve near-complete remission; a beneficial response correlates with the development of macrocytosis (mean corpuscular volume increased by 15 fl) perhaps indicating appropriate dosage and compliance (Witte et al. 1986). Cyclosporin may also be of value (Tindall et al. 1987), in a dose of 5 mg/kg in two divided doses. It is effective in 1–3 months, a little quicker than azathioprine, but less quickly than steroid therapy (Tindall et al. 1993). However, 35% of patients discontinued medication because of side effects, and in 10% significant nephrotoxicity developed.

Thoracic lymph duct drainage has been tried, and shown to be moderately effective (Mattell et al. 1976) but it has been superseded by plasma exchange. Its effect was maintained for only a day or two after its cessation, although there was some residual improvement. Other forms of treatment have included anti-lymphocytic or anti-thymocytic globulin (Leovey et al. 1975), splenic irradiation and total body irradiation (Engel et al. 1981b).

Plasma Exchange

In this technique 2–4 litres of the patient's plasma is exchanged with pre-warmed human purified protein fraction (50%) to which calcium and potassium have been added in physiological concentrations together with Dextran (25%) and Ringer-lactate (25%), using a cell separator. Plasma exchanges can be repeated as required, but in myasthenia a beneficial effect begins within a week after beginning plasma ex-

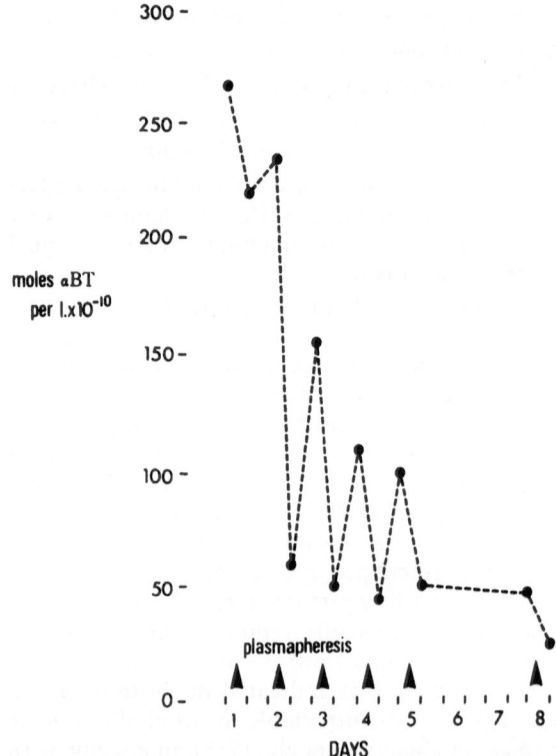

Fig. 12.7. Effect of daily plasma exchange in removing AChR antibody from the circulation in a patient with myasthenia. In this patient plasma exchange was carried out as part of the preparative procedure for thymectomy; there was a marked improvement in the patient's strength.

change. In severely ill patients daily exchanges have been used, resulting in a progressive benefit during this period, but generally five exchanges in a 2-week period are sufficient (Drachman and Kuncl 1994). Improvement reaches a maximum about 2 weeks after plasma exchange (Newsom-Davis et al. 1978), and may be maintained for 4–6 weeks (Pinching et al. 1976; Dau et al. 1977); it is associated with reduction in the level of the circulating ACh receptor antibody (Kornfeld et al. 1981) (Fig. 12.7) and decrease in the electrophysiological abnormality (Dau et al. 1977). Antibody-negative patients also respond to plasma exchange.

Immunosuppression using prednisone and azathioprine may result in a more sustained improvement (Pinching et al. 1976; Dau et al. 1977). Although the long-term value of plasma exchange is dubious (Newsom-Davis and Vincent 1979), it is a useful technique in acute fulminant myasthenia, and in the preparation of very weak patients for thymectomy. The technique seems to benefit patients before or after thymectomy and patients with or without thymoma seem to respond equally

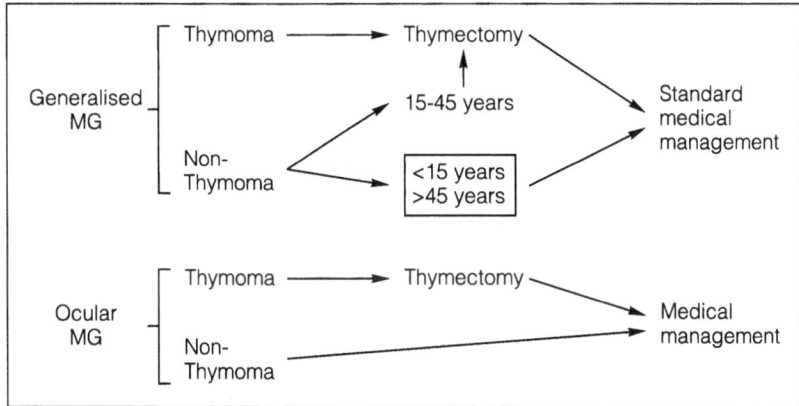

Fig. 12.8.   Flow diagram for treatment of myasthenia gravis.

well. Plasma exchange is of no benefit in congenital myasthenia (Pinching et al. 1976).

The main indications for plasma exchange are to produce a transient remission in myasthenic crisis, to prepare a patient for thymectomy, to control sudden deterioration during initiation of steroid therapy and, rarely, in the long-term management of very severely affected patients who have responded inadequately to other forms of treatment, including immunosuppressant drugs (Newsom-Davis 1979a).

Plasma exchange is not without complications, including septicaemia, air embolism, hypotension, cramps and localised thrombophlebitis, but most can be avoided with careful technique during the procedure.

Intravenous Immunoglobulin Therapy

This treatment is also effective, producing a beneficial response in 4–5 days in 85% of patients (Ferrero et al. 1993). It has been used especially in myasthenic crisis in a dose of 0.4 g/kg per day for 5 days. Clearly, this treatment is technically easier to administer than plasma exchange, and the response may be sustained for several weeks or months (Ferrero et al. 1993; Drachman and Kuncl 1994).

Recommended Treatment of Myasthenia Gravis

Our current scheme of management (Fig. 12.8) is as follows:

1. Establish diagnosis by clinical, electrophysiological and radiological techniques. AChR antibody levels are specific if raised.

2. Improve clinical status with anticholinesterase drugs. Use plasma exchange or IgG to obtain temporary improvement if necessary prior to thymectomy.

3. Thymectomy. We recommend this procedure in all but the elderly, children, or the most mildly affected patient. The operation may be deferred in patients with ocular myasthenia, but current evidence also supports thymectomy in these patients.

4. If there is no improvement after thymectomy, or if relapse occurs, improvement may be restored temporarily with plasma exchange. Immuno-suppressant drugs are useful in these patients. Steroids, given incrementally in daily dosage in hospital, produce a relatively rapid beneficial effect but long-term unwanted effects are both frequent and disabling and the dosage, even of alternate-day steroids, should be reduced to the minimum necessary, or the drug should be withdrawn, as soon as possible.

5. Azathioprine is useful in reducing the long-term steroid requirement, and is capable of producing remission or improvement when used alone. It should be continued indefinitely with regular blood counts and liver function tests. Azathioprine is much less toxic than steroid therapy. Cyclosporin may also be used.

Penicillamine-Induced Myasthenia Gravis

Several drugs may cause a reversible myasthenia-like disorder in patients in whom there is no previous evidence of disturbance of neuromuscular transmission, but D-penicillamine is the only drug known to induce myasthenic weakness *with* raised ACh receptor antibodies (Russell and Lindstrom 1978; Vincent et al. 1978a). Anti-striated muscle antibodies have been noted in high titre in some patients with D-penicillamine-induced myasthenia (Masters et al. 1977) and it has been suggested that the drug acts by binding AChR at motor end-plates, producing an immunogenic complex (Bever et al. 1982; Junel et al. 1986), rather than by unmasking the latent disease. Most cases have been associated with HLA Bw35, and DR1, but not with B8 or DR3. The latter are commonly found in idiopathic myasthenia gravis (Garlepp et al. 1983). The disease may affect limb or bulbar muscles. Improvement occurs during several months, associated with a fall in AChR antibody titres, when D-penicillamine is withdrawn (Fawcett et al. 1982). Many of the reported cases have occurred in patients treated with penicillamine for rheumatoid arthritis, but it has also been described during penicillamine therapy in scleroderma and in two patients with Wilson's disease. In one of the latter, the acetylcholine receptor antibody titres did not fall when penicillamine was withdrawn, suggesting that there was a fortuitous association between Wilson's disease and myasthenia gravis in this patient (Masters et al. 1977).

We have investigated one case of penicillamine-associated myasthenia gravis using single-fibre EMG (Case A of Vincent et al. 1978a). The findings were similar to those seen in spontaneously occurring mild myasthenia gravis. This patient, like the others reported, improved slowly when penicillamine was withdrawn (Fawcett et al. 1982).

Attempts to reproduce penicillamine-induced myasthenia gravis in the rat (Russell and Lindstrom 1978; Aldrich et al. 1979) have shown decremental responses to nerve stimulation, and small miniature end-plate potentials (MEPPs), but no circulating ACh receptor antibodies. These animals were obviously weak.

Lambert–Eaton Myasthenic Syndrome (LEMS)

This syndrome, which was first described by Lambert et al. (1956) and by Eaton and Lambert (1957) in patients with malignant tumours, especially small cell carcinoma of the lung, is characterised by weakness and fatiguability of proximal limb muscles, with relative sparing of extra-ocular and bulbar muscles. The first symptoms consist of weakness in proximal muscles, mainly in the legs, often accompanied by aching of these muscles. The weakness is usually *improved* by exercise but with continued exertion weakness again becomes evident. The tendon reflexes are diminished or absent in the legs, and dryness of the mouth is frequently noted. Further points of difference from myasthenia gravis include a male preponderance (2 : 1 (O'Neill et al. 1988)) and the age distribution of the disorder; 80% of reported cases have occurred in patients older than 40 years and the mean age of onset is about 55 years (O'Neill et al. 1988). The incidence of LEMS, at 0.4 per 100 000 is similar to that of myasthenia gravis, although the increased mortality in LEMS results in a lower prevalence of this condition.

Early descriptions of the association of carcinoma of the bronchus and myasthenic weakness were given by Henson et al. (1954) and Heathfield and Williams (1954). Cases have also been reported associated with carcinomas in other sites, including breast, prostate, stomach and rectum but these are uncommon associations (Henson 1974).

LEMS is usually found to be associated with carcinoma of the bronchus but the carcinoma may not be detectable until several months, or even years, after presentation of the myasthenic syndrome (Lambert and Rooke 1965). Lennon et al. (1982) found that 70% of men, and 25% of women with LEMS had or developed a carcinoma, usually small cell carcinoma of the bronchus. In a prospective study of 71 patients with small cell carcinoma 3% developed LEMS (Hawley et al. 1980). The youngest reported case is a child aged 9 years (Chelmicka-Schorr et al. 1979).

In some cases the syndrome is found without evident underlying disease, even after careful investigation and follow-up. In many of these an autoimmune disorder, such as thyroid disease (Guttmann et al. 1972) or treatment with certain drugs, such as neomycin, has been noted (McQuillen et al. 1968; Argov and Mastaglia 1979). The underlying cause of the disorder in both the groups of patients, i.e. those associated with neoplasia and those without, has been shown to be related to an autoimmune disorder (Lang et al. 1981). About one-third to a half of cases are non-neoplastic (O'Neill et al. 1988).

The prognosis is that of the underlying disorder but in the idiopathic group the outcome is uncertain; in the latter instances disability is slight and spontaneous remission may occur. A few patients have been reported who have shown clinical and EMG features both of myasthenia gravis and of myasthenic syndrome (Takamori and Gutmann

1971; Schwartz and Stålberg 1975b). Autonomic neuropathy, causing orthostatic hypotension, arrhythmias and impotence, all representing cholinergic defects, may occur rarely (Rubenstein et al. 1979; Manji et al. 1990).

Pathophysiology

Elmqvist and Lambert (1968) studied the defect in vitro in a biopsy of intercostal muscle from a patient with myasthenic syndrome associated with bronchogenic carcinoma. Intracellular recording showed that the frequency and size of the MEPPs was normal, but that the end-plate potentials (EPPs) were small (Lambert and Elmqvist 1971). Repeated nerve stimulation increased the size of the EPPs. These findings imply that each nerve impulse released fewer quanta of ACh than normal, but that the individual quanta were of normal size. Repetitive stimulation thus increased the number of quanta released by each nerve impulse. This abnormality is similar to that found in botulism but in the latter the MEPP amplitude is reduced (Brooks 1956).

Ishikawa et al. (1977) found that an extract from a lung tumour in a patient with myasthenic syndrome caused a reduction in ACh release in a frog nerve–muscle preparation. Gutmann et al. (1972) suggested an autoimmune basis for these cases, and Denys et al. (1979) found that plasma and IgG fraction from a patient with myasthenic syndrome produced a decremental response to slow rates of nerve stimulation and facilitation to fast rates when injected into laboratory animals, an observation confirmed by Lang et al. (1981).

These experimental findings indicated that the disease is associated with binding of an IgG antibody to nerve terminal immune determinants concerned with ACh transmitter release at the neuromuscular junction. Both quantal and nonquantal ACh release are impaired, a defect that could be due to a calcium-dependent effect at the ACh release sites (Lang et al. 1984).

In morphological studies of motor end-plates in LEMS Engel and Santa (1971) noted increase in size of the post-synaptic region, a phenomenon consistent with a presynaptic defect resulting in increased synthesis of post-synaptic ACh receptors, and a larger motor end-plate. Fukunaga et al. (1982), in a freeze-fracture study, found a reduced number of pre-synaptic active zones, representing sites of synaptic vesicle exocytosis (Heuser et al. 1979), and of active zone particles. The latter probably represent voltage-sensitive calcium channels in the pre-synaptic membrane of the motor end-plate (Pumplin et al. 1981). These sites may therefore represent the sites of immune attack in the disease. Sher et al. (1989) found circulating autoantibodies that interfere with neurotransmitter release at motor end-plates by downregulating pre-synaptic voltage-gated calcium channels. These antibodies are found in 30%–50% of cases of LEMS (Newsom-Davis 1993). These antibodies are more commonly found in autoimmune cases than in LEMS associated with small cell carcinoma (Leys et al. 1991). Low titres may be found in asymptomatic patients with small cell carcinoma of lung and in 67% of patients with rheumatoid arthritis or systemic lupus erythematosus (Leys et al. 1991). In LEMS patients with circulating antibody the antibody titre decreases as the patient improves with treatment. Of the four types of calcium channel recognised on the basis of their pharmacological and physiological characteristics (L, long-acting; T, transient; N, slowly inactivated; and P channels), antibodies to the L type channel seem important in the pathogenesis of LEMS (Lang et al. 1993). Small cell tumours express L, N or P type voltage-gated calcium channels (VGCCs) (Pancrazio et al. 1992). Motomura et al. (1995) found that antibodies to P type channels were particularly sensitive and may be the primary immunogenic target in the disease.

Other autoantibodies have been found in patients with LEMS. The overall frequency of organ-specific autoantibodies to thyroid, stomach and skeletal muscle in a series of 64 patients with LEMS was 45% (Lennon et al. 1982). The frequency of these antibodies was 52% in LEMS not associated with neoplasia, 28% in LEMS associated with tumour, and 17% in a control population of patients with other neurological disease. In HLA studies of five patients with the non-carcinomatous form of LEMS, Newsom-Davis et al. (1982) found that all five cases had the DR3 antigen and four showed the HLA-B8 antigen. These antigens have also been found in patients with LEMS associated with carcinoma (Ingram et al. 1984). It is thus possible that the disease arises in patients susceptible because of their HLA status. In the carcinoma-associated form of LEMS there is a common antigen in small cell neoplastic cells, and in cholinergic neurons. Small cell tumours have a neuro-ectodermal origin from the bronchial Kulchitsky cells, that show calcium-spike electrogenesis (Lennon et al. 1982).

Laboratory Investigations

Assay of voltage-gated calcium channels shows increased levels in up to 85% of cases (see above and Motomura et al. 1995). The CK is normal. Investigation should be directed toward the possible underlying cause. The chest X-ray, repeated from

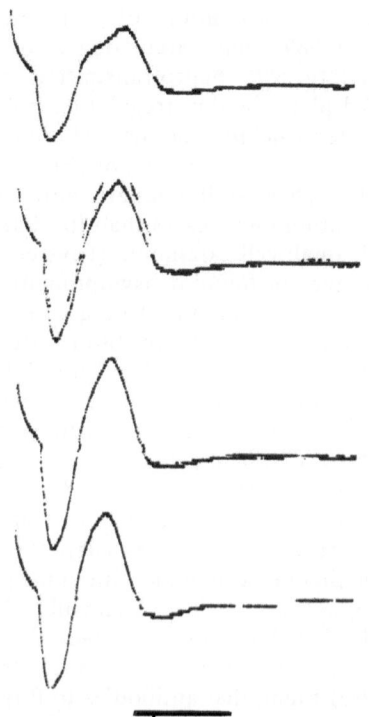

Fig. 12.9. Myasthenic syndrome (Lambert–Eaton) in a patient with small cell carcinoma of the lung. The initial response to stimulation of the ulnar nerve at a frequency of 10 Hz in the abductor digiti minimi is 3.5 mV amplitude, and the fourth response is 7.5 mV. Bar 10 ms.

time to time if necessary, and bronchoscopy with sputum cytology, are the most important investigations. Investigation of possible autoimmune disease is also important.

Electrophysiological Assessment

The diagnostic features (Oh 1989) are demonstrated with repetitive nerve stimulation (Fig. 12.9). The size of the initial evoked muscle action potential to supramaximal stimulation is smaller than normal; usually less than 4 mV (normal >10 mV). During nerve stimulation at 2 Hz there is usually a slight decrement of the fourth potential, findings similar to those recorded in myasthenia gravis. With faster rates of stimulation (>10 Hz) the size of the muscle action potential increases by a factor of two to six, or even more (Eaton and Lambert 1957; Elmqvist and Lambert 1968). The increase in size of the muscle action potential can also be demonstrated after exercise. Facilitation at fast rates of stimulation and following exercise is more prominent in abductor digiti minimi than in the trapezius or extensor digitorum brevis muscles (Ingram et al. 1984). The difference is partially due to the exceptionally low

amplitude of the initial MUAP in the abductor digiti minimi muscle. The potentiation following a tetanus is transient, and may be followed by post-tetanic exhaustion 2–4 min later (Kimura 1983).

Concentric needle EMG shows only minimal changes. With continued muscle contraction MUAPs show variations in amplitude and some polyphasic units may be noted. With single-fibre EMG many potential pairs show increased neuromuscular jitter, and impulse blocking. However, improvement in jitter, and reduction in the amount of impulse blocking occurs with higher innervation rates, a finding the opposite of that found in myasthenia gravis. Moreover, after a period of rest, the jitter increases, and blocking becomes *more* prominent in the myasthenic syndrome (Schwartz and Stålberg 1975c). Edrophonium hydrochloride, given intravenously, increases the amplitude of the initial response to repetitive stimulation (Henriksson et al. 1977) and slightly reduces the jitter in the myasthenic syndrome, and gives a transient clinical improvement (Schwartz and Stålberg 1975c). Axonal microstimulation single-fibre EMG in a patient with LEMS showed reduction in impulse blocking when the stimulation rate was increased from 1 Hz to 10 or 20 Hz (Trontelj and Stålberg 1991), together with a reduction in end-plate jitter. Stålberg and Trontelj (1994) noted that improvement in jitter in this experiment was less consistent because of the presence of variations in myogenic jitter, due to changes in velocity recovery function in muscle fibre membrane with changing stimulation rates.

In some cases there is an associated peripheral neuropathy (paraneoplastic neuropathy) and then the nerve conduction velocities may be slowed.

Muscle Biopsy

No specific abnormalities are observed in the muscle biopsy. Occasionally there may be an increase in interstitial nuclei, suggesting a sparse inflammatory cell response, and Type 2 fibre atrophy has been reported (Henriksson et al. 1977).

The characteristic abnormality of the motor endplates can be studied only with special techniques.

Management

The first step is to search for the underlying cause, usually autoimmune disease or a pulmonary neoplasm. Operative removal of the tumour can be hazardous because the neuromuscular transmission defect is often markedly worsened by muscle relaxant drugs and anaesthetics (Croft 1958; Wise and McDermot 1962; Kaeser 1984a), but there may be improvement in LEMS after successful treatment of small cell pulmonary cancers (O'Neill et al. 1988; Chalk et al. 1990). Lambert and Rooke (1965) also reported improvement after removal of tumour.

Various drugs have been tried in order to improve muscle strength. Neostigmine and pyridostigmine are generally of little benefit, probably because they do not improve ACh release at motor end-plates. Increased release of ACh can be promoted by calcium gluconate infusion, but longer-term benefit can be produced by oral guanidine (Lambert 1966; McQuillen and Johns 1967). Guanidine was shown to enhance ACh release following a nerve impulse in experimental work by Otsuka and Endo (1960), and in myasthenic syndrome it increases the amplitude of the initial MUAP to nerve stimulation, normalises the incremental response to rapid repetitive nerve stimulation and reduces the abnormalities found with single-fibre EMG (Henriksson et al. 1977). The beneficial effects of the drug may not be evident for several days. Unwanted effects may be severe; these include tingling, diarrhoea, chronic interstitial nephritis and pancytopenia from bone-marrow depression and the drug is, therefore, not much used (Cherington 1976).

Another drug, 4-aminopyridine, which similarly enhances ACh release at motor end-plates, has been used (Lundh et al. 1977). However, it may cause seizures, paraesthesiae and anxiety; a derivative, 3,4-diaminopyridine (3,4-DAP), which is less toxic and more potent in improving neuromuscular transmission, is useful (Lundh et al. 1984). Its beneficial effect is potentiated by anticholinesterase drugs (McEvoy et al. 1989). 3,4-DAP may also improve associated autonomic neuropathy, and is currently the drug of choice. McEvoy et al. (1989) reported that strength improved in the arms from 70% to 81% of normal, and in the legs from 45% to 65%, an improvement that was paralleled by electrophysiological improvement.

Plasma exchange and immunosuppressant drug therapy have also been shown to be of value both in carcinoma-associated and non-carcinimatous LEMS (Dau and Denys 1982; Ingram et al. 1984; Newsom-Davis and Murray 1984). Improvement begins within a few days of beginning plasma exchange therapy and the effect lasts for about 6 weeks. Immunosuppressant drug treatment seems to induce a more complete and sustained remission (Ingram et al. 1984) which may last for a year or more with continued azathioprine therapy (Newsom-Davis and Murray 1984). Steroid therapy also seems beneficial when combined with these drugs (Ingram et al. 1984;

Newsom-Davis and Murray 1984), or used alone (Streib and Rothner 1980). Steroids and azathioprine seem particularly useful in non-cancer cases if the response to 3,4-DAP is inadequate.

Differential Diagnosis

The myasthenic syndrome may be difficult to recognise clinically, especially in cachectic or ill patients. The differential diagnosis is from cachectic muscular atrophy, true myasthenia gravis, motor neuron disease, and other neuromuscular disorders of late onset, including myopathies and carcinoma-associated disorders such as carcinomatous neuropathy and polymyositis. Botulism should also be remembered (see below). These disorders can be distinguished by their clinical features, and by investigations, including EMG and nerve conduction studies, CK measurement and, if necessary, muscle biopsy. A few cases have been reported in whom myasthenia gravis and LEMS coexist as two separate autoimmune disorders: overlap myasthenic syndrome (Schwartz and Stalberg 1975b; Oh 1987).

Congenital Myasthenic Syndromes

In these rare disorders there is weakness and abnormal fatiguability. Several distinct syndromes have been delineated, which may present at birth or in infancy (Table 12.6). Acetylcholine receptor antibody is not present in the blood and there are no immune complexes present in the neuromuscular junctions (Engel 1984). In these disorders there are more or less typical features of myasthenia with extra-ocular and facial weakness, difficulty in swallowing and breathing at birth and fluctuations in the severity of weakness. The response to anticholinesterase drugs is variable. Most of these disorders represent mutations in genes controlling channel or receptor protein expression at pre- or post-synaptic sites in the motor end-plate (see Engel 1994 for review). The genetic basis of several syndromes is uncertain (Table 12.6). Engel (1994) has noted a number of so-far uncharacterised syndromes believed to be related to the recognised disorders.

Generally treatment is difficult because it is lifelong. Some cases are refractory to therapy and some improve transitorily. A combination of pyridostigmine and 3,4-DAP (5–20 mg tds or qds) is effective in patients with ACh receptor deficiency without a prolonged open time and in patients with defective

Table 12.6. Congenital myasthenic syndromes[a]

Pre-synaptic defects			
1. Defective ACh synthesis or mobilisation (Engel et al. 1981a)	Recessive	At birth	Decrement only after exercise (2 Hz)
2. Paucity of synaptic vesicles and reduced quantal release	?	Infancy	Decremental response at 2 Hz. Responds to anticholinesterase drugs
Pre- and post-synaptic defects			
1. End-plate ACh esterase deficiency (Engel et al. 1977)	Recessive ?	At birth	Decrement at all stimulation rates. Repetitive response to single nerve stimuli
Post-synaptic defects			
1. Slow (open) channel syndrome (Engel et al. 1982)	Dominant	Variable	Decremental response at slow rates (2 Hz). Repetitive response to single nerve stimuli
2. Prolonged open time	Sporadic	Infancy	Decremental or incremental response
3. AChR deficiency and short channel open time syndrome (Engel et al. 1993)	?	At birth	Decremental response at 2 Hz; variable facilitation or decrement at 20 to 50 Hz
4. Abnormal interaction of ACh and its receptor (Uchitel et al. 1993)	?	At birth	Decremental response at 2 Hz. Small MEPPs
5. High conductance fast channel syndrome	Recessive	Infancy	Decremental response at 2 Hz.

[a] See Engel (1994)

synthesis or release of ACh quanta (a pre-synaptic defect) (Palace et al. 1991).

Botulism

In developed countries botulism is very rare, but cases still occur in certain circumstances. The disorder is commoner in countries in which people live at high altitude, since water boils at a lower temperature at low barometric pressure, and the toxin produced by *Clostridium botulinum*, which may contaminate certain foods, especially fish and canned foods, is not then destroyed during cooking. The organism may also infect wounds (Wagen and Gutmann 1974).

Botulism was first described by van Ermengen in 1896, who isolated an anaerobic organism in his investigation of 23 musicians, three of whom died after eating raw salted ham at a wake in a Belgian village (Critchley and Mitchell 1990). Between 1950 and 1979, 336 outbreaks were reported in the USA (Feldman et al. 1981). Since 1979 the commonest form noted has been infantile botulism due to the ingestion of spores, and food-borne botulism has become less frequent (Pickett 1988). Food-borne botulism has mostly become a disease spread by cooked alkaline foods, such as vegetables, fruits and condiments (70%) rather than fish products (16%) or meat products (4%). In infantile botulism the organism replicates in the gut (Arnon 1980).

There are eight types of botulinum toxin, but most human cases are due to botulism A, B or E, and of these botulism type A is by far the most frequent.

The first symptoms may resemble those of food poisoning; viz, vomiting, diarrhoea, abdominal pain and dryness of the mouth. These may occur within a few hours of ingestion of contaminated food. Later, blurred vision and diplopia develop, with dysarthria and dysphagia, and generalised weakness follows. Many cases present with neuromuscular symptoms. Weakness may rapidly worsen in the day or two after onset and in severe cases death occurs from respiratory failure (Cherington 1974).

In wound botulism, in which toxin is slowly released into the circulation, the onset is slower (Wagen and Gutmann 1974). Ileus is common.

In infantile botulism the clinical presentation resembles that of adult cases, but a subacute onset of apathy and weakness may be difficult to characterise, and failure to thrive and constipation may be the major features. Unexpected sudden death may occur (Turner et al. 1978; Critchley and Mitchell 1990).

In adult botulism edrophonium, given intravenously, produces some improvement and may be a useful test. The disorder is not easy to diagnose without evidence of exposure to contaminated food, since a flaccid, arreflexic paralysis may be found, with involvement of external ocular muscles, and sometimes with pupillary involvement. Only the latter findings, the absence of sensory complaints, and the finding of a normal CSF protein allow clinical differentiation from Guillain–Barré syndrome.

Pathophysiology

Botulinum toxin prevents the release of ACh quanta at motor nerve terminals (Burgen et al. 1949). The toxin binds to the pre-synaptic terminal and is transported across the terminal membrane by a calcium-dependent process leading to destruction of the pre-synaptic terminal. Failure of neuromuscular transmission occurs because exocytosis of ACh-containing vesicles is prevented. Once the toxin has bound to the pre-synaptic terminal, it is endocytosed and becomes inaccessible to therapeutic antitoxin. Sprouting of pre-synaptic motor nerve terminals begins after about a week (Duchen 1970) and this becomes prominent in the following few weeks, resulting in proliferated motor nerve terminals. The muscle fibres become atrophied during the period of weakness and functional denervation; both fibre types are affected (Duchen 1970). These regenerative changes at the motor terminals induced by botulinum toxin have been shown to be related to increased numbers of ACh receptors at the post-synaptic membrane (Kao et al. 1976).

Electrophysiological Assessment

Abnormalities in the EMG examination are found in almost all cases, and are useful in diagnosis (Oh 1988). In about 50% of cases the resting CMAP amplitude is reduced. After exercise the CMAP is increased by 50%–170% in most patients, but the most prominent feature is an incremental response to repetitive stimulation at fast rates (50 Hz) of stimulation (Oh 1988). This abnormality is not as prominent as in Lambert–Eaton syndrome (Cherington 1974). In addition, there are striking variations in different nerve/muscle systems; for example, one limb may be normal and the other abnormal. In the early stages the responses to repetitive stimulation may be normal. There is a consistent relation between the clinical state and the amplitude of the CMAP (Cherington and Ryan 1970). In some patients there is a decrement at slow (2 Hz) rates of stimulation, but this is found in only about 10% of patients.

EMG reveals fibrillations in affected muscles, and the MUPs are typically small, and of short duration, resembling myopathic potentials. Single-fibre EMG reveals increased neuromuscular jitter and blocking, abnormalities that improve with increasing discharge rates (Schiller and Stålberg 1976; Cruz-Martinez et al. 1985). In vitro studies have revealed reduced MEPP amplitudes (Brooks 1956; Kao et al. 1976).

Management

Antitoxin may be given, but it is not clear if it has any effect once neurological manifestations have begun, since the toxin is already bound to nerve terminal receptors. There is a risk of anaphylaxis or serum sickness in about 10% of cases when this treatment is given. Infantile botulism is a self-limited disorder that does not require specific treatment apart from supportive measures, including ventilatory assistance, if required (Arnon 1980). Treatment with penicillin is of dubious value.

The main plan of management in adults rests on adequate respiratory support, if required, and measures to care for the paralysed patient. Recovery may be very slow, taking many months in severely affected patients, but in milder cases with only slight weakness recovery is more rapid. Guanidine is of some value in improving muscle strength in mild or moderately severe cases (Cherington 1974). 3,4-Aminopyridine has also been used (Ball et al. 1979), but may cause seizures. In the past a mortality as high as 23% has been recorded (Marson et al. 1974) but with modern intensive care this should now be much less and survivors can expect to recover completely.

Therapeutic Use of Botulinum Toxin

The paralytic effects of botulinum A toxin last for several weeks or months, and have been exploited in the management of certain muscle spasms, dystonia and spasticity. In this treatment selective weakness of certain muscles is induced by the direct injection of small, titrated doses of standardised botulinum toxin into affected muscle. Local injection reduces the CMAP amplitude and, in more distant muscles, increased neuromuscular jitter may be detected, with some impulse blocking, as a result of the effect of circulating botulinum toxin (Olney et al. 1988; Hamjian and Walker 1994). After injection the CMAP amplitude decreased within 48 hours and reached its nadir at 21 days (Hamjian and Walker 1994). Atrophy is quite marked by 6–7 weeks after injection and, after repeated injections into the same muscle, may become marked.

Treatment with botulinum toxin was introduced by Elston (1987) for idiopathic blepharospasm, and was rapidly extended to the management of hemifacial spasm (Jankovic et al. 1990), spasmodic tortocollis (Blackie and Lees 1990, laryngeal dystonia, oromandibular dystonia, focal limb dystonias, certain forms of strabismus and spasticity (Dunne et al. 1995). The value of this form of treatment was reviewed at a Consensus Development Conference held by the US National Institutes of Health (1991).

Toxins and Drugs Affecting Neuromuscular Transmission

There are many different toxins occurring in defence or attack behaviours of various species, such as snakes, spiders, scorpions, snails, sea anemones and fish, that interfere with the function of the neuromuscular junction. These toxins have different modes of action, and these have been used, in experimental neurophysiology, to investigate the component processes needed for neuromuscular transmission in mammals and other animals. These toxins may affect pre-synaptic processes, acetylcholine release, or post-synaptic processes (Table 12.7).

Table 12.7.   Toxins and drugs affecting neuromuscular transmission

	Toxin	Drug
Pre-synaptic		
Sodium channel	Tetrodotoxin ↓ Ciguatoxin ↑	
Potassium channel	Dendrotoxin ↑ Notoxin ↓	3,4-DAP ↑ Aminopyridine ↑
Calcium channels	Omega conotoxin ↓	Calcium channel blockers ↓ (e.g. verapamil) Magnesium ↓
ACh release	Atraxotoxin ↑ β bungarotoxin ↓ α latrotoxin ↑ ↓	Thallium ↓
Post-synaptic		
Binding of ACh to receptor	α bungarotoxin ↓ Cobratoxin ↓	Curare ↓ Succinylocholine ↑ ↓ Gallamine ↓
ACh receptor channels	α conotoxin ↓	Amantadine ↓ Procainamide ↓ Verapamil ↓
ACh esterase inhibitors	Fasciculin 2 ↑ (green mamba toxin)	

↓ Inhibition of normal function; ↑ enhancement of normal function

Toxins such as ciguatoxin that act on pre-synaptic neuromuscular junction *sodium channels* cause pain, cramp, tremor and autonomic instability. Electrophysiological studies reveal repetitive firing of motor unit action potentials (Fontana and Vital-Brasilo 1985). Tetrodotoxin causes paralysis. Both dendrotoxin and 3,4-diaminopyridine increase acetylcholine release by causing pre-synaptic blockade of *potassium channels*; this causes fasciculations and cramps due to repetitive firing of muscle fibres. Pre-synaptic *calcium channels* may be blocked by verapamil and certain other calcium channel blocking drugs, but this has no effect clinically or electromyographically in normal subjects. However,

these drugs may unmask or worsen the clinical symptoms in myasthenia gravis (Lee and Ho 1987). Nifedipine does not have this effect.

Magnesium is a competitive inhibitor of calcium uptake at pre-synaptic sites; magnesium infusion causes areflexia at 9–10 mEq/l and weakness at blood levels greater than 10 mEq/l in pre-eclamptic women. Drowsiness and coma occurs at higher levels, and respiratory depression and quadriplegia have been noted in infants and children with hypermagnesaemia. The CMAP is of reduced amplitude, there is a decremental response at low stimulus rates, and an incremental response after exercise, or at high repetitive stimulus rates (Swift 1979; Ramanathan et al. 1988). Magnesium infusion can umask myasthenia gravis by its effect on the neuromuscular junction (Bashuk and Krendl 1990). Motor and sensory conduction is normal.

Acetylcholine release is impaired by the toxin released from salivary glands of the American and Australian tick, causing tick paralysis (Cherington and Snyder 1968; Swift and Ignacio 1975), a form of generalised weakness that is relieved after the tick is removed. The paralysis is due, perhaps mainly, to an axonal neuropathy, with sensory symptoms and slightly reduced motor and sensory nerve conduction velocity (Swift and Ignacio 1975). *Black widow spider* venom (α-latrotoxin) causes increased release of ACh, leading to repetitive firing and muscle cramps, with systemic effects, e.g. vasoconstriction, hypertension and autonomic instability. Treatment is symptomatic (Howard and Gunderson 1980). Crotoxin, the venom of the South American rattlesnake, first depresses then increases ACh release until all transmitter is depleted. It also damages muscle mitochondria (Mebs 1989). The atraxotoxin from the Sydney funnel web spider causes similar effects to that of the black widow spider, causing repetitive firing (Sutherland 1978).

The major drugs affecting ACh receptors are *curare* and its derivatives, well-known for its use in poison arrows in South America, and in modern times as a muscle relaxant in anaesthesia. Curare causes a low-amplitude MAP with decremental responses during low-frequency repetitive stimulation. High-dosage causes complete blockade and paralysis. Curare markedly worsens myasthenia gravis (Hertel et al. 1977). The venom of the Formosan banded krait, α-bungarotoxin, irreversibly binds to the post-junctional ACh receptor causing flaccid paralysis with reduced CMAPs (Mebs 1989). Radioactive labelled α-bungarotoxin has been used to identify ACh receptors at motor end-plates and on the sarcolemma of muscle fibres. *Amantadine* blocks channels opened at the muscle end-plate after ACh receptor activation by ACh

Table 12.8. Drug-induced neuromuscular blockade

	Antibiotics	Antirheumatic drugs	Cardiovascular drugs	CNS drugs	Others
Drug-induced defect of neuromuscular transmission	Neomycin Streptomycin Kanamycin Gentamicin Polymyxin B Colistin	D penicillamine	Oxprenolol Trimethaphan	Phenytoin	
Aggravation or unmasking of Myasthenia gravis	(As above) Ampicillin Erythromycin Oxytetracycline	Chloroquine	Quinidine Propranolon Procainamide Veropamil	(As above) Lithium Chlorpromazine	Steroids Magnesium salts ACh esterase inhibitors Timolol
Post-operative respiratory depression	Neomycin Streptomycin Kanamycin Colistin				
Presentation of muscle relaxants	Lincomycin Clindamycin	Chloroquine	Quinidine Trimethaphan	Lithium Phenelzine Promazine	Ketamine Diazepam

From Argov and Mastaglia (1979).

itself. Opening these channels for longer than normal leads to repetitive firing of muscle fibres and weakness (Posa et al. 1990). Fasciculin 2, the toxin of the green mamba snake, causes fasciculations and muscle tremor from inhibition of acetylcholine esterase. Similar clinical effects are caused by *soman* and other organophosphates, originally developed as "nerve gases" for chemical warfare (Besser et al. 1990). Treatment requires neuromuscular blockade by pancuronium, with assisted ventilation.

Drugs that may Enhance Defective Neuromuscular Transmission in Myasthenia Gravis

Drugs may induce, unmask or aggravate myasthenia (Table 12.8). The most common problem, however, is the summation effect that various drugs show during the neuromuscular blockade induced by neuromuscular blocking drugs used during anaesthesia. The aminoglycoside antibiotics, e.g. neomycin, streptomycin, gentamycin, kanamycin and the polymyxins, are particularly likely to show this effect. These drugs may cause prolonged muscular relaxation and secondary apnoea after general anaesthesia, resulting in prolongation of postoperative respiratory depression. This effect can be partially antagonised by neostigmine and by calcium infusions (McQuillen and Engback 1973), which can also increase neuromuscular block in patients with idiopathic myasthenia gravis, as can quinine, procainamide and beta blockers (Kaeser 1984b). Streptomycin, propranolol, oxprenolol, metoprolol, atenolol and timolol may all produce myasthenia-type weakness in normal individuals, by an effect on the motor end-plate (Kaeser 1984b). The effect is more likely to occur in patients in whom the safety factor for neuromuscular transmission is reduced, particularly in motor neuron disease, some myopathies, polymyositis, polyneuropathy and multiple sclerosis.

Occasionally occult myasthenia gravis may be unmasked by these drugs, and this should be suspected particularly when the myasthenic effect is longlasting and severe. Similarly, the Eaton-Lambert myasthenic syndrome may be unmasked by neuromuscular blocking drugs, and by magnesium salt cathartics (Streib 1977). Phenytoin is a rare cause of exacerbation of myasthenia (Kaeser 1984b).

Trimethadione has been reported to cause myasthenia gravis (Booker et al. 1970) but the nature and specificity of this possible association has not been determined. Although procainamide may cause myasthenia-like weakness in patients with neurogenic disorders (see Niakan et al. 1981) it has not been reported to cause myasthenia gravis.

Chapter 13 Inflammatory Myopathies and Related Disorders

The term inflammatory myopathy encompasses a group of disorders characterised by muscular weakness, and often associated with clinical and pathological features suggestive of inflammation. The inflammatory myopathies, as a group of disorders, are the commonest of the acquired myopathies. Characteristically, muscular involvement is mainly proximal, although focal and distal presentations may occur. The syndrome may be acute, subacute or chronic.

Classification (Table 13.1) of the inflammatory myopathies depends on clinical, pathological and laboratory findings. Formerly, polymyositis and dermatomyositis were regarded as components of a spectrum of idiopathic inflammatory myopathies.

classification and to understanding pathogenesis. In addition, dermatomyositis and polymyositis may be associated with malignant disease. Accurate diagnosis is especially important in the inflammatory myopathies in determining appropriate treatment, since treatment may greatly modify the natural history of the disease.

The current classification of the inflammatory myopathies (Table 13.1) takes account of clinical features, clinical associations, data derived from laboratory and biopsy studies and response to treatment, and has superseded previous classifications.

Table 13.1. Classification of inflammatory myopathies

A. Idiopathic
   Polymyositis
   Dermatomyositis, of adults and childhood
   Dermatomyositis or polymyositis associated with connective tissue disease
   Inclusion body myositis
B. Paraneoplastic polymyositis
C. Polymyositis and myositis due to infection
D. Drug-induced polymyositis
E. Polymyositis associated with other disorders
F. Related disorders
   Eosinophilic syndromes
   Polymyalgia rheumatica

Table 13.2. Clinical characteristics of idiopathic inflammatory myopathies

	Polymyositis	Dermatomyositis	IBM
Age of onset	Adults	Childhood Adults	>50 years
Male : female ratio	1 : 1	1 : 2	3 : 1
Distribution of weakness	Proximal Arms weaker than legs	Proximal Arms weaker than legs	Proximal and distal
Cutaneous rash	–	Present	–
Evolution of illness	Variable	Acute/subacute	Chronic
CK levels	Raised ++	Raised ++	Normal/ raised +
Association with malignancy	±	+	None
Response to treatment	Good	Good	Poor

However, it is now recognised that these are clearly defined entities. The third major form of idiopathic inflammatory myopathy is inclusion body myositis (IBM). Clinical recognition of these three major forms of inflammatory myopathy is not always easy. Associated clinical features, particularly the age of onset and the presence of features of vasculitis or of other autoimmune disorder, are relevant both to

Idiopathic Inflammatory Myopathies

The first of the idiopathic inflammatory myopathies to be described was *dermatomyositis*. The earliest clinical description is attributed to Wagner (1863) and the term dermatomyositis was introduced by Unverricht in 1891. *Polymyositis*, without skin involvement, was first recognised by Hepp (1887). In 1903 Steiner defined dermatomyositis as "an acute, subacute or chronic disease of unknown origin characterised by a gradual onset with vague and indefinite prodromata followed by oedema, dermatitis and multiple muscle inflammation", a definition that remains appropriate today. The unique pathological features of *inclusion body myositis* were first recognised by Chou (1968) and the clinical syndrome was defined by Carpenter et al. in 1978.

Epidemiology

Idiopathic inflammatory myopathy has an annual incidence of 5–10/million (Medsgar et al. 1970; Dalakas 1991). Polymyositis shows no sex predominance but dermatomyositis is commoner in women than men (Rose and Walton 1966; Bohan et al. 1977). Inclusion body myositis is nearly three times commoner in men than in women (Lotz et al. 1989). Polymyositis is a disease of adults. Dermatomyositis shows a bimodal age distribution, with peak incidence rates for the childhood form between ages 5 to 14 years, and for the adult form between ages 45 to 64 years. Medsgar et al. (1970) noted that dermatomyositis was more frequent in black women (18/million) than in white women. Inclusion body myositis, however, is most common among white men.

Polymyositis and Dermatomyositis

These two disorders are closely related clinically but show differences in their pathology. Although for many years they were regarded as variations on a common theme, there are histological and immunological differences that suggest different mechanisms leading to these disorders.

Bohan and Peter (1975) and Bohan et al. (1977) suggested five major criteria for diagnosis of polymyositis/dermatomyositis (PM/DM):

1. Symmetrical proximal weakness progressing over weeks or months
2. Muscle biopsy findings of degeneration, regeneration and necrosis of muscle fibres, and interstitial mononuclear cell infiltration
3. Elevation of skeletal muscle enzymes in venous blood
4. Characteristic EMG findings
5. Typical cutaneous rash of dermatomyositis.

This approach determined the diagnosis and study of PM/DM until the advent of new immunological methods led to revision of the concept. In addition, the EMG criteria proposed in 1975 have also been modified in the light of subsequent experience and understanding of the causation of EMG abnormalities in these disorders.

Clinical Features of PM/DM

The pattern and progression of muscular weakness is similar in polymyositis and dermatomyositis. Clinically, the two disorders can be differentiated only by the presence of the characteristic rash in patients with dermatomyositis. This rash may be subtle and difficult to recognise, especially in artificial light.

Myopathy

The disease usually presents subacutely with proximal weakness affecting the upper and lower limbs, with involvement of the neck flexors and of the abdominal and paraspinal muscles. The pattern of weakness is variable. Although in most patients weakness is symmetrical and proximal, cases with striking asymmetry, even involving only the muscles of one limb, have been recorded (Stark 1978). Presentation with a facio-scapulo-humeral pattern of weakness has been recognised (Bates et al. 1973).

Weakness is usually more marked in proximal upper limb than lower limb muscles. The neck muscles and deltoids then appear weaker than the hip flexors or extensors. The patient's complaints reflect this distribution of weakness. Complaints of difficulty raising the arms, for example lifting objects on to a shelf, or combing the hair are common. The ability to climb or descend stairs, or to rise from a low chair is also affected. The neck flexor muscles are often severely affected so that the patient cannot easily lift the head from a pillow and may need to support the head with a hand when sitting. The neck flexors are accessory muscles for breathing and it is interesting to note that these muscles are also severely affected in myasthenia gravis, a disorder which may rarely be associated with polymyositis (Johns et al. 1971) and with dermatomyositis (Vasilescu et al. 1978a). Involvement of pharyngeal muscles is common, occurring in 30% of patients (Rowland et al. 1977). Dysarthria, however, is an unusual feature of the disease. Facial muscle involvement is uncommon. External ocular muscles are always spared.

Muscle pain and tenderness are often present in acute cases, but these features are less common in subacute and chronic cases (De Vere and Bradley 1975; Pearson and Bohan 1977). Affected painful muscles may be slightly swollen. Muscle pain may be especially common after exercise. Pain is often patchily located in affected muscles and it may be accompanied by areas of tenderness on palpation. When the disease is severe and rapidly progressive, symptoms and signs of systemic illness, especially malaise, lassitude, weight loss and fever, may be prominent. Muscular atrophy develops later in the course of the disease when the response to treatment has been unfavourable.

In the typical clinical presentation of idiopathic inflammatory myopathy there is a history of progressive or fluctuating muscle weakness, usually preferentially affecting shoulder girdle or neck muscles during a period of several weeks or months before presentation.

The cutaneous and muscular symptoms in dermatomyositis usually occur together, but either may precede the other by a month or so. Cutaneous manifestations may occur in isolation (Dawkins and Mastaglia 1973) but it is likely that most of the patients have muscular involvement (Layzer 1985b).

In the acute form of idiopathic inflammatory myopathy the patient presents within a month of the first symptom. There is rapidly progressive weakness in a proximal distribution, and oedema of muscle and sometimes also of subcutaneous tissues especially in the periorbital region, upper arms and thighs may be prominent features (Walton 1983). The muscles are painful both at rest and during movement. This muscle pain may be intense and is often associated with exquisite local tenderness (Venables et al. 1982). Dysphagia and involvement of respiratory muscles may develop. The latter may be so severe as to require ventilatory assistance. Cardiac involvement may occur. Myoglobinuria is often a feature and, when severe, it may lead to impairment of renal function. Most patients with acute presentation are ill, with features of systemic illness, especially fever, weight loss and lethargy. In some cases the onset of the disorder may be associated with viral illness or with malignancy (Urich and Wilkinson 1970).

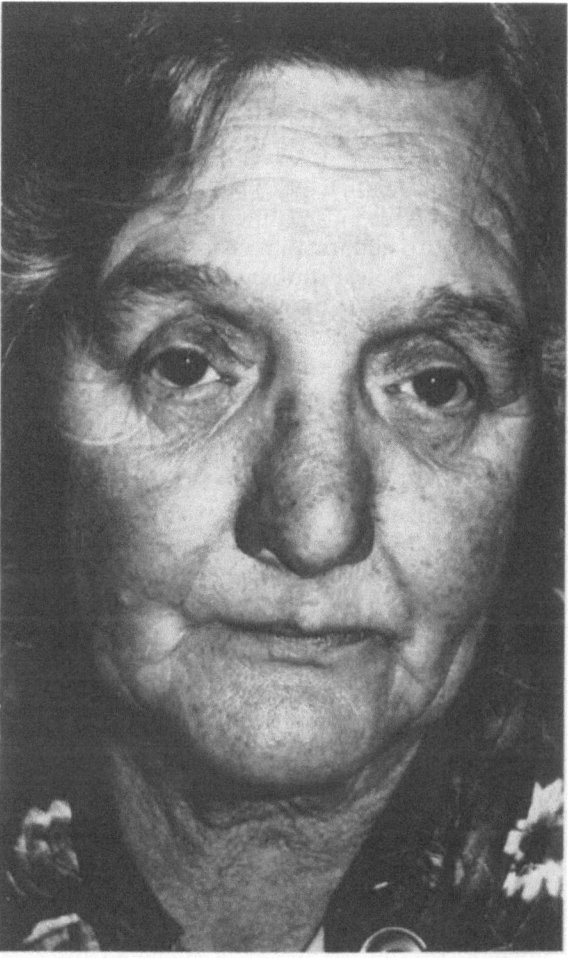

Fig. 13.1. Dermatomyositis. There is discoloration of the eyelids, cheeks and nose by a typically heliotrope and slightly oedematous rash.

Cutaneous Manifestations of Dermatomyositis

The skin rash in dermatomyositis may be florid or slight. It is characteristically a violaceous discoloration of skin exposed to light (Fig. 13.1) with dusky red patches on upper eyelids, cheeks, nose, knuckles, elbows and knees, and it usually blanches with pressure. The skin becomes scaly and atrophic and the nail beds appear shiny and reddened. In some cases the affected skin is oedematous. Telangiectasis is common in exposed skin and scleroderma-like inflexibility of the skin of the fingers and face

may occur. Small infarcts occur in the nail beds in some patients, as in other connective tissue diseases. The fingertips appear hyperaemic but ulcers may develop on the fingers. Cutaneous calcinosis may develop later.

Systemic Features

In about 5% of patients systemic features, such as weight loss and fever, dominate the clinical picture. Pulmonary disturbances, especially fibrosing alveolitis causing a diffusion defect, occur in an additional 5% of cases. An acute infiltrative pulmonary disturbance responds well to steroid therapy, but fibrosing alveolitis is refractory to treatment (Dickey and Myers 1984). The presence of anti Jo-1 antibody, which binds to histidyl components or RNA synthetase, is a marker for interstitial lung disease in PM/DM (Yoshida et al. 1983; Tazelaar et al. 1990). Oesophageal involvement, resembling that found in scleroderma, is found in about 30% of cases, but asymptomatic atonicity of the oesophagus is probably much more frequent. Cardiac involvement (Chapter 20) is a feature of most patients (Askari and Huettner 1982) but in the majority it is not recognised on routine clinical evaluation, although ECG abnormalities consisting of arrhythmias, conduction disturbances and tachyarrhythmias may develop in more than 50% of cases. Pericarditis may also occur, and this responds to steroid therapy. Pacemakers and anti-arrhythmic drugs may also be indicated in some patients.

Other features suggestive of multi-organ involvement may develop in some patients. Arthralgias may occur in up to 50% of cases (Pearson and Bohan 1977) and steroid-responsive joint effusions resembling those of rheumatoid arthritis may also develop. Raynaud's phenomenon occurs in about 30% of cases, and may precede the development of muscular symptoms by months or years (Rowland et al. 1977). These features are similar to those of mixed connective tissue disease, themselves sometimes associated with polymyositis, and it is usually an irrelevant exercise to try to classify patients with these features solely on the basis of the prior or later development of symptoms.

Juvenile (Childhood-Type) Dermatomyositis

Inflammatory muscle disease in childhood differs in several respects from that of adults. In the childhood or juvenile form cutaneous involvement is a characteristic feature, whereas in adults a rash is present in only 30% of cases (Bohan et al. 1977). Involvement of the gastro-intestinal tract with mucosal ulceration and perforation due to vasculitis is much more common in juvenile dermatomyositis than in the adult form (Banker and Victor 1966; Crowe et al. 1982). Intramuscular and subcutaneous calcinosis has been reported in up to 40% of patients with juvenile dermatomyositis and is functionally severe in 15% (Malleson 1982); in adults with inflammatory muscle disease calcinosis is rare.

The young person usually presents with weakness and tender muscles, often in association with fever and other features of systemic illness. The skin manifestations may be present from the onset or they may develop shortly afterwards; their severity does not correlate with the outcome. The rash consists of erythematous discoloration and oedema of the upper eyelids, periorbital region and cheeks with involvement of the extensor surfaces of the knuckles, elbows and knees. The mean age of onset

is about 7 years, ranging from the first year of life into the third decade (Carpenter et al. 1976; Malleson 1982). Proximal muscles are weak and tender in upper and lower limbs so that difficulty in rising and Gower's manoeuvre may be important early features. Weakness of neck flexion and of respiratory muscles is often prominent in childhood type dermatomyositis. Even at presentation the muscles may be atrophic and joint contractures, particularly in the arms, may be present. Dysphagia with pooling of secretion in the mouth develops in about 30% of patients, and oesophageal dysfunction is usually present in these cases (Metheny 1978; Pachman and Cooke 1980). Ulceration of the skin develops in about 6% of cases (Winkelmann 1982). Renal involvement with albuminuria or haematuria has also been recognised (Bitnum et al. 1964). ECG abnormalities occur, but overt cardiomyopathy is rare (Pachman and Cooke 1980). There is no association with interstitial lung disease (Pachman and Maryjowski 1984).

Myositis Associated with Autoimmune Disorders

The relation between myositis and connective tissue disorders is complex. While myositis may occur as a complication of these disorders, e.g. in rheumatoid arthritis, mixed connective tissue disease, systemic lupus erythematosus, polyarteritis nodosa (PAN) and scleroderma, clinical features suggestive of connective tissue disorder may also develop in patients initially presenting with polymyositis (see above). About 20% of cases of polymyositis and dermatomyositis show features of an associated connective tissue disease. Pearson and Bohan (1977) and Bohan et al. (1977) attempted to distinguish primary myositis and "overlap" myositis on the basis of the clinical features. In overlap myositis they included patients in whom the myositis either preceded or followed the development of generalised connective tissue disease (Table 13.3). The muscular symptoms in overlap myositis vary in severity and the possibility that they might result not from myositis, but from the effects of concurrent steroid therapy, joint disease or neuropathy, must always be considered.

Myositis Associated with Mixed Connective Tissue Disease

Mixed connective tissue disease (MCTD) is a disease, largely affecting women, that resembles a combination of SLE, polymyositis and scleroderma.

Table 13.3. Presenting features of primary polymyositis (52 patients) and overlap myositis (32 patients)

	Primary polymyositis	Overlap myositis
M : F ratio	1 : 2	1 : 9
Age of onset (mean)	47	35
Proximal weakness (%)	92	41
Arthralgias (%)	25	53
Raynaud's phenomenon (%)	17	47
Sclerodactyly (%)	2	44
Rash (%)	2	19
Myalgia (%)	25	41

From Bohan et al. (1977).

Non-specific features, especially non-erosive mild arthritis, puffy hands, impaired oesophageal motility and lymphadenopathy are common. Renal and pulmonary complications may develop and high titres of circulating antibody to extractable nuclear antibodies (anti-ENA) are found (Sharp et al. 1972; Nimelstein et al. 1980). Most patients with this syndrome have proximal weakness, myalgia, muscle tenderness and markedly raised blood CK levels (Isenberg 1984), and muscle biopsy features consistent with an inflammatory myopathy (Sharp 1981). Cutaneous features may resemble those of dermatomyositis or those of scleroderma.

Myositis Associated with Systemic Lupus Erythematosus (SLE)

In SLE myalgia and muscle tenderness are common, occurring in 30%–50% of patients (Dubois 1974; Isenberg and Snaith 1981), although a true necrotising myositis occurs in less than 10% of patients (Isenberg 1984). The presence of anti-SM ENA antibodies is particularly suggestive of SLE when found in patients with myositis (Bunch 1990).

Myositis Associated with Rheumatoid Arthritis (RA)

In RA muscular symptoms are commonly due to disuse from joint disease, or to steroid therapy. Myositis may develop as a rare complication of the disease, particularly in association with arteritis in the most severe clinical form of the disease. Typical polymyositis or nodular myositis may occur but interstitial myositis is more frequent. Rarely, polymyositis may be induced in RA during treatment with D-penicillamine (Morgan et al. 1981).

Weakness and muscle atrophy may be early features of RA, but these symptoms are not due to myositis.

Myositis Associated with Scleroderma

Myositis occurs in 10%–15% of patients with scleroderma and usually affects deltoid, pectoral and forearm muscles (Clements et al. 1978). The anterior tibial and forearm muscles may also be affected. Affected muscles show marked atrophy and necrosis of muscle fibres, which are replaced by dense collagenous connective tissue. In other patients proximal weakness is associated with fibre atrophy and fibrosis, without inflammatory myopathy. These muscular complications of scleroderma do not respond to steroid therapy (Clements et al. 1978). This syndrome has been associated with a specific antibody (Scl 70) directed against nucleolar protein complex (Genth et al. 1990).

Myosotis Associated with Other Autoimmune and Connective Tissue Diseases

Inflammatory myopathy is a feature of other autoimmune disorders. In PAN myalgia occurs in about 75% of patients but muscle biopsies are abnormal in only about 30% of patients, showing the features of necrotising vasculitis. Muscle fibre necrosis is a relatively uncommon feature (Lightfoot 1979). In *Sjögren's syndrome* about 10% of patients show features of mild, chronic, focal myositis (Pavlides et al. 1982; Ringel et al. 1979). Polymyositis may occur in association with myasthenia gravis (Johns et al. 1971; Oosterhuis 1983), either preceding or following the myasthenia. Namba et al. (1974) suggested that there might be an association between thymoma and inflammatory myopathy.

Inclusion Body Myositis (IBM)

This slowly progressive disorder predominantly affects men (3 : 1), with a mean age of onset of 56 years (Lotz et al. 1989). The mean duration of the disease from onset to diagnosis was 6 years in the series of 40 patients studied by Lotz et al. (1989). Muscular weakness can be proximal, distal or both, and is often asymmetrical (Fig. 13.2). There may be selective weakness and wasting of biceps, triceps, ilio psoas, quadriceps and tibialis anterior, and the fingers may be weak. In a third of patients distal weakness may be more striking than proximal weakness (Carpenter et al. 1978; Eisen et al. 1983a;

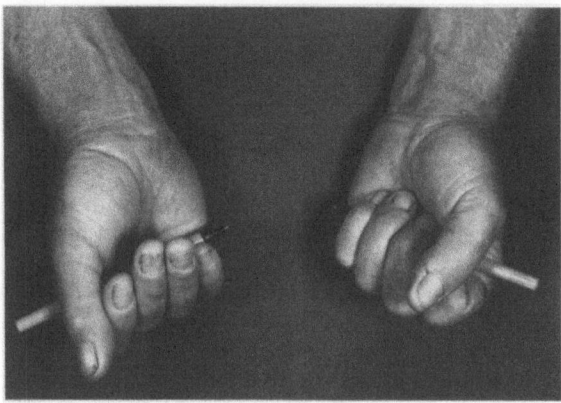

Fig. 13.2. Inclusion body myositis. There is asymmetrical distal weakness, often affecting the hands.

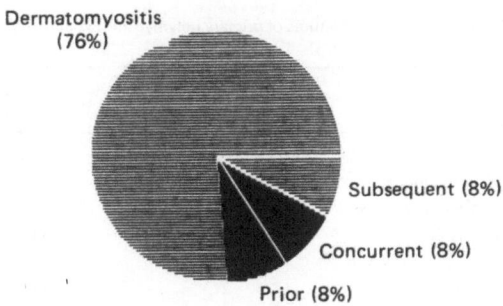

Fig. 13.3. Dermatomyositis and malignancy. In 76% of cases no malignancy was found but, in the others, malignant disease preceded, followed or was found concurrently with the dermatomyositis (after Callen 1984).

Lotz et al. 1989). The tendon reflexes are often decreased or absent; the knee jerks are almost always absent. Dysphagia occurs in about 40% of patients with IBM (Danon et al. 1982; Ringel et al. 1987). Lotz et al. (1989) attributed dysphagia to cricopharyngeal muscular dysfunction in five of their 40 patients and noted that this might be amenable to surgical treatment. Dysphagia is relatively less common in other inflammatory myopathies (Horowitz et al. 1986).

An association with hypertension was noted in almost 50% of cases of IBM by Lotz et al. (1989) and cardiac involvement was suspected in many others, consisting mainly of ischaemic heart disease (25%), rhythm disturbances and valvular disease. IBM has been related to a number of connective tissue diseases, e.g. SLE and Sjögren's syndrome, but no causative relationship has been established. The loss of tendon reflexes and distal weakness has been ascribed to an associated peripheral neuropathy but, if present, this is subclinical. There is no association between IBM and malignancy.

The true incidence of IBM is uncertain since most patients have been recognised when treatment of a progressive inflammatory myopathy with steroids has been unsuccessful, or following investigation in specialised referral centres. Dalakas (1991) noted that a third of steroid-unresponsive patients with inflammatory myopathy referred to the National Institutes of Health, Bethesda, had IBM. The slowly progressive clinical course of IBM resembles that of late onset limb girdle myopathy and it is likely that some patients described as myopathies in the past (e.g. Nevin 1936; Shy and McEachern 1951; Nattrass 1954) were suffering from IBM. The aetiology of this disease is unknown, and its classification as a form of inflammatory muscle disease, rather than degenerative muscle disease, remains controversial.

Paraneoplastic Dermatomyositis/Polymyositis

Because dermatomyositis and polymyositis have been associated with malignant disease (Brain and Henson 1958; Barnes 1976) it has been thought worthwhile to search for neoplasia in patients with these disorders. This association was noted in 1916 by Kankeleit. However, the risk of an association of these disorders with malignancy in patients younger than 40 years, especially in children, is very small (De Vere and Bradley 1975). In older patients, the incidence of malignancy in patients with polymyositis or dermatomyositis was noted to be about 20% by Mastaglia and Ojeda (1985a,b). The association has been found to be particularly strong with cancers of the lung and gastro-intestinal tract in men and with cancers of the breast and ovary in women (Barnes 1976; Callen 1984). The muscle disease and the cancer may present simultaneously or one may precede the other, but only rarely by more than a year. Dermatomyositis in patients older than 50 years has been particularly closely associated with cancer (Fig. 13.3). The controversy concerning the association of polymyositis and dermatomyositis with malignancy has been addressed more recently by Lakhanpal et al. (1986), who questioned this association. Sigurgeirsson et al. (1992) reported a population-based survey of all the in-patients with suspected dermatomyositis or polymyositis in Sweden in the years 1964–1983. The relative risk of malignancy in the 392 patients with dermatomyositis was 2.4 for males and 3.4 for females, but in the 396 patients with polymyositis the relative risk was only 1.8 for males and 1.7 for females. In the patients with dermatomyositis the mortality rate from cancer was higher than in those with polymyositis. The principal associated cancers were ovary (relative risk 8.2), pancreas, colon, bronchus and breast (relative risk 3.2). The incidence of cancers diagnosed before development of dermatomyositis was similar to that of cancers diagnosed after the onset of the muscle disease, as in the experience of Callen (1984) (Fig. 13.3). There is no association of malignancy with IBM (Callen 1988).

These findings suggest that patients presenting with dermatomyositis in particular should be kept under close surveillance if the initial investigation fails to reveal an underlying cancer. This investigation should comprise chest X-ray, mammography, pelvic and rectal examination and full blood count. Other investigations are probably not worthwhile, although CT of the abdomen is also often used in order to exclude lymphoma and pancreatic carcinoma.

Subacute Necrotising Myopathy

Necrosis of skeletal muscle, without an inflammatory reaction may occur as a remote association of carcinoma (Smith 1969; Urich and Wilkinson 1970; Swash 1974). The disorder has been differentiated from polymyositis by the absence of inflammatory response and by the widespread necrosis of muscle (Urich and Wilkinson 1970). However, it is probably a variant of acute polymyositis.

Aetiology of Inflammatory Muscle Disease

There is evidence that the pathogenesis of dermatomyositis and polymyositis differs. Dermatomyositis is characterised by complement-mediated autoimmune damage to the microvasculature (Kissel et al. 1986). Polymyositis is a cell-mediated autoimmune disorder, characterised by direct destruction of muscle cells by activated T cells (Engel and Arahata 1984; Arahata and Engel 1986). The immunological changes found in muscle biopsies in IBM are similar to those found in polymyositis (Engel and Arahata 1984).

The earliest and most characteristic feature of dermatomyositis is deposition of complement C5-9 membrane attack complex on the arterioles and capillaries in muscle and skin in five of 19 patients (Kissel et al. 1991). It is not known whether capillaries in other tissues are similarly involved. Cervera et al. (1991) showed IgG and IgM antibodies to endothelial cells in eight of 18 patients with dermatomyositis, six of whom also had interstitial lung disease. This deposition of complement is followed by necrosis of capillaries and ischaemic destruction of muscle fibres. In dermatomyositis there are endomysial cellular infiltrates; these consist of high proportions of B cells, with an increased ratio of CD4+ (helper) cells to CD8+ (suppressor-cytotoxic) T cells. The proximity of CD4+ cells to B cells and macrophages and the absence of lymphocytotoxic destruction of muscle cells is consistent with a humorally mediated mechanism. Peripheral blood lymphocytes produce immunoglobulin M in response to the presence of activated B and T cells (Cambridge et al. 1989). Childhood-type dermatomyositis shows a similar deposition of IgG on intramuscular capillaries (Whitaker and Engel 1972). Dermatomyositis has been associated with monoclonal gammopathy (Kiprov and Miller 1984).

Studies of HLA haplotypes have indicated an excess of HLAB8-DR3 in both childhood dermatomyositis (Pachman and Cooke 1980; Robb et al. 1988) and in adult dermatomyositis (Behan et al. 1978). These findings suggest a familial propensity to the disease associated with a genetic locus on chromosome 6.

In polymyositis and IBM the muscular disorder is the result of antigen-directed cytotoxicity mediated by cytotoxic T cells. Muscle cell destruction is associated with the presence of CD8+ cells and macrophages (Engel and Arahata 1984). The muscle fibres involved in this local inflammatory and cytotoxic process express major histocompatibility complex Class 1 (MHC-1) antigen, and the 65 kDa heatshock protein on their sarcolemma (Emslie-Smith et al. 1989; Hohlfeld et al. 1991). T cells in muscle in patients with polymyositis show cytotoxicity to autologous myotubes (Hohlfeld and Engel 1991). T cells expressing the γ/δ receptor may be especially important in this cytotoxic response to muscle cells (Hohlfeld et al. 1991). In IBM there is a threefold increase in the prevalence of the DR1 phenotype (Plotz et al. 1989).

Although a number of viruses have been implicated in the causation of inflammatory myopathies, for example picornavirus and Coxsackie virus in both polymyositis and dermatomyositis (Bowles et al. 1987; Rosenberg et al. 1989), and mumps virus antigen in IBM (Chou 1986; Nishino et al. 1989), these associations have not been confirmed as causative agents. Human retrovirus infections, both with HIV and HTLV-1, have been linked to the development of a polymyositis syndrome (Dalakas et al. 1986; Simpson and Bender 1988). The inflammatory cell infiltrate in HIV-associated polymyositis cannot be distinguished from that found in idiopathic polymyositis except that there are markedly fewer CD4+ T cells in HIV-associated myositis. Despite this similarity, HIV antigen has been detected only in macrophages in the latter disorder, rather than in muscle cells (Chad et al. 1990; Illa et al. 1991). HTLV-1 infection may produce a similar myositis, with CD8+ lymphocytes in the muscle and MHC-1 expression in muscle cells (Dalakas et al. 1992).

In both polymyositis and dermatomyositis there is an association with other diseases known to have an autoimmune basis, e.g. systemic lupus erythematosus, mixed connective tissue disease and myasthenia gravis, and in many of these disorders, as in dermatomyositis, there may be increased blood IgG levels with specific circulating IgG or IgM autoantibodies. Experimental models of autoimmune myositis have been produced by the use of autoallergic experiments with Freund's adjuvant (experimental allergic myositis) and these show similar cellular responses in the abnormal muscle to those found in the spontaneous human disease (Esiri and MacLellan 1974; Whitaker 1982). Polymyositis may be induced by D-penicillamine (Schraeder et al. 1972), a disorder that is self-limited. The pathogenesis of inflammatory myopathies associated with malignancies is not, as yet, understood, in that no specific autoantibody or cell-mediated response has been identified.

Laboratory Investigations

The blood CK is the single most useful test in the diagnosis of dermatomyositis, polymyositis and inclusion body myositis. The CK level is raised in most patients with polymyositis and dermatomyositis at presentation, but is less likely to be raised in patients in whom inflammatory myopathy is associated with other autoimmune disorders. It may reach a level as high as fiftyfold above the upper limit of normal in severe cases (Dalakas 1992). Some patients with inflammatory myopathy may have a normal CK at presentation (De Vere and Bradley 1975). A normal CK level does not therefore exclude active myositis. Further, during effective treatment or when the disease has become inactive the CK falls (Cane et al. 1989). In chronic polymyositis the CK may be normal in up to a third of cases (Trojaborg 1990). Serial CK measurements are useful in management since a rise in CK level may precede a clinical exacerbation of the disease by as much as 6 weeks (Bohan et al. 1977). Most of the elevated CK level consists of CK_{MM}, muscle-derived, isoenzyme (Zweig et al. 1980). An increase in the CK_{BB} isoenzyme in some cases has been ascribed to enzyme leakage from regenerating fibres (Zweig et al. 1980). In about a quarter of patients the blood CK_{MB} frac-

tion of CK is raised, usually due to release of CK_{MB} from regenerating muscle fibres rather than evidence of cardiomyopathy (Somer et al. 1976). Other enzyme tests are generally less widely useful. The serum glutamic-oxaloacetic transaminase (SGOT), serum glutamic-pyruvate transaminase (SGPT) levels are usually raised. Generally, if the SGOT is higher than SGPT a muscle disorder is likely; the converse suggests liver disease (Dalakas 1992). Carbonic anhydrase III, an enzyme specific to striated muscle, is also present in increased quantity in the serum in patients with active disease (Heath et al. 1983). The serum myoglobin level is raised in 50% or more of patients with active polymyositis, and may be raised in a third of patients in whom the CK level is normal (Nishkai and Reichlin 1977; Kagen 1977; Askmark et al. 1981). The disparity may relate to differing kinetics of release and breakdown of these substances in the blood. In IBM the CK level is raised in 80% of patients at diagnosis, but rarely to more than three times the upper limit of normal (Lotz et al. 1989).

The ESR is raised in about half the cases of inflammatory myopathy (Pearson and Currie 1974; Isenberg 1984). However, an elevated ESR is a non-specific finding since it is raised in many different disorders, and fluctuations in the ESR do not necessarily follow the clinical course. It is less likely to be raised in IBM than in dermatomyositis or polymyositis.

Serological studies reveal abnormalities that may sometimes be useful in diagnosis, especially in categorising patients with inflammatory myopathy associated with other autoimmune diseases. In patients in whom polymyositis complicates RA or SLE the humoral antibody abnormalities typical of these diseases may be found, e.g. rheumatoid factor and the presence of antinuclear antibody, but in patients with subacute inflammatory myopathy without other autoimmune diseases these tests are usually negative. Blood IgG levels are often increased in patients with mixed connective disease and polymyositis, but hypogammaglobulinaemia (Guiliano 1974) and monoclonal gammopathy (Kiprov and Miller 1984) may also be associated with the disease (see above). Circulating immune complexes have been detected in juvenile dermatomyositis (Spencer et al. 1979). In up to 70% of patients with polymyositis saline extractable antinuclear antibodies have been detected (Nishikai and Reichlin 1980). Of these the Jo-1 and PM-1 are relatively specific for polymyositis and dermatomyositis (Garlepp and Dawkins 1984) and the Jo-1 antibody is a marker for myositis associated with interstitial lung disease (Bernstein et al. 1984; Tazelaar et al. 1990). Antimyoglobin antibodies are found in about 70% of patients (Nishikai and Homma 1977) and anti-myosin antibodies have been found in up to 90% of patients with polymyositis (Wada et al. 1983).

Muscle Imaging

Radioisotope scanning using ^{99}mTc has been used to study the distribution of muscular involvement in polymyositis (Brown et al. 1976). With this technique the patchy involvement of proximal muscles is clearly seen, and during remissions the intensity of uptake of isotope is diminished.

CT imaging is not useful in management, although it demonstrates abnormalities with zones of reduced attenuation in chronic polymyositis. MR imaging shows patchy abnormalities even in acute cases but the appearances are not diagnostic, consisting of high intensity lesions in T2 weighted images that resolve during effective treatment. These investigations utilised a 1.5T magnetic field and may be useful in assessing the clinical course during treatment (Frazer et al. 1991; Fujino et al. 1991).

Electrocardiography

ECG abnormalities are frequent but symptomatic cardiac disease, e.g. arrhythmias, heart block and cardiac failure, is uncommon (Askari and Huettner 1982). The MB isoenzyme of CK is frequently raised, suggesting that cardiac muscle is involved (Askari and Huettner 1982) (see Chapter 20).

Electrophysiological Assessment

The EMG features of polymyositis and dermatomyositis vary according to the stage and activity of the disease (Mechler 1974). In the acute stage denervation potentials including fibrillation potentials and positive sharp waves (Fig. 13.4) are found in up to 80% of patients (Lambert et al. 1954). Streib et al. (1979) found fibrillation potentials in 93% of paraspinal muscles and 70% of proximal limb muscles. These features reflect the presence of focal necrosis or split fibres (Swash and Schwartz 1977; Sandstedt et al. 1982a). Cöers and Woolf (1959) found abnormal terminal axonal branches and motor end-plates in some muscle biopsies and Cöers et al. (1973) described collateral reinnervation and axonal branching near foci of cellular infiltration, suggesting that the innervation of muscle might be affected in some cases, a concept also consistent with the presence of clusters of small, pointed, NADH-dark fibres in some fascicles in biopsies taken in the acute stages of the disease.

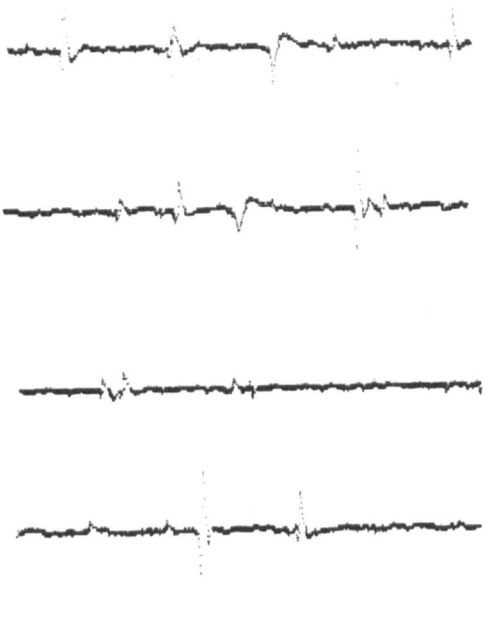

Fig. 13.4. Acute polymyositis. Prominent fibrillation potentials and positive sharp waves. Concentric needle EMG. Filters: 100 Hz and 10 kHz. Bar 20 ms.

Focal or segmental necrosis of fibres can lead to isolation of part of a fibre from its innervation and so to denervation of this part of the fibre (Hall-Craggs 1971; Ringel et al. 1976; Swash and Schwartz 1977). Denny-Brown (1960) showed that fibrillation potentials could be produced experimentally by cutting muscle fibres in such a way that parts of the fibres were separated from their innervation. However, denervation potentials may also be generated by regenerating fibres not yet sufficiently mature to have gained effective innervation, and active muscle fibre regeneration is a feature of the acute stage of the illness (see Schmalbruch 1976; Swash et al. 1978a).

Bizarre high-frequency potentials have often been associated with acute polymyositis. They occur at rest but may be induced by movement of the needle electrode or by volitional movement. Some of the repetitive discharges occur at low frequencies. Lambert et al. (1954) thought they were relatively specific for polymyositis but they also occur in a variety of other myopathies and neurogenic disorders (Emeryck et al. 1974). Partanen and Lang (1982) found bizarre high-frequency potentials only in chronic cases.

With conventional concentric needle EMG the abnormal potentials are typically of low amplitude (<1 mV) and of short duration (Fig. 13.5), as in

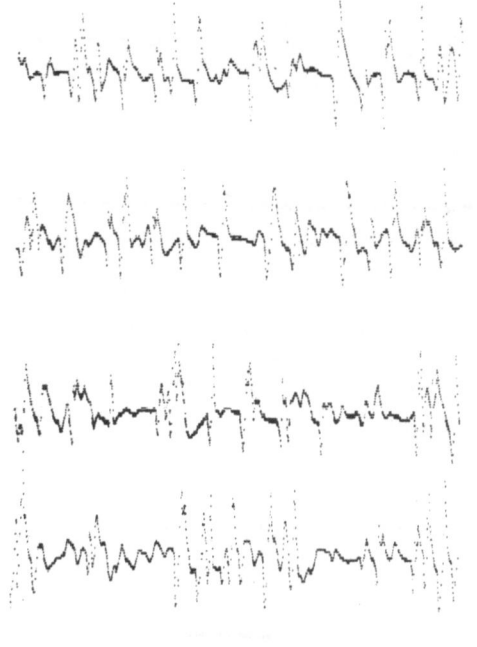

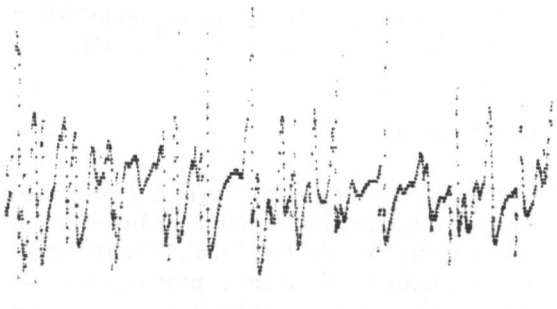

Fig. 13.7. Chronic polymyositis. Motor unit action potentials of normal or slightly increased amplitude. Concentric needle EMG. Filters: 100 Hz and 10 kHz. Bar 20 ms.

Fig. 13.5. Short-duration polyphasic motor unit action potentials in acute polymyositis. Concentric needle EMG. Filters: 100 Hz and 10 kHz. Bar 20 ms.

other myopathies. The duration of MUAPs varies in different muscles and at different ages (Chap. 2) and these factors must be taken into account. Some of the apparently short-duration polyphasic units contain late potentials (Fig. 13.6) of low amplitude (Borenstein and Desmedt 1974), a phenomenon which could be due either to delayed conduction in regenerating axonal sprouts, or to slowed propagation velocity in degenerate or small-diameter muscle fibres (Stålberg et al. 1974).

In adult idiopathic polymyositis, "myopathic" MUAPs are distributed in a characteristic, patchy manner in affected muscles, a distribution which is consistent with the similar patchy abnormality seen in biopsies of affected muscles. In childhood-type dermatomyositis, however, the EMG abnormality is usually more widely distributed but it may be very localised so that with even slight movement of the exploring electrode the abnormal potentials can no longer be recorded.

As the disease progresses the MUAPs become of larger amplitude and of longer duration (Fig. 13.7) (Mechler 1974). In acute polymyositis the MUAP amplitude is less than normal and the potentials tend to have a shorter duration than normal (Fig. 13.5). Even in the later stages some short duration low amplitude MUAPs are present, together with the larger amplitude potentials. The latter probably represent remodelled motor units, an interpretation supported by histological observations of fibre-type grouping in the late stages of the disease (Ringel et al. 1976; Swash et al. 1978a). Occasional large MUAPs are seen (Mechler 1974; Swash and Schwartz 1977). Using trigger-delay, the late components of MUAPs can be recorded, either with concentric needle or single-fibre EMG, especially in chronic polymyositis. These represent activity derived from fibres of small diameter, some of which are probably regenerating fibres (Swash and

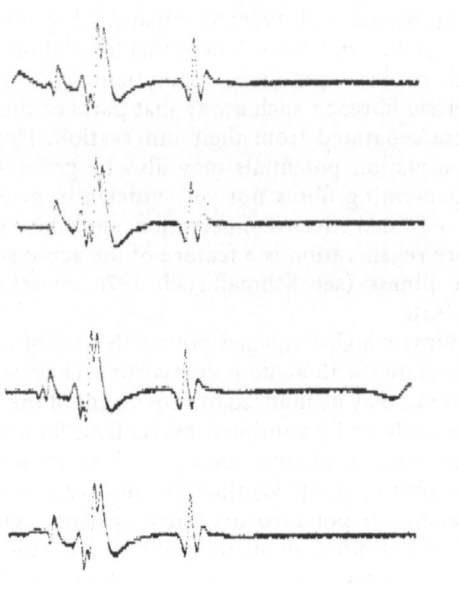

Fig. 13.6. Polymyositis. Polyphasic motor unit action potential showing a late component. Concentric needle EMG. Filters: 500 Hz and 10 kHz. Bar 4 ms.

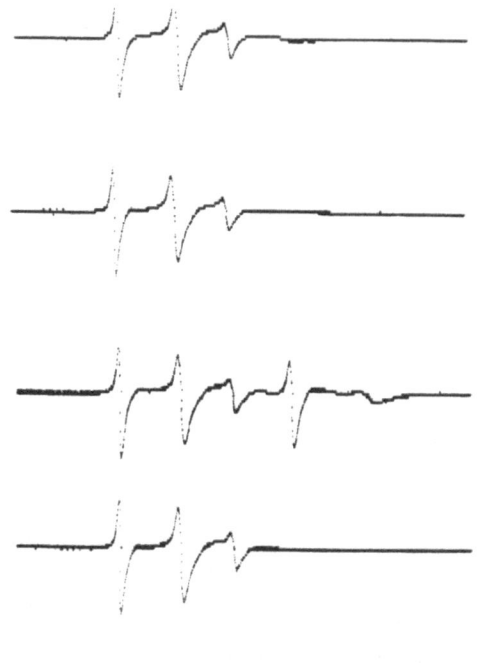

Fig. 13.8. Chronic polymyositis. Complex unit showing dispersed potentials and blocking of the last unit. Single-fibre EMG. Bar 2 ms.

Schwartz 1977; Partanen and Lang 1982). Uncini et al. (1990) found that non-polyphasic MUAPs were of short duration in acute and chronic polymyositis, but polyphasic MUAPs were of decreased duration but normal or of increased duration in the chronic stage.

In single-fibre EMG recordings the individual components of the MUP are dispersed, reflecting variations in propagation velocity in fibres of differing size within individual motor units (Fig. 13.8). There is often an increased jitter and blocking may occur (Henriksson and Stålberg 1978). With macro-EMG, the mean amplitude of the MUAPs recorded is reduced (Barkhaus et al. 1990).

The interference pattern in polymyositis is usually full with only moderate effort. This abnormal pattern of recruitment of motor units probably occurs as a compensatory phenomenon for loss of muscle fibres in individual motor units. More motor units must therefore be recruited during moderate effort to establish an isometric contraction at any required level of force. The interference pattern may be mildly reduced in wasted muscles; Trojaborg (1990) found that the recruitment pattern was full in 26 of 33 cases, and only mildly reduced in seven despite muscle weakness and wasting. The combination of large, polyphasic MUAPs and a reduced interference pattern may lead to an erroneous diagnosis of a primary neurogenic disorder. Turns

analysis demonstrates a higher ratio of turns to amplitude with increasing effort than in normal muscle (Stålberg et al. 1983). In a group of 153 patients with polymyositis and dermatomyositis Bohan et al. (1977) found small amplitude, short duration, polyphasic MUAPs in 90% of patients, fibrillation potentials, positive sharp waves and increased insertional activity in 74%, complex repetitive discharges in 78%, no abnormalities in 10% and abnormalities restricted to paraspinal muscles in 2% of patients.

Decremental, and occasionally incremental, responses may be found with repetitive nerve stimulation. The decremental response may define a group of patients in whom polymyositis co-exists with occult myasthenia gravis, but in other patients a decremental response may be found only at fast stimulation rates. Pestronk and Drachman (1985) found a reduced number of acetylcholine receptors in muscle fibres in patients with polymyositis. In addition serum and purified IgG from these patients accelerated the rate of degradation of acetylcholine receptors on healthy muscle fibres.

In IBM the electrophysiological features are similar to those found in dermatomyositis and polymyositis. However, in this disorder both small and large polyphasic potentials are prominent, a feature suggesting a neurogenic component. These features are also found in chronic polymyositis and they probably relate simply to the chronic course of IBM. Nerve conduction studies were abnormal in seven of 48 patients with IBM studied by Lotz et al. (1989). Three of these seven patients had diabetes mellitus. Joy et al. (1990) reviewed the electrophysiological features of IBM and found that only 37% of cases showed a mixed neurogenic and myopathic EMG. A myopathic pattern was found in 57% and a neurogenic EMG in 6%.

Muscle Biopsy

The pathological features of the main types of inflammatory myopathy are summarised in Table 13.4.

Idiopathic Polymyositis

The changes found in muscle biopsies in polymyositis vary according to the severity and duration of the disease, the effect of treatment and the muscle chosen for biopsy.

In acute idiopathic polymyositis (Table 13.5) inflammatory cell infiltrates are a major feature (Figure 13.9). These consist of aggregates of small lymphocytes together with macrophages, plasma cells and, occasionally, eosinophils. These cellular

Table 13.4. Pathological features of polymyositis, dermatomyositis and inclusion body myositis

	Polymyositis	Adult dermatomyositis	Childhood-type dermatomyositis	Inclusion body myositis
Muscle fibre necrosis	Single fibres	Single or groups	Single or groups Micro-infarcts	Rare single fibres
Perifascicular atrophy	–	Present	Prominent	–
Capillary numbers	Normal	Reduced	Reduced	Normal
Microvascular changes	–	Present	Frequent	–
Inflammatory cell infiltrates	Endomysial	Perimysial Perivascular	Perimysial Perivascular	Endomysial
CD8 + T cells	Common	Rare	Rare	Common
Rimmed vacuoles and filamentous inclusions in muscle fibres	–	–	–	Present

Table 13.5. Pathological and electrophysiological features of acute idiopathic polymyositis

Pathology	EMG
Inflammatory cell infiltration	Fibrillation potentials
Single fibre necrosis with phagocytosis	Positive sharp waves
	Complex high frequencypotentials
Regenerating (basophilic) fibres	
	Small polyphasic MUAPs of decreasedduration
"Moth-eaten" fibres	
Atrophy of both fibre types	Normal or slightly increased single-fibre EMG fibre density
Angular atrophic fibres	Jitter and blocking may occur
Increased central nucleation	Early recruitment of MUAPs

infiltrates occur mainly within fascicles in relation to necrotic fibres or to small intrafascicular blood vessels. In some biopsies focal intrafascicular cellular infiltrates are not seen, perhaps because of sampling error, but there may be a mild, diffuse increase in cellularity in the endomysium. The second major

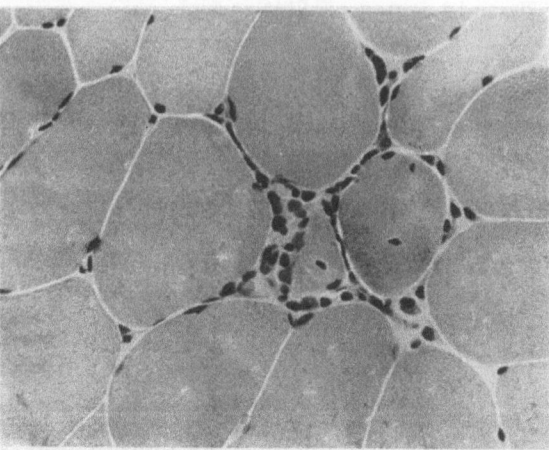

Fig. 13.9. Acute polymyositis. H and E, × 350. Two small regenerating fibres, marked by central nuclei, are surrounded by endomysial inflammatory cells.

feature is the presence of scattered necrotic muscle fibres (Fig. 13.10), occurring singly or in clusters with or without an active lymphocytic and macrophage response. These necrotic fibres are frequently pale and "ghost-like", unreactive in all enzyme preparations. Some have a brightly eosinophilic, hyaline appearance. Some abnormal fibres show histological features of regeneration, especially basophilia, even when surrounded by macrophages. Scattered atrophic fibres that may be dark in NADH preparations are common. There is usually an increase in central nucleation. "Moth-eaten" change is common in NADH and ATPase preparations. EM studies show loss of mitochondria, with disruption of myofibrillar architecture and Z-band streaming in these fibres. This feature is important in considering the diagnosis of inflammatory myopathy in those biopsies in which cellular infiltration is not prominent. If the diagnosis is suspected strongly on clinical criteria, and cellular infiltrates are not recognised in the biopsy, a second biopsy should be considered in order to establish the diagnosis (Dalakas 1991). Monoclonal antibody markers show that the lymphocytes in the biopsy consist of activated T cells, as well as macrophages, as described above (Arahata and Engel 1986).

In chronic polymyositis (Table 13.6) there are marked myopathic features, consisting of marked variation in fibre size with hypertrophic fibres, increased central nucleation, muscle fibre splitting, regenerating fibres and interstitial fibrosis (Fig. 13.11). Type 2 fibre atrophy is common, especially in patients who have been treated with steroids. These pathological features resemble those found in muscular dystrophies but two aspects of the pathology are important in recognising polymyositis in such biopsies. These are, firstly, the presence of an endomysial inflammatory cell infiltrate and, secondly, the focal distribution of the pathology. In addition, architectural changes in muscle fibres are prominent in polymyositis. In end-stage cases, however, the diagnosis can be very difficult.

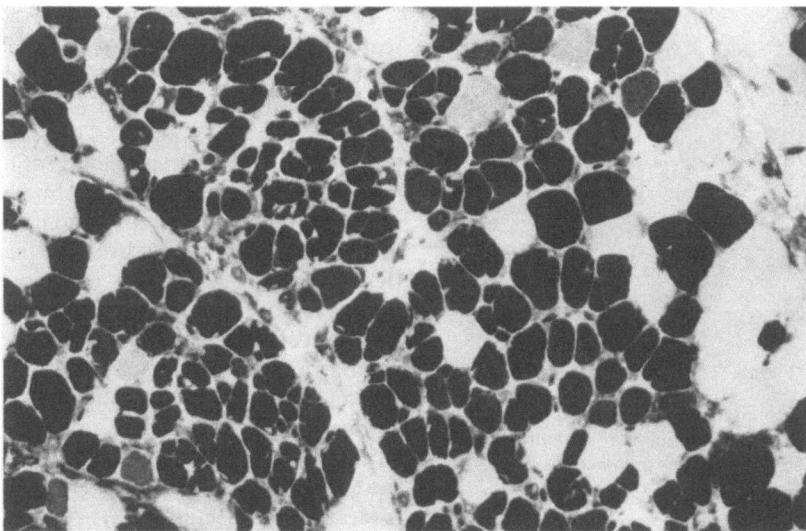

Fig. 13.10.   Acute polymyositis. ATPase, pH 4.3. TS. × 140. Widespread necrosis has occurred and has been followed by subendomysial regeneration. The fascicular borders of the zones of regenerating fibres can be clearly seen. To the right there is a fascicle of normal fibres.

Table 13.6.   Pathological and electrophysiological features of chronic polymyositis

Pathology	EMG
Myopathic features	Reduced interference pattern
Marked variation in fibre size	Polyphasic MUAPs of normal or increased amplitude
Hypertrophied fibres	
Central nucleation	MUAPs of increased duration
Fibre splitting	Increased jitter and blocking with single-fibre EMG
Regenerating and necrotic fibres	
Endomysial and perifascicular fibrosis	Increased fibre density with single-fibre EMG
Inflammatory cell exudates	
Focally distributed architectural changes in individual fibres	
Neurogenic features	
Fibre-type grouping (uncommon)	
Scattered, atrophic, pointed, NADH-tr-dark fibres	

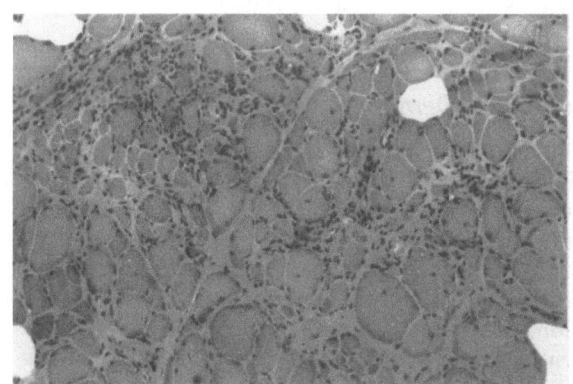

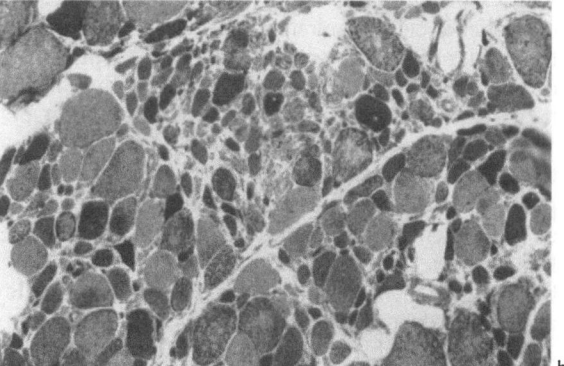

   Neurogenic features may be very prominent and may sometimes cause diagnostic confusion. Two varieties of neurogenic change occur. Clusters of isolated, small, pointed, NADH tr-dark fibres are usually seen, and small groups of fibres, up to about 15, of uniform histochemical type are found in discrete areas of the biopsy (Fig. 13.12). The latter abnormality is consistent with the EMG findings, especially polyphasic potentials of moderately increased amplitude, and the appearance of complex action potentials during single-fibre EMG, some containing late components. The fibre density

Fig. 13.11.   Chronic polymyositis, TS. × 140. **a** H and E. **b** NADH-tr. There is marked variability in fibre size and many fibres are conspicuously rounded. In the NADH-tr many smaller fibres are darkly reactive. There is some fibre-type grouping with architectural change and a marked increase in fibrous tissue. A diffuse inflammatory cell response is evident.

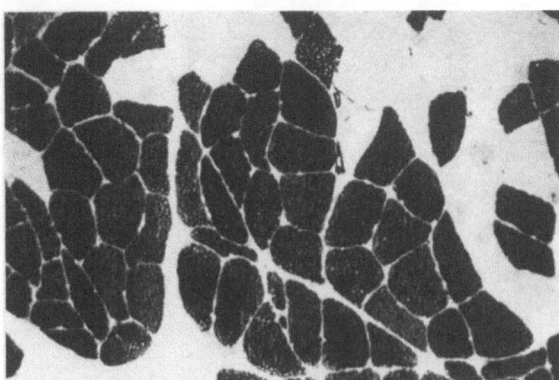

Fig. 13.12. Polyarteritis nodosa with polymyositis. ATPase, pH 4.3 × 140. There is fibre-type grouping. The features of polymyositis cannot be seen in the enzyme preparation.

is particularly increased in these patients (Table 13.4). The fascicular pattern is broken down in chronic polymyositis and the normal relationship of arterioles and capillaries within fascicles is also distorted by fibrous scarring and by the presence of increased amounts of adipose tissue.

Idiopathic Dermatomyositis

The histological features of adult and childhood dermatomyositis are similar, but differ from those found in polymyositis. The inflammatory cell infiltrates in dermatomyositis tend to be perivascular or in the interfascicular septa, rather than within fascicles as in polymyositis. Muscle micro-infarction, occurring within fascicles, is a characteristic feature of dermatomyositis. This is associated with necrosis of arterioles and capillaries. Ultrastructure studies of capillaries show undulating tubules in endothelial cells (Banker and Victor 1966), fibrous thrombi, particularly in children, and reduplication of the capillary basal lamina, suggesting that capillary regeneration has occurred (Carpenter et al. 1976; Emslie-Smith and Engel 1990). In childhood dermatomyositis capillary changes are particularly prominent with obliteration of their lumen, or even a "pipe-stem" like dilatation (Emslie-Smith and Engel 1991). Deposition of complement and IgG has been reported in muscle blood vessels in juvenile and adult dermatomyositis (Whitaker and Engel 1972; Kissel et al. 1986). The muscle micro-infarcts vary in extent with the vascular pathology (Banker 1975; Carpenter et al. 1976). All the fibres within a micro-infarct appear to be at the same stage of necrosis or regeneration. Indeed, regeneration will occur only if perfusion of the ischaemic zone is restored by arteriolar and capillary regeneration.

Perifascicular atrophy is also a characteristic feature, consisting of atrophic fibres at the periphery of fascicles (Fig. 13.13). Many of these abnormal fibres are rounded and show architectural or moth-eaten change (Fig. 13.13). These appearances are thought to result from ischaemia of the periphery of muscle fascicles. Moth-eaten fibres may be prominent generally in the biopsy and necrosis, phagocytosis and regenerating fibres are frequently noted. In clinically severe cases endomysial oedema is often a feature. In the childhood-onset form of dermatomyositis (Banker and Victor 1966) perifascicular atrophy is often particularly prominent.

Skin biopsies may also be helpful in diagnosis. The erythematous lesions show epidermal atrophy, with oedema of the upper dermis, degeneration of the basal cell layers and scattered inflammatory cell infiltrates, or vasculitic features. Calcification may be seen in childhood dermatomyositis.

Inclusion Body Myositis (IBM)

The characteristic histopathological features of IBM (Fig. 13.14) are basophilic granular inclusions located at the periphery of narrow vacuoles in muscle fibres (rimmed vacuoles), small rounded or angulated fibres often found in small groups, eosinophilic cytoplasmic inclusions and endomysial inflammation. In severely affected muscles there is extensive fatty and fibrous replacement of muscle tissue, but in less involved muscles the main feature of the disease may be the presence of scattered isolated fibres containing dark, basophilic rimmed vacuoles.

Rimmed vacuoles are not specific to IBM. They have also been reported in Welander's distal myopathy (Lindberg et al. 1991), in oculo-pharyngeal myopathy and in a rare hereditary vacuolar myopathy (Askanas et al. 1991). Nonetheless, rimmed vacuoles are an invariable feature of IBM, and are required for diagnosis of this condition (Lotz et al. 1989). In the cases of Lotz et al. (1989), 90% of biopsies showed rimmed vacuoles, endomysial infiltration and atrophic fibres, but cytoplasmic bodies were found in only 60% of cases. The rimmed vacuoles contain material that reacts positively in Sudan black B and acid haematoxylin preparations, but is negative for acid phosphatase. These vacuoles contain strong ubiquitin immunoreactivity localised to cytoplasmic tubulofilaments (Askanas et al. 1991) that is positive in Congo red preparations, suggesting the presence of amyloid (Mendell et al. 1991). Askanas et al. (1992) showed that this material, corresponding to the eosinophilic cytoplasmic inclusions, is β amyloid. These observations suggest that these filaments, which are 17–21 mm in diame-

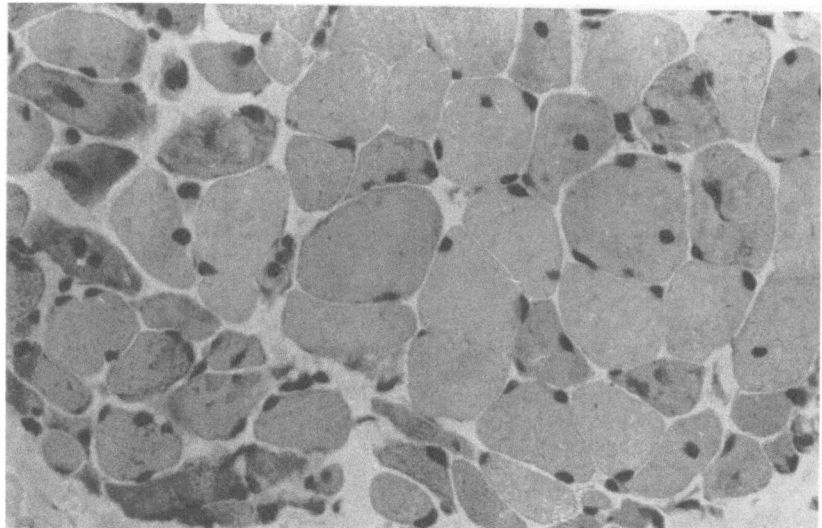

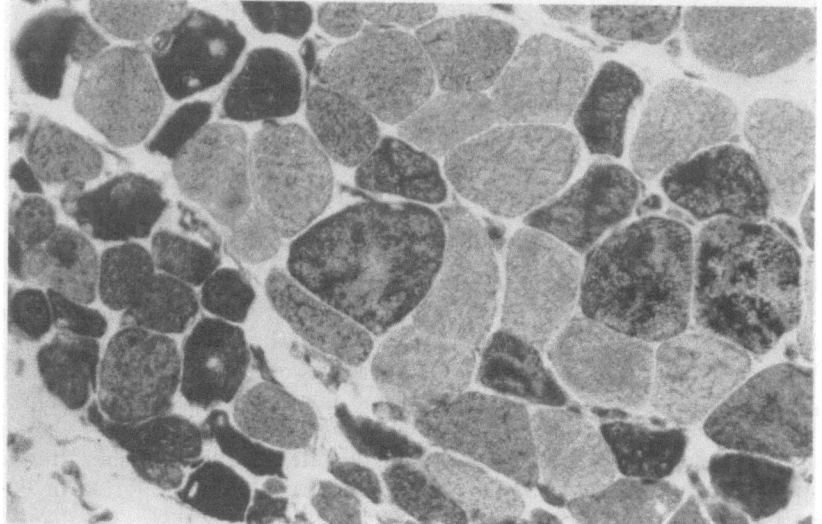

Fig. 13.13. Dermatomyositis. "Moth-eaten" fibres. TS. × 350. **a** Oil red 0. **b** NADH-tr. In these serial sections the moth-eaten appearance can be readily recognised in NADH-tr. Type 1 fibres are principally affected. The abnormal myofibrillar pattern can also be seen in the oil red 0 stain; central nucleation is also a prominent feature. There is marked perifascicular atrophy.

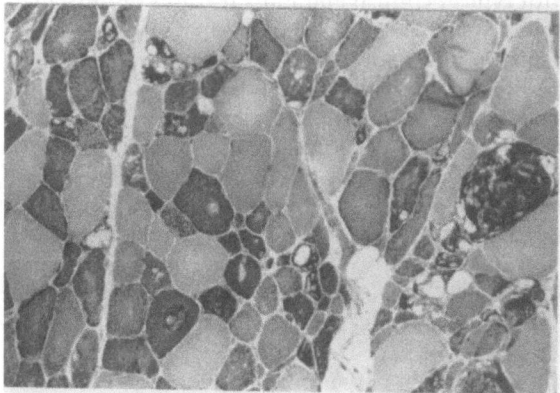

Fig. 13.14. Inclusion body myositis. NADH × 140. There is increased variation in fibre size, with prominent vacuolation and scattered dark angular fibres. The presence of inflammation cannot be assessed in this preparation.

ter, are derived by a degenerative process that resembles those found in other degenerative processes. Intranuclear fibrils 10–14 mm may also occur and this feature resembles that found in oculo-pharyngeal muscular dystrophy (Coquet et al. 1990).

The endomysial inflammatory cell response is similar to that of idiopathic polymyositis; perivascular inflammation is also common. Engel and Arahata (1984) reported that the exudate consists essentially of T cells and macrophages, most cells being cytotoxic T8 cells. Although small groups of atrophic fibres are commonly noticed, there is no histological evidence of fibre-type grouping or of other neurogenic features in muscle biopsies. Barolin et al. (1995) suggested that the inflammatory

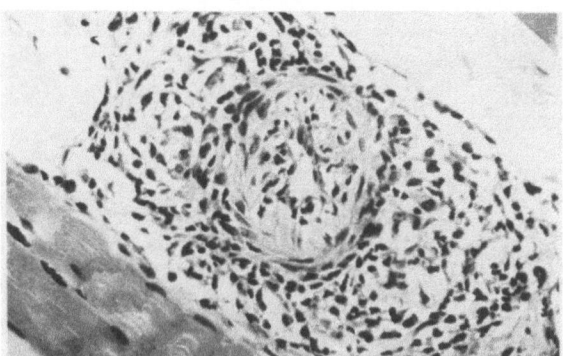

Fig. 13.15. Polyarteritis nodosa. H and E, × 350. In this biopsy a small artery shows intimal thickening with infiltration of its wall by macrophages and lymphocytes.

response in muscle biopsies of IBM was secondary, rather than a primary or cansative feature of the disease.

Chou (1986) suggested that mumps viral particles and antigens were present in the rimmed vacuoles, but subsequent work showed no evidence for viral involvement in IBM (Leff et al. 1992).

Other Inflammatory Myopathies

In polymyositis associated with other autoimmune diseases certain differences in the muscle pathology may be found. In *polyarteritis nodosa*, and Wegener's granulomatosis, the typical features of polymyositis are uncommon (Pearson and Bohan 1977) (Table 13.6). The major abnormality consists of small infarcts within muscle, involving the interstitial tissues, with prominent vasculitis often affecting arterioles, small arteries or veins. The media is most often affected and may become necrotic and eosinophilic (Fig. 13.15), leading to intimal involvement and thrombosis of affected vessels. Neutrophils and eosinophils are prominent in perivascular infiltrates, but later lymphocytes, plasma cells and macrophages predominate. The lesions vary in age and severity in different parts of the muscle. At least 30% of patients with polyarteritis nodosa show clinical signs of involvement of muscle. However, muscle biopsy is less useful in diagnosis than has been suggested (Wallace et al. 1958). Similar vascular involvement of arterioles on nerves leads to the classical presentation with mononeuritis multiplex (see Chap. 11).

In *rheumatoid arthritis* active polymyositis is relatively uncommon (Pitkeathley and Cromes 1966). Focal inflammatory changes in the muscle and emdomysium causing a focal nodular myositis may develop. Arteritis may also occur (Kim and Collins

1980). The differential diagnosis between polymyositis and muscle changes associated with rheumatoid disease may be difficult (Magyar et al. 1977). Disturbances of the innervation of muscle are relatively common (see Chap. 11).

In *systemic lupus erythematosus* polymyositis occurs in fewer than 10% of cases (Estes and Christian 1971; Foote et al. 1982). A sparse perivascular and endomysial infiltration may be present in 24% of cases at autopsy (Ropes 1976) but the CK is raised in only 4% of cases of SLE (Grigor et al. 1978). Vacuolar change may also occur.

In *mixed connective tissue disease* EMG findings typical of inflammatory myopathy are frequently found and the muscle biopsy similarly shows typical features of polymyositis (Singsen et al. 1977). The CK is often raised. *Scleroderma* is associated with stiffness, but only about 10% of patients show histological features of muscle involvement and this usually consists of replacement of muscle by collagenous tissue (Clements et al. 1978).

Clinical Variants of Inflammatory Myopathy

Localised nodular myositis is a rare disorder in which a painful mass develops, resembling a muscle tumour (Heffner et al. 1977). It may present as a multifocal problem which evolves into generalised polymyositis (Cumming et al. 1977; Allen et al. 1980). Calcification and new bone formation have been reported in the late stages (Lagier and Cox 1975).

Eosinophilic myositis is a form of polymyositis with typical clinical and EMG features of muscular involvement, but accompanied by features of systemic involvement, especially pericarditis, myocarditis with heart failure and heart block and a skin rash (Layzer et al. 1977; Stark 1979). The CK is raised and the eosinophil count in the blood is usually raised. In the muscle there is a prominent eosinophilic infiltrate. In some cases mononeuritis multiplex may develop so that the syndrome then resembles *Churg–Strauss syndrome* (Churg and Strauss 1951). *Eosinophilic fasciitis* is a related eosinophilic syndrome (Shulman 1975) in which thickening of skin is associated with muscle pain, contractures, hypergammaglobulinaemia and eosinophilia in the blood (Bjelle et al. 1980). The muscle biopsy shows round cell infiltration of the fascia, with only moderate numbers of eosinophils (Nassanova et al. 1979). Serratrice et al. (1990), in reviewing

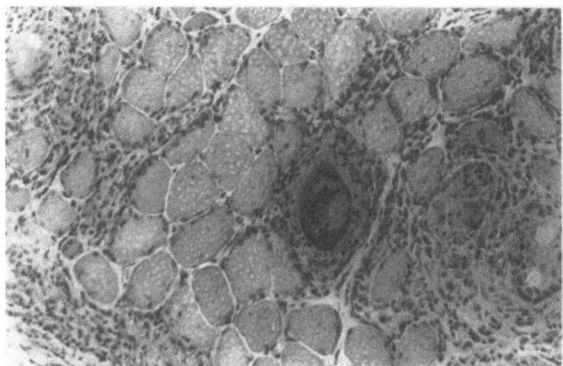

Fig. 13.16. Sarcoid myopathy. H and E, TS. × 350. A granulomatous inflammation with a giant cell can be seen in the muscle. Fibrosis and central nucleation are prominent.

this syndrome, noted the overlapping clinical features of diffuse and focal involvement of muscle, with fasciitis at the other end of the spectrum.

Granulomatous myositis is a rare syndrome. Granulomatous involvement of muscle occurs in about 50% of patients with sarcoidosis (Wallace et al. 1958), but this is frequently asymptomatic. Weakness or atrophy may develop and hypertrophy, especially of the calves, may be a feature. Muscle involvement usually indicates multisystem involvement by the disease. Initially small asymptomatic granulomas may be found, displacing muscle fibres (Hewlett and Brownell 1975). A skin rash resembling dermatomyositis may develop (Itoh et al. 1980) and a relapsing dermatomyositis syndrome has also been reported in association with sarcoidosis. The muscle biopsy in one such case showed non-caseating granulomatous myositis (Hart et al. 1988). Granulomatous myositis also occurs in association with Crohn's disease (Ménard et al. 1976). A granulomatous myositis has also been associated with thymoma, myasthenia gravis and autoimmune thyroid disease (Namba et al. 1974) and with viral and parasitic infections. Sarcoid myopathy as a clinical entity is very rare, amounting to only about 1% of all patients with sarcoidosis

Three clinical syndromes of muscular involvement have been reported in sarcoidosis. An *acute* form resembles polymyositis (Silverstein and Siltzbach 1969). A *nodular* form presents with pain, stiffness and muscle cramps and weakness and contractures may develop later (Douglas et al. 1973). A *chronic* myopathy with wasting and weakness is probably the commonest symptomatic form of sarcoid myopathy (Douglas et al. 1973). The muscle biopsy reveals non-caseating granulomata with muscle fibre destruction and mononuclear cell infiltration (Fig. 13.16).

Clinical Criteria for Diagnosis of Polymyositis

The diagnosis of inflammatory muscle disease is not always immediately evident. Bohan and Peter (1975) addressed this problem and suggested the clinical criteria listed in Table 13.7. When all four criteria are present a *definite* diagnosis of polymyositis or dermatomyositis can be made. When only three criteria are present the diagnosis is *probable*, provided that the clinical criteria are satisfied. In both these groups of cases treatment may be indicated if other causes, e.g. toxic or metabolic disorders of the syndrome can be excluded by investigation. In most cases satisfying fewer than two criteria, treatment should be deferred.

Table 13.7. Criteria for diagnosis of polymyositis and dermatomyositis

1. *Clinical*
   Proximal muscle weakness, usually symmetrical, progressing during weeks or months, with or without muscle pain. Dermatological manifestations may be present

2. *Pathological*
   Muscle fibre necrosis and regeneration, mononuclear cell infiltration. Perifascicular atrophy sometimes present

3. *Biochemical*
   Raised serum CK (MM isoenzyme), aldolase or myoglobulin levels

4. *EMG*
   Multifocal EMG features of myopathy; spontaneous activity often present at rest

Modified from Hudgson and Peter (1984).

Differential Diagnosis

Several diseases may show clinical and other features that mimic polymyositis. In polymyalgia rheumatica muscle pain with limitation of movement often occurs, and may be misinterpreted as muscle weakness. However, CK is normal and muscle biopsy shows only minimal abnormalities. Metabolic or endocrine muscle disorders, e.g. thyroid disease, exposure to myotoxic drugs such as alcohol, opiates and chloroquine should also be considered in excluding a diagnosis of polymyositis. However, autoimmune thyroid disease may rarely be associated with polymyositis and D-penicillamine treatment may induce polymyositis. Osteomalacic myopathy may be painful and progressive, leading to confusion with polymyositis, but appropriate investigation of calcium metabolism, together with muscle biopsy, which is usually normal, and the finding of a normal CK in most cases, enables this condition to be recognised. Genetic and metabolic disorders of muscle, e.g. acid maltase deficiency, McArdle's disease and mitochondrial disorders, can usually be recognised by their characteristic biochemical and pathological features. A family history of muscle disease strongly suggests one of the varieties of muscular dystrophy or spinal muscular atrophy rather than polymyositis. The clinical and pathological features of IBM in many ways resemble those of Welander's familial distal myopathy (Lindberg et al. 1991; Buchman and Cochran 1992). Myasthenia gravis may be difficult to differentiate from polymyositis, particularly since both sometimes occur together in the same patient. Evidence of granulomatous infestation in the biopsy also excludes the diagnosis, and eosinophilia in the blood or in the biopsy should always lead to consideration of infestation, polyarteritis nodosa or one of the eosinophilic syndromes. In chronic neurogenic muscle weakness, whether of spinal origin or due to peripheral neuropathy, the CK level may be moderately raised, but this should not lead to diagnostic confusion. A variety of muscle pain syndromes, mostly of undetermined origin but some following clinical viral infection, are found in clinical practice. These patients usually have normal muscle strength, normal CK levels and normal EMG characteristics but some have mild neurogenic changes of uncertain cause.

Treatment and Prognosis

Although steroid therapy is invariably used in the management of polymyositis its effectiveness has not been tested in controlled trials. Improvement has been reported in more than half of patients treated with steroid therapy (DeVere and Bradley 1975) but others have reported that only about one-third of patients were improved (Rowland et al. 1977) and Riddoch and Morgan-Hughes (1975) obtained improvement in only three of 18 patients. In 1966, however, Rose and Walton recorded a 14% mortality in a series of 40 cases of dermatomyositis, treated before corticosteroids became available. O'Leary and Waisman (1946) recorded a 50% mortality. Winkelmann et al. (1968) compared a group of steroid-treated patients with a group of patients managed at the Mayo Clinic before steroids were available and found that 38% of untreated patients recovered without treatment but 29% of the untreated patients died. In the steroid-treated group 64% improved or remitted, and these patients had an earlier remission. Before the advent of steroid

therapy one-third of children with juvenile dermatomyositis died, and another third were disabled by contractures. With steroid therapy the mortality of this disease has been reduced to 7% (Pachman and Maryjowski 1984) and residual disability is a problem in a further 16% of cases (Chalmers et al. 1982).

In adult polymyositis and dermatomyositis bed rest is required in the initial stages. Physiotherapy is useful in preventing muscle contractures, but muscle pain can be severe and splinting can be useful. Analgesics, local heat and range-of-motion exercises are beneficial. Dysphagia is occasionally severe and may require a semi-solid diet or even nasogastric tube feeding. Respiratory problems are relatively uncommon but, when severe, may necessitate intermittent positive pressure ventilation. It is thus important to monitor vital capacity and muscle strength by quantitative testing or by using the MRC scale, initially on a daily basis and later at less frequent intervals. Cardiomyopathy is usually subclinical, but may require specific management. Interstitial pulmonary fibrosis may develop insidiously in subacute or chronic cases.

Immunosuppression and antiflammatory drug treatment is the mainstay of therapy. Steroids are used initially, but other immunosuppressant drugs have a place. An initial dose of prednisolone of at least 60 mg daily, given as a single morning dose, is recommended for adult polymyositis and dermatomyositis (Dalakas 1989, 1991). If there is no response, judged clinically or by serum CK levels in the first 4 to 6 weeks of treatment, a higher dose should be used to a maximum of 2 mg/kg body weight. When improvement occurs the dose can be gradually reduced; usually a period of about 6 months treatment is required to reduce the dose to 7.5–10.0 mg daily (Ansell 1984). DeVere and Bradley (1975) suggested that a high dose should be maintained for the first 3 months whatever the clinical response. Reduction in steroid dosage is often best achieved by gradually changing to an alternate-day treatment regime after 4–12 weeks of daily therapy. This is believed to reduce the likelihood and severity of steroid-dependent unwanted effects (Warmolts and Engel 1972b). Treatment may need to be continued for several years, in relation to the clinical and biochemical features of disease activity. The cutaneous manifestations of adult dermatomyositis do not always remit concurrently with the muscular symptoms (Ansell 1984). Failure to respond to treatment may be an indication of the presence of an underlying malignancy.

In *childhood dermatomyositis* prednisolone 1–2 mg/kg body weight is used in divided doses, a daily dose that is usually slightly greater weight for weight to that used in adults. After 4–12 weeks, as in adults, and in milder cases from the outset, it is usually possible to proceed to a schedule of alternate-day treatment (Engel et al. 1971; Ansell 1984). The heliotrope rash varies from day to day and should not be used as a guide to changes in steroid dosage. Intensive physiotherapy is particularly important in children during the early stages, and a programme of graded rehabilitation is of great value. Exercises in the pool may be begun before weight bearing is possible and splints are often useful in the early stages to prevent contractures. Effective analgesia is usually necessary at this stage of the disease.

Granulomatous myositis merits treatment only if it is symptomatic. Steroid therapy is then indicated. In *mixed connective tissue disease* steroids and immunosuppressant drugs should be used as in acute polymyositis, and long-term treatment with alternate-day steroids may be required.

Immunosuppressant Drugs

In about 20% of patients PM/DM is not controlled with steroid therapy (Bunch 1990). In addition, some patients, for example patients with diabetes mellitus, active peptic ulceration, heart failure and post-menopausal women with osteoporosis, may be unable to tolerate treatment with steroids in high dosage for several weeks. In these patients immunosuppressive therapy may be given as primary treatment, and it seems likely that this type of treatment is beneficial in all patients with severe active polymyositis. Steroid therapy does not benefit IBM (Barolin et al. 1995), and immunosuppressant drugs and IV immunoglobulin (Amato et al. 1994) are also ineffective in this disease. In idiopathic PM/DM there is evidence that continued steroid and azathioprine treatment leads to a better long-term result with less functional disability and lower steroid requirement after three years treatment, than steroids alone (Bunch 1981). Methotrexate has been used in this way (Metzger et al. 1974) and this treatment, or chlorambucil, is successful in producing remission in some patients not responding to steroids (Sokoloff et al. 1971).

It is probably appropriate, therefore, to begin treatment with high doses of corticosteroids, and to add azathioprine in slowly increasing dosage as the prednisolone dose is tapered, i.e. 4–6 weeks after beginning steroids. An arbitrary dose of 50–150 mg azathioprine daily is used in adults, and 1–2.5 mg/kg body weight in children (Ansell 1984). Cyclophosphamide and methotrexate are more likely to lead to more serious unwanted effects than

azathioprine, but chlorambucil is also relatively easy to use in practice. Cyclophosphamide is probably the treatment of choice for fibrosing alveolitis complicating polymyositis (Plowman and Stableforth 1977). Cyclosporin has been used for acute dermatomyositis and polymyositis in uncontrolled studies (Zagel et al. 1984; Heckmatt et al. 1989; Lueck et al. 1991).

Plasma exchange has also been advocated but this treatment has not been effective in a double-blind trial (Miller et al. 1992). Other unvalidated forms of treatment include anti-lymphocytic globulin (Ansell 1984) and whole-body irradiation. The latter has been reported to be effective in several cases refractory to all other forms of treatment (Engel et al. 1981; Morgan et al. 1985). Intravenous immunoglobulin has been encouraging in uncontrolled studies (Lang et al. 1991).

Complications of Steroid Therapy

Long-term, high-dose steroid therapy leads to a number of well-recognised complications, e.g. hypertension, diabetes mellitus, osteoporosis leading to crush fractures of vertebrae, infections, cataract and bleeding from the upper gastro-intestinal tract. Various standard measures should be used to try to prevent and control these complications. Potassium supplements to prevent hypokalaemia and H_2 antagonists, e.g. cimetidine, are especially advocated. A particularly important complication is the development of steroid myopathy which may develop indolently, and mimic a failure of response of the underlying polymyositis, or even be misdiagnosed as relapse of the inflammatory myopathy. Askari et al. (1976) pointed out that this dose-dependent effect of steroid treatment (see Chap. 18) could be recognised by the development of increasing weakness without change in the serum CK, and could be confirmed by muscle biopsy. We use needle muscle biopsy in management to help decide this point, since a decision between the two possibilities has important implications for management. Prednisolone doses ranging from 15–100 mg daily for periods of 1 months to 5 years have been associated with steroid myopathy, presumably reflecting individual susceptibility.

Viral Myositis

Muscle is susceptible to viral invasion. Acute viral myositis usually presents with non-specific muscle aches and pains, often exacerbated by exercise, but not associated with weakness or with changes in muscle enzymes, e.g. CK in the blood. Several different viruses cause myositis, and the clinical syndrome although usually mild may be severe, with rhabdomyolysis (Table 13.8).

In children an acute infectious myositis, due to influenza A and B virus infection, predominantly affects the calf muscles, and resolves in 1–4 weeks (Mejlszenkier et al. 1973). The CK may be raised, and EMG changes and myoglobinuria may occur (Table 13.8) during the acute phase. The infection can be identified by rising blood antibody titres, and virus has been isolated by culture from muscle biopsies (Gamboa et al. 1979). In the acute stage the CK may be slightly raised (Friman 1976).

Table 13.8.   Syndromes of viral myositis

Benign acute myositis
    Influenza A and B
    Parainfluenza
    Adenovirus 2

Acute rhabdomyolysis
    Influenza A and B
    Coxsackie B5
    Echo 9
    Adenovirus 21
    Herpes simplex
    Epstein–Barr virus

Epidemic pleurodynia (Bornholm disease)
    Coxsackie B5 (also B1, B3 and B4)

Polymyositis syndrome
    HIV-1
    HTLV-1

Virus isolations from muscle in chronic polymyositis have been reported (Chou and Gutmann 1970; Kessler et al. 1980), including Coxsackie, influenza, hepatitis and unidentified viral particles (Tang et al. 1975). Despite these reports there is no evidence that typical idiopathic polymyositis or dermatomyositis is due to direct viral invasion (Leff et al. 1992), although the disease could nonetheless be initiated by viral infection.

Retroviruses and Inflammatory Myopathies

Although several retroviruses have been linked to inflammatory myopathies only two retrovirus infections are associated with human polymyositis; HIV-1 and HLTL-1 infections.

HIV-1 Polymyositis

In HIV-infected patients an inflammatory myopathy that in every way resembles idiopathic polymyositis has been reported. The polymyositis syndrome may be the presenting feature of HIV infection or may develop in association with other features of AIDS (Dalakas et al. 1986; Dalakas and Pezeshkpur 1988). In addition, HIV seroconversion may be associated with myalgia and myoglobinuria, suggesting that HIV may directly invade muscle cells early in the infection (Dalakas 1991). However, immunopathologic studies in muscle biopsies of patients with polymyositis associated with HIV and AIDS have shown that HIV antigen is detectable only in interstitial mononuclear cells, but not in muscle cells (Illa et al. 1991; Leon-Monzan et al. 1993). The endomysial inflammatory cell exudate consists predominantly of CD8+ cells. These cells and macrophages invade or approach muscle cells expressing MHC-1 antigen in the first stage of muscle cell destruction (Illa et al. 1991). These immunological features of HIV polymyositis are similar to those found in idiopathic polymyositis, suggesting that HIV infection can trigger the immune disturbance that leads to the development of the polymyositis syndrome. It has been proposed that this immune response results from molecular mimicry, since retroviral polypeptides coded for the *gag* gene react with certain anti-ribonuclear proteins in the cell.

Zidovudine Myopathy

The inflammatory myositis associated with HIV infection must be distinguished from zidovudine-related myopathy in which myalgia, weakness and a raised CK develop. This zidovudine-related myopathy is characterised by a myopathy with ragged-red fibres, in which there is proliferation of abnormal mitochondria. Zidovudine inhibits γ-DNA polymerase, a mitochondria-specific enzyme, and there is depletion of mitochondrial DNA in this syndrome. Improvement follows discontinuation of zidovudine therapy (Dalakas et al. 1990; Arnando et al. 1991). This myopathy develops in patients treated with zidovudine in a dose greater than 250 mg/day for more than 200 days (Mhiri et al. 1991).

HTLV-1 Polymyositis

HTLV-1 infection is particularly associated with tropical spastic paraparesis (TSP), a syndrome common in Jamaica and Japan in which a slowly progressive spastic paraplegia develops, sometimes associated with optic neuritis, demyelinating lesions in the brain (Cruikshank et al. 1992). Polymyositis is also associated with HTLV-1 infection occurring either alone or as a late complication of TSP (Cruikshank et al. 1992). Morgan et al. (1989)

reported seven patients with polymyositis associated with antibodies to HTLV-1, and noted that 85% of Jamaican patients with adult polymyositis had circulating HTLV-1 antibodies. The prevalence of positive HTLV-1 antibodies in Jamaican adults was 7%–18%. Dickoff et al. (1993) found perinuclear staining with immune HTLV-1 immunoglobulin in some remaining muscle fibres in a patient with polymyositis associated with TSP, and confirmed the presence of HTLV-1 antigen in muscle cells by the polymerase chain reaction. Inou et al. (1992) investigated 13 patients with HTLV-1 associated myelopathy by muscle biopsy. Six showed features of T lymphocyte predominant inflammatory myopathy and four showed neurogenic change. Myositis may be a common feature in HTLV-1 infection.

Bacterial Infections and Infestations of Muscle

Bacterial and other infections are rare causes of polymyositis, except in patients with septicaemia.

Pyomyositis

In the tropics pyomyositis is common, accounting for 4% of surgical admissions in East Africa (Horn and Master 1968). It is associated with trauma, malnutrition and acute viral infection. It has also been associated with diabetes mellitus. The condition presents with painful swelling of a muscle, usually quadriceps or glutei. Biceps and pectoral muscles are less commonly affected. The swelling is initially hard and woody but becomes fluctuant in a few days (Chiedozi 1979). There may be fever, leucocytosis and a raised ESR and creatine kinase. Muscle imaging reveals an enhancing lesion with a fluid density, and needle aspiration may reveal pus, often containing *Staphylococcus aureus* (85% of cases) (Shepherd 1983). In 5% of cases no organism can be found. In the tropics, anaerobic infection is also common (Banker 1986).

Pyomyositis has also been recognised in patients with HIV infection (Watts et al. 1987; Schwartzman et al. 1991).

Infestations

Infestation of muscle may follow invasion by a number of parasites, but these are uncommon in developed Western countries (see Banker 1986 for review). Muscular symptoms are prominent only in cysticercosis and trichinosis. In hydatid disease muscle invasion is usually asymptomatic. In *cysticercosis*, muscle infection by *Taenia soleum* causes pain and swelling, followed by hard, hypertrophied muscles, including the tongue. Other organs are involved including heart, eyes, brain and subcutaneous tissue. The calcified cysts are visible on plain X-rays. Urticaria and eosinophilia may be prominent features.

Trichinosis occurs from ingestion of infected meat. The larvae enter the circulation via the lymphatics of the intestine, and invade individual muscle fibres, producing characteristic coiled encysted larvae, which may calcify after several years. In the acute phase myalgia, periorbital oedema and swelling of affected muscles may be seen and death may occur from myocarditis, encephalitis or pneumonia. The EMG shows profuse fibrillation in affected muscles due to focal necrosis (Gross and Ochoa 1979). Later, fibrosis and contractures may develop. In the acute stages treatment with thiobendazole 50 mg/kg body weight per day, with steroids to prevent Herxheimer reaction, may be life-saving.

Toxoplasmosis may also involve muscle. Raised levels of IgM antibody specific to toxoplasma have been reported in 50% of patients with polymyositis (Magid and Kagen 1983) but the significance of this finding in relation to idiopathic polymyositis is doubtful. Myositis may also occur in *Plasmodium falciparum* malaria (De Silva et al. 1988; Swash and Schwartz 1993).

Other Infection of Muscle

A chronic proximal myopathy may complicate *Whipple's disease* (Swash et al. 1977). In a single case report the CK was normal but an EMG revealed myopathic features. The muscle biopsy showed mild Type 2 fibre atrophy with rare necrotic fibres. Endomysial macrophages contained PAS-positive membranous material similar to that found in a jejunal biopsy. Oral antibiotics and steroids resulted in improvement.

Kawasaki syndrome is an acute febrile illness, mainly affecting Japanese children under the age of 9 years. It is characterised by mucocutaneous inflammation and cervical adenitis, with fever and evidence of involvement of CNS, joints, cardiovascular system and muscle (Hicks et al. 1982; Feigin and Barron 1986). The CK level may be raised and the EMG abnormal (Koustros 1982). The vasculitic complication of this disorder may lead to involvement of muscle, and may be ameliorated by treatment with intravenous immunoglobulin (Newburger et al. 1986). The disorder has a seasonal incidence.

Borrelia burgdorfi and *Legionella* infections may involve muscle.

Drug-Induced Inflammatory Myopathies

Inflammatory myopathy can follow treatment with D-penicillamine and L-tryptophan. These myopathies are discussed in Chap. 19.

Polymyalgia Rheumatica and Giant Cell Arteritis

Polymyalgia rheumatica forms part of the differential diagnosis of polymyositis, although muscle strength is almost invariably normal. It presents with muscular pain and tenderness which is especially prominent in the early mornings. Pain and stiffness, especially in shoulder and pelvic girdles, is often relieved by activity; in polymyositis itself muscular pain is often induced or worsened by exercise. Polymyalgia rheumatica usually affects women older than 55 years. There may be a low-grade fever and patients often feel generally unwell. Symptoms similar to those of temporal arteritis, consisting of tenderness in the scalp, and in temporal and occipital vessels, may occur. The principal abnormality on investigation is the ESR, which is invariably greater than 70 mm/h. Liver function tests may be abnormal and there is often a polyclonal increase in serum globulins, particularly the alpha-globulin fraction. The CK is usually normal. In 40% of patients with the clinical features of polymyalgia rheumatica temporal artery biopsy shows giant cell arteritis (Fauchald et al. 1972). Of 182 cases reviewed prospectively by Behan et al. (1983) 8% had visual symptoms at presentation.

The EMG is often said to be normal (Dubowitz and Brooke 1973) but in our experience this is not the case. The main findings are increased insertional activity and a number of short-duration, low-amplitude polyphasic MUAPs. The interference pattern is full and generally the largest motor units are of normal amplitude, whereas in polymyositis even the largest MUAPs are of low amplitude (<1.5 mV). After treatment with steroids the EMG usually normalises. Muscle biopsy is not often performed in

polymyalgia rheumatica, but it usually shows abnormalities. These consist mainly of Type 2 atrophy with occasional moth-eaten and whorled fibres. Sometimes Type 2B fibres are preferentially affected. Lymphocytic infiltrates and central nucleation are not features of this disorder.

Patients with clinical features of polymyalgia rheumatica, irrespective of the findings at temporal artery biopsy, respond to low-dose steroid treatment, i.e. prednisolone 10–30 mg daily, but those with visual symptoms should be treated initially with higher doses, i.e. 60 mg prednisolone daily. In both groups treatment may need to be continued for several years and some patients require indefinite treatment. Treatment with low-dose steroids in polymyalgia may prevent the development of retinal complications (Behan et al. 1983). Non-steroidal anti-inflammatory drugs (e.g. indomethacin) are useful in controlling mild symptoms.

Graft Versus Host Myositis

Chronic graft versus host disease is a multisystem syndrome developing more than 100 days after allogeneic bone marrow transplanatation, either *de novo* or following the acute form of the disorder.

It consists of cutaneous manifestations, especially lichen planus and scleroderma-like changes, chronic liver disease, Sjögren's syndrome, gastro-intestinal manifestations (e.g. anal ulceration and diarrhoea), diffuse pulmonary fibrosis and recurrent bacterial infections (Ferrara and Deeg 1991). Polymyositis is an infrequent manifestation; there is subacute proximal weakness with some muscle pain and a normal or raised blood CK level. The muscle biopsy shows scattered necrotic, regenerating and, occasionally, vacuolated fibres. There is a prominent inflammatory cell infiltration in the endomysium and perimysium, consisting of histiocytes, cytotoxic T lymphocytes and plasma cells. There is fairly prominent perimysial fibrosis. IgG is deposited in some necrotic fibres. It is thought that these IgG deposits are part of the process of fibre necrosis, leading to immune-complex deposition (Reyes et al. 1983). Small blood vessels in the muscle biopsy show increased thickness of their walls, with reduplication of the basal lamina, and increased thickness of the endomysial cells (Urbano-Marquez et al. 1986). Graft versus host myopathy is steroid-responsive. Initial treatment with prednisolone in high doses has been recommended, e.g. 2 mg/kg body weight, together with azathioprine. Recovery has been recorded in a period of a few months (Reyes et al. 1983).

Chapter *14* Muscular Dystrophies

The term muscular dystrophy refers to a group of genetically determined myopathies characterised by progressive degenerative changes in muscle fibres, without primary abnormalities in the lower motor neuron. Most of these disorders are accompanied by marked structural abnormalities in muscle biopsies, with loss of muscle fibres and endomysial fibrosis. They are classified according to clinical, morphological and genetic characteristics. As the underlying genetic disorder has become better understood in each clinical syndrome, the classification has become more firmly based on the disturbance of cell protein expression that forms the primary defect.

A number of myopathies are characterised by X-linked inheritance. These vary in their clinical features. While progressive weakness and atrophy are major features of most of these disorders, in McLeod syndrome muscular involvement is subclinical (Swash et al. 1983). The most important of these disorders is Duchenne muscular dystrophy. Understanding of the underlying molecular genetics of Duchenne muscular dystrophy has led to a classification of X-linked myopathies that is based on the abnormality of protein expression in this and related disorders (Table 14.1).

Table 14.1. X-linked muscular dystrophies

Dystrophinopathies		*Protein*
Duchenne muscular dystrophy	Ch Xp 21.2	dystrophin
Becker muscular dystrophy	Xp 21.2	dystrophin
Myalgia/cramp syndrome	Xp 21.2	?
Emery–Dreifuss muscular dystrophy	Xq 27.3-q28	emerin
Scapulo-peroneal myopathy	?	?
McLeod myopathy	Xp 21 (1–2)	membrane transport protein
Centronuclear myopathy (infantile onset, severe form) (see Chap. 16)	Xq 28 ?	

The autosomal dominant and recessive muscular dystrophies form a heterogenous group of disorders characterised by progressive muscular weakness. The syndromes have usually been classified by their clinical features, although in some genetic loci have been recognised. The weakness may be limb-girdle in distribution, proximal or more widespread, as in facio-scapulo-humeral muscular dystrophy in which proximal involvement, affecting upper and lower limb girdles, and facial involvement occurs. Childhood or adult-onset syndromes are also recognised. These are listed in Table 14.2, with their genetic loci and protein products.

Table 14.2. Other muscular dystrophies: genetic loci and protein defects

	Locus	Protein	Dystrophin-related
Autosomal dominant			
Limb girdle syndrome			
Late onset type (LGMD-1A)	5q22-31	–	–
Early onset type (LGMD-1B)			
Facioscapulohumeral	4q	–	–
Welander's distal myopathy	14q	–	–
Oculopharyngeal muscular dystrophy	14q	–	–
Autosomal recessive			
LGMD-2A (Amish-Rénman type)	15q15-22	Calpain	No
LGMD-2B (Miyoshi distal myopathy)	2p13.3	–	–
LGMD-2C (secondary adhalin deficiency)	13q12	γ sarcoglycan	Yes
LGMD-2D (primary adhalin deficiency)	17q12-21	α sarcoglycan (adhalin)	Yes
LGMD-2E	4qt2	β sarcoglycan	?
Other LGMD syndromes	Unclassified		
Congenital muscular dystrophies			
Congenital muscular dystrophy with merosin deficiency	6q2	Merosin (laminin α 2 chain)	Yes
Fukuyama disease	9q31-33		
Other forms		–	–

X-Linked Muscular Dystrophies

Duchenne Muscular Dystrophy (DMD) (Psuedohypertrophic Muscular Dystrophy)

Duchenne muscular dystrophy (DMD) is one of the commonest of all the muscular dystrophies (Gardner-Medwin 1977), and was described by

Duchenne in 1868, although it was reported a few years earlier by Meryon (1852). It is usually first recognised by the age of 3 years, when it becomes apparent that the child has difficulty walking and learning to run or to climb stairs. Falls are frequently a presenting feature. Dubowitz (1995) found that 20% of cases were recognised before the age of 2 years and 72% before the age of 4 years. Duchenne muscular dystrophy is inherited as an X-linked recessive disorder, so that it is transmitted by females and expressed in males. Since more than one boy in any sibship may be affected the disease is often recognised at an earlier age in younger brothers of affected boys. In addition, the disease can be recognised by CK estimation in the first month of life (Bradley et al. 1993).

Pelvic girdle weakness is usually more evident than shoulder girdle weakness in the early stages. The neck flexors are also affected relatively early in the natural history of the disease. The gait is waddling and the lumbar lordosis is increased, with a forward tilt of the pelvis. Affected boys typically may never learn to run normally and, although they may be able to stand on one leg, they cannot hop. As the muscular weakness progresses difficulty rising from the floor, and then from a low chair, becomes obvious and the child begins to use his arms to help push his body off the floor, with the legs extended, in order to stand. The typical Gowers' manoeuvre (Gowers 1886) is seen in moderately advanced stages of the disease. Weakness of shoulder muscles develops later.

In most patients the disease is progressive; the ability to walk is usually lost by the age of 12 years and in 90% of cases death occurs by the age of 20 years (Emery 1987). In 15% of cases the disease appears milder and less rapidly progressive (Brooke et al. 1983). For a short period at about the age of 5–8 years there may be slight functional improvement, probably caused by the relatively rapid physical maturation which occurs at this age superimposed on the slowly progressive course of the disease. This is important because it may lead to an incorrect assessment of the natural history of the disease at this time. Rapid weakness becomes evident after the age of 8 years and 95% of patients require a wheelchair by the age of 12 years (Emery 1987). The tempo of the disease in relation to age and muscle strength has been investigated using rating scales and strength measurements by Scott et al. (1982).

Pseudohypertrophy is observed in most patients at some stage of the disease but is not an invariable feature. Pseudohypertrophy occurs most commonly in the calf muscles, deltoids and serratus anterior muscles but any muscle, including the tongue, may be affected. The enlarged muscles are often strikingly weak, but weakness is usually particularly prominent in hip flexors and extensors, quadriceps, anterior tibial, serratus anterior, pectorals, biceps and brachioradialis muscles. The external ocular muscles are always spared. The tendon reflexes are lost relatively early. As the disease progresses other features become apparent. Kyphoscoliosis and diminished ventilatory reserve, consisting of respiratory muscle weakness, best monitored by vital capacity measurements (Rideau et al. 1981), are common features and cardiomyopathy, as indicated by ECG changes, is almost invariable. Abnormal Q waves with prominent R waves are commonly seen in the ECG but tachycardia and cardiac failure also occur in some cases (see Chap. 20). Terminally, obesity or profound wasting may be found. Intellectual impairment has consistently been found; the mean IQ in most series has been about 85, although some children may show normal intellect (Worden and Vignos 1962; Marsh and Munsat 1974).

The gait abnormality does not result only from muscular weakness. Shortening of the Achilles tendon is very common, perhaps because of early weakness of the anterior tibial muscles, and the patient tends to walk on his toes, even before the age of 6 years. Contractures may also occur in the flexors of the elbows, the pronators of the forearm and the flexors of the hips and knees. These joint deformities can be lessened by proper support and physiotherapy.

Incidence and Inheritance

Duchenne muscular dystrophy occurs in about 1 in 3000 male births (Bradley et al. 1993). The prevalence of the disease is 3/100 000 of the total population (Gardner-Medwin 1970). Inheritance is always X-linked. The disease has been described in Turner's syndrome with an XO chromosome constitution (Emery and Walton 1967) and in girls with X-autosomal translocations (Zatz et al. 1981; Jacobs et al. 1981). A small proportion of females carrying the X-linked gene for Duchenne dystrophy show mild clinical signs of the disorder, consisting of asymmetrical hypertrophy of calf muscles or even slight proximal muscular weakness. It has been suggested that these manifestations of the disease in the carrier, although mild, are due to failure of suppression (Lyon's hypothesis) of the abnormal X chromosome (Moser and Emery 1974). It has been estimated that 30% of cases in boys are due to spontaneous mutation, i.e. their mothers are not carriers, a phenomenon leading to sporadic cases. However, in centres pursuing an active programme of education and carrier detection the proportion of sporadic cases has risen to about 70% (Thompson 1985).

The Genetic Defect and Dystrophin

In DMD there is a genetic defect on the short arm of the X chromosome at the Xp21.2 locus that results in the production of reduced amounts of dystrophin (Kunkel et al. 1989). The genetic locus was identified by Monaco et al. (1986) and the normal gene product that is absent or markedly reduced in amount in DMD was found by Hoffman et al. in 1987. The gene consists of 2.3 million base pairs, an enormous gene that occupies more than 1% of the X chromosome.

Dystrophin is one of a number of membrane proteins (Table 14.3) that are located in the membrane and act as structural proteins that maintain membrane dynamics and the relation of the membrane to the extracellular matrix. The extracellular matrix is composed of collagen, laminin and proteoglycans. The laminin complex binds to the sugar moieties of the glycoprotein dystroglycan at the muscle cell surface (Errasti and Campbell 1993). Beta dystroglycan spans the cell membrane and binds to the C terminal domain of dystrophin. The N terminus of dystrophin is linked to actin filaments which themselves link with the cell's internal cytoskeleton. Thus, this chain of structural proteins links the extracellular matrix to the internal structure of the muscle cell (Brown 1996). Sarcoglycans also span the muscle fibre membrane and interact with dystrophin at the cytoplasmic face of the membrane. One of these sarcoglycans is adhalin (Table 14.2). Syntrophins are another family of membrane associated proteins

that are linked to the C terminal region dystrophins (Brown 1996).

The gene encodes a 14 000 base pair mRNA for dystrophin, a 427 kDa rod-shaped protein that forms part of the cytoskeleton of the cell (Hoffman et al. 1987a) (Fig. 14.1). Dystrophin is located on the inner, cytoplasmic aspect of the plasma membrane at the I and M bands of the attachment of myofibrils to the muscle fibre membrane. This co-localises with the distribution of spectrin in muscle fibre membranes (Porter et al. 1992), although it amounts to only 5% of the cytoskeleton in muscle cell membranes (Ohlendieck and Campbell 1991). Dystrophin is therefore important in maintaining the linkage (Fig. 14.1) of cytoskeletal proteins to myofilaments and membranes (Ervasti and Campbell 1993). The N terminal end of the dystrophin molecule is attached to the subsarcolemmal actin cytoskeleton. The C terminal end of the molecule is attached to a 59 kDa protein located on the cytoplasmic surface of the plasma membrane that is itself linked by a transmembrane glycoprotein complex to a 156 kDa extracellular glycoprotein that binds a component of laminin in the extracellular matrix. These subsarcolemmal, transmembrane and extramembrane dystrophin associated glycoproteins (DAGs) form a functional unit (Ibraghimov-Beskrovnaya et al. 1992). Dystrophin deficient muscle permits the excessive inflow of calcium ion, leading to hypercontraction, focal necrosis and regeneration of muscle fibres. Dystrophin deficient muscle fibres are more vulnerable to injury and less able to sustain repair. A dystrophin-related protein, utrophin, has been identified at the myotendinous and neuromuscular junctions of normal adult human muscle (Lowe et al. 1989; Khurana et al. (1991). Utrophin production is upregulated in regenerating (Helliwell et al. 1992) and fetal muscle fibres (Karpati et al. 1993). This protein shows considerable molecular homology to dystrophin. Khurana et al. (1991) suggested that expression of utrophin in the sarcoplasm of fetal muscle prevents the onset of muscle fibre necrosis during gestation, DMD developing only as the level of utrophin declines after the third postnatal week. Unlike dystrophin, utrophin maps to human chromosome 6 (see Tinsley et al. 1992).

In DMD there is marked reduction in all the dystrophin-associated glycoproteins in muscle, but not in other tissues even through dystrophin is present in reduced quantities in these other tissues also (Ohlendieck et al. 1993). Abnormalities of dystrophin and its associated glycoproteins may account for the cardiomyopathy of Duchenne dystrophy. Specific defects of components of the dystrophin-associated glycoproteins, but not of

Table 14.3. Dystrophin and associated membrane proteins

	Size (kDa)	Chr	Disease
Dystrophin	427	Xp 21	DMD, BMD
Dystroglycans			
α-dystroglycans	153	3p21	
β-dystroglycans	43	3p21	
Sarcoglycans			
α-sarcoglycans (adhalin)	50	17q	Severe childhood autosomal recessive muscular dystrophy (LGMD-2D)
β-sarcoglycans	43	4q12	LGMD-2E
γ-sarcoglycans	35	13q12	LGMD-2C
δ-sarcoglycans	25	5q 33	LGMD-2F
Syntrophin			
α-syntrophin	59		
β_1-syntrophin	59	8q23	
β_2-syntrophin	59	16q23	
Laminin			
Merosin	90	6q2	Congenital muscular dystrophy
Utrophin	430	6	

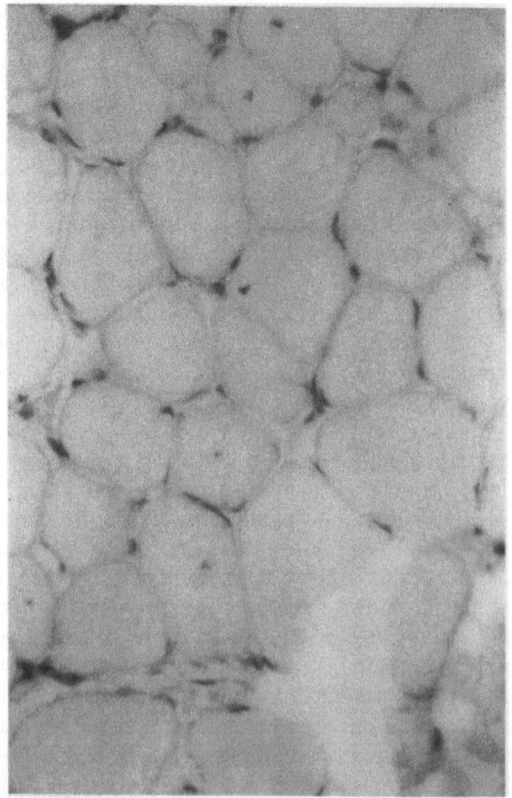

a

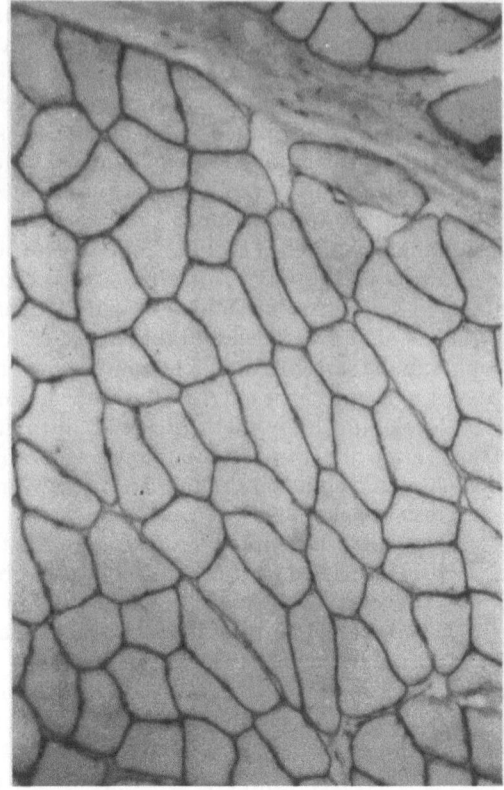

b

Fig. 14.1. **a** Normal dystrophin stain showing the membrane localisation of dystrophin × 360. **b** Absence of dystrophin in Duchenne muscular dystrophy (immunoperoxidase × 500).

dystrophin itself, have been found in childhood autosomal recessive muscular dystrophy and Fukuyama muscular dystrophy (Matsumara et al. 1993).

Analysis of DNA samples from patients with DMD with dystrophin cDNA and genomic clones has shown that about 65% of cases result from a loss of one or more exons of the dystrophin gene, which normally consists of more than 70 exons (Koenig et al. 1987, 1989; Kunkel et al. 1989; Hoffman 1991). A further 7% of cases have mutations in which exons are duplicated (Hu et al. 1990). The remaining 30% of cases have mutations which have not been identified, presumably because these point mutations are too small to detect easily within the large dystrophin gene (Hoffman 1991). In these cases point mutations may cause the production of a non-sense stop codon resulting in premature termination in dystrophin synthesis. This has been demonstrated in the mouse analogue of muscular dystrophy, the *mdx* mouse. Point mutations may also create or destroy splice sites, causing alternative splicing. A third mechanism of dysfunction in the gene caused by point mutations is downregulation of the muscle-specific promoter. In Becker muscular dystrophy 80% of cases have gene deletions. Deletions in the gene can be identified by Southern blot analysis and often also by polymerase chain reaction studies of exons in the dystrophin gene. About 80% of deletions detected by Southern analysis can be detected by polymerase chain reaction studies of DNA samples prepared from blood or other tissues (Multicenter Group 1992).

Patients with DMD and Becker muscular dystrophy (BMD) may have similar deletions in spite of the differing severity of the two diseases. This clinical difference has been explained by the suggestion that the abnormal dystrophin gene in DMD is unable to promote formation of a messenger RNA capable of producing dystrophin (Monaco et al. 1988), whereas in BMD dystrophin is produced that is abnormal in quantity or quality (Koenig et al. 1989). This suggestion has been called the "reading frame hypothesis" (Fig. 14.2). The presence of abnormal dystrophin in BMD, with a normal carboxyl terminus, is strikingly different from the situation in DMD, in which only a truncated and poorly immunoreactive dystrophin molecule is present. Indeed, in most fibres in DMD dystrophin immunoreactivity is absent (Vainzhoff et al. 1991b; Hoffman 1991).

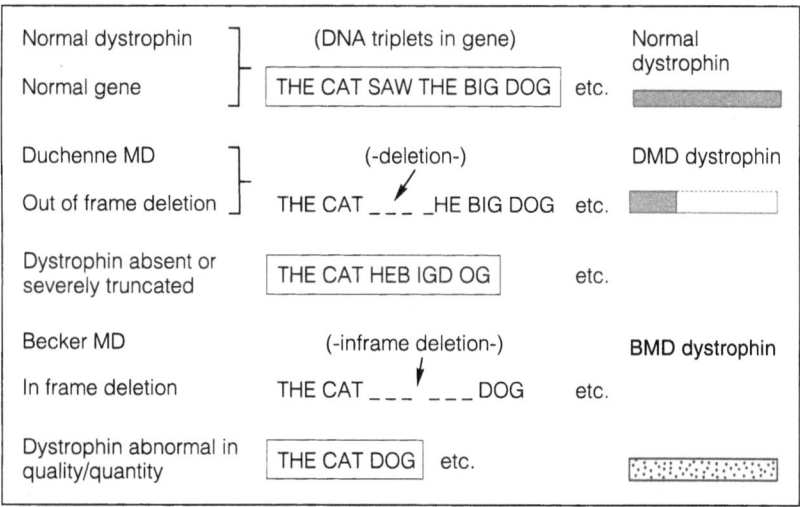

Fig. 14.2.   The reading frame hypothesis of the dystrophin abnormalities characteristics of Duchenne and Becker muscular dystrophies.

The genetic abnormality in inherited cases of DMD resembles in all respects that causing the disease in sporadic mutations. There seems to be no recognisable clinical correlation with the extent or location of the gene abnormality or exon deletion. Indeed, the range and location of exon deletions that have been recognised in the gene in DMD is remarkable. However, Hodgson et al. (1989), in a study of 218 patients with DMD, BMD or intermediate phenotypes, found that certain deletions, e.g. exons 33–34 and 33–35, occurred only in Becker disease. Deletions of exons 3–7 occurred in four patients with an intermediate phenotype and one with BMD. Hodgson et al. (1992) re-evaluated this problem and found that distal deletions were more likely to be associated with mental retardation than proximal deletions. Subsequently Davies (1993) has suggested that deletions in the carboxy terminal region are associated with severe disease phenotype, including mental retardation, and that deletions of the central rod domain are associated with a mild phenotype, some of these patients presenting only with exercise-induced muscle cramps. It has been suggested that three times more deletions occur distal to exon 40 than proximally (Perry 1992). Nudel et al. (1989) reported that the mRNA transcript of the dystrophin gene differs in brain and muscle in DMD patients.

Laboratory Investigations

The CK is raised in all cases of Duchenne dystrophy. The highest CK levels are found in the early stages. As the disease progresses the CK level gradually falls, although even in the terminal stages it never reaches the normal range. In the early stages the CK is usually greater than 10 times the upper limit of normal; levels lower than this should suggest the possibility of a different diagnosis. The CK is raised at birth, but reaches its peak values at 14–22 months, a time at which the first clinical signs of the disease become apparent (Heyck et al. 1966). The level of carbonic anhydrase III is also raised, and correlates with the CK level, being less raised in the later stages of the disease (Carter et al. 1983). The CK may also be raised (four or five times normal) at birth in normal infants (Zellweger and Antonik 1975), probably from the effects of trauma to muscles during delivery, but a confident preclinical diagnosis can be made on the CK level at the end of the first week after delivery (Beckmann 1977; Bradley et al. 1993). If the level of CK at 2 months of age is greater than 2000 IU/1 then Duchenne dystrophy is likely; if the level is less than 1000 IU/1 at this age the diagnosis is unlikely. Intermediate values require reassessment (Bundey 1985).

Density changes in CT scans of the lower limbs and pelvis have been used in monitoring progression of the disease. There are more marked zones of low density, representing fatty infiltration, in older boys. Certain muscles, especially adductor magnus, semimembranosus and tibialis anterior, show the most change during repeated observations. The most severely affected muscles, however, are gastrocnemius and quadriceps (Stern et al. 1984; Serratrice et al. 1985). Ultrasound studies, using the B-mode technique, have also been used to image muscle in the clinical investigation of the disease (Heckmatt et al. 1982, 1988). MR imaging can reveal a characteristic pattern of muscular

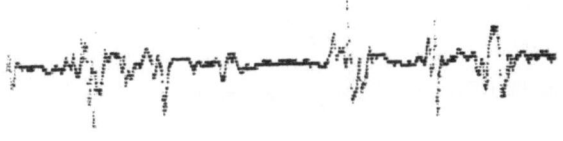

Fig. 14.3. Duchenne muscular dystrophy: Short-duration, low-amplitude polyphasic motor unit action potentials in a weak, wasted muscle. Concentric needle EMG. Filters: 100 Hz and 10 kHz. Bar 20 ms.

involvement with high T_1-weighted signal intensity in fast muscles (Suput et al. 1993). Magnetic resonance spectroscopy of forearm muscle in Duchenne dystrophy has shown reduced phosphocreatine levels but normal ATP content and normal intracellular pH (Newman et al. 1982; Griffiths et al. 1985).

Electrophysiological Assessment

The major electrophysiological abnormalities are found in weak, proximal muscles. Concentric needle EMG recordings usually show prominent spontaneous activity. On insertion of the electrode there is increased activity. Some of this is in the form of complex repetitive discharges. Fibrillation potentials are frequently recorded (Buchthal and Rosenfalck 1963). Desmedt and Borenstein (1976b) found fibrillation potentials in the deltoid muscles in seven of eight patients with Duchenne muscular dystrophy. Positive sharp waves are less commonly noted; they are usually only seen in the weakest muscles.

On volition 50% or more of the MUAPs are polyphasic in the deltoid muscle, but in distal muscles more than 60% of potentials are polyphasic (Desmedt and Borenstein 1976b). Many of the polyphasic motor units are of short duration (Buchthal and Rosenfalck 1963; Desmedt and Borenstein 1976), but using a trigger-delay line it has been found that about 30% of the polyphasic MUAPs are, in fact, of *long* duration, with late components occurring up to 50 ms after the first spike component of the unit (Desmedt and Borenstein 1976b). The MUAPs in Duchenne dystrophy are of lower amplitude than normal potentials, but the interference pattern is usually full, except in very weak and wasted muscles (Fig. 14.3).

With single-fibre EMG the MUAPs are complex and late components are sometimes recorded (Fig. 14.4). The fibre density is usually moderately increased; in five patients aged 5–12 years studied

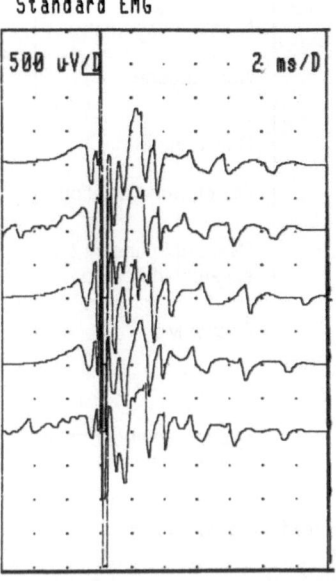

Fig. 14.4. Duchenne muscular dystrophy. Successive sweeps display 9–10 single-fibre action potentials. The last two potentials appear 12 ms after the first, triggering potential. Single-fibre EMG.500 μV and 2 ms/division.

by Schwartz et al. (1977a) the mean fibre density in the biceps brachii was 2.4 (range 1.8–3.0). Stålberg and Trontelj (1994) found that the mean fibre density in the extensor digitorum communis muscle in a group of seven patients aged 7–17 years was 3.5 (range 2.6–6.0). It is possible that the higher fibre density recorded by Stålberg and Trontelj was due to the greater mean age of their patients, whose disease was probably more advanced than in the patients studied by Schwartz et al. (1977a). In another study (Stålberg et al. 1974) of 16 cases of Duchenne dystrophy, the mean fibre density in the forearm muscles was 3.1 (range 2.0–4.9). Stålberg and Trontelj (1994) have suggested that in the late stages of the disease the fibre density, although still increased, is lower. An increased neuromuscular jitter has been noted in approximately 30% of MUAPs (Stålberg and Trontelj 1994) and the later components of the action potential are particularly likely to show this. Some of these components with a large jitter show impulse blocking. By contrast the neuromuscular jitter may be *less* than 5 μs in some potentials, a finding which has been presumed to correlate with fibre splitting (Stålberg 1977; Hilton-Brown and Stålberg 1983a). Paired blocking, that is simultaneous blocking of two or more components of an action potential, is seen only exceptionally in Duchenne dystrophy. Although paired blocking has been interpreted as nerve impulse blocking the phenomenon may also be due to impulse blocking in a single muscle fibre which has split into two or more fibres, innervated by a single axon. These EMG studies, particularly the comparison of data from single-fibre EMG, scanning EMG and macro EMG studies (Hilton-Brown and Stålberg 1983a,b), suggest that the fibre density is increased in focal zones within motor unit territories with zones of electrical silence representing fatty replacement and fibrosis.

The motor nerve conduction velocity in Duchenne muscular dystrophy is normal but the distal motor latency is increased in the common peroneal nerve (McComas et al. 1971c). McComas et al. (1971a), using an incremental stimulation/response technique to record motor units in superficial muscles, found a reduced number of motor units in the extensor digitorum brevis muscle in Duchenne dystrophy. They suggested that this observation indicated that Duchenne dystrophy has a neurogenic basis. However, McComas and his colleagues subsequently reported similar findings in a number of different myopathies, for example McArdle's disease (Upton et al. 1973) and thyrotoxicosis (McComas et al. 1974) as well as in a variety of neurogenic disorders, including motor neuron disease (McComas et al. 1971b). Their findings in Duchenne dystrophy have therefore led to controversy. Indeed, both Panayiotopoulos et al. (1974) and Ballantyne and Hansen (1974a,b) found that the number of motor units in Duchenne dystrophy was normal.

Studies have been made of the maximum isometric twitch tension and half relaxation time in Duchenne dystrophy. Both are abnormally prolonged. Edwards (1977) has reviewed the biochemical mechanisms underlying these abnormalities and has concluded that they do not represent specific physiological defects but, rather, are related to loss of functioning muscle mass.

Quantitative concentric needle EMG using turns/amplitude analysis at different forces of contraction show an increased ratio of potential reversals (turns) to mean amplitude at force levels 10% and 20% of maximum than at higher force levels, the opposite of the findings in neurogenic disorders. There was no detectable abnormality in the pattern of recruitment of motor units in this study (Fuglsang-Frederiksen et al. 1984a,b) and the results were consistent with selective involvement of low threshold units.

Muscle Biopsy

In most cases the diagnosis of Duchenne muscular dystrophy is evident from the clinical and genetic features, together with the markedly raised blood CK level. It might be thought that biopsy was unnecessary for diagnosis in such cases but, since there is no effective treatment, it is always important to establish the diagnosis beyond doubt. Although DNA studies will identify deletions in the dystrophin gene in the majority of patients muscle biopsy, with dystrophin immunostaining, provides the most reliable diagnostic test, and is the only reliable method of recognising Duchenne and Becker dystrophies (Hoffman et al. 1988). In Duchenne muscular dystrophy there is usually no dystrophin immunostaining detectable on muscle fibres; at most no more than 1% of fibres show detectable dystrophin at their rims (Fig. 14.5). In Becker muscular dystrophy, by contrast, there is a variation in the intensity of immunostaining in dystrophin-positive fibres, and a patchy rather than continuous distribution of dystrophin on muscle fibres. Nicholson et al. (1990) found three patterns in Duchenne muscular dystrophy. In 40% of cases dystrophin was absent, in 40% occasional dystrophin-positive fibres were present and 20% had weak dystrophin immunoreactivity in a high proportion of fibres. Nicholson et al. (1990) noted the variable features of Becker muscular dystrophy and also that in some patients dystrophin immunostaining was normal. Manifesting carriers showed a mosaic of dystrophin-negative and positive fibres (Nicholson et al. 1990). Ohlendieck et al. (1993) have shown that in Duchenne muscular dystrophy dystrophin-associated glycoproteins (DAGs), which are proteins that link the subsarcolemmal cytoskeleton with the extracellular matrix, and which are closely functionally related to dystrophin itself, are markedly reduced. This contrasts with the normal expression of these DAGs in other neuromuscular diseases. The abnormal expression of DAGs in Duchenne muscular dystrophy is a feature of all muscle fibres and is not restricted to necrotic fibres. No data are currently available about DAG expression in Becker muscular dystrophy. Specific defects of DAG expression are recognised in severe autosomal recessive muscular dystrophy and in Fukuyama muscular dystrophy, but in these disorders dystrophin expression is normal (see below). Utrophin is upregulated seventeen fold in Duchenne muscular dystrophy muscle fibres, possibly interacting with residual DAGs to bind the sarcolemmal membrane (Karpati et al. 1993).

The histological features of Duchenne dystrophy are usually easily recognised, with widespread abnormalities in the biopsy even in apparently early cases. The typical abnormalities consist of rounding of muscle fibres in transverse section, increased variability in fibre size with striking hypertrophy of some fibres and atrophy of others, increased central

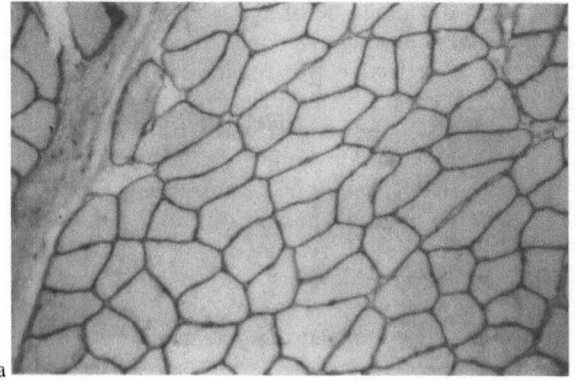

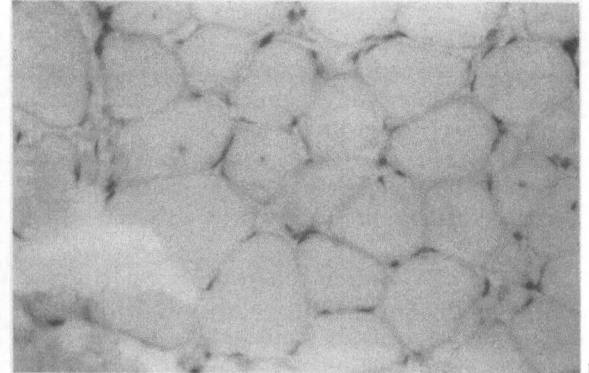

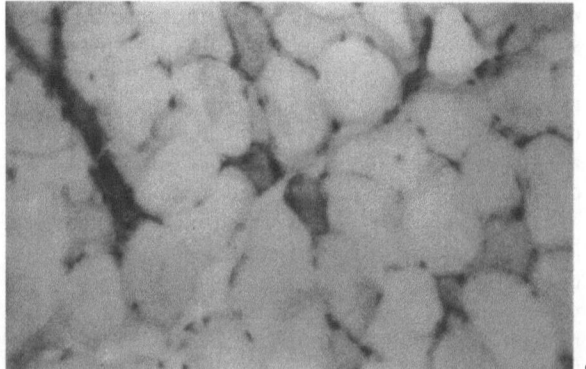

Fig. 14.5. Dystrophin staining. Immuno peroxidase method. **a** Normal membrane-located dystrophin. Note the homogeneous muscle fibre size. **b** Duchenne dystrophy: dystrophin is absent from the muscle fibre membranes. **c** Duchenne dystrophy: two regenerating muscle fibres express dystrophin in their membrane and cytoplasm.

nucleation, fibre splitting, the presence of degenerating and regenerating fibres, and increased amounts of fat and of endomysial and interfascicular fibrous tissue (Fig. 14.6).

A feature almost unique to Duchenne muscular dystrophy is the occurrence of opaque, *hyaline fibres*. These are rounded, large fibres which appear homogeneous and vitreous in haematoxylin and eosin stains, with loss of cross-striations in longitudinal sections. They stain darker than other fibres with this technique and with most other stains, including the Gomori and NADH-tr methods, and therefore have also been termed "opaque fibres" (Fig. 14.7). They often show calcium deposition at their periphery (Bodensteiner and Engel 1978) and have been thought by some workers to be artefactual, though others regard them as a form of necrosis (Walton 1973; Schmalbruch 1992). Serial sections of hyaline fibres may show adjacent necrotic segments with phagocytosis (Walton 1973). Uchino et al. (1985) have described abnormalities of structural proteins in these fibres consisting of reduced amounts of desmin and α-actinin. However, no abnormality or degradation of contractile proteins has been found in the disease (Neville and Harrold 1985). Opaque fibres represent focal zones of overcontraction,

associated with calcium influx. These fibres are intensely reactive in all enzyme reactions and are often of larger diameter than neighbouring fibres. They are sometimes present in large numbers, a finding suggesting that they represent a change that is reversible and does not necessarily progress to necrosis (Partridge 1993).

In some biopsies necrotic fibres are very prominent and there may be a sparse mononuclear cell infiltration, mostly consisting of macrophages and some T lymphocytes (Engel and Arahata 1984), around such fibres. Regenerating fibres are also prominent (Fig. 14.8), often being found in groups of small, round, basophilic, RNA-positive fibres containing vesicular cytoplasm and large nuclei with a dispersed chromatin pattern (Engel 1973). In longitudinal sections mononucleate myoblasts can sometimes be recognised in the early stages of regeneration, forming a continuous strand of regenerating sarcoplasm between the adjacent healthy parts of a fibre, "continuous" regeneration (Mastaglia and Kakulas 1969). In enzyme histochemical stains fibre-type differentiation is poorly developed (Fig. 14.9), partly because of the presence of increased numbers of Type 2C fibres; in most cases there is a relative deficiency of Type 2B fibres (Dubowitz and Brooke 1973). The two fibre types are equally

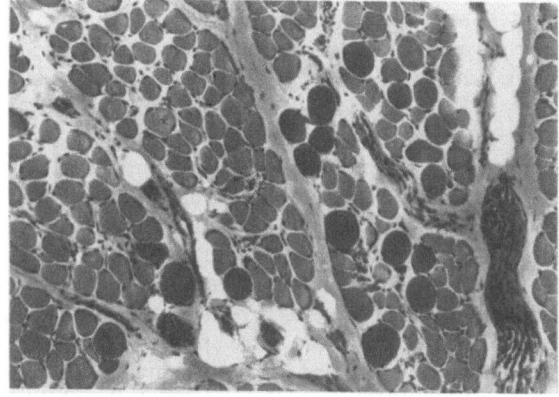

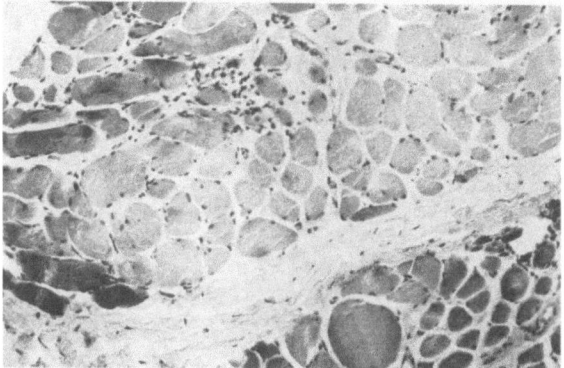

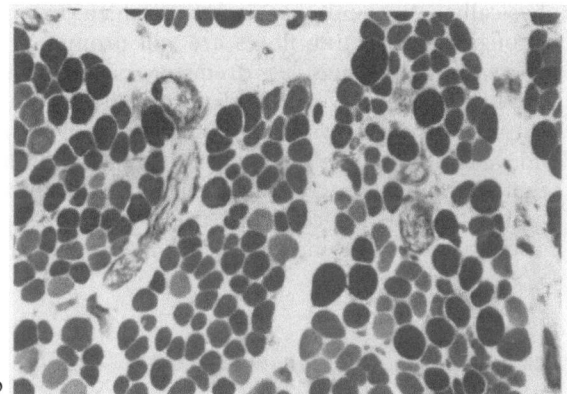

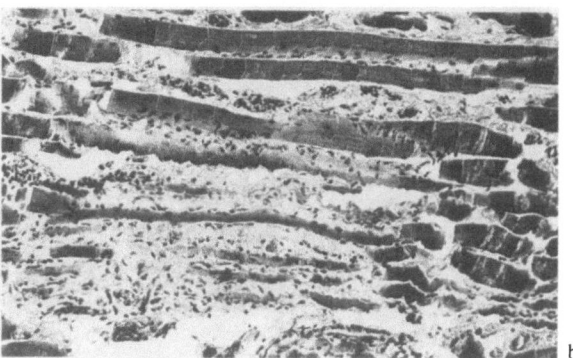

.8. Duchenne muscular dystrophy. H and E. × 140. n-embedded.) **a** TS. Variability in fibre size, rounded fibres, endomysial and inter-fascicular fibrosis and an enlarged, hyaline fibre. **b** LS. A zone of regenerative activity.

Fig. 14.6. Duchenne muscular dystrophy. × 180. **a** H and E. There is prominent endomysial and interfascicular fibrosis, the muscle fibres are rounded and vary in size, and there are many dark, rounded hyaline fibres. A nerve fibre bundle is present to the right. **b** ATPase pH 9.4 (inverted serial section). The muscle fibres show poor fibre-type differentiation, and there is some clustering of the two major fibre types. The rounded shape of the abnormal fibres is evident.

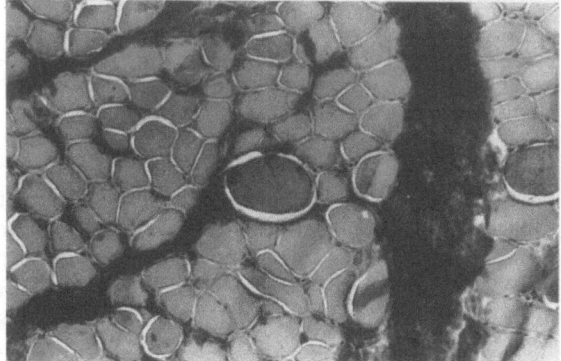

Fig. 14.7. Elastin van Gieson. TS. × 140. Duchenne muscular dystrophy. Dark strands of fibrous tissue are prominent in the thickened inter-fascicular and endomysial planes. There are two enlarged, rounded hyaline fibres and all the muscle fibres are unusually rounded.

involved in the sequence of necrosis and regeneration which characterises the disease (Engel 1977). The presence of 2C fibres may reflect the proportion of fibres in various stages of regeneration or delay in the process of regeneration (Nonaka et al. 1981b). Muscle protein synthesis is reduced (Rennie et al. 1982). Vrbova (1983) has suggested that the initial abnormality in the disease is delayed maturation of muscle fibres; i.e. immature muscle fibres might be less able to withstand motoneuronal activity than normal, particularly in the case of fibres maturing on the pathway to "fast" Type 2 fibres, and so might undergo "metabolic" necrosis because of inappropriate neural activity. However, the abnormalities in fibre type differentiation are more likely to reflect the interplay of regeneration and reinnervation in the course of the disease.

The histological features vary according to the stage of the disorder. In the early stages the biopsy shows relatively little abnormality. In male fetuses of 18–20 weeks gestation, presumed to have Duchenne dystrophy because the placental blood contained high concentrations of CK, there was an increased variation in muscle fibre diameter, with

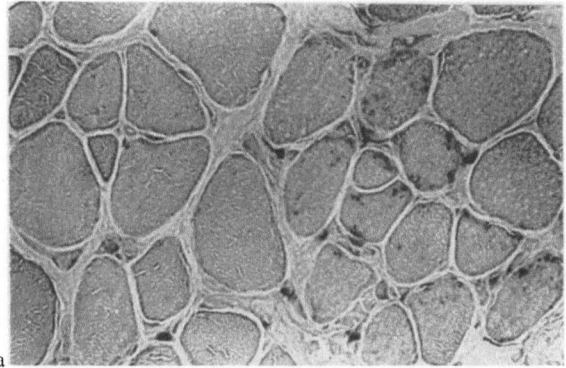

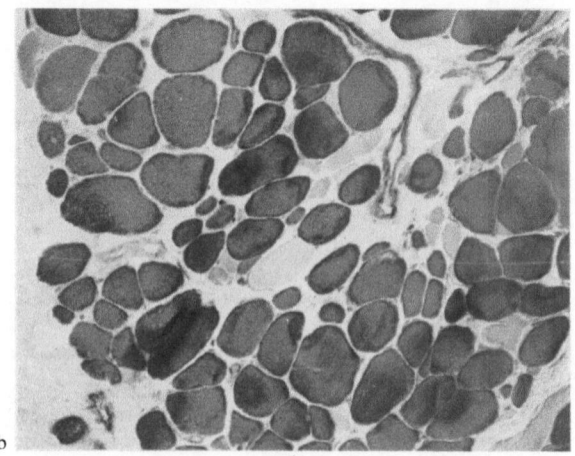

Fig. 14.9. Duchenne muscular dystrophy. **a** TS. × 350. Acid phosphatase; increased acid phosphatase activity is seen at the periphery of several smaller fibres. Note the endomysial fibrosis. **b** TX. × 140. Myosin ATPase, pH 4.3. Type 1 fibre predominance, variability in fibre size and several fibres of intermediate reactivity.

muscle biopsies in Duchenne dystrophy at various ages (Table 14.4) has been reviewed by Pearson (1963) and by Bell and Conen (1968). Biopsies taken early in the disease show more prominent degenerative features than at later stages. Degeneration is particularly marked in biopsies taken before the age of 4 years (Bell and Conen 1968), an age at which the disease may not be clinically apparent; necrotic fibres may occur in groups at this stage of the disease (Engel 1973) and regeneration is already a feature of the biopsy, as is central nucleation and fibre splitting. However, fibre splitting and central nucleation become more prominent between the ages of 5 and 7 years, an age at which the child is physically active and only slightly disabled. Later, although degenerating fibres are still prominent, regeneration becomes less frequent, particularly after the age of 9 years, and fibre splitting and central nucleation are also less frequently seen (Bell and Conen 1968). During the phase of regeneration segmental necrosis activates satellite cells to form myoblasts; satellite cells are three times more common than in normal muscle (Wakayama et al. 1979).

Table 14.4. Sequence of changes in muscle biopsies in Duchenne muscular dystrophy

	Early 1–5 years Ambulant	Moderately advanced 6–10 years Marked weakness	Late 10 years or older Chairbound
Hyalinised fibres	———————	———————	- - - - - - -
Fibre necrosis	———————	———————	- - - - - - -
Phagocytosis	———————	———————	- - - - - - -
Fibrosis	- - - - -	———————	———————
Rounded fibres	- - - - -	———————	———————
Regenerating fibres	———————	———————	
Central nucleation		———————	———————
Fibre splitting		———————	———————
Fibre hypertrophy		———————	———————
Fat replacement		- - - - - - -	———————
Poor fibre-type differentiation		———————	———————

hyaline fibres and an increase in the amount of connective tissue (Emery 1977; Mahoney et al. 1977). Emery and Burt (1980) have shown that the hyaline fibres in affected fetuses contain excess calcium. Bradley et al. (1972a) in a biopsy from a 2 1/2-week old boy with a CK of 1433 IU/1 found similar abnormalities. In a biopsy taken from the same boy at the age of 3 years, when the CK was 2160 IU/1, hyaline, necrotic and regenerating fibres, with increased endomysial fibrosis, were found, although even at this time there was not yet clear clinical evidence of the disease. In this case two older brothers had Duchenne dystrophy. In muscle from male fetuses aborted because of a high risk of Duchenne dystrophy, dystrophin was absent in muscle fibres from four of the six cases (Patel et al. 1988), but was present in all 16 muscle specimens from four other types of muscular dystrophy used as controls. The sequence of changes found in

In the terminal stages fat and fibrous connective tissue virtually replace the muscle fibres in most muscles (Fig. 14.10), although the external ocular muscles and the sphincter muscles are strikingly spared. In these later stages the CK level falls, although it scarcely ever reaches normal values. As the disease progresses the fascicular pattern is damaged and rearranged. Nerve fascicles are apparently spared but muscle spindles show necrosis and loss of intrafusal muscle fibres, with thickening of the spindle capsule and ultimately replacement by a fibrous scar (Swash and Fox 1976).

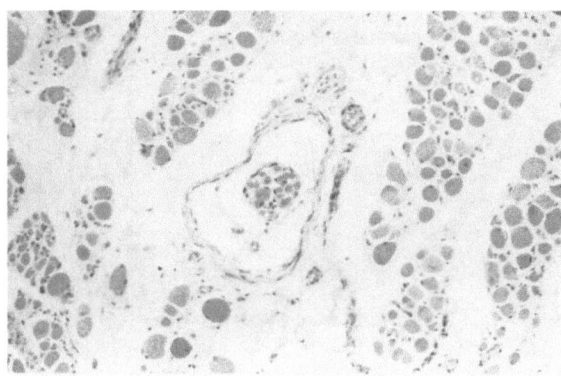

Fig. 14.10. Duchenne muscular dystrophy. TS. × 140. Autopsy. In the terminal stages the muscle fibres are small and rounded, and fibrosis is very marked. The muscle spindle shows similar abnormalities to the extrafusal muscle.

Coërs and Telerman-Toppet (1977) studied the terminal innervation in Duchenne dystrophy, with the supravital methylene blue technique, and found a marked enlargement of the termal innervation area giving an increased longitudinal scatter of motor end-plates. A dense innervation persists in muscles even when many muscle fibres have been lost so that there is an apparent excess of motor axons. However, there is no evidence of collateral sprouting of axons so that the terminal innervation ratio is *not* increased. Dubrovsky and Toratuto (1983) have shown that the capacity for reinnervation after denervation from plexus lesion in Duchenne dystrophy is normal.

Electron-microscopic studies of muscle in Duchenne dystrophy have shown abnormalities in the plasma membrane (Jones and Witkowski 1983). With transmission electron microscopy, breaks in the continuity of the plasma membrane extending for several micrometres have been reported (Mokri and Engel 1975; Carpenter and Karpati 1979). The basement membrane is always intact. This abnormality may be a very early change in the sequence of events leading to segmental fibre necrosis. In later stages there is loss of the Z disc, and mitochondrial alterations occur. Carpenter and Karpati (1979) found that these changes occurred in a few hours, but that the later phases of fibre necrosis continued over several days, being completed by phagocytosis. Mokri and Engel (1975) found that horseradish peroxidase in the extracellular fluid enters muscle fibres through the defective zones in the plasma membrane. Bradley and Fulthorpe (1978) made similar observations, using procion yellow, and found that the dye particularly penetrated hyaline and necrotic fibres. Carpenter and Karpati (1979) thought that the

membrane defects could lead to hypercontraction and hyalinisation of fibres, without the necessity for necrosis, as an artefact caused at the time of biopsy. Focal influx of calcium ions through defects in the plasma membrane will lead to segmental hypercontraction in some instances, and to focal fibre necrosis in others (see Fig. 14.11). With widespread dissolution of the plasma membrane a massive influx of calcium ions (Fig. 14.12) may occur leading to activation of endogenous proteases and, eventually, to muscle fibre necrosis (Carpenter and Karpati 1979).

Loss of areas of plasma membrane will thus lead to necrosis in some instances, but in others repair of the defect is possible by the production of a new membrane beneath the site of the original membrane. Carpenter and Karpati (1979) pointed out that evidence of repair of plasma membrane was uncommon in recently regenerated fibres. The morphological abnormalities in the plasma membrane are related to the absence of dystrophin and the abnormality in dystrophin-associated glycoproteins in the plasma membrane characteristic of DMD. These features explain the high CK levels found in Duchenne dystrophy even in patients in whom the biopsy shows relatively little evidence of fibre necrosis. Schotland et al. (1979) studied the membrane defect with the freeze–fracture technique. They found a reduction in the numbers of intramembrane particles in the two faces of the fractured membrane from dystrophic muscle fibres and extensive areas in which only a few particles were seen. In particular, the numbers of "square array" pits in the B face of the membrane were reduced. This abnormality (Rowland 1980a) may be a primary morphological defect in the disease (Schotland et al. 1980). Initial reports of similar changes in erythrocytes were not confirmed (Wakayama et al. 1982).

Pathological Features in Other Organs

Abnormalities in the ECG are frequent in patients with Duchenne dystrophy, but symptomatic heart disease is less common, occurring in fewer than 1% of cases and then only terminally (Griggs et al. 1977). Sinus tachycardia is common and sudden death may occur. Pathological examination shows much less involvement of cardiac than of skeletal muscles. The left ventricular muscle shows some fibrosis and the heart may be enlarged (Perloff et al. 1966). Myocardial muscle fibres do not undergo necrosis or other change.

Rosman and Kakulas (1966) examined the brains of 12 boys with Duchenne dystrophy. The brains were slightly smaller than normal and pachygyria

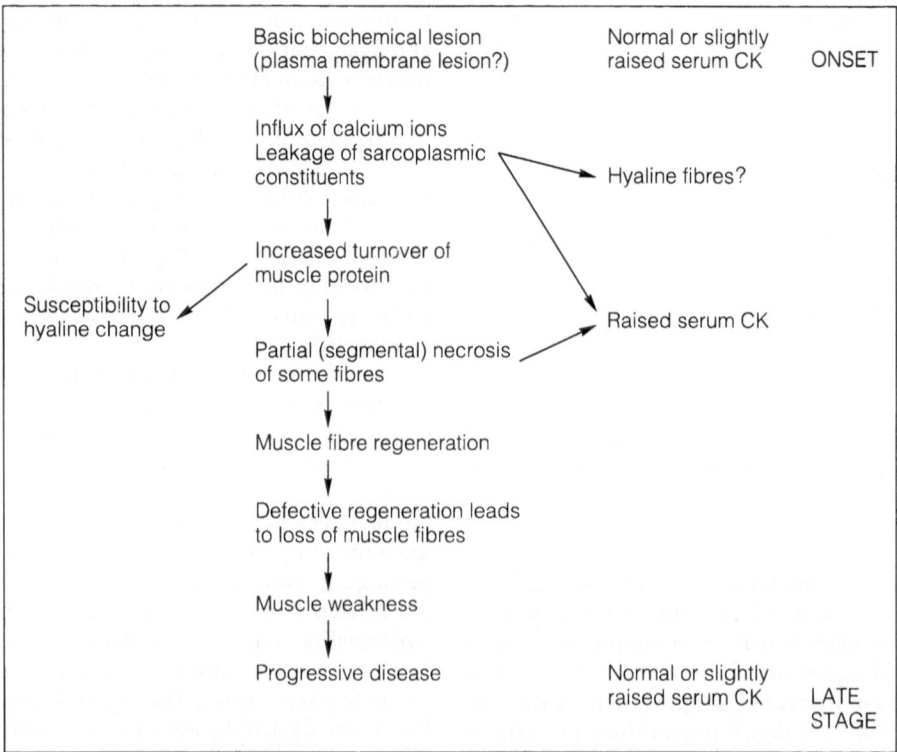

Fig. 14.11.   Course of Duchenne muscular dystrophy (from Pearson 1963).

and cortical heterotopias were seen in some cases, especially in those in whom mild mental deficiency had been recorded during life. Hodgson et al. (1992) noted that deletions of central axons in the dystrophin gene were especially likely to be associated with mental retardation. Because of the suggestion by McComas and his colleagues that the disease might have a neurogenic basis Tomlinson

et al. (1974) examined the spinal cord in five uncomplicated cases of Duchenne dystrophy; they found normal numbers of anterior horn cells, an observation that invalidated the hypothesis.

Diagnosis of Duchenne Muscular Dystrophy

In the majority of cases the diagnosis can be made from molecular studies, without the need for muscle biopsy (Miller and Wessel 1993). The diagnosis of Duchenne (or Becker) disease should only be suspected if the CK is greater than 1000 IU/1. The first step is to arrange for DNA analysis by polymerase chain reaction on a blood sample to detect deletions in the dystrophin gene. Southern blot analysis can be used to detect deletions and to establish exon–intron boundaries. If these studies are not informative muscle biopsy with dystrophin histochemistry and protein analysis should be performed.

Carrier Detection and Genetic Counselling

An important aspect of the management of a patient with Duchenne muscular dystrophy is to explain the implication of the diagnosis to the child's parents.

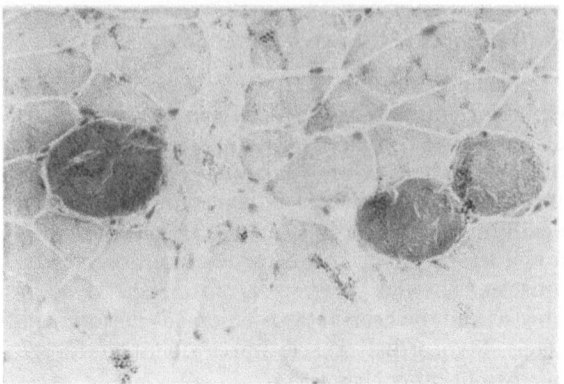

Fig. 14.12.   Duchenne muscular dystrophy. × 340. Alizarin red method for calcium. Three fibres stain intensely indicating increased calcium content; these are hyaline fibres.

The prognosis must be described and the objectives of physiotherapy and orthopaedic procedures explained. Since the disease is inherited as an X-linked recessive disorder, 50% of the male offspring of the parents of a boy with Duchenne muscular dystrophy will develop the disease and 50% of their female offspring will carry the gene. Two questions then arise: first, can carriers reliably be detected and second, is it possible to diagnose the disease in utero?

Carrier Detection. Carrier detection is important in the female siblings of known carriers, i.e. the sisters of mothers who have sons suffering from Duchenne dystrophy and girls who have brothers with the disease, and in possible carriers, i.e. the sisters and mothers of boys with Duchenne dystrophy whose brothers do not have the disease. *Definite carriers* (obligate carriers) are women who have two affected sons, or one affected son and another affected, close male relative. About 30% of cases of Duchenne dystrophy represent gene mutations so that although sisters of definite carriers have a 50% chance of carrying the gene, the risk is lower than this for sisters or daughters of *possible carriers*. Carriers of the disease usually show no clinical signs of dystrophy, but there is slight muscular weakness or calf hypertrophy, which may be unilateral, in about 8% of carriers (Moser and Emery 1974).

Formerly, carrier detection was based on pedigree analysis, supplemented by CK analysis and muscle biopsy. CK analysis is still a useful screening test, since the genetic abnormality is variable and may consist only of a point mutation which may be undetectable. Three blood samples should be taken for CK analysis, each at weekly intervals. The odds for carrier status should be assessed from the mean of these three CK values (Emery 1980). Clearly, the risk of carrier status is greater in the daughters of obligate carriers than in the daughters of possible carriers. About 70% of carriers will be detected by CK analysis (Emery 1987). The resting CK level is higher in pre-menarchal girls and post-menopausal women and is slightly reduced during pregnancy (Griggs et al. 1985). Since the CK level may rise slightly after exercise, exercise provocation tests have not proven reliable (Hausmanowa-Petrusewitz et al. 1977). Pedigree analysis and CK analysis can give a women a low risk of being a carrier. Only two of 94 boys born to a group of such women were affected by DMD (see Bundey 1992).

Although abnormalities in the EMG (Moosa et al. 1972) and muscle biopsy (Afifi et al. 1973; Ionanescu et al. 1975) have been reported in carriers of Duchenne dystrophy, these tests only rarely result in the detection of carriers not already recognised by CK studies. In an ECG study it was found that the R-S sum in lead V_1 was greater in carriers than in controls, and that the R/S ratio was abnormal in lead V_2 (Lane et al. 1980). These abnormalities can be incorporated as a conditional probability of carrier status in association with clinical and CK data according to a table of probability (Lane et al. 1980).

Manifesting carriers may show prominent myopathic change (Vainzof et al. 1991) although only 11% of females at risk of being carrier show abnormalities with conventional histochemical studies of muscle biopsies (Maunder-Sewry and Dubowitz 1981). Manifesting carriers may show a mosaic pattern of dystrophin positive and negative fibres (Vainzof et al. 1991a), but non-manifesting carriers nearly always show a normal distribution of dystrophin in the biopsy.

Identification of carriers is most accurately performed in at-risk women by direct identification of the gene abnormality on the X chromosome. In carriers with deletion mutations in the dystrophin gene the defect can be demonstrated by multiplex polymerase chain reaction studies in up to 95% of instances (Chamberlain et al. 1992). Point mutations in the gene can be detected by Western analysis (Bulman et al. 1991) and, having identified the point mutation, by PCR amplification and enzyme digestion (Yau et al. 1993). Both deletion and reduplication can be recognised in this way (Roberts et al. 1992). Linkage analysis, without direct identification of the mutation, can be analysed by detection of microsatellite repeat polymorphism within and flanking the dystrophin gene locus (Clemens et al. 1991). These authors were able to identify abnormalities in 97% of all families tested. These tests are all applicable on DNA samples obtained from venous blood.

Neonatal Screening and fetal and Neonatal Diagnosis

Diagnosis of DMD in the first month of life was introduced by Zellweger and Antonik (1975) by using a spot-screening technique for semi-quantitative measurement of CK level on blood taken by heel-prick. This procedure was initially regarded as of dubious benefit to patient and family, given the non-availability of effective treatment, but Bradley et al. (1993) have evaluated a screening programme of this type in South Wales. They found that the initial CK level was increased in 16 of 34 000 male newborn infants tested. In nine of these the CK was confirmed to be elevated at a second test on venous blood at 6 weeks of age. Of these nine male infants, five had deletions of exons in the dystrophin gene.

Muscle dystrophin analysis was consistent with DMD in the five boys subjected to muscle biopsy. Although there was a family history of DMD in only one family, the CK level was raised in seven of the nine mothers, a finding illustrating the value of CK testing in carrier detection. In two families older brothers were recognised as suffering from DMD following diagnosis in their newborn siblings.

Carter et al. (1993) designed their programme of neonatal screening for DMD in order to give families reproductive choice in future pregnancies, to enable them to avoid the experience of a delayed diagnosis, to plan for the future without a disabled child and to provide presymptomatic diagnosis in order to be available for possible future treatment. These are the four major aims of presymptomatic diagnosis in the newborn. Prenatal diagnosis is also possible by DNA analysis on samples of fetal blood or chorionic fetal tissue obtained at amniocentesis, but this technique has not been formally evaluated and is useful only for the purpose of recommending abortion, or in planning treatment should genetic therapy become available. Clerk et al. (1992) studied muscle obtained from low-risk and high-risk fetuses obtained at therapeutic abortion. Dystrophin stains were most reliable after 15 weeks gestation. Antibodies to the mid-rod region were most useful. This technique can establish phenotype in at-risk fetuses and is therefore useful for subsequent genetic counselling.

Management

No curative treatment is available. A wide variety of possible treatments, including pharmacological, physical and other methods have been tried, but none has been found to affect the inevitably fatal outcome of the disease (Dubowitz and Heckmatt 1980). However, the duration of the phase of active walking ability can be prolonged by physiotherapy, bracing, swivel rockers (Sibert et al. 1987) and appropriate orthopaedic procedures (Smith et al. 1987), such as tenotomy, performed to alleviate contractures (Spencer and Vignos 1962; Siegel 1977, 1978). Careful bracing can be particularly effective in preserving the ability to stand (Hyde et al. 1982) but whether this results in significant improvement in the overall behaviour and life pattern available to the affected boy is uncertain, and probably best decided on an individual basis in consultation with the child and his parents (Siegel 1977). Physiotherapy is not usually useful in restoring function in the weak foot with shortened Achilles tendon, but surgical treatment may be helpful (Siegel 1972) when proximal muscles are not too weakened. The equinus gait may be a functional compensation

maintaining forces acting about the knee within the range adequate for the weakened muscles, and thus tenotomy in some patients may have unexpectedly deleterious effects on gait.

Surgical correction of scoliosis is not usually recommended because of the progression inherent in the disease, together with impaired ventilatory reserve, but if scoliosis is rapidly progressive, surgical correction using the Luque procedure, which does not immobilise the costo-vertebral joints, can produce useful improvement with restoration of the ability to sit even in advanced cases of Duchenne dystrophy (Rideau et al. 1984). Inspiratory resistive training may improve ventilatory function and delay the onset of respiratory failure (DiMauro et al. 1985; Smith et al. 1987). Proper attention to posture, with frequent passive physiotherapy to prevent muscle shortening and contractures, is especially important when the affected boy becomes confined to a wheelchair (usually before the age of 11 years). The chair should be made to act as a passive spinal brace to prevent postural scoliosis.

Drug Therapy

The natural history of DMD is relatively stereotyped. The mean age at death is little different now from that in the time of Gowers more than a century ago (Emery 1987). Emery (1987) noted that 95% of affected boys were wheelchair-bound by the age of 12 years and the mean age of death was 16.8 years. Brooke et al. (1983) investigated the natural history of the disease, using a series of standardised measures of performance and muscle strength, and these data have been used subsequently in clinical trials of steroid therapy and of immunosuppressant drugs. Drachman et al. (1974) and Mendell et al. (1989) showed that prednisone was effective in improving muscle strength and muscle mass when used orally in a dose of 0.75 mg/kg per day. This effect was observed within 10 days and reached a plateau after 3 months treatment. Griggs et al. (1993) have since shown that this effect was maintained for at least 18 months and was associated with a 36% increase in muscle mass. Smaller doses were less effective. This beneficial effect of prednisone is probably due to decreased muscle catabolism, perhaps by mitigating proteolysis in muscle (Moxley et al. 1990). The clinical improvement was not accompanied by any significant reduction in blood CK levels or by increased dystrophin expression in the muscle (Mendell et al. 1989). Griggs et al. (1993) recommended that prednisone should be used in ambulatory patients older than 5 years and continued indefinitely provided that side effects were not severe. Dubowitz (1991) suggested that prednisone treatment for 10 days each month might be effective without causing steroid side effects.

Although azathioprine is ineffective (Griggs et al. 1993), cyclosporine A therapy was followed by improvement in tetanic force and in maximal voluntary force in anterior tibial muscles within 14 days of its commencement (Sharma et al. 1993). The mechanism of this effect is unknown but it appears not to be due to specific effects on inflammatory cell infiltrates in muscle, associated with fibre necrosis (Kissel et al. 1993).

Dantrolene therapy, which inhibits calcium release from the sarcoplasmic reticulum, significantly reduced blood CK levels during the first year of treatment but without affecting the clinical deterioration characteristic of the disease in historical controls (Bertorini et al. 1991).

Myoblast Transfer and Gene Therapy

Partridge et al. (1989) showed that injection of normal cultured mouse myoblasts into the muscle of the *mdx* dystrophic mouse was followed by the appearance of dystrophin-positive fibres in the host muscle. Similar attempts to treat human DMD by transferring as many as 5 billion normal, cultured human myoblasts with or without immunosuppressant therapy, however, have not been accompanied by clinical improvement in controlled double-blind studies (Partridge 1991; Dubowitz 1992). Uncontrolled studies showed variable results, not suggestive of practical clinical application (Huard et al. 1992). Gussoni et al. (1992) reported that about 10/1000 fibres were dystrophin-positive after myoblast transfer, a proportion no greater than the numbers of revertant dystrophin-positive fibres in control muscles.

Gene therapy, by inserting dystrophin genome into cultured myoblasts taken from patients with DMD or BMD, poses technical problems and ethical dilemmas that are currently unresolved.

Becker-Type Muscular Dystrophy

A slowly progressive form of X-linked muscular dystrophy has been described (Becker and Kiener 1955; Becker 1962). The patient develops proximal weakness in a similar distribution to that found in Duchenne muscular dystrophy, with enlargement of the calves and sometimes with shortening of the Achilles tendons, but the onset of the disease is later, weakness being first observed usually between

the ages of 6 and 18 years. The best clinical discriminant between Becker and Duchenne disease is the age of wheelchair-dependence; 95% of Duchenne patients are in a wheelchair by the age of 12 years, but 97% of Becker's dystrophy patients are still mobile at this age (Emery and Skinner 1976). The mean age of wheelchair-dependence is 27 years and the mean age of death is 42 years (Emery and Skinner 1976; Bradley et al. 1978). The ECG may show similar abnormalities to those found in Duchenne dystrophy (see Chap. 20). Pes cavus is common, but contractures are less common (Gardner-Medwin 1980). Muscle cramp is common. The face is usually spared. Scoliosis is rare. Mental retardation is uncommon. Because of its relatively late onset and slow progression the disease is easily mistaken for limb-girdle muscular dystrophy. Hoffman et al. (1989) found that two-thirds of their 54 cases of BMD presented with limb weakness, but that the others presented with myalgia, increased CK levels, myoglobinuria, malignant hyperthermia or ankle tendon contractures. Clinically apparent cardiomyopathy is present in 15% of patients under 16 years, and in 73% of those older than 40 years (Nigro et al. 1995). This is usually a dilated cardiopathy, and does not correlate with the severity of skeletal muscle involvement.

The CK level is usually raised, ranging to as much as 30 000 IU/l, with a mean value of about 5000 IU/l and median value 3610 IU/l (Hoffman et al. 1989). The highest levels are found in the early stages of the disease.

Genetic Correlations

The severity of the Becker phenotype can be related to the quantity of dystrophin expressed in the muscle biopsy. Those with less than 10% of the normal adult quantity of dystrophin had a severe form of BMD and were wheelchair-bound between the ages of 12 and 20 years, and those with 20% or more had a less severe phenotype, becoming wheelchairbound after the age of 20 years (Hoffman et al. 1989). However, there is also an abnormality of dystrophin quality in BMD, resulting from the in-frame deletion in the dystrophin gene that characterises BMD, and this also influences clinical severity, although no clear correlation of the clinical features with the molecular pathology has yet emerged. Molecular genetic studies have identified gene deletions in 72% of sporadic BMD patients, a similar proportion to that found in familial cases (Norman et al. 1989). Applying molecular genetic analysis with cDNA probes for dystrophin gene deletions in male patients with a diagnosis of limb-girdle dystrophy revealed that 27% in fact had BMD.

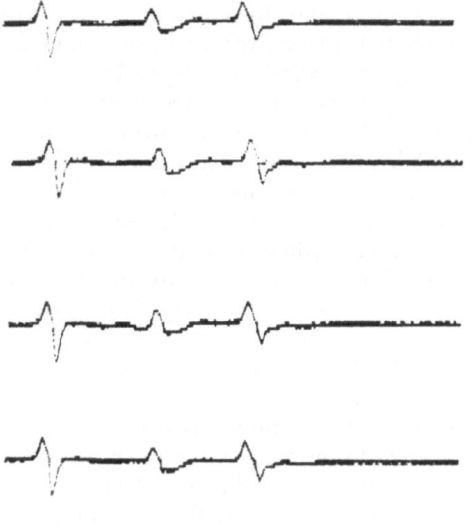

Fig. 14.13. Becker-type muscular dystrophy: a motor unit action potential recorded with single-fibre EMG showing three dispersed components. The complex is 10 ms in duration. Bar 4 ms.

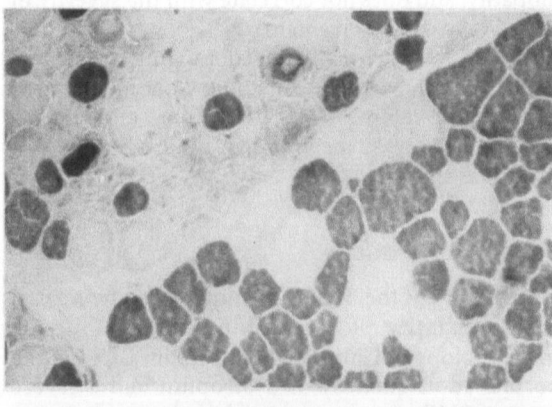

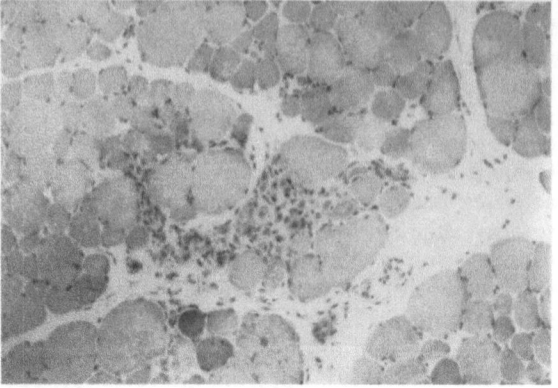

Fig. 14.14. Becker muscular dystrophy. H and E, × 180. The abnormality resembles that of Duchenne muscular dystrophy with marked regenerative fibre clusters.

These patients had an earlier age of diagnosis than other patients with limb-girdle weakness, had calf hypertrophy, and had CK levels five times higher than the limb-girdle dystrophy patients (2500 versus 500 IU/l) (Norman et al. 1989). Arikawa et al. (1991) identified five men and two women with dystrophinopathies in a group of 41 cases of limb-girdle dystrophy syndrome. The two women proved to be manifesting carriers of DMD. Thus about 40% of male patients with limb-girdle syndromes may suffer from BMD (Norman et al. 1989).

These data are important in genetic counselling, carrier detection and neonatal screening in the Becker and limb-girdle syndromes since they imply the necessity for dystrophin gene studies both in men and women with the limb-girdle syndrome.

Electrophysiological Assessment

The EMG is usually myopathic but about 10% of cases may show a "mixed" pattern (Hoffman et al. 1989) with fibrillation potentials and positive sharp waves and, on volition, polyphasic MUAPs of both high and low amplitude. These units recorded by concentric needle EMG were usually of short duration in the patients reported by Bradley et al. (1978) but with single-fibre EMG late units are found (Fig. 14.13). The interference pattern is reduced.

The CT scan shows enlargement of calf muscles with reduced attenuation, with involvement of thigh musculature (De Visser and Verbeeten 1985).

Muscle Biopsy

There are differences between the changes found in the muscle biopsy in Becker and Duchenne dystrophy (Bradley et al. 1978). In Becker dystrophy the muscle fibres are usually not rounded and hyaline fibres are rare, in contrast to the two most typical features of Duchenne dystrophy. Hypertrophy, fibre splitting and central nucleation, atrophic and angular fibres and clumps of pyknotic nuclei are common in older cases of Becker dystrophy (Fig. 14.14), whereas in Duchenne dystrophy they are less common. At the early stages of the two diseases, however, these distinctions are less clear. Fibrosis is as much a feature of Becker dystrophy as it is of Duchenne dystrophy. Angulated fibres are a feature of BMD and these may cause confusion with neurogenic disease (Bradley et al. 1978). Inflammatory cell infiltrates are rather more prominent in BMD than DMD.

Dystrophin immunostaining in BMD reveals that more than 3% of muscle fibres are dystrophin-positive (Hoffman et al. 1989). In some biopsies most or all of the fibres may be dystrophin-positive, but the distribution of dystrophin in the fibre membrane is discontinuous and patchy, or if present in normal quantity is itself abnormal. Hoffman et al. (1989) introduced the concept of abnormalities in quantity and/or quality in describing these features. Abnormalities in dystrophin quality refer to reduction in size of the dystrophin molecule, which is normally 400 kDa.

Management and Carrier Detection

Since Becker dystrophy is only slowly progressive no active measures are necessary in management until the later stages when tenotomy and physiotherapy may be very useful in alleviating deformities and maintaining mobility. The diagnosis can be confirmed when older male relatives have a similar disorder. Assessment of the heart is important, since cardiomyopathy is a potentially serious feature of BMD (see Chap. 20).

Carrier detection can be accomplished, as in Duchenne dystrophy, by the detection of raised CK levels in female first-degree relatives, but this method is not as reliable in Becker dystrophy as in Duchenne dystrophy (Emery et al. 1967). Aston et al. (1984) found raised CK levels in 42% of 31 obligate carriers of Becker muscular dystrophy, indicating that the test has some value. The Becker type of muscular dystrophy usually appears as a homogeneous entity in affected families but in some families both the Duchenne and Becker types of muscular dystrophy occur (Furukawa and Peter 1977) and rare cases of intermediate severity have been described (see Bradley et al. 1978). Manifesting carriers of BMD are rare but may present with mild weakness and a raised CK, together with calf hypertrophy (Ionanescu et al. 1989). Genetic testing has superseded the CK determinations.

Other Dystrophinopathies

There are a number of less severe clinical syndromes that have recently been shown to be due to abnormalities in dystrophin expression, associated with exon deletions in the dystrophin gene on Xp 21.2. These, therefore, are all present in male patients. Some were formerly regarded as distinct clinical syndromes, for example quadriceps myopathy, but others represent less well-defined or less characteristic clinical syndromes, for example familial X-linked myalgia and cramps.

Quadriceps Myopathy

A form of hereditary myopathy restricted to the quadriceps muscles was first described by Bramwell

(1922) and there have been a few subsequent reports of a similar disorder (Denny-Brown 1939; Turner and Heathfield 1961). Van Wijngaarden et al. (1968) described two brothers with clinical involvement apparently restricted to the quadriceps muscles but with EMG abnormalities widely distributed in other muscles. The CK level may be raised as much as 10 times normal (Swash and Heathfield 1983). The restriction of this myopathy to the quadriceps muscles may be more apparent at the early stages of the syndrome, since a limb-girdle muscular dystrophy develops later in the natural history of the disorder (Espir and Matthews 1973; Swash and Heathfield 1983). It is important to consider the possibility that chronic polymyositis (Turner and Heathfield 1961), spinal muscular atrophy and diabetic amyotrophy may present in this way. Sunohara et al. (1990) showed that this syndrome of quadriceps myopathy is a limited form of BMD with abnormalities in the dystrophin gene and partial expression of dystrophin in the muscle fibre membrane. This is consistent with recognition that all reported cases have occurred in men.

X-Linked Myalgia and Cramps

Kuhn et al. (1979) and Hoffman et al. (1989) recognised that one presentation of BMD was with myalgia, cramps and a raised CK level. Gospe et al. (1989) reported a family in which nine affected male members had muscle cramps, myalgia and a raised CK level (up to 20 times normal). In all there was well-developed musculature with calf hypertrophy but without muscular weakness. EMG and single-fibre EMG studies were normal. A quadriceps biopsy showed rounded muscle fibres, frequent fibre splitting and increased numbers of internalised sarcolemmal nuclei. In this family there was a deletion in the proximal third of the dystrophin gene and dystrophin expression was of normal quantity, but was truncated. The myalgia in this variant of BMD may respond to prednisone therapy, in a dose of 15–40 mg daily (Higuchi et al. 1993).

X-Linked Myoglobinuria

A family of 19 males in four generations, with obligate transmission through females has been reported in which severe muscle cramps and dark urine was induced by exercise. There was marked elevation of CK, mild weakness and myopathic EMG changes. A muscle biopsy showed mild myopathic features. The female carriers showed mild elevation of CK and were subject to mild cramps. Muscle from an affected male propositus showed abnormal

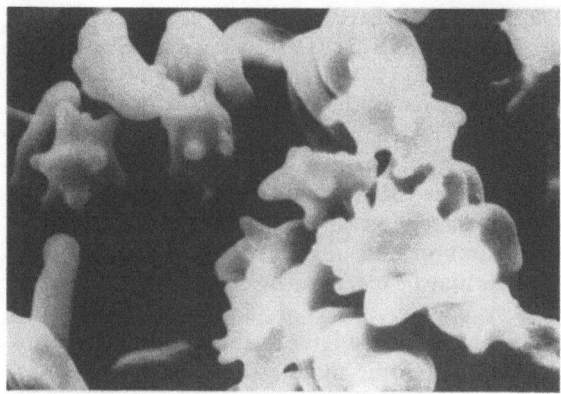

Fig. 14.15. McLeod's syndrome. Acanthocytes shown by scanning electron microscopy.

dystrophin (Fischbeck et al. 1988; Gospe et al. 1989). Hoffman et al. (1988) noted that myoglobinuria was sometimes a presentation of BMD.

Mabry Syndrome

This variant of DMD/BMD with long survival, mild disability and cardiac involvement, reported in a large family in Kentucky, has not been confirmed in other studies (Mabry et al. 1965; Ringel et al. 1977) and is probably a mild form of BMD.

Animal Models of Dystrophinopathies

There are several animal models of human DMD/BMD. The X-linked muscular dystrophy mouse (*mdx*) is biochemically and genetically homologous with human DMD. The muscle fibres in the *mdx* mouse lack dystrophin but the disease is less severe, with a peak of muscle necrosis between the third and fourteenth post-natal weeks. The affected animals are never severely weakened and eventually grow to be larger and stronger than wild strains of mice (Hoffman et al. 1987a; Coulton et al. 1988). Several mutations in the dystrophin locus have been identified (Partridge 1991).

The canine X-linked muscular dystrophy is also biochemically homologous with the human disease and, unlike the *mdx* mouse, the dogs develop weakness, contractures and respiratory problems. Eventually the muscles become wasted, fibrotic and calcified (Valentine and Cooper 1991).

Studies of the mechanisms underlying progression in the dog and clinical recovery in the mouse may be helpful in directing attention to possible roles of utrophin and dystrophin-related or associated proteins in stabilising the human disease. A transgenic mouse derived by gene transfer of the

human dystrophin gene into the *mdx* mouse, produced by injecting the human gene into the pronuclei of fertilised ova, offers another experimental approach (Wells et al. 1992).

Other X-Linked Muscular Dystrophies

Several additional forms of X-linked muscular dystrophy have been described. All are rare. They include McLeod's syndrome (Swash et al. 1983), Emery–Dreifuss syndrome (Emery and Dreifuss 1966), X-linked scapulo-peroneal myopathy (Thomas et al. 1975) and X-linked myotobular myopathy (van Wijngaarden et al. 1969).

McLeod's Syndrome

McLeod's syndrome is a rare X-linked recessive phenotype characterised by acanthocytosis (Fig. 14.15) and weakened red blood cell antigenicity in the Kell blood group system. The blood CK level is raised and the EMG and muscle biopsy show mild myopathic features. However, there is no weakness or pseudohypertrophy and the patients themselves are clinically normal. The occurrence of this combination of myopathy and Kell blood group suggests an association within the genetic loci on the short arm of the X chromosome near or overlapping with the locus for Duchenne muscular dystrophy, and the genetic locus has been identified at Xp21(1–2) (Bertelson et al. 1988). The Kell blood group is also associated with chronic granulomatous disease, in which an abnormality of leukocyte function impairs the ability to destroy ingested bacteria (Segal and Peters 1976), but the allelic relation of Kell antigenicity and chronic granulomatous disease is such that the blood CK level is normal in most patients with the latter disease (Swash et al. 1983). There are a number of other acanthocytic neuromuscular syndromes, some with abetalipoproteinaemia, in many of which the CK level is raised (Estes et al. 1967), but these are autosomal recessive or dominant disorders with a different pathogenesis.

In McLeod's syndrome the dystrophin gene at Xp21–2 is normal and there is normal expression of dystrophin in muscle (Carter et al. 1990; Ho et al. 1996). There is no evidence of any interaction between the Kell red cell antigen and dystrophin in the expression of the McLeod phenotype, and the pathogenesis of the mild myopathy that may occur in this disease is unknown. Ho et al. (1996) reported a point mutation in exon 2 of the McLeod gene causing a frame shift and an abnormal protein.

The McLeod syndrome is of historical importance, however, because Francke et al. (1985)

described a patient with DMD, McLeod's syndrome and chronic granulomatous disease in whom there was deletion of part of the X chromosome at Xp21. DNA from this patient was used to derive the PERT clones within the dystrophin gene that led to characterisation of the dystrophin gene itself. Nonetheless, the McLeod locus (Xk) for the Kell protein has been mapped at a position some thousands of kilobases from the DMD locus and is unrelated to it.

Emery–Dreifuss Muscular Dystrophy

In 1961 Dreifuss and Hogan described a large family in Virginia in which an X-linked muscular dystrophy occurred, beginning in early childhood and characterised by contractures of the Achilles tendons, causing a toe-walking gait, elbow and posterior cervical muscle contractures, slowly progressive muscular wasting and weakness in a predominantly humero-peroneal distribution in the early stages, and cardiomyopathy with conduction defects (Emery and Dreifuss 1966). The disorder was probably first described in 1902 by Cestan and Lejonne but it is rare and only about 200 cases have been described in about 30 families (Emery 1989; Shapiro and Specht 1991). The lower limbs are affected more than the upper limbs but less than 10% of cases lose the ability to walk. Survival into middle age is usual unless cardiomyopathy intervenes and sudden death occurs (Case Records 34–1992). Calf hypertrophy is not a feature and there is no mental impairment. Sudden death occurred in 30 of 73 cases reviewed by Merlini et al. (1986) but this can probably be prevented by regular cardiac assessment and insertion of a ventricular demand pacemaker. Atrial fibrillation and atrioventricular conduction block are the main features (Waters et al. 1975; Hara et al. 1987). In some cases, however, ventricular dysfunction develops leading to cardiac failure (Bialer et al. 1991) and cardiac transplantation has been reported (see Chap. 21). The blood CK level is moderately raised (Emery 1989) and the EMG shows myopathic features with some spontaneous activity (Cruz-Martinez and Dutheil 1989). The muscle biopsy shows Type 1 atrophy in mildly affected muscles, often with Type 2 fibre predominance. In more severe cases there is a dystrophic appearance with fibre degeneration and muscle fibrosis. Dystrophin immunolocalisation is normal (Hoffman et al. 1988). Some biopsies show atrophic, dark fibres, with features suggesting fibre-type grouping. The disorder has been localised to the Xq27.3-q28 locus, close to the loci for red–green colour blindness and for factor VIII coagulation deficiency (Cole et al. 1992). The defective protein product of this locus is called emerin. Some cases exhibiting autosomal dominant inheritance have been reported (Miller et al. 1985). Neurogenic features are more prominent in these dominantly inherited cases.

Carriers are generally asymptomatic with a normal CK level but they are at a high risk of cardiac complication with advancing age. They should undergo careful cardiac monitoring (Merlini et al. 1986).

X-Linked Myotobular Myopathy

This X-linked disorder is similar to centronuclear myopathy but presents a more severe clinical syndrome. It is described in Chap. 16.

Limb-Girdle Muscular Dystrophy

The term limb-girdle muscular dystrophy was introduced by Walton and Nattrass (1954) in a study of 105 cases of muscular dystrophy in North-East England. They recognised that the earlier classification of pelvi-femoral muscular atrophy (Leyden-Möbius type), scapulo-humeral onset myopathies (Erb's type) and late-onset myopathy was complex and difficult to utilize in clinical practice. They proposed that facio-scapulo-humeral muscular dystrophy was a separate clinical entity but that the remaining syndromes should be grouped together as forming a recognisable clinical syndrome. However, it was recognised in subsequent studies that the clinical syndrome of limb-girdle muscular dystrophy did not represent a single nosological entity but rather comprised a number of different disorders with similar clinical presentations (Munsat 1977). A simple classification of these syndromes (Table 14.5) is that of Jerusalem and Steb (1992). The severe childhood onset auto-

Table 14.5. Clinical classification of limb-girdle syndromes

1. Autosomal-recessive muscular dystrophy of childhood
   Pelvi-femoral type (Leyden–Möbius)
   Scapulo-humeral type (Erb)
   Bethlem myopathy
   Rigid spine syndrome
   Severe childhood form

2. Autosomal-dominant early-onset type with contractures (Bethlem type)
   Autosomal-dominant late-onset type (Nevin)

3. Limb-girdle syndromes of defined cause

Muscular dystrophies are separately classified (see below).
After Jerusalem and Steb (1992).

somal recessive muscular dystrophy (SCARMD) syndromes are sub-classified by their chromosomal locus, and by the feature of primary or secondary adhalin deficiency (Table 14.2). The clinical phenotype of these syndromes (LGMD types 2c and 2D) are variable.

The Clinical Syndromes

Limb-girdle muscular dystrophy usually presents in the second or third decade, although the onset may be delayed until middle life. Both sexes are equally affected. It consists of progressive muscular weakness and atrophy, usually first apparent in the pelvic girdle musculature (Walton and Nattrass 1954). The weakness and wasting is often asymmetrical initially and the rate of progression is variable from case to case. In some patients the disease may apparently become arrested but most patients become unable to walk about 20 years after the onset of the disease. Contractures may then occur. Pelvi-femoral myopathy was recognised in natives of Berne, Switzerland, and in their Amish and Hutterite kindred in North America (Shokeir and Kobrinsky 1976). The prognosis is generally similar in cases beginning early or later in life. Skeletal deformities, even in the advanced stages of the disease, are unusual. Pseudohypertrophy occurs in some patients. Certain proximal muscles, especially biceps and periscapular muscles in the upper limbs, may show striking atrophy at a stage when other muscles are relatively less severely affected. Muscle cramps are not a feature of the disorder but skeletal pain, presumably resulting from weakness of axial muscles, is common. Although the cranial muscles are typically spared, there may be mild bilateral facial weakness. The tendon reflexes are usually present, but may be difficult to elicit; however, the triceps reflex is usually relatively brisk. Life expectancy is slightly reduced. Death may occur from pulmonary complications in those with involvement of respiratory muscles. The prognosis is probably somewhat better in patients presenting with shoulder-girdle weakness. Cardiomyopathy, however, is not a feature of this syndrome, and intelligence is normal.

The incidence of limb-girdle dystrophy is uncertain, perhaps because of difficulties in diagnosis and thus of case ascertainment, but Morton et al. (1963) estimated that the incidence was 6.5/100 000. This estimate may err on the high side, and Gardner-Medwin et al. (1971) suggested an incidence of less than 1/100 000. Yates and Emery (1985) reported a prevalence of 3/million for the adult-onset form of limb-girdle muscular dystrophy, consisting of 11 subjects in only 10 families in Scotland. In Denmark Leth et al. (1985) found a prevalence of 36.5/million, but included all age ranges on their population. Panegyres et al. (1990) in a review of 33 patients noted that 18 had a slowly progressive symmetrical proximal limb weakness with elevated CK, abnormal muscle biopsy and myopathic EMG findings. The remaining patients included a group with facial weakness and a group with distal involvement. Although it has been suggested that limb-girdle dystrophy is not a definite entity (see Munsat 1977), this view is not supported by the recent clinical investigations which suggests a number of underlying genetic syndromes. It is important to exclude cases in which a recognisable disorder is present, for example late-onset glycogenosis, periodic paralysis and mitochondrial disorders.

In recent years it has become increasingly apparent that many cases formerly classified by their clinical, electromyographic and pathological features as limb-girdle muscular dystrophy were misdiagnosed and that many, perhaps more than half, of the patients were in fact suffering from chronic spinal muscular atrophy of juvenile onset (Kugelberg–Welander disease) or adult-onset (Mastaglia and Walton 1971a,b; Tomlinson et al. 1974). The clinical features of spinal muscular atrophy and of limb-girdle muscular dystrophy may be very similar and unless careful EMG and histological studies, including enzyme histochemical stains, are made the two disorders may be virtually indistinguishable. The presence of cramps and of action or post-exercise fasciculations in patients with spinal muscular atrophy are important diagnostic points.

In the younger patients Becker muscular dystrophy, or manifesting carriers of Duchenne muscular dystrophy (Jerusalem and Steb 1992) may be difficult to exclude, particularly if calf muscle hypertrophy is a feature. In some cases the differentiation can be made by the genetic background since Becker muscular dystrophy is inherited as an X-linked disorder. The muscle biopsy and CK level may also be useful (see below).

Laboratory Investigations

The CK level is moderately increased; it is rarely as high as 10 times the normal range (Panegyres et al. 1990; Jerusalem and Steb 1992). Blood lactic dehydrogenase levels may also be raised. There are no specific biochemical abnormalities and no association with other biochemical disorders has been noted.

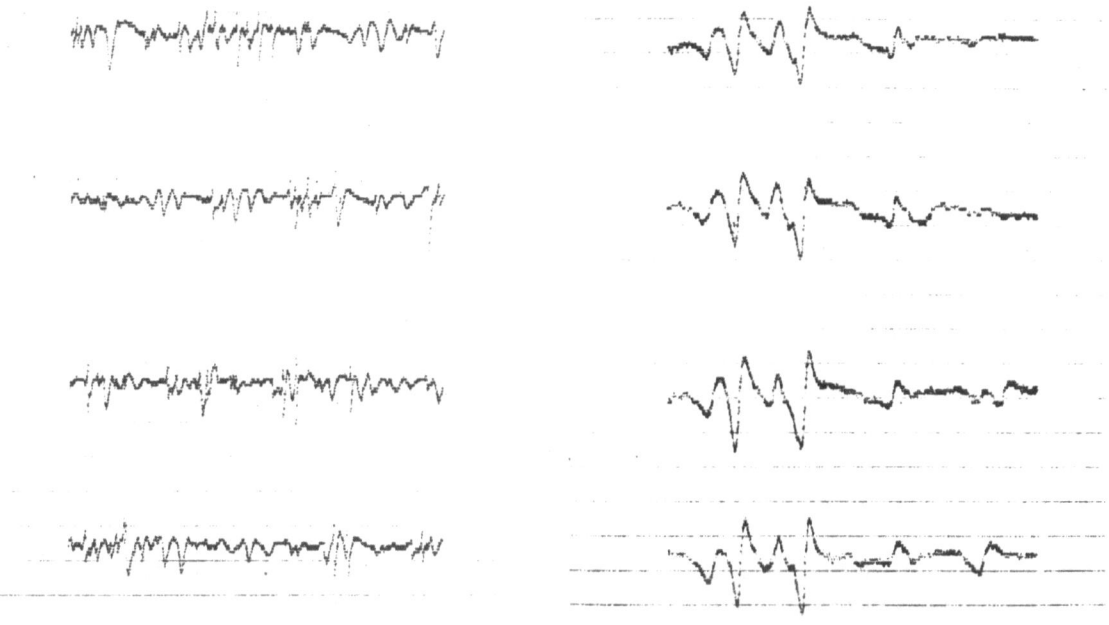

Fig. 14.16. Limb-girdle muscular dystrophy: concentric needle EMG recording of maximal voluntary activity. The interference pattern is full. A number of short-duration units can be recognised, and the maximal amplitude is 1 mV. Filters: 100 Hz and 10 kHz. Bar 20 ms.

Fig. 14.17. Limb-girdle muscular dystrophy: a complex motor unit action potential of long duration (10 ms). Note that without the use of the delay line the early components of this potential would not be recognised. Concentric needle EMG. Filters: 500 Hz and 10 kHz. Bar 2 ms.

Electrophysiological Assessment

There are no specific EMG features. Concentric needle EMG reveals typical myopathic short-duration polyphasic MUAPs of low amplitude (Fig. 14.16), often with a full interference pattern. Complex repetitive discharges may be present, but myotonia is absent and fibrillation potentials are sometimes recorded (Lang and Partanen 1976). These myopathic abnormalities are usually most prominent in the more severely affected proximal muscles (Fig. 14.17). In some patients, particularly those with distal involvement, a mixed myopathic and neurogenic pattern may be found (Panegyres et al. 1990).

With single-fibre EMG the neuromuscular jitter may be increased in some motor units, although it is usually normal. Some motor unit potentials may show an abnormally low jitter (<5 μs), a finding thought to represent recordings from split fibres. Impulse blocking is uncommon. The fibre density is increased in weak muscles and late potentials are sometimes recorded. Stålberg et al. (1974) found a mean fibre density of 2.1 in the extensor digitorum communis and 1.9 in biceps brachii (Stålberg 1977). These fibre density values are much smaller than those recorded in the X-linked muscular dys-

trophies, and in the spinal muscular atrophies, the main area of diagnostic difficulty (Shields 1984). Nerve conduction velocity studies are normal (Hayward 1980).

Muscle Biopsy

Muscle biopsy shows the general features of a myopathy; indeed limb-girdle muscular dystrophy shows no characteristic histological features (Schmalbruch 1992). There is often considerable variation in fibre size with very hypertrophied fibres, even up to 200 μm or more, and small fibres. Internal nuclei are prominent, especially in the hypertrophied fibres, and fibre splitting is seen in some fibres, especially in more severely involved muscles and in the later stages of the disease (Dubowitz and Brooke 1973). Degenerative and regenerative changes are common, both necrotic fibres and, less commonly, basophilic fibres being seen in the biopsy (Fig. 14.18). Ring fibres are also commonly seen, perhaps as a manifestation of mechanical injury to fibres resulting in fracture of peripheral myofibrils. Sarcoplasmic masses are usually found in such fibres. Later in the course of the disease, fibre splitting and fibrosis are more

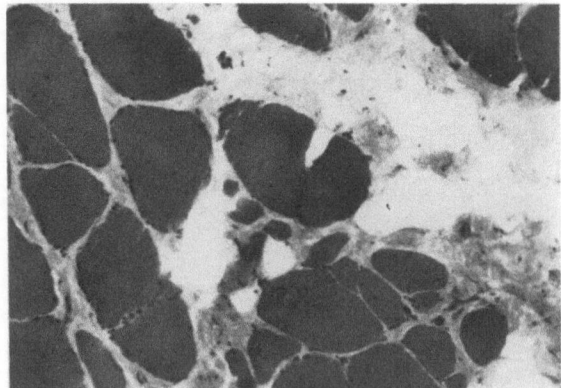

Fig. 14.18. Limb-girdle muscular dystrophy. H and E, × 180. There is fibrosis and fibre splitting is prominent.

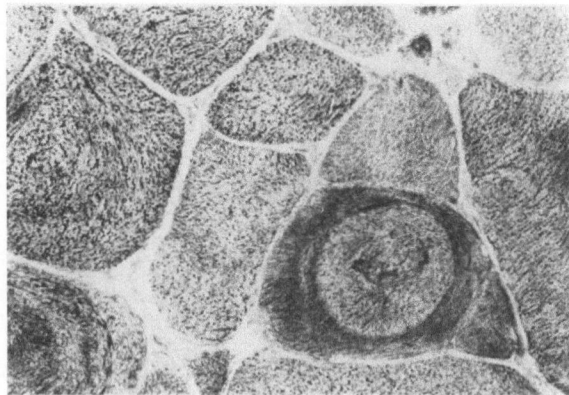

Fig. 14.19. Limb-girdle muscular dystrophy: whorled fibres. NADH, × 500.

prominent. Fibre splitting is usually found in relation to centrally situated muscle nuclei as in other disorders in which this phenomenon occurs (Schwartz et al. 1976a; Swash and Schwartz 1977). With enzyme histochemical stains whorled fibres are seen, especially in the NADH-tr preparation (Fig. 14.19) and fibre splitting may be seen to result in clusters of small fibres of similar histochemical type (see Dubowitz and Brooke 1973; Swash and Schwartz 1977). In some fibres vacuoles which appear red in Gomori preparations may be seen. A recessive form of limb-girdle dystrophy with rimmed vacuoles resembling inclusion body myositis has been reported (Argov and Yarom 1984), a disorder which clinically has features that resemble scapulo-peroneal dystrophy.

All fibre types show atrophy and hypertrophy (Dubowitz and Brooke 1973). Fibre-type grouping is not a feature of the disorder. Further, small pointed NADH-dark fibres are not commonly seen, except in the late stages. These probably represent failed reinnervation of split fibre fragments (Schwartz et al. 1976a; Schmalbruch 1992). The absence of these features is important since it represents the most useful histological feature by which chronic limb-girdle dystrophy can be distinguished from chronic spinal muscular atrophy, in which secondary myopathic features may be so prominent as to lead to diagnostic confusion (see Schwartz et al. 1976a). In the earliest stages the biopsy may only show increased variability in fibre size, with increased central nucleation and fibre splitting. Later a dystrophic pattern emerges, with giant fibres and hyalinised and necrotic fibres.

Ultrastructural studies reveal a variety of morphological changes including myofibrillar abnormalities, myelin fibres and other lipid filled vacuoles, degenerative changes in mitochondria, enlargement of nuclei and evidence of regenerative activity. The basal lamina may be redundant or reduplicated. Dystrophin immunostaining is important, especially in sporadic cases, in order to recognise Becker dystrophy and manifesting female carriers of Duchenne muscular dystrophy.

Histological studies are important and should always be carried out as part of the diagnostic evaluation in order to exclude other specific, biochemical or morphological disorders which might also present with proximal weakness.

The pattern of innervation has been little studied in limb-girdle dystrophy. Coërs and Woolf (1959) found evidence of sprouting occurring terminally and subterminally in motor end-plates but reported that the functional terminal innervation ratio was normal, a finding indicating the absence of more proximal axonal sprouting.

Differential Diagnosis

Diagnosis depends on the exclusion of other disorders, particularly those disorders such as chronic spinal muscular atrophy and Becker X-linked recessive muscular dystrophy which might easily be confused with limb-girdle muscular dystrophy. Since limb-girdle muscular dystrophy is essentially a syndrome, probably heterogeneous in aetiology, it must be recognised that in the future a variety of causes will be found important and so the syndrome will become less of an enigma. Glycogenosis, especially acid maltase deficiency, muscle carnitine deficiency and polymyositis, must all be excluded and the combination of clinical assessment, CK estimation and EMG and muscle biopsy is thus important in all such cases. It is, of course, particularly important to exclude polymyositis since effective treatment is available for this condition (see Chap. 13). Clinically overt cardiomyopathy is not a feature of typical limb-girdle muscular dystrophy.

Management

The management of patients with limb-girdle muscular dystrophy is symptomatic. Simple measures, such as physiotherapy and attention to the provision of aids to daily living, such as a wheelchair when appropriate, are all important in alleviating disability when this becomes severe. No specific treatment for the disorder itself is available. In some patients there is early and severe diaphragmatic involvement resulting in alveolar hypoventilation with morning headache, somnolence or confusion. Assisted ventilation at night is useful in relieving these symptoms.

Genetic counselling is difficult because of the frequency of sporadic cases. CK estimation in unaffected family members does not provide evidence about the carrier state in this disorder and there is thus no reliable method available for carrier detection. In many cases autosomal recessive inheritance may be suspected, as has been documented in Amish and Hutterite communities (Shokeir and Kobrinsky 1976) and in a form of the disease affecting children in Tunisia (Ben-Hamida et al. 1983). Dominant inheritance has also been described but this is uncommon (Bethlem and van Wijngaarden 1976). Chromosomal loci for some of these syndromes are recognised (see Table 14.2 and below). If X-linked inheritance is recognised or possible, e.g. in sporadic male cases, a dystrophinopathy should be suspected.

Distinctive Clinical Types of Limb-Girdle Muscular Dystrophy

The different types that have been recognised are listed in Table 14.4.

Leyden–Möbius Pelvi-Femoral Myopathy

This was the first-recognised syndrome. The disorder is sporadic, only 20% of cases having a family history of the disease. Muscle weakness begins in the second decade in the pelvic girdle muscles and slowly progresses, later involving the upper limbs but not the face. Mobility is impaired, but walking may still be possible 20 years after the onset. In some patients the disease seems to arrest.

There is wasting of affected muscles. The CK is about six times normal (Shields 1986). Older accounts of the disease, e.g. Jackson and Strehler (1968); Bradley (1979), are difficult to interpret since some of these phenotypes probably resulted from spinal muscular atrophy. Some of these cases may represent LGMD Type 2B, localised to chromosome 2 p 13.3 (Bashis et al. 1994).

Erb's Scapulo-Humeral Myopathy

This disorder consists of a progressive syndrome of weakness and wasting affecting peri-scapular, shoulder-girdle and humeral muscles but often sparing deltoids, sternomastoids and intraspinati. The face is only rarely involved and then only very mildly, a feature separating this disorder from facio-scapulo-humeral muscular dystrophy. Frequently, scapulo-humeral myopathy also involves pelvic girdle musculature as the disease progresses. The disorder is autosomal recessive in inheritance and begins at any age from childhood to the fourth decade. There is little disability until late in the course.

Late-Onset Dominant Limb-Girdle Dystrophy (LGMD-IA)

This syndrome (Table 14.2) is a slowly progressive disorder, generally affecting pelvic more than upper limb girdle muscles. The disorder begins in the third or fourth decade. Facial muscles are spared. Families with this disorder have been described by Henson et al. (1967), Schneiderman et al. (1969) and Marconi et al. (1991). Cases limited to women (Henson et al. 1967; Swash et al. 1970) or men (DeCoster et al. 1974) have been described, all with autosomal dominant transmission. The CK is only slightly raised. In a number of reports rimmed vacuoles have been described, a feature resembling inclusion body myositis (see Chap. 13). CT scans have showed progressive loss of muscle tissue in the posterior compartment of the leg, with relative preservation of the anterior compartment, during an 8-year period (Marconi et al. 1991).

Autosomal Dominant, Early-Onset Type with Contractures (Bethlem Myopathy)

The disease begins in infancy or early childhood with limb-girdle muscle weakness (Bethlem and van Wijngaarden 1976) of slow progression. There are contractures of fingers, elbows and ankles. Life expectancy is normal and most patients can live a relatively normal life. There is no cardiac involve-

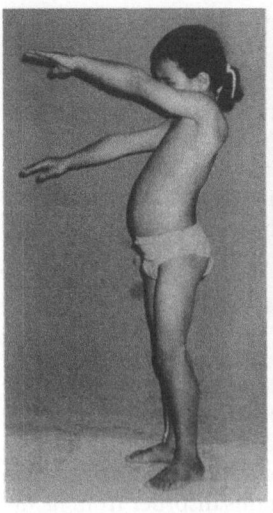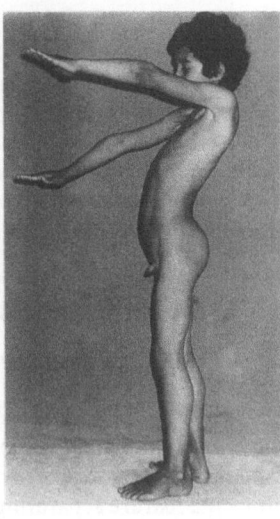

Fig. 14.20. Autosomal recessive muscular dystrophy of childhood. This Tunisian brother and sister have a severe muscular dystrophy syndrome associated with deficiency of the cytoskeletal protein adhalin, a member of the dystrophin-associated membrane glycoprotein group. (Illustration kindly supplied by Dr. F. Hentati; Tunis.)

ment. Although first reported in three Dutch families, cases have been reported in other countries, including French Canada (Mohire et al. 1988). The disorder is inherited as an autosomal dominant trait probably on chromosome 21q, at the telomeric region. Muscle biopsies in this benign syndrome show increased variation in fibre size and increased central nucleation with some fibre splitting and giant fibres, but no necrosis or regeneration and no neurogenic features (Mohire et al. 1988).

Rigid Spine Syndrome

In 1965 Dubowitz described a syndrome of proximal muscle weakness beginning in infancy or early childhood, mainly affecting boys and progressing over a period of several years with gradually increasing limitation of flexion of the neck and trunk, leading to rigidity of the spine, scoliosis, forward tilting of the trunk and hyperextension of the neck. The sternomastoids, pelvic girdle and pectoral girdle muscles are weak and there may be a cardiomyopathy with complete heart block and ventricular hypertrophy in some cases (Dubowitz 1965; Goebel et al. 1977). Poewe et al. (1985) reported four cases and reviewed the 18 cases in the literature to that date. Fourteen were male. All had contractures of the spine, 14 had scoliosis, five had cardiomyopathy and five had restricted ventilation. The CK was increased to no more than six times normal in 14 cases. The EMG was myopathic and the biopsy

showed increased variation in fibre size with increased central nucleation and frequent small atrophic fibres. Proliferation of fibrous tissue was prominent and Type 2 fibre predominance was usually present, sometimes with Type 1 fibre atrophy (Goebel et al. 1977). Death may occur before age 30 years from right heart failure. This syndrome has some clinical similarity to Emery–Dreifuss syndrome (Mohire et al. 1988), but is sporadic without a clear pattern of inheritance.

Autosomal Recessive Muscular Dystrophy of Childhood

A severe progressive muscular dystrophy of childhood onset (Table 14.2), usually between 3 and 12 years of age, that resembles Duchenne muscular dystrophy, (Fig. 14.20) was first reported in 93 children from the Maghreb in Tunisia by Ben Hamida et al. (1983). Hypertrophy of the calf muscles is a frequent feature in the early stages and the triceps brachii are also sometimes hypertrophied. Later, weak muscles become atrophic. In the early stages the CK is as high as 4000–10 000 IU/l. The disease differs strikingly from Duchenne dystrophy in that it occurs equally in both sexes, is often associated with parental consanguinity and is not associated with intellectual impairment. Survival is variable, walking ability being lost as early as age 12 years or as late as the fourth decade. Survival into the seventh decade has been noted. The later the onset the slower the progression, and the lower the CK levels. Cardiac involvement, if it occurs, is subclinical. In some cases the clinical syndrome is benign.

The muscle biopsy shows marked myopathic change, with fibre atrophy and hypertrophy, fibre-splitting, Type 1 fibre predominance. Most Type 2 fibres were Type 2A. No hyaline fibre change was observed (Ben Hamida et al. 1983). Clusters of necrotic fibres were seen. Dystrophin is expressed normally in muscle fibre membranes, but there is a deficiency of the 50 kDa dystrophin-associated membrane glycoprotein, called adhalin after the Arabic word for muscles, in this disorder (Matsumura et al. 1992). Autopsy studies showed normal spinal cord and motor neurons (Ben Hamida and Hentati 1989).

Shields (1986) noted that this autosomal recessive form of muscular dystrophy in Tunisia was probably identical with the syndrome reported in 37 patients in two Amish kindreds by Jackson and Strehler (1968). However, most Amish patients are linked to chromosome 15 (Table 14.2): some of these show adhalin deficiency (Workshop 1995). A similar disorder has been reported in other parts of North Africa (Salih et al. 1983; Faraq and Teebi 1990) and it is possible that some cases of Duchenne-like dystrophy reported in females also represent this syndrome (Gardner-Medwin and Johnstone 1984). Tomé (Workshop 1995) has investigated biopsies from 66 cases, 30 of which were European patients of Mediterranean origin. Adhalin deficiency may be primary (LGMD 2D), or secondary to another membrane disorder (LGMD 2C). Othmane et al. (1992) linked the syndrome to the pericentric region of chromosome 13q. This genotype is associated with secondary adhalin deficiency. In the cases with primary adhalin deficiency there is linkage to chromosome 17q 21. Further heterogeneity is suggested by cases of adhalin deficiency not linked to chromosome 13 or 17.

The incidence in certain regions of Tunisia may be as high as 7/100 000 births (Ben Hamida et al. 1983).

Congenital Muscular Dystrophy

The term congenital muscular dystrophy is used to describe a heterogeneous group of disorders, some of which are progressive, others non-progressive and yet others severe and fatal. The term was introduced to describe a muscular syndrome presenting at birth with weakness of limb, trunk and facial muscles, hypotonia and joint deformities (Banker et al. 1957; Rotthauwe et al. 1969; Donner et al. 1975; Fig. 14.21). The concept that muscular dystrophy could present as arthrogryposis multiplex congenita seems to derive from Batten (1903). The term congenital muscular dystrophy was introduced by Howard (1908). Arthrogryposis congenita multiplex is a syndrome that may result from myopathic or neurogenic disease (Banker et al. 1957). For example, cases of meningomyelocele, myotonic dystrophy and fibre type dysproportion have been cited (see Banker et al. 1957) as causes. However, this term has now largely been superseded by the term congenital muscular dystrophy, and joint deformities resulting from congenital nervous system malformations are recognised by their underlying cause.

In the *benign type*, often referred to as the Batten–Turner type (Turner and Lees 1962), there is flaccid weakness from birth, with a non-progressive course. The CK is usually normal, and the EMG shows myopathic changes. The hypotonia improves with age but mild proximal weakness develops with contractures of fingers and wrists. One such family

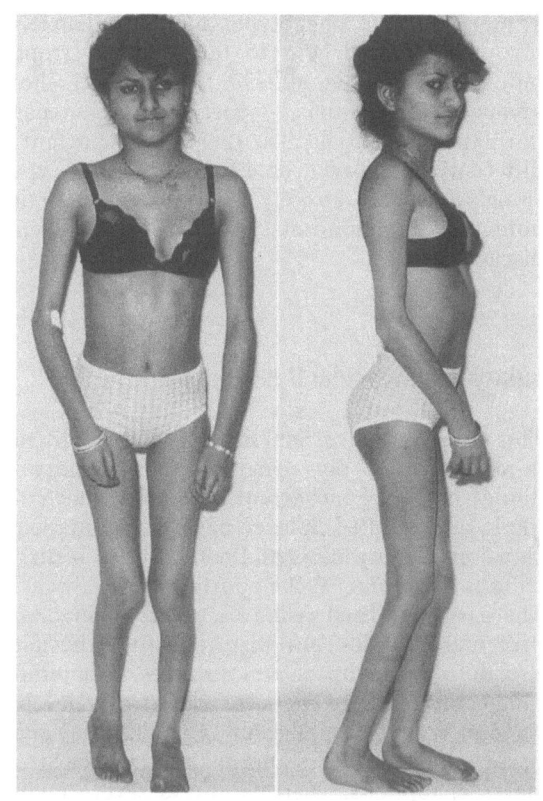

Fig. 14.21. Congenital muscular dystrophy with joint contracture. The disorder was present at birth, and is relatively non-progressive.

has been described in a Palestinian family in Israel (Mahjneh et al. 1992). In these cases merosin distribution in muscles fibres is normal (Philpot et al. 1995).

Merosin Deficiency Myopathy (Table 14.2)

Merosin is an extra-cellular matrix protein, the subunit of laminin. In merosin deficiency congenital muscular dystrophy there is severe congenital weakness, with inability to walk unsupported. In some cases the disorder is life-threatening (Zellweger et al. 1992). There are contractures, and MR scans of the brain show abnormal cerebral white matter, with sparing of the basal ganglia and cerebellum. The mental status, however, is normal. The CK is increased to 1000–2000 IU/l. The disorder has been mapped to chromosome 6q2 (Hillaire et al. 1994). The muscle biopsy shows variation in fibre size, increased endometrial fibrous tissue and a few necrotic fibres (Tomé et al. 1994). Congenital muscular dystrophy without merosin deficiency has a more benign phenotype. Merosin deficiency myopathy is analagous to the dy/dx dystrophic mouse (Asahata et al. 1993). The EMG shows myopathic potentials, sometimes with sparse fibrillation potentials: it is therefore important to differentiate this syndrome from Type 1 or Type 2 spinal muscular atrophy. Sensory nerve action potentials are abnormal in merosin deficiency disease.

Fukuyama Muscular Dystrophy

This is a progressive, fatal muscular dystrophy that is often evident in utero by the presence of diminished fetal movements. About a quarter of mothers of affected children have had spontaneous abortions (Fukuyama et al. 1960; 1981). At birth the child is hypotonic, sucks poorly and cries weakly. There is generalised weakness, especially involving proximal muscles but also affecting the face. Pseudohypertrophy of calf muscles is common. Mild contractures of knees and elbows may develop. Tendon reflexes are absent. Generalised seizures occur in half the cases and death may occur from status epilepticus. There is always severe mental retardation and all milestones are delayed. Only a small proportion of affected children ever stand or take a few steps and death usually occurs by age 10 years. CT brain scans show a paucity of cerebral gyri, with ventricular dilatation and decreased white matter density (Kamoshita et al. 1976). In Japan this disorder is second to Duchenne dystrophy in incidence (2 : 1) affecting one in every 18 000 young people (Takeshita et al. 1977). The disorder has been linked to chromosome 9q 31–33 (Toda et al. 1993).

The CK is raised, 10–50 times above normal. The cholesterol is elevated. There may be myoglobinuria.

Pathology

In the CNS there are neuronal heterotopias with polymicrogyria and lissencephaly. The abnormalities involve cerebral hemispheres and, particularly, the cerebellum. The cerebral white matter volume is reduced with ventricular enlargement. In skeletal muscle there are dystrophic changes with rounded fibres and prominent proliferation of connective tissue. Muscle fibre necrosis is prominent and some inflammatory cell infiltrates are present associated with this. Type 1 fibre predominance may be present and there is often an excess of Type 2c fibres.

Expression of dystrophin in skeletal muscle fibres is normal or near-normal (Matsumura et al. 1993); a few muscle fibres show reduced and patchy staining. There is a marked reduction in the amount of dystrophin-associated glycoproteins (DAG) present in the muscle, especially of the 43 kDa DAG (Matsumura et al. 1993). This failure of expression of DAGs in muscle cell membranes and also in the brain is a common feature of Duchenne muscular dystrophy, severe autosomal recessive childhood onset muscular dystrophy and Fukuyama muscular dystrophy (Beggs et al. 1992; Matsumura et al. 1993; Ohlendieck et al. 1993). Thus these disorders are all associated with membrane disturbances.

Congenital Myopathy with Abnormal Accumulation of Desmin

A number of families have been described in which a congenital myopathy, presenting at birth with hypotonia and weakness and with subsequent delayed motor milestones or increasing weakness, develops. In these cases muscle biopsy has shown sarcoplasmic accumulation of desmin intermediate filaments (Fardeau et al. 1978; Pellissier et al. 1989; Prelle et al. 1992). The biopsy shows subsarcolemmal eosinophilic material which contains intermediate filaments at electron microscopic examination. Western blot studies and immunocytochemistry has revealed that these filaments are desmin and that, in one case, this was associated with co-storage of dystrophin. This co-storage suggests that these two proteins, both structurally related to α-actinin, are in close structural and functional relationship to each other (Prelle et al. 1992).

Facio-Scapulo-Humeral Muscular Dystrophy

A slowly progressive form of muscular dystrophy, facio-scapulo-humeral muscular dystrophy is usually first recognised in the first or second decade of life. The classical description of the clinical features is that of Landouzy and Déjérine (1885), after whose names the disease is sometimes known. Morton et al. (1963) thought it an uncommon disorder but most clinical studies have revealed a prevalence of 1 in 20 000 (Lunt and Harper 1991). It is inherited as an autosomal dominant trait located on the distal part of the long arm of chromosome 4 (Wijmenga et al. 1990). Weiffenbach et al. (1992)

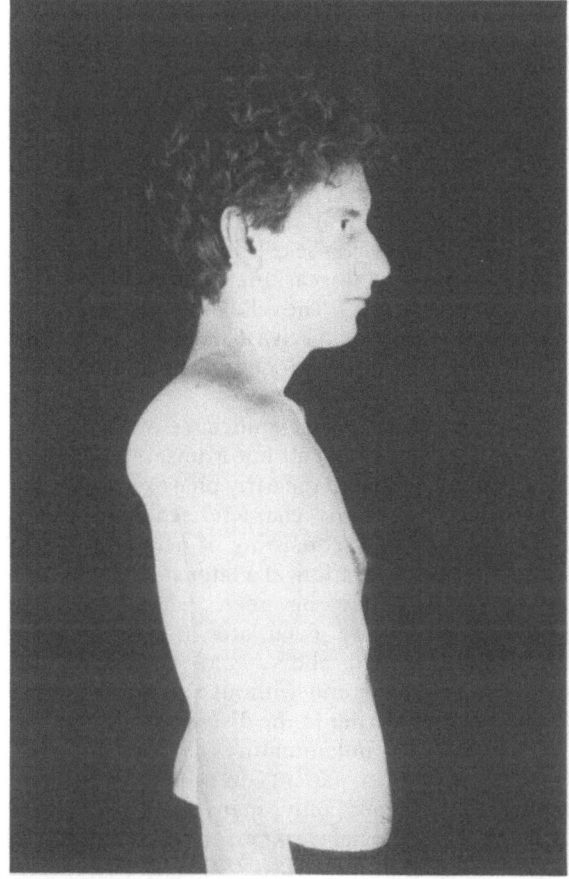

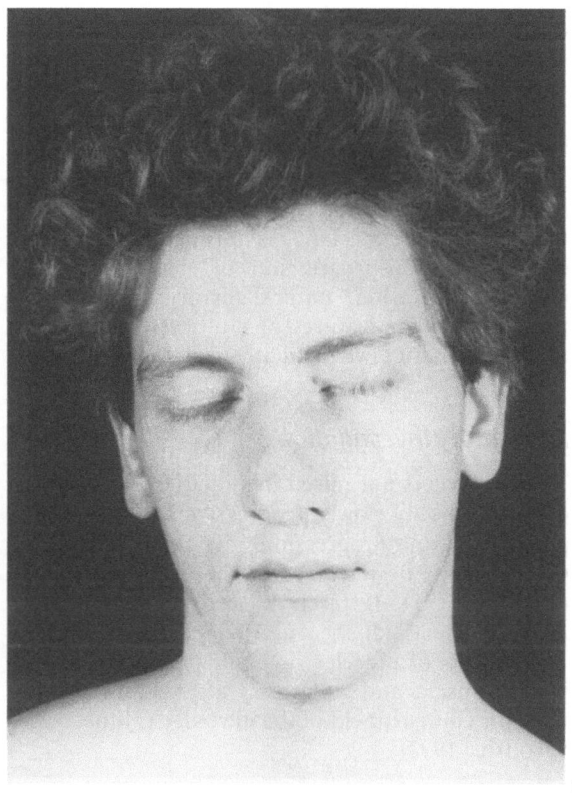

a

b

Fig. 14.22. Facio-scapulo-humeral muscular dystrophy. There is **a** scapular winging and atrophy of the humeral muscles, and **b** weakness of facial muscles, including eye closure.

localised the gene more precisely to 4q35. There is a wide spectrum of clinical presentation between and within families and even in monozygotic twins (Tawil et al. 1993). There is evidence for anticipation and an association of deletion size and severity has been reported (Tawil et al. 1996). In the classical form, which is the most common, weakness begins simultaneously in the face and in the shoulder-girdle musculature before the third decade. As in limb-girdle dystrophy the biceps brachii and periscapular muscles are particularly severely involved (Fig. 14.22). Facial weakness is insidious in onset and the patient usually notices difficulty in whistling or using a straw before weakness of eye closure becomes apparent. The pelvic muscles are involved somewhat later and weakness of anterior tibial muscles is particularly characteristic, with a resultant footdrop. The combination of pelvic girdle weakness and footdrop produces a characteristic gait disorder. The weakness is usually symmetrical and it is accompanied by wasting of the weakened muscles. Pseudohypertrophy is not a feature of the disease but relatively uninvolved muscles, for example the

anterior deltoid muscles, may appear hypertrophied. The sternal head of the pectoralis major muscle is almost invariably severely involved giving an unusual upward-curving fold to the anterior axillary line. The shoulder-girdle weakness weakens scapular fixation so that during arm abduction and elevation the scapulae ride upwards and may even become visible anteriorly. The trapezius and posterior neck muscles are spared. The tendon reflexes are usually diminished early in the disease. There is often a very pronounced lumbar lordosis.

A variant of the disorder is a form noted by Landouzy and Déjérine (1885) in their original description, in which facial involvement may be apparent in childhood without weakness of other muscles until middle age. Further, subclinical cases, in which facial weakness is evident with only minimal weakness of the limb muscles, are common in relatives of patients with the established form of the disease. A variety of muscular dystrophy in a facio-scapulo-humeral distribution is found in infancy, usually in the first 2 years of life, in which there is severe limb weakness; it has been regarded as a variant of facio-scapulo-humeral muscular dystrophy as one or other of the parents usually shows signs of mild weakness in the same distribution. However, in these infantile cases the disorder is a serious one; mobility is often lost by the age of 10 years (Hanson and Rowland 1971; Brooke 1977). The classical form of facio-scapulo-humeral dystrophy, on the other hand, is relatively benign and life expectancy is normal in most cases. Periods of non-progression of the disease are common in its long natural history. Cardiomyopathy and other features of multisystem involvement are absent (Tyler and Stephens 1950).

Laboratory Investigations

The CK level is not raised in all patients. Since the disorder is only slowly progressive and may show periods without progression, it is possible that the CK may only be raised when the disease is active (Hughes 1971). It rarely exceeds five times the normal value (Padberg et al. 1991).

CT scans of muscles reveal hypertrophy of the psoas muscle and decreased attenuation of the anterior compartment of the lower leg (Munsat and Serratrice 1992).

Electrophysiological Assessment

The findings with concentric needle EMG are somewhat variable. Fibrillation potentials are not uncommonly found and pseudo-myotonic bursts may be recorded. During voluntary activation typical myopathic MUAPs are usually seen but in some patients large units and a reduced interference pattern, suggestive of a neurogenic disorder, may be found (Munsat et al. 1972). With single-fibre EMG the motor unit fibre density was normal in biceps brachii, a severely involved muscle, in three patients studied by Stålberg (1977) but this result requires further investigation since an increase in fibre density would be expected in a severely involved muscle, particularly in a disorder in which large units can be recorded with concentric needle EMG.

Muscle Biopsy

Muscle biopsy shows an increased variability in fibre size, but there are many hypertrophied fibres and the mean fibre diameter may be increased. Atrophic fibres are less prominent but small angular fibres, strongly reactive in oxidative enzyme techniques, are frequently seen. Central nucleation and fibre splitting are uncommon in this disease and other muscle-fibre degenerative changes are

also infrequent. Moth-eaten and whorled-fibre change may be seen in some fibres, often particularly in Type 1 fibres (Dubowitz and Brooke 1973). Van Wijngaarden and Bethlem (1971) reported lobulated fibres, consisting of peripheral zones of reorganisation of the intermyofibrillar network, in some cases but this feature is not specific for facio-scapulo-humeral myopathy. A striking cellular response consisting of lymphocytes, macrophages and occasional plasma cells is a feature of some cases. The cellular response is found in an interfascicular, perivascular and endomysial location and it may appear densely nodular (Munsat et al. 1972).

Interpretation of the significance of the inflammatory change is difficult but Munsat et al. (1972) have suggested that in the early phase of the disease the muscle biopsy is characterised by minimal myopathic changes consisting of necrosis, phagocytosis and regeneration; at a later stage inflammatory changes may be seen with prominent regenerative activity. Even later, the more typical features, described above, may be found with increasing fibrosis and without the inflammatory changes found earlier in the disease. Brooke (1977) has noted that inflammatory changes are particularly found in patients in whom limb-girdle weakness develops only many years after the development of facial weakness. However, the cases reported by Munsat et al. (1972) were all younger than 25 years. Another interpretation of inflammatory changes is that the patients were suffering from a chronic form of polymyositis, a possibility excluded by the family history in two of the cases studied by Munsat et al. (1972), although van Wijngaarden and Bethlem (1971) have noted that weakness in a facio-scapulo-humeral distribution may occur in a number of other neuromuscular disorders.

Differential Diagnosis

Weakness in a facio-scapulo-humeral distribution may occur not only in facio-scapulo-humeral muscular dystrophy itself but in a number of other disorders. These include cases of limb-girdle muscular dystrophy and spinal muscular atrophy in which mild facial weakness may occur and in which inheritance may also be dominant (Fenichel et al. 1967), polymyositis (Rothstein et al. 1971; Bates et al. 1973), myasthenia gravis, myotubular myopathy, nemaline myopathy, central core disease and mitochondrial myopathy (van Wijngaarden and Bethlem 1971). These disorders may be recognised to some extent by their clinical features or their mode of onset and by the presence or absence of a family history, but other investigations including EMG and muscle biopsy may be necessary.

In patients in whom the clinical syndrome of facio-scapulo-humeral weakness is incomplete, diagnosis may be very difficult and confusion with limb-girdle dystrophy or with scapulo-peroneal dystrophy is especially likely to occur. The extensor digitorum brevis muscle may be spared both in facio-scapulo-humeral muscular dystrophy and in scapulo-peroneal muscular dystrophy and the two disorders are probably closely related, if indeed, they are not variations of the same disorder (Serratrice et al. 1969).

Management

The disorder is generally only slowly progressive and functional disability is often not severe. Patients usually learn a variety of compensatory or trick movements which enable them to remain independent and able to care for themselves even when weakness of some muscle groups, for example biceps, periscapular and tibialis anterior muscles, is very severe. In those patients in whom inflammatory changes are present in the muscle biopsy it might be thought that steroid therapy would be helpful. Prednisone has been tried in such patients without clinical benefit other than short-term improvement, although in one study the CK level progressively decreased during the 4 months of treatment (Munsat et al. 1972; Munsat and Bradley 1977). Steroid treatment therefore is not indicated. External bracing to improve footdrop and to stabilise weakened spinal muscles may be useful, but only light appliances can be used because of the severe proximal weakness (Siegel 1977). Surgical fixation of the scapula to the rib cage may improve shoulder elevation, although this procedure is not without risk since it restricts ventilatory expansion of the rib cage.

Scapulo-Peroneal Muscular Dystrophy

Weakness in a scapulo-peroneal distribution is a relatively common feature of a number of different neuromuscular disorders. For example, it is found in limb-girdle dystrophy, facio-scapulo-humeral dystrophy, nemaline myopathy and central core disease. Scapulo-peroneal muscular dystrophy, however, is a discrete but uncommon entity (Kaeser 1965; Ricker and Mertens 1968). Scapulo-peroneal

muscular dystrophy exists as X-linked (Thomas et al. 1972) and autosomal dominant or sporadic traits (Munsat and Serratrice 1992). The latter is clearly defined but the former probably represents a misclassification.

The disease usually presents with involvement of the legs but the clinical picture in the X-linked and autosomal dominant forms differs. The autosomal dominant form generally runs a more benign course (Fig. 14.23). The onset may be in infancy or in adult life (Thomas et al. 1975). Either the peroneal or the shoulder-girdle muscles may be first affected and there is marked variability even within individual families both in the pattern of involvement and in the rate of progression of the disease. There is usually mild facial weakness, with diminished or absent tendon reflexes. The occurrence of mild facial weakness suggests a relationship between dominantly inherited scapulo-peroneal muscular dystrophy and facio-scapulo-peroneal muscular dystrophy, especially since the expression of the latter disorder is so variable. Indeed, Serratrice et al. (1982) suggested that there was a continuum between these disorders. Genetic studies may resolve this issue. The course is slow, with periods of stable, non-progressive weakness. Most patients remain ambulant and the life span is normal.

The X-linked form of scapulo-peroneal weakness (Rotthauwe et al. 1972; Thomas et al. 1975), a more severe disease usually beginning in the first decade of life with muscular contractures, particularly of the gastrocnemius group and later of the muscles of the neck and other limb muscles, has been described. Muscle weakness develops in the second decade, particularly involving deltoids, pectorals, upper arm muscles and the extensors of the hands, fingers and feet, but pelvic girdle muscles and other shoulder girdle muscles are usually spared. Cardiomyopathy is usual in these cases, but is not a feature of the autosomal dominant form, and death often occurs in middle age from the cardiac involvement. This X-linked syndrome probably represents Emery–Dreifuss syndrome (see above).

Laboratory Investigations

The CK level is occasionally slightly raised in autosomal dominant scapulo-peroneal muscular dystrophy. The electro-cardiogram is normal.

Electrophysiological Assessment

The typical features of a myopathic disorder are found with concentric needle EMG (Thomas et al. 1975).

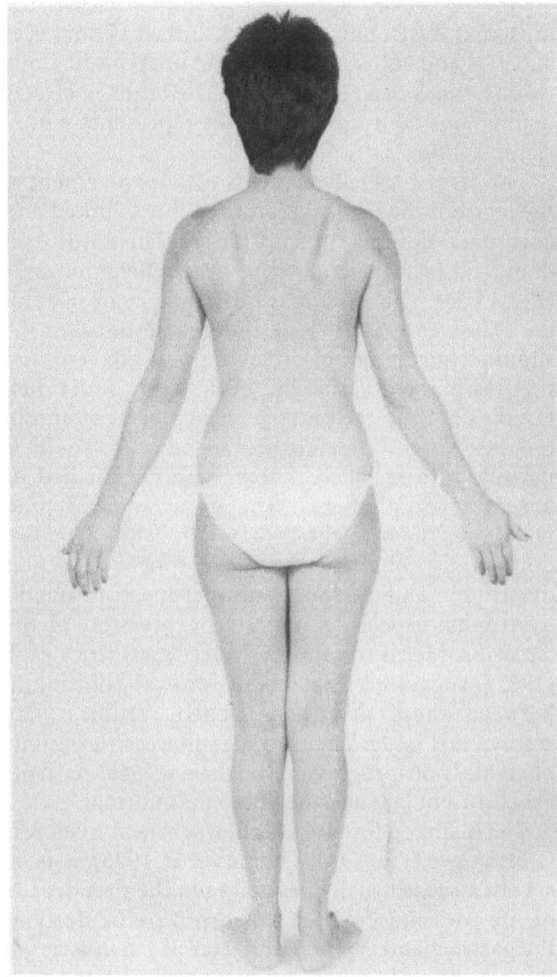

a

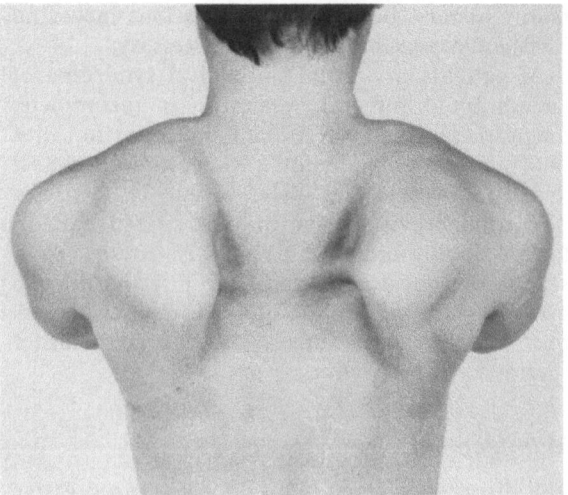

b

Fig. 14.23. Scapulo-peroneal muscular dystrophy. There is marked scapular winging **a**, which is best seen during elevation of the arms, **b**.

affecting peripheral nerves, perhaps at a proximal level, or even of anterior horn cells and posterior root ganglia (Schwartz and Swash 1975), and varying modes of inheritance are given in different reports. The differential diagnosis from other neurogenic disorders is discussed in Chap. 6. As noted above, the separation of scapulo-peroneal muscular dystrophy from facio-scapulo-humeral muscular dystrophy may be artificial. X-linked inheritance suggests Emery–Dreifuss syndrome in which cardiomyopathy is prominent.

Distal Myopathies

Primary muscle disease with a distal distribution of weakness involving upper or lower limbs is uncommon. Several distinct syndromes have been recognised. In many, the presentation initially suggests a neurogenic disorder, but electrophysiological and histopathological assessment clearly indicates the primary nature of the myopathic process. In distal myopathies there is no sensory disturbance, no evidence of a central nervous system disorder, especially cervical cord disease, and there is no clinical or EMG evidence of myotonia. If any of these features are present a diagnosis other than distal myopathy is likely. The first report of distal myopathy was by Gowers (1902).

The distal myopathies can be classified according to mode of inheritance (Table 14.6).

Muscle Biopsy

The muscle biopsy shows the typical features of a myopathy, with increased variability in fibre size, degenerative changes, central nucleation and, in more advanced cases, fibrosis and fatty infiltration of the muscle. Inflammatory and neurogenic features have not been described in these cases.

Differential Diagnosis

Weakness in a scapulo-peroneal distribution may also be due to a neurogenic disorder and spinal muscular atrophy may present with this distribution of muscular weakness (Emery et al. 1968; Meadows and Marsden 1969). Neurogenic weakness in a scapulo-peroneal pattern may also occur in association with distal sensory impairment, which may also affect the hands (Davidenkow 1939); the syndrome may be due to a degenerative process

Table 14.6. Distal myopathies

Autosomal dominant inheritance
   Infantile and juvenile syndromes
   Welander's distal myopathy

Autosomal recessive (or sporadic) types
   Distal muscular dystrophy
   Distal myopathy with rimmed vacuoles

After Buchman and Cochran 1992.

Welander's Distal Myopathy

A hereditary, late-onset, distal myopathy with dominant inheritance was first recognised in Scandinavia by Welander (1951) who reported 249 cases in 72 families in Sweden. The disorder began between the ages of 20 and 77 years (mean 47 years), pursued a slowly progressive course and was more common in men (male to female ratio: 3:2). The weakness began in the intrinsic muscles of the hands and feet, and in the extensors of the fingers and toes, with subsequent involvement of hand and wrist, and toe long extensor muscles. The long flexor muscles were always spared. More proximal muscles may be involved to some extent later, but cranial muscles are spared. Cardiomyopathy developed in many patients. Subsequently similar cases have been described from other countries, although many have been sporadic, or have shown autosomal recessive inheritance, with differences in age of onset and pattern of weakness (Milhorat and Wolff 1943; Markesbery et al. 1974; Scappetta et al. 1984). Borg et al. (1987a) found that autonomic function was normal, but that subtle abnormalities in sensory thresholds could be detected in automated tests (Borg et al. 1987b).

Investigations

The CK level is usually normal in the familial Scandinavian cases. EMG assessment shows myopathic potentials with normal motor and sensory conduction velocity. Complex repetitive discharges may be recorded. Fibrillation potentials may be present (Scappetta et al. 1984). The ECG may be normal, or may show features consistent with cardiomyopathy.

Muscle Biopsy

In the familial Scandinavian cases Edstrom (1975) found Type 1 atrophy in normal or slightly weak muscles. In more severely affected muscles there was poor fibre-type differentiation, with a predominance of Type 2C fibres, increased central nucleation, fibre

splitting and vacuolisation and phagocytosis (Welander 1951; Edstrom 1975). Thornell et al. (1984) found that residual fibres in weak muscles contained fetal myosin, and in ultrastructural studies there were non-specific changes in myofibrillar organisation with some autophagic vacuoles, and evidence of regeneration and necrosis. This finding was confirmed by Borg et al. (1989), who also noted abnormalities in sural nerve biopsies.

In the sporadic cases similar abnormalities occur, although vacuolar changes are often more prominent both in light microscopy and ultrastructural studies (Markesbery et al. 1974). The vacuoles may have a rimmed appearance in light microscope preparations.

Infantile and Juvenile Distal Myopathy Syndromes

Two large families have been described, one with an infantile onset, dominantly inherited disorder in 18 members of one family (Magee and De Jong 1965) and the other of juvenile onset in 19 members of a Dutch family (Biemond 1966). The family described by Magee and De Jong (1965) presented with footdrop and later developed mild weakness of finger and hand extension. Van der Does de Willebois et al. (1968) described a similar disorder, but affected individuals had hypertrophied calves. The family described by Biemond (1966) showed both neurogenic and myopathic features as determined by the investigations available at that time, and its precise classification is difficult.

Distal Myopathy with Rimmed Vacuoles

This recessive disorder usually begins in the second or third decade with distal weakness in the legs, leading to difficulty walking. A steppage gait disorder develops, followed by weakness of flexion of the neck, and of the arms. Later there is marked proximal weakness and wasting but facial, bulbar and intercostal muscles are not clinically involved. The CK is moderately elevated and the EMG shows myopathic features. Sensory and motor nerve conduction velocities are normal. Many of the cases described have been Japanese (see Nonaka et al. 1981a, 1985; Sunohara et al. 1989).

Pathology

The major abnormality consists of rimmed vacuoles, found in both fibre types. The vacuoles are rimmed by basophilic granules that are acid-phosphatase positive, and negative in PAS and oil red 0 lipid preparations. There is Type 1 fibre predominance, with increased numbers of Type 2C fibres. There is no inflammatory response (Nonaka et al. 1981b, 1985). Electron microscopy shows autophagic vacuoles, lamellar bodies and filamentous inclusions. Although these changes resemble those found in inclusion body myositis, they differ in the absence of inflammation and in their clinical association with the autosomal recessive syndrome of relatively early onset.

Rimmed vacuoles themselves occur in a number of different neuromuscular syndromes, including inclusion body myositis, polymyositis, Bethlem myopathy and Kugelberg–Welander disease. They represent an autophagic process rather than a specific feature of any disorder.

Distal Muscular Dystrophy

Distal muscular dystrophy may be autosomal dominant or sporadic (Markesbery et al. 1974, 1977). Miyoshi et al. (1986) described 17 cases of recessive inheritance in eight families. The disorder developed in young adults with distal atrophy mainly involving gastrocnemius and soleus, causing impairment of standing on tiptoe. The forearms become atrophic, with weak hand grip, but the small hand muscles are spared. More proximal weakness develops later. The CK is markedly raised (20 to 100 times normal) and the EMG is myopathic with normal nerve conduction.

Pathology

The changes are especially marked in gastrocnemius and soleus, with only mild changes in gluteus maximus and quadriceps (Miyoshi et al. 1986). Extensive fatty infiltration and fibrosis, fibre hypertrophy and atrophy, fibre necrosis and regeneration are prominent, and some opaque fibres are present. Type 1 fibre predominance may develop. There is no inflammation or grouped atrophy.

Prognosis and Nosology

This syndrome is slowly progressive. Limb girdle muscular dystrophy (LGMD2B) is a proximal onset disorder that has the same chromosomal locus (Ch 2p 13.3, Bashir et al. 1994; Bejaoui et al. 1995) as Miyoshi myopathy, although the latter has a striking distal onset and progression. Both are autosomal recessive.

Vacuoles in Muscle Disease

In light microscopic preparations vacuoles in muscle fibres may contain stainable material or appear empty (Carpenter and Karpati 1984). Small vacuoles, 5–10 μm in diameter, often arise from cellular constituents, e.g. microtubules or sarcoplasmic reticulum, but larger vacuoles are of uncertain origin. The specific histological features of vacuoles have been used to characterise certain muscle diseases, some of which are due to specific metabolic defects, such as acid maltase deficiency. Others, for example rimmed vacuoles, have less specificity (see above). These vacuoles are listed in Table 14.7.

Ocular Myopathies

The classification of chronic progressive external ophthalmoplegia has been controversial because of differences of opinion about the clinical, pathological and physiological features of the various disorders in which this symptom is a major feature (Drachman 1968; Bastiaensen 1978). Danta et al. (1975) classified their patients into a group with ptosis and ophthalmoplegia only, another in which ptosis and ophthalmoplegia were associated with weakness of other muscles including nuchal, facial and limb muscles and a third with other manifestations. Differing manifestations occur even in the same family. Patients with oculo-pharyngeal weakness must also be recognised. The cases thus fall into three groups; *oculo-pharyngeal muscular dystrophy* (Victor et al. 1962), *progressive external ocular ophthalmoplegia* alone (Kiloh and Nevin 1952) and *oculocraniosomatic neuromuscular disease* (Kearns and Sayre 1958; Olson et al. 1972). This clinical classification needs to be considered in the light of the finding that the majority of cases presenting with progressive external ophthalmoplegia (PED) show ragged red fibres in biopsies of limb muscles.

Progressive External Ophthalmoplegia (PEO)

Progressive ocular myopathy without other signs was the first form of the ocular myopathies to be recognised (van Graefe 1856). Danta et al. (1975) found that half of their cases fell in this group. The first sign of the disease is usually ptosis, often beginning unilaterally. Ophthalmoplegia and ptosis only rarely begin at the same time; the first sign of

Table 14.7. Vacuoles in muscle disease[a]

Vacuole	Disease	Contents
Lysosomal (autophagic)	Batten's disease	Ceroid lipofuscin in stacked lamellae
	Acid maltase deficiency	Glycogen and membranous whorls
	Oculopharyngeal muscular dystrophy	Glycogen and membranous whorls
	Distal myopathy (recessive form)	Membranes, glycogen, myeloid bodies
	Chloroquine myopathy	Lipopigments and membranous whorls
	Inclusion body myositis	Membranous whorls, filaments and glycogen
Peroxisomes	Lafora disease	Polyglucosans
Microtubular	Periodic paralysis	Membranes and calcified debris or empty vacuoles
	Sarcotubular myopathy	Empty vacuoles
Sarcoplasmic spaces	Other glycogen storage diseases	Glycogen
	Centronuclear myopathy	Lipofuscin, nuclei, glycogen
	Polysaccharide storage myopathy	Polysaccharide deposits
Lipid	Lipid storage disease	Neutral lipid
Granular degenerative	Sporadic distal myopathy	Degenerative myofibrillar products

impairment of ocular motility is impaired upward gaze, usually symmetrical. The patient may turn the head to direct gaze. Diplopia is rare, probably because of the very slow progression; the course is typically very slow. The disease usually begins in the third decade, although in the cases studied by Danta et al. (1975) the onset was later. Cases in which the disorder is present at birth have also been recognised. Some patients develop mild facial and trigeminal weakness and in about 25% of cases weakness of upper limb musculature may also develop late in the natural history of the disease (Kiloh and Nevin 1952; Danta et al. 1975; Croft et al. 1977). The tendon reflexes are often absent even when limb muscles are not clinically involved. The pupils are always spared. Women are more commonly affected than men (Danta et al. 1975).

Biopsies of limb muscles reveal ragged red fibres, a feature characteristic of mitochondrial myopathy, in the majority of cases (Serratrice and Pellissier 1987). The ocular muscles themselves show abnormalities of fibre size, shape and number but the precise delineation of the ocular muscle abnormality is difficult because of the special features of these muscles in normal subjects. Ragged red fibres have been recognised in external ocular muscles in PEO (Mikol et al. 1976), in addition to limb muscles (Engel 1971). The clinical finding of facial and limb weakness in about 25% of cases suggests that these cases are suffering from oculopharyngeal muscular dystrophy (see below), an interpretation that is supported by the absence of ragged red fibres in these patients. However, muscle fatigue and weakness may also be a feature of mitochondrial myopathy. Another important differential diagnosis, especially in a patient with ptosis and ophthalmoplegia is myasthenia gravis. However, in PEO the

ocular abnormalities do not vary during the day and do not worsen with effort. In addition they are not responsive to anticholinesterase tests, e.g. the Tensilon test. Myotonic dystrophy must also be considered in the differential diagnosis of PEO and a central abnormality in the brain stem must always be excluded. Thyroid eye disease is also part of the differential diagnosis.

In summary, PEO is a syndrome due either to a mitochondrial disorder or a manifestation of oculopharyngeal muscular dystrophy (see Serratrice and Pellissier 1987).

Oculo-Pharyngeal Muscular Dystrophy

In this disorder progressive external ophthalmoplegia is associated with dysphagia. The latter becomes apparent after the former. The onset is in the third or fourth decade. Weakness of the external ocular musculature is frequently asymmetrical at first, but progresses to virtually complete external ophthalmoplegia with paralysis of levator palpebrae muscles during many years (Fig. 14.24). Involvement of facial, trigeminal and lower cranial muscles is present, even in the early stages, but becomes prominent later, with involvement of the shoulder and pelvic girdle muscles; areflexia is then common. Dysphagia can be very severe; Roberts and Bamforth (1968) found dysphagia in 11 of 17 patients they examined and showed that the dysphagia was due to inadequate and incoordinate contraction of the pharyngeal sphincters and of the striated muscle in the upper third of the oesophagus. In some of their patients there was widespread involvement of limb and trunk muscles with marked wasting.

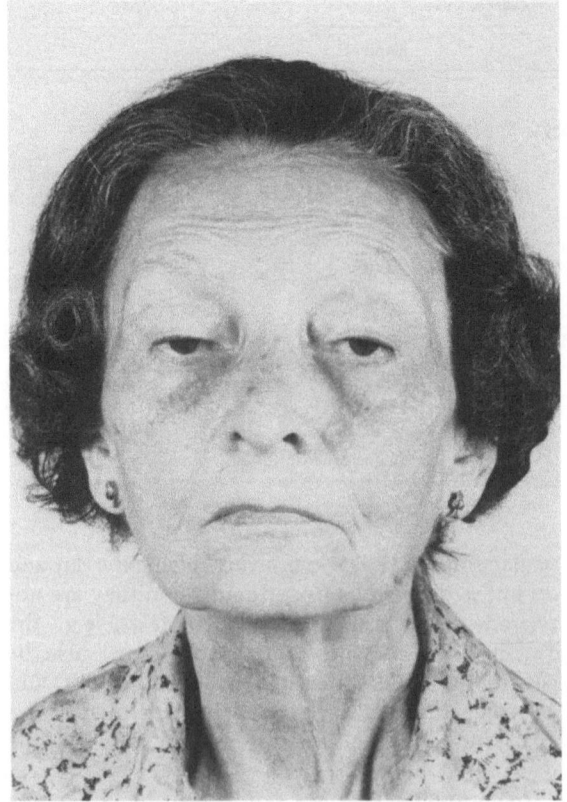

Fig. 14.24. Oculo-pharyngeal muscular dystrophy. There is ptosis, and external ophthalmoplegia with only slight involvement of other cranial muscles and of the pectoral girdle musculature.

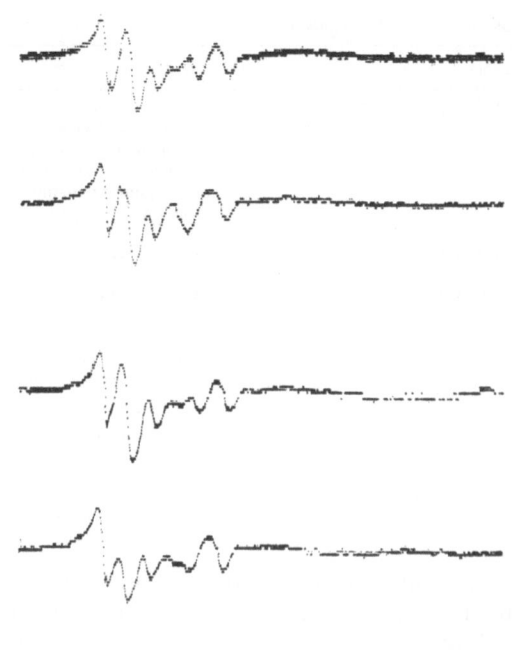

Fig. 14.25. Oculo-pharyngeal muscular dystrophy. Single-fibre EMG recording showing a complex, stable motor unit action potential. Bar 2 ms.

The disease has been particularly carefully studied in several French-Canadian kindreds (Barbeau 1966). In them dysphagia may become incapacitating, leading to weight loss (Bray et al. 1965). The disease is usually inherited in an autosomal dominant pattern and sporadic cases are rare; cardiac involvement has not been noted.

There are five essential criteria for the diagnosis: PEO, prominent dysphagia, autosomal dominant inheritance, typical inclusions (see below) and absence of ragged red fibres (Rowland 1992b).

Investigations

The CK is normal or only slightly raised (Barbeau 1966). The CSF protein is normal in both PEO and oculo-pharyngeal muscular dystrophy (Danta et al. 1975; Barbeau 1966). The EMG shows minor myopathic features in limb muscles. Complex units may be prominent (Fig. 14.25). The muscle biopsy shows mild myopathic features, with increased variability in fibre size; atrophy more commonly affects Type 1 than Type 2 fibres. Small angular fibres, more frequently Type 1 than Type 2, which are dark with NADH stains, are common, but the significance of this finding is unclear. Internal nuclei are common and Type 2 fibres may be hypertrophied. The presence of 8 μm thick unbranched intranuclear filaments appears to be a specific abnormality (Fig. 14.26), restricted to muscle fibre nuclei (Tomé and Fardeau 1980; Martin et al. 1982; Coquet et al. 1983). The origin of these fibrils is unknown. They form intranuclear inclusions seen by electron microscopy in about 5% of muscle nuclei, but also detectable by phase contrast microscopy. Small rimmed vacuoles may be present, usually in Type 1 fibres. The rim, which is red in Gomori and basophilic in haematoxylin and eosin stains, defines a lucent, punched-out area in the fibre (Dubowitz and Brooke 1973; Little and Perl 1982; Bouchard et al. 1989). Non-specific mitochondrial abnormalities may occur (Julien et al. 1974) but ragged red fibres are not a feature.

A neurogenic syndrome, probably representing a variety of inherited motor neuropathy allied to the

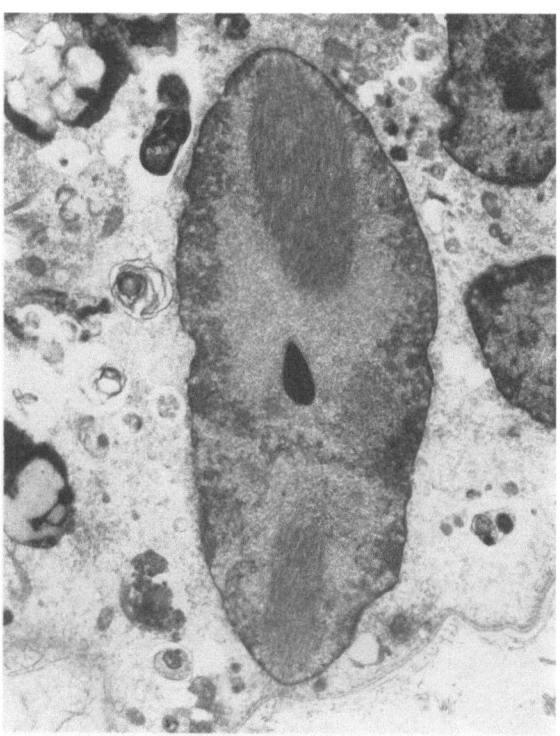

Fig. 14.26. Intranuclear fibrillary inclusion in oculo-pharyngeal muscular dystrophy. Electron micrograph, × 18 600.

spinal muscular atrophies has been reported (Matsunaga et al. 1973; Schmitt and Krause 1981).

Management

The main problem is cachexia with recurrent pulmonary infections associated with dysphagia. This may necessitate tracheotomy and gastrostomy.

Oculo-Cranio-Somatic Neuromuscular Disease

Chronic progressive external ophthalmoplegia may be associated with other clinical manifestations, including retinitis pigmentosa, heart block and cardiomyopathy, reduced tendon reflexes, cerebellar ataxia, deafness, mental retardation and corticospinal signs. In addition the stature may be short and the CSF protein is usually raised. This syndrome was first recognised by Kearns and Sayre (1958) but the full range of associated clinical manifestations has been recognised more recently (Berenberg et al. 1977). The disorder is usually recognisable before the age of 15 years; the external ophthalmoplegia is followed by the recognition of pigmentary retinal degeneration and heart block, but other features are less conspicuous at this stage. The CT scan may show calcification of the basal ganglia (Seigel et al. 1979). Abnormalities in mitochondrial metabolism have been recognised in these patients, including many with progressive ocular myopathy, and these disorders are discussed in Chap. 17.

Dropped head syndrome

This clinical syndrome, in which there is selective weakness of neck extensor muscles, occurs in polymyositis, myasthenia gravis, Guillain–Barré syndrome and as an isolated myopathic disorder (Suarez and Kelly 1992). Isolated neck extensor myopathy is an uncommon sporadic disorder presenting in the elderly. Its cause is unknown, and the disorder is not generalised. Rarely amyotrophic lateral sclerosis may present in this way (Katz et al. 1996).

The myotonic syndromes consist of a number of different conditions in all of which the clinical phenomenon of myotonia occurs (Table 15.1). Becker (1971, 1977) ascertained the prevalence of the various myotonic syndromes in West Germany and noted the overwhelming predominance of myotonic dystrophy in 80% of the patients surveyed, although it is likely that his results were biased by reliance on hospital-based cases. Myotonic dystrophy is the most common of the adult-onset muscular dystrophies, occurring in 1 in 8000 people (Harper 1989). Myotonia congenita occurs in about 4 in 100 000 people.

Table 15.1.   Genetic classification of the myotonias

Chloride channel diseases	Ch7q
Myotonia congenita	
Autosomal dominant (Thomsen)	
Autosomal recessive (Becker)	
Sodium channel disease	Ch17q
Hyperkalaemic periodic paralysis	
Paramyotonia congenita	
Potassium sensitive myotonia congenita (myotonia fluctuans)	
Protein kinase-related disease	Ch19q
Myotonic dystrophy	
Other myotonic syndromes	
Schwartz–Jampel disease	
Andersen's syndrome	
Drug-induced myotonia	

From Ptacek et al. (1993).

The Phenomenon of Myotonia

Myotonia is a persistent contraction of a muscle, or of a group of fibres in a muscle, observed after the cessation of voluntary contraction or in response to a mechanical stimulus, such as percussion of the muscle. It is often most easily recognised in small hand muscles, facial muscles or tongue but, in severely affected subjects, percussion of the deltoid may induce it (Fig. 15.1). The clinical phenomenon of myotonia is accompanied by an easily recognised EMG feature, the "dive bomber" phenomenon (see Chap. 2 and below). In some of the myotonic disorders, such as myotonia congenita, myotonia may be the only, or the major, manifestation of the disease but in others it is only one of several other manifestations, as in myotonic dystrophy. Myotonia is variable in severity even in affected subjects and it is characteristically accentuated by cold, and after a period of rest. Continued activity may thus lessen its severity.

Clinical Tests for Myotonia

Myotonia is not always easily demonstrable or obvious but its recognition is very important in diagnosis. Myotonic stiffness is most likely to be induced by activity at its onset but relieved by continued exercise. The most useful test is forced hand grip: the patient's hand fails to relax immediately after gripping the observer's hand and this is immediately obvious. Sometimes the patient uses a characteristic unwinding movement of the fingers in order to unclasp the hand. Myotonia may also be elicited in the hand by a sharp tap delivered to the thenar minence: the resultant dimple slowly flattens and the thumb may even abduct slightly during the myotonic contraction induced by the blow. Percussion-myotonia may also be induced in the tongue, and in other muscles, in some patients. Myotonia can often be observed in the face and eyelids by prolonged contraction after forced eye closure or forced facial movement. Denny-Brown and Foley (1941) noted that myotonic persistence of a contraction does not follow a blink of the eyes or a tendon reflex but requires more forceful eyelid closure or limb muscle contraction to elicit it. Further, the myotonic contraction is always only a small proportion of the mechanical intensity of the preceding contraction that elicited it. These two features suggest that not every nerve impulse to an affected muscle can initiate myotonia and that myotonia does not involve all the fibres in a muscle

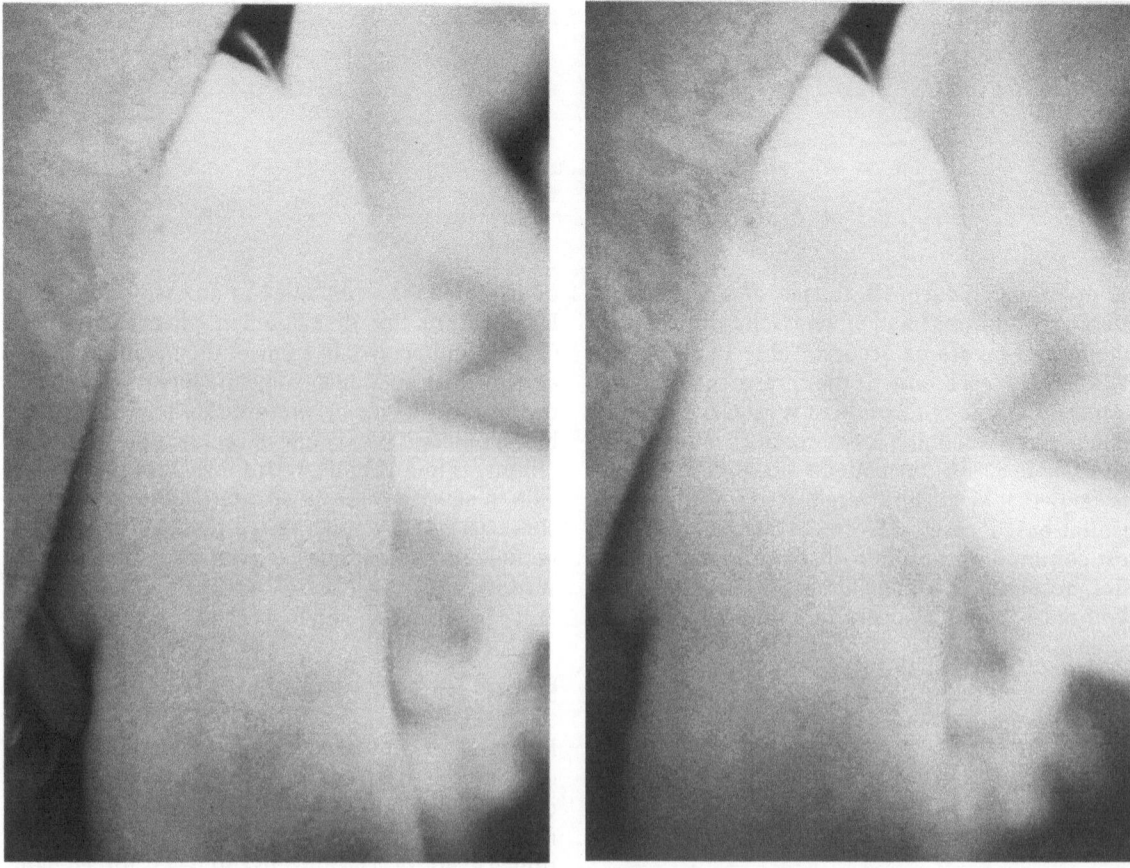

Fig. 15.1.   Recessive myotonia congenita. A fascicle of the deltoid shows slow relaxation after percussion.

at any one moment. In some patients myotonia, rather than being relieved by repeated movement, is worsened (*paradoxical myotonia*).

When recording with a concentric needle EMG electrode the myotonic burst can be detected immediately after cessation of voluntary contraction. The discharge frequency increases gradually to 100 or 150 Hz and then decreases. The amplitude increases and decreases with the changing discharge frequency. This variation produces the characteristic "divebomber" sound in the loudspeaker. The discharge often lasts for up to about 500 ms, but much longer bursts may occur and they may recur after a short interval of a few milliseconds. This myotonic activity can be induced by needle movement or by voluntary contraction. The waveforms may be either positive potentials or negative spikes with a small initial positive phase (Kimura 1983). Single electrical shocks applied to a nerve will not elicit a myotonic discharge but repetitive stimulation, particularly at more rapid rates, will produce myotonia in the muscle supplied by the nerve (Denny-Brown

and Foley 1941). This pattern of stimulation mimics the discharge rates of anterior horn cells during voluntary movement. Neither nerve block with procaine nor curarisation of a muscle will inhibit myotonia in an affected muscle, showing that the abnormality is in the muscle fibres themselves (Denny-Brown and Nevin 1941; Denny-Brown and Foley 1941; Landau 1952).

Repetitive nerve stimulation may induce weakness and reduction in the amplitude of the compound muscle action potential, especially in myotonic dystrophy (Aminoff et al. 1977). Exercise may have a similar effect (Streib et al. 1982). Brown (1974) found that electrical stimulation of myotonic muscle also produces a decremental response, implying reduced membrane excitability during continuous activation.

With single-fibre EMG the myotonic discharges consist of action potentials satisfying the criteria for single-fibre action potentials. The shape of these potentials changes continuously during the recording. In the early part of the discharge the potentials are of high amplitude and have a short rise time but later they are smaller with a slower rise time (Stålberg and Trontelj 1994). Taizzo and Lehmann-Horn (1990) showed that electrical afteractivity, following contraction or tetanus in isolated bundles of muscle fibres in recessive Becker myotonia congenita, correlated with slowed relaxation (stiffness). In earlier experiments Denny-Brown and Nevin (1941) suggested that this myotonic afterspasm was due to motor unit discharge, occurring as a reflex phenomenon, but this explanation is no longer accepted.

Pathophysiology of Myotonia

The occurrence of myotonia in a number of different diseases indicates that it may result from several different underlying abnormalities. The EMG evidence shows that the phenomenon is due to trains of action potentials representing the repeated discharge of single muscle fibres. The frequency of the discharges initially increases but then decreases and stops, producing the characteristic dive-bomber-like sound. The amplitude of the potentials similarly increases and then decreases.

The physiology of myotonia has been studied in man and also in the myotonic goat, a form of autosomal dominant myotonia congenita (Brown and Harvey 1939). The phenomenon is due to increased instability of the muscle fibre membrane leading to repetitive firing following a single stimulus, or a short period of contraction. The myotonic repetitive firing does not occur spontaneously, but is always initiated by an external event or by voluntary contraction. In clinical electromyography this may be the mechanical stimulus of the proximity of the tip of the recording electrode. Normal muscle fibres show slight intrinsic instability of their membrane potentials. There is a small steady-state sodium current in resting muscle which tends to depolarise the membrane, and a similar but more longlasting effect results from the accumulation of potassium within the tubular system. Both these unstabilising, depolarising effects are normally countered by the stabilising effect of current generated by the conductance of chloride ion into the muscle fibre.

Chloride Channel Myotonia

In the myotonic goat, chloride conductance is greatly reduced (Bryant 1969). This causes slight depolarisation of the resting membrane potential so that only a small increase in sodium conductance is necessary to initiate an action potential. The repeated train of action potentials may be generated in this unstable state if there is a sufficient inward flow of current from sodium conductance or potassium accumulation in the tubules to sustain it. When the resting membrane potential rises toward the end of the train of discharges the potential amplitude and firing rate decrease and the discharge ceases (Bryant 1977). The critical abnormality is thus of chloride conductance.

In myotonia congenita both the chloride and the potassium conductance are lower than normal (Lipicky et al. 1971), but in the myotonic goat from which the hypothesis described above was derived the potassium conductance is mildly increased and the chloride conductance reduced (Bryant and Morales-Aquilera 1971). Barchi (1975) showed that repetitive firing may be induced by reducing the intracellular chloride ion concentration. Genetic studies of the "arrested development of righting response" (ADR) mouse, a model of the recessive form of myotonia congenita, have revealed mutations in a voltage-gated muscle chloride channel gene. These mutations consisted of insertions (missense mutations) resulting in disrupted transcription of exons encoding membrane-spanning segments of this channel (Steinmeyer et al. 1991a, 1991b). This gene is located on chromosome 6 in the mouse. Subsequently, mis-sense mutations of this gene, on human chromosome 7q35, have been identified in human myotonia congenita, both in the recessive and dominant forms (Steinmeyer et al. 1991b; Abdalla et al. 1992). The abnormal gene results in the formation of non-functional chloride channels.

Sodium Channel Myotonia

A role of sodium channel dysfunction in myotonia was suggested by the observation that sodium channel neurotoxins produce repetitive action potentials in muscle fibres, associated with reactivation of sodium channels before the membrane has fully repolarised following generation of an action potential (Strichartz et al. 1982). Nearly 10 years later it was recognised that hyperkalaemic periodic paralysis and paramyotonia congenita shared a common genetic locus with the gene encoding the adult isoform of the muscle sodium channel (Fontaine et al. 1990; Ebers et al. 1991). This observation strongly suggested that in these disorders the phenomenon of myotonia was due to abnormal inactivation of the sodium channel (Ptacek et al. 1993).

Voltage-dependent sodium channels are highly conserved across species and tissues. They are membrane proteins consisting of a single large poly-peptide of 260 kDa. The conserved regions include components that function in voltage-sensitive gating, inactivation and ion selectivity. The sodium channel protein has four internally repeated domains (D1–D4), each containing six membrane spanning segments (S1–S6). The S4 segment probably functions as a voltage sensor that controls opening of the channel pore during membrane depolarisation. This S4 segment is the site of two of the recognised mutations that underlie paramyotonia congenita (Stuhmer et al. 1989).

In myotonic dystrophy there is abnormal regulation of sodium channels, which open at membrane potentials that have no effect in normal muscle. The intracellular sodium concentration is increased, sodium conductance is altered, and potassium conductance is normal. The resting membrane potential of skeletal muscle fibres is lowered (Rudel and Lehmann-Horn 1985). In hyperkalaemic periodic paralysis and paramyotonia congenita there is also increased sodium conductance across muscle fibre membranes. In the former disorder the membrane channel abnormality is sensitive to increased extracellular potassium concentration, and in the latter it is sensitive to cooling (Lehmann-Horn et al. 1987; Rudel et al. 1989). In hyperkalaemic periodic paralysis, abnormal activation of the pathological sodium channels may cause inactivation of the normal sodium channels resulting in paralysis (Cannon et al. 1991; Lehmann-Horn et al. 1991). Myotonia fluctuans is a third sodium channel myotonic disorder, with potassium sensitivity, but without weakness. Myotonia is exacerbated by exercise, but not by cold (Ricker et al. 1990, 1994).

Protein Kinases and Myotonic Dystrophy

A defect in protein kinase activity, suspected from genetic linkage date, may explain many of the clinical manifestations of myotonic dystrophy. The myotonia may result from altered phosphorylation of voltage-dependent sodium channels in muscle (Brook et al. 1992). Myotonia is more severe in myotonia congenita than in myotonic dystrophy.

Myotonic Dystrophy

Myotonic dystrophy, described in 1909 by Steinert and by Batten and Gibb, is a multisystem disorder inherited as a dominant trait (Harper 1979). It is the

commonest of the adult-onset muscular dystrophies. The lifetime occurrence risk for the disease is about 1 in 8000 (Harper 1989), but prevalence and incidence are difficult to determine because the disease varies greatly in its severity and in the penetrance of its various major features (Table 15.2) (Caughey and Myrianthopoulos 1963). Todorov et al. (1970) found that the incidence at birth was 13.5/100 000. Myotonic dystrophy is the commonest inherited muscle disease of adults. The common form usually becomes evident between the ages of 20 and 25 years, although there is a congenital form of the disease (described below). The first muscular symptom is usually myotonia, but other stigmata of the disorder are usually obvious before myotonia becomes troublesome and it is not uncommon for patients to present with bilateral posterior subcapsular cataracts, or with infertility (Harper 1989). Cataracts may present in the first decade but more usually between the ages of 25 and 50 years. Polgar et al. (1972) found cataracts in 85% of their patients and this figure is in agreement with larger surveys in Denmark (Thomasen 1948) and Switzerland (Klein 1958). Slit-lamp examination may reveal an even higher incidence of cataract (Dark and Streeten 1977).

Table 15.2. Multi-organ abnormalities in myotonic dystrophy

Skeletal muscle:	weakness, wasting and myotonia
Heart:	heartblock arrhythmias and sudden death benign mitral valve prolapse
Eye:	cataract, ptosis, slowed saccades retinal degeneration, ophthalmoparesis
CNS:	low IQ, personality disorder, abnormal MRI
Skin:	frontal balding, calcifying epithelioma
Smooth muscle:	motility disorder of oesophagus, colon, gall bladder and uterus weak anal sphincter
Endocrine:	testicular atrophy, insulin resistance
Skeletal:	cranial hyperostosis small pituitary fossa
Respiratory:	hypersomnolence and sleep apnoea

The presentation is variable and incomplete manifestations of different distributions are common even within kinships (Pryse-Phillips et al. 1982). Bundey (1983) suggested that patients with infantile onset showed prominent facial and mild limb weakness, patients with onset between the ages of 4 and 20 years showed severe limb and less marked facial involvement. Later onset cases seemed not to show constant features. The general appearance is usually characteristic and the disease can often be recognised at a glance, from the typical stance and facial

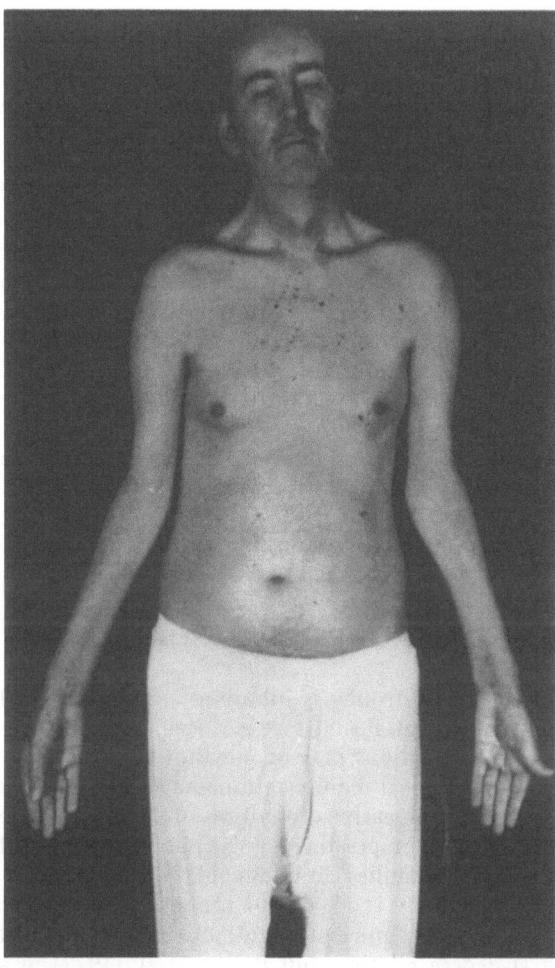

Fig. 15.2. Myotonic dystrophy. The facies is myopathic, the sterno-mastoids are atrophic and there is baldness, and predominantly distal atrophy in the arms. The smile is inverted.

appearance (Fig. 15.2). The face is long, the lower jaw often seeming to be hanging down so that the lips are parted. Ptosis is an almost constant feature and the lips may form a characteristic "inverted smile". There is marked wasting of the muscles of mastication, producing striking hollowing of the temporal fossae and of the cheeks. The patient's head may be tilted slightly backwards to compensate for the ptosis and this enables the wasting of the sterno-mastoids to be noticed. The neck is then curved forwards producing a swan-like posture. The neck flexors are weaker than the neck extensors. Frontal baldness, especially in men, and cataract may also be obvious, but the latter may only be evident with ophthalmic examination or with a slit lamp. In the limbs, wasting may be prominent in distal muscles, especially forearm muscles and anterior tibial and calf muscles, but small hand muscles

are usually spared until the late stages of the disease (Walton 1963). The ankle jerks are diminished or absent in some cases. These features suggest a neuropathic component in the disease, and this is prominent in some families (Spaans et al. 1986).

Although presentation with muscular stiffness, or difficulty relaxing grasp, perhaps brought to the patient's notice by contact with a cold object, is a well-known phenomenon, weakness of grip and difficulty in walking because of weakness of foot dorsiflexors are more common presenting complaints. Cataract and infertility may also be initial complaints and other patients are first recognised because of presentation with diabetes mellitus, or hirsutism. Myotonia is not as prominent a feature as in myotonia congenita, and as weakness becomes more severe during the course of the disease, myotonia usually becomes less evident. It may then only be demonstrable in the more proximal muscles.

Although ECG abnormalities are very common in the disease (De Wind and Jones 1950; Reeves et al. 1980), symptomatic cardiomyopathy is delayed until the later stages of the disease when Stokes–Adams syncope and cardiac failure may develop. Heart block is the commonest treatable cardiac complication. Sudden death is common in patients with atrial and ventricular tachyarrhythmias and may occur in young people with the disease during exercise (Editorial 1992). Reeves et al. (1980) found that 17% of patients with myotonic dystrophy had mitral valve prolapse, a finding supported by Streib et al. (1985) who suggested that the valvular abnormality was due to thoracic deformities rather than to primary valvular disease. Other aspects of the multisystemic involvement so characteristic of the disease in its major form include dysphagia and recurrent pulmonary infection due to involvement of striated muscle in the pharyngeal sphincters and of the smooth muscle of the oesophagus (Harvey et al. 1965; Hughes et al. 1965). Smooth muscle of the lower gastro-intestinal tract, producing megacolon, and of the urinary bladder and uterus may also be affected. Alveolar hypoventilation, often associated with hypersomnia and decreased ventilatory response to hypoxia, may occur in the disease. This is associated with poor diaphragmatic function perhaps because of myotonia and weakness of both diaphragm and intercostal muscles (Jammes et al. 1985). Endocrine involvement may include hypothyroidism, primary gonadal failure and abnormalities of glucose and insulin metabolism (Huff et al. 1967), occasionally with frank diabetes mellitus (Marshall 1959). Mental defect may be associated with the disease and it has often been observed that patients with myotonic dystrophy make poor social adjustments, often appearing poorly cared for and unkempt. Only 24 of Thomasen's (1948) 101 cases were of normal intelligence. Progressive mental decline occurs in some patients. Portwood et al. (1986) showed that patients with paternal inheritance were of normal intelligence but those with maternal inheritance had significantly lower scores in all cognitive tests. There was no difference between affected men and women. The tendon reflexes are usually absent or diminished in affected distal muscles.

Special care is required in women with the disease during pregnancy. Increased muscle weakness, with respiratory dysfunction may develop, perhaps due to diaphragmatic displacement. There is an increased risk of spontaneous abortion during the first trimester. Labour may be prolonged or ineffective and retained placenta, neonatal deaths and placenta praevia are all more frequent than normal (Harper 1989).

The neuromuscular disorder is progressive and usually leads to severe disability within 15–20 years of the onset. However, there is considerable variation in the natural history of the disorder, even within affected sibships, and patients with minor manifestations of the disease often develop little weakness or other disability, suggesting that the disease may be only partially expressed in these cases. In general, the earlier the presentation the more rapid the progression. However, only 10% of patients become wheelchair-bound (Harper 1989).

Congenital Myotonic Dystrophy

The clinical manifestations of this form of the disease differ from those of the commoner, adult-onset variety. The abnormality can be recognised at birth or in the neonatal period. The main features are hypotonia with difficulty in sucking and swallowing. There may be severe respiratory distress and the diaphragm is elevated (Chudley and Barunada 1979). There is marked facial weakness so that the mouth appears triangular in shape and the eyes cannot be closed fully. Clubbed-foot deformity is often present. There is a high incidence of hydramnios and the mother may have noted that fetal movements were weak and infrequent. Myotonia is not demonstrable, even by EMG, until the second year of life or later. Mental retardation is a common feature; in infants surviving the neonatal period there is gradual improvement in strength during the first 2–3 months of life.

Congenital myotonic dystrophy occurs in children born to affected mothers, even though the mother may be only mildly or minimally affected.

Paternal transmission of neonatal-onset myotonic dystrophy is very rare, occurring in only three of 70 cases studied by Harper (1975). Later studies have suggested that all congenital cases are associated with maternal inheritance (Moxley 1992). Harper (1975) suggested that the most likely explanation for the weakness and hypotonia at birth in congenital myotonic dystrophy is a maternal intra-uterine factor affecting those individuals already carrying the dominant gene for myotonic dystrophy (see also Harper and Dyken 1972; Harper 1979). This phenomenon has been termed genomic imprinting. As surviving affected children grow up the more typical manifestation of myotonic dystrophy may develop (Pruzanski 1966). Congenital myotonic dystrophy occurs in 10% of the children of affected mothers. In dystrophic mothers who have given birth to an affected child, 31% of subsequent children will be affected (Koch et al. 1991).

Genetic Aspects

Myotonic dystrophy is inherited as an autosomal dominant trait. Penetrance is variable so that clinical manifestations may or may not be severe. The variable clinical manifestations have been used in studies of the early recognition of stigmata of the disease in attempts to recognise possible carriers of the gene in families (Bundey et al. 1970; Polgar et al. 1972). Bundey et al. (1970) found that lenticular opacities were present in 16% of clinically normal first-degree relatives but Polgar et al. (1972) in a study of 39 first- and second-degree relatives not known to have the disease found that 41% showed clinically diagnostic signs of myotonic dystrophy and half of these showed EMG evidence of myotonia. Only 29% had lenticular opacities. Thus clinical examination is a practical method of assessing the gene frequency in a family and identifying those members of a family at risk of developing or transmitting the disease.

The gene for myotonic dystrophy was mapped to the long arm of chromosome 19 by linkage to the loci for ABH blood secretor antigens, the Lutheran and Lewis blood groups, and to the third component of complement C3 (McKusick 1982; Davies et al. 1983; Roses et al. 1983), and near to the genes for the apolipoproteins C2 and E (Shaw et al. 1985; Lunt et al. 1986). The mutation segregates to a single locus at chromosome 19q13.3 in every population studied (Harper 1989). The mutation causing the disease consists of an unstable DNA sequence of cytosine-thymine-guanine trinucleotide repeats (CTG repeats) at this locus. This triplet is repeated 5–40 times in normal subjects, but 50 to several thousand times in DNA from patients with the disease (Buxton et al. 1992; Brook et al. 1992). The severity of the disease phenotype is related to increasing numbers of CTG repeats (Fu et al. 1992). In addition, the phenomenon of genetic anticipation, in which the disease seems to occur earlier and often more severely, in successive generations (Penrose 1948) has been correlated with increasing numbers of CTG repeats at Ch19q13.3 in successive generations. Increasing numbers of CTG repeats seem to be generated during meiosis. Rare instances of reduction in the size of the CTG repeat into the normal range during transmission from an affected parent to asymptomatic children have been described (Brunner et al. 1993). The original mutation event may have been the insertion of this unstable DNA onto the 13.3 region of Ch19q leading to the enlargement of this allele in subsequent generations (Harley et al. 1992). A similar molecular mechanism of inheritance, involving trinucleotide repeats, occurs in Kennedy's X-linked bulbo-spinal muscular atrophy, and in the fragile X syndrome of mental retardation.

In myotonic dystrophy the deduced amino acid sequence of the gene locus is a protein, myotonin, analogous to a serine-threonine specific protein kinase, dependent on cyclic AMP, that may be important in phosphorylation of ion channels in cell membranes, thus accounting for the myotonia, and for the multi-organ involvement so characteristic of the disease. There is no genetic relationship between myotonia congenita and myotonic dystrophy; Höweler et al. (1980) described the separate inheritance of these two diseases in a single, large Dutch family.

Direct identification of the CTG repeat in myotonic dystrophy is possible using a specific molecular probe p5B1.4. This probe identified 108 of 112 patients with the disease, and provides a tool for improved ascertainment of asymptomatic cases in genetic counselling of family members in families with the disease (Shelbourne et al. 1993).

Laboratory Investigations

The CK level is slightly raised in some adult cases, but it may be normal. It is usually normal in the congenital form of the disease. The level of the muscle-specific enzyme carbonic anhydrase III (CAIII) was raised in all 33 patients with myotonic dystrophy studied by Mokuno et al. (1986), but the CK level was elevated in only 12 of their patients. This relatively specific elevation of CAIII may reflect selective involvement of Type 1 fibres in myotonic dystrophy (Mokuno et al. 1986).

A number of other abnormalities have been described. Of these, hypogammaglobulinaemia is the most easily recognised. Increased catabolism of IgG was reported by Wochner et al. (1966). The glucose tolerance curve may be flattened or diabetic in type and levels of insulin in the blood are often high, indicating decreased responsiveness of insulin receptors since insulin antibodies are not present (Huff et al. al. 1967; Stuart et al. 1983). This insulin resistance is probably related to abnormality of the insulin receptor. However, the insulin receptor maps to chromosome 19p and is therefore not homologous with the gene for myotonic dystrophy. Red blood cell membranes are abnormal, showing disturbed ion transport (Appel and Roses 1977), and erythrocyte survival may be abnormal (Sydow et al. 1985). Membrane-associated defects in neutrophil function have also been described (Seay et al. 1978). The general abnormality consists of primary atrophy of the seminiferous tubules, with secondary overproduction of pituitary gonadotrophins. No consistent alteration of thyroid function has been found (Moxley 1992).

Radiological abnormalities of the skull have been reported, including hyperostosis of the skull and a small sella turcica (Walton and Warrick 1954). CT brain scans may show ventricular enlargement. MR brain scans frequently show white matter lesions that may resemble multiple sclerosis. In addition, Huber et al. (1989) described abnormalities in white matter in the anterior temporal lobes that appeared to be specific for the disease, and that could be correlated with behavioural and intellectual disturbances. These lesions have been associated with slowed smooth pursuit eye movements (Bollen et al. 1992). The sequence of atrophic change in muscles, sometimes preceded by hypertrophy of individual muscles has been investigated by CT scanning (Bulcke and Baert 1982).

Electrophysiological Assessment

Typical EMG evidence of myotonia is usually present in the adult cases. In mild cases it may only appear when the muscle is cooled (Buchthal and Rosenfalck 1963). In neonatal-onset myotonic dystrophy myotonic discharges are not evident until the second year of life or later. The myotonic discharges in myotonic dystrophy are rarely as prominent as in myotonia congenita (Fig. 15.3). Pseudo-myotonic discharges may also be recorded. In contrast to the clinical difficulty in eliciting myotonia in weak, wasted muscles, electrical evidence of myotonia is more prominent in such muscles (Streib and Sun 1983). Myotonia is nearly

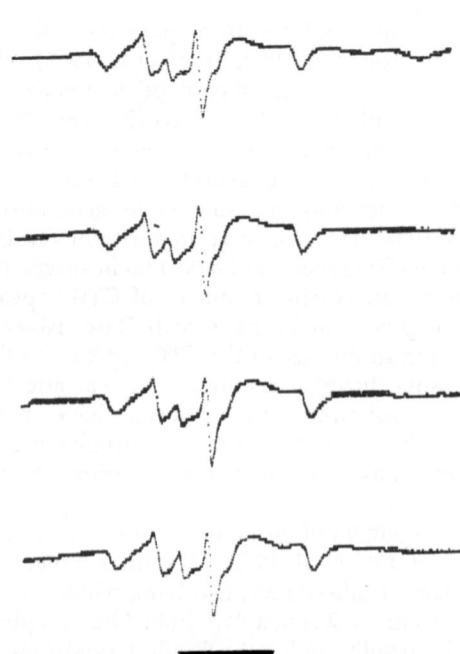

Fig. 15.4. Myotonic dystrophy. A stable, complex motor unit action potential. Concentric needle EMG. Filters: 500 Hz and 10 kHz. Bar 2 ms.

always found in distal hand muscles and periorbital muscles, and in the extensor compartment of the leg but, in biceps brachii, deltoid and vastus medialis myotonia is found in only about half of the patients examined (Streib and Sun 1983). Random spontaneous activity, similar to fibrillation potentials, is seen at rest in some muscles, but there is doubt as to the origin of these potentials since, unlike fibrillation potentials, they persist when the muscle is cooled (Buchthal and Rosenfalck 1963). Sampling with concentric needle electrodes during voluntary activity reveals short-duration polyphasic motor unit action potentials of low amplitude (Fig. 15.4), as in other myopathies. With single-fibre EMG the fibre density is usually increased; this abnormality is more prominent in the forearm extensor muscles than in the biceps brachii. The neuromuscular jitter may be increased (Fig. 15.5) (Stålberg and Trontelj 1994). The anal sphincter is also involved, with myotonia and an increased incidence of faecal incontinence (Eckardt and Nix 1991).

The motor conduction velocity may be slightly slowed. The mean motor conduction velocity was reduced by 15% in a group of patients studied by Panayiotopoulos and Scarpalezos (1976), a similar reduction in motor conduction velocity to that found in patients with spinal muscular atrophy in this study. Both the distal motor latency and F wave conduction velocity have also been reported to be

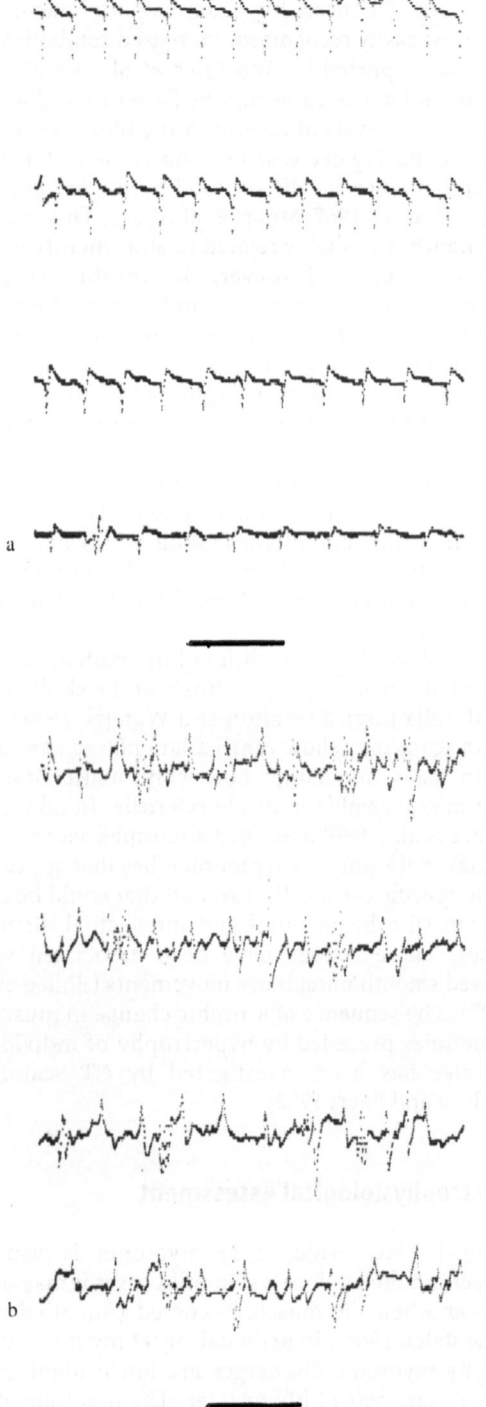

Fig. 15.3. Myotonic dystrophy. Concentric needle EMG. Filters: 100 Hz and 10 kHz. Bars 20 ms. **a** Myotonia: a gradual decrease in frequency and amplitude of the myotonic response is characteristic in its later part. **b** Voluntary activity showing short duration, small, polyphasic motor unit action potentials. Myotonia can be recognised superimposed on this voluntary activity.

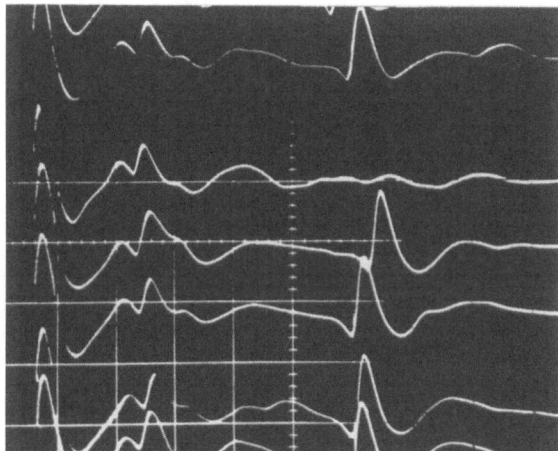

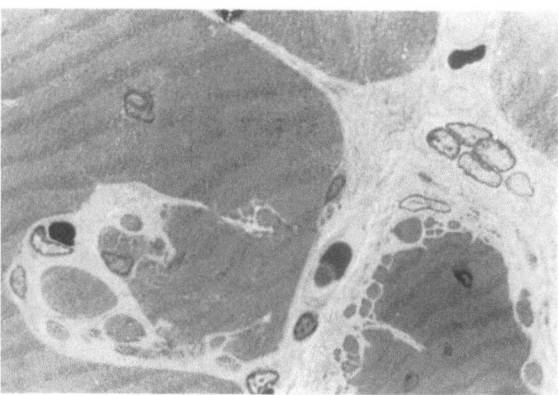

Fig. 15.7. Myotonic dystrophy. Toluidine blue. × 560. TS. Fibre splitting is seen in association with centrally placed nuclei, but it is prominent at the edge of the fibres. One fibre shows increased clear sarcoplasm at its rim: sarcoplasmic masses.

Fig. 15.5. Myotonic dystrophy. Single-fibre EMG recording showing a complex unit with increased jitter of the two later components, and blocking of the last component. Grid 2 ms.

slowed (Panayiotopoulos and Scarpalezos 1976). The abnormalities were not related to the presence or absence of diabetes. Estimations of the number of motor units in the extensor digitorum brevis muscle have consistently shown a reduced number in myotonic dystrophy (McComas et al. 1971d; Ballantyne and Hansen 1974b). Increased sensory thresholds in psychophysical tests were found by Jamal et al. (1986). These studies indicate that there must be a neural lesion in the disorder, although there has not been thorough histological evaluation (but see Swash 1972). In this context it may be important that peripheral neuropathy has been reported as a rare associated feature in myotonic dystrophy (Paramesh et al. 1975; Borenstein et al. 1977) and Refsum et al. (1967) found a raised CSF protein in nine of 16 cases.

After a period of activation the compound muscle action potential is of lower amplitude and repetitive stimulation similarly causes a reduction in CMAP amplitude that is more marked at high stimulus frequencies (Aminoff et al. 1977; Streib et al. 1982). This abnormality is a feature of all myotonic syndromes, although not an invariable finding.

Electroencephalography may also show abnormalities, consisting of increased amounts of mild diffuse slow activity (Barwick et al. 1965).

Muscle Biopsy

The characteristic abnormality in muscle in adult-onset myotonic dystrophy consists of the presence of large numbers of internal nuclei (Fig. 15.6), often occurring in long chains when studied in longitudinal section, together with sarcoplasmic masses and ring-fibres. In addition there is increased variability in fibre size, with increased endomysial and interfascicular fibrous tissue. Individual necrotic or regenerating fibres are rarely seen, but very small fibres may be prominent, containing dense pyknotic nuclei, in more advanced cases often resembling the small angular fibres found in classical neurogenic disorders. Moth-eaten fibres may also be a feature and fibre splitting (Fig. 15.7) may be present. Indeed, ring-fibres themselves (Fig. 15.8) represent a form of localised splitting of some of the myofibrils in a fibre, the displaced myofibril coming to lie in a spiral around the edge of the fibre, or traversing part of its cross-sectional diameter. This displacement of a myofibril results in the isolation of a

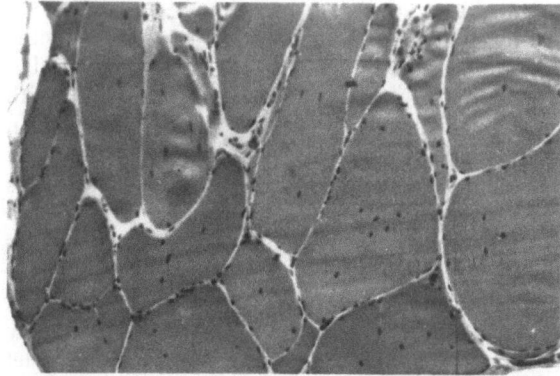

Fig. 15.6. Myotonic dystrophy. H and E. × 560. TS. All fibres contain multiple centrally located nuclei. Fibre splitting is present.

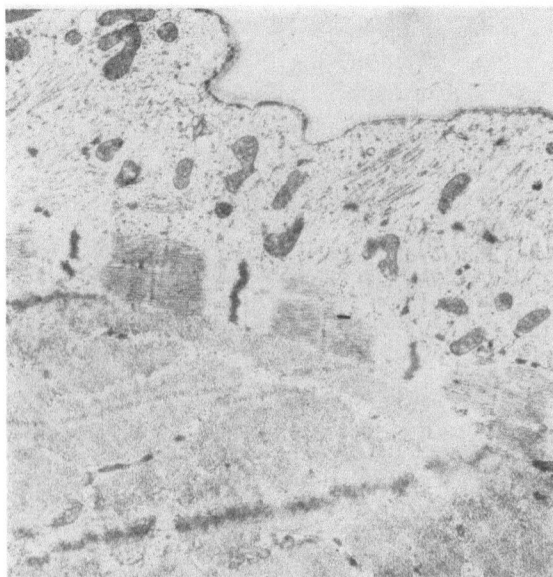

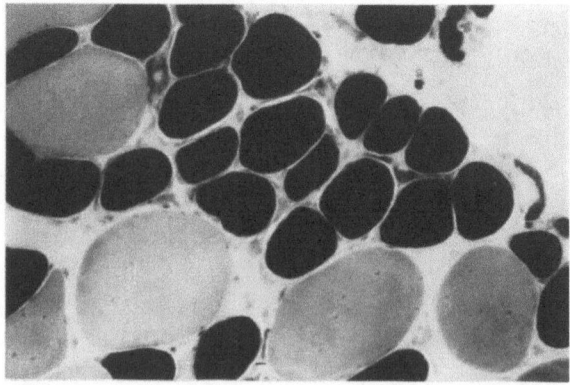

Fig. 15.9. Myotonic dystrophy. ATPase pH 4.3. × 350. Type 1 fibres are small and Type 2 fibres are slightly hypertrophied. The Type 1 fibres are clustered into a small group, and all the fibres are slightly rounded. (Reproduced with permission from Schwartz et al. 1977a, and the Journal of the Neurological Sciences.)

Fig. 15.8. Myotonic dystrophy. Electron micrograph. TS. × 9000. A myofibril has become displaced and, running at 90° to the longitudinal axis of the fibre, has come to encircle it. There is a zone of granular sarcoplasm between the displaced myofibril and the edge of the fibre.

zone of sarcoplasm in the subsarcolemmal region, resulting in a "sarcoplasmic mass".

With enzyme histochemical techniques Type 1 fibres often appear smaller than Type 2 fibres (Fig. 15.9), either because the Type 1 fibres are smaller than normal or, in some cases, because Type 2 fibres have undergone hypertrophy (Brooke and Engel 1969c). Casanova and Jerusalem (1979) found that Type 1 fibres were smaller than normal in 70% of cases. The disparity between Type 1 and Type 2 fibres is an early feature of the disorder, appearing in biopsies taken at a stage in the disease when the only other definite abnormality is increased central migration and proliferation of muscle fibre nuclei. In more advanced cases the disparity in size of Type 1 and Type 2 fibres may no longer be evident, the histological appearance then having become dominated by the dystrophic changes.

In the congenital form of the disease Type 1 hypotrophy becomes more prominent with increasing age. Karpati et al. (1973) noted, in a study in which a patient was biopsied at 18 months and 4 years of age, that Type 1 fibres had increased in size by 30% in the second biopsy, but Type 2 fibres had increased in size by 45%. In addition, they noted more prominent acid phosphatase activity, located subsarcolemmally, in the first than in the second biopsy. Ultrastructurally, these areas showed disorganised myofilaments and dense-cored tubular

structures, features of *sarcoplasmic masses*. In electron-microscopic preparations mitochondria and myofilaments are absent from these regions (Aicardi et al. 1974).

Sarcoplasmic masses are devoid of myofibrils but contain myofilaments, triads, mitochondria and glycogen particles. They show prominent acid phosphatase activity and are also rich in glycolytic and oxidative enzymes (Samaha et al. 1967; Schroder and Adams 1968). Klinkerfuss (1967) interpreted sarcoplasmic masses as foci of regeneration because they contained disorganised myofilaments and large numbers of ribosomes and polysomes. Although sarcoplasmic masses are particularly prominent in myotonic dystrophy they are not a unique feature of the disorder. Other non-specific abnormalities, such as cytoplasmic masses and finger-print inclusions, commonly occur (Schroder and Adams 1968; Tomé and Fardeau 1972).

Electron microscopic studies of adult-onset cases have shown destructive changes in the myofilaments, beginning in the A band and encroaching on the I band (Klinkerfuss 1967). Swelling and disorganisation of the sarcoplasmic reticulum, with less specific changes in the T tubes, have been recognised as an early and prominent change (Mussini et al. 1970). Myofibrillar degeneration is seen only in the more advanced cases.

In the abnormal muscles of myotonic dystrophy the muscle spindles show characteristic abnormalities (Fig. 15.10). The principal abnormality consists of the presence of an excessive number of unusually thin intrafusal muscle fibres (See Fig. 3.32) (Daniel and Strich 1964), each probably derived by longitudinal splitting from a parent intrafusal muscle fibre (Swash 1972; Swash and Fox 1975a). The normal dif-

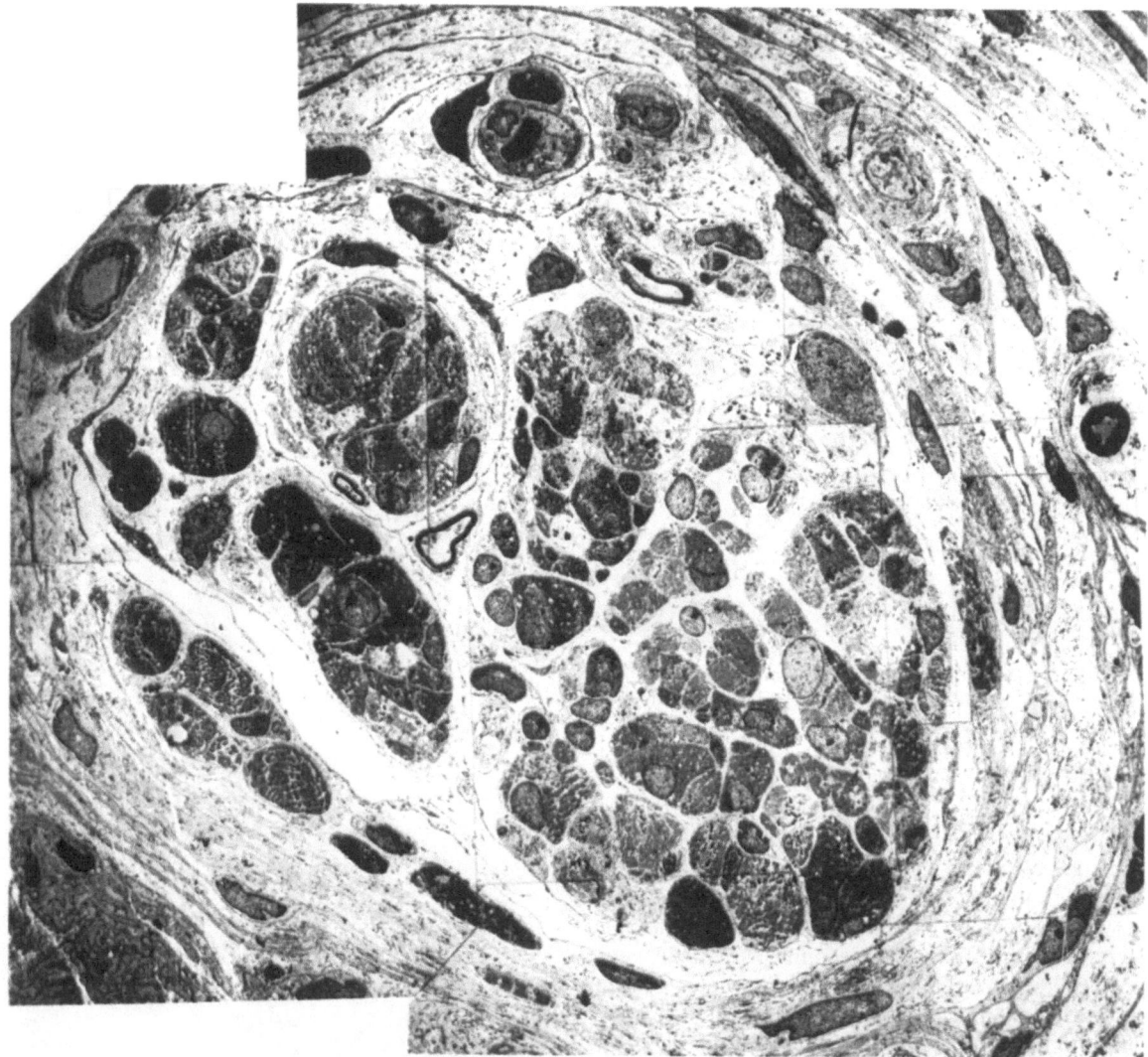

Fig. 15.10. Myotonic dystrophy. EM montage. TS. In this muscle spindle there is an increased number of intrafusal muscle fibres, formed by fragmentation and regeneration. The spindle capsule is thickened.

ferentiation between nuclear bag and nuclear chain fibres is lost, all the fibres appear of uniform histochemical type (Heene 1973) and the capsule of affected spindles is thickened. As the disorder progresses the intrafusal muscle fibres show myopathic changes and degenerate (Fig. 15.11), leading to fibrosis of the spindle lumen and capsule. Even then, however, the spindle abnormality is patchily distributed within any given muscle. The spindle abnormality has been shown in a congenital-onset case biopsied at the age of 18 months, in which increased acid phosphatase activity was present in several of the abnormal intrafusal muscle fibres (Karpati et al. 1973 Fig. 5b). Both the motor and sensory innervation (Fig. 15.12) of affected muscle

spindles is abnormal (Swash 1972; Swash and Fox 1975a,b; Stranock and Newsom-Davis 1978). The fusimotor abnormality precedes the abnormality of sensory innervation and the development of intrafusal fibre splitting (Swash 1972) and is additional evidence for an independent neurogenic component in myotonic dystrophy.

With the supravital methylene blue impregnation the terminal innervation of extrafusal muscle fibres is often seen to be abnormal. The terminal arborisations are expanded and there is prominent axonal ramification leading to innervation of several adjacent muscle fibres. The terminal innervation ratio (TIR) is increased in about a third of cases, but never to a large degree (Coërs et al. 1973). These

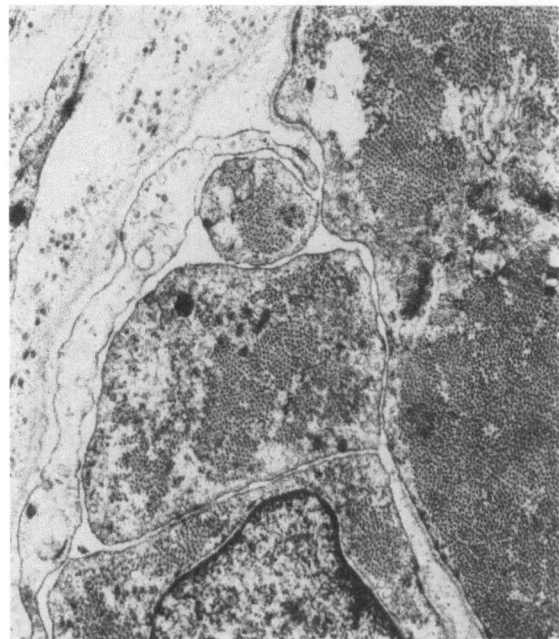

Fig. 15.11. Myotonic dystrophy. Electron micrograph. TS. × 30 000. Degenerative changes in the myofilaments in these intrafusal muscles are widespread. Adjacent fibre fragments are separated only by plasma membrane.

changes also lend weight to the concept of a neural disorder in myotonic dystrophy but Coërs et al. (1973), like Allen et al. (1969), thought that they were different from those seen in classic neurogenic disorders and might represent hyperneurotisation of individual muscle fibres. The fine structure of the motor end-plate is also abnormal. The nerve terminal shows an increased mitochondrial area and decreased density of synaptic vesicles, changes similar to those seen in polymyositis and steroid myopathy, but the post-synaptic region is normal. The changes are probably not specific (Engel et al. 1973). Intra-muscular nerve bundles in this study showed no ultrastructural abnormalities.

Management

Myotonia itself is not usually a sufficient problem to require drug treatment but phenytoin therapy is useful in some patients in whom muscular stiffness is a persistent complaint. Procainamide and mexiletine are also used and may relieve the myotonia to some extent. Other drugs such as tocainide have potentially serious cardiac unwanted effects. These drugs are all class I anti-arrhythmic drugs.

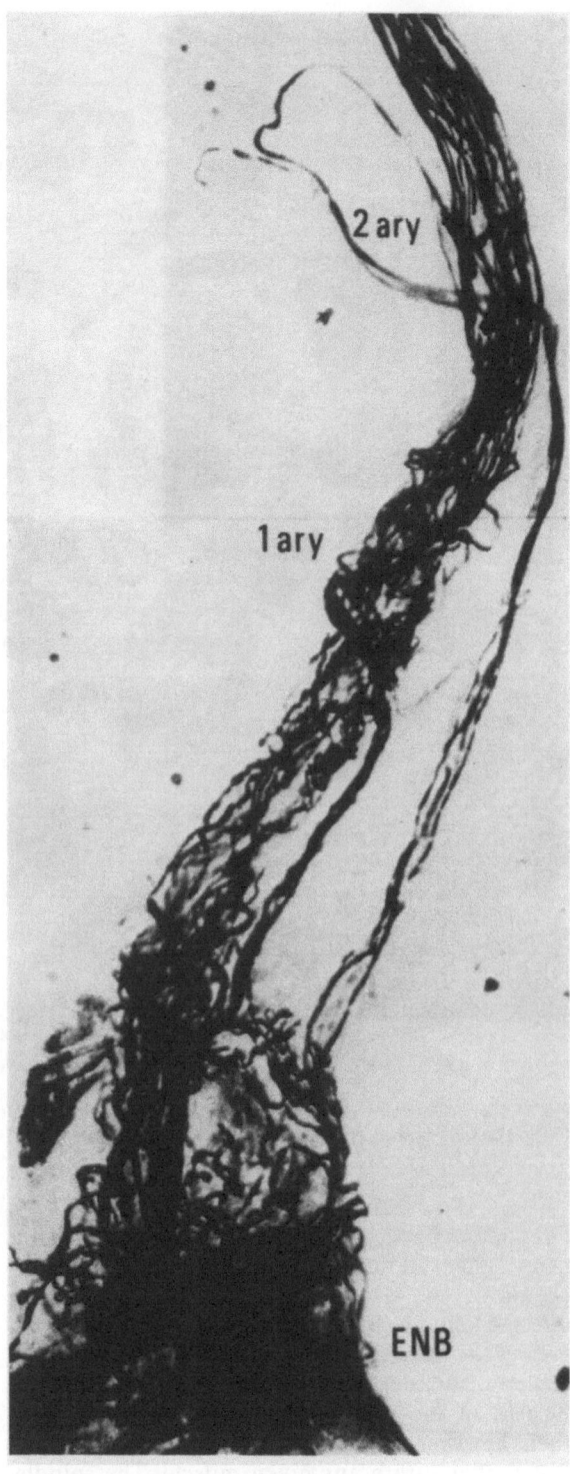

Fig. 15.12. Myotonic dystrophy. Teased muscle spindle. Ranvier's gold chloride. The pattern of innervation is grossly abnormal, the intrafusal nerve fibres having formed a tangled web of fibres. 1ary, primary sensory ending; 2ary, secondary sensory ending. (Reproduced with permission from Swash (1972) and the editor of *Brain*.)

Cataracts may seriously impair vision and require surgical excision. The distal leg weakness itself impairs gait, leading to a steppage gait; light splints support dorsiflexion and improve the gait pattern. Complete heartblock or arrhythmias should be treated by anti-arrhythmic drugs, e.g. mexiletine or nifedipine, or may require cardiac pacing The ECG should be checked annually to forestall the development of life-threatening cardiac complications. Similarly, ventilation may become impaired, due to diaphragmatic, intercostal and accessory respiratory muscle weakness and, in some patients, nocturnal intermittent positive pressure ventilation may be necessary to prevent hypoxia and sleep apnoea. Patients with myotonic dystrophy may develop a psychotic mental state and this is sometimes associated with ventilatory failure. The forced vital capacity (FVC) should be greater than 40 ml/kg.

Dysmotility in the gut is rarely a problem, but gastric retention may lead to vomiting through the achalasic oesophagus, with an attendant risk of inhalational pneumonia. Dysphagia may be troublesome. Anaesthesia is a potential hazard, both because of the oesophageal disorder, the muscular disorder and the cardiac involvement. Patients with myotonic dystrophy are sensitive to suxamethonium and long-acting neuromuscular blocking agents, and thiopentone anaesthesia may cause prolonged respiratory depression. Monitoring for arrhythmias is indicated during and after anaesthesia, and pre-operative assessment should include ECG and pulmonary function tests (Aldridge 1985).

Genetic Counselling

The proportion of symptomatic patients in families with myotonic dystrophy increases with increasing age and most, if not all, gene carriers can be detected by clinical examination, including EMG and slit-lamp examination for cataract by age 40 years (Bundey 1974; Harper 1989; Brunner et al. 1991). However, DNA analysis now plays the major role in genetic counselling; (Southers et al. 1992, Harper 1996). Direct determination of the number of CTG repeats on chromosome 19q provides firm data concerning gene carrier status. This information is especially important in women because of the potentially severe manifestation of congenital myotonic dystrophy. The p5B1.4 probe identified the mutation in 108 of the 112 unrelated patients studied by Shelbourne et al. (1993). This test is also useful in that it will identify the rare instance of children of fathers with the disease inheriting a *shorter* CTG repeat sequence and perhaps even escaping the disease.

Proximal Myotonic Myopathy (PROMM)

This is a multisystem, autosomal dominant disorder that is distinct from myotonic dystrophy, although there are many clinical similarities (Thornton et al. 1994; Ricker et al. 1994, 1995). Patients with PROMM often notice proximal myotonia and muscle pain, rather than the distal weakness and myotonia so characteristic of myotonic dystrophy. Proximal weakness develops, especially in the thighs. Cataracts are a feature, as in myotonic dystrophy. The mental state in PROMM is normal. Muscle atrophy is not a major feature. Facial weakness and distal limb weakness is not found in PROMM. The striking features of PROMM are the combination of proximal weakness and myotonia with pain, which may be severe. The weakness varies in severity over periods of hours or days. The disease is only slowly progressive, and there is variability in the phenotype within families. Rhabdomyolysis followed surgery in one patient (Moxley 1996), and cardiac arrhythmias have been noted. The CK is mildly elevated in some patients and, as in myotonic dystrophy, the gamma glutamyl transferase level (α GT) may be raised (Ricker et al. 1995). EMG reveals myotonia, but this may not be a prominent abnormality. High frequency discharges were reported by Ricker et al. (1995). The muscle biopsy shows nonspecific myopathic features will increased central nucleation and Type 2 hypertrophy.

Genetic analysis shows no abnormality in CTG repeats in the myotonia gene (19q 13.3), further evidence for the distinct nature of this disorder (Thornton et al. 1994).

Carbamazepine therapy may relieve muscle pain, but there is no other treatment.

Non-Dystrophic Myotonic Syndromes

Several different inherited forms of myotonia, without progressive myopathic weakness, are recognised (Table 15.3). Both the dominant and recessive forms of myotonia congenita are linked to chromosome 7q and represent abnormalities of chloride channels. A genetically distinct form of dominant myotonia congenita, responsive to acetazolamide treatment, is linked to the sodium channel locus on chromosome 17q (Ptacek et al. 1992). The clinical phenotypes of the chloride channel and sodium channel types of autosomal dominant myotonia congenita appear identical with the exception that the latter responds to acetozolamide (Ptacek et al. 1993).

Table 15.3. Non-dystrophic myotonic syndromes

	Age of onset	Distribution of myotonia	Myotonia induced by	Muscle hypertrophy	Weakness	Severity	Inheritance
Myotonia congenita (Thomsen's)	Congenital (birth or infancy)	Generalised, especially leg muscles	–	Variable	–	Usually mild	Autosomal dominant
Myotonia congenita (Becker's)	Usually 4–12 years	Generalised	–	Proximal muscles	Proximal muscles and hands	Variable, may be severe	Autosomal recessive
Paramyotonia congenita	Congenital	Face, hands	Cold, and repetitive movements	–	Hands	Periodic	Autosomal dominant
Hyperkalaemic period paralysis	Congenital	Face, hands	Repetitive movements	–	Mainly legs	Periodic	Autosomal dominant
Proximal myotonic myopathy	20–60 years	Proximal	–	–	Proximal, Mainly legs	Mild	Autosomal dominant
Myotonia fluctuans	2nd decade	Local or generalised	Exercise and oral potassium	–	–	Periodic may be severe	Autosomal dominant

Autosomal Dominant Myotonia Congenita

This is a benign disorder characterised by myotonia, first recognised shortly after birth or during infancy. The disorder is inherited as an autosomal dominant trait. It was first described by Dr Thomsen in 1876 in 20 members of his own family in four generations and was sufficiently severe to lead Thomsen to campaign for recognition of the disorder to prevent his son's conscription into the army. Myotonia is often first apparent in infancy when the child's cry is noted to sound strangled and the face is seen to relax in a delayed fashion after crying. The disorder is usually mild and is not progressive. It affects the legs more than the arms. Later in life myotonia congenita can be suspected by the presence of muscular hypertrophy, although the muscles often appear of normal bulk. The patient's major complaint, however, is usually of muscular stiffness induced by movement and relieved by continued exercise. Muscular stiffness (myotonia) is thus most troublesome at the start of a period of exercise or movement. Rarely myotonia induced by movement may be so sudden and severe that it leads to falls. Variations in this clinical picture, including the presence of painful muscular contractions and unusually marked cold dependency with facial involvement, have been reported in a few families by Becker (1977).

The muscles may be mildly weak when first tested, at a time when myotonia is severe. When the muscles have been "warmed-up" by exercise muscular strength is normal (Zwarts and van Weerden 1989). The myotonia tends to become less severe with increasing age. It can usually be induced by percussion and by electrical stimulation. The disease is rare (Becker 1971), occurring in 0.25–4/100 000 of the population in Germany (Becker 1977), and is genetically distinct from myotonic dystrophy (Höweler et al. 1980). Many cases may be unrecognised. Disability follows in only about 1% of cases (Bundey 1985).

The clinical features of the major disorders associated with symptomatic myotonia are summarised in Table 15.3. Becker (1977) and Ricker et al. (1990) described a form of dominant myotonia congenita with muscle pain associated with myotonic contracture and marked variation in severity from time to time. They termed this form of the disorder myotonia fluctuans.

Autosomal Recessive Myotonia Congenita

This syndrome has a similar incidence to the dominantly inherited myotonia congenita. Becker (1977) estimated an incidence of 2/100 000 and a carrier frequency of about 1%. The disease becomes apparent between the ages of 4 and 12 years and most cases present before age 6 years. It tends to become non-progressive, as a cause of disability, in adult life. Muscular hypertrophy is more striking than in the dominant form, but proximal muscles are mainly affected, especially thigh, buttock and shoulder-girdle muscles, and may be somewhat weak (Fig. 15.13). About 60% of patients develop some permanent weakness, especially of forearm and sterno-mastoid muscles. These features resemble those of myotonic dystrophy, and pes cavus and reduced reflexes may also occur, but the lens opacities so characteristic of myotonic dystrophy do not occur. Some male patients have reduction of potency, with small testes. Weakness may be quite transient, developing during initial effort after a

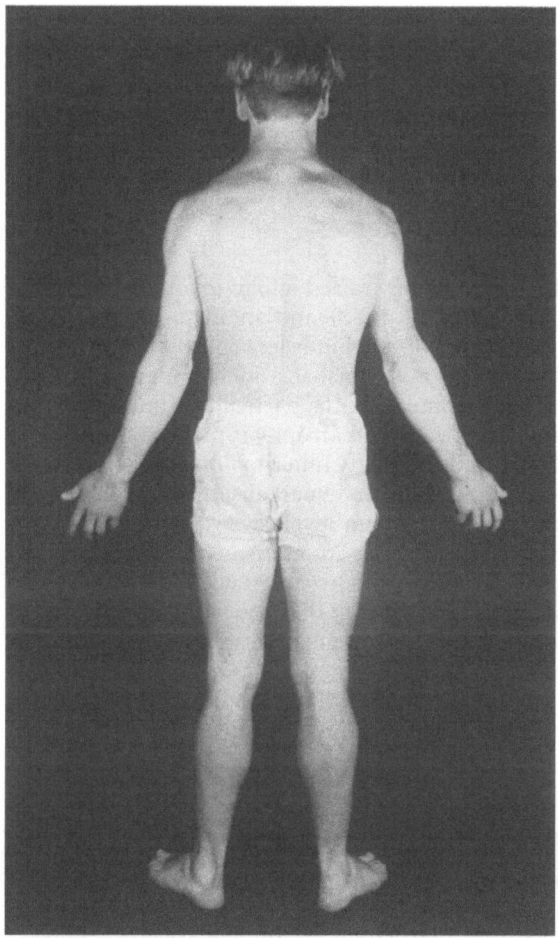

Fig. 15.13. Recessive myotonia congenita. Muscular hypertrophy develops as a result of the myotonia.

muscles and is aggravated by cold (Thrush et al. 1972). Myotonia may also be induced by movement, i.e. repetitive muscular contraction, in paramyotonia congenita, a phenomenon unique to this disorder that was termed *paradoxical myotonia* by Eulenberg. A characteristic feature of paramyotonia congenita is the response of muscles to cooling. EMG in a warm muscle may be normal or may show myotonic discharges, both at rest and following voluntary contraction. Cooling the muscle will provoke muscle stiffness (Eulenberg 1886), the phenomenon termed *paramyotonia* to distinguish it from myotonic stiffness. Paramyotonia is a phenomenon of much longer clinical duration than classical electrical myotonia and is accompanied by weakness of the stiff, inexcitable, cooled muscle. There is an abnormality both of excitability of the muscle membrane and of relaxation of the muscle fibre. The period of weakness following paramyotonia may last for several hours (Magre 1966; Lehmann-Horn et al. 1981). Myotonia induced by exercise, a form of true myotonia accompanied by electrophysiological features of myotonia in EMG recordings (Nielsen et al. 1982), may be followed by mild to moderate weakness of gradual onset and recovery during a period of up to several hours. Nielsen et al. (1982) noted that in myotonia congenita cooling produced prominent clinical and electrophysiological myotonia, an important point of difference from paramyotonia congenita.

Patients with paramyotonia congenita may have episodes of weakness that are not associated with muscle cooling. In some these episodes can be induced by potassium-loading. This feature had led to the suggestion that paramyotonia congenita is closely related to hyperkalaemic periodic paralysis, a disorder in which myotonia is also a feature (Table 15.3). Although paramyotonia is a benign disorder which may improve with increasing age, mild weakness may be a permanent feature, even between attacks of paramyotonia, in the later stages of the disease. Muscle fatigue is also a feature of paramyotonia congenita, a component of the disease also explained by the membrane defect in sodium channel function (Table 15.1).

period of rest, but usually disappears during continued activity. Thus, the clinical picture of a person with large, hypertrophied muscles, but with mild weakness, may be characteristic. Becker (1977) noted that there was an excess of more severely affected boys than girls in his cases. The myotonia is not cold-sensitive and is not associated with abnormal potassium homeostasis.

Paramyotonia Congenita

Eulenberg described this disorder in 1886 in six generations of a family with autosomal dominant inheritance, myotonia, paradoxical myotonia, post-myotonic weakness, weakness after vigorous exercise and cold provoked muscle stiffness. The condition is generally first recognised in childhood. The myotonia is most prominent in facial and hand

Hyperkalaemic Periodic Paralysis

This disorder is dominantly inherited, and usually presents in childhood with transient episodes of weakness (Gamstorp 1956). Becker (1977) used the term paralysis periodica paramyotonica to describe patients with hyperkalaemic attacks associated with cold-induced paramyotonia and weakness. Rest after exercise often induced attacks of weakness.

Myotonia can be induced by fist-clenching or percussion but is often particularly prominent in the periorbital muscles (van der Meulen et al. 1961). Missed meals may also provoke an attack of weakness and tingling or pain in the legs may precede weakness (Bradley 1969). Weakness invariably begins in the legs and arms and respiratory muscles are spared. The weakness reaches a peak in 30–60 min. and recovery is complete in a few hours. Death has not been recorded in an attack. During attacks the blood potassium is usually raised. Recovery can be hastened by exercise and can be localised to muscles used in exercise (Ricker et al. 1986).

The observation that myotonia in hyperkalaemic periodic paralysis may be worsened by cold led to the suggestion that this disorder might be related to paramyotonia congenita (Layzer et al. 1967a). However, some families with hyperkalaemic periodic paralysis do not have myotonia (McArdle 1962; Lehmann-Horn et al. 1983). Genetic linkage studies suggest that hyperkalaemic periodic paralysis and paramyotonia congenita are allelic disorders of the skeletal muscle sodium channel. The nature and site of the altered amino acid in the sodium channel subunit structure determines the phenotype, which may consist of either disorder or an intermediate phenotype with features of both rare disorders. Each family thus shows a consistent disorder (Barchi 1992). The other potassium disorders of muscle, hypokalaemic and normokalaemic periodic paralysis, do not show linkage to the sodium channel on chromosome 17q.

Myotonia Fluctuans

Myotonia fluctuans is the third myotonic syndrome associated with a mutation in muscle sodium channels. It has been recognised in only four families (Ricker et al. 1990, 1994). It is an autosomal dominant disorder, with onset in the second decade, characterised by myotonia of fluctuating severity, but without periodic weakness. The myotonia is not induced by cold exposure but is increased by exercise, it tends to develop 20–40 min after exercise. Recovery may occur in 30–60 min, or the myotonia may last all day. Sometimes, it is generalised leading to temporary immobilisation. Oral potassium loading can also induce an attack of myotonia. The CK level is raised. There is no association with malignant hyperthermia. The physiological basis for the induction of myotonia, with potassium sensitivity, but without muscular weakness, is uncertain (Ricker et al. 1994). The muscle biopsy shows slightly increased central nucleation and increased range of fibre diameter, with absence of Type 2B

fibres in some patients. DNA analysis has revealed mutations in exon 22, and in exon 14 of the sodium channel gene on chromosome 17q.

Laboratory Investigations in Inherited Myotonic Syndromes

The CK is usually raised in paramyotonia congenita (Thrush et al. 1972) and in myotonia fluctuans (Ricker et al. 1990), but is less abnormal in recessive generalised myotonia, in which it may be slightly raised in some patients, particularly those in whom distal weakness and atrophy is present (Kuhn et al. 1979). In dominantly inherited myotonia congenita the CK is normal. In hyperkalaemic periodic paralysis blood potassium levels are raised in attacks of exercise-induced or spontaneous generalised weakness, but normal between attacks. The CK may be slightly raised during the recovery phase. The ECG is normal in all these genetically determined myotonic syndromes, unless there is hyperkalaemia at the time of the recording. No other abnormalities have been reported.

Electrophysiological Findings in Inherited Myotonic Syndromes

The main EMG feature of these disorders is myotonia (Fig. 15.14) which may be so marked that analysis of MUAPs is difficult. Abnormal MUAPs have been reported only in recessive generalised myotonia, where myopathic potentials may be seen in proximal muscles and also in wrist and finger extensors and anterior tibial muscles (Sun and Streib 1983; Swash and Schwartz 1983b). In dominant myotonia congenita MUAPs are normal; the myotonia often predominates in the lower limb muscles. The electrical features of the myotonia, however, do not differ in different clinical syndromes. Intense

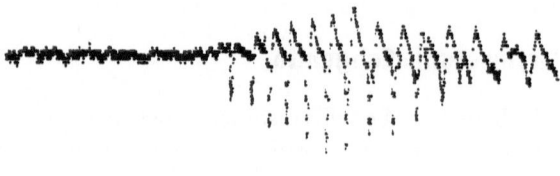

Fig. 15.14. Myotonia. Waxing and waning of the amplitude of the potential is evident in this recording from a patient with myotonia congenita. Concentric needle EMG. Filters: 100 Hz and 10 kHz. Bar 20 ms.

voluntary effort may produce distinctive abnormalities. In both myotonia congenita and paramyotonia congenita fatigue occurs, but a definite dropout of voluntary MUAPs occurs only in patients with paramyotonia. Patients with myotonia congenita can produce a full recruitment pattern immediately after a rest of a few seconds, but the recruitment pattern in patients with paramyotonia congenita is poor after a similar rest period.

In patients with paramyotonia there is relative electrical silence for 5–7 s after exercise even with needle movement (Subramony et al. 1983). Cooling may also induce fibrillations in paramyotonia but usually causes cessation of myotonia, weakness and electrical silence (Nielsen et al. 1982). Burke et al. (1974b) found that electrical nerve stimulation did not produce myotonia in paramyotonia congenita, as it does in myotonia congenita. They also noticed that myotonia became more difficult to elicit as the muscle under test fatigued, and that EMG evidence of myotonia subsided *before* the muscle relaxed completely, indicating an early electrical or membrane-dependent component and a later mechanical or contractile component. Lehmann-Horn et al. (1981) found that cooling caused depolarisation of the resting membrane potential of paramyotonic muscle from –80 mV to –40 mV; this was associated with slow (2 Hz) myotonic discharges. Later, with further cooling, the muscle fibres became inexcitable, with weakness and fatiguability (see also Haynes and Thrush 1972).

In hyperkalaemic periodic paralysis fibrillation potentials, positive sharp waves and complex repetitive discharges have been recorded between attacks (McArdle 1962; Layzer et al. 1967a) in addition to true myotonia (van der Meulen et al. 1961). The resting membrane potential, recorded with intracellular microelectrodes, is lowered during attacks of weakness and the muscle fibres are inexcitable to electrical stimulation at this time (Creutzfeldt et al. 1963; Brooks 1969), representing depolarisation block of muscle fibres (see chap. 19).

In myotonia fluctuans prominent myotonic activity may be seen, and this is enhanced after exercise when continuous fibrillation-like activity may be a feature. The MUPs themselves are normal (Ricker et al. 1994).

A decremental response to repetitive stimulation occurs in all forms of these inherited myotonic syndromes, as well as in myotonic dystrophy (Aminoff et al. 1977). This phenomenon was investigated by Brown (1974), who noted that the decremental response was more prominent at higher stimulation rates (10 Hz) than at slower rates, when the muscle was rested. At continued 10 Hz stimulation the response slowly increases in size after the initial

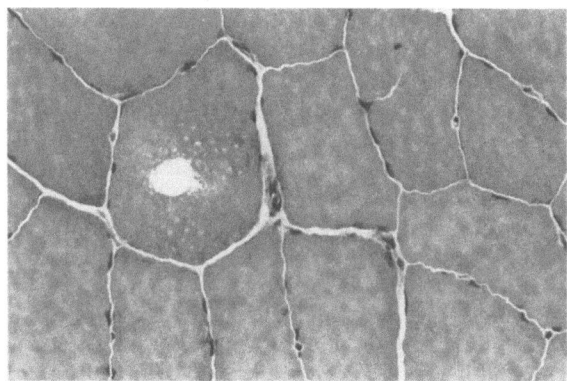

Fig. 15.15. Myotonia congenita. TS. H and E. × 140. There is hypertrophy of both fibre types and central nucleation is slightly increased with fibre splitting. A necrotic fibre is present. Mean diameter: Type 1, 92 μm; Type 2, 102 μm.

decrement so that it approaches the amplitude of the first response (Aminoff et al. 1977). Not all patients show this decremental/incremental response; it is particularly marked in recessive generalised myotonia (Aminoff et al. 1977) and Lundberg et al. (1974) noted a similar abnormality in one patient with paramyotonia congenita after 20 s stimulation at 10 Hz. In this patient the pretest amplitude of the evoked response was not attained until 20 s after cessation of the repetitive stimulation. In myotonia congenita decremental responses were found only in patients with weakness (Aminoff et al. 1977).

Motor and sensory nerve conduction velocity is normal in all non-dystrophic forms of inherited myotonia. Complex repetitive discharges, occurring in bursts, were reported by Lundberg et al. (1974) in paramyotonia congenita. Single-fibre EMG recordings in paramyotonia congenita have shown an increased neuromuscular jitter that sometimes increased until complete neuromuscular block occurred, but in other potentials an initially increased neuromuscular jitter would normalise within a few seconds of beginning a contraction (Lundberg et al. 1974). The motor unit fibre density was slightly increased in this patient. In myotonia congenita the fibre density and jitter are normal, but in recessive generalised myotonia, in association with myopathic potentials, the fibre density is increased (Swash and Schwartz 1983b), and the jitter is increased in about 10% of recordings.

Muscle Pathology

The most prominent abnormality is hypertrophy of muscle fibres (Fig. 15.15), slightly more evident in recessive generalised myotonia than in the dominantly inherited myotonia congenita. Central nucleation is slightly increased, but chains of nuclei and sarcoplasmic masses are not present (Swash and Schwartz 1983b). Scattered atrophic and degenerative fibres are a feature of recessive generalised myotonia. Type 2B fibres are absent in some cases of myotonia congenita (Crews et al. 1976) and are also absent in recessive generalised myotonia (Zellweger et al. 1980). Scattered necrotic fibres can be seen in recessive generalised myotonia, but not in dominant myotonia congenita. Tubular aggregates and vacuoles have been reported in dominant myotonia congenita and in paramyotonia congenita (Schroder and Becker 1972) but not in recessive generalised myotonia, an observation that may be related to hyperkalaemia. Subsarcolemmal filamentous bodies were reported in dominant myotonia congenita by Kuhn et al. (1979). In paramyotonia congenita Thrush et al. (1972) noted the presence of undifferentiated fibres with central nucleation, and some central vacuoles. Fibre splitting may be prominent. They also found expansion of motor end-plates on hypertrophied fibres and some multiple end-plate formation. The pattern of innervation in myotonia congenita is normal (Coërs and Woolf 1959). Muscle spindle morphology and innervation in recessive generalised myotonia is normal (Swash and Schwartz 1983b). The pathology of hyperkalaemic periodic paralysis includes vacuolar change, tubular aggregates and mild myopathic features resembling the changes found in other periodic paralysis syndromes.

Treatment of Myotonic Syndromes

Various drugs are used in the management of myotonia. For chronic therapy phenytoin has been recommended (Munsat 1967; Griggs 1977), but quinine and procainamide have also been used, although both of these drugs theoretically disturb atrio-ventricular cardiac conduction. In some patients (Griggs 1977) acetazolamide (Diamox) may be useful and occasional patients are said to respond to diazepam, thiazides or baclofen (Karli and Bergstrom 1974). Phenytoin, quinine and procainamide are thought to act by stabilising muscle fibre membranes, decreasing net sodium influx during membrane depolarisation. Acetazolamide, however, causes kaliuresis, reducing extracellular potassium levels and so increasing the resting membrane potential. Brooke

(1977) stated that acetazolamide made myotonia worse in paramyotonia congenita. Class 1 cardiac antiarrhythmic drugs, such as tocainide, verapamil and mexilitene (Streib 1986) have been tried and tocainide 1200–1600 mg/day is probably the most effective drug. It stabilises the muscle membrane by an action on the sodium channel. Side effects include nausea, irritability and action tremor, but the problems resolve when dosage is reduced (Rudel et al. 1980; Streib 1986). Unfortunately, tocainide has potentially serious cardio-toxic effects and mexilitene, phenytoin or quinine are the drugs of choice. The mechanisms of action of Class 1 drugs have been reviewed by Roden and Woosley (1986), who noted other serious unwanted effects, particularly agranulocytosis, that limit the usefulness of tocainide. These drugs modify myotonia by prolonging the refractory period of sodium channels, thus preventing repetitive discharges of muscle fibres. Verapamil (Cook and Henderson-Tilton 1984) and nifepidine may also be of value (Grant et al. 1987).

Since succinylcholine and anticholinesterase agents may aggravate myotonia (Kaufman 1960; Paterson 1962) d-tubocurarine is preferable as a muscle relaxant during anaesthesia of patients with myotonia of any cause (Caughey and Myrianthopoulos 1963). Potassium-sparing diuretics, such as spironolactone, and potassium supplements may also aggravate myotonia.

Differential Diagnosis

Myotonia congenita must be distinguished from other disorders in which myotonia occurs. In infancy congenital myotonic dystrophy is usually a serious disorder with weakness, hypotonia and a characteristic facies (see below). Further, the mother usually shows stigmata of the disease. In older children or adults neuromyotonia must be considered as an explanation for the muscular stiffness and can be recognised by the presence of MUAPs, rather than single muscle fibre potentials, with EMG (Chap. 2). Myotonia congenita must also be distinguished from typical myotonic dystrophy and this may be difficult, especially in recessive generalised myotonia in which distal atrophy may be a feature. The diagnosis of a genetic myotonic syndrome can be made by muscle biopsy and by the absence of the other characteristic features of myotonic dystrophy, especially cataract, frontal baldness etc. Genetic testing with specific markers can be used to establish diagnosis and heredity in doubtful cases and for genetic counselling.

Schwartz–Jampel Syndrome

Although chondrodystrophic myotonia (Schwartz and Jampel 1962) has been characterised as a disorder associated with myotonia the muscle fibre discharges at rest are continuous and of high frequency and low voltage. They also differ from typical myotonic discharges in that they do not wax and wane; in some reports they were not blocked by curare, an observation suggesting that in these cases these discharges were originating in the muscle fibres, like true myotonia. Discharges blocked by curare resemble neuromyotonia. The spontaneous activity recorded in Schwartz–Jampel syndrome therefore seems to be of several types (Cao et al. 1978). The electrical activity does not disappear with sleep, a point of difference from Isaac's syndrome and from stiff man syndrome (Spaans et al. 1990). Benzodiazepines have no effect.

The clinical features of the disorder consist of muscular stiffness and hypertrophy with persistent electrical discharges in muscle and multiple ocular, facial and skeletal deformities. Blepharophimosis is a characteristic feature (Schwartz and Jampel 1962). There is often dwarfism and mental retardation may occur (Fowler et al. 1974; Farrell et al. 1987). Most cases are familial, probably autosomal recessive, but with variable expression. The presence of many of the clinical features of Schwartz–Jampel syndrome in other disorders has suggested that the disorder may not be homogeneous in character (Fitch et al. 1971).

Electrophysiological Assessment

The main features consist of the myotonia and pseudomyotonia discussed above (Black et al. 1972). Nerve conduction studies are normal (Cao et al. 1978). Study of individual motor unit potentials is difficult because of the presence of continuous spontaneous activity (Cao et al. 1978). Repetitive stimulation results in delayed relaxation due to after discharges (Fowler et al. 1974).

Muscle Biopsy

The most prominent abnormality is fibre hypertrophy, with increased variation in fibre size, increased central nucleation and occasional small angulated fibres, degenerative fibres and fibres showing fibre splitting. The atrophic fibres are often Type 1 and may occur in small groups. The hypertrophied fibres may be strikingly rounded (Fariello et al. 1978). There is sometimes increased interfascicular and endomysial fibrous tissue. There may be scattered morphological changes, such as vacuolation and focal hyaline change in some fibres (Spaans et al. 1990). In one of the patients described by Fowler et al. (1974) there was a diffuse increase in sarcoplasmic staining for acetylcholinesterase. The motor end-plates, however, were not studied in this case. Nonetheless, the abnormality in acetylcholinesterase distribution suggests that the entire surface of the muscle fibre membrane may retain its sensitivity to acetylcholine, as in fetal muscle, and not show regional specialisation of acetylcholine receptor activity in the motor end-plate region as in normally innervated muscle. It may therefore represent an abnormality of the trophic response to innervation (Fowler et al. 1974) and could lead to abnormal excitability and prolonged depolarisation of the muscle fibre membrane as a whole.

Ultrastructural studies have shown dilatation of the endoplasmic reticulum, an abnormality which has also been shown in cutaneous fibroblasts (Fowler et al. 1974).

Management

In some cases the spontaneous activity decreases with phenytoin therapy, presumably because the drug is effective in the treatment of neuromyotonia. Procainamide may be helpful in those cases in which true myotonia is a feature.

Drug-Induced Myotonia

Myotonia may be acquired, for example in myxoedema and in hypokalaemic paralysis, and may occur after treatment with drugs which interfere with lipid metabolism in muscle fibre membranes, such as 20,25-diazocholesterol, monocarboxylic aromatic acids, 2,4-dihydroxy acetate, clofibrate and triparonol (Winer et al. 1966; Seiler et al. 1975; Bryant 1977). It has been suggested that the underlying membrane defect in these experimental and drug-induced myotonias is an accumulation of desmosterol (Ramsay et al. 1978) and it is of some interest that these drugs may also induce cataracts. Desmosterol accumulation leads to an abnormality of chloride conductance (Chalikian and Barchi 1982). These experimental studies led Barchi (1982) to suggest that myotonia could arise from low membrane chloride conductance, from changes in the physical properties of muscle fibre membranes, and from specific abnormalities in the sodium conductance system.

Muscle Contracture Induced by Exercise

Brody and Dudley (1969) described a single case of a young man who had noted painless muscle stiffness induced by exercise, which could be so severe that he would fall during running. The stiffness was more prominent in cold weather and was painless unless he continued his efforts to exercise in the face of the muscular stiffness. Investigation revealed that the muscle contractions were electrically silent, thus resembling the painful cramps of McArdle's disease, and so were not due to myotonia but to a defect in the relaxation phase of muscle fibre contraction. Evidence was presented that the underlying cause was defective re-uptake of calcium by the sarcoplasmic reticulum, perhaps from a selective defect of "relaxing factor". In addition, an abnormally high production of lactate was demonstrated at rest, a finding thought to be due to increased calcium-dependent phosphorylase activity. Although somewhat similar changes in calcium re-uptake in the sarcoplasmic reticulum have been found in muscular dystrophy and other disorders (Samaha and Gergely 1969), no similar cases have been reported.

Chapter **16**   Childhood Myopathies

The childhood myopathies are a group of slowly progressive or non-progressive myopathies, often presenting in the neonatal period or in infancy with weakness and reduced muscle tone. These disorders are defined by their pathological features. They form a subgroup of the "floppy infant syndrome" (Dubowitz 1980). The first of these disorders was described by Shy and Magee (1956) as a congenital non-progressive myopathy, a term that has replaced the older designations amyotonia congenita and benign congenital hypotonia (Walton 1956).

The clinical syndrome consists of reduced resistance of joints to passive movements and increased range of movement of joints. Affected infants usually show reduced spontaneous movements, and older children have delayed motor development milestones. These features can result from myopathies, including metabolic disorders such as glycogen storage disease, or from neurogenic disease, for example spinal muscular atrophy or motor neuropathy. However, similar clinical features are also found in children with disorders of the central nervous system, especially cerebral palsy, birth trauma, and hypoxic injury. Metabolic encephalopathies may also cause hypotonia. Additional causes include connective tissue disease, e.g. mucopolysaccharidosis and Ehlers–Danlos syndrome, Prader-Willi syndrome and reversible metabolic diseases, e.g. rickets and hypothyroidism. In a few cases the syndrome is not associated with any underlying cause and with increasing maturity the hypotonia resolves (Dubowitz 1980).

In the congenital myopathies, as a group, there is slowness in achieving motor milestones, the palate is often highly arched and there may be associated skeletal deformities. Although most of these myopathies are inherited the gene locations are not yet characterised in many of them. Some are very rare (Table 16.1). Laboratory investigations are not usually helpful; CK levels are often normal. The EMG is useful in establishing that weakness is due to muscle disease and is thus an important step in the decision to perform a muscle biopsy. Diagnostic criteria have been suggested for nemaline myopathy, central core disease and minicore disease, based on the clinical and pathological features and on the genetic information (Table 16.1) (Middleton and Moser 1994).

Central Core Disease

This was the first of the benign myopathies of childhood to be characterised as a separate entity and is probably the most common. Shy and Magee (1956) defined central core disease by its histological features and described the clinical features. They reported five patients in three generations of a single family in whom hypotonia was recognised shortly after birth. There was delay in achieving motor milestones, such as walking, with mild and non-progressive weakness of proximal limb musculature. Sometimes weakness may be more generalised and mild weakness of face and neck musculature may be evident (Gonatas et al. 1965). Occasionally the onset of the disease may be delayed until childhood (Bethlem et al. 1966; Dubowitz and Roy 1970). Congenital dislocation of the hip is a frequent feature and there may be kyphoscoliosis, increased lumbar lordosis and pes cavus (Armstrong et al. 1971). In cases observed in adult life weakness remains only slight. The tendon reflexes are normal or slightly reduced. The disorder has almost always been reported as showing a dominant pattern of inheritance, as in the original report (Shy and Magee 1956), but sporadic cases have also been recognised. Patterson et al. (1979) have described a family in which some affected members showed progression of the disease, and others developed it in adult life. Malignant hyperpyrexia has also been associated with central core disease (Denborough et al. 1973; Frank et al. 1980). In central core disease the genetic locus is on the proximal long arm of

Table 16.1. Congenital myopathies: clinical and genetic features

Myopathy	Inheritance	Gene location	Dysmorphisms	Ocular muscle weakness	Facial weakness	Pain, cramp, stiffness	Muscle wasting	cardiomyopathy
Central core disease	AD	19q 13.1	+++	+	+	+		
Multicore disease	Variable		++	+	+			+
Nemaline								
infantile onset	AD	1q 21-23	+++	++	+++		++	
adult onset	AD					++	+++	++
Myotubular								
infantile onset	X-linked recessive	xq 28		++	++			++
adult onset	AD		++	++	++		++	
Congenital fibre-type disproportion	AD		++++		+++	+		
Other rare syndromes								
Fingerprint	?AR		++				++	
Reducing body			+++	+	+			+
Sarcotubular								
Tubular aggregates			+			+++		+
Desmin storage	AD	+						
Cytoplasmic body	AD					++	+	
Zebra body								
Trilaminar body	(only one case described)				.	++	+	
Lysis of myofibrils	?AR		++					
Cap disease	(only one case described)		++					

AD, autosomal dominant; AR, autosomal recessive.

chromosome 19 (13q 19.1) adjacent or identical to the locus for the ryanodine receptor, the underlying membrane defect in malignant hyperpyrexia (Kausch et al. 1991; Zhang et al. 1993). Since susceptibility to malignant hyperpyrexia is found in most but not all cases of central core disease the genetic defect may not be identical in the two disorders (Bodensteiner 1994).

Laboratory Investigations

The CK is usually normal, but may be raised in cases of later onset (Patterson et al. 1979).

Electrophysiological Assessment

The EMG usually reveals mild myopathic changes, consisting of polyphasic MUAPs of short duration in a proportion of the units sampled. In some patients the units may be of long duration and the interference pattern may be reduced (Dubowitz and Roy 1970). The single-fibre EMG fibre density may be increased (Cruz-Martinez et al. 1979). Motor nerve conduction velocity is normal. EMG recordings can be normal.

Muscle Biopsy

In haematoxylin and eosin preparations the abnormality is very slight. Scattered atrophic, or hypertrophied fibres may be seen but central nucleation

and degenerative or regenerative changes in single muscle fibres are rare (Dubowitz and Roy 1970). Connective tissue is normal. However, in the modified Gomori preparation many fibres show a sharply defined bluish central region. These abnormal cores (Fig. 16.1) are found almost invariably in Type 1 fibres, and there is usually Type 1 fibre predominance in the biopsy. NADH-tr preparations show that the central cores are unreactive but in myosin ATPase and phosphorylase preparations there may be increased enzyme activity within them. Central cores can also be readily demonstrated in PAS preparations, in which they stain relatively lightly, and in formalin-fixed material they can be demonstrated as light zones with the PTAH technique. Cores vary in size but may be as large as half the area of affected fibres, and they may be centrally or eccentrically located. Most fibres contain only a single core but individual fibres may contain one or several cores. Thornell et al. (1983) showed accumulation of desmin (Fardeau and Tomé 1994) in and surrounding cores. There is a trend for cores to be present in a larger proportion of Type 1 fibres in the biopsies of affected parents than in their offspring (Dubowitz and Roy 1970; Morgan-Hughes et al. 1973).

In the family described by Patterson et al. (1979) it was noted that in one patient, in whom biopsies were performed 18 months apart, there was an increase in Type 1 fibre predominance, an observation that suggests that Type 2 muscle fibres became reinnervated by Type 1 axons.

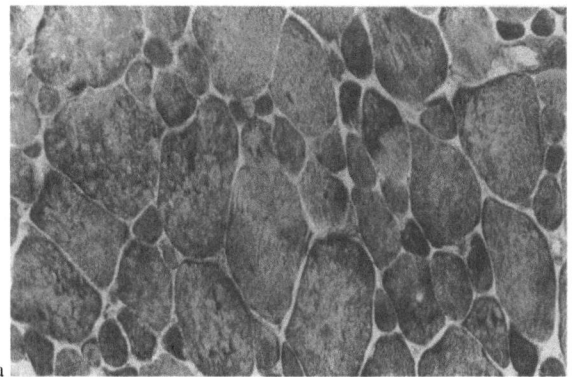

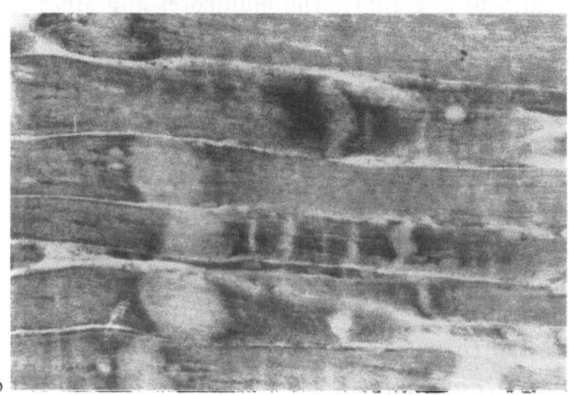

Fig. 16.1. Central core disease. TS. × 140. **a** NADH-tr **b** ATPase. Type 1 fibres contain pale zones (cores unreactive in NADH-tri and ATPase preparations. The margin of these non-reactive cores is slightly dark with NADH-tr, but this dark rim is not as prominent as in target fibres (see Fig. 3.21). Cores unreactive for ATPase are termed *unstructured*, and cores reactive for ATPase are termed *structured*. **b** Shows relatively normal sarcomeres, which are slightly contracted in relation to the adjacent normal sarcomeres. Unstructured cores show disorganisation of myofibrils within the cores.

The differentiation between cores and target fibres has led to confusion because of the recognition of two types of core; structured and unstructured (Neville and Brooke 1973). In central core disease structured cores are easily differentiated from target fibres. In the former the central core area has altered myofibrils which retain their cross-striations although their sarcomeres may be contracted and their associated mitochondria are absent. In the latter the myofibrillar pattern is distorted. With the light microscope structured cores show increased staining for myosin ATPase, but target fibres are negative with this technique. In addition, target fibres may be found both in Type 1 and Type 2 fibres, and central cores, unlike targets, extend throughout the length of affected Type 1 fibres, as far as this point can be ascertained.

Unstructured cores, however, are more difficult to differentiate from target fibres. The myosin ATPase reaction shows an almost unstained central zone similar to that shown in NADH-tr preparations, and the darkly staining edge of the central area of abnormality seen in ATPase preparations of target fibres is absent. Even with electron microscopy unstructured cores and targets appear similar and the term "core-targetoid" fibres has been proposed in order to circumvent this apparently artificial distinction (Engel et al. 1966). Isaacs et al. 1975) found structured and unstructured cores in the biopsies of two cases of central core disease.

Causation and Associated Features

The similarity of central cores to targets, the selective involvement of Type 1 fibres, the finding of an increased terminal innervation ratio in intra-vital methylene blue studies (Telerman-Toppet et al. 1973; Isaacs et al. 1975), the frequent occurrence of pes cavus and reduced tendon reflexes and the experimental replication of core-like fibres in the cat 3–5 weeks after denervation (Engel et al. 1966) has led to the suggestion that central core disease may represent an abnormality of the differentiation of muscle fibres occurring during development, possibly from a neurogenic cause acquired in utero. However, this explanation does not account for the suggestion that the number of cores may increase with age. Schmitt and Volk (1975) noted a sequence of changes in the central regions of muscle fibres after denervation in man, in which lesions resembling unstructured cores seemed to develop from an initial targetoid appearance. In rare cases rod bodies have been found in association with central cores, but this is probably a non-specific finding (Isaacs et al. 1975). However, in one family, the affected mother's biopsy showed both cores and rod bodies and her daughter's biopsy showed only cores (Afifi et al. 1965). Cores may develop experimentally in rat muscle following tenotomy (Shafiq et al. 1969; Baker and Hall-Craggs 1980), and Bethlem et al. (1978) suggested that cores, miniature cores, rods and focal loss of cross-striations (see below) all have a common origin.

Multicore Disease

Rarely, multiple cores have been seen in all Type 1 fibres (Engel et al. 1971). This disorder may be genetically distinct, being inherited as an autosomal recessive character, and is probably more severe clinically. The infant is floppy at birth, with reduction in muscle bulk especially of the upper limbs. Contractures may be present and external ocular movements may be restricted or there may be external ophthalmoplegia. The disorder may be progressive, even in late-onset variants (van Wijngaarden et al. 1977; Swash and Schwartz 1981). Respiratory failure may occur with respiratory tract infections (Fitzsimons and Tyer 1980; Swash and Schwartz 1981). Multicore disease has also been reported in adults (Bonnette et al. 1974). Ben Hamida et al. (1987) described a patient in whom "multi-minicore disease" was associated with rigid spine syndrome. Cardiac abnormalities are common including septal defects and cardiomyopathy.

Investigations

The EMG shows myopathic features, with normal motor nerve conduction velocity. The fibre density is increased and some potentials show an increased neuromuscular jitter (Swash and Schwartz 1981). The CK is normal. The ECG may be abnormal in patients with heart block or cardiomyopathy (Shuaib et al. 1988).

Pathology

Central cores are longer than multicores (minicores), typically extending for at least several hundred μm (Shy and Magee 1956) but multicores are short (Currie et al. 1974), although there is overlap in the transverse diameters of core and multicore lesions (Bethlem et al. 1978). In central core disease each fibre usually contains only one core lesion (Bethlem et al. 1966; Telerman-Toppet et al. 1973), and the abnormality is almost restricted to Type 1 fibres but in multicore disease the abnormality is found in both fibre types. However, cases have been reported in which typical cores, multicores and focal loss of cross-striations co-existed in the same biopsy and even in the same fibre (Bethlem et al. 1978). The distinction between multicores and focal loss of cross-striations rests on the presence of vesicular nuclei in and around the latter lesions, and on the larger size of the former. Bethlem et al. (1978) suggested that focal loss of cross-striations represented a late stage in the evolution of multicore lesions and that in congenital multicore disease the lesions remained in the multicore phase. However, there was no relation between age and the presence of focal loss of cross-striations as might have been expected if these lesions were derived from multi-

cores. The biopsies of the two patients reported by Swash and Schwartz (1981) and some of those reported by Bethlem et al. (1978) showed both multicores and areas of focal loss of cross-striations. Martin et al. (1986) reported a similar case.

Areas of focal loss of cross-striations tend to occur in adjacent zones of different muscle fibres. It has been postulated that this distribution of lesions might be due to their proximity to small blood vessels (Bethlem et al. 1978) but it might equally well be explained by local stresses within the muscle, and no abnormality in morphology or distribution of capillaries has been detected (Swash and Schwartz 1981). The multicores and areas of focal loss of cross-striation show Z band streaming, and smearing, sparse mitochondria and abnormalities in the tubular system (van Wijngaarden et al. 1977). In cases in which multicores are associated with focal loss of cross-striations, failure of fibre-type differentiation may also be a feature (Swash and Schwartz 1981).

Management of Central Core and Multicore Disease

When disability is modest no active measures are necessary. Infants with congenital dislocation of the hip, or kyphoscoliosis may require treatment, as indicated, for these features of the disorder. Respiratory failure is a serious but uncommon complication that may accompany infection but management with ventilatory assistance is effective and recovery of muscle strength develops (Swash and Schwartz 1981). The onset of adolescence may be accompanied by improvement in strength. Intellect is unaffected in these disorders.

Nemaline Myopathy

There are three forms of this disease, a severe neonatal syndrome which is usually fatal (Schmalbruch et al. 1987), an infantile-onset syndrome, and an adult-onset disorder. Shy et al. (1963) and Conen et al. (1963) described two infants aged 4 years with generalised hypotonia, proximal muscular weakness, absent tendon reflexes, weakness of facial and pharyngeal muscles with a high palate and high-arched pectus excavatum. These features have suggested a primary neurogenic cause for nemaline myopathy, but all investigations nonetheless support its current classification as a myopathy. Motor milestones are delayed. Respiratory difficulties may be prominent in infancy, but the disorder varies greatly in severity from case to case (Kurtonen et al. 1972). Sometimes death occurs from respiratory failure (Shafiq et al. 1967). These clinical features have subsequently been recognised in other cases, but may also be seen in other congenital myopathies of childhood. One in five affected children die in the first 5 years of life. Hopkins et al. (1966) pointed out that nemaline myopathy had previously been termed Krabbe's universal muscular atrophy.

In an adult-onset form, that is less common than the infantile-onset disorder, weakness may be present in a proximal distribution, especially affecting the legs (Engel and Resnick 1966; Heffernan et al. 1968), or in a scapulo-peroneal distribution with footdrop (Feigenbaum and Munsat 1970). This syndrome may be very mild, and recognised only on presentation with cardiomyopathy, or in a genetic investigation of a family following recognition of the disease in a child (Meier et al. 1984). The adult-onset form may be a different disease, given its different clinical course (Shimomura and Nonaka 1989).

The disease is usually dominantly but may be recessively inherited (Spiro and Kennedy 1965). Kondo and Yuasa (1980), however, suggested that it is always dominantly inherited. A locus on chromosome 1q 21–23 has been reported (Laing et al. 1992). Biopsies of parents of affected children may show sparse rod bodies (Arts et al. 1978), but a more constant feature is Type 1 fibre predominance and atrophy (Bender and Willner 1978).

Investigations

The CK may be mildly elevated, but is often normal. With concentric needle EMG typical myopathic MUAPs are found. In five cases studied with single-fibre EMG the fibre density was moderately increased (2.4 to 2.9) (M.S. Schwartz, unpublished observations). Motor conduction is normal. Wallgren-Patterson et al. (1989) noted the development of neuropathic features on EMG during follow-up, possibly due to remodelling of the motor unit during the disease.

Muscle Biopsy

In most cases the muscles sampled, both at biopsy and at autopsy, show little abnormality apart from

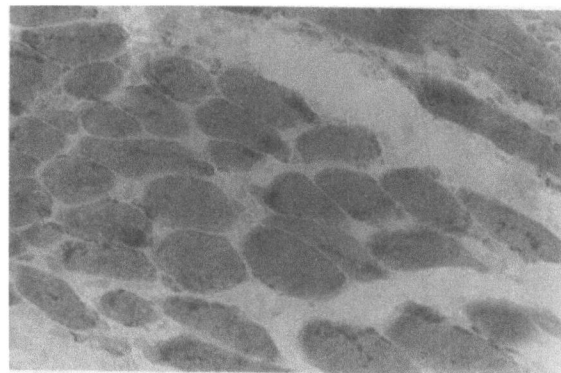

Fig. 16.2. Gomori trichome. TS. × 360. Rod bodies. Peripherally placed collection of rod-like structures, stained red in this preparation, are the characteristic feature of nemaline myopathy. Almost all the fibres are affected.

the presence of nemaline (rod) bodies. Shafiq et al. (1967) found increased variability in fibre size, disruption of the fascicular structure, degeneration of individual fibres and proliferation of perimysial and endomysial fibrous tissue in autopsied cases but these changes were unusually severe. There may be Type 1 fibre predominance and the Type 1 fibres are often smaller than normal.

Rod bodies are difficult to see in haematoxylin and eosin stains, but they may be seen with phase-contrast microscopy (Hudgson et al. 1967). They are best demonstrated in frozen sections with the modified Gomori technique, in which they appear as short, bright-red structures often arranged in subsarcolemmal clusters (Fig. 16.2). They may also be recognised as pale areas. They vary in number from case to case and from muscle to muscle, and even from fibre to fibre in individual muscles. There is no correlation between the number of rods found in a muscle and the degree of weakness. Type 1 fibres are mainly affected. Intrafusal fibres may also be affected. Rods have also been recognised as intranuclear inclusions (Engel and Oberc 1975). In some cases there is failure of differentiation of fibre types (Nienhuis et al. 1967; Karpati et al. 1971).

With electron microscopy the rod bodies, 3–6 μm in length and 1–3 μm in width, can sometimes be seen to originate from the Z disc. They consist, in transverse sections, of a tetragonal array of filaments continuous with thin filaments (actin) of the myofilaments (Engel 1966a). Individual rods may extend over several sarcomeres and they may then replace normal elements of muscle (Fig. 16.3).

The main component of rod bodies is α-actinin, which is also the main protein component of the Z disc (Jennekens et al. 1983). Desmin, the structural protein of the intermediate filaments of muscle

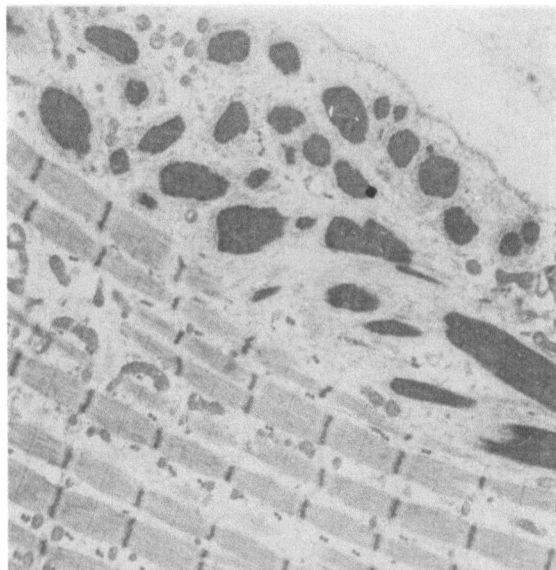

a

fibres, tends to accumulate at the periphery of rod bodies (Thornell et al. 1983). α-Actinin probably holds the actin filaments to the Z line in normal muscle (Stromer et al. 1976). Rod body formation results from derangement of the control mechanism that restricts α-actinin to the Z disc in normal myofilaments (Morris et al. 1990).

Rarely, rod bodies have been associated with cores and minicores in the same biopsy (Vallat et al. 1982). Rod bodies have also been described in the heart in a patient presenting with cardiac failure, with a family history of sudden death; in this case the typical features of nemaline myopathy were found in a quadriceps muscle biopsy (Meier et al. 1983).

Rod bodies are not a feature specific to nemaline myopathy. They also occur in normal extra-ocular muscle (Mukano 1969), central core disease (Afifi

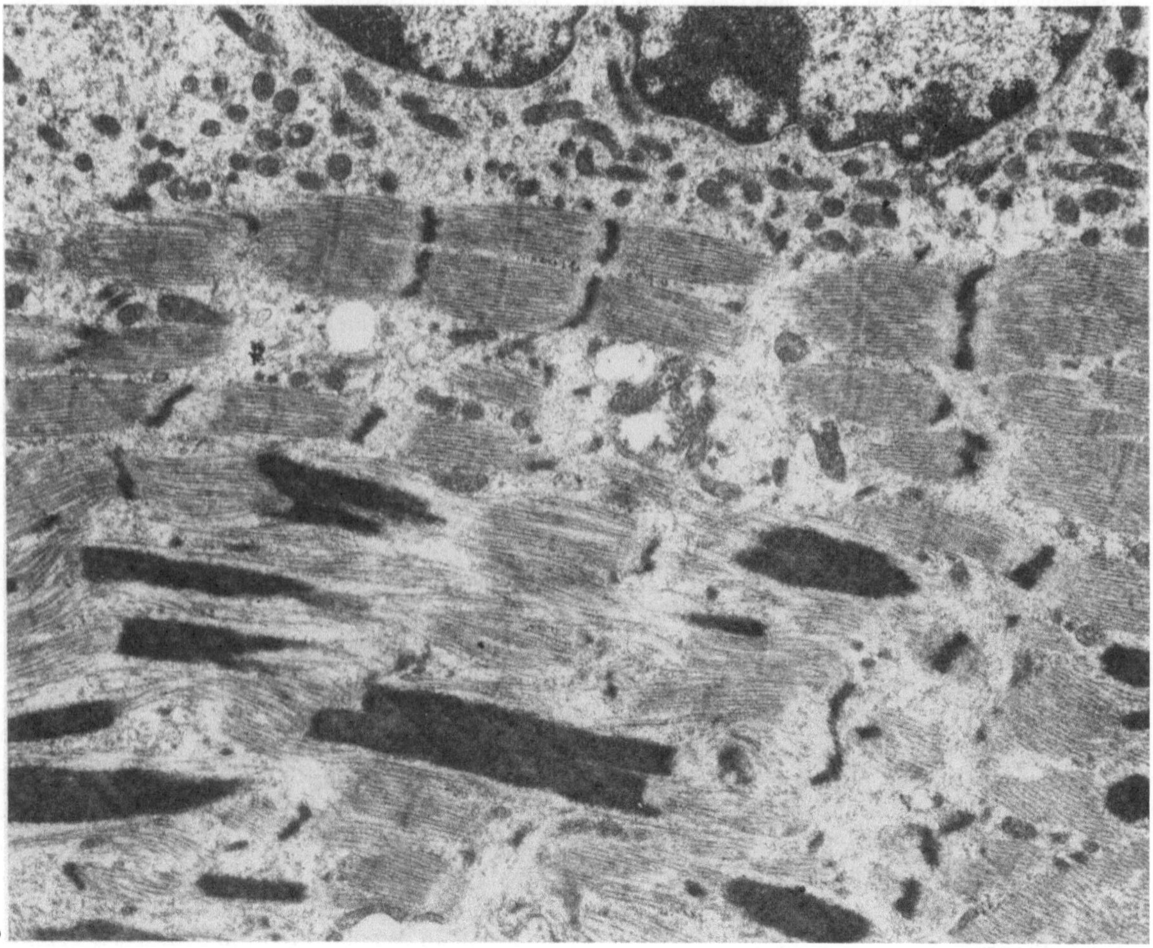

b

Fig. 16.3a,b.   Electron micrography, LS. Rod body myopathy. In these two micrographs the tendency for rod bodies to accumulate at the periphery of affected fibres, in a zone of myofibrillar disruption, can be seen. In addition, the origin of rod bodies from Z band material is also apparent.

et al. 1965), other myopathies (Dubowitz and Brooke 1973), denervation (Mair and Tomé 1973), polymyositis, after tenotomy in the cat (Engel et al. 1966), and even in schizophrenia (Meltzer et al. 1973). In these conditions, however, rods are found less frequently than in nemaline myopathy itself in which most of the fibres in a biopsy may contain rod bodies, and they are usually diffusely located in affected fibres rather than mainly in the subsarcolemmal zone, as in nemaline myopathy itself.

Management

In affected infants the major life-threatening problem is respiratory embarrassment from weakness of pharyngeal and other muscles. The myopathy, however, may be mild and no special measures are then required. Cardiomyopathy has also been described (Meier et al. 1983), and is potentially fatal, when cardiac transplantation is offered.

Myotubular (Centronuclear) Myopathy

Myotubular myopathy (Spiro et al. 1966), also known as centronuclear myopathy (Sher et al. 1967), is a rare disorder usually characterised by hypotonia with delayed motor milestones in infancy. Three forms of the disease have been recognised (Table 16.2). In cases with neonatal onset, there is generalised weakness and hypotonia which may progress rapidly leading to death from cardio-pulmonary failure before the age of 18 months. There is often facial weakness (Fig. 16.4) and external ophthalmoplegia. Cardiomyopathy may be a feature (Verhiest et al. 1976). Bilateral talipes and dislocation of the hips may be present (Heckmatt et al. 1985) and myotonic dystrophy must be excluded by EMG and by clinical and genetic analysis of the family, especially the mother. All these early-onset cases are

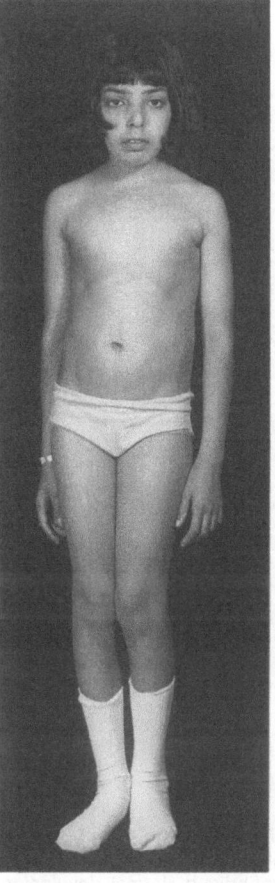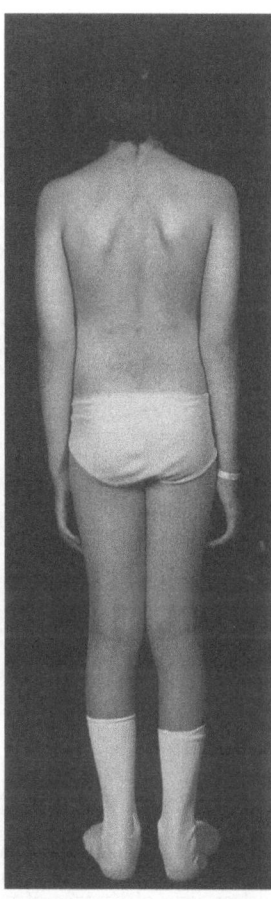

Fig. 16.4. Myotubular myopathy. This young girl has mild facial and limb-girdle weakness with hypotonia. Muscular atrophy is not a major feature.

inherited as X-linked recessive traits (Barth et al. 1975; Askanas et al. 1979).

Other cases of early infantile onset may have a slower course with severe disability (van Wijngaarden et al. 1969), and the ultimate disability may be relatively slight. The extra-ocular and facial and neck muscles may be involved (Bethlem et al. 1969). The tendon reflexes may be absent.

A form of the illness beginning in later childhood is more benign (Serratrice et al. 1978b), and in an adult-onset group of cases, in which inheritance may be dominant, the disease begins in the second decade or later and runs a benign course (McLeod et al. 1972). In one family of four affected sisters this form of the disease was associated with diabetes mellitus (Swash et al. 1970). Calf muscles may be hypertrophied.

De Angelis et al. (1991) reviewed 288 cases and noted a 90% mortality in the neonatal X-linked recessive form. The variable prognosis, and the vari-

Table 16.2. Types of myotubular (centronuclear) myopathy

Onset	Genetics	Clinical features
Neonatal	X-linked	Diffuse weakness Respiratory weakness Fatal outcome
Infancy and early childhood	Variable	Ophthalmoplegia Delayed motor milestones Mild generalised weakness
Late onset	Dominant	Proximal weakness

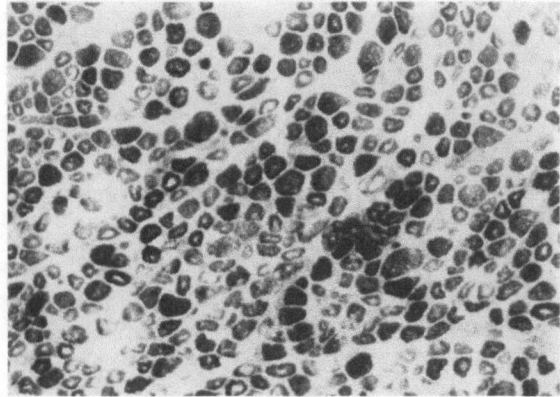

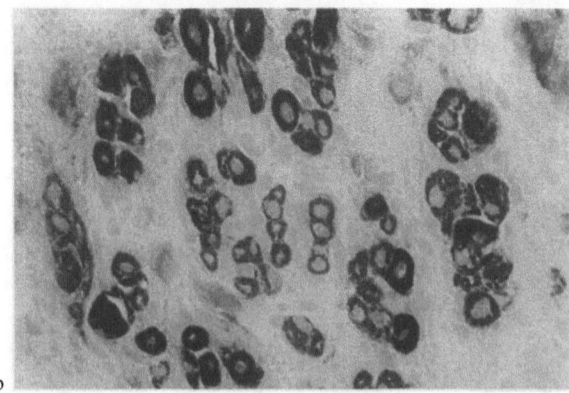

Fig. 16.5. a Myotubular myopathy. ATPase pH 4.3. × 350. Most fibres show a central zone of non-reactivity, consisting of a perinuclear zone of absence of myofibrils. **b** Normal developing muscle fibres in biceps brachii of an aborted fetus (8 weeks gestation). Myotubes are normal developing muscle fibres at this stage of development.

able degree of weakness of other muscles appears to be related principally to the age of onset of the disease. Parents of severely affected children may show minor clinical and pathological features (Brooke 1977), but the mode of inheritance differs in the different types (Tables 16.1 and 16.2). The X-linked form (Table 16.2) has been mapped to chromosome Xq 28 (Lehesjoki et al. 1990).

Investigations

The CK is usually moderately raised in the late onset forms (Serratrice et al. 1978b), but may be normal in the early onset disease (Barth et al. 1975).

With concentric-needle EMG typical myopathic short-duration polyphasic MUAPs are found. Fibrillation potentials have been reported in neonatal and juvenile forms (Spiro et al. 1966). The motor nerve conduction velocity is normal. The EEG may be abnormal, and seizures have been

described in the early infantile onset form (PeBenito et al. 1978).

Muscle Biopsy

The principal feature of the biopsy is the presence of a large proportion of fibres with central nuclei. Central nuclei are found in both Type 1 and Type 2 fibres but Type 1 fibres are predominantly affected. In addition, the Type 1 fibres are usually smaller than normal (selective hypotrophy of Type 1 fibres). In some cases only Type 1 fibres seem to be affected by the disease. The central nuclei are surrounded by a relatively clear zone of sarcoplasm which contains glycogen granules, increased numbers of mitochondria and lipid vacuoles, but in which myofibrils are absent. This zone does not stain in myosin ATPase preparations but is deeply stained in oxidative enzyme reactions such as NADH-tr preparations (Fig. 16.5). This central zone contains RNA and glycogen (Fardeau and Tomé 1994). It may extend through part or all of the length of the fibre. Other focal degenerative changes in individual fibres are only rarely seen in light- or electron-micrographs. Hypertrophied fibres may show fibre-splitting and Z-band streaming is found (Bill and Cole 1979). Fetal vimentin and desmin may be present (Sarnat 1990), and an increased number of Type 2C fibres, suggesting delayed maturation (Sasaski et al. 1989). The extra-ocular muscles are similarly affected in the infantile-onset form. The peripheral nerves and spinal cord are normal (Bradley et al. 1970).

The central, perinuclear clear zones suggest a similarity to central cores, but the latter do not contain nuclei (Edstrom et al. 1982). The features of myotubular myopathy have led to discussion of the similarities of these fibres to normal fetal myotubes (Spiro et al. 1966), but clinically identical cases may not show the perinuclear clear area described above, and the term centronuclear myopathy is thus preferable. In the parents of affected children it may be possible to find increased central nucleation, or rare myotubes (van Wijngaarden et al. 1969) and these parents usually show some clinical signs of the disease, illustrating the familial nature of the disorder (Edstrom et al. 1982). The combination of small Type 1 fibres with central nuclei may also lead to confusion with myotonic dystrophy, especially since the nuclei may be located in long rows (see Chap. 15).

Outcome

Severely affected infants succumb to cardio-respiratory complications. In the older onset cases disability is variable.

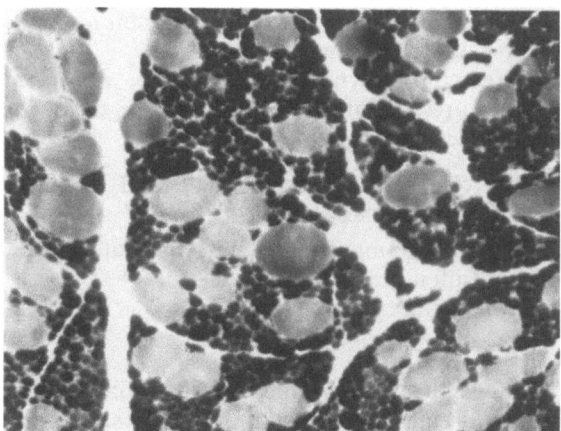

Fig. 16.6. Fibre-type disproportion. ATPase × 450. The small dark Type 1 fibres are atrophic and predominant, and the larger, pale Type 2 fibres are slightly hypertrophied.

Controversies in Aetiology

Spiro et al. (1966) thought that myotubular myopathy represented the persistence of fetal myotubes into post-natal life. However, the abnormal fibres in these children are larger than those found in fetal life and most authors have not regarded them as true myotubes. In addition, the abnormal muscle fibres do not contain fetal myoglobin (Munsat et al. 1969a). A neurogenic aetiology has also been suggested, particularly since the tendon reflexes are usually absent, and Engel et al. (1968) suggested that a selective defect of the motor innervation of Type 1 fibres might explain the pathological features. However, this suggestion has not been supported by clinical, electrophysiological or subsequent pathological studies (Bradley et al. 1970) and the cause of the disease remains unknown. Generally, the maturation defect hypothesis is supported (Fardeau and Tomé 1994), perhaps associated with a defect in the organisation of the cytoskeleton. In normal development myofibre nuclei are peripherally located by 24 weeks gestational age.

Congenital Fibre-Type Disproportion

In this syndrome the infant presents with hypotonia (floppy infant syndrome) and generalised muscular weakness which may be mild or severe. Respiratory difficulties may occur in the more severe cases in the first year of life. Contractures occur in half the cases and congenital dislocation of the hip in a third

(Brooke 1973, 1977). Kyphoscoliosis, varus and valgus deformities of the foot and a high-arched palate may also be noted (Clancy et al. 1980).

The hypotonia and weakness tend to worsen during the first 2 years but later some improvement may occur and this is sometimes quite marked (Cavanagh et al. 1979b). Only three of Brooke's (1977) 12 patients attained normal strength. Although birth weight is usually normal most patients fail to grow normally, remaining short and strikingly thin; most are below the third percentile for weight (Glick et al. 1984).

The weakness is greater proximally than distally and may also involve the face. The tendon reflexes are usually diminished. The pattern of inheritance is not clear, but in most families an autosomal dominant pattern has been reported (Kinoshita et al. 1975). Autosomal recessive inheritance has been reported, however.

Laboratory Investigations

The CK may be mildly raised. No ECG abnormalities have been described.

Electrophysiological Assessment

The EMG shows small, short-duration myopathic potentials together with other potentials of larger amplitude. Complex repetitive discharges, positive sharp waves and fibrillation potentials have been described in some patients (Kimura 1983). The nerve conduction velocity is normal (Brooke 1977). Thus, the EMG may suggest denervation.

Muscle Biopsy

The characteristic feature of the biopsy is that the mean diameter of the Type 1 fibres is at least 12% smaller than the mean diameter of the Type 2 fibres (Fig. 16.6). In the younger patients the Type 1 fibres are often of *normal* size, but the Type 2 fibres, particularly the Type 2B fibres, are larger than normal. Thus, the Type 1 fibres are usually not atrophic (Brooke 1973; Dubowitz and Brooke 1973). Occasionally, there may be increased central nucleation, moth-eaten or whorled fibres, and rod bodies in some fibres but these features are not prominent (Fardeau et al. 1975). Angulated fibres, or fibre-type grouping do not occur, but in more than half the patients Type 1 fibre predominance is a feature. The nosology of this syndrome has been questioned on the basis that small Type 1 fibres are not specific to any disorder, but the clinico-pathological correlation is characteristic (Martin et al. 1976; Fardeau and Tomé 1994).

Differential Diagnosis

Disorders in which atrophy of Type 1 fibres is a feature may be confused with fibre-type disproportion if the clinical features are not known. These disorders include myotonic dystrophy, spino-cerebellar degeneration and nemaline myopathy. Since rods occur in some fibres in fibre-type disproportion differentiation may be difficult. Myotubular myopathy with Type 1 fibre hypotrophy and congenital muscular dystrophy, in which Type 2 fibres may be large, may also lead to confusion. However, the additional clinical and pathological features should allow a diagnosis to be made. Very rarely a biopsy will show uniformly Type 1 fibres, without other abnormality, in the clinical context of a congenital myopathy, and without evidence of neurogenic change (Oh and Danon 1983). This is believed to be a separate entity.

Management

The liability to respiratory infection in the first year of life may need special measures. Contractures should be treated and spinal deformities, which may be congenital, may need special orthopaedic management. In most cases strength improves with increasing maturity.

Other Rare Syndromes

Other congenital myopathies (Table 16.1) have been described, but are much less common, or seem to be characterised by less specific pathological features. In some only a few individuals or families have been described. The older term (minimal change myopathy; Dubowitz 1995) is a non-specific description that encompassed many of these syndromes.

Myopathy with Tubular Aggregates

Tubular aggregates represent the major structural abnormality in this disorder. Although tubular aggregates occur in other conditions, such as periodic paralysis, toxic myopathies, hypoxia and in congenital myasthenic syndromes (Fardeau and Tomé 1994), in these disorders there are additional

clinical or pathological features that indicate the specific underlying diagnosis.

Three clinical syndromes have been associated with the presence of tubular aggregates as the major pathological finding:

1. Exercise-induced cramps, pain and weakness (Morgan-Hughes et al. 1970)
2. Progressive muscle weakness without cramps, but with myalgia (Rokhamm et al. 1983)
3. Congenital myasthenic syndrome (Morgan-Hughes et al. 1981).

In the first syndrome, the disorder begins in adult life or in childhood, with *cramps or muscle pain*, which may be longlasting, on exertion. Muscle weakness gradually becomes evident. There is no myoglobinuria and clinical examination reveals no abnormality. There is no wasting, myotonia or fasciculation. The serum electrolytes are normal (Rosenberg et al. 1985; Martin et al. 1991). This disorder is sporadic without a known genetic basis.

In the second syndrome there is *slowly progressive weakness*, with some myalgia, but without muscle cramp or fatiguability. There is no change in symptoms after exercise. Three families have been described (Pierobon-Bormioli et al. 1985; Fardeau and Tome 1994). This syndrome is inherited as an autosomal dominant or recessive trait.

Congenital myasthenic syndrome with tubular aggregates is poorly characterised. The underlying defect in neuromuscular transmission responded to treatment with neostigmine and with prednisolone therapy and seemed to be due to decreased affinity of acetylcholine receptors. There was no anti-acetylcholine receptor antibody detected in venous blood (Morgan-Hughes et al. 1981). The relationship of this defect in neuromuscular transmission is not understood. The EMG showed increased neuromuscular jitter and blocking, and decremental responses of 15% at 3 Hz supramaximal stimulation. The pattern of inheritance of this syndrome is unclear.

Pathology

The tubular aggregates consist of intensely staining basophilic, irregularly shaped manes of material in the cytoplasm of the muscle fibre. These aggregates are bright red in Gomori trichrome, positive in NADH and negative in cytochrome oxidase and succinic dehydrogenase preparations. They are also negative in ATPase preparations. Immunostaining reveals positive reactions with sarcoplasmic reticulum ATPase, calcium pump protein, heat shock protein and calciquestrin (Falviati et al. 1985;

Martin et al. 1991). These features indicate an origin from sarcoplasmic reticulum.

Ultrastructural studies show that the tubules are densely packed, and oriented at right angles or longitudinal to the myofibrils. The tubules are 60–80 nm in width and arranged in hexagonal arrays. Each tubule contains a core of 25–30 nm, separated from the wall by a narrow clear zone. The mechanism of production of these tubular aggregates is not understood, but presumably represents a sarcoplasmic response to injury, perhaps metabolic in type.

Treatment

No therapy is available for the muscle cramp, muscle pain or weakness. The myasthenic syndrome associated with tubular aggregates seems to respond to steroids and to anti-cholinergic medication (Morgan-Hughes et al. 1981).

Desmin Storage Myopathies

A number of disorders have been reported in which desmin storage in muscle fibres is a feature (Fardeau et al. 1978). Desmin is a normal cytoskeletal protein, forming intermediate filaments in all muscle cells. It is prominent in regenerating muscle fibres, and is particularly prominent in the Z bands, where it maintains the alignment of adjacent myofibrils. Desmin is therefore found in nemaline rod disease and is also present in increased amounts in infantile myotonic dystrophy and in myotubular myopathy (Sarnat 1993). Desmin accumulation is therefore relatively non-specific (Thornell et al. 1980). Osborn and Goebel (1983) noted that desmin was a feature of cytoplasmic bodies.

Fardeau et al. (1978) described a family in which a myopathy and cardiomyopathy was associated with accumulation of electron-dense granular and filamentous material between the myofibrils and under the sarcolemma, later shown to be desmin (Rappaport et al. 1988). Subsequent reports have noted weakness, often more distal than proximal with or without cardiomyopathy, with pharyngeal, truncal and cervical involvement. Hypertrophic cardiomyopathy may develop. The age of onset ranges from childhood to adult life. The EMG is myopathic (Edstrom et al. 1980) and the CK is usually raised (Fardeau and Tomé 1994). Most cases appear to be autosomal dominant.

Pathology

The morphological appearance is variable. There are zones of absence of oxidative enzyme activity, e.g. NADH, in the sacroplasm, especially in split fibres, peripheral dense, inclusion body-like areas that stain red in Gomori are prominent and amyloid deposits and accumulation of sarcoplasmic dystrophin may be seen (Prelle et al. 1992). Rimmed vacuoles and centrally placed nuclei may be features. Electron microscopy reveals dense material between adjacent myofibrils, often in register with Z lines. This material stains strongly positive in immunoreactions for desmin. Ovoid, desmin bodies may develop at the periphery of the fibres.

Treatment and Outcome

No specific treatment is available, and the prognosis is uncertain. Sarnat (1993) has argued that desmin storage is always non-specific, a view that is difficult to accord with the severe disability found in cardiac and skeletal muscle in some cases of desmin storage myopathic syndromes (Martoni et al. 1994).

Cytoplasmic Body Myopathy (Spheroid Body Myopathy)

Cytoplasmic bodies are small round bodies that stain purple-red with Gomori trichrome (MacDonald and Engel (1969). They consist of a tangle of 3–7 nm fine filaments surrounded by a halo of radially oriented filaments, with an outer shell of disorganised myofibrils. Although they occur in various disorders, e.g. polymyositis, myotonic dystrophy and denervation, they are a feature of a childhood-onset myopathy, presenting with proximal weakness (rarely distal weakness), atrophy, fatigue and cramp. Most cases present in adults, and respiratory problems may be evident. The quadriceps and calf muscles may be hypertrophied. Adult cases are mostly mild, but infantile-onset cases are severe with reduced life expectancy (Patel et al. 1983).

The CK is slightly increased, and the EMG is usually myopathic. The cytoplasmic bodies are often predominant in Type 1 fibres, affecting up to about 30% of fibres in the biopsy.

Myopathy with Lysis of Myofibrils in Type 1 Fibres

Cancilla et al. (1971) described a brother and sister with a non-progressive myopathy with lysis of myofibrils in Type 1 fibres. There was hypotonia at birth, with delayed milestones and slowly progressive weakness. A 50-year-old patient described by

Sahgal and Sahgal (1977) had been weak since the age of 6 years with a scapulo-peroneal distribution.

Fingerprint Body Myopathy

This disorder is characterised by a non-progressive or slowly progressive myopathy, which begins at birth or in infancy, and is associated with sarcoplasmic fingerprint-like inclusions (Engel et al. 1972), seen mainly in Type 1 fibres consisting of concentrically arranged lamellae, in an area of amorphous matrix material. They are probably composed of cytoskeletal proteins (Fardeau and Tomé 1994). Fingerprint bodies are also found in myotonic dystrophy and oculo-pharyngeal dystrophy (Goebel 1986).

Reducing Body Myopathy

Brooke and Neville (1972) described two infants with hypotonia, proximal weakness, joint contractures and ptosis. This disorder is non-progressive and may affect adults as well as children. The muscle biopsy shows Type 1 fibre predominance and subsarcolemmal eosinophilic, round or oval bodies that stain pink in H and E, and purple in Gomori trichrome. They are negative in NADH and positive in menadione linked α-glycerophosphate dehydrogenase, RNA, glycogen and sulphhydryl groups. The origin of these "reducing bodies" is unknown, but ultrastructurally they consist of granules and tubular filaments (Tomé and Fardeau 1975, Oh et al. 1983).

Sarcotubular Myopathy

Only two cases have been described (Jerusalem et al. 1973), with consanguinity. There was a microvacuolar myopathy affecting Type 2 fibres consisting of membrane derived from sarcoplasmic reticulum.

Zebra Body Myopathy

Two cases have been described. Lake and Wilson (1975) and Reyes et al. (1987) reported a congenital onset myopathy with weakness and hypotonia in which leptofibrils (zebra bodies) with a 270 nm periodicity were present. Other myopathic features including fibre splitting and vacuolar change were present.

Trilaminar Disease

Ringel et al. (1978) described a patient with increased muscle tone and weakness and contractures, in whom the CK was greatly raised. A trilaminar appearance of muscle fibres was found in the Gomori and NADH dehydrogenase preparations. This disorder may be central in origin.

Myopathy with Cylindrical Spirals

Bove et al. (1980) described a disorder of infantile onset with cramp, percussion myotonia and stiffness in muscles. The cylindrical spirals consist of tubular profiles arranged in parallel circles near the sarcolemma, perhaps derived from T tubules.

Cap Disease

A boy with a severe congenital myopathy was found to have abnormal peripheral crescents in most fibres. The EMG was myopathic and nerve conduction normal (Fidzianska et al. 1981).

Hyaline Body Myopathy

This is a non-progressive myopathy with onset in infancy, in which hyaline bodies are found in Type 1 fibres. These consist of undefined amorphous granular material (Barolin et al. 1994a). In reporting two cases Barolin et al. (1994a) suggested that this disorder was closely related to myopathy with lysis of myofibrils in Type 1 fibres.

Rigid Spine Syndrome

This is a rare, sporadic disorder of childhood commencing between the ages of 1 and 7 years. It is characterised by limitation of flexion of the whole spine due to shortening of the axial extensor muscles (Dubowitz 1965). Scoliosis occurs and may be progressive. Contracture of the hands and feet may be a feature. Muscle weakness is not a major feature. The CK level is normal or slightly raised, and the EMG and muscle biopsy both show myopathic features, particularly in the paraspinal extensor muscles, where fat replacement and fibre necrosis, with increased connective tissue may be prominent. Fibre-type disproportion has been reported, but the rigid spine syndrome probably does not represent a nosological entity, but is a clinical description of the syndrome (Van Munster et al. 1986).

Arthrogryposis Multiplex Congenita

This clinical syndrome consists of congenital restriction of joint movement, involving at least two joints, usually with talipes equinovarus and flexion deformity of the wrists; distal joints are especially severely affected but knees and elbows are also frequently involved. The postural deformity appears to be due to immobility in utero associated with muscular weakness. The latter may be due either to neurogenic or myopathic (Banker et al. 1957) disease including meningomyelocele, multiple congenital deformities and congenital muscular dystrophies. Myotonic dystrophy, congenital fibre-type disproportion and congenital myasthenia have also been recorded as causes of this syndrome and anterior horn cell degeneration may also present in this way. The various disorders are discussed in the appropriate sections of this book.

Chapter 17

Inherited Metabolic Myopathies

The inherited metabolic myopathies consist of a group of genetically determined muscular disorders, of varying severity, characterised by muscular weakness and associated with biochemical defects of muscle metabolism (Fig. 17.1). In some, a fixed or progressive myopathy develops, but in others there are recurrent episodes of muscular weakness, or cramps and stiffness associated with exercise; sometimes myoglobinuria occurs in these episodes. In many of these disorders there are features of involvement of other systems. The severity of the clinical syndrome often varies according to the age of onset, reflecting the severity and distribution of the enzyme deficiency, so that infantile and adult-onset types of a disorder may present with strikingly different clinical features.

There are six separate categories of inherited metabolic myopathies (Table 17.1).

Table 17.1. Categories of inherited metabolic myopathies

Glycogen storage diseases
Myoadenylate deaminase deficiency
Mitochondrial and lipid storage myopathies
Familial periodic paralysis
Malignant hyperthermia
Other disorders

Glycogen Storage Diseases

Seven types of glycogenosis have been recognised, each with a distinct enzyme deficiency, but muscular involvement does not occur in all of them (Table 17.2). Myopathy is prominent among other manifestations in acid maltase deficiency (Type II glycogenosis), in debrancher enzyme deficiency (Type III glycogenosis), in myophosphorylase deficiency (Type V glycogenosis: McArdle's disease) and in phosphofructokinase deficiency (Type VII

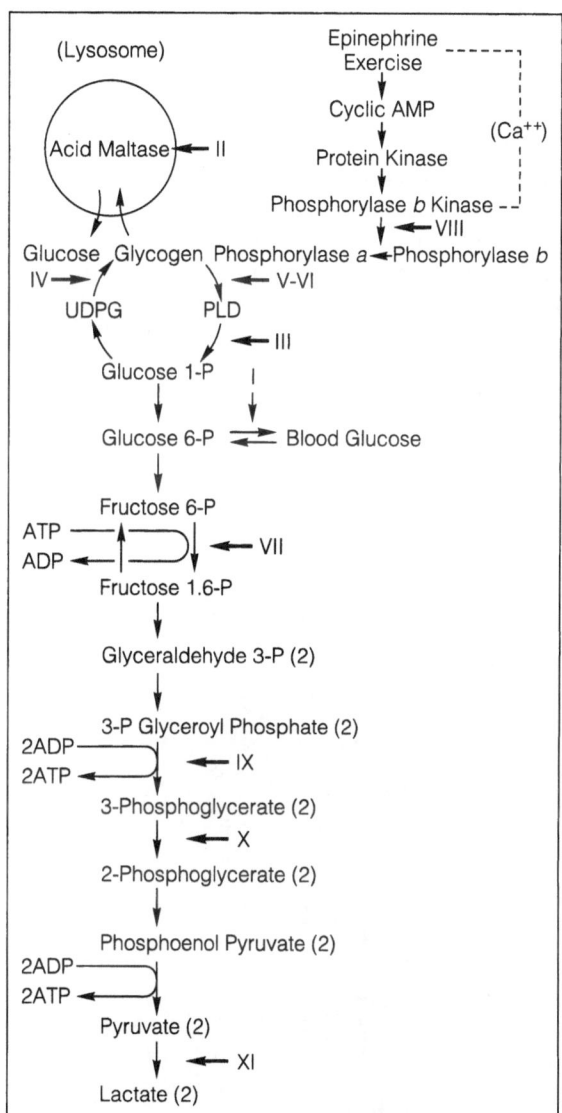

Fig. 17.1. Glycogen metabolism. Type II, acid maltase deficiency; Type III, debrancher enzyme deficiency; Type IV, brancher enzyme deficiency (Andersen's disease); Type V, phosphorylase deficiency (McArdle's disease). (From Cornelio and Di Donato 1985.)

Table 17.2. Clinical features of glycogenoses

Type		Enzyme deficiency	Genetic locus	Histochemically demonstrable	Muscle involvement	Other systems
I	von Gierke's disease	Glucose-6-phosphatase		No	No	Liver, kidney
II	Pompe's disease	Acid maltase (α1,4-glucosidase)	17q 23-25	Yes	Infantile-onset severe weakness, fatal Adult-onset limb-girdle weakness	Heart, kidney CNS Heart
III	Cori–Forbes disease Limit dextrinosis	Debrancher enzyme (amylo-1,6-glucosidase)		No No	Infantile-onset hypotonia Adult-onset limb-girdle weakness	Heart, liver, hypoglycaemia –
IV	Andersen's disease Amylopectinosis	Brancher enzyme (amylo-1,4,1,6-transglucosidase)		Yes Yes	Infantile-onset muscle wasting Adult-onset limb-girdle weakness	Liver –
V	McArdle's disease	Myophosphorylase	11q 13	Yes Yes	Infantile-onset severe weakness Adult-onset exercise intolerance, cramp and fatigue	– –
VI	–	Liver phosphorylase		No	No	Liver
VII	Tarui's disease	Phosphofructokinase	1q 32	Yes	Childhood-onset exercise intolerance, cramps and fatigue	–

glycogenosis), but only in the last two diseases are muscular symptoms the major manifestation (Fig. 17.2). Muscular symptoms may also occur in Type IV glycogenosis (Andersen's disease). Weakness, fatigue and muscle pain on exercise occur in several of these syndromes and in a number of other enzyme defects of glycolysis (Table 17.3).

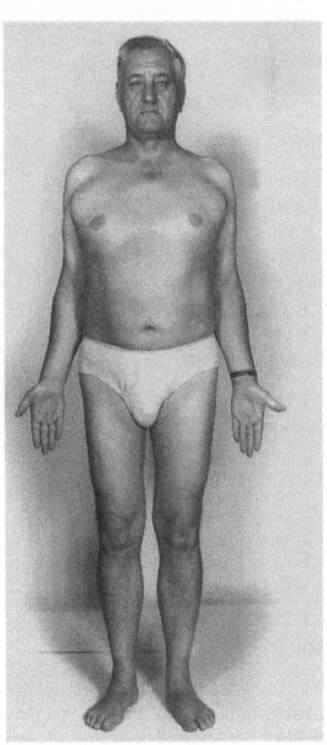

Fig. 17.2. Adult-onset acid maltase deficiency. There is slight atrophy of deltoids and quadriceps, but the calf muscles are prominent. There was respiratory involvement with diaphragmatic weakness that required ventilatory assistance and led to death.

Table 17.3. Enzyme defects in glycolytic metabolism associated with muscular fatigue, weakness, stiffness and pain on exercise

Debrancher enzyme deficiency	Type IV
McArdle's disease	Type V
Phosphofructokinase deficiency (Tarui et al. 1965)	Type VII
Phosphorylase b kinase deficiency (Ohtani et al. 1982)	Type VIII
Phosphoglycerate kinase deficiency (Bresolin et al. 1984)	Type IX
Phosphoglycerate mutase deficiency (Di Mauro et al. 1981)	Type X
Lactate dehydrogenase M subunit deficiency	Type XI

Acid Maltase Deficiency (Pompe's Disease) (Type II Glycogenosis)

Acid maltase (α1,4-glucosidase) deficiency is a rare autosomal recessive disorder. Since there may be slight deficiency of the enzyme in muscle lymphocytes, cultured fibroblasts (Di Mauro et al. 1984) and in the urine (Mehler and Di Mauro 1976) of heterozygotes, carriers of the gene can sometimes be detected by enzyme assay (Engel and Gomez 1970). The enzyme deficiency was first recognised by Hers (1963). There are three clinical forms of the disease: a severe infantile form, in which death usually occurs from cardio-respiratory failure before the second birthday, a milder form in which proximal weakness develops in early childhood (Engel et al. 1973), and a milder adult-onset variety (Engel 1970; McComas et al. 1983).

In the severe infantile form (Pompe's disease) the disorder usually becomes evident a few months after birth with generalised progressive muscular weakness, hypotonia, cardiomegaly and hepatomegaly. In addition enlargement of the tongue usually occurs. Respiratory difficulties are prominent (Newsom–Davis et al. 1976) and the muscles feel firm and of normal bulk, despite the weakness and hypotonia. Death occurs from cardiac failure before the age of 2 years. The ECG may show a short PR interval, with increased QRS voltage and signs of left ventricular hypertrophy.

The childhood-onset form is less severe than the infantile form. Motor milestones are delayed after the initial period of development, i.e. after about age 18 months. There is proximal muscular weakness with shortening of Achilles tendons leading to toe-walking, a rubbery texture to the muscles, proximal weakness and a waddling gait. The calf muscles are often enlarged, a feature that resembles Duchenne muscular dystrophy (Engel et al. 1973). There is no cardiomegaly. Death occurs in 30% of cases in childhood from respiratory muscle weakness (Di Mauro 1979; Matsuishi et al. 1984). In both the infantile and childhood-onset forms massive glycogen storage may occur, leading to muscle masses and causing organomegaly.

The adult-onset form of the disease (Fig. 17.2) begins in the third or fourth decade with slowly progressive proximal weakness and wasting, mainly affecting the pelvic girdle muscles. This disorder thus represents a biochemically defined form of the limb-girdle syndrome (Hudgson et al. 1968). Weakness of the diaphragm and intercostal muscles is prominent in 35% of cases, and may be the presenting feature of the disease (Rosenow and Engel, 1978; Sivak et al. 1981). Some of these patients have particular problems breathing during sleep because of diaphragmatic weakness and may require nocturnal ventilation (De Jager and Meinesz 1983; Swash et al. 1985). Hypertrophy of the calf muscles with absent tendon reflexes has been observed (Engel 1970). Involvement of the heart may be evident in the terminal stages of the disease (van der Walt et al. 1987). A scapulo-peroneal presentation has been described (Barolin et al. 1993).

In some families there is marked variation in the clinical phenotype (Loonen et al. 1981a) or even adult and infantile onset cases occurring in the same family, perhaps due to allelic diversity (Hoefsloot et al. 1990).

Laboratory Investigations

Acid maltase activity is absent or reduced in muscle in all three forms of the disease (Engel et al. 1973). Engel et al. (1973) found that there was acid maltase deficiency in liver biopsies of five adults with the disease in whom there was no abnormality of liver function, but in whom muscular weakness was severe. The enzyme defect is generalised in both the childhood and adult forms of the disease, as shown by muscle and liver biopsies and studies of skin fibroblasts, leucocytes and urine (Di Mauro 1979).

In heterozygotes there is a partial deficiency of acid maltase in muscle but the levels overlap with those found in some normal controls (Engel et al. 1973). Urinary enzyme assay may also be useful (Mehler and Di Mauro 1976). Mehler and Di Mauro (1976) found low residual levels (mean 7%) of acid maltase activity in muscle and other tissues from patients with the adult-onset form of the disease, but absent enzyme activity in the infantile form. This observation and the very rare appearance (Hoefsloot et al. 1990) of the adult and infantile forms in the same family suggests that they are genetically distinct. In addition, in the adult form neutral maltase activity is normal in muscle and liver, whereas in the childhood form neutral maltase activity is decreased only in the liver, and in the infantile form it is reduced in heart, liver and muscle (Angelini and Engel 1972). However, a small amount of residual acid maltase activity is present in muscle in childhood and adult onset cases, but not in the infantile form (Mehler and Di Mauro 1977), and this seems to explain the later onset and milder course of the former disorders. Differences in residual acid maltase activity seem more evident in fibroblasts and muscle cultures than in muscle biopsy specimens (van der Ploeg et al. 1988). In a post-mortem study of a case of adult-onset acid maltase deficiency the residual activity of acid maltase was lower in muscle than in other tissues, an observation which may account for the relative susceptibility of muscle in this disease (Di Mauro et al. 1978b), rather than differences in neutral maltase activity (van der Ploeg et al. 1989).

The CK is raised in all forms of the disease, but the CK levels overlap between the three clinical forms, although they are generally lower in adult cases. The ECG shows very large QRS complexes, with a short PR interval in some cases (Lenard et al. 1974), but in others it is normal (Swash et al. 1985).

Definitive diagnosis requires biochemical analysis of muscle or lymphocytes. Prenatal diagnosis can be achieved by electron microscopy of amniotic fluid cells, which contain autophagic vacuoles containing glycogen (Hug et al. 1984). Trophoblast cell biopsies can be used to measure enzyme levels.

Electrophysiological Assessment

Similar abnormalities are found in each of the three clinical forms, but they are more widespread in the infantile-onset cases. In adults some muscles may be normal, especially more distal muscles (Swash et al. 1985). Fibrillation potentials, positive sharp waves and bizarre high-frequency potentials occur (Hogan et al. 1969; Engel et al. 1973). Myotonic discharges have been reported, without clinical myotonia. In adults the EMG abnormalities may be

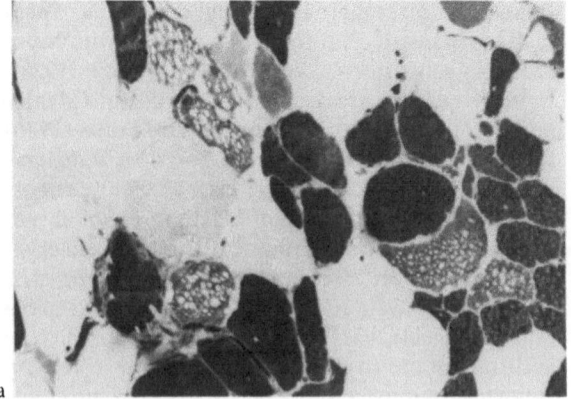

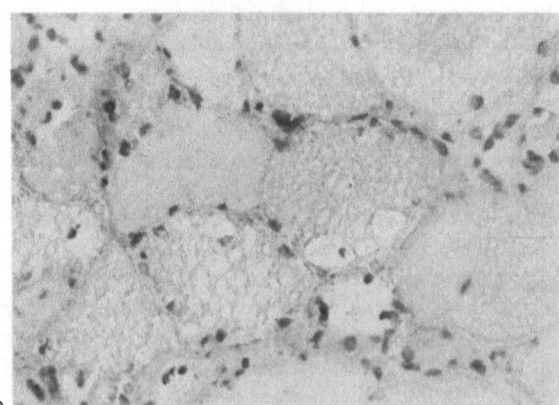

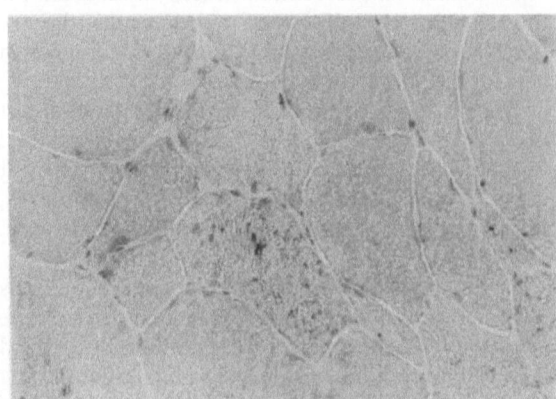

Fig. 17.3. Type II glycogenesis (adult-onset acid maltase deficiency). **a** ATPase, pH 4.3. × 140. Vacuolated, intermediate-type fibres are seen (Type II B), but Type II A fibres are also affected. There is marked variation in fibre size. **b** PAS. × 350. Vacuoles are prominent in some fibres, and these vacuoles are faintly PAS-positive. **c** Acid phosphatase. × 350. Vacuoles are filled with punctate, positive reactivity indicating increased lysosomal activity.

most marked in the paraspinal muscles (Rosenow and Engel 1978). During voluntary activation short-duration polyphasic MUAPs are often recorded. Motor and sensory nerve conduction is normal,

and there is no abnormality of neuromuscular transmission.

Muscle Biopsy

The major change is a vacuolar myopathy (Fig. 17.3); this is more prominent in the infantile variety and the vacuoles are larger in these cases. In the clinically unaffected muscles of adults only rare vacuoles are seen (Swash et al. 1985). The disease progresses in subsequent biopsies (Swash et al. 1985). However, these histologically normal muscles also show markedly reduced acid maltase activity (Di Mauro et al. 1984). In severely affected muscles the normal histological pattern of the muscle is distorted, the muscle fibres being rounded, variable in size and often surrounded by excessive fibrous tissue. The vacuoles themselves contain glycogen, recognised by the strong reaction in the PAS stain, and are also strongly reactive for acid phosphatase (Fig. 17.3), showing their lysosomal derivation (Engel 1970).

In infants nearly all the muscle fibres in a biopsy are affected, whereas in adults the abnormality is less marked. The relative sparing of distal muscles is confirmed at autopsy (van der Walt et al. 1987). Intrafusal muscle fibres in muscle spindles are involved (van der Walt et al. 1987).

Autopsy also reveals some involvement of smooth muscle in the gut, of Schwann cells in peripheral nerves, and of cardiac muscle.

The autophagic nature of the vacuoles is confirmed by electron microscopy which shows glycogen granules packed free in the sarcoplasm in whorled, membrane-bound glycogen bodies, and in autophagic vacuoles (Engel 1970; Engel et al. 1973). These vacuolar changes can be reproduced in tissue culture from affected patients (Askanas et al. 1976). The limiting membrane of the vacuoles resembles the sarcolemma expressing dystrophin, spectrin and vinculin (Vita et al. 1994a). This was not evident in vacuoles in an infantile-onset case and Vita et al. (1994) speculated that defective exocytotic processes might be important in the accumulation of debris on the cell cytoplasm in this disorder. Nerve twigs in muscle biopsies are normal.

Other Pathological Features

Glycogen accumulation occurs in other organs in the infantile and childhood forms of the disease. Schwann cell involvement described by Araoz et al. (1974) was confirmed by van der Walt et al. (1987). Glycogen deposition is also seen in the central nervous system including cerebral cortex and anterior horn cells (Crome et al. 1963). Glycogen deposition in the anterior horn cells may explain the fibrillation potentials and other neurogenic features found with EMG. Demyelination in the CNS is not a feature. Cardiac muscle shows gross vacuolar changes with glycogen deposition in the infantile form, and similar, less marked features are found in the heart in the adult form (van der Walt et al. 1987). Smooth muscle may be involved.

Genetics

All three forms are autosomal recessive with a genetic locus on chromosome 17q 23–25 (Solomon et al. 1979). They are probably allelic. The infantile forms have only been recognised in the same family in one instance (Loonen et al. 1981a). Heterozygotes, e.g. parents of affected patients, are unaffected clinically, but show reduced levels of acid maltase activity in fibroblasts and leucocytes. All three clinical phenotypes show reduced enzyme activity (Loonen et al. 1981a). Restriction fraction length polymorphisms have also been used for identification of heterozygotes (Tzall et al. 1990).

Management

There is no effective treatment. Engel et al. (1973) thought that carbohydrate restriction resulted in slight improvement in mild adult cases. Treatment with a high-protein diet has been tried in a case of infantile onset with slight benefit (Slonim et al. 1983). Treatment with thyroid hormone, progesterone and vitamin A has been tried without consistent improvement (Di Mauro et al. 1984). Respiratory problems can be improved by inspiratory resistance training for 15 minutes twice a day (Martin et al. 1983), but ventilatory assistance, particularly during sleep (Swash et al. 1985) may be necessary, and may even result in some improvement in muscle strength, or non-progression of limb weakness for several years (Newsom-Davis et al. 1976; De Jager and Meinesz 1983). Trend et al. (1985) recommended domiciliary ventilatory support using a rocking-bed system or tracheostomy with intermittent positive pressure ventilation, and noted that the muscle disorder seemed to remain static or to progress more slowly with this treatment. Enzyme replacement therapy is not yet a practicable therapy.

Lysosomal Glycogen Storage Disease with Normal Acid Maltase Activity

A few cases have been described of a disorder resembling acid maltase deficiency in which acid maltase activity is normal. Dworzak et al. (1994) reported a family and reviewed 12 cases in the literature. This syndrome has mostly been reported in boys, with severe cardiomyopathy, mental retardation seizures, and a mild myopathy (Danon et al. 1981; Byrne et al. 1986). The CK is markedly elevated, up to 10 times normal. The EMG is myopathic and the muscle biopsy shows a vacuolar myopathy. The vacuoles contain debris, glycogen and acid phosphatase as in acid maltase deficiency itself. Female cases seem to show less marked mental retardation. The biochemical basis of this syndrome, presumed to be an unclassified glycogenosis, is unknown. Dworzak et al. (1994) suggest that patients presenting with hypertrophic cardiomyopathy should have a muscle biopsy, in order to consider this diagnosis.

Debrancher Enzyme Deficiency
(Limit Dextrinosis) (Type III Glycogenosis)

Type III glycogenosis, like Type II glycogenosis, affects both liver and skeletal muscle, but it is a more benign disorder than Type II glycogenosis. The infantile-onset form is an autosomal recessive disorder characterised by hypotonia and weakness, with hepatomegaly (Murase et al. 1973). Affected subjects are usually mentally unimpaired. The liver involvement may lead to hepatomegaly, fasting hypoglycaemia and seizures (Di Mauro et al. 1984). The metabolic error, a deficiency of amylo 1,6-glucosidase, prevents breakdown of the inner part of the glycogen molecule, only the outer chains being accessible, resulting in the accumulation of glycogen with short outer chains (Illingworth et al. 1956). Despite the metabolic error infants with the disease may show improvement as they enter adolescence, the liver becoming of normal size. In some cases the liver may be involved without muscular weakness (Brandt and De Luca 1966).

In an adult-onset form of the disease, fatiguability may be the first indication of the disorder. The disorder is predominent in men. Weakness begins in the third or fourth decade but onset in the sixth decade has been described (Yang et al. 1991) in spite of the complete absence of debrancher enzyme. Half the patients have atrophic muscles affecting distal muscles of the legs and hands. Cramps may be a feature but myoglobinuria does not occur. The heart may be involved, with cardiac failure (Cornelio et al. 1984; Cornelio and Di Donato 1985). This syndrome may resemble motor neuron disease or peripheral neuropathy. In some patients the hepatic disorder of childhood resolves but muscular involvement becomes apparent in adult life (Di Mauro et al. 1979; Smit et al. 1990).

Laboratory Investigations

The metabolic error can be detected in muscle, skin and liver. Debrancher enzyme deficiency can also be detected in leucocytes. The CK is raised. The heart is involved and the ECG shows a short PR interval and large QRS complexes. Other laboratory tests may be abnormal. A diabetic glucose tolerance curve, fasting hypoglycaemia and a lack of response of blood glucose to adrenaline or glucagon may be found (Brunberg et al. 1971; Murase et al. 1973). In addition, in 50% of cases there is no rise of venous lactate after ischaemic forearm exercise (Brunberg et al. 1971), and in 40% the response is decreased (Cornelio and Di Donato 1985). Prenatal diagnosis can be achieved by biochemical studies of cultured amniocytes exposed to a glucose-free medium (Yang et al. 1990). The characteristic abnormal polysaccharide can be detected.

Electrophysiological Assessment

The EMG shows fibrillations, positive sharp waves, complex repetitive discharges at rest and myopathic motor unit potentials on volition. These features are similar to those found in acid maltase deficiency, but not as pronounced, and true myotonia is not a feature (Di Mauro et al. 1979). In half the cases motor nerve conduction is slower than normal (Cornelio et al. 1984).

Muscle Biopsy

The muscle fibres are disrupted by a marked vacuolar change. The vacuoles are coarse, and located in a subsarcolemmal and intermyofibrillar distribution. They contain glycogen and are thus positive with PAS, but do not contain acid phosphatase. However, there is some lysosomal accumulation of glycogen in this disorder. Glycogen is also found in increased quantities in the sarcoplasm, particularly beneath the sarcolemma. In some patients the vacuoles are more abundant in Type 2 fibres. Ring fibres and multicore-like structures occur. Biochemical analysis reveals glycogen accumulation, to four to six times normal, and debrancher enzyme activity of only 4%–11% of normal (Di Mauro et al. 1984). This enzyme defect appears to be present in all tissues, allowing prenatal diagnosis from fibroblast cultures. Glycogen is also found in axons and Schwann cells of intra-muscular nerves (Ugawa et al. 1986). The CNS is also affected.

Management

Fasting hypoglycaemia is an important aspect of the disease in affected infants and frequent low-carbohydrate feeds, with a high-protein intake, are important at this stage, and may lead to some clinical improvement in severely affected infants (Fernandes and van de Kamer 1968). This treatment is not effective in adults with the disease, although a high-protein diet is recommended.

Type IV Glycogenosis

This is a very rare form of autosomal recessive glycogenosis, due to deficiency of the brancher enzyme amylo 1,4 → 1,6-transglucosidase. It may be associated with muscular weakness and wasting but affected infants are gravely ill with hepatosplenomegaly, hepatic failure and failure to thrive. Cardiomyopathy may be a feature. The CK is normal. The glycogen content of muscle is normal, unlike that in other forms of glycogenosis, but amylopectin may be found at autopsy (Brown and Brown 1966). McMaster et al. (1979) showed abnormal polysaccharide deposits of granular and filamentous material in vacuoles in muscle biopsies of half the cases. Death usually occurs before the age of 4 years.

An adult-onset form of this disorder has been described, but is incompletely documented. Only one case showed possible reduction of brancher enzyme in muscle (Ferguson et al. 1983). The heterogeneity of these cases raises doubt on the relation of amylopectin storage disease to brancher enzyme defects in adult cases presenting with myopathy (Fig. 17.2).

Adult polyglucosan body disease is a disorder of late onset (older than 60 years) with upper and lower motor neuron signs, sphincter problems, neurogenic bladder and, in half the cases, dementia (Cafferty et al. 1991). Some of these cases have brancher enzyme deficiency in leucocytes and brain, although it is usually normal in muscle in these patients (Bruno et al. 1992). The molecular basis for the phenotypic difference between brancher enzyme deficiency disease of Andersen type and polyglucosan storage disease in brain or muscle is uncertain.

Myophosphorylase Deficiency
(McArdle's Disease) (Type V Glycogenosis)

McArdle's disease is restricted to striated muscle. Like most of the other glycogenoses it is an autosomal recessive disorder. The gene for myophosphorylase is located on chromosome 11q 13.

The main clinical features (McArdle 1951) are cramps and muscular stiffness on exertion; occasionally myoglobinuria may occur after such an episode in about 50% of cases. Easy fatiguability may be an early manifestation in childhood and adolescence, cramps and weakness on exercise with transient myoglobinuria becoming evident in the second and third decades, when the diagnosis is usually made. Myopathic weakness and wasting may appear later in life (Schmid and Mahler 1959), usually affecting arms more than legs (Nixon et al. 1966). About a third of patients, especially older patients, have fixed muscular weakness. Some patients with late-onset McArdle's syndrome, in the fifth or sixth decade, describe progressive weakness without cramp or myoglobinuria (Engel et al. 1963; Pourmand et al. 1983). Fatigue, tiredness, or poor stamina without more specific symptoms may be the presenting feature (Di Mauro et al. 1984). The disease begins in childhood in 84% of cases, and 55% have a positive family history. In the typical presentation, pain can occur on exercise in any muscle, even the jaw musculature; rest rapidly relieves muscular pain unless exercise has been severe and continued when pain may be prolonged. Sometimes muscular pain and swelling, with weakness, may persist for several days after vigorous exercise. In such cases myoglobinuria may lead to acute renal failure (Grunfeld et al. 1972). Renal failure develops in about 50% of patients developing acute muscle necrosis after exercise (Di Mauro and Bresolin 1986a).

Muscular pain and fatigue may sometimes disappear after a brief halt, or slowing of exercise rate, allowing exercise to be resumed at the initial rate, provided muscular stiffness has not occurred. This has been called the "second-wind" phenomenon and has been related to increased blood flow in the muscle with exercise and to the level of plasma free-fatty acids (Perkow et al. 1967; Braakhekke et al. 1986). Between attacks of weakness or muscular pain examination is normal, except in older patients in whom muscular weakness and atrophy may be detectable (Schmid and Mahler 1959). Mental clouding or seizures may occur in 5% of patients as a consequence of metabolic alkalosis developing during exercise (Hagberg et al. 1982).

Although the typical form of McArdle's disease is usually manifest in young adults, rare instances of later and earlier onset cases have been reported. Di Mauro and Hartlage (1978) have described an infant with a severe myopathy associated with complete lack of myophosphorylase who died at the age of 13 weeks; an affected sister was described later by Miranda et al. (1979), in whom cardiac involvement was a feature. Late onset of the disease (at age 49 years) was described in a family with deficiency of myophosphorylase by Engel et al. (1963). It has been suggested that this variability in severity could be explained by genetic differences between cases (Di Mauro et al. 1977). This possibility is also raised by the male preponderance of cases (2.4 : 1). In some patients no phosphorylase enzyme protein can be demonstrated in muscle by immunological or electrophoretic methods but in others the enzyme protein can be demonstrated but it is inactive or only partially active (Rowland et al. 1963; Dreyfus and Alexandre 1971; Feit and Brooke 1976; Di Mauro et al. 1977). Roelofs et al. (1972) demonstrated myophosphorylase activity in regenerating and in cultured muscle fibres from patients with McArdle's disease. They explained this phenomenon on the basis that cultured adult and fetal muscle contain myophosphorylases of different isoenzymic type and regenerative fibres express myophosphorylase activity of fetal type. In culture, McArdle's disease muscle fibres contain only the fetal isoenzyme, but by 4 months of gestation normal muscle contains both fetal and adult isoenzymes (Di Mauro et al. 1978a). Fetal myophosphorylase is identical with brain phosphorylase (Crerar et al. 1988). Phosphorylase is not seen in satellite cells. Phosphorylase activity in tissues other than muscle in McArdle's disease is normal.

Genetic Basis of McArdle's Disease

The disorder is inherited as an autosomal recessive trait, on chromosome 11q 13. Apparent dominant transmission in some families probably represents the presence of homozygotes and manifesting heterozygotes in the same family (Schmidt et al. 1987).

There are three human phosphorylase isoenzymes, characteristic of skeletal muscle, liver and brain, localised to chromosomes 11, 14 and 10 or 20 (see Tsujino et al. 1993a). Genetic analysis of 40 patients with myophosphorylase deficiency has revealed point mutations in exons 1, 5 and 14 (Tsujino et al. 1993). Lebo et al. (1990) found no deletions in the gene. The most common point mutation is a substitution of thymidine for cytosine at codon 49 in exon 1. Only 12% of patients do not show a point mutation. Tsujino et al. (1993a) proposed that the diagnosis can be established in 90% of patients by studying genomic DNA from leucocytes. Some patients had more than one mutation in the gene, a finding that might account for phenotypic variation. Most patients lack immunologically detectable myophosphorylase protein in muscle, indicating that mis-sense mutations are important in pathogenesis.

Biochemical Basis of the Syndrome

Absence of functional myophosphorylase results in a block in carbohydrate metabolism so that ATP synthesis is impaired (Fig. 17.1). Free fatty acids and other lipid fuels must therefore be used for energy metabolism at rest and during exercise. With more intense exercise this source of energy is insufficient to replace the absent or abnormal anaerobic glycolytic pathway and fatigue develops as ATP and creatine phosphate stores are exhausted. Fatigue may be due to impaired excitation–contraction coupling due to excessive accumulation of ADP. The latter may activate endogeneous proteases, via a calcium-dependent pathway, leading to cell death (Haller et al. 1985). The mechanism of cramp and muscle pain is uncertain. Magnetic resonance spectroscopy of muscle at rest and during exercise have shown that the normal reduction in intracellular pH during anaerobic exercise does not occur. During aerobic exercise creatine phosphate levels fall, indicating the severe abnormality in energy metabolism. Even slight anaerobic exercise causes a marked fall in creatine phosphate levels (Ross et al. 1981; Edwards et al. 1982; Borgi et al. 1983). Glycogen accumulates because of the block in glycolysis. The ratio of glycogen/creatine phosphate signal areas in the ^{13}C NMR spectroscopy signal was 12.9 in McArdle's disease and 2.0 in normal subjects, in calf muscle at rest (Jelenson et al. 1991).

Patients with McArdle's syndrome experience a "second wind" phenomenon after a few minutes of exercise. The second wind is also experienced, of course, by normal subjects and athletes during prolonged aerobic exercise. During the initial phase of exercise the patient with McArdle's syndrome utilises free glucose, alanine and other amino acids since the pathway for phosphorylation of muscle glycogen is not available (Wahren et al. 1973). Amino acid utilisation is accompanied by increased venous blood ammonia levels. Ammonia production is a feature of the period of metabolic stress in the muscle (Braakhekke et al. 1986); as the second-wind phase of adaptation commences blood-borne glucose and fatty acids become available as energy sources. This process occurs after a delay comparable to that found in normal subjects who can, however, exercise more vigorously or for longer before the second-wind change in metabolism occurs. During the adaptation phase of the second-wind phenomenon heart rate, cardiac output and muscle blood flow are increased, thus supplying more glucose and free fatty acid (FFA) substrate to muscle, as a substitute for muscle glycogen. During this phase there is an increase in surface recorded EMG activity. This parallels fatigue and probably represents recruitment of more motor units (Braakhekke et al. 1986)

Myophosphorylase deficiency represents abnormality in the muscle content of the active enzyme phosphorylase a, which is produced by the action of phosphorylase b kinase on the inactive precursor phosphorylase b. Phosphorylase b kinase deficiency (Glycogenosis Type VII) is described below.

Laboratory Investigations

The CK is usually raised, and becomes much higher during periods of muscular discomfort or weakness, or after exercise. The ECG is normal. Transient or, rarely, more longlasting uraemia may occur if myoglobinuria is severe.

The metabolic basis of the disorder has been used in diagnosis. The muscle is unable to degrade glycogen to lactic acid during exercise because of the phosphorylase deficiency. This abnormality is best shown by the lack of rise in the level of lactate in venous blood following ischaemic exercise of the forearm. Ischaemic exercise is necessary in order to ensure that muscular contraction is dependent on glycogen breakdown during the test. It must be recognised that this ischaemic exercise test is not specific for the diagnosis of McArdle's disease since deficient lactate production will occur also in phosphofructokinase deficiency (Type VII glycogenosis), in Type III glycogenosis, and during the acute phase of alcoholic myopathy (Perkoff et al. 1966). Abnormal results have also been reported in myasthenia gravis, polymyositis and muscular dystrophy.

Standardised Ischaemic Lactate Test

Munsat (1970) has devised a standardised form of McArdle's (1951) test which is generally used. Ischaemia is produced by inflating a sphygmomanometer cuff to 200 mmHg, or well above systolic blood pressure above the elbow. The hand is rhythmically and vigorously clenched and unclenched at a rate of 60/min for 1 min. The cuff is then deflated. Blood is drawn from the antecubital vein of this arm at 1-, 3-, 5-, 10- and 20-min intervals after cessation of exercise. It is useful to study a control subject at the same time. The peak lactate level in normal subjects occurs 1–5 min after cessation of exercise, and it should increase by more than 100% of a control value taken prior to exercise; the level of this peak will depend on the work done during the period of exercise. In patients with McArdle's disease negligible or only minor rises in venous blood lactate are observed (Gruener et al. 1968; Layzer 1985a). In addition, nearly all patients with McArdle's disease experience painful contractures and cramps during the test, and the CK will rise if this occurs. This is a useful clinical predictor of a positive ischaemic lactate test.

Coleman et al. (1986) identified only five abnormal tests in 70 patients examined for cramp and fatiguability. Three had myophosphorylase deficiency and two others had myoadenylate deaminase deficiency and a mitochondrial myopathy respectively. A reduced response was found in some patients with debrancher enzyme deficiency (glycogenosis Type III).

Electrophysiological Assessment

The EMG is usually normal, although in more advanced cases mild myopathic changes may be seen. Fibrillation potentials may be found, probably indicating necrosis of muscle. The motor nerve conduction velocity is normal. Voluntary activity sometimes produces a contracture; these contractures, unlike ordinary cramps, are electrically silent, showing that they result from contracture of muscle without a neural influence. Repetitive stimulation of a motor nerve at fast rates may produce a rapid decremental response, the amplitude of the evoked muscle action potential decreasing by as much as 75%. This is not necessarily associated with a contracture (Dyken et al. 1967; Cochrane et al. 1973).

Muscle Biopsy

The most characteristic change is the absence of muscle phosphorylase, but in some cases myophosphorylase is present, although in a reduced amount and in an inactive form (see above). There is an increased amount of sarcoplasmic glycogen, often located in small subsarcolemmal accumulations. Necrotic or small fibres occur particularly in those cases in which there is a history of myoglobinuria, and moth-eaten fibres may also be found. Ultrastructural studies confirm the presence of increased glycogen; lysosomal vacuoles are not present. Biochemical examination of the muscle biopsy confirms the absence of myophosphorylase activity.

Regenerating fibres in the biopsy, for example after an episode of myoglobinuria, may show phosphorylase activity (Roelofs et al. 1972; Mitsumoto 1979). Mild non-specific changes in motor nerve terminals have been reported with methylene blue stains, but the terminal innervation ratio is normal (Cochrane et al. 1973).

Management

There is no specific treatment. Supplemental glucose and fructose have been recommended to improve exercise tolerance but no clear benefit has been demonstrated in long-term use (McArdle 1974). Glucagon may improve exercise performance temporarily (Mineo et al. 1984). Patients should be advised to avoid sudden strenuous exercise, to stop exercise when pain or cramp develops and to try to limber up gradually before exercise is expected, in order to encourage the second-wind phenomenon. Slonim and Goans (1985) described improved endurance, but no change in strength, in a patient treated with a high protein diet. Jensen et al. (1990) found improved energy kinetics with NMR spectroscopy following a high-protein diet maintained for 6 weeks.

Phosphofructokinase Deficiency
(Type VII Glycogenosis)

This syndrome closely resembles phosphorylase deficiency (Tarui et al. 1965) because the enzyme defect is situated in the same enzymatic metabolic chain (Fig. 17.1) (Di Mauro et al. 1984). The enzyme is necessary for the phosphorylation of fructose phosphate to fructose 1,6-diphosphate. Thus the abnormal muscle cannot utilise glucose. The disorder is recessively inherited with a gene location on chromosome 1q 32. Episodes of nausea and vomiting may occur, a feature which may allow the disorder to be distinguished from McArdle's syndrome on clinical criteria (Layzer et al. 1967b). The disorder begins in childhood with fatiguability, cramp and myoglobinuria. Muscle weakness is less prominent in adults, but is progressive and fatal in the infantile-onset form (Amit et al. 1992) with terminal respiratory failure.

Laboratory investigations are similar to those found in McArdle's disease, including the absence of a rise in venous lactate after exercise, and an increased CK, but the muscle biopsy shows normal phosphorylase activity. Histochemical stains for phosphofructokinase, however, reveal no activity (Bonilla and Schotland 1970) and this can be confirmed by biochemical evaluation of the muscle biopsy (Tarui et al. 1965). Polyhedral, PAS-positive inclusions consisting of masses of 6–8 nm filaments similar to those found in brancher enzyme deficiency (glycogenosis Type IV) occur in up to 10% of fibres. This material resists diastase digestion (Agamanolis et al. 1980). The bilirubin level is raised due to haemolysis. In addition, the uric acid level may be increased and gout has been reported

(Di Mauro et al. 1984). The EMG and nerve conduction studies are normal (Layzer et al. 1967b).

A reduction of the erythrocyte phosphofructokinase level can be found in the heterozygous parents of patients with the disease (Layzer et al. 1967b).

No treatment is available. Glucagon did not improve exercise tolerance (Mineo et al. 1984), because the metabolic defect is downstream from the entry of glucose into the glycolysis cycle.

Other Defects of Glycolysis

Other defects of glycolysis, phosphoglycerate kinase (PGK) deficiency, phosphoglycerate mutase (PGAM) deficiency, lactate dehydrogenase (LDH) M subunit deficiency are all rare, and all present with exercise intolerance and myoglobinuria.

Phosphorylase b Kinase Deficiency (Type VIII Glycogenosis)

There are four principal syndromes: liver disease, liver and muscle disease, a myopathy and a cardiomyopathy (van der Berg and Berger 1990). All are autosomal recessive disorders. The clinical phenotypes are not clearly associated with specific mutations in the multimeric enzyme, which is made up of four subunits, one of which is calmodulin which has calcium binding functions, and directly activates the enzyme.

Ohtani et al. (1982) described a child with hypotonia and myopathy who was unable to walk. In other cases the onset was less severe with muscle stiffness, myalgia and weakness, with episodic myoglobinuria. A late onset case, a man aged 58 years, has also been described (Clemens et al. 1990; Di Mauro and Servidei 1993).

Phosphoglycerate Kinase (PGK) Deficiency (Type IX Glycogenosis)

This disorder consists of a rare syndrome characterised by seizures, haemolytic anaemia and mental retardation (Di Mauro and Bresolin 1986b). Exercise intolerance, muscle cramp and myoglobinuria occurred in one patient (Di Mauro et al. 1983a) with a pure muscle syndrome. Only four cases have been reported. The resting CK may be increased; the ECG is normal. There is no rise in venous blood lactate with ischaemic exercise. The muscle biopsy shows minor, non-specific abnormalities, but the phosphoglycerate kinase activity, an enzyme involved in terminal glycolysis below the phosphofructokinase reaction (Fig. 17.1) is markedly reduced (Di Mauro et al. 1983a; Tonin et al. 1993). Genetic heterogene-

ity has been recognised in the enzyme defect in the four reported cases with myopathy (Di Mauro and Servidei 1993). Phosphoglycerate kinase has been linked to a genetic locus on chromosome xq 13, and Type IX glycogenosis is inherited as an X-linked recessive disorder (Di Mauro et al. 1983a).

Phosphoglycerate Mutase Deficiency (Type X Glycogenosis)

This uncommon disorder, initially reported in five Afro-Americans, has an autosomal recessive pattern of inheritance with a locus assigned to chromosome 7p 12–13 (Edwards et al. 1989; Tsujino et al. 1993b). A caucasian case has also been described (Vita et al. 1994). There is exercise intolerance, cramps and recurrent myoglobinuria. The muscle biopsy can show increased glycogen content and tubular aggregates (Kissel et al. 1985). The ischaemic lactate test may produce a lower than normal response. Phosphoglycerate mutase, like CK, exists in muscle and brain isoforms and in Type X glycogenosis only the M isoform is abnormal, accounting for sparing of other tissues, including the heart. The B isoform is associated with a chromosome 10 locus (Sakoda et al. 1988). During exercise there is accumulation of phosphorylated monoesters in muscle, with intracellular acidosis (Duboc et al. 1987), with slow recovery (see Vita et al. 1994b).

Lactate Dehydrogenase Deficiency (Type XI Glycogenosis)

Six patients with LDH deficiency have been reported, five with exercise intolerance and recurrent myoglobinuria, and one an asymptomatic woman, identified by blood screening (Tsujino et al. 1994). The disorder can be detected by observing failure of the blood LDH level to rise commensurately with the CK level during an episode of myoglobinuria (Kanno et al. 1980). The normal rise in venous lactate with ischaemic exercise is impaired. Boone et al. (1972) assigned this disorder to a locus on chromosome 11p 15.4. There is genetic heterogeneity in the reported cases, with deletions and amino acid substitutions reported in the genome resulting in frame shift or non-sense mutations (Tsujino et al. 1994). The gene location is at 11p 15.

Myoadenylate Deaminase Deficiency

This enzyme deficiency has been described in more than 130 patients (Sabina et al. 1989). A primary deficiency has been described, presenting with fatiguability, cramps or muscle pain following exercise. A secondary deficiency has been associated with a number of other neuromuscular disorders, e.g. Duchenne muscular dystrophy, inflammatory myopathies, myotonic dystrophy and Werdnig-Hoffman SMA Type 1 (Sabina et al. 1992). The clinical heterogeneity associated with myoadenylate deficiency has led to difficulties in classification (Fishbein 1985), and in clearly establishing a phenotypic relationship to the enzyme defect.

The primary deficiency is inherited as an autosomal recessive trait, linked to a locus on the short arm of chromosome 1 (Sabina et al. 1990). The gene has been cloned and sequenced (adenosine monophosphate deaminase – amp *amp* 1 gene: see Sabina et al. 1992). The carrier frequency for mutation in the gene probably approaches 20% (Fishbein 1985). The mutations are probably point mutations or base pair rearrangements. In secondary myoadenylate deaminase deficiency, although there may be marked muscle destruction associated with the underlying disease, the enzyme deficiency probably results from altered gene expression.

In primary myoadenylate deaminase deficiency the residual enzyme activity is less than 2% of the control mean, the CK level is normal. The muscle biopsy is usually normal, but rarely occasionally angular regenerating fibres may occur (Sabina et al. 1992).

Mitochondrial Myopathies and Related Disorders

The concept of mitochondrial myopathy has emerged from an apparently heterogenous group of diseases, since the recognition of a specific pathological feature, the ragged-red fibre, in the muscle biopsy. This group of diseases is characterised by structural and biochemical abnormalities in the mitochondria. Classification of clinical syndromes in relation to the biochemical abnormalities has proved difficult, or even elusive, and not all these syndromes are accompanied by the finding of ragged-red fibres on muscle biopsy. They may also be defined according to abnormalities recognised in the mitochondrial genome but this has also proved to have an inconstant relationship to clinical phenotype. Indeed, some disorders of mitochondrial metabolism appear to result from defects in nuclear DNA, since these same aspects of mitochondrial structure and function are determined not by mitochondrial genes but

by nuclear genes. Marked overlap therefore exists in the clinical findings from case to case, and there is considerable genetic as well as phenotypic heterogeneity. Nonetheless, certain clinical syndromes can be recognised (Table 17.4).

Table 17.4. Disorders with prominent mitochondrial abnormality considered not to be due to mitochondrial metabolic disorder

Some cases of progressive external ophthalmoplegia
Oculopharyngeal dystrophy
Myotonic dystrophy
Facio-scapulo-humeral syndrome
Inclusion body and idiopathic polymyositis
Other myopathies with >1% ragged-red fibres

In 1962 Luft et al. reported a patient with fatiguable weakness in whom there was a hypermetabolic state due to a defect in the control of oxidative phosphorylation in skeletal muscle mitochondria. In this patient energy generated by abnormal mitochondria was dissipated as heat. The mitochondria were large, with distorted cristae and paracrystalline inclusions. Abnormal aggregates of mitochondria were soon recognised in muscle biopsies of other patients, not associated with a raised metabolic rate (Shy et al. 1966), and the characteristic ragged-red fibres demonstrated by the Gomori trichrome stain were described by Olson et al. (1972). These patients presented with extraocular or limb weakness, with fatiguability, variable lactic acidosis, mental retardation, seizures and cardiomyopathy, a cluster of features often termed oculo-cranio-somatic syndrome (Kearns–Sayre syndrome) (Chap. 14). The classification of mitochondrial disorders was extended by the recognition of the complex, multisystem, hereditary disorders with defects of the mitochondrial respiratory chain, in which cerebral and cerebellar features co-existed with myopathy (Spiro et al. 1970), and by descriptions of non-progressive mitochondrial myopathies with defects in mitochondrial ATPase, or cytochrome metabolism (see Schotland et al. 1976; Morgan-Hughes et al. 1982). Di Mauro et al. (1985) have recognised three groups of mitochondrial myopathies, those with defective substrate utilisation, defects of respiratory complexes and defects of phosphorylation–respiration coupling.

Several clinical syndromes are associated with *mitochondrial* disorder. In one, there is *encephalopathy, lactic acidosis and stroke*-like syndromes (Pavlakis et al. 1984) – MELAS, and in another there is familial *myoclonic epilepsy with ragged-red fibres* – MERRF (Fukuhara et al. 1980; Pavlakis et al. 1984). There are a number of clinical syndromes with myopathy only, syndromes with cerebral dysfunction and syndromes with chronic progressive external ophthalmoplegia (Morgan-Hughes et al. 1982; Petty et al. 1986a,b). In Petty and colleagues' (1986a,b) experience 73% of patients with mitochondrial disorders had muscle weakness induced by exercise; the remaining 27% presented with central manifestations, including ataxia, dementia, deafness, involuntary movements and seizures.

Disorders in which mitochondrial abnormalities are often found, but in which the primary disorder is considered not to be due to mitochondrial metabolic disturbance are shown in Table 17.4.

Principles of Mitochondrial Metabolism

Mitochondria consist of a matrix space bound and enclosed by a convoluted inner membrane, and a less convoluted outer membrane (Green 1983). Mitochondria contain enzymes that mediate the oxidation of pyruvate, glucose and fatty acids to produce energy, as ATP, and carbon dioxide and water as waste products. Thus the prime function of mitochondria is to produce energy, at great speed, from the principal products of digestion of foodstuffs, or mobilised food stores, e.g. glycogen and fat.

There are five principal steps (Di Mauro 1993) in mitochondrial metabolism:

1. Transport across the inner and outer mitochondrial membranes; this involves a set of carriers or translocases.
2. In the mitochondrial matrix metabolites are oxidised. Pyruvate is oxidised by the pyruvate dehydrogenase complex, and fatty acids by the beta-oxidation pathway.
3. Acetyl CoA, the product of both pyruvate and fatty acid oxidation, are oxidised further in the Krebs cycle.
4. The reducing equivalents of metabolism in the Krebs cycle are processed along a chain of proteins, the electron transport (respiratory) chain, embedded in the inner mitochondrial wall. This process consists of several cycles of oxidation (reduction reactions in which the final product is water).
5. The energy released in these reactions is used to pump protons across the mitochondrial membrane, from its matrix to the cytosol of the cell. This electrochemical proton gradient is used to synthesise ATP at three sites along the respiratory chain, which are the sites of oxidation/ phosphorylation coupling.

This description of mitochondrial metabolism leads naturally into a classification of mitochondrial myopathies (Table 17.5), based on disordered metabolism, and allows phenotypic variability around the basic biochemical disturbances. Of course, in clinical practice, the clinical phenotype is paramount, and the biochemical disorder underlying the clinical presentation is very difficult to predict (Rowland 1994a).

Table 17.5. Biochemical disorders of mitochondria associated with myopathy

1. Defects of transport
    CPT deficiency
    Carnitine deficiency

2. Defects of substrate utilisation
    Pyruvate carboxylase deficiency
    Pyruvate dehydrogenase complex deficiency
    Defects of β oxidation

3. Defects of the Krebs cycle
    Fumarase deficiency
    α-ketoglutarate dehydrogenase deficiency

4. Defects of oxidation/phosphorylation coupling
    Luft's syndrome

5. Defects of the respiratory chain
    Complex I deficiency (NADH ubiquinone oxidoreductase)
    Complex II deficiency (succinate ubiquinone oxidoreductase)
    Complex III deficiency (ubiquinone cytochrome C oxidoreductase)
    Complex IV deficiency (cytochrome C oxidase)
    Complex V deficiency (mitochondrial ATPase)
    Combined defects of respiratory chain components

From Di Mauro (1993)

Principles of Mitochondrial Genetics

Mitochondria contain their own, unique DNA, arranged as a circular, double-stranded mtDNA molecule, 16,569 base pairs in length (Anderson et al. 1981). This mitochondrial genome is exclusively maternally inherited (Giles et al. 1980). mtDNA encodes 13 structural proteins, all subunits of respiratory chain subcomplexes, together with two ribosomal RNAs (rRNAs) and 22 transfer RNAs (tRNA) essential for translation of the genetic code into structural proteins. Mitochondria are believed to be a feature of eukaryotic cells following a symbiotic fusion of bacteria and protocells in past millennia (Rosenberg 1994).

Mitochondrial DNA differs from nuclear DNA in several respects. It utilises a different genetic code. It contains no introns. It is liable to mutations more commonly than nuclear DNA. It is present in each mitochondrion, sometimes in up to 10 copies, so that each cell contains hundreds or more copies of the mitochondrial genome. It is transmitted by maternal inheritance, because the sperm contains little or no cytoplasm and therefore no mitochondria. The mitochondrial DNA consists of heavy and light strands, containing their own separate replication origins. Expression of mitochondrial genes relies on mitochondrion-specific protein synthesis, controlled by the interplay of nuclear-encoded transcriptional and translational factors, with tRNAs and rRNAs synthesised from corresponding mitochondrial genes. Thus mitochondrial DNA contains both protein-encoding and protein-synthesizing genes.

After fertilisation of the ovum, cell division occurs resulting in the development of the multicell stages of zygote development. During these successive cell divisions, the daughter cells will receive populations of mitochondria in a process of random selection. Mutant mitochondria present in the parent cell will thus pass in varying numbers to daughter cells. This could result in a mitochondrial population consisting wholly of normal mitochondria, wholly of abnormal mitochondria (homoplasmy) or a mixed population (heteroplasmy).

The phenotypic expression of a mtDNA mutation depends on the severity of the defect of oxidative phosphorylation that results, in relation to the energy requirements of the tissue containing the mutation. In addition the level of mutant mtDNA varies in different tissues, and with time (Poulton et al. 1993, Poulton 1996). This concept allows understanding of the phenotypic variation found in different members of a family and, since there is a gradual decline in oxidative phosphorylation with increasing age (Trounce et al. 1989), it also explains the late age of onset of some mitochondrial myopathies and other mitochondrial syndromes.

Several features of the clinical genetics of mitochondrial disorders stand out. Since inheritance is maternal it, in some respects, resembles the pattern of X-linked traits; however, *both* sexes are affected. The phenotypic expression of a mitochondrial disorder is dependent on the relative proportion of mutant and normal ("wild-type") mtDNA genomes, and a critical number of mutant mtDNA genomes must be present to cause expression of the disease (the "threshold effect"). There is a risk that all the children of an affected mother will be affected, a risk modified only by the threshold effect caused by the mutant mtDNA content of mitochondria in the ovum. Thus more of an affected woman's offspring are affected by mitochondrial disorder than by an autosomal dominant gene.

Despite the importance of mtDNA it must be recognised that 90% of all mitochondrial proteins are encoded by nuclear DNA. This requires transport of proteins from cytoplasm into mitochondria by a complex translocational process, requiring involvement of peptides and receptor proteins at the mitochondrial surface, together with the action of heat shock proteins (HSP70) as part of the conformation of these large molecules (Schatz 1991; Di Mauro 1993; Schapira and Di Mauro 1994).

Genetic Defects in Mitochondrial Diseases

Mitochondrial disorders are important in the pathogenesis of a number of different syndromes involving muscle, brain, kidney, the visual system, the auditory system and in ageing. In addition, mitochondrial disease may result in episodic metabolic disturbances, usually characterised by lactic acidosis, and often with seizures, myoclonic epilepsy and stroke-like syndromes. Renal disease, e.g. Pearson's syndrome, may also result from mitochondrial disorder.

These disorders result, in most cases, from deletions, duplications and point mutations in mitochondrial DNA, or from abnormalities in nuclear DNA controlling the mitochondrial genome and showing Mendelian inheritance. Examples of the latter include carnitine palmitoyl transferase deficiency, causing carnitine deficiency, and fumarase deficiency (Table 17.6).

Table 17.6. Classification of mtDNA defects in mitochondrial disease

Deletions of mtDNA	Kearns–Sayre syndrome Sporadic progressive external ophthalmoplegia with ragged-red fibres Pearson's syndrome
Point mutations of mtDNA	MERRF MELAS Leber's hereditary optic neuro retinopathy Myopathy and cardiomyopathy
Defects in nuclear DNA	Carnitine palmitoyl transferase deficiency Fumerase deficiency

Not all patients with the same mutation have the same clinical syndrome, and not all the patients with a defined syndrome have the same mutation in mtDNA (Moraes et al. 1993). Thus, not all patients with Kearns–Sayre syndrome show an abnormality in mtDNA; deletions are a feature in only about 60% (Moraes et al. 1993; Rowland 1994a).

Ragged-Red Fibres

Ragged-red fibres consist of fibres in which there is a subsarcolemmal rim of irregular bright red, or reddish-blue material in sections stained with the modified Gomori technique (Fig. 17.4a). In the later stages of the abnormality the whole fibre may contain a reticulated network of this red material. The abnormal material (Fig. 3.24) stains positively

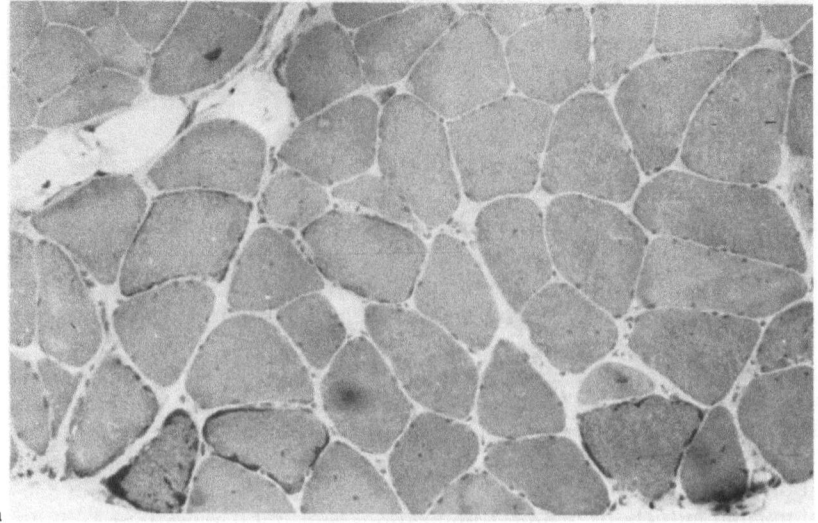

a

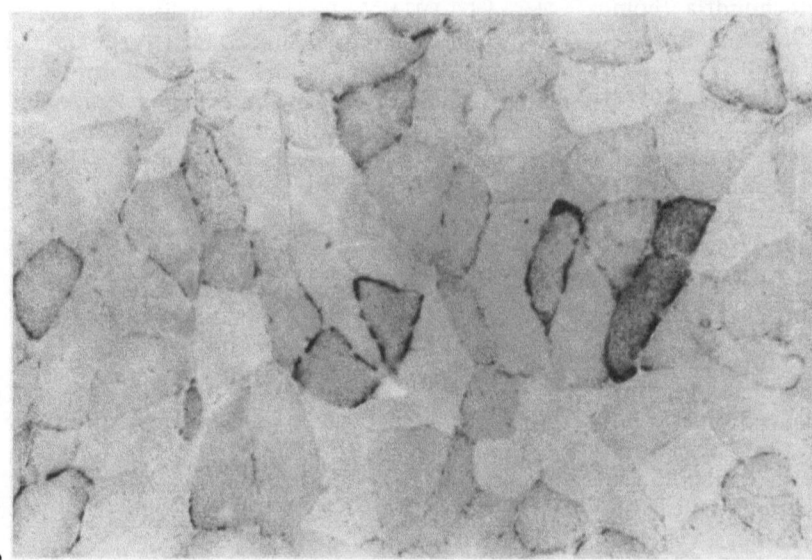

b

Fig. 17.4. (a) Ragged-red fibres. Gomori trichrome. × 140. Several fibres show the characteristic peripheral abnormality; shown in more detail in Fig. 3.24. (b) Succinic dehydrogenase × 140. This enzyme is localised in mitochondria and demonstrates the sub-sarcolemonal accumulation of abnormal mitochondria.

in oxidative and other mitochondrial stains (Fig. 17.4b) can be stained with neutral lipid techniques and is negative in myofibrillar stains such as in the myofibrillar ATPase reactions. This abnormality has been found in 1%–20% of fibres in biopsies of patients with mitochondrial disorders, and is virtually restricted to Type 1 fibres (Olson et al. 1972). Ragged-red fibres are found commonly in oculocranio-somatic syndrome and in the other forms of chronic external ophthalmoplegia. The non-specific nature of the finding of ragged-red fibres in a muscle biopsy is shown by their occurrence in other disorders, including cases of myopathy without ophthalmoplegia (Black et al. 1977; Kamieniecka 1977), carnitine deficiency, and polymyositis (Swash et al. 1978b), but in most of these cases other histo-

logical abnormalities have been observed. Ragged-red fibres occur in up to 3% of muscle fibres in biopsies of elderly subjects. In cases with cytochrome c oxidase deficiency absence of cytochrome c oxidase (COX) can be demonstrated in ragged-red fibres, and in other Type 1 fibres that appear otherwise relatively normal (Johnson et al. 1983). Not all ragged-red fibres are COX-negative. In MELAS syndrome ragged-red fibres are present, but are cox-positive. In Kearns–Sayre syndrome and in progressive external ophthalmoplegia Degoul et al. (1991) noted a relationship between the cytochrome oxidase activity in muscle and the amount of mtDNA deleted from the mitochondrial genome.

Ragged-red fibres are not seen in muscle biopsies of mitochondrial disorders *not* involving the respiratory chain. Thus, they are not a feature of carnitine palmitoyl transferase deficiency, fumarase deficiency and Luft's disease.

With the electron microscope the characteristic feature of ragged-red fibres is the mitochondrial abnormality. The mitochondria appear large, may assume unusual shapes and are present in increased number in zones corresponding to the light microscopical abnormality. These abnormal mitochondria contain striking rectilinear arrays of double membranes resembling crystals, located between the inner and outer mitochondrial membranes (Fig. 3.24 and 17.5). These paracrystalline crystals consist of deposits of mitochondrial creatine kinase (Stadhouders et al. 1990). These abnormal mitochondria may also contain osmiophilic dense bodies. The muscle fibres themselves show disarray of myofibrils and there is an excess of lipid droplets. Other degenerative changes may be seen. Similar mitochondrial abnormalities may be observed in other organs in a variety of other disorders unrelated to the progressive opthalmoplegias.

Ragged-red fibres represent the morphological expression of a longstanding, progressive degenerative process, associated with mitochondrial metabolic defect dependent on an imbalance between energy requirement and oxidation/phosphorylation efficiency of the muscle fibre (Morgan-Hughes et al. 1977, 1979; Di Mauro 1993). The abnormality has been reproduced in tissue culture (Askanas and Engel 1977), a finding which could indicate either horizontal or vertical transmission of the abnormality. The whole range of ultrastructural abnormality found in mitochondrial myopathies has been reproduced experimentally by respiratory toxins, e.g. crotoxin (rattlesnake venom) and 2–4 dinitrophenol (Shah et al. 1982).

Abnormal proliferation of mitochondria in brain and choroidal arterioles, as well as in blood vessels in muscle, as shown by SDH activity, has been recognised in MELAS (Sakuta and Nonaka 1989; Hasegawa et al. 1991).

Mitochondrial Disorders Affecting Muscle

The clinical and biochemical features of the identified mitochondrial disorders show no consistent correlation (Petty et al. 1986a), and correlation with genetic defects in mtDNA or nuclear DNA is also imprecise (Hammans and Morgan-Hughes 1994). The biochemical abnormalities can be classified as defects in the transport, or utilization of substrate, defects in the Krebs cycle, defects of oxidation/phosphorylation coupling and defects in the respiratory chain (Table 17.5). These disorders can be related to the pathways illustrated in Figs. 17.6, 17.7 and 17.8. Of these disorders defects in the respiratory chain are the most common.

Defects of Fatty Acid Transport: Lipid Disorders of Muscle

Fatty acids are an important fuel for muscle. The transport system through the inner mitochondrial membrane requires carnitine, and the enzyme carnitine palmitoyl transferase (CPTase).

Defects of Carnitine Utilisation

These myopathies are characterised by the accumulation of neutral lipid in muscle fibres (Engel et al. 1970), and sometimes by degenerative changes in muscle fibres, including the presence of ragged-red fibres. The disorders may also be classified as mitochondrial myopathies because they are due to defects of mitochondrial metabolism, and some are accompanied by characteristic morphological changes in mitochondria in affected fibres. Although lipid deposition may occur in muscle fibres in a number of neuromuscular disorders only in two instances, viz, carnitine deficiency and carnitine palmitoyl transferase deficiency, have the underlying biochemical defects been recognised. Harriman and Reid (1972), in a review of the distribution of excessive lipid droplets in 139 muscle biopsies, noted that increased numbers of lipid droplets were found in Type 1 fibres in steroid myopathy, alcoholic myopathy and in some cases of diabetic neuropathy and myasthenia gravis. Excess lipid droplets in Type 2 fibres were rare; scattered single fibres with excess lipid were particularly in Duchenne dystrophy.

Carnitine Metabolism. Carnitine (α-trimethylamino-β-hydroxybutyrate) is distributed in all tissues, except the brain. About 50% of ingested carnitine is taken up by muscle (Yue and Fritz 1962), and 95% of total body carnitine is stored in muscle. Carnitine is thus important in metabolic pathways in muscle. Plasma carnitine is derived from dietary sources, from synthesis in the liver, and perhaps by release from tissue stores. In the liver endogenous synthesis of carnitine occurs from lysine (Tanphaichitr and Broquist 1974). The main role of carnitine is in the transport of long-chain fatty acids into mitochondria (Fig. 17.7). In the mitochondrial matrix fatty acids undergo beta-oxidation and, because of its role in fatty acid transport, carnitine is important in energy metabolism in muscle. Active

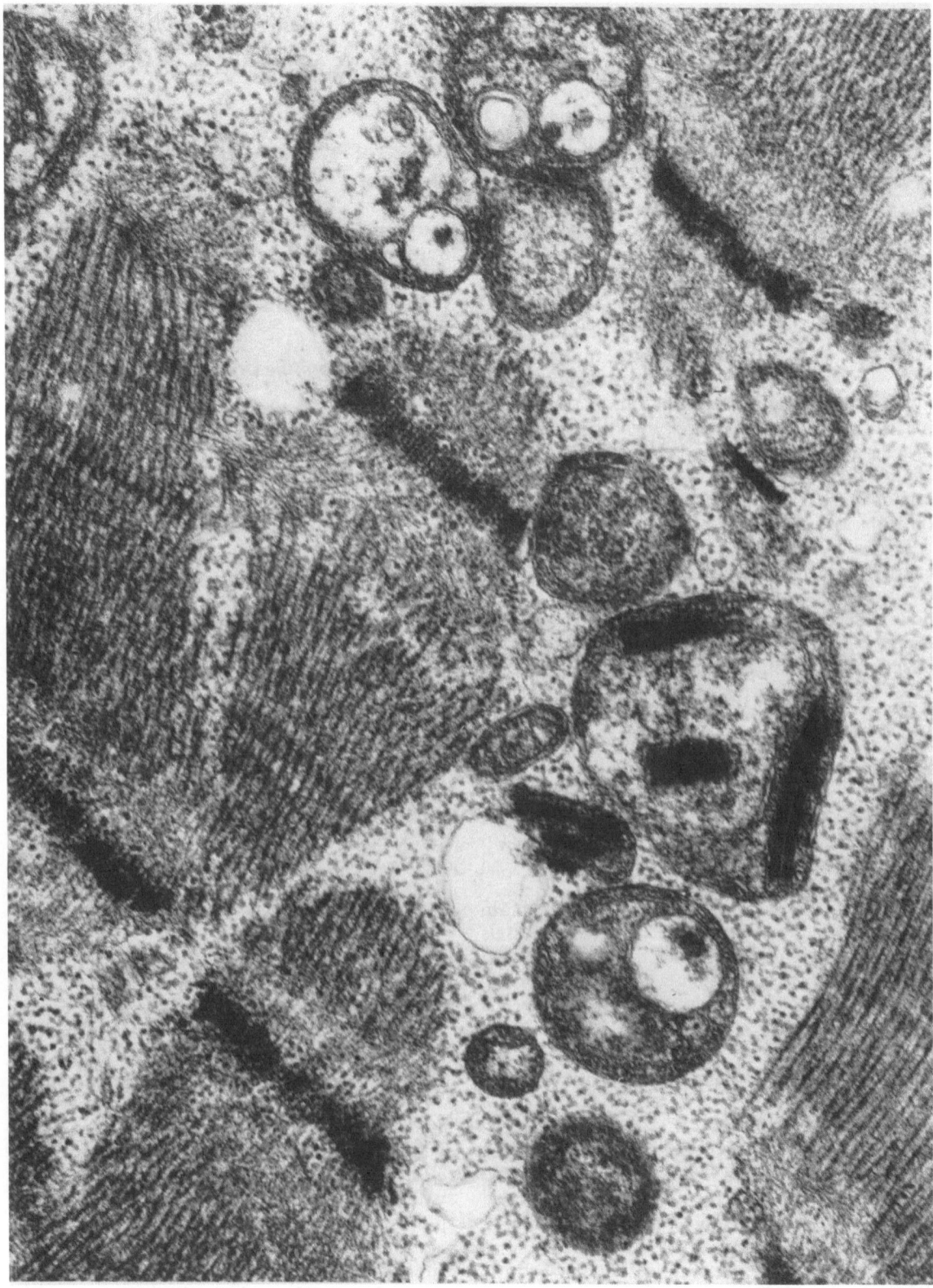

Fig. 17.5. Ragged-red fibre. Electron micrograph × 30 000. The mitochondria show a variety of paracrystalline inclusions and osmiophilic dense bodies, and their cristae are destroyed.

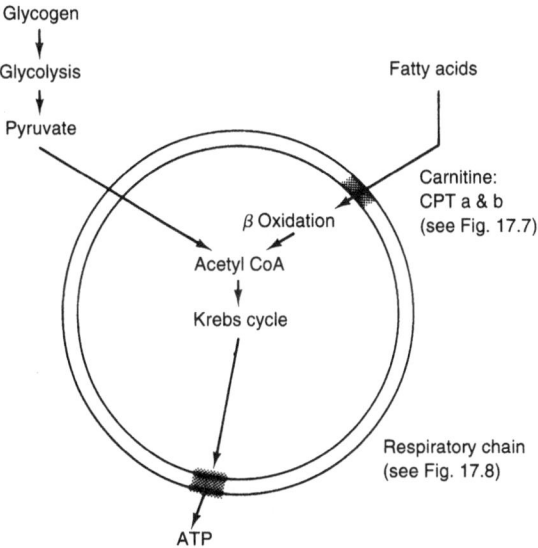

Fig. 17.6. Metabolic pathways for ATP synthesis in the mito-chondrion. CPT a & b: carnitine palmitoyl transferase a and b.

reabsorption of carnitine occurs in the proximal renal tubules (Hoppel 1992). Carnitine is important not only in the transport of long chain fatty acids into cells and into the mitochondrial matrix, but also in buffering the acyl CoA/COASH ratio, scavenging potentially toxic acyl CoA groups and in the oxidation of peroxisomal fatty acids and branched chain fatty acids (Hoppel 1992).

An enzyme, carnitine palmitoyl transferase, catalyses the reversible reaction of long-chain fatty acyl groups (palmitoyl CoA) and carnitine. Carnitine palmitoyl tranferase (CPTase) exists in two forms; CPTase I acts at the outer surface of the inner mitochondrial membrane to form palmitoyl carnitine which then crosses to the inner surface, where CPTase II acts, releasing carnitine and palmitoyl CoA (Hoppel and Tomec 1972; Van Dyke et al. 1975).

The importance of carnitine transport of fatty acids in muscle mitochondrial metabolism is evident from consideration of the fact that, at rest and with a normal diet, fatty acid oxidation provides more than half the energy needs of mammalian skeletal muscle. During fasting or prolonged exercise, fatty acid oxidation becomes indispensable to energy supply.

Carnitine Deficiency Syndromes. Three forms of this syndrome have been described.

1. *Myopathic carnitine deficiency.*

In this syndrome carnitine deficiency is restricted to skeletal muscle. The disorder is characterised by slowly progressive muscular weakness, with onset in childhood. (Engel and Angelini 1973). Onset in adult life has also been described (Markesbery et al. 1974; Cornelio and Di Donato 1985). The myopathy is proximal, often with striking involvement of paraspinal neck and jaw muscles, which are both weak and atrophic. The tendon reflexes are decreased or absent. The patient may appear thin and small, with a considerable lumbar lordosis, but without muscle tenderness. Gowers' manoeuvre is often evident (Van Dyke et al. 1975). The disorder is progressive, and there may be tachycardia and ventricular enlargement, suggesting cardiac involvement. Mental retardation is not a feature of this form of the disease (Willner et al. 1979). Other tissues are spared and there is no increased excretion of organic acids in the urine (Di Donato et al. 1992). Plasma free fatty acid levels are normal. This primary myopathic form of carnitine deficiency usually responds to treatment with oral L-carnitine supplements, 100 mg/kg per day (Engel 1986). Parental muscle carnitine levels may be slightly low (Van Dyke et al. 1975).

2. *Systemic carnitine deficiency.*

Delineation of primary and secondary systemic carnitine deficiency syndromes is clinically difficult,

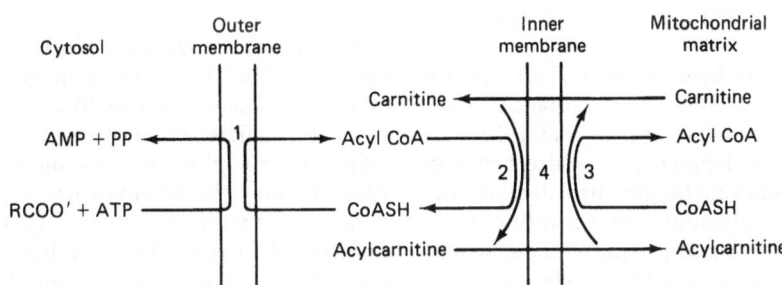

Fig. 17.7. Transport of long-chain fatty acids into mitochondria. (From Cornelio and Di Donato 1985). 1, Thiokinase; 2, Carnitine palmitoyl transferase I; 3, Carnitine palmitoyl transferase II; 4, Carnitine-acylcarnitine translocase; RCOO′, long-chain fatty acids; PP, pyrophosphate.

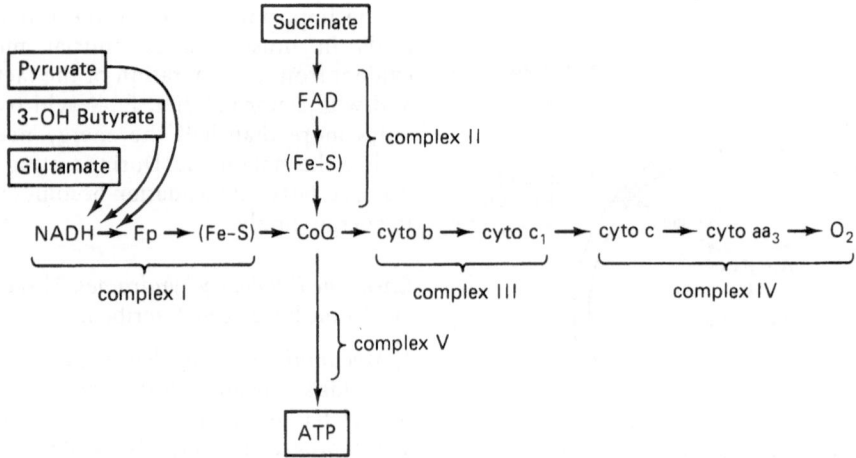

Fig. 17.8. Electron transfer chain and oxidative phosphorylation; this system is located in the inner membrane of the mitochondrion. It consists of an electron transfer process that releases energy for ATP synthesis using pyruvate, 3-hydroxybutyrate, glutamate or succinate or substrates. The location of the various complexes isolated by detergent treatment of the inner membrane, and associated with various clinical syndromes, is indicated on the figure.

and the earlier literature difficult to interpret, since recognition of the development of severe systemic carnitine deficiency in metabolic acidaemias was delayed.

Primary systemic carnitine deficiency, with cardiomyopathy, is an autosomal recessive disorder that presents with progressive dilated cardiomyopathy in childhood. Hypoketotic hypoglycaemic episodes, and skeletal muscle symptoms, e.g. exercise intolerance and fatigue, are features, and hypotonia is marked. Plasma carnitine levels are less than 10% of normal, and carnitine levels are low also in heart, liver and muscle. The muscle biopsy shows small lipid droplets in Type 1 fibres. There is no dicarboxylic aciduria, perhaps because long-chain fatty acids cannot be broken down in cells to these smaller molecules (Treem et al. 1988). Treatment with L-carnitine supplements 2–6 g/day produces dramatic and sustained improvement (Matsuishi et al. 1985; Angelini et al. 1992). This disorder is due to a defect of sodium-linked membrane transport of carnitine in muscle, intestinal mucosa and renal tubules.

Consanguinity has been a feature of several reported cases. In one fatal case parental carnitine levels were 65% of normal (Cornelio et al. 1977).

Systemic carnitine deficiency may also occur in association with other metabolic disorders, occurring as a secondary phenomenon. Carnitine levels are low in muscle, liver and plasma (Rebouche and Engel 1983). Patients present with skeletal myopathy, cardiomyopathy, or both, and with episodic vomiting, encephalopathy and hepatomegaly, and with hypoketotic hyperglycaemic episodes and a syndrome resembling Reye's syndrome (Karpati et al. 1975; Boudin et al. 1976; Chapoy et al. 1980). Many of these patients have a defect of β oxidation of fatty acids, most commonly due to medium-chain or multiple acyl CoA dehydrogenase deficiency (Turnbull et al. 1984; Di Donato et al. 1986). Treatment with L-carnitine is less effective than in other carnitine deficiency syndromes and the syndrome may be fatal, often before age 25 years (Cornelio et al. 1977).

3. Secondary systemic carnitine deficiency.

Carnitine deficiency (Editorial 1990) is frequently found in patients with renal failure, often those treated with dialysis, and treatment with sodium valpo rate. Therapy with pivampicillin may also cause carnitine deficiency (Holme et al. 1989). This deficiency may produce weakness and fatigue. It probably results from metabolic disturbances in fatty acid metabolism as well as from loss of carnitine by excretion or by binding.

Laboratory Investigations. The CK is usually mildly raised in those forms of carnitine deficiency with myopathy. The ECG is usually abnormal in systemic carnitine deficiency, showing evidence of ventricular hypertrophy, and of conduction abnormalities, and may also be abnormal in muscle carnitine deficiency. In the severe form (systemic carnitine deficiency) abnormalities of liver function, with raised liver enzymes, may be found. In addition the episodes of lactic acidosis may be recognised and hypoglycaemia may be a feature at this time. Fasting induces a marked increase in liver enzyme levels, and in the CK, and may provoke hypoglycaemia and acidosis if continued for longer than 1–2 days. These abnormalities are not a feature of restricted muscle carnitine deficiency.

Electrophysiological Assessment. The EMG shows myopathic potentials without specific features, and the nerve conduction velocity is normal.

Muscle Biopsy. The main abnormality is the presence of excess numbers of lipid droplets in Type 1 fibres (Fig. 17.9). Type 2 fibres, especially Type 2A fibres (Willner et al. 1979), may also contain more lipid droplets than normal muscle but lipid droplet accumulation in these fibres is not as marked as in Type 1 fibres. The latter may become atrophic. The lipid droplets are larger than normal droplets and are especially densely distributed in the subsarcolemmal region, often closely related to muscle mitochondria. They contain neutral lipid, which is visible as unstained spaces in the haematoxylin and eosin stain, as red droplets in oil red O and Sharlach R preparations, and as reddish-brown material in Gomori stains. They may also be visible in NADH-tr preparations, and this technique may also demonstrate an increase in mitochondrial number. Sometimes acid phosphatase activity can be seen in the subsarcolemmal regions. Muscle fibre size is normal or slightly smaller than normal and some cases may show an increased number of small fibres. With the electron microscope lipid droplets are present in columns between the myofibrils. There is usually an excess of mitochondria which may be abnormally shaped, and these may contain paracrystalline inclusions (ragged-red fibres). This abnormality has been reported mainly in systemic carnitine deficiency (Karpati et al. 1975; Boudin et al. 1976; Engel et al. 1977a).

The carnitine level can be determined by quantitative analysis of muscle biopsy tissue.

Other Pathological Features. In the systemic form, carnitine levels can be determined in the liver biopsy, and histologically the liver may show fat accumulation within hepatocytes, especially if an episode of liver dysfunction has recently occurred. Renal epithelial cells and myocardial muscle fibres may also show fat accumulation, as may circulating leucocytes (Markesbery et al. 1974; Boudin et al. 1976).

Management. Prednisone, given in high dosage, has been reported to lead to dramatic clinical improvement (Engel and Siekert 1972) in systemic carnitine deficiency, although not all cases respond to this treatment. Supplemental dietary L-carnitine

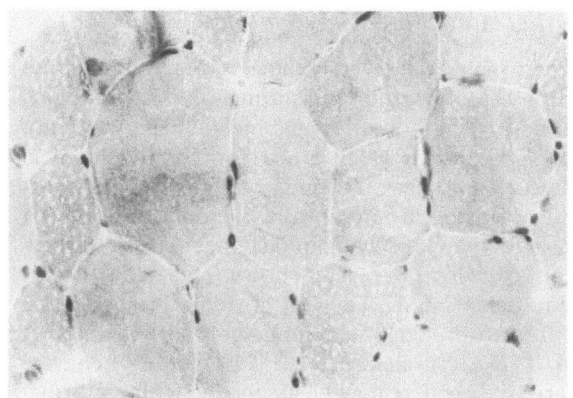

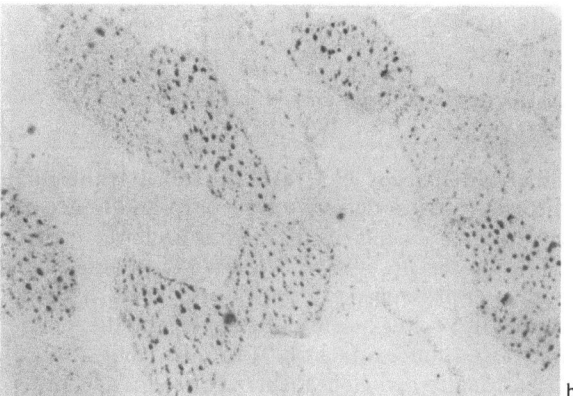

Fig. 17.9. Carnitine deficiency myopathy. **a** H and E, × 350. Unstained, rounded vacuoles of varying size are seen in some fibres; these are all Type 1 fibres. **b** Oil red O, × 350. The vacuoles are stained intensely in this neutral lipid preparation.

(100 mg/kg body weight) has also been tried and has led to improvement in both systemic and muscle carnitine deficiency (Matsuishi et al. 1985; Angelini et al. 1992) and also in secondary carnitine deficiency syndromes, although the extent of this improvement is variable (Karpati et al. 1975; Angelini et al. 1976), and some cases do not respond (Willner et al. 1979). Supplemental carnitine increases plasma carnitine levels, but not muscle carnitine levels, suggesting that in these cases of muscle carnitine deficiency there is a defect of transport of carnitine from plasma into muscle fibres (Karpati et al. 1975). Oral carnitine treatment has usually been accompanied by supplements of medium chain triglycerides. Life-threatening episodes of acidosis and hypoglycaemia in the systemic form should be treated with glucose infusion, correction of acidosis and carnitine supplementation. Propranolol may be helpful in muscle carnitine deficiency (Martyn et al. 1981). Riboflavin supplements have also been recommended (Cornelio and Di Donato 1985).

Other Lipid Storage Myopathies

There have been several reports of other myopathies with excess neutral lipid in muscle fibres in which abnormalities of carnitine metabolism were not present, and in which the underlying biochemical defect is unknown (Miranda et al. 1979). Before carnitine metabolism was understood a number of cases of myopathy with lipid storage were described, some of which were later shown to be due to carnitine deficiency (Bradley et al. 1969; Bradley et al. 1972b), although others remain obscure (Salmon et al. 1971; Jerusalem et al. 1975). These uncharacterised disorders may be associated with abnormal mitochondria in some instances (Salmon et al. 1971; Miranda et al. 1979).

Carnitine Palmitoyl Transferase (CPTase) Deficiency

CPTase deficiency is a rare, recessively inherited disorder, due to defective transport, and hence of β-oxidation of fatty acids. It has a characteristic clinical presentation with cramps and muscular pain after prolonged exertion, fasting, fever, high fat intake and cold exposure. Ibuprofen and diazepam may also induce attacks of weakness (Zierz 1994). Occasionally myoglobinuria may occur. Weakness is not a feature unless rhabdomyolysis occurs and in severe attacks weakness may last for days. Reversible renal failure may accompany the rhabdomyolysis. CPT deficiency is the commonest cause of rhabdomyolysis (Tonin et al. 1990). About 60 cases have been reported (Zierz 1994). Although of autosomal recessive inheritance, the disorder is commoner in boys by 5 : 1 (Cornelio and Di Donato 1985). The symptoms have usually commenced in the second or third decade (Di Mauro and Di Mauro 1973; Bank et al. 1975). Contracture of muscle does not occur and fatiguability is not a feature although muscle pain and cramp limit exercise tolerance. The second-wind phenomenon does not develop in these patients, presumably because of the defective utilisation of free fatty acid. Short intensive exercise is normally tolerated. The muscles are usually normal between attacks.

Laboratory Investigations. The CK is normal but may rise to >50 000 IU/l in an episode of rhabodmyolysis. The CK may also rise after a provocative fasting and exercise test; this may also lead to detectable myoglobinaemia and myoglobinuria. Fasting does not lead to marked ketoacidosis, as occurs in systemic carnitine deficiency. The plasma triglycerides may be increased (Bank et al. 1975) or normal (Carroll et al. 1978). Ischaemic exercise is

accompanied by a normal rise in venous blood lactate (Bank et al. 1975), an important differential point from the glycogenoses. The activity of CPTase can be assayed in the muscle biopsy. Little data is yet available on CPTase I and CPTase II levels in patients with the syndrome, but Scholte et al. (1979) have described a patient with CPTase II deficiency in muscle and leucocytes, in whom CPTase I was normal. This patient developed muscle pain and myoglobinuria with strenuous exercise. In other patients CPTase II has usually been abnormal (Cornelio and Di Donato 1985). The gene for CPTase II is located on chromosome 1 p11–13, and several mutations have been identified at this locus (Di Donato 1994).

Assays of CPTase activity in muscle of affected patients range between 0 and 30% of normal; in asymptomatic or heterozygotic people the level of CPTase activity is about 50% of normal (Mengihi et al. 1991). Levels of CPTase activity in liver are also often abnormal, although no abnormality of liver function can be detected.

Electrophysiological Assessment. The EMG is normal between periods of exercise. The ECG is normal.

Muscle Biopsy. No abnormality can be detected. Electron microscopy may show a very slight increase in lipid droplets (Bank et al. 1975).

Management. A high-carbohydrate and low-fat diet will usually prevent muscular symptoms; however, no more specific treatment is available (Cumming et al. 1976). Carbohydrate supplements before exercise may help prevent muscular symptoms. Fasting should be avoided. Rhabdomyolysis may lead to acute renal failure, which is reversible.

Defects of Substrate Utilisation

There are three uncommon symdromes, all with systemic features, in which muscular involvement is relatively minor (Table 17.5).

In *pyruvate decarboxylase deficiency*, the severe neonatal form presents with seizures, hypotonia and dysmorphic features with lactic acidosis. In the infantile form, which resembles Leigh's syndrome, seizures are associated with ataxia, ophthalmoplegia, optic atrophy and mild lactic acidosis. In a benign form intermittent ataxia and exercise intolerance may respond to thiamine supplements (Di Mauro et al. 1992).

Pyruvate carboxylase deficiency causes two syndromes. In one hepatomegaly and metabolic acidosis lead to death in the first 3 months. A milder form progresses more slowly, leading to death in childhood.

In *defects of β-oxidation* (Di Donato 1994), liver dysfunction leads to metabolic encephalopathy, non-ketotic hypoglycaemia and dicarboxylic aciduria. There is failure to thrive, hypotonia and retardation. Long chain, medium chain and short chain acyl CoA dehydrogenase deficiencies, and combinations of these defects, have been described (Di Mauro et al. 1992). One form, glutaric aciduria, may respond to riboflavin supplements (multiple acyl CoA dehydrogenase (MAD) deficiency (De Visser et al. 1986)).

Defects of the Krebs Cycle (Table 17.5)

Fumarase deficiency exists in several forms, but less than 10 cases have been described. A fatal encephalopathy may occur with microcephaly and hypomyelination and a more slowly progressive infantile onset has been described. Muscle is not clinically affected (Zinn et al. 1986).

In *α-ketoglutarate dehydrogenase deficiency* there is lactic acidosis and predominant extrapyramidal features, with hypotonia. Muscle is not clinically involved.

Defects of Oxidation/Phosphorylation Coupling

This was the first of the metabolic disorders of energy transport to be recognised, but it appears to be exceptionally rare. Luft et al. described two patients in 1962, with euthyroid hypermetabolism due to uncoupling of oxidative phosphorylation (Di Mauro et al. 1976). There was heat intolerance, hyperthermia, sweating, polyphagia, polydipsia and mild fatiguability beginning in childhood. The basal metabolic rate (BMR) was increased, but thyroid function was normal. The disorder is due to a defect in energy production and its coupling to muscle contraction.

Defects of the Respiratory Chain

The various components of the respiratory chain (electron transport chain) produce molecular oxygen for energy metabolism (Fig. 17.7). When the concept of mitochondrial neuromuscular disorders, especially myopathies, was first enunciated (Shy et al. 1966; Morgan–Hughes 1982), it was expected that elucidation of the underlying biochemical and enzymatic disorders would form the basis of classification. However, the clinical syndrome proved heterogenous (see Rowland 1994a). Similarly, a cytogenetic classification (Holt et al. 1988) cannot readily be used as the basis for a clinically useful classification (Rowland 1994a), although certain mtDNA deletions, for example, are associated with some of the major syndromes.

Adults with mitochondrial myopathies most frequently have defects of the respiratory chain localised to complex I (Petty et al. 1986a). However, the clinical syndrome shown by these patients variably includes a multisystem disorder, and lactic acidosis, in addition to myopathy. Defects of complex II are uncommon. Complex III defects produce variable phenotypes, and similarly variable phenotypes, including myopathy with acidosis, renal tubular acidosis and Leigh's syndrome. In some patients multiple defects of the electron chain have been described (Harding and Holt 1989).

In about a third of patients no abnormality in mtDNA can be recognised. This reflects both the difficulty in searching for point mutations in the mitochondrial genome, and heteroplasmy, that is, the presence of a population of mitochondria with deleted mtDNA, and another population of mitochondria with normal mtDNA, in the same cell. The variability in clinical phenotype is also partly explained by segregation of mtDNA mutations or deletions in certain tissues, e.g. brain, kidney, marrow, muscle or retina (see Rowland 1994a for discussion).

Investigations in the Diagnosis of Suspected Mitochondrial Disease

The most useful investigation is muscle biopsy, which may reveal ragged-red fibres (see above). The cytochrome oxidase technique is useful since it may demonstrate focal cytochrome oxidase deficiency in fibres that otherwise appear normal. Electron microscopy may reveal subsarcolemmal accumulation of abnormal mitochondria. In patients with mitochondrial encephalopathy, ragged-red fibres may be infrequent or absent, and conversely ragged-red fibres may be found in non-mitochondrial diseases, especially in the elderly, polymyositis, glycogen storage disease and muscular dystrophies. Usually there are less than 3% of ragged-red fibres in these situations.

The blood CK is normal, or only slightly increased in mitochondrial myopathies. Brain imaging is useful, either with CT or MR, in demonstrating calcification of the basal ganglia, atrophy of the brain or cerebellum and, sometimes, stroke-like lesions (Seigel et al. 1979; Rowland et al. 1991). In Kearns–Sayre syndrome 80% of cases show abnormal CT brain scans.

The ECG and echocardiogram may show abnormalities, and renal, endocrine and liver function tests may also be abnormal. A useful clinical screening test for mitochondrial disease is the finding of raised venous blood lactate and pyruvate levels at rest and, especially, following aerobic exercise (Petty et al. 1986a). Indeed, many patients with mitochondrial myopathy experience rapid fatigue, weakness and acidosis when attempting aerobic exercise. The CSF lactate may also be elevated, and the CSF protein is elevated in almost all cases of Kearns–Sayre syndrome (Berenberg et al. 1977).

Clinical Syndromes of Mitochondrial Myopathies and Related Disorders

There are a number of core clinical syndromes, from which clinical variations occur (Table 17.7).

Table 17.7   Mitochondrial disorders: clinical phenotypes

Myopathy
    With progressive external ophthalmoplegia
    With Kearns–Sayre syndrome
    With cardiomyopathy
    With other syndromes
        MELAS
        MERRF

Encephalomyopathy
    MERRF
    MELAS
    Associated with Kearns–Sayre syndrome

Neuropathy
    NARP
    Associated with Kearns–Sayre syndrome

Cardiomyopathy
    With myopathy

Leigh's syndrome

Leber's optic atrophy

Deafness

Renal disease (Pearson's syndrome)

Anaemia

Liver Disease

Others
    e.g. multiple symmetrical lipomas
    Migraine headache
    Recurrent ketoacidotic coma

MERRF, myoclonic epilepsy with ragged-red fibres; MELAS, mitochondrial encephalopathy, lactic acidosis and stroke-like episodes; NARP, neurogenic weakness, ataxia and retinitis pigmentosa.

Kearns–Sayre Syndrome (KSS)

In 1958 Kearns and Sayre described a sporadic syndrome consisting of a triad of progressive external ophthalmoplegia, atypical pigmentary retinopathy and heart block. Both sexes are equally affected. The syndrome had probably been described as long ago as 1886, by Bristowe, in four patients with external ophthalmoplegia, one of whom had Stokes–Adams attacks. The core feature of KSS is myopathy, since the presence of ragged red fibres was one of the defining features used to related the syndrome to the general group of mitochondrial myopathies. However, the syndrome is more correctly defined by its clinical features (Table 17.8). In addition to the clinical features noted in Table 17.8, a number of other clinical signs may be apparent (Berenberg et al. 1977). Patients with KSS are usually of small stature. There may be sensorineural deafness, extensor plantar responses, delayed puberty, occasional seizures and a mild sensory neuropathy, with impaired vibration sense in the extremities. The syndrome develops gradually over several years.

Table 17.8.   Clinical features of Kearns–Sayre syndrome

Major features
Progressive external ophthalmoplegia
Pigmentary retinopathy
Onset before age 20 years

Minor features
Ataxia
Cardiac conduction defect (usually complete heart block)
CSF protein >1 g/1

The first manifestation is usually ptosis or ophthalmoplegia, sometimes with deafness. Ptosis almost always precedes ophthalmoplegia. Cardiomyopathy with conduction defects develops 5 to 20 years later, and pigmentary retinal degeneration is also often delayed for up to 20 years after the development of ophthalmoplegia (Berenberg et al. 1977; Petty et al. 1986a). CT of the brain reveals intracranial calcification in the basal ganglia and thalamus, with attenuation of central white matter (Seigel et al. 1979). Hypoparathyroidism may also be a feature (Dewhurst et al. 1986).

Progressive External Ophthalmoplegia (PEO)

Presentation with slowly progressive ptosis and ophthalmoplegia is usually characteristically of childhood onset. The disorder is insidiously progressive and often affects upgaze more than other ocular movements. Rowland et al. (1991) found that of 40 patients with ragged-red fibres on muscle biopsy four had PEO alone and 11 had PEO with limb weakness. Petty et al. (1986a) noted that three of 52 patients with PEO had ptosis alone, one had PEO without ptosis and 48 had both. Ocular move-

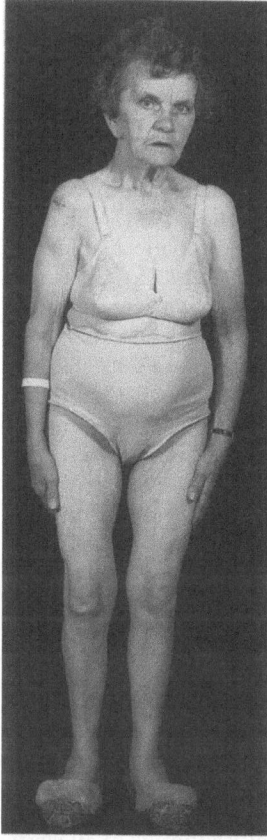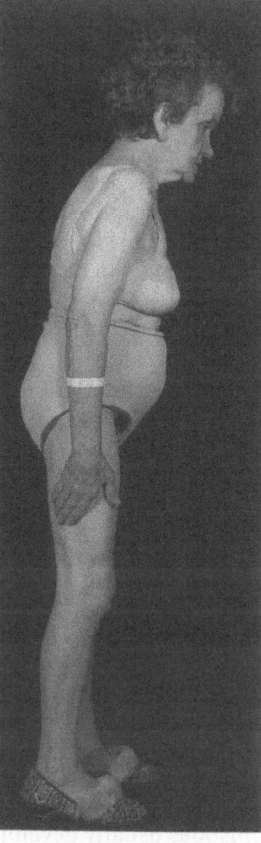

Fig. 17.10. Mitochondrial myoencephalopathy. This patient presented in middle life with mild muscle weakness, prominent fatigue and a confusional state that worsened with exercise, probably because of associated lactic acidosis (Morgan-Hughes et al. 1982).

ments were disconjugate in 18, and 19 had diplopia. PEO may also be associated with heart block (Kearns–Sayre 1958, Rowland et al. 1991). Encephalopathic features may also occur sometimes, including dementia, seizures, myoclonus, stroke-like episodes and, especially, fatigue. Indeed, a diagnosis of myasthenia gravis is sometimes suspected. The prognosis is good with regard to life expectancy, and most patients develop only mild disability (Rowland et al. 1991).

Myopathies

Limb weakness, often with exercise intolerance, or subjective fatigue, may be the only clinical manifestation of mitochondrial disease. Petty et al. (1986) found that weakness was the presenting symptom in 18 of 66 patients with mitochondrial disease, but was detectable on examination in as many as 47 of the 66. Weakness is mild, and usually most evident

in the proximal upper limb muscles. About 50% of patients with mitochondrial myopathy complain of fatigue. Some patients develop acidotic, hyperlactic acidaemic dyspnoea and fatigue during aerobic exercise, but this is evident only in the more severe cases. (Fig. 17.10). PEO and other associated features of mitochondrial myoencephalopathy (Morgan–Hughes et al. 1982) may be present. The majority of cases of mitochondrial myopathy are not familial (Hammans and Morgan–Hughes 1994).

Genetics of KSS, PEO and Myopathies

PEO is associated with deletions of mitochondrial DNA. Indeed, all patients with deletions have had PEO, although not all patients with PEO have had deletions (Holt et al. 1988; Moraes et al. 1989; Hammans and Morgan–Hughes 1994). In the auto-somal dominant form of PEO a combination of mitochondrial DNA deletions and a nuclear DNA abnormality that mapped to chromosome 10q 23.3–24.3 has been reported (Suomalainen et al. 1995). The majority of patients with KSS have deletions of mtDNA in muscle, but not in blood (Moraes et al. 1989; Hammans and Morgan–Hughes 1994). About 70% of patients with PEO show deletion of mtDNA. In KSS deletions have been reported in cerebral cortex (Shanske et al. 1990). In mitochondrial myopathy point mutations have been noted, for example in base pair bp 3243 tRNA, but families with multiple mtDNA deletions have also been described (Hammans et al. 1991; Ohno et al. 1991).

Electrophysiological Assessment

Concentric needle EMG in patients with KSS show myopathic potentials in about half the patients studied (Kamieniecka and Schmalbruch 1978). Single-fibre EMG (Krendel et al. 1987) showed an increased fibre density and neuromuscular jitter in 13 of 16 patients with CEO. Repetitive nerve stimulation studies are normal, allowing electrophysiological differentiation from myasthenia gravis (Brust et al. 1974).

Motor conduction is usually normal, but mild slowing may be found, mainly in the legs (Petty et al. 1986a), in patients with associated clinical or subclinical neuropathy, e.g. KSS (Drachman 1968; Berenberg et al. 1977). F wave latencies may be increased. Sensory conduction is usually normal, but the SNAPs may be absent or of low amplitude (Yiannakis et al. 1986; Mizusawa et al. 1991).

Muscle Biopsy

The morphological hallmark is the ragged-red fibre (see above).

Nerve Biopsy

There is axonal degeneration, e.g. in KSS, in those mitochondrial disorders characterised by neuropathy. In sural nerve biopsies Schröder (1993) reported axonal degeneration with some evidence of regeneration, and secondary segmental demyelination, in KSS. Schröder (1993) also reported prominent mitochondrial abnormalities in Schwann cells in MELAS, with less prominent axonal pathology. Curiously, abnormal mitochondria were more prominent in Schwann cells myelinating thin axons. Abnormal Schwann cell mitochondria were also a feature in sural nerves of patients with KSS.

Encephalomyopathies

Two major syndromes, MELAS and MERFF (Table 17.7), are recognised (Shapira et al. 1977). KSS also sometimes shows encephalopathic features (see above). There is considerable overlap in the clinical features (Table 17.9).

Table 17.9. Features of mitochondrial myopathies

	KSS	MERRF	MELAS
PEO	+		
Retinal degeneration	+		
Heart block	+		
CSF protein >1 g/l	+		
Myoclonus		+	
Ataxia	+	+	
Weakness	+	+	+
Episodic vomiting			+
Cerebral blindness			+
Focal signs			+
Seizures	+	+	
Dementia	+	+	+
Short stature	+	+	+
Deafness	+	+	+
Lactic acidosis	+	+'+	
Family history	+	+	
Ragged-red fibres	+	+	+
Spongy degeneration	+	+	+
mtDNA deletion	+		
mtDNA point mutation	+	+	

The boxed areas represent the core features.
From Di Mauro (1993).

MERRF

Myoclonic epilepsy with ragged-red fibres (MERRF) is characterised by myoclonus, seizures, cerebellar ataxia and ragged-red fibres in the muscle biopsy (Tsairis et al. 1973; Fukuhara et al. 1980). The age of onset varies from childhood to adult life and the disorder may progress slowly or rapidly, even in the same family. Associated features include those of mitochondrial disorders, including deafness, limb weakness, dementia, headache, optic atrophy and peripheral neuropathy. Cardiomyopathy and mental retardation have also been reported (see Hammans and Morgan–Hughes 1994). Electrophysiological studies may reveal atypical spike and wave activity on the EEG (So et al. 1989a). Giant cortical sensory evoked potentials have been reported (Rosing et al. 1985). MERRF shows an exclusively maternal pattern of inheritance, and 70%–80% of cases have mutations in bp 8344 tRNA^{Lys} (Hammans et al. 1991; Zeviani et al. 1991b). Additional mutations have been described in some cases. The genetic defect was found in leucocyte mtDNA in six of six cases by Hammans et al. (1991). Abnormal mitochondria have been identified in vascular smooth cells in MERRF (Coquet et al. 1993).

MELAS

Mitochondrial encephalopathy, lactic acidosis and stroke-like episodes (MELAS) was first described by Pavlakis et al. (1984). Myopathy is also a feature (Table 17.9). The encephalopathy may manifest as dementia with or without seizures. The stroke-like episodes usually develop before the age of 40 years, and are often not in a single vascular territory, suggesting a metabolic rather than vascular cause. The stroke-like episodes are usually followed by complete recovery. There may be lactic acidosis, and ragged-red fibres are usually present on muscle biopsy. Most patients are of short stature, and recurrent headaches, with vomiting, are a typical feature. In a third of cases there are cerebellar signs, and hearing loss and limb weakness in more than two-thirds. About 40% of cases have a family history of the disease (Hirano and Pavlakis 1994). Seizures may be an initial symptom, often associated with recurrent vomiting, headache and anorexia. Seizures may be focal or show secondary generalisation. All patients eventually show cognitive decline (Koo et al. 1993).

MELAS is associated with bp 3243 tRNA in some patients (Koo et al. 1993). The genetic abnormality was found in leucocyte mtDNA in 10 of 11 patients with MELAS (Hammans et al. 1991). Estimates of the frequency of this mutation range from 20% to 80% (Hammans et al. 1991; Hammans and Morgan–Hughes 1994). The mitochondria in cerebral blood vessels are abnormal (Ohama et al. 1987), but muscle capillaries are normal (Koo et al. 1993). Brain imaging shows infarct-like lesions in the occipital regions that often extend anteriorly, that do not conform to vascular territories, and that vary from time to time. Later, brain calcification may develop (Koo et al. 1993). It has been concluded that these strokes result from localised metabolic dysfunction, rather than brain ischaemia (Morita et al. 1989). The muscle biopsy shows ragged-red fibres in most patients. The prognosis is poor.

Other Syndromes

There are many additional mitochondrial disorders, as listed in Table 17.7). Most of these have little or no neuromuscular involvement.

In maternally inherited mitochondrial myopathy and cardiomyopathy affected family members present with exercise intolerance and exertional dyspnoea, and some die from congestive heart failure (Zevrani et al. 1991). Muscle biopsy in five affected and 10 asymptomatic individuals showed ragged-red fibres and/or COX-negative fibres, and a 3260 mutation in all but one of these family members (Zeviani et al. 1991a). Other syndromes, e.g. NARP (neurogenic muscle weakness, ataxia and retinitis pigmentosa (Holt et al 1990)), are uncommon, and ragged-red fibres are not found in this disorder.

Genetic Counselling in Mitochondrial Myopathies

In mitochondrial disorders genetic counselling is imperfect. It is important to ascertain the diagnosis and the nature of the underlying defect, to consider the prognosis, and to try to determine the risk of occurrence in other family members. Knowledge of the presence of mtDNA deletions and mutations is relevant in considering these questions. The difficulties in calculating recurrence risks in mitochondrial disease are summarised in Table 17.10.

Table 17.10. Difficulties in calculating the risk of recurrence in mitochondrial myopathies

Mitochondrial disease is sporadic, maternally inherited or follows Mendelian autosomal inheritance

Pedigree data is insufficiently complete in literature

Phenotype/genotype correlations are inexact

Mutations or deletions of mtDNA occur only in <60% of cases

Mitochondrial disorders have age-dependent penetrance

Phenotype and severity varies in individual families

Degree of heteroplasmy in tissues does not predict clinical severity

After Hammans and Morgan-Hughes (1994).

There are several principles that should be remembered in considering risks to individuals:

1. Males, whether or not affected, do not transmit mitochondrial disease, and cannot be genetic carriers
2. Both sexes are affected by mitochondrial diseases. In some conditions, e.g. Leber's optic neuropathy, males are affected more than females
3. Females may be symptomless carriers. All daughters of an affected or carrier female may transmit or develop the disorder. All sons are at risk of being affected
4. The proportion of offspring affected in variable.

Genetic testing has led to the following conclusions:

1. Analysis of muscle mtDNA is preferable to blood, because even large deletions may not be detected by Southern blot analysis of leucocytes, and point mutations are generally found in higher proportion in muscle than in blood (Hammans and Morgan-Hughes 1994). Lack of phenotype/genotype correlation means that screening for all recognised mutations and deletions is required.

2. Single mtDNA deletions are usually sporadic (Degoul et al. 1991; Hammans and Morgan-Hughes 1994).

3. Multiple mtDNA deletions are uncommon, but should not be overlooked.

4. Point mutations of mtDNA are not necessarily associated with consistent phenotypes (see above). The bp 8344 tRNA Lys mutation is generally associated with the MERRF phenotype, with variable additional features, and can be detected in blood or muscle (Hammans et al. 1991). The risk of development of the MERRF phenotype in people with this mutation ranges between 50% and 85%, but can occur at any age. The risk of transmission by heteroplasmic females is undefined, and probably variable. The risks for people with the bp 3243 tRNA mutation, which has a wide clinical spectrum, are similar.

5. Patients with mitochondrial myopathies without known mtDNA mutations probably represent hitherto undescribed mtDNA mutations. The recurrence risk for offspring of such women is about 10%–20% (Hammans and Morgan-Hughes 1994). For affected males it is less than 2%, reflecting the possibility of nuclear genome-dependent mitochondrial disorders.

6. Prenatal testing is difficult unless there is a recognised correlation in the family between heteroplasmy and the phenotype. Advice to women of child-bearing age must include recognition of the likely development of progressive disability and

possible dependence as well as the risk to any off-spring of development of the clinical syndrome.

Periodic Paralysis

Periodic paralysis consists of a group of disorders characterised by a common feature, the occurrence of episodes of acute and reversible weakness of the limbs (Westphal 1885). Weakness varies in severity and distribution, but often affects limited groups of muscles and may be asymmetrical. The weakness usually persists for several hours but may last for days. The legs are usually affected first, and the arms and cranial musculature are involved later. Weakness is always more severe proximally than distally and muscles of mastication, swallowing and respiration are usually relatively spared. Even in severe attacks movement of the fingers is usually possible. External ocular muscles are spared. Death in an attack is extremely rare.

The tendon reflexes are diminished in weak muscles. These disorders are inherited as autosomal dominant traits. In addition to these primary, genetically-determined forms of periodic paralysis (Table 17.11), acquired, secondary periodic paralysis can occur (Table 17.12). The association with hypokalaemia was first recognised by Biemond and Daniels (1934), Aitken et al. (1937) and Herrington (1937).

Table 17.11. Classification of primary (genetic) periodic paralysis

Genetic		
Sodium channel disorders		
Hyperkalaemic periodic paralysis	AD	Ch 17q 13.1-13.3
Normokalaemic periodic paralysis	AD	–
Paramyotonia congenita	AD	Ch 17q 13.1-13.3
Dihydropyridine receptor (voltage-gated calcium channel) disorder		
Hypokalaemic periodic paralysis	AD	Ch 1q 31-32
Thyrotoxic periodic paralysis	?	–

AD, autosomal dominant.

Table 17.12. Acquired potassium-related muscle weakness syndromes

Potassium depletion
Diuretic drug therapy
Gastro-intestinal disease
Renal disease
Alcoholism
Adrenal insufficiency
Barium carbonate poisoning
Laxative abuse syndrome
Potassium retention
Renal failure

All the primary, inherited forms of periodic paralysis have been found to be due to mutations in the genes coding for membrane ion channel proteins (Table 17.11). In the sodium channel disorders myotonia is a feature (see Table 15.1 and discussion of myotonia in hyperkalaemic periodic paralysis in Chapter 15). This group of conditions is due to mutations at the 13.1–13.3 position on chromosome 17q, the different phenotypes resulting from different mutations in the muscle sodium channel gene at this locus (Tahmoush et al. 1994).

Hypokalaemic Periodic Paralysis

This is the commonest form of periodic paralysis. It is inherited as an autosomal dominant disorder, with complete penetrance but with reduced expression in women such that some affected women are asymptomatic, or may have only one lifetime experience of an episode of weakness. This accounts for previous descriptions of an increased prevalence of the disorder in men (Johnsen 1981). The attacks of weakness are associated with a fall in blood potassium levels.

The disease can be recognised at a very early age, especially in affected children of parents known to have the disease, and it may even be evident in the first few years of life. Most cases begin before the second decade. As affected patients become older the attacks lessen in severity and frequency but some fixed, myopathic proximal weakness may develop in the fourth decade sufficient to cause severe disability in some cases. The development of permanent weakness is independent of a history of attacks of periodic paralysis, and is common in older patients (Links et al. 1990).

An attack of weakness may become evident on waking, the patient being unable to move in severe attacks. Attacks are often provoked by a heavy carbohydrate meal, and cold or anxiety are other recognised precipitants. Rest after exercise induces an attack on some occasions, but attacks can sometimes be aborted by mild exercise ("working off" the attack). Other recognised precipitating factors include steroid therapy, e.g. ACTH and mineralo-corticoids, and alcoholism (Martin et al. 1971; Rubenstein and Weinapel 1977). During an attack the weak muscles may ache. The frequency of attacks of weakness varies from once in a lifetime to several per week. Attacks may last from 2 hours to a day or more. Cardiac arrhythmia may sometimes develop, but respiration is usually unimpaired even though accessory respiratory muscles may be weak, and coughing is impaired. Asymmetrical weakness, or weakness restricted to one limb, is frequent.

Usually muscles affected toward the end of an attack of weakness are the first to recover. During the hypokalaemic phase the R wave of the ECG is tall, and the T wave becomes diphasic or inverted, reflecting the hyperpolarisation of cardiac myocytes (Fontaine 1993). The PR interval may be increased and U waves appear.

The genetic locus for hypokalaemic periodic paralysis on chromosome 1 is near the gene encoding the skeletal muscle dihydropyridine receptor (Fontaine et al. 1994; Ptacek et al. 1994b). This receptor acts as a voltage gated, calcium-sensitive ion channel and is involved in excitation–contraction coupling in muscle. There is no current evidence for locus heterogeneity in the mutation.

Carriers may note fluctuations in muscle detection, and abnormalities in muscle propagation velocity have been noted in these, and asymptomatic carriers in an affected family (van der Hoeven et al. 1994). In spontaneous attacks of hypokalaemic periodic paralysis weakness is usually first noted at venous blood potassium levels of about 3.0 mmol/l and becomes marked at 2.5 mmol/l. Normal subjects do *not* become weak until their blood potassium falls to less than 2.5 mmol/l. The blood potassium remains low during the period of paralysis and rises with recovery, suggesting that the paralysis is due to an increase in the amount of potassium in the muscle fibres (Grob et al. 1957). During attacks there is also increased permeability of muscle fibre membranes to sodium so that the muscle fibre surface membrane is unable to propagate an action potential and the sarcoplasmic reticulum also functions abnormally leading to a failure of excitation–contraction coupling (Engel and Lambert 1969).

At rest the serum potassium is normal, but in an attack the serum potassium level is low. Weakness and a fall in serum potassium may be induced by a glucose load, given as 100 g glucose orally, or by an insulin provocation test in which 100 g glucose given orally is combined with 20 IU soluble insulin given subcutaneously. The glucose/insulin test may also be performed by giving the glucose and the insulin intravenously. Since weakness induced by this test may occasionally be severe it is wise to begin with glucose alone, since this is a less potent stimulus, and glucose and insulin together may produce life-threatening cardiac arrhythmia if the blood potassium falls to very low levels (Rowland and Layzer 1975). It is important to avoid intravenous glucose infusions in patients known to suffer from the condition. Anaesthesia itself may also provoke attacks of weakness, perhaps due to the stress of anaesthesia rather than from a drug effect. Carbohydrates, alcohol, stress, cold and glucocorticoid steroid hormones may also induce an attack, and even a large carbohydrate meal may be enough to produce a diagnostic attack of weakness.

Electrophysiological Assessment

Between attacks motor and sensory nerve conduction studies are normal. During attacks the CMAP is reduced, progressively, as paralysis develops, but sensory conduction and SNAPs remain normal (Campa and Sanders 1974). As the muscle fibres become electrically inexcitable with a falling blood potassium level, propagation of the action potential is slowed and twitch tension decreases (Engel and Lambert 1969; Gordon et al. 1970). Van der Hoeven et al. (1994) studied a large Dutch pedigree using a muscle electrode technique to measure muscle fibre conduction (propagation) velocity and found abnormalities both in affected patients and in carriers; most of the latter had complained of fluctuations in muscle strength. Fibrillation potentials have been recorded in the early part of an attack (Shy et al. 1961). In the development of an attack of weakness the first abnormality is an increased proportion of short-duration, low-amplitude polyphasic potentials, followed by a reduction in the number of voluntarily activated motor units and, eventually, virtual absence of MUPs (Campa and Sanders 1974). During recovery the CMAP gradually returns to normal amplitude (Warner et al. 1993). Because the propagated conduction velocity in muscle fibres is slowed (Zwarts et al. 1988) when there is hypokalaemia, the distal motor latency is increased (Warner et al. 1993).

EMG tests can be used to assess the patient after provocative exercise. After 5 minutes of maximal voluntary contraction the CMAP and muscle twitch tension are reduced to as much as 50% of normal, an abnormality that may persist for 30 to 40 minutes (Engel et al. 1965; McMannis et al. 1986). During an attack repetitive nerve stimulation at 25 Hz shows a 50% increase on the CMAP amplitude at the fourth potential, indicating that muscle exercise during an attack may improve muscle fibre membrane conductance (Campa and Sanders 1974).

Myotonia is generally thought not to be a manifestation of hypokalaemic periodic paralysis, although lid lag has been described (Resnik and Engel 1967).

Muscle Biopsy

Biopsies taken between attacks of weakness usually show little or no abnormality unless there is some degree of fixed weakness. In patients with fixed weakness (Links et al. 1990) there are often large vacuoles in some or many muscle fibres (Fig. 17.11).

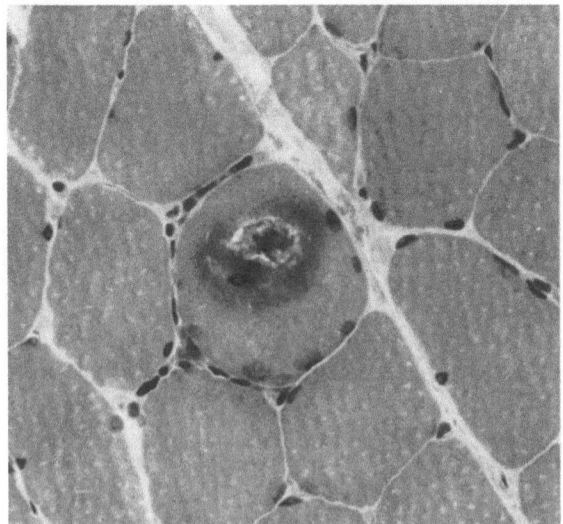

Fig. 17.11. Familial hypokalaemic periodic paralysis. TS. Gomori. × 350. One fibre is swollen and rounded. It contains a central granulovacuolar zone.

These vacuoles are situated in the central part of muscle fibres. In haematoxylin and eosin stains the vacuoles appear empty but they usually contain traces of PAS-positive material. Electron microscopy (Fig. 17.12) reveals that the vacuoles are membrane bound and continuous with the sarcoplasmic reticulum and T tube system (Howes et al. 1966; Engel 1970b). Other non-specific tubular abnormalities have also been described (Bradley 1969). Tubular aggregates have been seen in Type 2 fibres both between attacks and, less prominently, during the attacks (Brooke 1977). These represent abnormalities in the sarcoplasmic tubular system. In severe attacks some fibres become necrotic, and the typical sequence of necrosis, ingestion by macrophages and basophilic regeneration, usually subsarcolemmal, then occurs. In biopsies of patients with longstanding periodic paralysis Weller and McArdle (1971) demonstrated calcium salts (hydroxy-apatite) in the vacuoles and in the muscle fibres themselves. The vacuoles themselves are usually more prominent in older patients. The fixed myopathy found in

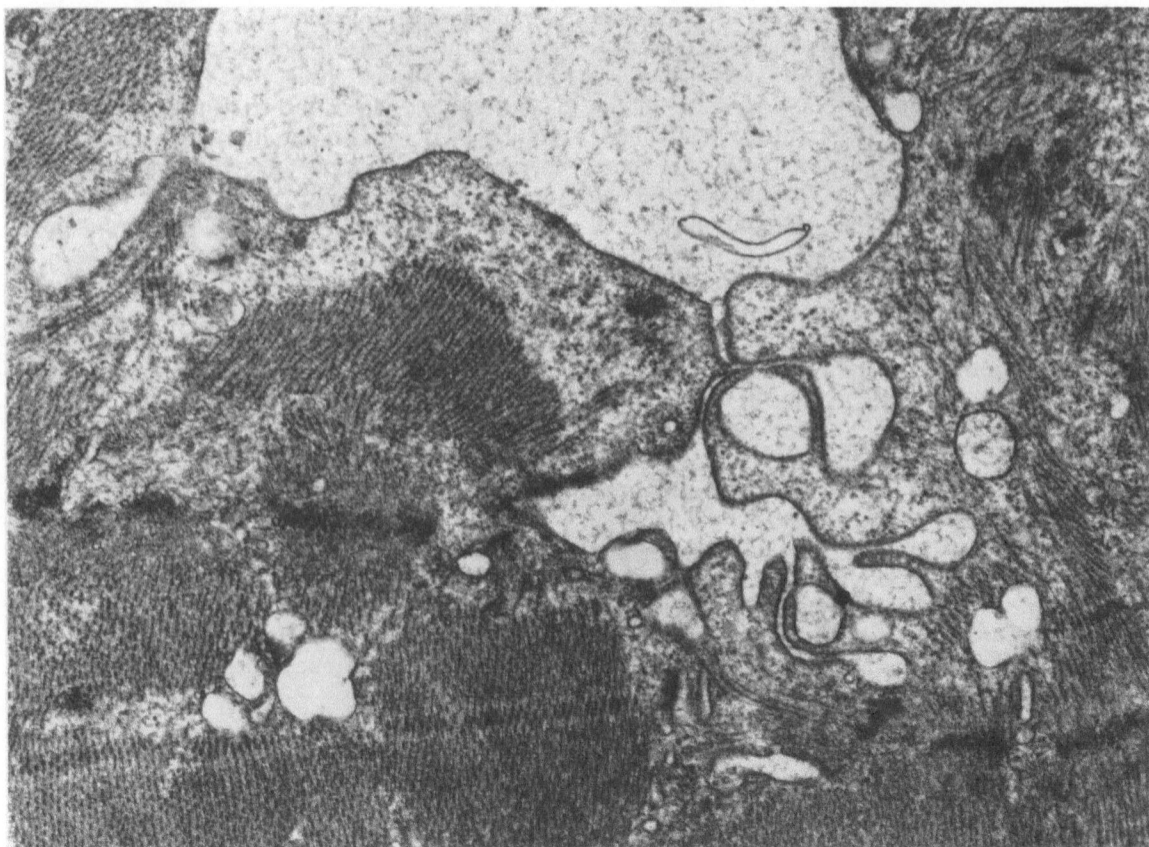

Fig. 17.12. Familial hypokalaemic periodic paralysis. TS. EM. × 9000. The fibre is disrupted by vacuoles limited by a single layer of membrane. They contain an amorphous material, thought to consist of mucopolysaccharide since it is PAS-positive, and are continuous with tubules of the sarcoplasmic reticulum. In addition there are several small cores of myofibrillar damage.

some patients with hypokalaemic periodic paralysis is also associated with the typical non-specific features of a myopathy, including variability in fibre size, central nucleation, single-fibre necrosis and regeneration and increased endomysial fibrous tissue. However, even in these cases there may be vacuolation of fibres and this is then an important clue to the diagnosis.

During attacks of weakness vacuoles may or may not be present.

Biochemical Features

Apart from hypokalaemia, no specific features are found. The CK is usually normal between attacks, but may rise in severe attacks and in the late, myopathic phase of the disease. Rhabdomyolysis and myoglobinuria do not occur.

Hyperkalaemic Periodic Paralysis and Paramyotonia Congenita

Hyperkalaemic periodic paralysis, called adynamia episodica hereditaria by Gamstorp (1956), affects men and women equally, and begins in early childhood. The disorder is characterised by reversible attacks of muscle weakness, as in hypokalaemic periodic paralysis, lasting from a few minutes to several hours, usually reaching their most severe at 30–40 minutes and resolving in 1–3 hours (McArdle 1974). The weakness may be focal and often involves a limb that has been used actively. These episodes usually occur during the day, at an interval after heavy exercise, but may commence during sleep. Attacks can sometimes be delayed or aborted by continued mild exercise but this, if unsuccessful, may lead to a more severe attack (Layzer et al. 1967a). Attacks may also develop after exposure to cold, with excitement, after alcohol or ingestion of potassium salts (Bradley 1969). In contrast to weakness with hypokalaemic periodic paralysis carbohydrates have a prophylactic effect, and meals only induce attacks if they contain a substantial potassium load. As in hypokalaemic periodic paralysis, permanent muscle weakness may develop in the fourth decade (Bradley et al. 1990).

Three clinical variants of hyperkalaemic periodic paralysis have been recognised, each type from within affected individual families. These are with myotonia, with paramyotonia and without myotonia. Permament weakness is mostly found in family members in which the paralytic element of the disorder, rather than the myotonia, predominates. Myotonia is usually most evident in the eyelids, rarely in limb muscles, but can be demonstrated relatively easily electrophysiologically. This myotonia can be induced by cold (Van der Meulen et al. 1961) but, unlike other forms of myotonia, is not relieved by exercise; indeed, it may be worsened by exercise (Eulenberg's paradoxical myotonia).

In hyperkalaemic periodic paralysis with myotonia, weakness is due to depolarisation block of the muscle membrane. In the form without myotonia it is due to inexcitability of the muscle membrane (Ricker et al. 1989a). The relationship between these various forms of hyperkalaemic periodic paralysis, myotonia and paramyotonia is discussed in Chapter 15.

Laboratory Assessment

In spontaneous attacks of hyperkalaemic periodic paralysis moderate weakness occurs with venous serum potassium levels of 5.0 mmol/l and severe paralysis with levels of 7.0 mmol/l which leave normal subjects unaffected (McArdle 1974). During these attacks potassium is leaking from the muscles into the circulation. Abnormal calcium metabolism in the sarcoplasmic reticulum may also be involved in the genesis of the paralysis and myotonia (McArdle 1974).

In *hyperkalaemic* periodic paralysis an oral potassium load (12 g potassium chloride) may precipitate an attack of weakness associated with hyperkalaemia (Griggs 1977). It is important to recognise that the serum venous potassium may fall with insulin and glucose, or rise with potassium loading in normal subjects, and it is the combination of the demonstration of an association between a change in the serum potassium and an increase in weakness that is important in establishing the diagnosis.

The ECG is normal between attacks but may show features of hypokalaemia (prominent U waves, flattened T waves, prolongation of the PR interval, and bradycardia) or of hyperkalaemia (tall, slender T waves, tachyarrhythmia). Lisak et al. (1972) described symptomatic cardiac arrhythmias leading to syncope in a case of hyperkalaemic periodic paralysis, and death may occur if the potassium level is very high.

The CK is normal between attacks, but may be raised in attacks of weakness and also in the later stages of the disease, if permanent weakness develops.

DNA Analysis

Hyperkalaemic periodic paralysis, in its various forms, paramyotonia congenita, and myotonia fluctuans (Ricker et al. 1994) are usually due to mutations in a gene encoding the muscle sodium channel (see Chapter 15). Ptacek et al. (1994a) have described several mutations in humans, and in horses, causing this syndrome, all involving the sodium channel gene (Rudolph et al. 1992). Since genotype/phenotype correlations can be established relatively accurately (Feer et al. 1993; Ptacek et al. 1994a) DNA testing is the preferred diagnostic test (Nadkarni et al. 1994).

Electrophysiological Assessment

In all forms of hyperkalaemic periodic paralysis sensory nerve conduction studies are normal. In addition, repetitive nerve stimulation at slow rates is normal. In hyperkalaemic periodic paralysis, without myotonia or paramyotonia, EMG between attacks is normal. During attacks the MUPs decrease in amplitude and duration, and eventually disappear when the muscle becomes inexcitable, and paralysed (Bradley et al. 1990).

In the form of the disease associated with myotonia, fibrillation potentials, positive sharp waves and myotonic discharges are recorded between attacks (van der Meulen et al. 1961; Layzer et al. 1967a). During attacks abnormalities in MUPs develop as in the pure form of the disease. Ischaemia, induced by a tourniquet, may induce Trousseau's sign and Chvostek's sign, indicating neural hyperexcitability (Segura and Petajan 1979). Lundberg et al. (1974) found that rapid rates of nerve stimulation delivered to a test muscle produced a decremental response, when there was associated myotonia, more marked at fastest rates, and suggested this could be used to differentiate the hypokalaemic and hyperkalaemic form of periodic paralysis. The resting membrane potential of muscle fibres in hyperkalaemic periodic paralysis, recorded with microelectrodes, is lowered during attacks of weakness, and the muscle fibres are inexcitable to electrical stimulation at this time (Creutzfeldt et al. 1963; Brooks 1969), representing depolarisation block of muscle fibres.

Muscle Biopsy

In hyperkalaemic periodic paralysis the muscle biopsy usually shows little abnormality. Tubular aggregates are noted, especially in the later stage of the disease, in Type 2 fibres. Vacuolation may be evident only at electron microscopy, which shows some dilatation of T tubules (Pearson 1964; Bradley 1969).

Normokalaemic Periodic Paralysis

This disorder was described by Poskanzer and Kerr (1961) and Meyers et al. (1972). Poskanzer and Kerr

(1961) described 21 members of one family who had periodic paralysis without changes in the serum potassium. Attacks were precipitated by exercise and by ingestion of potassium salts. Some of these cases have subsequently been shown to have hyperkalaemic periodic paralysis (Brooke 1977). DNA studies on these patients are not available, but this disorder may not be a distinct entity. However, Bradley (1969) noted that two of his cases seemed to be normokalaemic.

Management of Periodic Paralysis Syndromes

Although weakness may be severe in acute episodes death is uncommon (Johnsen 1981), probably because respiratory and bulbar muscles are usually spared. Sometimes an acute attack of weakness may be so severe as to necessitate treatment. In acute hypokalaemic paralysis oral potassium, 20–100 mmol, is the safest form of treatment; intravenous potassium is also effective and may be necessary to produce improvement. Doses of 20 mmol/h are usually effective, but some patients require up to twice this dose (Pullen et al. 1967). Prophylactic oral potassium supplements at bedtime were the mainstay of management. Acetazolamide 250–750 mg daily (Griggs et al. 1970) or the longer-acting carbonic anhydrase inhibitor, dichlorphenamide, (McArdle 1962, 1974) 50 mg daily are now used. In two reports (Dalakas and Engel 1983; Thompson and Hutchinson 1984) improvement in a fixed, progressive proximal myopathy occurred during a year-long regime of acetazolamide, and no further acute attacks of hypokalaemic paralysis developed. Carbonic anhydrase inhibitors decrease the movement of potassium across cell membranes and produce a metabolic acidosis, but carry the risk of the development of renal calculi (Howlett 1975). Although acetazolamide and dichlorphenamide have both been used effectively, chlorothiazide seems equally effective and is probably less hazardous (Layzer et al. 1967b).

Patients should be advised to avoid sudden glucose or carbohydrate loads in their diet and should be encouraged to exercise mildly every day and to avoid sudden strenuous exercise. Salt restriction and a low-carbohydrate diet are also important in prevention of attacks of weakness. Meals should be small and taken late in the day. The possibility that direct action of insulin on muscle fibre receptors may be important in the causation of attacks of weakness, especially in view of the effect of insulin on potassium metabolism in the cell, led to attempts to block pancreatic insulin release with diazoxide. Although this treatment seemed effective (Johnson et al. 1981) in clinical trials, this drug is too hazardous for practical application in the periodic paralyses.

Acute episodes of hyperkalaemic paralysis can be treated with high-carbohydrate food or fluids. In severe cases, when vomiting may be a problem, intravenous glucose, sodium chloride, bicarbonate and insulin may all be effective (Griggs 1977) and intravenous calcium gluconate may also be useful. However, most attacks are of brief duration and treatment is usually not necessary. In severe attacks salbutamol, given by inhalation, may be effective (Wang and Clausen 1976). Acetazolamide is useful both in preventing attacks and in lessening the severity of attacks (McArdle 1962). Cardiac arrhythmias, which may be lethal, may occur in severe attacks when the potassium level is very high (Lisak et al. 1972).

Thyrotoxic Periodic Paralysis

This unusual disorder is particularly common among Oriental men (MacFadzean and Yeung 1967; Cheah et al. 1975), but rare cases have been reported in other races (Layzer and Goldfield 1974). In Japan and China about 2% of patients with hyperthyroidism develop periodic paralysis. There is a male preponderance of nearly 20 to 1 (Ferreiro et al. 1986). The clinical features of the periodic weakness closely resemble those of primary hypokalaemic periodic paralysis, including sparing of ocular and respiratory muscles. The blood potassium level is usually decreased, but may be normal, during attacks. In the intervals between attacks the potassium level is normal. The pathology of this form of periodic paralysis resembles that of hypokalaemic periodic paralysis (Fig. 17.10), but tubular aggregates may be more prominent. Treatment with potassium supplements is beneficial in the attacks, and propranolol is effective in preventing attacks (Conway et al. 1974). Acetazolamide, however, in contradistinction to primary hypokalaemic periodic paralysis, may precipitate attacks of weakness. The definitive treatment consists in the establishment of the euthyroid state. Attacks of weakness then cease, except in rare instances (Ferreiro et al. 1986). Jackson and Barohn (1992) used the exercise test described by McMannis et al. (1986) to monitor the effect of treatment of hyperthyroidism in a case of thyrotoxic periodic paralysis.

Thyrotoxicosis enhances sodium conductance and the activity of the sodium/potassium pump, even in normal subjects, indicating an effect on sodium channels in muscle.

Other Forms of Hypokalaemic Myopathy

Weakness, with similar vacuoles in muscle fibres, may occur with profound hypokalaemia (Table 17.12) due to excessive diuretic therapy (Lawson et al. 1979), renal disease or liquorice ingestion, and also in some patients with severe acute alcoholism. Barium carbonate poisoning of the water supply produced an epidemic form of hypokalaemic paralysis in China in 1943 (Pa Ping disease) and cases have been reported in other countries (Ku et al. 1943). Barium competes for potassium conductance channels in muscle fibres (Layzer 1982). In these instances the precipitating cause is usually obvious and there is no family history. The myopathy resolves when potassium replacement is begun. Hyperkalaemia (Table 17.12) is less likely to cause muscle weakness.

Malignant Hyperpyrexia Syndrome

Malignant hyperpyrexia is a rare disorder in which rapid-onset and often fatal hyperpyrexia occurs unexpectedly during anaesthesia (Denborough and Lovell 1960). Shortly after the induction of anaesthesia there is a rapid and uncontrollable rise in body temperature, associated with rigid contraction of all skeletal muscles, cyanosis, acidosis and tachycardia (Ellis and Halsall 1980). The hyperthermia and myoglobinuria may also be precipitated by severe physical stress, resembling heat-stroke (Denborough 1982). The major feature of the syndrome is the rapid rise in body temperature, which may reach 44 °C or more. The mortality rate corresponds to the level of the pyrexia. Temperatures of 39 °C or less are associated with 100% survival, but death is inevitable if the temperature reaches 44 °C. Although pyrexia may begin within minutes of induction of anaesthesia it may be delayed for as long as 4 hours, or even occur in the recovery room after anaesthesia has ended. Hyperpyrexia is thought to develop only during anaesthetics more than 10 min in duration, but it may not occur on one occasion but then develop in another. The condition is life-threatening because of the profound metabolic disturbance that occurs, with hyperpyrexia, rhabdomyolysis, hyperkalaemia and metabolic acidosis, factors that lead to multiorgan failure.

The first sign of the development of the syndrome is tachycardia and tachypnoea; rigidity follows and later hypotension, bradycardia and cardiac arrhythmia develop as fever becomes severe. The blood calcium falls as rigidity becomes prominent, and hyperkalaemia and myoglobinuria may develop. The blood CK rises as high as 50 000 IU/ml (Isaacs and Barlow 1974).

The syndrome is particularly likely to occur in susceptible individuals when succinylcholine or volatile anaesthetics, such as halothane, enflurane and isoflurane (Ellis and Heffron 1985) are used (Denborough and Lovell 1960), particularly when both are used (Nelson and Flewellen 1983). Other anaesthetic agents have been suspected, but not confirmed as causative (Harriman et al. 1973). The muscle rigidity may commence with succinylcholine administration. Nitrous oxide anaesthesia is thought to be safe and narcotics, barbiturates, diazepam, droperidol and ester-class local anaesthetics are also safe. Pancuronium, a non-depolarising muscle relaxant, is also safe (Nelson and Flewellen 1983).

Susceptibility is inherited (Denborough and Lovell 1960) as a dominant trait. The overall incidence is about 1:50 000 anaesthetics (Ellis et al. 1972). In children an incidence of 1:15 000 anaesthetics has been noted (Schwartz et al. 1984). Only 34 cases were recorded in the UK between 1967 and 1976 (Ellis and Halsall 1980). Denborough et al. (1982) noted that 30% of children dying of sudden infant death syndrome had a parent with positive susceptibility tests for malignant hyperpyrexia syndrome.

Some of the patients who have developed the syndrome have been noted to show mild myopathic features on examination after recovery, such as thigh hypertrophy, lumbar lordosis and mild weakness of proximal muscles in the legs. However, there is no clinical or pathological evidence to support the existence of a specific "hyperthermia myopathy" (Figorella–Branger et al. 1993). Patients who recover from an episode of hyperpyrexia may show massive myoglobinuria with a high CK, and develop renal failure, although recovery may eventually be complete.

Denborough et al. (1973) and Isaacs and Barlow (1974) noted an association of malignant hyperthermia with central core disease. This clinical observation has been confirmed by the discovery that both these disorders are linked to the same genetic locus on chromosome 19q 13.1. The gene product of this locus is the ryanodine receptor (McCarthy et al. 1990; MacLennan et al. 1990; Quane et al. 1993). The ryanodine receptor is the major receptor in a calcium release pathway concerned with initiation of contraction. A defect in this pathway could therefore result in uncoupling of excitation from contraction in the pathway from depolarisation of the sarcolemma to calcium release from the terminal cisternal membrane of the sarcoplasmic reticulum

(Nelson and Butler 1992). A second locus on chromosome 17q 11.2–24 has been reported (Denfel 1992).

It is of interest that a similar disorder has been reported in Landrace and Pietrain pigs (Hall et al. 1972; Anderson and Jones 1976), and in these animals histological studies show an appearance suggestive of a myopathy (Gallant et al. 1986). In the pig, stress hyperpyrexia is an autosomal recessive disorder in which there is a single amino acid substitution in the ryanodine receptor gene (Fujii et al. 1991). This mutation is rare in humans (Gillard et al. 1991).

Screening for Susceptibility

Malignant hyperpyrexia is suspected in a family when an episode of malignant hyperpyrexia occurs in a patient. Unfortunately, the episode may have been fatal. There has, therefore, been a need for the development of a reliable screening test to ascertain susceptibility or non-susceptibility in relatives. Ascertainment requires a test other than anaesthesia. In the pig disorder, malignant hyperthermia can be triggered by stress or by increased temperature but, in humans, anaesthesia is the only recognised triggering factor. However, abnormalities unrelated to malignant hyperthermia have been reported, including unexplained sudden death (Raukler et al. 1985) and acute rhabdomyolysis (Haverkort-Poels et al. 1987).

The disorder has been associated with central core disease, and associations have also been reported with King–Denborough syndrome, a combination of dysmorphic skeletal and facial abnormalities and a non-progressive myopathy (McPherson and Taylor 1981), and X-linked muscular dystrophy (Heimann-Patterson et al. 1986). The CK is raised in some patients susceptible to malignant hyperthermia, but 20% of patients surviving an episode have a normal CK afterwards (Rowland 1984). In some families the CK is normal in all probands (Moulds and Denborough 1974b), and Paasuke and Brownell (1986) found that CK levels could be used neither to exclude nor confirm susceptibility, and suggested that CK levels had no place in the determination of susceptibility. Amaranath et al. (1983) screened 1800 patients by CK measurement prior to anaesthesia and found one patient with a raised CK and a history of malignant hyperthermia, one patient with a normal CK who developed hyperpyrexia under anaesthesia and 108 patients with raised CK levels whose anaesthetic proceeded uneventfully. CK levels in population studies tend to be higher in black males than white males and, to a lesser extent, in black females compared with white females

(Meltzer and Holy 1974). However, the finding of a raised CK should prompt consideration of the presence of an underlying myopathy.

The in vitro provocation test has become the standard test for susceptibility. This consists of measuring the isometric tension in a strip of muscle excised at biopsy and placed in a bath of oxygenated modified Ringer's solution at body temperature (see Ellis et al. 1972; Britt et al. 1982). Changes in tension occurring in response to a variety of anaesthetic agents can be measured, and contracture observed, if it occurs. It is particularly important to test halothane and succinylcholine, but caffeine and other anaesthetic agents may also be tested (Ellis et al. 1972; Moulds and Denborough 1974b). The test is carried out according to slightly different protocols in Europe and North America. The normal response to halothane is less than 0.2 g contraction force with 2% halothane and for caffeine is less than 0.2 g contracture at 2 mmol/1 caffeine (European MH Group 1984). The North American data are described by Larach (1989). Halothane-induced contraction can be reversed in this in vitro system by the addition of procaine to the bath (Moulds and Denborough 1974b). This test has proved reliable as a screen for susceptibility when positive but it is, inevitably, uncertain whether a negative test entirely excludes susceptibility to this potentially lethal syndrome. False negative results are found in less than 2% of cases (Isaacs and Badenharst 1993) and false positives probably also occur. A test using both caffeine and halothane in the perfusate may be more sensitive (Nelson et al. 1983). A ryanodine contracture test has also been developed (Hopkins et al. 1991).

Molecular genetic testing for susceptibility is not appropriate, since even in the same family the genetic mutation may be heterogeneous and several families have been reported in North America and Europe in which the ryanodine receptor mutation was excluded (Levitt et al. 1991), accounting for lack of concordance between genetic testing and muscle contraction tests (Mackenzie et al. 1991). The presence of a second locus for susceptibility on chromosome 17q (Denfel 1992) is further evidence for genetic heterogeneity. It is possible that 38P MR spectroscopy, to assess energy metabolism in muscle during contraction, and in response to inhaled anaesthetics, in non-invasive studies, may be developed to replace these tests for susceptibility (Reiss et al. 1991).

Pathophysiology of the Rise in Temperature

Despite investigation, using the in vitro provocation test, the cause of the rapid rise in temperature after exposure to anaesthetic drugs is not yet fully understood. Heat is produced in muscle during an attack and this is invariably accompanied by rigid muscular contraction, although lesser degrees of rigidity may be present in some cases (Isaacs and Barlow 1974). The rapid heat production so characteristic of the syndrome (1 °C increase/5 min) suggests that uncoupling of excitation–contraction coupling is initiated by the anaesthetic agents. This could be due to decreased reuptake of calcium ions by sarcoplasmic reticulum, increased uptake of calcium ions by sarcoplasm itself (muscle cells), from the extracellular fluid or, perhaps, release of calcium ions from calcium-dependent muscle cell mebranes into the sarcoplasm. Moulds and Denborough (1974b) suggested that the latter mechanism was the most likely, the rapid rise in temperature occurring from muscle contraction induced by calcium ions released from sarcoplasmic reticulum itself. Severe metabolic acidosis develops during the attack, with increased oxygen consumption (Nelson and Flewellen 1983). Calcium release in muscle cells, presumably because of abnormality in the ryanodine receptor, leads to activation of phosphorylase b and of myosin ATPase, with accelerated glycolysis, muscle contraction, uncoupled phosphorylase and excessive heat production.

Associated Disorders

Malignant hyperpyrexia has been associated with a number of different disorders. A definite association with central core disease was recorded by Denborough et al. (1973) and confirmed subsequently (Ohtani et al. 1985). However, although frequent this association is not universal, possibly because there is genetic heterogeneity between these two disorders (Romero et al. 1993). Other disorders are listed in Table 17.13.

Table 17.13. Disorders that have been associated with malignant hyperthermia

Definite
Central core disease
King–Denborough syndrome

Possible
Mitochondrial disorders
Duchenne & Becker muscular dystrophy
Myotonic dystrophy
Schwartz–Jampel syndrome

In those disorders in which the association is indefinite, care should be exercised during anaesthesia, but specific testing for susceptibility is probably unnecessary (Brownell 1988).

Electrophysiological Assessment

Mild myopathic features may occur after an attack. Unless there is an underlying or co-existent disorder the EMG is usually normal.

Muscle Biopsy

The muscle usually shows minor abnormalities in susceptible subjects studied in health. There may be slightly increased variability in fibre size, increased central nucleation, increased numbers of sarcolemmal nuclei and some fibre splitting. Further, moth-eaten fibres may be observed (Harriman et al. 1973). Figarella-Branger et al. (1993) studied 120 patients with malignant hyperpyrexia. No specific abnormality or "malignant hyperpyrexia phenotype" (Harriman et al. 1973) was observed. Ten of the 120 biopsies showed rhabdomyolysis. Other changes included those of specific disorders, e.g. central core disease found in five biopsies, mitochondrial myopathy in seven, myotonic dystrophy in one. In 71 biopsies the histology was normal.

Ultrastructural studies performed in biopsies taken in acute episodes in two fatal cases showed rupture of mitochondria, crystalline inclusions between the myofibrils, dilated sarcoplasmic reticulum and T tubules, and decreased glycogen content. However, another case studied 10 hours and again 4 months after the onset of hyperpyrexia showed scarcely any abnormality (Schiller and Mair 1974).

Management of Hyperpyrexia

In an attack of hyperthermia induced during anaesthesia it is important, as a life-saving measure, to lower the body temperature. The three major procedures are to stop the anaesthetic, cool the patient and give dantrolene to reverse the muscle contraction. Anaesthesia must be discontinued and 100% oxygen given. Cooling is begun by all possible means, including cold water bathing and increasing airflow over the exposed body. Gastric, peritoneal and rectal lavage have also been used. The metabolic acidosis must be reversed by bicarbonate infusions and hyperkalaemia may be so severe as to warrant treatment with glucose and insulin infusion. Calcium gluconate may be necessary to reverse the hypocalcaemia. The rigidity itself is difficult to reverse quickly.

Dantrolene is the treatment of choice because of its action on the sarcoplasmic reticulum (Harrison 1975). A dose of 2.5 mg/kg IV is usually effective, but larger doses may be necessary (Kolb et al. 1982). Steroids are usually given. Curare may be used to reverse the effect of succinylcholine, but it has no effect on halothane-induced hyperpyrexia (Harrison 1971). Procainamide may be useful (Kalow et al. 1970) and procaine infusion has also been used (Harrison 1971).

After recovery from an attack renal function and urinary output must be monitored because of the risk of renal failure, due to myoglobinuria or from other factors associated with hyperpyrexia or electrolyte imbalance. Intense muscular weakness and wasting may develop after recovery from a severe attack, indicating severe muscle necrosis, and prolonged physiotherapy and rehabilitation may then be necessary (Isaacs and Barlow 1974). A search for susceptibility among relatives is then indicated.

If anaesthesia becomes necessary in a susceptible subject halothane and succinylcholine must be avoided. Thiopentane sodium, nitrous oxide and d-tubocurarine are probably the safest agents (King and Denborough 1973); dantrolene may be given orally for 1–3 days before anaesthesia in a dose of 4–8 mg/kg/day as prophylaxis. The last dose should be given 2 hours before anaesthesia (Harrison 1975; Nelson and Flewellen 1983). The role of neuroleptic anaesthetic agents, such as ketamine, is uncertain. Local, regional or spinal anaesthetics are preferred to volatile anaesthetic agents when anaesthesia is necessary in persons known to be at risk.

Neuroleptic-Malignant Syndrome

In neuroleptic-malignant syndrome hyperthermia, hypertonicity of skeletal muscles resembling severe extrapyramidal rigidity, fluctuating consciousness and instability of the autonomic nervous system consisting of pallor, sweating, tachyarrhythmia and labile hypertension occur. Involuntary movements, dystonia and tremor may occur and seizures may be a feature (Guzé and Baxter 1985). These clinical features develop during a period of 1 to 3 days in patients taking phenothiazines, butyrophenones, tricyclic antidepressants, monoamine oxidase inhibitors, lithium, tetrabenazine and L-Dopa (Heyland and Souve 1991). It has especially been related to dopamine-depleting agents (Burke et al. 1981). It may develop after cessation of antiparkinsonian drugs. The onset of the syndrome is not related to the duration or dosage of neuroleptic therapy. It may persist for up to 2 weeks after stopping oral neuroleptic medication or even as long as a month after depot therapy. The syndrome develops in 0.5%–1% of all patients exposed to neuroleptic drugs, but especially in young men (Kellam 1987).

Muscular involvement is reflected in rhabdomyolysis with myoglobinuria and renal failure. The CK level is greatly raised (Caroff 1980). Physical exhaustion and dehydration may be precipitating factors.

The neuroleptic-malignant syndrome resembles the malignant hyperthermia syndrome in that heat production seems to originate in muscle, but differs in that there is a CNS abnormality, the disorder is of gradual onset and the muscle rigidity in patients with neuroleptic-malignant syndrome show a normal flaccid paralytic response to curare. This is not a recommended test, however, because of the risk of a hyperthermic response to this drug in patients susceptible to malignant hyperpyrexia.

Neuroleptic-malignant syndrome is not familial. The factors conferring susceptibility are not understood, but the brain is histopathologically normal, as are EEG, CT brain and CSF studies (Guzé and Baxter 1985).

Muscle Biopsy

Martin and Swash (1987) carried out muscle biopsy 1 hour after death in one patient and found glycogen depletion and scattered "ghost fibres" and muscle fibre necrosis. They suggested that the source of hyperthermia, therefore, was uncoupled oxidative phosphorylation in muscle, perhaps triggered by dopamine-based brain dysfunction. The nature of this link is uncertain.

Management

It is essential to discontinue neuroleptic medication as soon as the diagnosis is suspected. Dantrolene, amantadine and bromocriptine have been used successfully (Guzé and Baxter 1985). Symptomatic treatment may require management of hypertension and renal failure. Death may also occur from respiratory failure due to aspiration or tachypnoeic, but ineffective, hyperventilation, and mechanical ventilation may be necessary. Muscle relaxation can be achieved with muscle relaxants, such as pancuronium (Renwick et al. 1992).

The mortality ranges from 20%–30% (Guzé and Baxter 1985).

Myoglobinuria and Rhabdomyolysis

This syndrome consists of muscle pain, often with weakness, associated with dark-coloured urine and a markedly raised CK level. In severe cases there

Table 17.14. Causes of myoglobinuria

Metabolic
Myophosphorylase deficiency (Glycogenosis Type V: McArdle's syndrome)
Phosphofructokinase deficiency (Glycogenosis Type VII)
Hypokalaemic periodic paralysis
Carnitine palmitoyl transferase deficiency
Malignant hyperpyrexia myopathy
Other systemic disorders, e.g. diabetic acidosis

Toxic
Alcohol, carbon monoxide and barbiturate poisoning
Liquorice excess (hypokalaemia)
Heroin myopathy
Chloroquine, amphotericin B, and epsilon amino caproic acid-induced acute toxic myopathies
Exposure to industrial toxins (Haff's disease)
Various biological toxins, e.g. hornet stings, Malaysian sea-snake bites, etc.

Fever
Heat exhaustion and heat-stroke
Malignant hyperpyrexia
Neuroleptic-malignant syndrome

Exertion-related
Marathon running, long-distance skiing
Compartment syndromes
Status epilepticus
Electric shock injury

Trauma and ischaemia
Crush injuries
Volkman's ischaemic contracture
Anterior tibial syndrome
Major arterial occlusion

Acute polymyositis and *acute necrotising myopathy* associated with carcinoma

Infections
Viral infections, especially influenza A and B, coxsackie, infectious mononucleosis
Typhoid fever
Gram-negative infections
Toxic shock syndrome

Idiopathic rhabdomyolysis

may be renal failure. This syndrome has many causes (Table 17.14). Myoglobinuria is a feature of muscular disorders in which myoglobin, a protein with a molecular weight of 17 KDa, is present in the urine in sufficient amounts to give it a pink-red colour, turning to brown when exposed to light for several hours. Myoglobinuria occurs when there is relatively significant necrosis or injury to skeletal muscle. In normal muscle there is about 1–2 mg myoglobin/g muscle; since myoglobinuria is only detectable to the naked eye when present in a concentration of more than 1 mg/ml it is necessary for at least 15 g of muscle to undergo necrosis before myoglobinuria occurs (Knochel 1982; Layzer 1985b). Myoglobinuria thus implies rhabdomyolysis (Bowden et al. 1956).

Acute attacks of rhabdomyolysis with myoglobinuria are characterised by muscle pain, swelling and weakness. Myoglobinuria tends to persist for 3 to 5 days after the onset of the attack, and begins within 24 hours of the first muscular symptom. It is fairly common for rhabdomyolysis to be precipitated by unduly vigorous or prolonged muscular exertion, e.g. in military recruits. Muscle strength returns quite rapidly, but may require several days in severe attacks. In severe attacks renal tubular damage may develop, leading to renal failure or even anuria. This may be accompanied by hyperkalaemia, hyperphosphataemia and metabolic acidosis (Hed 1955), and may require dialysis. Renal failure usually recovers with appropriate management, but there may be permanent sequelae, especially after recurrent attacks. The CK is markedly raised concomitantly with the rhabdomyolysis, and remains elevated for several days after the myoglobinuria has resolved. Myoglobinuria does not occur without a raised blood CK level. Rarely, disseminated intravascular coagulation may complicate myoglobinuria and rhabdomyolysis (Rowland and Penn 1972).

Myoglobinuria has many causes (Table 17.14), and the muscle biopsy, while demonstrating muscle necrosis and regeneration, may reveal the specific features of the underlying metabolic disorder (Tonin et al. 1990). Nonetheless, in many cases, the aetiology remains uncertain. Focal areas of muscle damage or necrosis can be demonstrated by radioisotope scanning, or by CT scanning, and this may be helpful in differential diagnosis (Chaikin 1980; Vukanovic et al. 1980). This may be especially important when rhabdomyolysis follows crush injury, or Volkmann's ischaemic contracture, since recovery of function may depend on decompression of compartmental necrosis, in order to prevent permanent avascular necrosis and secondary damage to the innervation of affected muscles.

The term idiopathic rhabdomyolysis is used to embrace a group of patients, usually young men, with recurrent myoglobinuria developing after exercise, sometimes leading to permanent wasting and weakness after severe attacks, and with a familial background of similar illness in about 30% of cases (Type I disorder). In a second group exercise was not a factor, but intercurrent illness could lead to an attack; either sex was affected (Type II disorder). This classification has been superseded, but in a proportion of cases of acute rhabdomyolysis with myoglobinuria no cause can be found after investigation (Layzer 1985b). Tonin et al. (1990) reviewed 77 biopsies from patients with myoglobinuria. Sixty of these were men. Exercise was the main precipitating factor, both in patients with and those without an enzymopathy. Eight enzymes were studied and about half the patients had abnormalities. Carnitine palmitoyl transferase deficiency was found in 17,

myophosphorylase deficiency in 10, phosphorylase kinase deficiency in four, myoadenylate deaminase deficiency in three, phosphoglycerate mutase deficiency in one and combined CPT and MAD deficiency in one patient. In patients in this study with suspected but unproven myoglobinuria, enzyme deficiencies were found in a similar proportion. The high proportion of abnormalities in this study, however, probably reflects selection of patients referred to the muscle centre at Columbia University, New York.

Viral causes of rhabdomyolysis are probably relatively common. In most, influenza A infection has been incriminated (Josselson et al. 1980). In these patients the illness is self-limited and there is no evidence of preceding inflammatory myopathy or autoimmune disease. In adult cases the prognosis is good but in one series of affected children there was a 30% mortality (Savage et al. 1971). Two-thirds of survivors had multiple episodes of myoglobinuria, suggesting the possibility of an unrecognised metabolic disorder in these patients.

Myoglobinuria in crush injuries probably results from stretching of muscle, which increases membrane permeability to calcium ions leading to hypercontraction and protease activation. In traumatic muscle injury intramuscular pressure may exceed intra-arterial pressure within a few minutes, an effect exacerbated by hypotensive, hypovolaemic shock (Better and Stern 1990).

After strenuous exercise (Clarkson et al. 1987) the CK level rises to a maximum at 6 hours, although muscle soreness reaches a peak at about 24 hours.

Electrophysiological Assessment

Spontaneous fibrillations, without fasciculations, may be prominent in the early stages, and short-duration polyphasic units of low amplitude with a full interference pattern may be recorded during the recovery phase. The EMG may remain abnormal for several months after a severe attack (Haase and Engel 1960).

Muscle Biopsy

In the early stages there is massive necrosis of muscle fibres. In some biopsies every fibre may be necrotic. The necrosis is often subendomysial, the basal laminar scaffold being preserved, and sometimes normal fibres are seen scattered sparsely among the necrotic fibres. In some forms, e.g. drug-induced necrotising myopathies with myoglobinuria, multiphasic changes may be seen with some fibres showing necrosis and others undergoing regeneration, or in various stages of maturity. Individual fibres thus show a variety of changes ranging from hyaline necrosis, phagocytosis, subendomysial regenerating crescents with prominent basophilia and lipid droplets, fibres of varying size and marked basophilia, and fibres showing less variability in fibres size with excess central nucleation. The capillary network surrounding the muscle fibres is usually normal. Electron microscopic studies add little further information except that the typical mitochondrial abnormality of mitochondrial myopathy may be seen. Motor end-plates are usually normal. Biochemical studies are indicated.

Biopsies made after recovery should be utilised for biochemical studies of enzyme deficiency, especially of the enzymes discussed above (Tonin et al. 1990).

Management

Exposure to any causative agent, if known, should be removed, e.g. in drug-induced myoglobinuria. In other instances, as in hyperpyrexic myopathy, the causative factors can often be readily identified and avoided in future. Limitation of exercise should be advised in idiopathic paroxysmal myoglobinuria, and in metabolic myopathies. Many patients with metabolic causes have recurrent attacks of myoglobinuria and exercise is the most frequent inducing factor.

In acute attacks muscle pain can be relieved by splinting the limbs, and by simple analgesics such as aspirin. Renal failure is a serious complication usually heralded by oliguria, prominent myoglobinuria and hyperkalaemia. Renal failure is likely when myoglobinuria occurs at a concentration greater than 1 mg/1 urine. Dialysis may be necessary and recovery of renal function usually occurs in a few days or weeks. Life is rarely threatened by respiratory failure in this group of disorders. Recovery is usually complete. Fasciotomy is useful in very severe compartment syndromes in which the intramuscular pressure is raised.

Chapter 18 — Endocrine Myopathies

Chapter **18**

Myopathies are associated with a number of different endocrine disorders (Table 18.1). In these "endocrine myopathies" the onset of weakness is insidious, proximal muscles are predominantly affected and recovery generally occurs when the endocrine disorder is corrected. In addition to myopathies occurring with endocrine disease, myopathic weakness may also occur when certain hormones are used in treatment. For example, long-term steroid therapy often leads to a steroid-dependent proximal myopathy. In most instances the myopathy associated with endocrine disease is a minor part of the clinical disorder but sometimes, as in some patients with thyrotoxic myopathy, muscular symptoms may be a presenting feature of the endocrine disorder. Occasionally endocrine myopathies may show more complex clinical features as in thyrotoxic myopathy in which myasthenic weakness may sometimes occur.

Table 18.1. Endocrine myopathies

Thyroid myopathies
Hyperthyroidism
Hypothyroidism

Parathyroid disorders
Hyperparathyroidism
Hypoparathyroidism

Adrenal disorders and steroid myopathy
Cushing's syndrome (hyperadrenalism)
Steroid therapy
Addison's disease

Pituitary disorders
Acromegaly

Thyroid Myopathies

Thyroid hormone affects metabolism in complex and incompletely understood ways, modifying energy, lipid and protein metabolism and having effects on mitochondrial oxidation. Impaired thyroid hormone homeostasis, resulting in either reduced or increased thyroid activity, produces recognised clinical syndromes but these effects are relatively more evident in some tissues, e.g. skeletal and cardiac muscle, and adipose tissue, than in others. In addition, the clinical syndromes resulting from relatively reduced or excess thyroid hormone secretion differ in infants, adults and aged individuals. Muscle is commonly affected in both hyperthyroidism and hypothyroidism, but the relative severity of the muscular abnormality varies from patient to patient. In addition, hypokalaemic periodic paralysis may complicate hyperthyroidism, especially in Oriental people, and myasthenia gravis may be associated with the disease, as part of the autoimmune disturbance. The incidence of hyperthyroidism in myasthenic patients is about 5% but myasthenia complicates hyperthyroidism in only 0.5% of patients (Kissel et al. 1970) (Table 18.2). About 5% of myasthenic patients are hypothyroid. Thyroiditis is found at autopsy in 19% of myasthenics (Becker et al. 1964).

Some of the syndromes noted in Table 18.2, e.g. myokymia in hyperthyroidism and myasthenic syn-

Table 18.2. Neuromuscular complications of thyroid disease

Hyperthyroidism
Hyperthyroid myopathy
Bulbar myopathy
Hypokalaemic paralysis
Myokymia

Hypothyroidism
Hypothyroid myopathy
    (Kocher-Debré-Semelaigne and Hoffmann syndromes)
Polyneuropathy and nerve entrapment syndromes

Other
Exophthalmic ophthalmoplegia
Myasthenia gravis
Myasthenic syndrome

drome in hypothyroidism, are not fully elucidated. Thyroid ocular myopathy (exophthalmic ophthalmoplegia) is a feature of autoimmune thyroiditis (Graves' disease) and often develops or intensifies during the recovery phase of hyperthyroidism.

Hyperthyroid Myopathy

Muscular weakness is a common, but usually inapparent feature of hyperthyroidism. Few patients with hyperthyroidism present with muscular weakness. Ramsay (1966) found that half his patients had a history of muscular weakness; the most common symptom was difficulty in climbing stairs. Most patients with thyrotoxicosis have difficulty in getting up from the squatting position. In 4% of patients with hyperthyroidism weakness was the presenting feature of the disease and in 17% weakness and thyrotoxic symptoms began together. On examination 82% of the patients had weakness or wasting of muscles. Seven per cent of the patients had signs of involvement of external ocular muscles. Muscles of the shoulder girdles, especially supraspinatus, triceps and deltoid, were more commonly affected than muscles in the pelvic girdle or legs, but this is often not symptomatic. Atrophy of small periscapular and shoulder girdle muscles may be marked in some patients. The tendon reflexes are usually normal or even increased (Ramsay 1966, 1974).

Muscle twitches, often resembling fasciculation, are uncommon. Puvanendran et al. (1979a) noted fasciculation in 12% of a group of unselected patients with hyperthyroidism, but Ramsay (1974) recorded a higher incidence. These fasciculations are electrophysiologically similar to fasciculations recorded in neurogenic disorders (Daube 1979). The combination of wasting, weakness, hyperreflexia and fasciculations may sometimes lead to the erroneous diagnosis of motor neuron disease, and in some patients this diagnostic difficulty may be heightened by the presence of extensor plantar responses (Garcia and Fleming 1977). These features are all reversible with treatment of the hyperthyroidism. Myokymia (Harman and Richardson 1954) consisting of muscle twitching of an undulating continuous character in face, tongue, limb and trunk muscles has been recorded, even during sleep. This activity consists of repetitive discharges of several motor units, not abolished by brachial plexus block, but abolished by curare (Harman and Richardson 1954). Muscle cramps may also occur but these are relatively uncommon in hyperthyroidism.

Bulbar involvement is uncommon in hyperthyroid myopathy but a few cases of predominant bulbar myopathy associated with thyrotoxicosis have been recorded (Weinstein et al. 1975), and Gaan (1967) described a chronic form of *hyperthyroid bulbar myopathy*. Improvement occurred in these cases when the hyperthyroidism was corrected; there was no response to edrophonium hydrochloride and no decrement was noted with 2 Hz repetitive stimulation.

In acute severe thyrotoxicosis there may be striking involvement of bulbar and external ocular muscles in addition to the more typical periscapular and upper limb weakness. This *"acute thyrotoxic myopathy"* probably represents myasthenia gravis occurring in association with thyrotoxic myopathy (Gaan 1967). However, myasthenia gravis is rare in patients presenting with thyrotoxicosis or thyrotoxic myopathy (Kissel et al. 1970), although thyrotoxicosis occurs in 5% of patients with myasthenia gravis during the course of their disease (Millikan and Haines (1953).

In Japan *hypokalaemic periodic paralysis* has been noted in about 4% of men with thyrotoxicosis (Okinaka et al. 1957) and a similar association has been observed in Hong Kong in Chinese men with thyrotoxicosis (McFadzean and Yeung 1967). In Oriental women the association is much less evident, and it is extremely rare in non-Oriental patients with thyrotoxicosis (McFadzean and Yeung 1967; Brody and Dudley 1969). Nearly all these instances of periodic paralysis are sporadic. A *polyneuropathy* has also been reported in association with thyrotoxicosis (Feibel and Campa 1976). Very rarely polymyositis may be associated with Hashimoto's thyroiditis.

Thyroid eye disease does not necessarily parallel thyroid function, and may occur in euthyroid patients. It is probably due to a cell-modulated immune response against orbital muscle antigens, with an associated deposition of immune complex in these muscles. The primary abnormality is thought to be an autoimmune response to thyroid-stimulating hormone (TSH) receptors in the external ocular muscles (Havard 1979). It has been suggested that thyroglobulin and acetylcholinesterase have similar antigenic determinants, thus accounting for a cross-reaction of anti-thyroglobulin antibody with certain motor end-plates (Ludgate et al. 1986; Swillons et al. 1986). Thyroid eye disease, hyperthyroidism and diffuse goitre, and localised pretibial myxoedema form the characteristic features of Graves' disease. Only about 10% of patients with thyroid eye disease have normal thyroid function. Thyroid eye disease is uncommon in Hashimoto's thyroiditis (Amino et al. 1980), a feature consistent with the probable differing aetiology of this disorder and Graves' disease.

Investigations

The serum CK is usually normal, or reduced (Graig and Smith 1965); the serum myoglobin is also normal (Kasai 1979). In thyroid storm, the CK may be high, with severe weakness, rhabdomyolysis and myoglobinuria (Bennett and Huston 1984). The Achilles reflex shows a shorter contraction and relaxation time than normal, but this test is not of diagnostic value (Rives et al. 1965). The most important test, however, is assessment of thyroid function. Since there is nearly always clinical evidence of thyrotoxicosis these tests serve to confirm the presence of hyperthyroidism. Only in thyroid eye disease can thyroid function tests prove confusing since in 10% of patients they will reveal euthyroidism. In these patients there is an abnormal response to the T3 suppression test, or to the TRH stimulation test (Tamai et al. 1980). CT scanning of the orbit may be useful since it may show enlargement of one or several external ocular muscles, but similar findings may develop in idiopathic orbital myositis, leukaemic infiltration of the orbit and lymphoma of the orbit (Trokel and Hilal 1979).

Concentric needle EMG shows myopathic potentials in almost all patients with hyperthyroid myopathy. The severity of the EMG changes correlates with the clinical evidence of muscle involvement, and is more marked in the more severely affected proximal muscles (90% of cases) than in distal muscles (Ramsay 1965). Some subclinical cases of hyperthyroid myopathy may be revealed by EMG. Fasciculation potentials may be recorded at rest. When the hyperthyroidism is treated the EMG abnormality normalises (Satoyoshi and Kinoshita 1970). Decremental responses to nerve stimulation at low frequencies, with facilitation resembling the Lambert–Eaton myasthenic syndrome, have been reported by Puvanendran et al. (1979b). Cardiomyopathy, with an abnormal EMG, may be present.

Muscle Biopsy

The pathological features of thyrotoxic myopathy are not specific. They consist of atrophy of muscle fibres, with slight increase in endomysial connective tissue and fat, and a mild excess of sarcolemmal nuclei (see Ramsay 1965). Muscle fibre atrophy is not type-specific. Muscle fibre necrosis, or regeneration, is unusual, but central nucleation may be excessive. Lymphorrhages may occur in some patients. On the whole, the muscle biopsy is surprisingly normal in relation to the severity of the weakness and atrophy evident clinically. Electron microscopy reveals only non-specific changes, although giant mitochondria have been reported

(Engel 1972). In the rare periodic paralysis syndrome occurring in association with thyrotoxic myopathy the muscle biopsy may show vacuolation, as is found in familial hypokalaemic paralysis, but the biopsy in such patients has often shown remarkably little abnormality (Resnick et al. 1969; Brooke 1977). Thyrotoxicosis may not be obvious clinically in these patients.

Pathophysiology of Hyperthyroid Myopathy

Hyperthyroid myopathy represents a functional disturbance, with accompanying electrophysiological abnormality, but without structural change or increase in serum CK level. In hyperthyroidism there is a hypermetabolic state with increased turnover of protein, and also increased metabolism of carbohydrate and lipid. This abnormality is not located solely in the mitochondria and does not consist of uncoupling of oxidative metabolism from excitation/contraction. However, ATP is expended more rapidly than normal and a greater oxidative capacity may be needed to generate ATP than in normal tissues (Wiles et al. 1979). Weakness in hyperthyroidism probably results from the interaction of several factors, including reduced membrane excitability and a lower contraction time because of more rapid relaxation (Wiles et al. 1979). These changes may be associated with increased numbers of active Na–K pumps in skeletal muscle membranes in hyperthyroidism (Kjeldsen et al. 1984). Celsing et al. (1986) found that the proportion of Type 1 fibres in muscle increased after 10 months treatment of hyperthyroidism, the capillary density decreased, glycogen content decreased and hexokinase activity decreased.

Management

Treatment of the underlying hyperthyroidism results in reversal of the myopathy in 4–12 weeks. No special measures are necessary if medical treatment is begun, but surgical thyroidectomy should be avoided in patients with significant myopathy because there is a risk of anaesthetic difficulty associated with bulbar weakness and some patients, as in patients with myasthenia gravis, show unexpected sensitivity to the effects of muscle relaxants leading to difficulty in establishing adequate pulmonary ventilation in the post-operative period. Further, the associated cardiac disorder, with or without arrhythmia, may be an additional hazard. Beta-adrenergic blockade is said to be useful in improving strength in some patients with thyrotoxic myopathy (Pimstone et al. 1986).

Hypothyroidism

Muscular symptoms are common in hypothyroidism; these consist of weakness, cramp, muscle stiffness and pain, enlargement of muscles and myoedema. Muscle fatigue is a common and easily overlooked symptom, which may be a presenting feature (Wilson and Walton 1959). These features rarely occur together. Muscle pain is probably the commonest feature, occurring in up to half of patients with hypothyroidism. Proximal weakness is a feature in about 25% of patients (Rao et al. 1980). Several overlapping neuromuscular syndromes have been described in hypothyroidism. The Kocher–Debré–Semelaigne syndrome (Najjar 1974) is a disorder found in cretinous children in which the muscles are hypertrophied and muscular contraction and relaxation are slowed (infant Hercules syndrome). The muscles feel abnormally firm. These muscular effects may be reversed by effective treatment. In some patients, particularly in hypothyroid adults, muscle cramps and painful spasms, often induced by exertion, may accompany muscle hypertrophy; this is called Hoffmann's syndrome (Norris and Panner 1966). Mild myopathic proximal weakness develops gradually during months or years in adult hypothyroidism, often with cramp and muscle pain. Weakness is accompanied either by atrophy or hypertrophy (Nickel et al. 1961) and may be limited to neck muscles (Katz and Pate 1980). Myoedema consists of a local knot of contraction induced in a muscle by percussion. The localised contraction persists for up to a minute. The phenomenon is not specific for hypothyroidism since it is also found in cachexia, ageing and in some normal subjects (Nickel et al. 1961), although it is of shorter duration than in hypothyroidism, usually lasting only a few seconds. Hypothyroidism is also accompanied by fatigue and cold intolerance.

Two-thirds of patients with hypothyroidism have increased relaxation time of the Achilles reflex, a finding that is relatively specific for hypothyroidism if cooling of muscle, drugs such as propranolol and quinidine, and local oedema are excluded (Waal and Manning 1969). Slowed relaxation of the ankle jerk is therefore useful in the diagnosis of hypothyroidism (Chaney 1924; Lambert et al. 1951). Lambert et al. (1951) showed that both the contraction and relaxation phases of the ankle jerk were delayed, suggesting that both contractile and relaxation processes were abnormal (Rao 1971). Khaledi et al. (1983) suggested that quadriceps force measurements and ankle jerk recordings were more useful than clinical examination in detecting hypothyroid myopathy. The ankle jerks are often reduced related to coincidental hypothyroid neuropathy. Other features of myoedema, including coarseness of the skin and facial features, loss of scalp and eyebrow hair, irregularity of menstruation, weight gain and vitiligo may be important clues to diagnosis. Further, carpal tunnel syndrome is often associated with myxoedema in adults. This association may be more frequent than is usually realised. Gelberman et al. (1980) found that 12% of patients with carpal tunnel syndrome had hypothyroidism.

Laboratory Investigations

The CK is usually raised, perhaps because the enzyme is cleared more slowly than normal from plasma (Fleischer et al. 1965; Karlsberg and Roberts 1978; Klein et al. 1980). The serum myoglobin may be raised (Kasai 1979). Diagnosis rests on the demonstration of hypothyroidism by thyroid function tests. Since muscular cramps are a major feature of the clinical presentation this symptom should suggest the diagnosis and lead to appropriate investigation of thyroid function. The blood TSH level is always raised in patients with primary thyroid failure, and is therefore a useful test in the assessment of myxoedema. The ECG may show ischaemic changes, and the cardiac rate is usually slow. Immunological disturbances, such as a mildly raised ESR, and circulating autoantibodies, suggest a diagnosis of Hashimoto's thyroiditis.

Electrophysiological Assessment

Conventional EMG studies may show increased insertional activity, with complex repetitive discharges in about 30% of patients (Waldstein et al. 1958). There is no evidence of myotonia. On volition typical polyphasic myopathic potentials of short duration are usually found in weak muscles. The interference pattern is full. Similar EMG abnormalities are found in childhood and adult-onset cases. Rao et al. (1980) found polyphasic potentials in 90% of patients with hypothyoidism, but only 20% of his patients had detectable weakness.

In cretinism the motor and sensory nerve conduction velocity is usually slowed (Moosa and Dubowitz 1971) and similar slowing of nerve conduction may sometimes be noted in adult myxoedema myopathy (Shirabe et al. 1975). These EMG and nerve conduction abnormalities improve with treatment. Carpal tunnel syndrome and tarsal tunnel syndrome (Schwartz et al. 1983) can be recognised by slowed motor and sensory conduction velocity in the median and medial plantar nerves.

Myoedema is electrically silent and is probably due to persistence of calcium ions in the sarcoplasmic reticulum leading to local prolongation of active contraction (Mizusawa et al. 1983).

Muscle Biopsy

The histological features are similar in the various forms of hypothyroidism. There is moderate variation in fibre size; in the Kocher–Debré–Semelaigne syndrome hypertrophic fibres may be prominent. Central nucleation is more common than in normal muscle, especially in Type 2 fibres; there may be Type 2 fibre atrophy (McKeran et al. 1975, 1979; Wiles et al. 1979). Type 1 predominance may be a feature (McKeran et al. 1975; Wiles et al. 1979). Ring fibres and sarcoplasmic masses may occur (Afifi et al. 1974). Basophilic inclusions have been reported in Type 1 fibres (Ho 1989). Degenerating and regenerating fibres are unusual but have been reported (Shirabe et al. 1975). Ultrastructural studies show prominent aggregation of mitochondria in the sub-sarcolemmal regions (Godet-Guillain and Fardeau 1970). These may contain rectangular inclusions. Similar mitochondrial changes have been produced after thyroidectomy in the rat (Gustafsson et al. 1965). The sarcoplasmic reticulum is often dilated and tubular aggregates may be seen. Myofilamentous changes, with Z-band disarray, are often noted (Afifi et al. 1974). These changes are not specific for hypothyroid myopathy, but represent non-specific myopathic abnormalities. Glycogen content may be increased in electron microscopic studies (Norris and Panner 1966; McKeran et al. 1981), but some PAS-positive crescents are resistant to diastase (Scarlato and Spinnler 1967). Acid maltase activity may be reduced (McDaniel et al. 1977), sometimes quite markedly (Hurwitz et al. 1970).

Nerve Biopsy

Although neuropathy is not usually a major feature of hypothyroidism nerve biopsy may show the features of segmental demyelination, often in a restricted paranodal distribution. Electron microscopy shows a tendency to onion-bulb formation and naked axons. The larger nerve fibres are particularly susceptible (Shira be et al. 1975). Glycogen deposition may be noted in the Schwann cell cytoplasm (Dyck and Lambert 1970). This neuropathy is thus thought to be a primary disorder of Schwann cells. A mucinous deposit, showing metachromasia with toluidine blue, has been reported in the endoneurium of sural nerve biopsies (Nickel et al. 1961). The carpal tunnel syndrome in myxoedema is due to thickening of the transverse ligament, perhaps by a similar mucinous infiltration (Murray and Simpson 1958).

Management and Course

Treatment with thyroid hormone usually induces remission of the myopathy, and of the neuropathy. Treatment must be begun with small incremental doses of L-thyroxine or tri-iodothyronine because of the risk of cardiac and other vascular complications. It may take a year or more before full replacement doses can be used and the patient's symptoms have resolved. The ECG must be carefully assessed during treatment.

Parathyroid Disorders

Hyperparathyroid and hypoparathyroid states cause neuromuscular symptoms as part of the more major systemic features of these syndromes.

Hyperparathyroidism

The classical findings in primary hyperparathyroidism reflect the hypersecretion of parathyroid hormone; plasma calcium is raised and plasma phosphorus is lowered. There is an increase in the level of alkaline phosphatase, derived from bone, in the blood, and the urinary calcium excretion is raised. Most patients present with confusion, renal stones or other renal disorders, such as renal failure, resulting from the hypercalcaemia. Neuromuscular symptoms are mild and may be inapparent.

In parathyroid crisis, myopathic weakness may become much more evident (Lemann and Donatelli 1964); in such patients stupor and seizures may develop (Swash and Rowan 1972).

In hyperparathyroidism weakness is rare, occurring in only three of 76 patients in the series of Frame et al. (1968), and in 7% of Lafferty's series (1981). Patten et al. (1974a) and Mallette et al. (1975) reported a few patients with neurogenic weakness and abnormal calcium metabolism but these cases were heterogeneous. The tendon reflexes may be increased (Turken et al. 1989). There may be a rapid response to removal of a parathyroid tumour in primary hyperparathyroidism even in a few days (Frame et al. 1968; Patten et al. 1974).

Hypoparathyroidism

The major feature is tetany with carpopedal spasm (Trousseau's sign), and irritability of facial muscles to percussion over the facial nerve (Chvostek's sign). Hypoparathyroid myopathy is very rare (Snowdon et al. 1976) but the CK level may be raised (Kruse et al. 1982), even in the absence of weakness. Hypoparathyroidism has been associated with Kearns–Sayre syndrome, but the relation of muscle weakness to the underlying mitochondrial disorder or to the hypocalcaemia is difficult to determine (Pellock et al. 1978; Dewhurst et al. 1986). EMG recordings show spontaneous, repetitive firing of motor units, often occurring in doublets or triplets at rates approaching 100 Hz. Fasciculations have been reported. Muscle biopsy shows only minor abnormalities (Kruse et al. 1982).

Adrenal Disorders and Steroid Myopathy

Muscle weakness may complicate hypoadrenalism and hyperadrenalism, but the latter disorder, especially when due to administration of steroid hormone in the treatment of a variety of other diseases, is far more common.

Hyperadrenalism and Steroid Myopathy

Proximal weakness and wasting is common in patients with Cushing's syndrome and in patients treated with steroids for prolonged periods. As many as 90% of patients with Cushing's syndrome have muscular weakness (Urbanic and George 1981). The myopathy is usually of insidious onset, especially when associated with Cushing's syndrome, but in some patients treated with steroids the muscular symptoms develop relatively rapidly, and wasting and muscular pain may become apparent in less than a month (Askari et al. 1976). The rapidity of development of steroid-dependent myopathy, and its severity, are related to the dose of steroids given, but there is individual variation in susceptibility. In some patients clinical evidence may appear within 10 days of starting steroid treatment at high dose levels. The muscles in such patients may be tender to palpation and the distinction between steroid myopathy and active polymyositis in patients receiving steroids for treatment of polymyositis can be difficult (Askari et al. 1976). Severe muscle pain is not a feature.

The weakness is usually more severe in the legs, especially in quadriceps, than in the arms, and is almost entirely proximal in distribution. There are usually other clinical signs of steroid therapy or hyperadrenalism, particularly a high facial colour, facial puffiness, increased body adipose tissue and acne vulgaris. Impaired glucose tolerance and hypertension may also be associated features, especially in Cushing's syndrome and during chronic steroid therapy. The tendon reflexes are present.

Laboratory Investigations

Steroid myopathy occurs as a result of glucocorticoid excess. Glucocorticoids inhibit protein synthesis in muscle, due to interference with incorporation of amino acids into muscle cell proteins (Bullock et al. 1968; Clark and Vignos 1979), and also have a catabolic effect on muscle proteins (Goldberg and Goodman 1969). This is reflected in increased levels of urinary creatine; the blood creatine may also be increased, especially during glucocorticoid therapy (Perkoff et al. 1959). The CK is almost invariably normal although it may approach the upper limit of normal during the active phase of the disorder. Askari et al. (1976) found that the urinary creatine excretion was the best indicator of steroid myopathy. They commented that a raised urinary creatine excretion, with normal CK, in a patient treated with steroids for polymyositis, indicated steroid myopathy rather than relapse of polymyositis.

Steroid myopathy is probably due to the protein catabolism associated with glucocorticoid hormones.

Electrophysiological Assessment

EMG is normal even in severe cases. Twitch and tetanus contraction tensions are normal, implying that excitation–contraction coupling and membrane excitability are normal (Ruff et al. 1982).

Muscle Biopsy

The main feature in light-microscopic preparations is atrophy of both fibre types, usually particularly prominent in Type 2 fibres (Pleasure et al. 1970). Type 2B fibre atrophy is especially prominent even in patients treated with steroids, without clinical evidence of myopathy (Carpenter and Karpati 1984). Necrosis and vacuolation of muscle fibres may occur (Dubowitz and Brooke 1973). Lipid droplets and glycogen accumulations are prominent features (Fig. 18.1), usually in Type 1 more than Type 2 fibres (Prineas et al. 1968). With the electron microscopy (Fig. 18.2) enlarged degenerate mitochondria, dilatation of the sarcoplasmic reticulum, marked thickening of the basement membrane and loss of myofibrils have been described (Engel 1966b; Afifi et al. 1968). Glycogen accumulation may also be a feature.

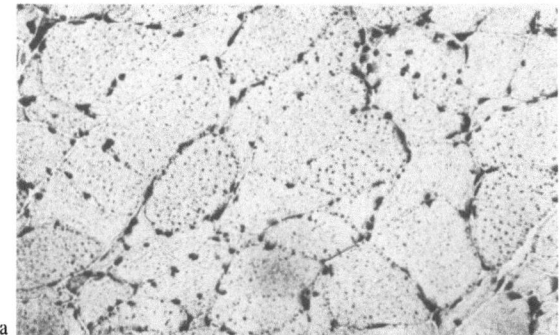

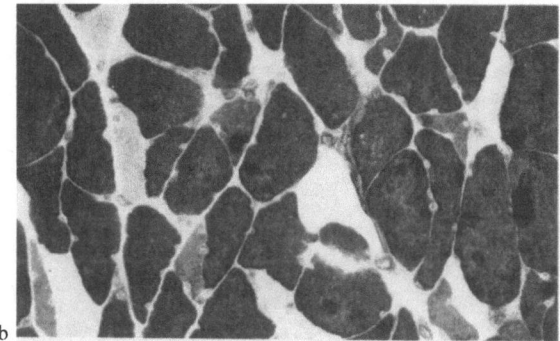

Fig. 18.1. Steroid myopathy. **a** Oil red O. TS. × 360. Lipid droplets are prominent, especially in the larger Type 1 fibres. **b** ATPase pH 4.3. The dark Type 1 fibres are predominant, and the Type 2 fibres are atrophic.

This myopathy has been studied experimentally, particularly in the rabbit. Vignos et al. (1976) found alterations in the contractile properties of muscle, related to changes in myosin or other contractile protein elements of the fast-twitch/glycolytic fibres (Type 2 fibres). Afifi et al. (1977) found that high doses of hydrocortisone (20 mg/kg per day) were necessary to produce a marked histological abnormality in rabbit muscles. These changes included fibre fragmentation and phagocytosis, variation in fibre size and vacuolation of fibres.

Management

Reduction of steroid dosage or treatment of Cushing's disease results in rapid improvement in mild cases of steroid myopathy but in some severely affected patients recovery may be protracted. Recovery occurs within 1–4 months of discontinuing steroids, or utilising a non-fluorinated systemic steroid (Askari et al. 1976). Similar recovery follows treatment of idiopathic Cushing's syndrome. The dose of steroid implicated in steroid-dependent myopathy is not large. For example, 1.5–6 mg dexamethasone daily for 3–12 weeks may be sufficient to induce a myopathy (Afifi et al. 1968; Askari et al.

1976). Prednisone, 15–100 mg daily for periods ranging from 1 month to 5 years has also been associated with steroid myopathy. The variability of these dose regimens illustrates the role of individual susceptibility in development of steroid myopathy. Further, additional factors, such as poor nutrition, recovery from other muscular diseases, especially polymyositis, and cachexia and disuse atrophy may be important contributory factors in the development of muscular wasting and weakness in patients taking steroids. Activity may be important in preventing steroid-induced muscle atrophy (Hickson and Davis 1981).

Hypoadrenalism (Addison's Disease)

This disorder is often associated with asthenia and fatiguability. Muscle cramps and contractures may occur. Some patients show wasting of proximal muscles. When hypokalaemia is present attacks of intermittent flaccid paralysis resembling periodic paralysis may occur (Duc et al. 1970).

Short-duration motor units, without polyphasia or spontaneous activity, were noted by Buchthal and Rosenfalck (1963) in two cases.

The features of muscle biopsies have not been described.

Conn's Syndrome

In primary aldosteronism about two-thirds of patients present with muscle weakness, as part of their clinical syndrome. This is probably due to hypokalaemia (Conn et al. 1964), and episodes of hypokalaemic paralysis may also occur. These symptoms remit after removal of the adrenal adenoma, when the blood potassium returns to normal.

Pituitary Disorders

Acromegaly

In the early stage of acromegaly the muscles may be hypertrophic and stronger than normal (Marie 1886; Maranon and Richet 1937) but later in the disease, although the muscles may not appear very atrophic, they feel flabby to palpation (Cushing 1912) and proximal weakness may become evident. Atrophy develops only in the more advanced stages of the untreated disease (Adams et al. 1962). Fatigue was a common complaint in the later stages of

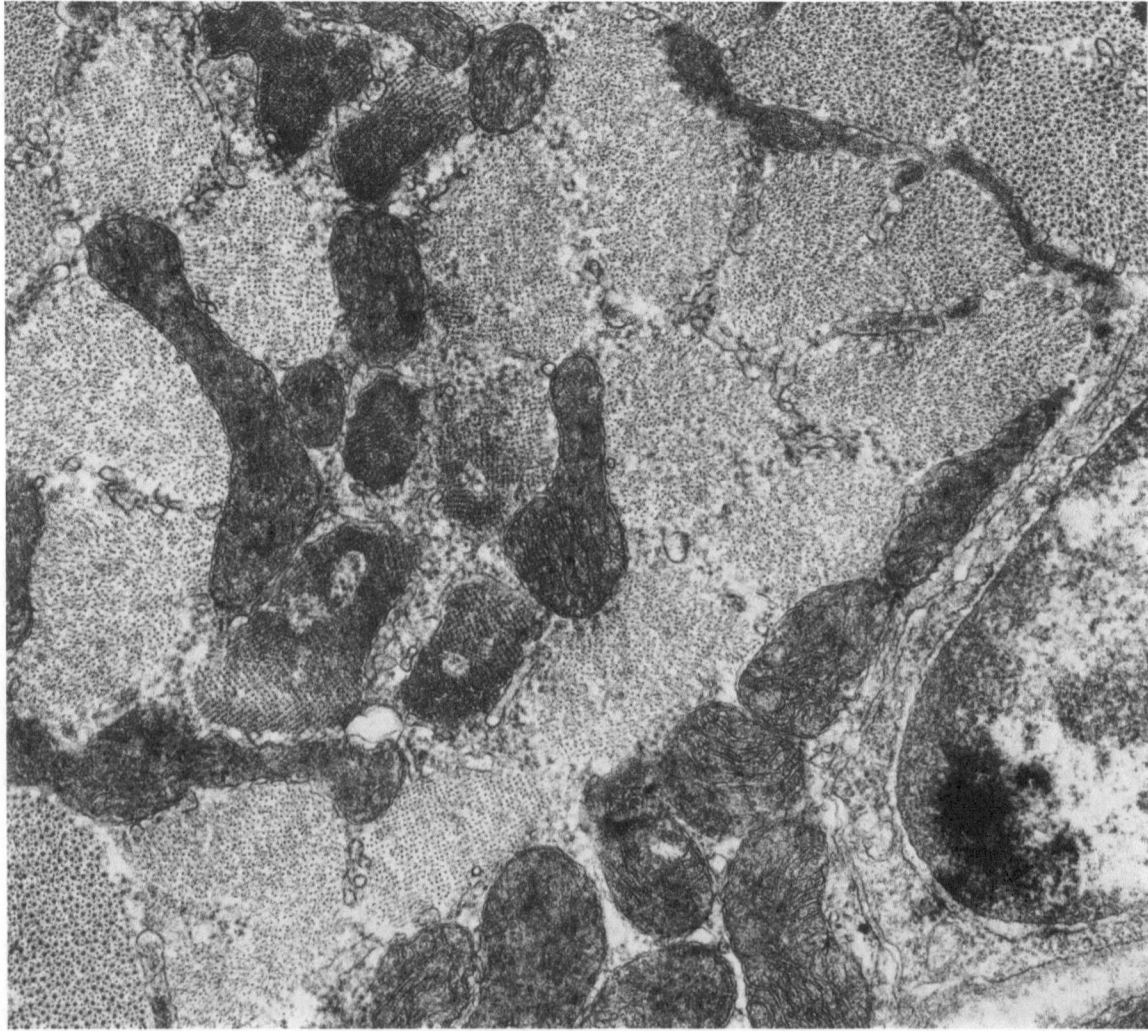

Fig. 18.2. Steroid myopathy. Electron micrograph. TS. × 45 000. The mitochondria are enlarged and, in some, the cristae pattern is disturbed. The tubules of the endoplasmic reticulum are enlarged and unusually prominent. Glycogen granules can be seen between the myofibrils. The latter show variations in morphology related to varying sectional planes, in relation to Z band and actin/myosin lattices.

untreated acromegaly (Cushing 1912). Carpal tunnel syndrome and diabetes mellitus are commonly associated with acromegaly. Pickett et al. (1975) noted that about 50% of patients with acromegaly had muscle weakness at presentation. Muscle wasting is uncommon.

Laboratory Investigations

The CK is slightly increased in about 20% of cases of acromegaly (Pickett et al. 1975). The diagnosis can be confirmed by the finding of a raised level of growth hormone in the blood, but the level of growth hormone does not correlate well with the severity of the myopathy (Nagulesparen et al. 1976). The duration of the disease, however, bears a closer relation with the degree of muscular weakness (Pickett et al. 1975).

Electrophysiological Assessment

At rest there is usually no spontaneous activity. In most patients conventional EMG shows only slight abnormalities. On volition short-duration polyphasic MUAPs may be noted (Fig. 18.3) but this is not a prominent abnormality. Mastaglia et al. (1970a) found decreased duration of MUAPs in proximal muscles. Single-fibre EMG studies have shown a

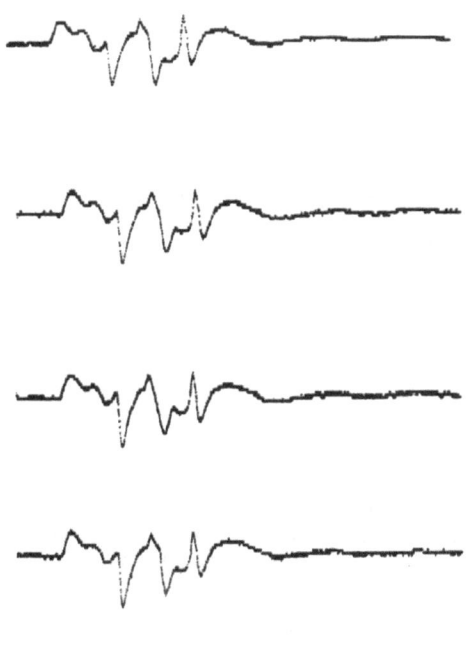

Fig. 18.3. Acromegaly. A complex, stable, motor unit action potential. Concentric needle EMG. 500 Hz. 10 kHz. Bar 2 ms.

normal neuromuscular jitter (Lundberg et al. 1970) but the fibre density may be slightly raised. The nerve conduction velocity is usually normal, although slowed median nerve conduction velocity across the carpal tunnel is frequently encountered because of the associated carpal tunnel syndrome. The presence of diabetic mellitus, also often associated with acromegaly, may lead to diabetic neuropathy with a resulting mixed myopathic and neurogenic EMG disturbance, and with mildly slowed nerve conduction. Stewart (1966) reported a hypertrophic neuropathy in patients with acromegaly, unrelated to associated diabetes. Low et al. (1974) found electrophysiological evidence of peripheral neuropathy, with slowed motor and sensory nerve conduction unrelated to nerve entrapment, in 11 patients with acromegaly. In six of these patients diabetes mellitus was considered not to be the underlying factor because the glucose tolerance test was normal or only minimally disturbed. As in the case of acromegalic myopathy, this neuropathy was unrelated to growth hormone levels.

Muscle Biopsy

In the muscle the main feature is the presence of hypertrophic and atrophic fibres. In earlier studies the biopsy was thought to be normal (Adams et al. 1962; Lundberg et al. 1970) but quantitative enzyme histochemical studies have shown hypertrophy of Type 1 fibres (Mastaglia et al. 1970a) and atrophy of Type 2 fibres, particularly of Type 2A fibres (Nagulesparen et al. 1976). Some atrophic Type 1 fibres, and hypertrophied Type 2 fibres may also be seen. These hypertrophic changes may persist for years, even after normal levels of growth hormone have been restored by appropriate treatment of the pituitary adenoma. Greenbaum and Young (1950) produced an increase in muscle bulk in rats treated with growth hormone and, in two other studies, the myofibrillar area was increased, with increased muscle protein synthesis (Goldberg 1969). These findings indicate that fibre hypertrophy may be a specific effect of growth hormone on muscle. Only rare necrotic fibres undergoing phagocytosis have been observed (Nagulesparen et al. 1976). Tubular aggregates have also been found in the biopsy (Mastaglia 1973).

Nerve Biopsy

Sural nerve biopsies show a reduction in the number of myelinated nerve fibres with segmental demyelination. There is an increased amount of subperineurial and endoneurial tissue. The fascicular area is increased. Electron microscopy has shown small onion bulbs, and clusters of small regenerating myelinated fibres may be seen (Low et al. 1974).

Course

The proximal weakness shows little improvement in the first few weeks after treatment, but some improvement may be evident a year later in some patients. About half of the patients reviewed by Pickett et al. (1975) showed clinical and EMG improvement a year after surgery. Improvement was not related to normalisation of levels of growth hormone which occurred in all patients.

Carcinoid Myopathy

Carcinoid syndrome results from the effects of high circulating levels of serotonin (5-hydroxytryptamine). Argentaffin tumours of the gut, especially of the ileum, secrete serotonin and, if there are hepatic metastases, serotonin may enter the systemic circulation causing diarrhoea, blue discoloration of the face, flushing attacks and tricuspid and pulmonary valvular heart disease, leading to intractable heart failure. There have been two reports of proximal myopathy associated with this syndrome (Berry et al. 1974; Swash et al. 1975) and a third report of a polymyositis-like syndrome in a patient with a carcinoid tumour (Green et al. 1964). Carcinoid myopathy is thought to be due to a direct toxic effect of serotonin on skeletal muscles. Myopathy has been noted only after several years of carcinoid syndrome, and has been associated with muscular weakness and atrophy, and with slight muscular tenderness and a tendency to develop cramps.

Laboratory Investigations

The urinary 5-hydroxyindole acetic acid excretion is markedly raised (Swash et al. 1975) and blood serotonin levels may be raised (Berry et al. 1974). The CK may be slightly raised.

Electrophysiological Assessment

EMG studies have revealed a reduced interference patteren with numerous short-duration, low-amplitude, polyphasic MUAPs typical of a myopathy. No spontaneous activity is recorded.

Muscle Biopsy

Advanced Type 2 fibre atrophy with less marked atrophy of Type 1 fibres, and scattered necrotic fibres, has been reported (Swash et al. 1975). No more specific features have been found.

Management

Improvement has been noted with anti-serotonin drugs, including cyproheptadine and methysergide (Berry et al. 1974; Swash et al. 1975). This effect of cyproheptadine has been reproduced experimentally during serotonin infusion in rat nerve–muscle preparations (Patten et al. 1974b). In these experiments serotonin was shown to induce more marked weakness in the rat anterior tibial muscle, which contains numerous Type 2 fibres, than in the predominantly Type 1 soleus muscle, suggesting that serotonin has a relatively specific adverse effect on Type 2 fibres.

Chapter 19

Drug-Induced Toxic and Nutritional Myopathies

With the exception of steroid myopathy, which is almost invariably iatrogenic (Swash and Schwartz 1983a) (see Chap. 18), drug-induced myopathies are relatively rare. Muscle is thus relatively less susceptible to drug effects than peripheral nerve (see Chap. 11). The most useful, practical classification of drug-induced myopathies is by mode of clinical presentation. This approach was adopted by Lane and Mastaglia (1978). The diversity of the syndromes tends to lead to a complex classification (Kakulas and Mastaglia 1992) but this overlaps with diseases having a recognised metabolic basis in which drug effects play a causative role, e.g. malignant hyperpyrexia (Table 19.1). These syndromes to some extent overlap.

Muscle Pain, Stiffness and Cramp

These symptoms are often the first feature of muscular involvement. They may occur in response to treatment with a variety of drugs and are frequently rapidly reversible. When severe, the symptoms may be associated with muscle tenderness and a raised blood CK level, features that imply rapid destruction of muscle cells. However, similar symptoms can arise in inflammatory myopathies, with vascular involvement, and when energy metabolism is compromised. The latter is a feature of alcoholic myopathy (Hudgson 1984) and perhaps with other causative drugs, e.g. lithium which interferes with sodium/potassium-dependent membrane potentials of muscle cells and so causes weakness.

Acute Rhabdomyolysis

Muscle pain, stiffness and cramp may be premonitory symptoms of acute necrosis of muscle (Fig. 19.1), leading to severe flaccid paralysis, muscle tenderness and swelling and rhabdomyolysis. The latter may be complicated by renal failure; indeed,

Table 19.1. Clinical syndromes of drug-induced myopathies

Syndrome	Causative drugs
Muscle cramp	Lithium, cimetidine, salbutamol, clofibrate, danazol
Acute rhabdomyolysis (with renal failure)	Heroin, phencyclidine, epsilon aminocaproic acid, drug-induced coma
Malignant hyperpyrexia	Inhalational anaesthetic agents (see Chap. 17), succinylcholine
Neuroleptic malignant syndrome	Dopamine-blocking neuroleptic drugs (see Chap. 17)
Inflammatory myopathy	Penicillamine, procainamide (see Chap. 13), hydralazine, phenytoin
Acute hypokalaemic paralysis	Diuretics, purgatives, amphotericin, carbenoxolone
Injection myopathy (focal myopathy)	Antibiotics, pentazocine, pethidine
Subacute *painful* myopathy	Alcohol, clofibrate, epsilon aminocaproic acid, emetine
Chronic *painless* myopathies	Corticosteroids (see Chap. 18), chloroquine, cyclosporin

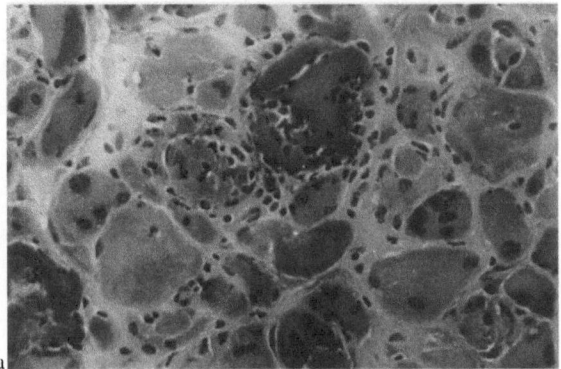

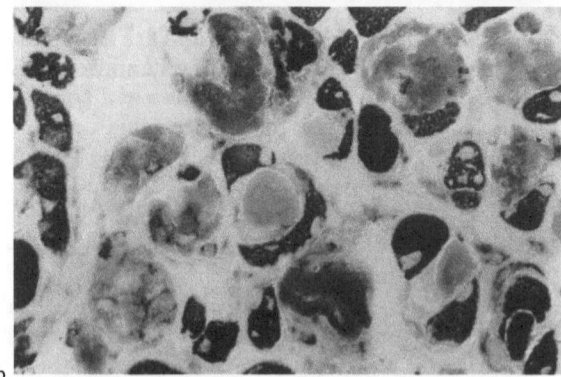

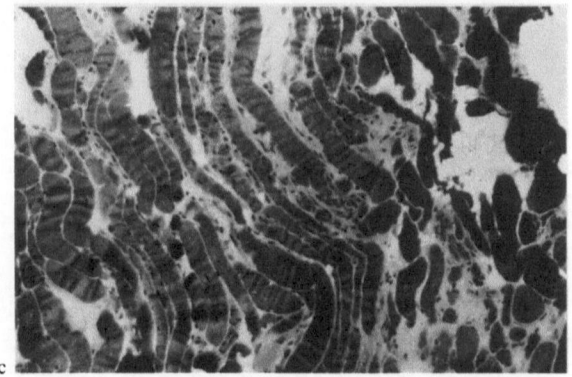

Fig. 19.1. Acute toxic myopathy due to ε-aminocaproic acid (EACA). TS. × 350. **a** H and E. There is widespread necrosis of muscle fibres. Macrophages can be seen within several fibres and there is a sparse lymphocytic response. Some endomysial nuclei are enlarged and vesicular. **b** ATPase. pH 4.3. Peripheral crescents of enzyme-positive, regenerating muscle fibres are evident adjacent to necrotic fibres. These crescentic and necrotic zones are contained within individual endomysial tubes and thus represent regeneration from myoblasts derived from satellite cells. **c** H and E. × 140. In this needle biopsy taken 1 month after EACA therapy was stopped regeneration has occurred. Most fibres, however, are small and many contain centrally placed nuclei. Adipose tissue is also present, represented by clear spaces.

renal failure may dominate the clinical presentation. Weakness is usually predominantly proximal and axial in distribution, as in the acute myopathy that was induced by ε-aminocaproic acid (Korsan-Bengsten et al. 1969; Kennard et al. 1980). This complication occurred after a few days treatment, or was delayed for weeks or months. Acute muscle necrosis may occur after only a single intravenous dose of heroin, perhaps particularly in drug abusers who have been abstinent for several months (de Gans et al. 1985). Recovery from the acute necrotising myopathy occurs gradually, in weeks or months, depending on the severity of the myopathy (Lane et al. 1979). Treatment consists of withdrawal of the causative drug, and passive and active physiotherapy to maintain full movement of affected limbs. Some cholesterol-lowering agents, e.g. clofibrate and lovastatin, may cause a syndrome of muscle pain, weakness and rhabdomyolysis (London et al. 1991). The myopathy may occur within days of starting the drug, or after as long as several months treatment, and recovery commences rapidly when the offending drug is stopped (Smith et al. 1970; Abourizk et al. 1979; Pearce et al. 1990). Several of these drugs cause myotonia, especially diazocholesterol (see Chap. 15).

Ischaemic contracture of muscle, similar to that described by Volkmann as a complication of certain injuries to the limbs, sometimes occurs after recovery from carbon monoxide or barbiturate poisoning. Occasionally muscle necrosis is sufficiently extensive to result in myoglobinuria and renal failure. Disability from paralysis and contracture in affected vascular compartments of limb muscles is usually severe since, during the necrosis, oedematous swelling often results in secondary pressure and ischaemic damage to the innervation of affected muscles (Howse and Seddon 1966).

Inflammatory Myopathy

This is a very infrequent complication of drug therapy. Penicillamine treatment most commonly causes myasthenia gravis but may also cause inflammatory myopathy when used in the treatment of both rheumatoid arthritis and Wilson's disease (Carroll et al. 1987). Procainamide may also produce inflammatory myopathy. The myopathy is mild, but steroid therapy may be necessary, in addition to cessation of penicillamine or other drugs, in order to induce remission (Morgan et al. 1981). There may be a more widespread vasculitis, of which muscle involvement is only a part. Recovery occurs slowly (Schraeder et al. 1972; Fernandes et al. 1977). Sulphonamides, propyl cimetidine, hydralazine and phenytoin have also been reported as inducing inflammatory myopathy (Kakulas and Mastaglia 1992).

Tryptophan-Induced Eosinophilia-Myalgia Syndrome

This multisystem syndrome was first recognised in the USA in 1989 (CDC 1989). L-tryptophan is a naturally occurring amino acid which was promoted as a natural cure for insomnia, depression and premenstrual symptoms in a dose of 1.5 g/day, about twice the natural dietary intake. Most patients developing the eosinophilia-myalgia syndrome (EMS) took tryptophan for a few weeks, or for as long as several years; some developed the syndrome after stopping tryptophan. Tryptophan became available in 1974 and, by 1990, there were 1269 cases in the USA. EMS consists of a syndrome in which the eosinophil count in the blood is more than 1×10^9 cells/l, incapacitating myalgia and a variety of other symptoms affecting skin, subcutaneous tissue and fascia (Medsgar 1990). Cutaneous manifestations include alopecia, maculo-popular or urticarial rash, and induration of subcutaneous tissue and fascia leading to contractures. Myalgia may be accompanied by weakness, but the CK level is usually normal and weakness is thought to result mainly from involvement of the peripheral nervous system. Sensorimotor neuropathy, even leading to respiratory failure and death, and resembling Guillain–Barré syndrome, may develop. Two-thirds of patients have pulmonary symptoms, including dyspnoea, at presentation. The ESR is normal (Hertzman et al. 1990; Silver et al. 1990).

EMS shares many clinical features with eosinophilic fasciitis and localised forms of scleroderma. There are also clinical similarities with the Spanish toxic oil syndrome (Deighton 1990).

The EMG has often shown a mixed pattern of myopathic and neurogenic abnormalities (Martin et al. 1990) but typical short-duration, low-amplitude, polyphasic myopathic features have also been noted (Tanhelco et al. 1992). Martin et al. (1990) reported electrophysiological evidence of peripheral neuropathy in four of their 10 cases, three of whom also showed myopathic change in EMG studies. Six of nine patients had absent sensory MAPs in the sural nerves (Smith and Dyck 1990).

Pathology

The muscle biopsy reveals perimysial infiltration by mononuclear cells and, rarely, eosinophils. Muscle fibre necrosis in zones of muscle, suggestive of vasculopathy, may be seen. Immunohistochemical studies show that the mononuclear cell infiltrates consist of T lymphocytes. Fibre-type grouping has not been reported (Martin et al. 1990; Tanhelco et al. 1992). Sural nerve biopsies showed axonal degeneration, mononuclear epineural and perivascular inflammation, inflammatory vasculopathy and some features of axonal regeneration. Skin and fascia may be involved with scleroderma-like changes.

Management

The prognosis in severe cases is poor. Most deaths have occurred in patients taking large doses; usually after the ingestion of more than 2000 g of L-tryptophan. The neuropathic component may be very severe, with disabling ascending sensorimotor neuropathy, including facial involvement, requiring assisted ventilation. L-tryptophan withdrawal is followed by slow improvement during several months. Steroid therapy has been tried but there is no proof of its efficacy.

The cause of EMS remains uncertain but contamination of L-tryptophan with another metabolite has been suspected (Belangra et al. 1990). Slutsker et al. (1990) reported involvement of a single manufacturer as the source of EMS.

Mitochondrial Myopathy

AZT (zidovudine) may lead to a mitochondrial myopathy, associated with deletion of mitochondrial DNA, during treatment of patients with HIV infection (see Chap. 13).

Acute Hypokalaemic Paralysis

Severe hypokalaemia, from any cause, may present with muscular weakness. Diuretics, amphotericin B, liquorice ingestion (Gross et al. 1966) or carbenoxolone therapy, purgatives and alcohol (Martin et al. 1971; Rubenstein and Weinapel 1977) have been noted to induce this syndrome. Liquorice contains glycyrrhizic acid, a potent mineralo-corticoid substance that promotes sodium retention and potassium loss in the kidney, and across cell membranes (Valeriano et al 1983). The weakness is reversed by potassium replacement, and it is more likely to occur when there is chronic potassium depletion, as in patients on chronic diuretic therapy. In mild cases changes in the resting membrane potential lead to decreased excitability of the muscle fibre membrane and so to weakness. In severe cases, when there is rapid and marked hypokalaemia, muscle fibre necrosis with increased blood CK levels and, rarely, rhabdomyolysis, may develop.

Blocking Agent/Corticosteroid Myopathy

This is a severe generalised disorder, with marked proximal weakness and wasting that develops in the context of a period of several days treatment with neuromuscular blocking agents, such as pancuronium, and steroids, e.g. in the management of status asthmaticus with positive pressure ventilation. On cessation of treatment with the blocking agent severe myopathic weakness becomes evident, with areflexia and muscle atrophy. Facial and bulbar muscles may be slightly involved. Recovery occurs over a period of weeks or months.

Muscle biopsy shows striking abnormalities consisting of fibre atrophy, centrally located zones of pallor in muscle fibres in ATPase preparations, which were negatively reactive in NADH and dark blue in Gomori preparations, and a few scattered necrotic fibres. Semithin sections showed loss of thick A bands in the central parts of affected muscle fibres, some of which were devoid of striated myofilaments, and loss of mitochondria. Electron microscopy showed marked loss of thick myofilaments and abnormalities in mitochondrial size, shape and distribution. There was no inflammation and no abnormality in muscle capillaries was seen (Danon and Carpenter 1991).

Selective loss of thick filaments has been produced experimentally in rats by combining denervation with high doses of steroids (Rouleau et al. 1987) and by tenotomy (Karpati et al. 1971).

Injection (Focal) Myopathy

Even needle injuries to a muscle, perhaps from concentric needle EMG (Engel 1967; Chrissian et al. 1976), may be sufficient to cause an increase in the blood CK level and focal necrosis and regeneration of muscle fibres in the region of the needle track. The effects of needling of muscle are usually clinically unimportant since the CK level rarely rises above the normal range. Cherington et al. (1968) noted that although the CK may rise 50% immediately after needle EMG, it does not exceed the normal range in normal subjects. However, in myopathic subjects it may increase more markedly. Sandstedt (1981), using frequency analysis of the EMG, found "myopathic"

changes in 21% of muscles a week after previous concentric needle EMG examination.

Drug injections into muscle may cause more extensive local trauma and haemorrhage, and the injected drug may have local myotoxic effects, including necrosis, e.g. paraldehyde, chlorpromazine and cephalosporin antibiotics. Repeated injections, for example of narcotics, antibiotics or phenothiazines (Bergeson et al. 1982) may lead to fibrosis and contractures. The CK may be raised even several days after a single injection of chlorpromazine (Meltzer et al. 1970). Pentazocine therapy has been particularly incriminated (de Lateur and Halliday 1978). Narcotic-induced fibrosis may produce disabling contractures (Levin and Engel 1975). Muscle stretching, physiotherapy or even surgical treatment may be required.

Subacute or Acute Painful Myopathy

These include myopathies associated with alcoholism and with treatment with clofibrate ε-aminocaproic acid and emetine (Sugie et al. 1984). These drugs are relatively infrequently used, so that these complications are rare. Cyclosporin therapy in renal transplant patients may lead to weakness and myalgia 5–25 months after beginning treatment. This complication is rare, occurring in less than 0.2% of treated patients, but muscle cramps are common (Fernandez-Sola et al. 1990; Arrelano and Krupp 1991).

Chronic Painless Myopathy

This is probably the most common clinical syndrome of drug-induced myopathy, because of the frequency of muscle weakness and atrophy in patients treated with *steroid* drugs (see Chap. 18).

Chloroquine may also produce myopathy (Hughes et al. 1971). In this syndrome muscular weakness is diffuse, but affects lower limbs more than upper limbs, with facial involvement. Cardiomyopathy may also develop. The EMG shows myopathic changes, with some myotonic discharges, and the biopsy shows a vacuolar myopathy consisting of autophagic vacuoles laden with membranous debris (Mastaglia et al. 1977). The CK may be slightly raised. Pathologically there may be evidence of neuropathy, but chloroquine myopathy and neuropathy seem not to co-exist. Retinopathy may also develop with chloroquine toxicity. Related drugs, e.g. other 4-aminoquinoline drugs, may also cause myopathy (Hughes et al. 1971). This myopathic complication resolves, like steroid myopathy, when the toxic drug is withdrawn.

Myopathy has also been reported as a complication of treatment with β blocker drugs (Forfar et al 1979), rifampicin (Jenkins and Emerson 1981) and cyclosporin (Goy et al. 1989).

Toxic Myopathies

These are acquired myopathies with a metabolic basis, caused by ingested agents. Only alcoholic myopathy is common.

Alcoholic Myopathy

Alcoholics may develop proximal muscle weakness. Acute and chronic syndromes are recognised.

Acute alcoholic myopathy varies in severity. In severe cases there is a history of a recent, heavy binge of drinking often ceasing abruptly before the onset of muscular symptoms (Hed et al. 1962). The syndrome consists of myalgia, rhabdomyolysis with myoglobinuria and an increased CK level (Perkoff et al. 1966; Perkoff 1972; Walsh and Conomy 1977). The muscular symptoms may be relatively localised, affecting shoulders more than hips, sometimes involving bulbar and facial muscles (Weber et al 1981), and often with painful calves, thighs and buttocks. The disorder may mimic deep vein thrombosis in the legs (Walsh and Conomy 1977). In mild cases there may be only slight muscle tenderness and a raised blood CK level.

The rhabdomyolysis and myoglobinuria may lead to renal failure (Hallgren et al 1980). Recovery occurs in 2–8 weeks, but repeated attacks may follow recurrent alcoholic debauches, with the development of permanent weakness.

In acute alcoholic myopathy the EMG shows myopathic features, often with fibrillation potentials. The muscle biopsy shows muscle fibre necrosis. This may be widespread, but it is often associated with scattered regenerating fibres. Muscle biopsies carried out during the recovery phase show regenerative activity sometimes with poor enzyme reactivity in the ATPase preparations (Martinez et al. 1973) and, rarely, there may be some inflammatory infiltrates, mainly consisting of macrophages.

The cause of acute alcoholic myopathy is uncertain, but experimental evidence suggests that ethanol has direct myotoxic effects. In both humans and rats ethanol has been shown to cause an increase in blood CK (Haller and Drachman 1976; Lane and Radoff 1981; Spargo 1984). In starved rats ethanol can induce muscle fibre necrosis (Haller

and Drachman 1976). In humans fed alcohol in high dosage for a month ultrastructural studies showed destruction of mitochondria and myofilaments (Rubin et al. 1976), changes similar to those found in the naturally occurring disease (Klinkerfuss et al. 1967).

Acute myopathy may also develop in alcoholism in association with *alcohol-induced hypokalaemia*. In this syndrome sweating, vomiting or diarrhoea develop during a prodromal period of several days, followed by severe proximal weakness, even quadriplegia. Rhabdomyolysis and myoglobinuria develop in severe cases, sometimes leading to renal failure (Martin et al. 1971; Rubenstein and Weinapel 1977). The CK level is markedly raised, depending on the severity of the myopathy. The muscle biopsy shows a vacuolar myopathy with scattered necrotic fibres. Treatment with intravenous and oral potassium supplement leads to rapid improvement, with recovery in 2 to 7 days.

The *chronic form of alcoholic myopathy* is less well defined than the acute disorder. Urbano-Marquez et al. (1989) found that 42% of a group of chronic alcoholics had weak deltoid muscles, and biopsies of these muscles showed myopathic change. However, clinically significant weakness in chronic alcoholics usually affects the legs more than the arms, and electrophysiological studies show a mixed picture of myopathy (Ekbom et al. 1964b) and of neuropathy (Faris and Reyes 1971). Indeed, neuropathy often seems the dominant syndrome, and many patients also have other complications of alcoholism, including seizures, cerebellar ataxia and amnesia syndrome. Cardiomyopathy is also frequent (Rubin et al. 1976; Rubin 1979). The CK level is normal or raised. Karttinen et al. (1970) found that the CK level was raised in 43% of a group of chronic alcoholics.

The muscle biopsy shows mild myopathic changes, including degenerating and regenerating fibres, and fibrosis (Klinkerfuss et al. 1967) with striking Type 2B fibre atrophy (Hamid et al. 1981; Slavin et al. 1983). There may also be features of neurogenic change (Faris and Reyes 1971).

Abstention from alcohol is followed by slow recovery that is often partial (Perkoff et al. 1966; Pittman and Decker 1971).

Pathogenesis

The cause of acute and chronic myopathy is uncertain. Experimental evidence suggests that alcohol is myotoxic (see above). Spargo (1984) found a fourfold increase in blood CK levels following a single intraperitoneal dose of ethyl alcohol in rats. Haller et al. (1984) showed that the toxic effect of alcohol on muscle was independent of changes in the blood potassium level. Haller and Drachman (1980) found that the myotoxic effect of alcohol in the rat was manifest only when the rats were fasted for 24 hours during their 3-week exposure to ethanol. Teravainen et al. (1978) noted no myotoxic effects without concomitant fasting. Perkoff et al. (1966) showed impaired production of lactate during ischaemic exercise in chronic alcoholics and correlated this with low phosphorylase levels in skeletal muscle. Bollaert et al. (1989) has confirmed the glycogenolytic abnormality reported by Perkoff et al. in 1966. The effects of ethanol on oxidative enzyme activity and membrane ion transport are complex and probably also contribute to ethanol myotoxicity.

Management

Correction of hypokalaemia is effective in the management of the hypokalaemic form of alcoholic myopathy (Martin et al. 1971). Renal failure requires appropriate management and treatment of myoglobinuria. Abstinence from alcohol is essential to prevent further episodes of acute myopathy and to prevent the development of chronic myopathy. Once established, the patient is unlikely to recover fully. It may be difficult to exclude coincidental alcoholic neuropathy in the latter group and this may account, in part, for the poor prognosis of this syndrome. The reason for development of neuropathy in some patients and myopathy in others is unknown; a similar problem concerns the specificity of development of the various central nervous system complications of alcoholism.

Microbial Toxic Myopathy

Acute myopathic weakness with raised CK levels may be a feature of several systemic disorders, particularly in Weil's disease (Ho and Scully 1980), typhoid fever (David and Tolayma 1978), and other infections including Legionella, mixed enteric organisms, Aspergillus infections and toxic shock syndrome related to the presence of staphylococcal infection in vaginal tampons (Tanner et al. 1981). Other staphylococcal infections, and staphylococcal puerperal sepsis, in which staphylococcal exotoxin gains access to the circulation, may cause an acute, severe illness with fever, hypotension, rash, myalgia and gastro-intestinal disturbance. The CK level may be very high, reaching 10 000 IU/l. This syndrome is potentially fatal, and recovery may be protracted (see Layzer 1985b). Clostridial infection may also cause focal lysis of muscle, due to the effect of its

α-toxin, lecithinasec, on the muscle fibre membrane (Strunk et al. 1967).

Envenomation Myopathies

The venoms of a number of snakes, spiders and wasps can cause acute rhabdomyolysis, severe weakness and myoglobinuria. Some envenomation myopathies are potentially fatal, usually as a consequence of renal or cardiac failure. The Elapid snakes, including tiger snakes, sea snakes, Jameson's mamba and crotalid snakes, including prairie rattlesnakes, South American rattlesnakes, the western diamondback rattlesnake and the jumping viper of Costa Rica have venoms in which specific myotoxins have been identified (Kakulas and Mastaglia 1992). The effect of sea snake venom is characteristic of these envenomation myopathies.

The sea snake bite is usually no larger than a pinprick, with no local reaction and little pain. Two to eight hours after the bite painful muscles, slurred speech, dysphagia, ptosis, opthalmoplegia, ascending paralysis and myoglobinuria develop. These symptoms may be followed by renal and cardiac failure and respiratory insufficiency but most patients recover (Auerbach 1991).

Chemical Poisons Causing Myopathy

Although a number of chemical compounds can cause muscle necrosis experimentally, there are few examples of chemical toxins causing myopathy in clinical practice. Triethyltin poisoning in the rat can lead to core formation, 2, 4-dinitrophenol can cause ragged-red fibres and mitochondrial inclusions, iodoacetates and fluoracetates, which block lactate production, can cause muscle necrosis and organophosphates, which characteristically cause axonal neuropathy in humans, can cause necrosis of muscle fibres after exposure to high doses. This myotoxic effect begins in the end-plate region and may be due to increased neurotransmitter release (Wecker et al. 1978; Good et al. 1993).

Toxins from plants occasionally cause acute necrotising myopathy in cattle, for example senna, but human toxicity has not been documented.

Nutritional Myopathies

These are rare disorders in developed countries.

Vitamin E Deficiency

Vitamin E deficiency causes a necrotising myopathy in the rat, chicken, duck and in domestic pets

(Machlin et al. 1978) and in the Rottnest quokka, an Australian marsupial rodent-like creature. In man, chronic vitamin E deficiency occurs in patients with chronic cholestatic jaundice, and in malabsorption syndromes. In human vitamin E deficiency, sensorimotor neuropathy is the main feature, and myopathy is uncommon (Tomasi 1979; Lazaro et al. 1986). Muscle biopsies show dense, subsarcolemmal bodies, probably lysosomal in origin (Neville et al. 1983) that stain pink in trichrome and purple in haematoxylin and eosin preparations. They are autofluorescent. These bodies are associated with lipofuscin accumulation. In most cases the myopathy appears subclinical in severity, although peripheral neuropathy may be severe and disabling.

Protein-Calorie Malnutrition

The muscular wasting and weakness that accompanies severe, chronic protein-calorie malnutrition in famine-afflicted zones of Africa and India may be associated with myopathic features, and also with some neurogenic change (Dastur et al. 1982). Whether this is more marked than would be expected in cachexia due to starvation is uncertain.

Tropical Sprue and Coeliac Disease

In Southern India a third of patients with tropical sprue had proximal weakness and atrophy, a myopathic EMG pattern and scattered necrotic fibres with Type 2 atrophy in the muscle biopsy (Iyer et al. 1973). There was a similar abnormality in 12% of patients with untreated coeliac disease (Banerji and Hurwitz 1971). The CK is normal in this syndrome. It is possible that this myopathic involvement was secondary to impaired calcium and vitamin D metabolism associated with the malabsorption (Banerji and Hurwitz 1971).

Osteomalacic Myopathy

Proximal muscle weakness, often associated with muscular tenderness or aching, is common in patients with osteomalacia and other metabolic bone diseases (Dastur et al. 1975), but is relatively infrequent in hyperparathyroid states or in hypercalcaemia from other causes, e.g. malignant bone disease. Investigation of the disorder in man has revealed only minor morphological changes in muscle biopsies, including atrophy of muscle fibres, more marked in Type 2 than in Type 1 fibres (Schott and Wills 1975). Although usually considered to be myopathic in origin (Prineas et al. 1965; Skaria et al. 1975), it has been suggested that the muscular weakness associated with osteomalacia and secondary hyperparathyroidism is due to a neurogenic disorder (Mallette et al. 1975). This suggestion is no longer accepted. The precise biochemical abnormality leading to muscular weakness in these patients is uncertain (Schott and Wills 1976). Vitamin D deficiency in osteomalacia reduces calcium uptake, protein synthesis and, by causing a reduction in the ATP stores, may cause weakness and fatiguability in metabolic bone disease (Pleasure et al. 1979). Anticonvulsant medication, especially phenytoin therapy, has been associated with osteomalacic myopathy because of inhibition of calcium transport in the gut and complex effects on bone mineralisation.

Clinical Features

Muscular weakness and muscle pain, with tenderness, occurs in about half of patients with osteomalacia, but in fewer than 10% of patients whose metabolic bone disease is due to primary hyperparathyroidism (Smith and Stern 1967). Muscular weakness may be a presenting feature of patients with metabolic bone disease. In those with nutritional rickets it is an almost invariable presenting symptom. The weakness is proximal and nearly always more severe in the legs than in the arms. It is often associated with bone pain and tenderness, but this pain may be described as being situated deeply within the legs and it is often more prominent after exercise. Muscle wasting often occurs. There is usually a typical waddling, myopathic gait, and hyperactive tendon reflexes. Weakness is usually insidious in onset and progressive, often over a period of months or years. Other symptoms, including loss of height and small stature, diarrhoea, finger clubbing, and renal colic may occur. Hypertension, peptic ulcer and renal failure may also develop.

Laboratory Investigations

Secondary hyperparathyroidism usually results from renal failure, but may be due to vitamin D deficiency. The plasma calcium is often low and parathyroid hormone levels are raised. The raised alkaline phosphatase is an indication of the metabolic bone disease. Steatorrhoea is a common cause of vitamin D deficiency, leading to this syndrome. Anticonvulsant drugs interfere with hepatic vitamin D metabolism and may also cause secondary hyperparathyroidism with osteomalacia and muscle weakness.

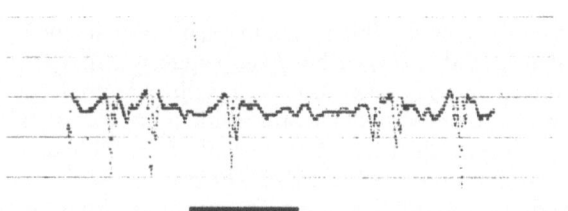

Fig. 19.2. Short-duration, low-amplitude, polyphasic motor unit action potentials in osteomalacic myopathy. Concentric needle EMG. 100 Hz. 10 kHz. Bar 20 ms.

In myopathy associated with osteomalacia the CK is usually normal or only slightly raised. It is important to recognise that since osteomalacic myopathy may be associated with a high or a low blood calcium, there is no direct relationship between the calcium level and the severity of the muscular weakness.

Electrophysiological Assessment

With conventional EMG studies in hyperparathyroidism the insertional activity is often increased. Fibrillation potentials are occasionally noted. During activation short-duration polyphasic MUAPs are prominent even in mild cases (Fig. 19.2) but the fibre density, studied by single-fibre EMG, was normal in two cases we have studied. These EMG abnormalities rapidly reverse with appropriate treatment.

Muscle Biopsy

Even in patients with prominent weakness the changes in the muscle biopsy may be very slight. Prineas et al. (1965) reported scattered atrophic fibres in the biopsy of one case. Others (Ekbom et al. 1964a; Smith and Stern 1967; Dastur et al. 1975) described non-specific fibre atrophy (Serratrice et al. 1978a) with fatty infiltration and subsarcolemmal nuclear proliferation. Ekbom et al. (1964) observed degeneration of single muscle fibres.

Schott and Wills (1975) noted atrophy of Type 2 fibres in two biopsies and in one of these, Type 2B fibres were predominantly affected.

In an experimental study of osteomalacic myopathy in the rat Swash et al. (1979b) found that Type 2B fibre atrophy was the main feature, although increased central nucleation, fibre splitting and a few motheaten fibres were also observed. Scattered small rounded fibres were also a feature. Weakness in osteomalacia is not readily explained by loss of muscle bulk but must depend on abnormalities in calcium transport within the muscle cells. Calcium transport in the sarcoplasmic reticulum is probably dependent on the presence of an active metabolite of vitamin D, 1,25-dihydroxycholecalciferol, formed in the kidney from circulating 25-hydroxycholecalciferol (Currie et al. 1974). Disturbance of calcium transport leads to abnormal excitation–contraction coupling and so to muscle-fibre weakness and atrophy. The fibre atrophy found in this disorder thus resembles disuse atrophy (Swash et al. 1979b). Vitamin D is best regarded as a calcium-related hormone.

Management

Treatment with vitamin D_2 (ergocalciferol) or vitamin D_3 (cholecalciferol) causes an increase in plasma calcium and phosphorus, and a reduction in alkaline phosphatase levels, together with a gradual improvement in muscle strength, and healing of bone lesions with reduction in muscle pain. Oral treatment with 2000–4000 IU daily for 6–12 weeks is adequate, followed by daily supplements of 200–400 IU. Treatment for as long as 6 months may be necessary. Calcium supplements are necessary only if there is dietary malabsorption. Ultraviolet dermal treatment has been used. In hypophosphataemic rickets, in which there is renal loss of phosphate, "megadoses" of vitamin D are necessary. Patients with anticonvulsant drug-induced osteomalacia, associated with myopathy, have low blood calcium levels. Treatment with high doses of vitamin D is necessary, together with calcium supplements.

20 # Cardiomyopathy in Neuromuscular Disorders

The term cardiomyopathy was introduced by Brigden (1957) to indicate myocardial disease not due to myocardial ischaemia or volume/pressure overload of the heart. In clinical practice a functional classification of these myocardial disorders has evolved (Table 20.1). This classification has practical value, although some patients may show features of more than one functional category, e.g. congestive (dilated) cardiomyopathy associated with disorders of conduction or rhythm (Davies 1984). *Congestive cardiomyopathy* implies cardiac failure with impaired ventricular contraction but in some patients ventricular dilatation occurs without cardiac failure. In *hypertrophic cardiomyopathy* a failure of diastolic compliance combined with abnormally rapid or disorganised ventricular contraction may cause functional obstruction to ventricular outflow. In *restrictive* cardiomyopathy the ventricular myocardium is stiff and non-compliant in diastole, due to endocardial thickening, e.g. in endomyocardial fibro-elastosis and in Loeffler's syndrome, or to pericardial disease, e.g. constrictive pericarditis. *Abnormalities of atrio-ventricular conduction or of cardiac rhythm* may also lead to cardiac symptoms, including syncope and heart failure.

Table 20.1. Clinical classification of cardiomyopathies

Congestive cardiomyopathy
  Primary
  Secondary to other disorders

Hypertrophic cardiomyopathy

Restrictive cardiomyopathy
  Endocardial
  Pericardial

Disorders of atrioventricular conduction or rhythm

Involvement of the heart is a well-recognised feature of many neuromusclar diseases. In some,

cardiac involvement may be severe and may even lead to death from congestive failure or arrhythmia but in others cardiac involvement is slight or even subclinical (Tables 20.2 and 20.3).

Table 20.2. Primary diseases of muscle associated with cardiac involvement

Genetically determined myopathies
a. Muscular dystrophies
  Duchenne (an X-linked dystrophinopathy)
  Becker (an X-linked dystrophinopathy)
  Emery-Dreifuss (X-linked)
b. Myotonic dystrophy
c. Metabolic myopathies
  Mitochondrial cytopathies
  Glycogen storage diseases
  Periodic paralyses
  Malignant hyperpyrexia
d. Myopathies of childhood
  Nemaline myopathy
  Myotubular myopathy
  Central core disease

Acquired myopathies
a. Inflammatory myopathies
b. Endocrine myopathies
c. Drug-induced myopathies
d. Infections and infestations

In all these disorders congestive (dilated) cardiomyopathy may occur and in some (Table 20.3), atrioventricular block may develop and, as in

Table 20.3. Neurogenic disorders with cardiomyopathy

Genetically determined polyneuropathies
1. Spinocerebellar degenerations
    Friedreich's ataxia
2. Peripheral neuropathies
    Refsum's disease
    Familial amyloid polyneuropathy (FAP)
    Acute intermittent porphyria

Acquired polyneuropathies
Guillain-Barré syndrome
Diphtheria
Diabetic neuropathy
Alcoholic neuropathy

Kearns–Sayre syndrome, this may be the presenting feature. The earliest abnormality is sinus bradycardia, representing dysfunction in a "sick" sinoatrial node. Atrial flutter may develop causing tachycardia, and as the disease progresses first-degree heart block, right bundle branch block and QRS prolongation representing abnormal intraventricular conduction, and complete heart block may develop (Table 20.4).

Table 20.4. Neuromuscular disorders with atrioventricular conduction block

Myotonic dystrophy
Kearns–Sayre syndrome
Scapulo-peroneal syndrome
Limb-girdle muscular dystrophy
Polymyositis

Afrer Perloff (1981b)

Cardiac involvement is a potentially serious feature of most of these neuromuscular diseases. Cardiomyopathy may be the presenting feature, or may become a major clinical problem. In some it may be a cause of death and in reversible acquired diseases such as Guillain–Barré syndrome it is therefore important to recognise cardiomyopathy as a complication of the disease prior to any serious cardio-circulatory event. In most of the disorders, however, the pathological change in the myocardium is relatively non-specific, consisting of fibrosis, fat replacement, non-specific loss of conducting fibres in the bundle of His, non-specific foci of macrophages and lymphocytes and evidence of necrosis of individual muscle fibres. Necrosis of muscle fibres is particularly a feature of congestive cardiomyopathies, but its features are virtually indistinguishable from those of ischaemic heart disease. A number of more specific abnormalities may be found, e.g. inflammatory changes in cardiomyopathy or polymyositis and amyloid deposition in the cardiomyopathy of hereditary amyloid neuropathy (Davies 1984). Other less specific features include hypertrophy of the media of the coronary arteries with luminal narrowing and scarring of the postero-lateral wall of the left ventricle (Perloff et al. 1967).

Although cardiomyopathy is a relatively frequent feature of neuromuscular diseases, Fairfax (1977) found that of 984 patients with chronic atrioventricular block only six had evidence of an underlying neuromuscular disorder (Lambert and Fairfax 1977). Similarly, most cases of cardiomyopathy presenting to cardiologists show features consistent with primary congestive cardiomyopathy, hypertrophic obstructive cardiomyopathy or restrictive cardiomyopathy (Perloff 1981a).

Primary Diseases of Muscle and Cardiomyopathy

The muscular dystrophies are relatively uncommon inherited disorders of muscle, characterised by a progressive course and by degenerative changes in skeletal muscle fibres. Classification of these disorders depends on clinical, genetic and histological criteria (Table 20.2).

X-Linked Dystrophinopathies

Cardiac involvement is common in these disorders. In both Duchenne and Becker muscular dystrophy the severity of cardiomyopathy does not correlate with the severity of skeletal muscle disease.

Duchenne Muscular Dystrophy

Cardiac involvement is common, occurring in 80% of boys with the disease (Hunsacker et al. 1982), usually manifested as tachycardia, arrhythmia and cardiac failure (Nigro et al. 1990). The cardiac problems become more prominent and frequent as the disease progresses (Boland et al. 1996), but are often masked by the severity of the disability caused by the skeletal muscle weakness and, especially, by ventilatory difficulties related to kyphoscoliosis and intercostal muscle weakness. These thoracic deformities may result in a prominent left sternal impulse and a loud pulmonary second sound. In the preclinical stage, even in early childhood, the ECG is often abnormal (Slucka 1968). The precordial R waves are tall, with increased R/S wave amplitude ratio and deep Q waves in the lateral precordial leads, and in leads I and aVL (Fitch and Auger 1967; Nigro et al. 1990). Some female carriers of the gene also show ECG abnormalities (Lane et al. 1980), and dilated cardiomyopathy has been reported in carriers (Kamakura et al. 1990). Conduction defects may also occur. Hypertrophic cardiomyopathy has been described in the early stages of the disorder. The latter consists of ectopic atrial rhythms, short PR interval and paroxysmal rapid heart action. Ventricular tachycardias also occur and, rarely, sudden death may occur (Perloff 1984). In the later clinical stages a dilated cardiomyopathy commonly develops. In a third of cases this is associated with pulmonary insufficiency with nocturnal oxygen desaturation and hypercarbia. The cardiomyopathy is associated with predilection for involvement of the posterobasal and lateral walls of the left ventricle (Sanyal et al. 1980). Although about 80% of patients with Duchenne disease have cardiomyopathy, death due to heart disease occurs in only 10%.

Histopathological studies (Perloff 1984; Wakai et al. 1988) of the heart show fatty infiltration and mild fibrosis in the sinus and AV nodes. Papillary muscle degeneration may lead to mitral valve prolapse. Fibrous replacement and vacuolar degeneration of muscle fibres, with fatty infiltration of the heart muscle and of the peripheral conduction system, occur. There are abnormalities in the distribution of dystrophin in cardiac myocytes (Schmidt-Achert et al. 1992).

Becker Muscular Dystrophy

This mild form of dystrophinopathy causes less disability, presents later than Duchenne muscular dystrophy, and may have a nearly normal life expectancy. Cardiac involvement is therefore clinically important, and may be the presenting feature of the disease (Quinlivan and Dubowitz 1992). Dilated cardiomyopathy, bundle branch block, tachyarrhythmia or complete heart block may develop. Subclinical cardiomyopathy is very common in Becker muscular dystrophy, and the severity of cardiac involvement is unrelated to age, or to the severity of skeletal muscle disease (Palmucci et al. 1992). The prognosis of Becker dystrophy is variable, some patients having a normal life expectancy. About 30% of patients develop dilated cardiomyopathy and congestive failure (Quinlivan and Dubowitz 1992). Steare et al. (1992) found that although 89% of their patients were symptom free, 74% had abnormal ECGs. In 42% there was RBBB, and echocardiography showed left ventricular dilatation and hypokinesis. Nigro et al (1995) found that 82% of patients older than 40 years had clinically evident myocardial damage. In Becker disease all four cardiac chambers may be affected by dilation, and the disorder is often more severe than in Duchenne disease. Dystrophin staining of the myocardium in Becker dystrophy reveals abnormally patchy staining (Anan et al. 1992). Cardiac transplantation has been used in five patients with Becker dystrophy; two of these patients returned to work (Quinlivan and Dubowitz 1992).

Other Dystrophinopathies

In a family with fatal X-linked dilated cardiomyopathy Muntoni et al. (1993) found that the first exon in the dystrophin gene, and the muscle promoter region were deleted. In this family there was only mild muscular involvement, consisting only of a raised CK level and mildly increased variability in fibre size with increased central nucleation in a needle muscle biopsy. There was no muscular weakness or hypertrophy and the EMG was normal. Dystrophin immunostaining in muscle was normal, but the heart muscle was not examined. Taubin et al. (1993) showed abnormal n-terminal epitopes of the dystrophin molecule in cardiac, but not in skeletal muscle, in families with cardiomyopathy and raised muscle CK levels, but without skeletal muscle weakness. Some of these patients had slightly hypertrophied calves. These syndromes illustrate the heterogeneity of the clinical expression of different deletions within the dystrophin gene at the Xp21 locus.

Emery–Dreifuss Syndrome

This is a rare X-linked (Ch Xq28) disorder in which muscular weakness and wasting develop in a predominantly humero-peroneal distribution during childhood. There are contractures of the elbows, posterior neck muscles and Achilles tendons. Cardiac involvement is invariable. The early cardiac features consist of premature atrial contractions and sinus bradycardia. Later, permanent atrial standstill, atrial fibrillation or flutter develop. There is a risk of A-V block, and sudden death occurs in as many as 50% of patients (Merlini et al. 1986). Cerebral emboli and stroke may also occur. Since most patients have no cardiac symptoms prior to sudden death, cardiac monitoring and follow-up is indicated, and implantation of a pacemaker has been recommended if the heart rate falls below 50/min. Histologically, the heart shows hypertrophy, fibrosis and fatty replacement (Hara et al. 1987).

Myotonic Dystrophy

The disease may sometimes present with cardiomyopathy rather than with the typical manifestations of myotonia, distal weakness and atrophy, and other features.

ECG abnormalities occur in 90% of patients (Church 1967), particularly impaired conduction in the bundle of His. The commonest ECG abnormalities are increased PR and ST intervals. Oram (1981) found that the PR interval was almost always greater than 0.2 ms, and the P wave was small in standard lead 1. Pathologically, the heart may show little abnormality apart from patchy fibrosis and fatty infiltration in the conducting system (Nguyen et al. 1988). These changes lead to delayed and re-entrant conduction and arrhythmias (Perloff et al. 1984). It has been recommended that patients with myotonic dystrophy should be reviewed annually, including

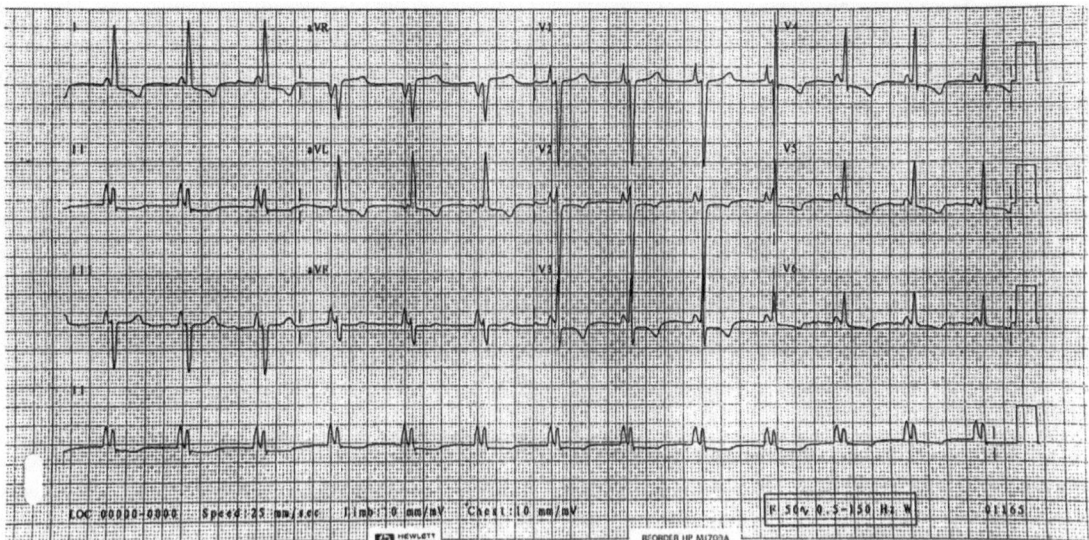

Fig. 20.1. Mitochondrial cytopathy. There is an ectopic sino-atrial pacemaker, with a short PR interval, and a cardiomyopathy with abnormal ventricular repolarisation, associated with abnormal ST segments and inverted waves. In addition, there is an interventricular conduction defect.

ECG studies. Patients with cardiac symptoms, e.g. dizziness or syncope, should have 24-hour monitoring and, if abnormalities are revealed intracardiac electrophysiological studies may be useful (Hawley et al. 1991). As many as 30% patients die suddenly, with Stokes–Adams syncope, conduction block and ventricular arrhythmias (Editorial 1992). Pacing may be required (Hawley et al. 1991). Mitral valve prolapse, due to stretching of the valve annulus, was reported in 17% of a series of patients by Reeves et al. (1980) and Streib et al. (1985).

In addition to the cardiac manifestations, sleep apnoea relates to the progressive involvement of respiratory muscles in the disease, and this complication may be clinically associated with symptomatic cardiomyopathy (Chang et al. 1993).

Mitochondrial Cytopathies

Cardiomyopathy may develop in many of the defects of mitochondrial oxidative phosphorylation, whether due to deletions or point mutations in the mitochondrial DNA or tRNA genes respectively. The clinical syndromes include cardiomyopathies associated with skeletal myopathies of infantile or later onset, or characteristic multisystem disorders such as MELAS, MERRF and Kearns–Sayre syndrome (Petty et al. 1986a; Berenberg et al. 1977). The conduction system is particularly affected (Fig. 20.1), leading to complete heart block, but overt cardiomyopathy with heart failure and dilated cardiomyopathy is unusual. Treatment with a pacemaker, however, is often necessary, e.g. in Kearns–Sayre syndrome (Berenberg et al. 1977). The sequence of abnormality includes left bundle branch block, bifascicular block and then complete block, in a period of 7 years in the case described by Lambert and Fairfax (1977).

A family has been described in which inherited dilated cardiomyopathy was associated with multiple deletions in mitochondrial DNA, but without neurological disease (Suomalainen et al. 1992).

Scapulo-Peroneal Syndrome

Cardiomyopathy is a feature of the X-linked form of scapulo-peroneal myopathy (Rotthauwe et al. 1972) with complete heart block and cardiac failure. Heart block may develop early in the illness, necessitating cardiac pacing (Lambert and Fairfax 1976). In the autosomal dominant form cardiac involvement is unusual (Thomas et al. 1977).

Periodic Paralysis

During hyperkalaemia, due to potassium release from muscle cells, the ECG shows high-peaked T waves and, during hypokalaemia the converse ECG change is seen. In either form of periodic paralysis

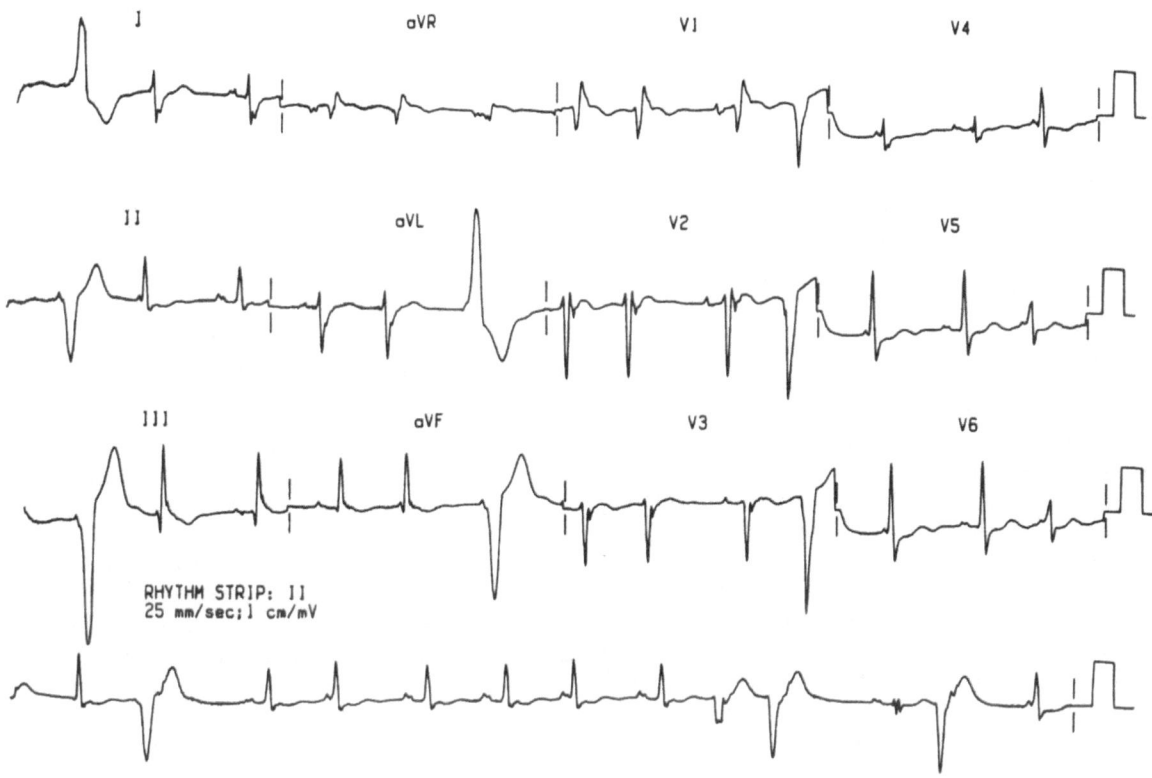

Fig. 20.2. ECG in polymyositis. This patient developed congestive heart failure during treatment. The ECG shows tachycardia, frequent ventricular extra systoles, and abnormal QRS complexes.

ventricular arrhythmias may occur, believed to originate in the left ventricle, that revert with mild exercise, but not necessarily with potassium supplements (Lisak et al. 1972; Karpawich et al. 1987). Death from cardiac arrest was reported by Levitt et al. (1972).

Glycogenoses

In Pompe's disease, the infantile-onset form of Type II glycogenosis associated with acid maltase deficiency, cardiac involvement is one of the features of the systemic involvement that is characteristic of the disease. Cardiomegaly and heart failure are evident and death usually occurs from cardiorespiratory failure before the second birthday. The ECG shows very large QRS complexes, with a short PR interval in some cases of the adult-onset form of the disorder (Lenard et al. 1974), but in others it is normal (Swash et al. 1985). In Pompe's disease the ventricular myocardium is greatly thickened, and is much stiffer than normal (Oram 1981), and sudden death in infancy is common. The heart may also be involved, with cardiac failure, in the adult-onset

form of Type III glycogenosis (Cornelio and Di Donato 1985).

In McArdle's disease (Type IV glycogenosis) the ECG may resemble that of Pompe's disease, with large QRS complexes and T wave changes. However, unlike Pompe's disease, the PR interval is normal or increased (Oram 1981).

Inflammatory Myopathies

Cardiac involvement, including congestive heart failure, pericarditis, myocarditis and arrhythmia, has been reported in polymyositis and dermatomyositis at any stage of the disease (Gottdiener et al. 1978). Although it has been suggested that as many as 50% of patients with polymyositis have serious cardiac manifestations such as congestive failure, clinically significant features of cardiac disease are uncommon in unselected series of patients (Haupt and Hutchins 1982). Asymptomatic ECG abnormalities occur in many cases, perhaps as many as 50% (Askari and Huettner 1982), consisting of tachyarrhythmias (Fig. 20.2) and conduction defects, but the most sensitive index of cardiac involvement is an increased blood level of CK_{MB}. Serum cardiac troponin T levels may also be a sensitive index of cardiac involvement (Kobayashi et al. 1992). Most patients with clinically significant cardiac involvement are elderly, or have a history of several months of muscular weakness. The cardiomyopathy usually improves with treatment with steroids and immunosuppressant drugs but, occasionally, it may be fulminant, acute and fatal (Bhan et al. 1990). Transplantation may be the only form of treatment feasible in these cases.

Autopsy studies of the heart have revealed widespread myocardial necrosis with focal areas of relative sparing and evidence of regeneration. In some cases infiltration with mononuclear cells has been recorded (Gottdiener et al. 1978).

Similar cardiac complications may occur in other collagen–vascular diseases, especially in systemic lupus erythematosus and scleroderma. Oram and Stokes (1961) found that 11 of 49 patients with scleroderma had cardiac involvement as a presenting feature, but conduction block is particularly common in the terminal stages (Roberts 1981). Necrosis and fibrosis of the nodal tissue occurs less frequently in systemic lupus erythematosus, and in polyarteritis (see Davies et al. 1985).

Inclusion Body Myositis

This disorder is a non-vasculitic form of inflammatory myopathy recognised as distinct from other forms of myositis only in the last decade. Lotz et al. (1989) found cardiac abnormalities in 22 of their series of 40 patients. These consisted of ECG evidence of rhythm disturbances, conduction defects and ischaemic change. Two were in cardiac failure and one had hypertrophic cardiomyopathy. Eighteen were hypertensive. The average age at diagnosis was 64 years, and the specificity of these features in this disorder is uncertaon.

Neurogenic Disorders with Cardiomyopathy

Neurogenic weakness may result from genetic or acquired disease of anterior horn cells, or from genetic or acquired disease of peripheral nerves (Table 20.3). The spinal muscular atrophies, most of which are inherited as autosomal recessive disorders, do not involve the heart, and the commonest inherited type of peripheral neuropathy, the heredi-

tary motor and sensory neuropathies (HMSN; Charcot-Marie-Tooth disease) also spare the heart.

Friedreich's Ataxia

In his original description in 1863 Friedreich noted cardiac abnormalities at autopsy in three of his six subjects. The incidence of cardiac signs and symptoms in the early stages of the disease is low, however, despite the finding of ECG changes in about 80% of patients (Harding 1981). These ECG abnormalities consist of inverted T waves, right axis deviation and abnormal ST segments. However, cardiac disease is often the cause of death (Child et al. 1986). The most common cardiac symptom is exertional dyspnoea, a symptom which is limited in its expression by the immobility that usually develops as the disorder progresses. Most patients are restricted to a wheelchair by age 25 years. Hewer (1968) reported death from heart failure in 46 of his 82 fatal cases, and evidence of cardiac dysfunction during life in 60 patients. The mean age at death is 37 years. Echocardiography commonly reveals concentric left ventricular hypertrophy and asymmetrical septal hypertrophy (Pentland and Fox 1983). In contrast to idiopathic hypertrophic cardiomyopathy malignant ventricular arrhythmias are rare. Dilated cardiomyopathy is uncommon and may represent a different form of the disease, in which atrial and ventricular arrhythmias occur (Harding and Hewer 1983).

Refsum's Disease

This rare autosomal recessive disorder is characterised by peripheral neuropathy, ataxia, deafness, ichthyosis, night blindness, pes cavus and cardiomyopathy, with storage of a lipid, phytanic acid, in the tissues. Congestive heart failure, arrhythmias and acute left ventricular failure tend to develop in relation to relapses in the neuropathy, and may lead to sudden death, perhaps associated with autonomic involvement. The heart shows patchy fibrosis (Skjeldaal et al. 1992).

Family Amyloid Polyneuropathy (FAP)

In this dominantly inherited group of disorders amyloid fibrillar protein is deposited in many tissues, including the heart. The main feature in the Portuguese (Type I) form of the disease is progressive peripheral neuropathy with distal pain and sensory loss. There are prominent autonomic disturbances, including impotence, diarrhoea, incontinence, hypotension and pupillary abnormalities. In other forms, e.g. Type II FAP, carpal tunnel syndrome is the mean presenting feature. Cardiac manifestations consist of constrictive or congestive cardiomyopathy. The importance of cardiomyopathy varies in different mutations of the transthyretin gene (Ch 18.1) (Kyle and Dyck 1992). In one such mutation in Denmark (MET 111) cardiomyopathy is the major feature of the disease (Husby et al. 1985).

Guillain–Barré Syndrome (GBS)

The autonomic nervous system is frequently affected in this acute post-infective polyneuropathy. This may lead to sudden death, probably due to cardiac arrhythmia (Lichtenfeld 1971). Most patients show sinus tachycardia, due to relative overactivity of the sympathetic innervation of the heart. Vagal involvement is shown by loss of normal sinus arrhythmia and by fluctuations of blood pressure, leading to hypertension and arrhythmias that may presage sudden death (Winer and Hughes 1988). The most common problem is sinus bradycardia or asystole occurring after tracheal suction in ventilated patients. The ECG shows atrial and ventricular arrhythmias, often with inverted T waves (Hughes 1991). Cardiac monitoring is advisable in patients with GBS sufficiently severe to warrant assisted ventilation.

Alcoholic Myopathy

The cardiomyopathy associated with alcoholism is often associated with alcoholic myopathy but relatively rarely accompanies alcoholic neuropathy, and is not necessarily found in patients with hepatic cirrhosis, suggesting that it is due to the alcohol itself, and not to any associated vitamin deficiency. In thiamine deficiency the ECG is usually normal even in the presence of congestive heart failure. In alcoholic congestive cardiomyopathy the ECG shows pathological Q waves and T wave changes consisting of pointed, dimpled or sharply inverted waves (Regan 1973; Rubin 1979). The functional capacity of the heart is reduced long before clinical abnormalities become apparent (Rubin 1979). Mural thrombi are common in the grossly dilated alcoholic heart and anticoagulant therapy is indicated to prevent pulmonary and systemic embolisation. Demakis et al. (1974) noted that almost 50% of patients with alcoholic cardiomyopathy died within 3 years.

Diphtheria

Sudden death from cardiac arrhythmia is a well-known feature of diphtheria. Two-thirds of patients with the disease develop myocarditis but this is clinically apparent in only about 10% of cases. The development of arrhythmias or heart block is common in those with cardiac involvement and is frequently fatal. Congestive failure is rare. Fibrosis may develop leading to permanent cardiac problems (Good 1948; Kurdi and Abdul-Kader 1979). Cardiac involvement is classically evident 3–5 weeks after recovery from the infection, and may occur without involvement of the peripheral nervous system.

Endocrine Myopathies

In *hypothyroidism* the heart rate is slow, and the QRS complexes are of low voltage. The PR interval is prolonged. There may be some features of restrictive cardiomyopathy, especially affecting the right ventricle, with pericardial effusion. Part of the ECG change may be due to changes in skin resistance in the disease. Associated ischaemic heart disease, or metabolic change in myocardial cells due to the hypothyroidism, is a risk factor during normalisation of cardiac function with thyroid replacement therapy.

In *hyperthyroidism* the characteristic features are tachycardia and atrial fibrillation. Rarely, left ventricular failure may occur, due to the cardiomyopathy and the high-output state associated with the hypermetabolism.

In *acromegaly* the heart is markedly enlarged, especially involving the left ventricle. Individual muscle fibres are enlarged and there is myocardial fibrosis. Heart failure occurs in two-thirds of the patients, and arrhythmias and heart block also occur.

Carcinoid syndrome is rarely associated with skeletal muscle disease but damages the heart by causing thickening of the tricuspid and pulmonary valves, leading to heart failure.

Skeletal Muscle in Primary Cardiomyopathies

Skeletal muscle function may be abnormal in patients with primary cardiomyopathies. Cafario

Table 20.5.   Need for cardiological investigation and intervention

Diagnosis	Presentation	Risk	Cardiological management
Duchenne dystrophy	Weakness	Sudden death Cardiac failure Tachyarrhythmia	Diuretics, vasodilators and glycosides
Becker dystrophy	Weakness, Cardiac failure	Dilated cardiomyopathy Tachyarrhythmia RBBB	Diuretics, vasodilators and glycosides Cardiac transplantation
Emery-Dreifuss	Muscular syndrome and cardiac failure	Sudden death A-V block	Regular assessment Pacemaker, ?Transplantation
Myotonic dystrophy	Muscular syndrome and cardiac failure	Stokes–Adams syncope and ventricular arrhythmia	Annual ECG and echocardiogram Intracardiac physiology Pacemaker
Mitochondrial cytopathy	Neuromuscular syndrome and heart block or cardiac failure	Heart block	Annual ECG Pacemaker ?Transplantation
Polymyositis	Muscular syndrome	Sudden death Cardiac failure	Glycosides and diuretics Regular cardiac assessment Transplantation
Friedreich's ataxia	Neurological syndrome	Cardiac failure Heart block Sudden death	Glycosides and diuretics
Refsum's disease	Neurological syndrome	Sudden death Left heart failure	Glycosides and diuretics
Guillain–Barré syndrome	Acute neuropathy	Tachycardia hypo- and hypertension, Sudden death	Cardiac monitoring during ventilation

et al. (1989) studied skeletal muscle in patients with idiopathic dilated and hypertrophic cardiomyopathies. They found abnormalities of myopathic type in electromyographic (EMG) studies in 35% of patients in both groups. Nine patients had muscle biopsies and all were abnormal, showing mild myopathic changes, including central cores in Type 1 fibres.

These findings must be assessed in relation to the observation that in patients with congestive heart failure, of any cause, skeletal muscle is abnormal, probably as a result of disuse, hypoxia, underperfusion and increased venous pressure. There is atrophy of Type 1, slow twitch fibres and of Type 2B fibres, features typically associated with disuse atrophy.

In 51 patients with familial or non-familial dilated cardiomyopathy none showed a dystrophin gene defect (Michells et al. 1994). Muntoni et al. (1993) noted that dilated cardiomyopathy associated with a raised blood CK_{MM}, in patients of either sex, could be due to an X-linked dystrophinopathy. In some families with familial idiopathic hypertrophic cardiomyopathy there is a mutation in the cardiac B myosin heavy chain gene MYH7, an abnormality that allows predictive genetic testing (Watkins et al. 1992).

Conclusions

There is marked variation in the clinical features and in the severity of cardiomyopathies associated with neuromuscular disease. This complication in this group of disorders has usually been neglected by clinicians. There is a place for regular assessment of vulnerable patients (Table 20.5) in order to prevent sudden death from arrhythmia, and to treat cardiac failure, especially in myotonic dystrophy, Becker dystrophy, and the mitochondrial disorders. Cardiac transplantation has begun to be used in Becker and Emery–Dreifuss dystrophies.

The molecular pathogenesis of these cardiomyopathies is currently poorly understood, but there are sufficient similarities to some of the inherited idiopathic cardiomyopathies to suggest that investigation of the former may lead to better understanding of the latter.

Chapter 21   Miscellaneous Disorders

Stiff Man Syndrome

The stiff man syndrome (Moersch and Woltman 1956) is a disorder characterised by the gradual development of symmetrical stiffness or rigidity of axial and proximal limb muscles. The rigidity is usually associated with spasms of muscular contraction often provoked by sensory or emotional stimuli. The rigidity consists of a board-like contraction which lessens during sleep. There are no other neurological signs. Other causes of muscular rigidity, including metabolic disorders, polymyositis and chronic tetanus (McQuillen et al. 1967) must be excluded.

Most of the early reported cases were men, usually in their fourth or fifth decade (Gordon et al. 1967), but the disorder is, in fact, equally common in either sex (Thompson 1993). It usually comes on insidiously over a period of weeks or months. Stiffness occurs in brief episodes at first, becoming more persistent later. Axial muscles are usually involved earlier and more severely than limb muscles. Examination shows persistent, maintained contraction of muscle groups. The face and distal limb muscles are usually spared but most other muscles are involved and dysphagia may occur. The spine is rigid and may be hyperextended. The abdominal muscles are contracted. Attempts to contract muscles voluntarily, or passive movement induced during examination, often evoke intense, painful muscular spasms which begin in the part moved and spread to all muscle groups. These spasms of contraction may last several minutes before gradually lessening; the so-called jerking stiff man syndrome (Leigh et al. 1980). Other stimuli, including pain, a full bladder and emotional distress, will also induce painful spasms and copious sweating in the attacks. Spasticity and extra-pyramidal rigidity are absent, and the plantar responses are flexor. No other abnormality is found in the nervous system; the external ocular muscles are spared. The rigidity is reduced, or even absent, during sleep and

it is also abolished by neuromuscular blocking drugs. No fasciculations or involuntary movements are observed.

The stiff man syndrome is a rare disorder, and there has been much discussion as to whether it represents a single nosological entity (Gordon et al. 1967). It has been associated with diabetes mellitus (Howard 1963), thyrotoxicosis (Werk et al. 1961) and multiple pituitary hormone deficiencies (George et al. 1984). Solimena et al. (1990) noted that two-thirds of patients had diabetes mellitus with auto-antibodies to pancreatic B cells, together with antibodies to GABA-ergic neurons. Whiteley et al. (1976b) described a similar disorder due to a form of progressive encephalomyelitis with rigidity, a syndrome previously reported by Kasperek and Zebrowski (1971) and by Lhermitte et al. (1973).

The stiffness is thought to result from an imbalance between facilitating long-latency spinal reflex pathways and the inhibitory effects of GABA in the spinal cord grey matter (Thompson 1993). Antibodies against GABA-ergic neurons have been detected in 60% of patients, and these have been identified as anti-glutamic acid decarboxylase (GAD) antibodies, the same antibodies that are often detected in Type I diabetes mellitus (Gorin et al. 1990; Solimena et al. 1990). Johnstone and Nussey (1994) found that some of these anti-GAD antibodies were IgG class antibodies.

Laboratory Tests

Most investigations yield normal results but CSF lymphocytosis with a slightly raised protein has been noted in those cases ascribed to viral encephalomyelitis (Whiteley et al. 1976; Howell et al. 1979). Two cases of progressive encephalomyelitis with rigidity in whom anti-GAD antibodies were found have been described, suggesting that the inflammatory response in this disorder might be auto-immune in origin (Meinck 1992). Bateman et al. (1990) reviewed the relation of subacute myoclonic spinal neuronitis to paraneoplastic disease. Folli et al. (1993) reported three patients with breast cancer associated with antibodies against a 128 KDa brain protein antigen. These patients did not have anti-GAD antibodies.

Electrophysiological Assessment

The characteristic finding is continuous motor unit activity in all muscles sampled, despite attempts at relaxation. The action potentials themselves are of normal configuration and amplitude (Moersch and Woltman 1956). Nerve blocks abolish this motor unit activity (Valli et al. 1983). Nerve conduction velocities are normal. Howard (1963) showed that this ongoing motor unit activity was reduced by diazepam administration. It is presumed that the most likely cause for the excessive motor unit activity is abnormal function in interneurons and their descending spinal reflex control (see above and Meinck et al. (1984)).

Exteroceptive reflexes, e.g. blink reflexes and abdominal reflexes, are of shortened latency and longer duration than normal, indicating an increased excitability of motor cells in brain stem and spinal cord, and repetitive firing of these neurons. This is probably due to decreased inhibition from a disorder of descending brain-stem systems which usually exert a net inhibitory influence on brain stem and spinal motor neuron excitability (Meinck et al. 1984; Meinck and Conrad 1986). In another patient Leigh et al. (1980) commented on the association of myoclonus of brain-stem origin with features of stiff man syndrome. However, in the typical cases of this rare syndrome myoclonus is absent (Moersch and Woltman 1956).

Pathology

No characteristic abnormality has been noted in muscle biopsies, except in those cases in which polymyositis has become apparent as the diagnosis after this investigation. A few degenerate fibres and slight fibrosis have also been reported. In typical stiff man syndrome no abnormality is detected in the CNS (Thompson 1993).

In the cases due to progressive encephalomyelitis perivascular lymphocytic infiltration with gliosis in the spinal cord and brain stem have been noted, with diffuse neuronal loss in the anterior horns, especially in the cervical region, and degeneration of the dorsal columns and anterior spino-thalamic tracts (see Whiteley et al. 1976b). These findings corroborate the suggestion that the rigidity is due to uninhibited tonic discharge of anterior horn cells, perhaps due to selective loss of spinal internuncial neurons – a form of "spinal rigidity".

Management

The spasms but not the rigidity can sometimes be relieved by diazepam or baclofen but in some cases no effective therapy can be found (Whiteley et al. 1976b). The prognosis in these cases is poor but occasionally the disorder may enter a non-progressive phase, with residual severe disability.

Drugs, such as clonidine, tizanidine and methylamphetamine, that produce α-adrenergic stimulation may lead to reflex suppression and muscular relaxation (Meinck and Conrad 1986). Tizanidine 0.3 mg daily in two divided doses was effective in reducing the rigidity in the patient described by Meinck and Conrad (1986). Sodium valproate and baclofen may also be effective in some cases (Spehlmann et al. 1981; Miller and Korsvick 1981). Plasma exchange, used with prednisolone, has been reported effective in some cases (Brasher and Phillips 1991), evidence for an autoimmune aetiology.

Continuous Muscle Fibre Activity Syndrome (Isaacs' Syndrome) and Neuromyotonia

Neuromyotonia and continuous muscle fibre activity are the same phenomenon; there is continuous activity of motor units. The disorder may occur in association with peripheral neuropathy (see below) or as an isolated phenomenon, sometimes inherited.

Table 21.1. Isaac's syndrome (neuromyotonia)

Sporadic acquired neuromyotonia
Associated with neuropathy
Chronic inflammatory demyelinating neuropathy
Paraneoplastic neuropathy
Hereditary motor and sensory neuropathy
Dominantly inherited Isaac's syndrome

In continuous muscle fibre activity syndrome (Isaacs 1961; Isaacs and Heffron 1974) there is muscular contraction resulting in a stooped posture with stiffness of the arms and legs. The wrists are often flexed, and the fingers extended. The feet are plantar flexed and an equinus deformity may develop. The muscular contraction underlying these abnormal postures is not modified by sleep, but movement may lead to transient increase or decrease in the amount of stiffness. In the early stages of the disorder stiffness may only develop following exercise. The syndrome seems to continue for many years but gradual improvement may occur

(Isaacs and Heffron 1974). The disorder is very rare (Welch et al. 1972). Sweating is prominent, perhaps due to heat generated in the contracting muscles. Unlike stiff man syndrome, pain is not a feature of Isaacs' syndrome. Reflexes are usually absent, either because of inhibition of the spinal stretch reflex by the continuous muscle activity or due to an underlying peripheral neuropathy (Thompson 1993).

Sometimes the affected muscles show continuous waves of undulating muscular contraction; this is particularly evident in the earlier stages of the syndrome. This *myokymia* is thus part of the syndrome of continuous muscle fibre activity if it is generalised, and there are earlier descriptions of such patients (Gardner–Medwin and Walton 1969; Lutschg et al. 1978).

The syndrome can occur with, or without, an associated peripheral neuropathy. The latter may be due to hereditary motor and sensory neuropathy, CIDP, toxic neuropathy or of unknown cause. Some cases are inherited (Ashizawa et al. 1983; Auger et al. 1984); in these there is no associated neuropathy. In the latter cases nerve biopsies are normal (Auger et al. 1984). Of 40 cases reviewed by Newsom–Davis and Mills (1993) five had an associated thymoma, two myasthenia gravis, two a raised AChR antibody level and one was induced by D-penicillamine therapy (Reeback et al. 1979). Passive transfer of IgG into mice resulted in increased efficacy of neuromuscular transmission with an enhanced resistance to *d*-tubocurarine (Sinha et al. 1991). ACh quantal release was increased in these mice, suggesting that there was an antibody present reactive against pre-synaptic potassium channels (Shillito et al. 1995).

Terminology

It is difficult to separate cases described in the literature as neuromyotonia, for example those described by Reeback et al. (1979) and by Lance et al. (1979), from those described variously as continuous muscle fibre activity (Isaacs 1961), or as myokymia (Gardner–Medwin and Walton 1969; Hughes and Matthews 1969; Welch et al. 1972). The term neuromyotonia was introduced by Mertens and Zschoke (1965). It may develop during infancy or even in the newborn (Black et al. 1972), and laryngeal spasm has been reported. Using intraneural recordings in two siblings with neuromyotonia associated with Charcot–Marie–Tooth disease (Lance et al. 1979; Vasilescu et al. 1984) showed that there was hyperexcitability of both sensory and motor nerve fibres. Proximal procaine nerve blocks reduced, but did not abolish, the amount of neural activity recorded in these fibres. Warmolts and Mendell (1980) have suggested that neuromyotonia results from repetitive discharges in motor nerves induced by afferent or efferent impulses passing along the nerve toward a damaged segment. Reeback et al. (1979) studied two patients with symptomatic neuromyotonia, one associated with penicillamine therapy given for rheumatoid arthritis and the other in a patient with Guillain–Barré syndrome associated with Hodgkin's disease. The former responded to phenytoin 300 mg daily and the latter to carbamazepine 800 mg daily. In neuromyotonia (see Chap. 2) motor units discharge at rapid rates, even approaching 200 Hz, thus suggesting that the activity does not represent neuronal firing. The amplitude of the activity shows a decrement during continuous recordings. Neuromyotonia differs from myokymia in that the latter consists of grouped action potentials, followed by electrical silence, occurring in a repetitive, even rhythmic sequence.

The term neuromyotonia is now used to describe the clinical phenomenon interchangeably with Isaac's syndrome, recognising that there are a variety of acquired forms, and also an inherited syndrome.

Electrophysiological Assessment

Concentric needle EMG reveals bursts of MUAPs firing at varying speeds: up to 50 Hz or even 200 Hz. Some units tend to fire in doublets or triplets. The MUAPs usually have a normal duration and amplitude although low-amplitude units, and polyphasic units of increased duration, may be found (Welch et al. 1972). Following voluntary activity this spontaneous activity becomes briefly less evident. Sometimes trains of motor unit activity can be correlated with myokymia. Single-fibre EMG shows the continuous motor unit activity. The fibre density was increased in two of three patients examined. The neuromuscular jitter was increased and some potentials showed impulse blocking (Stålberg and Trontelj 1994). The motor and sensory nerve conduction velocities may be mildly slowed, and the terminal motor latencies are increased (Wallis et al. 1970) in patients with an associated or causative neuropathy. Fibrillation and fasciculation potentials are noted in up to 75% of patients.

The spontaneous motor unit activity is abolished by curare, but not by spinal anaesthesia. Peripheral nerve blocks with procaine do not modify the muscle activity if the nerve blocks are applied proximally. However, motor point infiltration with procaine will reduce the muscle fibre activity recorded by EMG (Wallis et al. 1970). These observations suggest that the defect is situated in the terminal parts of the motor axons. This suggestion is in accord with the immune transfer experiments described above (Sinha et al. 1991). In some cases the excess excitability may be generated at nodes of Ranvier in the distal innervation (see Newsom-Davis and Mills 1993).

Muscle and Nerve Biopsy

Muscle biopsies show increased variability in fibre size, with fibre-type grouping and scattered small, pointed denervated muscle fibres. Sural nerve biopsies may show evidence of some segmental demyelination (Wallis et al. 1970; Welch et al. 1972) in patients with peripheral neuropathy. The terminal arborisation of the motor nerves shows excessive branching, with proliferative terminal branching of some motor end-plates (Isaacs and Frere 1974).

Management

The muscular stiffness can sometimes be relieved by phenytoin (Isaacs 1961) or by carbamazepine (Lance et al. 1979). Spontaneous remission has been reported (Isaacs and Heffron 1974). Immunosuppressant therapy with prednisolone and azathioprine has been reported as successful (Sinha et al. 1991) and plasma exchange is also helpful (Newsom–Davis and Mills 1993).

Rippling Muscle Disease

This autosomal dominant disorder was first recognised by Torbergson in 1975. It consists of electrically silent rippling contractions passing across muscles in a characteristic lateral rolling cadence induced by mechanical stimulation, voluntary contraction or exercise. Patients present with muscle cramp, stiffness and pain. Muscular hypertrophy may develop, particularly of the calves. Percussion of a muscle may induce localised contractions, persisting for up to 20 seconds, accompanied by a short burst of EMG activity. There is no electrical myotonia. The CK may be increased, up to 17 times normal. Muscle biopsy shows mild non-specific abnormalities. The rippling muscle waves are propagated at a velocity of 0.6 m/s, only 10% of the propagation velocity of the muscle fibres (Ricker et al. 1989b). A family described by Stephan et al. (1994) showed a gene locus at chromosome 1q 41, although other families did not map to this locus. The disorder is believed to be due to defective myofibrillar contraction. There is no neural, membrane or excitation-contraction compling abnormality recognised. Dantrolene may be effective in reducing muscle stiffness.

Restless Legs Syndrome

Ekbom described this syndrome in 1944. The syndrome arises in adults, and continues indefinitely. It consists of unpleasant crawling or itching paraesthesiae felt deeply in the legs and thighs. These sensations are induced by repose and are relieved by movement so that the patient's legs appear restless. Cramp may be a feature. Periodic movements occur during sleep, consisting of rhythmic movements of one or both legs, with awakening. These movements distress both the patient and their partner. Ekbom's syndrome occurs in a variety of mild neuropathies, but especially in uraemic patients (Callaghan 1966; Thomas et al. 1971; Thomas 1978) and in diabetes (Gorman et al. 1965). Some cases are familial, with a dominant pattern of inheritance; there are no clinical features of neuropathy in these cases. In most cases, however, there is no evident aetiology.

Spillane et al. (1971) reported patients, with electrophysiological evidence of mild peripheral neuropathy or root lesions, in whom the paraesthetic sensations were induced by rest, and relieved by movement, which they termed "painful legs and moving toes", an observation which serves to deepen the confusion surrounding the nosology of Ekbom's syndrome. Some cases have been associated with anaemia. The symptoms may be relieved by chlorpromazine 50–100 mg at night, and by clonazepam 0.5 mg b.d. The latter treatment was effective in 14 of 15 patients with restless legs complicating uraemia (Read et al. 1981). L-Dopa has also been reported effective (von Scheele 1986). L-Dopa has been proposed as treatment of first choice, although the results are variable. Carbamazepine was more effective than placebo in 274 patients treated by Telstaad et al. (1984), although placebo itself was also effective.

Chronic Fatigue Syndrome

Epidemiological surveys suggest that fatigue is a common symptom, only second in frequency to respiratory symptoms in community surveys (Hanney 1978). Point prevalence rates for fatigue were 14.3% for men and 20.4% for women in the USA (Chen

1986) and 20% and 30% in the UK (Cox et al. 1987). David et al. (1991) noted that these responses reflected the design of the questionnaire, and the question asked, and that fatigue and chronic fatigue syndrome were probably different qualitatively and quantitatively.

Sharpe et al. (1991) defined chronic fatigue syndrome as chronic, severe fatigue, of 6 months duration or more, that is disabling, in the absence of neurological signs; myalgia, psychiatric symptoms and previous viral infection are common, but not necessary, associated features. The term chronic fatigue syndrome itself was introduced by Holmes et al. (1988). The US Center for Disease Control has used the diagnostic system of Holmes et al. (1988) comprising two major criteria (fatigue, and the absence of a cause), 11 minor criteria and three physical criteria (Table 21.2).

Table 21.2. CDC criteria for chronic fatigue syndrome

Major criteria
1. Persistent or relapsing debilitating fatigue for >6 months
2. Absence of a recognised organic aetiology for fatigue

Minor criteria
1. Mild fever
2. Sore throat
3. Painful lymph nodes in neck or axillae
4. Unexplained generalised muscle weakness
5. Myalgia or muscle discomfort
6. Prolonged fatigue (>24 hrs) after moderate exercise
7. Generalised headaches
8. Migratory arthralgia without joint swelling or redness
9. Neuropsychological complaints; e.g. depression, poor concentration, photophobia
10. Sleep disturbance
11. Rapid onset of the syndrome

Physical examination
1. Low grade fever
2. Non-exudative pharyngitis
3. Palpable or tender lymph nodes

After Holmes et al. (1988).

David et al. (1990) surveyed 611 people consecutively attending a general practice, only one of whom fulfilled these strict criteria, although 11.5% had symptoms of fatigue, with other of the features noted by Holmes et al. (1988) for more than three months. Pawlikowska et al. (1994) reported that only 1.4% of patients with excessive tiredness themselves considered they had the chronic fatigue syndrome. The prevalence in the general population is unknown; however, Lloyd et al. (1990) reported a prevalence of 40/100 000 in New South Wales, Australia. Since fatigue is such a common symptom in apparently normal people some more rigorous definition of fatigue as a symptom in isolation is needed before it can be recognised as a discrete symptom. Fatigue was recognised as a problem in clinical practice in the past; indeed there are many

reports in the literature at the turn of the century (Wessely and Thomas 1990). An epidemic of fatigue, termed benign myalgic encephalomyelitis, at the Royal Free Hospital in London in 1955 (Medical Staff 1957; Ramsay 1986) led to attempts to characterise a non-epidemic, non-infectious fatigue syndrome, and consequent polarisation of views, with extensive involvement of the media and of patient-activist groups in a discussion characterised by polemic, intense belief in the syndrome and rejection of the concept by many physicians. Maclean and Wessely (1994) noted that the popular view of the syndrome, reinforced by the media, is biased toward an organic origin, and tends to be critical of medical disbelief.

Associated Features

Chronic fatigue syndrome is accompanied by a number of striking associated features, including an over-representation of upper social classes, noted not only in modern times (Wessely 1990) but more than a hundred years ago (Savage 1875; see Wessely and Thomas 1990). Ramsay (1986) at the Royal Free Hospital noted an over-representation of healthcare professionals among patients that was also noted in 1880 (Wessely and Thomas 1990).

An association with viral infection is commonly reported but, since viral infection occurs in 90% of the population annually, this simple association is likely to be non-causative (Wessely and Thomas 1990). Several viral infections, however, are characterised by post-viral fatigue, e.g. Epstein-Barr virus (EBV) and Coxsackie virus infections. However, titres of antibodies to these and other viruses are not more common in patients with chronic fatigue syndrome than in the general population (Straus et al. 1985, 1988) and fatigue is not a regular accompaniment of viral infections, nor does it persist after EBV infection for longer than a few weeks. Landay et al. (1991), however, found evidence of immune activation, as a non-specific response, and increased titres of antibody to early antigen of EBV in 51% of patients, but in only 15% of controls. Coxsackie virus infection, similarly, may cause fatigue, but there is little or no convincing evidence that such infections can be incriminated in the pathogenesis of the chronic fatigue and neuropsychiatric disorder so characteristic of the chronic fatigue syndrome (Wessely and Thomas 1990).

Neuropsychiatric Features

Psychiatric disorder is common in patients with chronic fatigue syndrome. The commonest psychiatric disorder in these patients is depression, occurring in about 50% of cases, and somatisation (13%), minor depression (6%), phobia (2%), anxiety disorder (4%) and conversion disorder (2%) also occur. No psychiatric diagnosis was apparent in only 23% of cases (Wessely and Powell 1989). Clearly, causation in chronic fatigue syndrome associated with depression can be in either direction, but fatigue is itself a well-established symptom in depressive illness.

Neurophysiological Assessment

Conventional motor and sensory nerve conduction studies are normal (Thomas 1987). Conventional EMG is also normal. Single-fibre EMG studies showed varying abnormalities in neuromuscular jitter (Jamal and Hansen 1985; Roberts 1990), but no evidence of impulse blocking, a feature suggesting that the interpretation of jitter in these studies needs reassessment. Fatigue could only be correlated, as in myasthenia gravis, with impulse blocking but not with increased jitter. Central motor conduction time is normal (Waddy et al. 1990), as are standard evoked potential studies (Prasher et al. 1990). Lloyd et al. (1991) showed no difference in isometric force, maximal twitch force, twitch contraction time, or in central activation in subjects with chronic fatigue compared with normals and concluded that neither poor motivation nor muscle contractile failure are important in "fatigue" as a symptom in these patients. Repetitive stimulation is normal at both low and high rates of motor nerve stimulation.

Magnetic resonance spectroscopic studies have shown no consistent abnormality in muscle at rest, or after fatiguing exercise (Arnold et al. 1984). Sometimes co-contraction of agonists and antagonists is seen during "fatigue", implying a psychogenic origin for a factitious complaint of fatigue. The CK is normal in chronic fatigue syndrome.

Management

Organically determined treatments are not effective. Thus antibiotics, antiviral treatments, vitamin supplements, special diets and other energy-enhancing treatments do not cause improvement. Treatment consists of three components. Compassion and understanding are essential and continuing requirements. Attempts to "shame" the patient into recovery are counter-productive. Underlying depression or other psychiatric disorder, together with any evident precipitating causes should be managed conventionally. Important precipitating life events should be explored. Tricyclic antidepressants, which are also effective in the treatment of insomnia, form the mainstay of treatment. Rest, particularly

bedrest, should be avoided, since it simply serves to increase the underlying loss of muscle conditioning and physical fitness that leads to early fatigue on modest effort. By contrast, a graded exercise programme under the supervision of a physiotherapist or aerobics gymnasium will often produce sustained improvement, although some patients are refractory to all attempts to help them (Newham and Edwards 1979; Bonner et al. 1994). Much difficulty is often experienced in raising the patient's level of confidence so that they can return to ordinary activities or to employment without overwhelming stress and lapse back into fatigue, inactivity and a sick-role. Studies of outcome in the long term (Wilson et al. 1994) show that only 6% of patients were fully recovered after 3 years, 40% found social activity impossible, 20% were unable to perform any physical activity and 25% were in receipt of disability benefit. Vercoulen et al. (1996) reported only a 3% recovery, and 17% improvement, 18 months after diagnosis the mean duration of symptoms was 4–5 years. The only significant predictors of prognosis were primary psychiatric diagnosis during the illness, a long duration of illness, and a strong conviction that the illness represented physical disease (Wilson et al. 1994). These were both predictors of poor outcome.

Primary Fibromyalgia and Overuse Syndromes

Yunus (1983) defined primary fibromyalgia as a disorder characterised by generalised aches and pains, or prominent stiffness involving at least three anatomical sites without evident cause, but with consistent tender points. In many respects this clinical syndrome overlaps chronic fatigue syndrome, but localised tenderness is more marked, and there may be generalised pain (Wolfe et al. 1990). Nineteen of 27 patients with chronic fatigue syndrome studied by Goldenberg et al. (1990) met the diagnostic criteria for fibromyalgia. There may be an association with anxiety, depression, fatigue, headache, vague sensory symptoms, insomnia and irritable bowel syndrome. Many patients note a relation to changes in the weather, and some ascribe these, or similar symptoms, to overuse or repetitive strain in affected muscle groups or joints (Fry 1986; Lederman and Calabrese 1986). The disorder predominantly affects women, and painful trigger points are found in muscles or tendinous insertions (Yunus et al. 1981; Yunus 1983; Bengtsson 1986).

Bengtsson et al. (1986) found ragged-red fibres, moth-eaten fibres, focal inflammatory cell infiltrates and regenerating fibres in biopsies taken from tender points in about half of their 57 patients. Similar changes were observed by Bartels and Danneskiold–Samsøe (1986). Oxygen electrode studies showed reduced tissue oxygenation at these trigger points (Lund et al. 1986). Nerve conduction and EMG studies are normal (Simms and Goldenberg 1988). Management requires explanation, sympathy, longitudinal support, treatment with tricyclic antidepressants and graded increasing physical activity. There is frequently conflict with a desire to obtain or continue with disability payments, whether obtained from the state, the employer or from private insurers, and if this secondary gain is powerful the prognosis, as in chronic fatigue syndrome, is likely to be poor.

Disuse

Immobilisation of a joint results in striking muscular atrophy. This is particularly prominent in the quadriceps when the knee has been immobilised; measurable atrophy of the vastus medialis is apparent after only a few days. Further, full recovery of bulk and strength in this muscle may never occur. The pathogenesis of this disuse atrophy is not yet fully understood. Gibson et al. (1987) noted that the cross-sectional area of the mid-thigh decreased by 17% after immobilisation for 6 weeks following fracture of the tibia; Dastur et al. (1979) found that eight weeks immobilisation caused a 50% reduction in fibre size in this muscle. Tenotomy also leads to rapid muscle atrophy, probably because of lack of muscle tone by contraction against the tendon attachment. It has been thought that the Type 2 fibre atrophy which occurs in patients with rheumatoid arthritis, osteomalacia, thyroid disease, corticosteroid therapy and a number of other neuromuscular disorders (Dubowitz and Brooke 1973) might be due to disuse rather than to a specific effect of these metabolic disorders in muscle.

Studies of the histology of disuse atrophy in the quadriceps after knee injury or immobilisation by plaster casts have shown marked atrophy of Type 1 fibres during the first month (Edstrom 1970, Gibson et al. 1987) but atrophy of both fibre types after 2 to 6 months of immobilisation (Sargeant et al. 1977). Immobilisation increases the ratio of Type 2B to Type 2A fibres (Andersen and Henriksson 1977). Gibson et al. (1988) found that during disuse protein breakdown was normal, but protein synthe-

sis was reduced, leading to loss of muscle bulk. This could be prevented by daily low intensity electrical stimulation of muscle. Goldspink (1977) found that stretch of an immobilised muscle tended to reduce disuse atrophy. Functional impairment is relatively slight, however, as shown in an ingenious one-leg cycling experiment (Sargeant et al. 1977). Stokes and Young (1984) have proposed that rehabilitation programmes should be tailored to these relatively selective patterns of muscle fibre atrophy after disuse, joint injury or joint surgery. In the latter, an inhibitory effect, probably due to joint pain, results in greater muscle wasting than in simple disuse, an effect described by John Hunter in 1835.

Disuse atrophy is most evident in quadriceps. However, it rarely leads to loss of more than 25%–30% of the normal bulk of a muscle, whereas in denervation virtually the whole of a muscle may be lost. In the latter situation, however, muscle fibres are lost; in disuse atrophy the fibres are simply smaller than normal.

In patients with paralysis from central nervous system lesions, e.g. hemiplegia or cervical cord injury, including surgical myelotomy, denervation changes, including EMG abnormalities, e.g. fibrillation potentials (Spaans and Wilts 1982) and histological abnormalities, e.g. target fibres and scattered, angulated atrophic fibres (Segura and Sahgal 1981). After CNS lesions spontaneous EMG activity suggestive of denervation first appeared after 2–3 weeks, and had gradually resolved about 6 months later (Spaans and Wilts 1982). The cause of this lower motor neuron dysfunction in patients with upper motor neuron lesions is obscure, but is believed to be related to trans-synaptic changes, perhaps involving trophic factor abnormalities at the anterior horn cell level. This might cause abnormalities in axonal transport that could lead to lower motor neuron dysfunction (Spaans and Wilts 1982).

In many respects, disuse atrophy resembles the effects of denervation, since there is a reduced resting membrane potential (Albuquerque and McIsaac 1970), reduced propagation velocity possibly due to fibre atrophy (Stålberg and Trontelj 1994), and sprouting of intramuscular nerve fibres (Snider and Harris 1979). It is possible some of these effects reflect upregulation of trophic factor release.

Cachexia

Muscular atrophy in cachexia differs from that found in disuse because although there may be severe loss of muscle bulk, this is not associated directly with disuse, but results from protein catabolism within the muscle. Cachexia usually occurs in malnutrition, chronic infections or cancer and these may themselves cause nutritional disorders (such as vitamin deficiency) or secondary effects on muscle (as in the myopathies associated with malignant disease). Pure cachectic muscular atrophy is thus difficult to define. Muscular atrophy in cachexia usually recovers relatively quickly when nutrition is restored.

The muscle shows a variety of minor histological changes, including scattered fibre necrosis, lipid accumulation, central nucleation and slight endomysial fibrosis but the specificity of these changes is doubtful. These problems have been reviewed by Tomlinson et al. (1969); Emery et al. (1984) reported that protein synthesis in skeletal muscle was reduced sixfold in patients with cachexia due to cancer. This could not be wholly explained by poor food intake (see Brennan 1977), and may be partly due to insulin resistance in muscle so that protein synthesis cannot be increased normally after feeding (Lundholm et al. 1978). Malnutrition, and the other causes of cachexia noted above, leads in addition to increased protein breakdown, the combination of decreased protein synthesis and increased catabolism causing rapid muscle atrophy. In cancer, the muscle atrophy may, in part, be due to a hypermetabolic state.

Protein-calorie malnutrition retards the development of large myelinated nerve fibres and leads to mild segmental demyelination, features perhaps accounting for some of the hypotonia and weakness associated with malnutrition (Chopra et al. 1986).

Ageing

Many aged people show mild to moderate degrees of muscular atrophy. This is usually particularly evident in the arm musculature, and in the quadriceps, but both proximal and distal muscles are affected. Muscle fibre diameter is slightly decreased (Halban 1894). Weakness is not complained of by most elderly people but the maximum tension developed during isometric twitch contraction of the extensor hallucis brevis was 30% less in patients older than 60 years than in young patients (Campbell et al. 1973; Bosco and Komi 1980). Further, Burke et al. (1953) found that grip strength fell by almost a half between the ages of 25 and 79

years. These changes in muscular performance are accompanied by mild distal impairment of fine cutaneous sensibility so that the thresholds for two-point discrimination in the fingers, and for vibration sense in the toes are impaired. Fasciculations are not a feature of the muscular wasting but it is often noticeable that muscular contraction occurs with a peculiar fascicular pattern in the elderly. Exercise programmes in the elderly, however, result in increased muscle bulk even in very aged people.

Electrophysiological Assessment

Wagman and Lesse (1952) noted that ulnar nerve motor conduction velocity was reduced by about 10% in subjects older than 60 years. In addition, Buchthal and Rosenfalck (1966) found that sensory conduction velocity, in both the median and ulnar nerves, was 15% slower in subjects older than 70 years. The amplitudes of the sensory action potentials recorded in these nerves at the level of the wrist were reduced by about 60%. However, certain peripheral nerves, particularly the common peroneal motor conduction and the sural sensory conduction velocities, do not show changes with increasing age (Rosenfalck 1975). The distal motor latency increases in most nerves in the elderly, especially those in the hand.

With concentric needle EMG the mean duration of MUAPs is increased by about 25% in the biceps brachii and first dorsal interosseous muscles by the age of 70 years. The other small hand muscles, however, show much less marked changes with age. Similar changes are found in the quadriceps and tibialis anterior muscles as in the biceps brachii (Rosenfalck 1975). Single-fibre EMG also reveals changes in aged subjects. The fibre density begins to increase in the seventh decade and in the ninth decade it is about twice that found in young subjects. At age 75 years the fibre density in extensor digitorum communis is 2.1, but at age 20 years it is 1.5 (Thiele and Stålberg 1975; Stålberg and Trontelj 1994). Fibrillations are not a feature of normal aged subjects. However, many elderly people have subclinical nerve compression or entrapment syndromes and EMG signs of denervation may be found in the territory of affected nerves, especially the median and common peroneal nerves.

Campbell et al. (1973) found a reduction in numbers of motor units in the extensor digitorum brevis of subjects over the age of 60 years, but this finding was probably due to associated damage to the small motor nerve branches supplying this muscle, caused by pressure injury from the subject's shoes. They also found that in this muscle twitch tensions developed more slowly in elderly than in younger subjects; this phenomenon has also been observed in other muscles in the aged.

Muscle Biopsy

A number of changes have been found in the muscles of the aged, especially those older than 65 years. However, these studies have mainly been carried out at autopsy and the effects of intercurrent disease, and wasting, have not been thoroughly controlled. Furthermore, in most of the studies there is little clinical information as to the presence of neurological disease, such as occult diabetic neuropathy or cervical and lumbar spondylosis. The studies have shown disseminated neurogenic atrophy and, occasionally, grouped denervation atrophy. Wohlfart (1939, 1957) suggested that the changes were due to loss of motor nerve fibres or anterior horn cells, a suggestion supported by Duncan's (1934) counts of ventral root fibres in rats aged 800 days, and by Gardner (1940), who found a 27% reduction in the number of nerve fibres in the ventral roots at the T8 and T9 levels in subjects aged 70 to 79 years. Rubinstein (1960) noted increased fat and fibrous tissue in the muscles of aged subjects with excess lipofuscin in the muscle fibres, and Tomlinson et al. (1969) found denervation changes in muscle from cachectic and demented subjects but not in three of seven elderly subjects who died suddenly. There is evidence of a reduction in number of

muscle fibres in aged muscles and a relative increase in Type 1 fibres from 40% in young men to 65% in men over 60 years, in the vastus lateralis muscle (Larsson et al. 1978).

In studies of muscle spindles Swash and Fox (1972) described a loss of intrafusal muscle fibres, with thickening of the spindle capsule and slight fibrosis of the peri-axial space of the spindles. Moore et al. (1971) found a slight reduction in muscle fibre diameter in senescence and Type 2 fibre atrophy has been reported (Tomanga 1977). However, these changes could be due, at least in part, to disuse (Payton and Poland 1983) and it is possible that they might be prevented by adequate exercise programmes in the elderly population. Thus myofibrillar protein synthesis is not impaired in normal elderly subjects.

Changes in Nerves with Age

In addition to the loss of motor axons found in elderly subjects, described above, there is a reduction in the number of sensory axons with increasing age. This has been shown in the sural nerve by Ochoa and Mair (1969) and by Arnold and Harriman (1970). Nerve sprouting at axon terminals is also less efficient than in younger subjects (Pestronk et al. 1980) and there may be retraction of axon terminals from motor end-plates (Gutmann and Hanzlikova 1976).

References

Abarbanel JM, Frisher S, Osimani A (1986) Primary amyloidosis with peripheral neuropathy and signs of motor neuron disease. Neurology 36: 1125–1127

Abdalla JA, Casley WL, Cousin HK et al. (1992) Linkage of autosomal dominant myotonia congenita (Thomsen's disease) to the TCRB gene locus on chromosome 17q 35. Neurology 42: 1426 (abstract)

Abourizk N, Khalil BA, Bahuth N et al. (1979) Clofibrate-induced muscular syndrome. J. Neurol Sci 42: 1–9

Abramsky O, Brenner T, Lisak RP et al. (1979) Significance in neonatal myasthenia gravis of inhibitory effect of amniotic fluid on binding of antibodies to acetylcholine receptor. Lancet ii: 1333–1335

Abramsky O, Webb C, Teitelbaum D et al. (1975) Cellular immune response to peripheral nerve basic protein in idiopathic facial paralysis (Bell's palsy). J. Neurol Sci 26: 13–20

Abu-Shakra SR, Cornblath DR, Avila OL et al. (1991) Conduction block in diabetic neuropathy. Muscle Nerve 14: 858–862

Achari AN, Anderson MS (1974) Myopathic changes in amyotrophic lateral sclerosis. Neurology 24: 477–481

Ackil AA, Shahani BT, Young RR et al. (1981) Late response and sural conduction studies: usefulness in patients with chronic renal failure. Arch Neurol 38: 482–485

Ackroyd RS, Finnegan JA, Green SH (1984) Friedreich's ataxia. Arch Dis Child 59: 217–221

Adams CBT, Logue V (1971) Studies in cervical spondylotic myelopathy. I. Movement of the cervical roots, dura and cord and their relation to the course of the extrathecal roots. Brain 94: 557–568

Adams CR, Ziegler DF, Lin JT (1983) Mercury intoxication simulating amyotrophic lateral sclerosis. JAMA 250: 642–643

Adams RD, Denny-Brown D, Pearson CM (1962) Diseases of muscle, 2nd edn. Cassell, London

Adrian ED, Bronk DW (1929) The discharge of impulses in motor nerve fibres. II. The frequency of discharge in reflex and voluntary contraction. J Physiol (Lond) 67: 119–151

Afifi AK, Al-Gailany AM, Salman JM et al. (1977) Nerve and muscle in steroid-induced weakness in the rabbit. Arch Phys Med Rehabil 58: 143–148

Afifi AK, Bergman RA, Harvey JC (1968) Steroid myopathy: clinical, histological and cytologic observations. Johns Hopkins Med J 123: 158–174

Afifi AK, Bergman RA, Zellweger H (1973) A possible role for electron microscopy in detection of carriers of Duchenne type muscular dystrophy. J Neurol Neurosurg Psychiatry 36: 643–650

Afifi AK, Najjar SS, Mire-Salman J et al. (1974) The myopathology of the Kocher-Debré-Sémélaigne syndrome. J Neurol Sci 22: 445–470

Afifi AK, Smith JW, Zellweger H (1965) Congenital non-progressive myopathy: central core disease and nemaline myopathy in one family. Neurology 15: 371–381

Agamanolis DP, Askari AD, Di Mauro S et al. (1980) Muscle phosphofructokinase deficiency: two cases with unusual polysaccharide accumulation and immunologically active enzyme protein. Muscle Nerve 3: 456–467

Aguayo AJ, Attiwell M, Trecorten J et al. (1977) Abnormal myelination in transplanted Trembler mouse Schwann cells. Nature 265: 73–75

Aguayo AJ, Nair CPV, Bray GM (1971) Peripheral nerve abnormalities in the Riley–Day syndrome: findings in a sural nerve biopsy. Arch Neurol 24: 106–116

Aicardi J, Castelein P (1979) Infantile neuroaxonal dystrophy. Brain 102: 727–748

Aicardi J, Conti D, Gontieres F (1974) Les formes néonatales de la dystrophie myotonique de Steinert. J Neurol Sci 22: 149–164

Aita JF, Synder DH, Reichl W (1974) Myasthenia gravis and multiple sclerosis: an unusual combination of diseases. Neurology 24: 72–75

Aitken R, Allot EN, Castleden LIM et al. (1937) Observations in a case of familial periodic paralysis. Clin Sci 3: 47–57

Alberca R, Montero C, Ibáñez A et al. (1980) Progressive bulbar paralysis associated with neural deafness. Arch Neurol 37: 214–216

Albers JW, Allen AA II, Bastron JA et al. (1981) Limb myokymia. Muscle Nerve 4: 495–504

Albers JW, Danofrio PD, McGonagle TK (1985) Sequential electrodiagnostic abnormalities in acute inflammatory demyelinating polyradiculoneuropathy. Muscle Nerve 8: 528–539

Albert ML (1974) Carbamazepine for painful post-traumatic paresthesia. N Engl J Med 290: 693

Albuquerque EY, McIsaac RJ (1970) Fast and slow mammalian muscles after denervation. Exp Neurol 26: 183–202

Albuquerque EY, Rash JE, Mayer RF et al. (1976) Electro-physiological and morphological study of the neuromuscular function in patients with myasthenia gravis. Exp Neurol 51: 536–563

Al-Din N, Anderson M, Eeg-Olofsson O et al. (1994) Neuro-ophthalmic manifestations of the syndrome of ophthalmo-plegia, ataxia and areflexia. Acta Neurol Scand 89: 87–94

Aldrich MS, Kim YI, Sanders DB (1979) Effects of D-penicillamine on neuromuscular transmission in rats. Muscle Nerve 2: 180–185

Aldridge LM (1985) Anaesthetic problems in myotonic dystrophy. Br J Anaesth 57: 1119–1130

Alexander MP, Emery ES, Korner FC (1976) Progressive bulbar paresis in childhood. Arch Neurol 33: 66–68

Alexander WS (1966) Phytanic acid in Refsum's syndrome. J Neurol Neurosurg Psychiatry 29: 412–416

Al Hakim M, Katirji MB (1993) Femoral mononeuropathy induced by the lithotomy position: a report of 5 cases and a review of the literature. Muscle Nerve 16: 891–895

Allbrook D (1981) Skeletal muscle regeneration. Muscle Nerve 4: 234–245

Allbrook DB, Aitken JT (1951) Reinnervation of striated muscle after acute ischaemia. J Anat 85: 376–390

Allen DE, Johnson AG, Woolf AL (1969) The intramuscular nerve endings in dystrophia myotonica: a biopsy study by vital staining and electron microscopy. J Anat 105 1–26

Allen I, Mullaly B, Mawhinney H et al. (1980) The nodular form of polymyositis: a possible manifestation of vasculitis. J Pathol 13: 183–191

Allen IV, Dermott E, Connolly JH et al. (1971) A study of a patient with the amyotrophic form of Creutzfeldt-Jakob disease. Brain 94: 715–724

Allen N, Mendell JR, Billmaier DJ et al. (1975) Toxic polyneuropathy due to methyl-n-butyl ketone. Arch Neurol 32: 209–218

Al-Lozi MT, Pestronk A, Yee WC et al. (1994) Rapidly evolving myopathy with myosin deficient muscle fibers. Ann Neurol 35: 273–279

Aloisi M, Pierobon-Bormioli S, Schiaffini S (1974) Cell multiplication and histochemical changes in compensatory muscle hypertrophy. In: Hausmanowa-Petrusewick K, Jedrejowska H (eds) Structure and function of normal and diseased muscle and peripheral nerve. Polish Medical Publishers, Warsaw, pp 27–32

Altenkirch H, Mager J, Stoltenburg G et al. (1977) Toxic polyneuropathies after sniffing a glue-thinner. J Neurol 214: 137–152

Alter M, Schaumann B (1976) Hereditary amyotrophic lateral sclerosis: a report of two families. Eur Neurol 14: 250–265

Amadio PC (1992) The Mayo Clinic and carpal tunnel syndrome. Mayo Clin Proc 67: 42–48

Amaranath L, Lavin TJ, Trusso RA et al. (1983) Evaluation of creatine phosphokinase screening as a predictor of malignant hyperthermia. Br J Anaesth 55: 531–533

Amato AA, Barohn RJ, Jackson CE et al. (1994) Inclusion body myositis: treatment with intravenous immunoglobulin. Neurology 44: 1516–1518

American Association of Electrodiagnostic Medicine (1992) Guidelines in electrodiagnostic medicine. Muscle Nerve 15: 229–253

Amino N, Yuasa T, Yabu Y et al. (1980) Exophthalmos in autoimmune thyroid disease. J Clin Endocrinol Metab 51: 1232–1234

Aminoff MJ, Goodin DS, Barbaro NM et al. (1985a) Dermatomal somatosensory evoked potentials in unilateral lumbosacral radiculopathy. Ann Neurol 17: 171–176

Aminoff MJ, Goodin DS, Parry GJ et al. (1985b) Electrophysiologic evaluation of lumbosacral radiculopathies: electromyography, late responses and somatosensory evoked potentials. Neurology 35: 1514–1518

Aminoff MJ, Layzer RB, Satya-Murti S et al. (1977) The declining electrical response of muscle to repetitive nerve stimulation in myotonia. Neurology 27: 812–816

Amit R, Bashan N, Abarbanel JM et al. (1992) Fatal familial infantile glycogen storage disease: multisystem phosphofructokinase deficiency. Muscle Nerve 15: 455–458

Anan R, Higuchi I, Ichinari K et al. (1992) Myocardial patchy staining of dystrophin in Becker's muscular dystrophy associated with cardiomyopathy. Am Heart J 123: 1088–1089

Andersen H, Nielsen JF, Kamp-Nielsen V (1994) Inability of insulin to maintain normal nerve function during high frequency stimulation in diabetic rat tail nerves. Muscle Nerve 17: 80–84

Andersen P, Henrikssen J (1977) Training-induced changes in the subgroups of human Type 2 skeletal muscle fibres. Acta Physiol Scand 99: 123–125

Anderson IC, Jones EW (1976) Porcine malignant hyperthermia: effect of dantrolene sodium on in vitro halothane-induced contraction of susceptible muscle. Anaesthesiology 44: 57–61

Anderson MH, Fullerton PM, Gilliatt RW et al. (1970) Changes in the forearm associated with median nerve compression at the wrist in the guinea pig. J Neurol Neurosurg Psychiatry 33: 70–79

Anderson R, Blom S (1972) Neurophysiological studies in hereditary amyloidosis with polyneuropathy. Acta Med Scand 191: 233–239

Anderson S, Bonkier AT, Barrel BG et al. (1981) Sequence and organisation of human mitochondrial genome. Nature 290: 457–465

Andrade C (1952) A peculiar form of peripheral neuropathy: familial atypical generalised amyloidosis with special involvement of the peripheral nerves. Brain 75: 408–427

Andrade C, Araki S, Block W et al. (1970) Hereditary amyloidosis. Arthritis Rheum 13: 902–915

Andres PL, Finison LJ, Conlon MPH et al. (1988) Use of composite scores (megascores) to measure deficit in amyotrophic lateral sclerosis. Neurology 38: 405–408

Andres PL, Hedland W, Finison L et al. (1986) Quantitative motor assessment in amyotrophic lateral sclerosis. Neurology 36: 937–941

Angel RW, Hoffmann WW (1963) The H reflex in normal, spastic and rigid subjects. Arch Neurol 9: 591–596

Angelini C, Engel AG (1972) Comparative study of acid maltase deficiency. Arch Neurol 26: 344–349

Angelini C, Lücke S, Cantarutti F (1976) Carnitine deficiency of skeletal muscle: report of a treated case. Neurology 26: 633–634

Angelini C, Martinuzzi A, Vergani L (1992) Treatment with L-carnitine of the infantile and adult form of primary carnitine deficiency. In: Ferrari R, Di Mauro S, Sherwood G (eds) L- carnitine and its role in medicine. Academic Press, London, pp 139–153

Angus-Leppon H, Burke D (1992) The function of large and small nerve fibres in renal failure. Muscle Nerve 15: 288–294

Ansell BM (1984) Management of polymyositis and dermatomyositis. Clin Rheum Dis 10: 205–213

Antel JP, Arnason BGW, Fuller TC et al. (1976) Histocompatibility typing in amyotrophic lateral sclerosis. Arch Neurol 33: 423–425

Appel SH, Elias SB (1979) Anti-acetylcholine receptor antibodies in myasthenia gravis. In: Dau PE (ed) Plasmapheresis and the immunobiology of myasthenia gravis. Houghton Mifflin, Boston, pp 52–58

Appel SH, Roses AD (1977) Membranes and myotonia. In: Rowland LP (ed) Pathogenesis of human muscular dystrophies. Excerpta Medica, Amsterdam, pp 747–761

Appenzeller O, Atkinson R (1984) Autonomic disorders: assessment and management. In: Asbury AK, Gilliatt RW (eds) Peripheral nerve disorders. Butterworths, London, pp 58–91

Appenzeller O, Kornfeld M, MacGee J (1971) Neuropathy in chronic renal disease. Arch Neurol 24: 449–461

Aquilonius SM, Askmark H, Gillberg PG et al. (1984) Topographical localisation of motor end-plates in cryosection of whole human muscles. Muscle Nerve 7: 287–293

Arahata K, Engel AG (1986) Monoclonal antibody analysis of mononuclear cells in myopathies. I. Quantitation of subsets according to diagnosis and sites of accumulation and demonstration and counts of muscle fibres invaded by T cells. Ann Neurol 16: 193–208

Arahata K, Hayashi Y, Koga R et al. (1993) Laminin in animal models for muscular dystrophy Proc Jpn Acad 69 (Ser B): 259–264

Araoz C, Sun CN, Shenefelt R et al. (1974) Glycogenosis Type II: Pompe's disease. Neurology 24: 739–742

Archer AG, Watkins PJ, Thomas PK et al. (1983) The natural history of acute painful neuropathy in diabetes mellitus. J Neurol Neurosurg Psychiatry 46: 491–499

Argov Z, Mastaglia FL (1979) Drug-induced peripheral neuropathies. Br Med J i: 663–666

Argov Z, Yarom R (1984) Rimmed vacuole myopathy sparing the quadriceps: a unique disorder in Iranian Jews. J Neurol Sci 64: 33–43

Argov Z, Bank WJ, Maris J et al. (1986a) Treatment of mitochondrial myopathy due to complex III deficiency with vitamins K_3 and C: a ^{31}P NMR follow-up study. Ann Neurol 19: 598–602

Argov Z, Soffer D, Eisenberg S et al. (1986b) Chronic demyelinating peripheral neuropathy in cerebro-tendinous xanthomatosis. Ann Neurol 20: 89–91

Argyropoulos CJ, Panayiotopoulos CP, Scarpalezos S (1978) F and M wave conduction velocity in amyotrophic lateral sclerosis. Muscle Nerve 1: 479–485

Arikawa E, Hoffman EP, Kaido M et al. (1991) The frequency of patients with dystrophin abnormalities in a limb-girdle patient population. Neurology 41: 1491–1496

Armon C, Daube JR, Windebank AJ et al. (1990) How frequently does classic amyotropic lateral sclerosis develop in survivors of poliomyelitis. Neurology 40: 172–174

Armstrong RM, Knigsberger R, Mellinger J et al. (1971) Central core disease with congenital hip dislocation: a study of two families. Neurology 21: 369–376

Arnando E, Dalakas MC, Shanske S et al. (1991) Depletion of muscle mitochondrial DNA in AIDS patients with Zidovudine-induced myopathy. Lancet 337: 508–510

Arnason BGW (1975) Inflammatory polyradiculoneuritis. In: Dyck PJ, Thomas PK, Lambert EH (eds) Peripheral neuropathy, vol 2. Saunders, Philadelphia, pp 1110–1148

Arnason BGW, Asbury AK (1968) Idiopathic polyneuritis after surgery. Arch Neurol 18: 500–507

Arnason BGW, Chelmica-Szare E (1972) Passive transfer of experimental allergic neuritis in Lewis rats by direct injection of sensitized B lymphocytes into sciatic nerve. Acta Neuropathol (Berl) 22: 1

Arnason BGW, Soliven B (1993) Acute inflammatory demyelinating polyradiculoneuropathy. In: Dyck PJ, Thomas PK (eds) Peripheral neuropathy, 3rd edn. Saunders, Philadelphia, pp 1437–1497

Arnold DL, Matthews PM, Radda GK (1984) Metabolic recovery after exercise and the assessment of mitochondrial in human skeletal muscle in vivo by use of ^{31}P NMR. Magn Res Med 1: 307

Arnold N, Harriman DGF (1970) The incidence of abnormality in control human peripheral nerve studies by single axon dissection. J Neurol Neurosurg Psychiatry 33: 55–61

Arnon SS (1980) Infant botulism. Ann Rev Med 31: 541–560

Arrelano F, Krupp P (1991) Muscular disorders associated with cyclosporin. Lancet 337: 915

Arts WF, Bethlem J, Dingemans KP et al. (1978) Investigation on the inheritance of nemaline myopathy. Arch Neurol 35: 72–77

Arts WF, Busch HFM, van den Brand HJ (1983) Hereditary neuralgic amyotrophy. J Neurol Sci 62: 261–279

Asbury AK (1973) Renaut bodies. A forgotten endoneurial structure. J Neuropathol Exp Neurol 32: 334–343

Asbury AK (1977) Proximal diabetic neuropathy. Ann Neurol 2: 179–180

Asbury AK (1984) Uraemic neuropathy. In: Dyck PJ, Thomas PK, Lambert EH et al. (eds) Peripheral neuropathy, 2nd edn, vol 2. Saunders, Philadelphia, pp 1811–1825

Asbury AK, Cornblath DR (1990) Assessment of current diagnostic criteria for Guillain–Barré syndrome. Ann Neurol 27: 541–524

Asbury AK, Fields HZ (1984) Pain due to peripheral nerve damage: an hypothesis. Neurology 34: 1587–1590

Asbury AK, Gilliatt RW (1984) The clinical approach to myopathy. In: Asbury AK, Gilliatt RW (eds) Peripheral nerve disorders. Butterworths, London, pp 1–20

Asbury AK, Aldredge H, Hershberg R et al. (1970) Oculomotor palsy in diabetes mellitus: a clinico-pathological study. Brain 93: 555–556

Asbury AK, Arnason BGW, Adams RD (1969) The inflammatory lesion in idiopathic polyneuritis. Medicine (Baltimore) 48: 173–215

Asbury AK, Arnason B, Karp H et al. (1978) Criteria for the diagnosis of Guillain–Barré syndrome. Ann Neurol 3: 565–566

Asbury AK, Gale MK, Cox SC et al. (1972) Giant axonal neuropathy: a unique case with segmental neurofilamentous masses. Acta Neuropathol 20: 237–247

Asbury AK, Victor M, Adams RD (1963) Uraemic polyneuropathy. Arch Neurol 8: 413–428

Ashizawa T, Butler IJ, Harati Y et al. (1983) A dominantly inherited syndrome with continuous motor neuron discharges. Ann Neurol 13: 285–290

Ashworth B, Smyth GE (1969) Relapsing motor polyneuropathy. Acta Neurol Scand 45: 342–350

Ashworth B, Tait GBW (1971) Trigeminal neuropathy in connective tissue diseases. Neurology 21: 609–614

Askanas V, Engel WK (1977) Diseased human muscle in tissue culture: a new approach to the pathogenesis of human neuromuscular disorders. In: Rowland LP (ed) Pathogenesis of human muscular dystrophies. Excerpta Medica, Amsterdam, pp 856–871

Askanas V, Engel WK, Alvarez RB et al. (1992) Beta amyloid protein immunoreactivity in muscle of patients with inclusion body myositis. Lancet 339: 560–561

Askanas V, Engel WK, Di Mauro S et al. (1976) Adult-onset acid maltase deficiency: morphologic and biochemical abnormalities reproduced in cultured muscle. N Engl J Med 294: 573–578

Askanas V, Engel WK, Reddy NB et al. (1979) X-linked recessive congenital muscle fibre hypotrophy with central nuclei: abnormalities of growth and adenylate cyclase in muscle tissue cultures. Arch Neurol 36: 604–609

Askanas V, Serdarogen P, Engel WK et al. (1991) Immuno-localisation of ubiquitin in muscle biopsies of patients with inclusion body myositis and oculopharyngeal muscular dystrophy (OPMD). Neurosci Lett 130: 73–76

Askari AD, Huettner TL (1982) Cardiac abnormalities in polymyositis-dermatomyositis. Semin Arth Rheum 12: 208–219

Askari A, Vignos PJ Jr, Moskowitz RW (1976) Steroid myopathy in connective tissue disease. Am J Med 61: 485–492

Askmark H, Osterman PO, Roxin LE et al. (1981) Radioimmunoassay of serum myoglobin in neuromuscular diseases. J Neurol Neurosurg Psychiatry 44: 68–72

Ask-Upmark E (1950) Amyotrophic lateral sclerosis observed in 5 persons after gastric resection. Gastroenterology 15: 257–259

Aston JP, Kingston HM, Ramasamy I et al. (1984) Plasma pyruvate kinase activity in Becker muscular dystrophy. J Neurol Sci 65: 307–314

Astrom KE, Webster H de F, Arnason BG (1968) The initial lesion in experimental allergic neuritis: a phase and electron microscopic study. J Exp Med 128: 469–496

Auerbach PS (1991) Marine envenomations. N Engl J Med 325: 486–493

Auger RG (1979) Hemifacial spasm: clinical and electrophysiologic observations. Neurology 29: 1261–1272

Auger RG (1994) Diseases associated with excess motor unit activity (AAEM minimonograph 44). Muscle Nerve 17: 1250–1263

Auger RG, Daube RJ, Gomez MR et al. (1984) Hereditary form of sustained muscle activity of peripheral nerve origin causing generalised myokymia and muscle stiffness. Ann Neurol 15: 13–21

Austin JH (1958) Recurrent polyneuritides and their corticosteroid treatment. Brain 81: 157–192

Austin J, Armstrong D, Fouch S et al. (1968) Metachromatic leucodystrophy (MLD) VIII. MLD in adults. Arch Neurol 18: 225–240

Austin J, Armstrong D, Shearer L (1969) Metachromatic form of diffuse cerebral sclerosis. V. nature and significance of low sulfatase activity. Arch Neurol 13: 593–614

Axelrod FB, Pearson J (1984) Congenital sensory neuropathies. Am J Dis Child 138: 947–954

Baer RD, Johnson EW (1965) Motor nerve conduction velocities in normal children Arch Phys Med Rehabil 46: 698–704

Bailey RO, Ritaccio AL, Bishop MB et al. (1986) Benign monoclonal IgA kappa gammopathy associated with polyneuropathy and dysautonomia. Acta Neurol Scand 73: 574–580

Baker JH, Hall-Craggs ECB (1980) Recovery from central core degeneration of the tenotomised rat soleus muscle. Muscle Nerve 3: 151–159

Ball AP, Hopkinson RB, Farrell ID et al. (1979) Human botulism caused by *Clostridium* botulinum Type E: the Birmingham outbreak. QJM 48: 473–491

Ballantyne JP, Hansen S (1974a) Computer method for the analysis of evoked motor unit poentials. J Neurol Neurosurg Psychiatry 37: 1187–1194

Ballantyne JP, Hansen S (1974b) New method for the estimation of the number of motor units in a muscle. II. Duchenne, limb-girdle and facio-scapulo-humeral and myotonic muscular dystrophies. J Neurol Neurosurg Psychiatry 37: 1195–1201

Ballin RHM, Thomas PK (1968) Hypertrophic changes in diabetic neuropathy. Acta Neuropathol (Berl) 11: 93–102

Banerjee TK, Mostofi MS, Us O et al. (1993) Magnetic stimulation in the determination of lumbosacral motor radiculopathy. Electroencephalogr Clin Neurophysiol 89: 221–226

Bannerji NK, Hurwitz LJ (1971) Neurological manifestation in adult steatorrhoea (probable gluten enteropathy). J Neurol Sci 14: 125–141

Bank WJ, Di Mauro S, Bonilla E et al. (1975) A disorder of lipid metabolism and myoglobinuria. N Engl J Med 292: 443–449

Banker BQ (1960) The experimental myopathies. Res Publ Assoc Res Nerv Ment Dis 38: 197–233

Banker BQ (1975) Dermatomyositis of childhood: ultrastructural alterations of muscle and intramuscular blood vessels. J Neuropathol Exper Neurol 34: 46–75

Banker BQ (1986) Parasitic myositis and other inflammatory myopathies. In: Engel AG, Banker BQ (eds) Myology. McGraw-Hill, New York, pp 1467–1524

Banker BQ, Engel AG (1994) Basic reactions of muscle. In: Engel AG, Franzini-Armstrong C (eds) Myology, 3rd edn. McGraw-Hill, New York, pp 832–888

Banker BQ, Victor M (1966) Dermatomyositis (systemic angiopathy) of childhood. Medicine (Baltimore) 45: 261–289

Banker BQ, Victor M, Adams RD (1957) Arthrogryposis multiplex due to congenital muscular dystrophy. Brain 80: 319–334

Bannister RG, Davies B, Holly E et al. (1979) Defective cardiovascular reflexes and supersensitivity to sympathetic drugs in autonomic failure. Brain 102: 163–176

Baquis GD, Kelly JJ, Lieberman A et al. (1991) Adult metachromatic leucodystrophy and pes cavus foot deformity. Muscle Nerve 14: 784–785

Barbeau A (1966) The syndrome of hereditary late onset ptosis and dysphagia in French Canada. In: Kuhn E (ed) Symposium über progressive Muskeldystrophie-Myotonie-Myasthenie. Springer, Berlin Heidelberg New York, pp 102–109

Barchi RL (1975) Myotonia: an evaluation of the choloride hypothesis. Arch Neurol 32: 175–180

Barchi RL (1982) A mechanistic approach to the myotonic syndromes. Muscle Nerve 5: 560–563

Barchi RL (1992) The non-dystrophic myotonic syndromes. In: Vinken PJ, Bruyn GW, Klawans HL (eds) Handbook of clinical neurology, vol. 62. Elsevier, Amsterdam, pp 261–286

Bardwick PA, Zvaiflen NJ, Gill GN et al. (1980) Plasma cell dysplasia with polyneuropathy, organomegaly, endocrinopathy, M protein and skin changes: the POEMS syndrome. Medicine (Baltimore) 59: 311–322

Barilla E, Sciacco M, Tanji K et al. (1992) New morphological approaches to the study of mitochondrial encephalomyopathies. Brain Pathol 2: 113–119

Barker AT, Freeston IL, Jalinous R et al. (1986) Clinical evaluation of conduction time measurements in central motor pathways using magnetic stimulation of the human brain. Lancet I: 1325–1326

Barkhaus PE, Nandedkar SK, Sanders DB (1990) Quantitative EMG in inflammatory myopathy. Muscle Nerve 13: 247–253

Barnemann A, Schmalbruch H (1992) Desmin and vimentin in regenerating muscles. Muscle Nerve 15: 14–20

Barnes BE (1976) Dermatomyositis and malignancy: a review of the literature. Ann Intern Med 84: 68–76

Barolin RJ, Amato AA, Sahenk Z et al. (1995) Inclusion body myositis. Neurology 45: 1302–1304

Barolin RS, Brumback RA, Mendell JR (1994a) Hyaline body myopathy. Neuromusc Disord 4: 256–262

Barolin RS, Jackson CE, Rogers SJ et al. (1994b) Prolonged paralysis due to non-depolarising neuromuscular blocking agents and corticosteroids. Muscle Nerve 17: 647–654

Barolin RJ, McVey AL, Di Mauro S (1993) Adult acid maltase deficiency. Muscle Nerve 16: 672–676

Bartels EM, Danneskiold-Samsøce B (1986) Histological abnormalities in muscle from patients with certain types of fibrositis. Lancet i: 755–757

Barth PG, van Wijngaarden GK, Bethlem J (1975) X-linked myotubular myopathy with fatal neonatal asphyxia. Neurology 25: 531–536

Bartolome M, Erill S, Laporte J et al. (1974) Iatrogenic neurological syndromes: hormonal drugs. In: Subirana A, Espadaler JM (eds) Neurology. Excerpta Medica, Amsterdam, pp 8–27

Barwick DD, Osselton JW, Walton JN (1965) Electroencephalographic abnormalities in hereditary myopathy. J Neurol Neurosurg Psychiatry 28: 109–114

Bashis R, Strachan T, Kaers S et al. (1994) A gene for autosomal recessive limb-girdle muscular dystrophy maps to chromosome 2p. Hum Molec Genet 3: 455–457

Bashuk RG, Krendl DA (1990) Myasthenia gravis presenting as weakness after magnesium administration. Muscle Nerve 13: 708–712

Basmajian JV (1978) Muscles alive. Williams and Wilkins. Baltimore, p 495

Barson JA, Thomas JE (1981) Diabetic polyradiculopathy: clinical and electrophysiologic findings in 105 patients. Mayo Clin Proc 56: 725–732

Bastiaensen LAK (1978) Chronic progressive external ophthalmoplegia. Staflen, Leyden

Bateman DE, Weller RO, Kennedy P (1990) Stiff man syndrome: a rare paraneoplastic disorder. J Neurol Neurosurg Psychiatry 53: 695–696

Bates D, Stevens JC, Hudgson P (1973) "Polymyositis" with involvement of facial and distal musculature: one form of the facio-scapulo-humeral syndrome? J Neurol Sci 19: 105–108

Batten FE (1903) Three cases of myopathy, infantile type. Brain 26: 147–148

Bauer M, Bergstrom R, Ritter B et al. (1977) Macroglobulinaemia, Waldenström and motor neuron syndromes. Acta Neurol Scand 55: 245–250

Bauermeister W, Jabre JF (1992) The spectrum of concentric macro EMG correlations. Part I. Normal subjects. Muscle Nerve 15: 1081–1084

Bauman TD, Gelberman RH, Mubarak SJ et al. (1981) The acute carpal tunnel syndrome. Clin Orthop 156: 151–156

Baylan SP, Paik SW, Barnett AL et al. (1981) Prevalence of the tarsal tunnel syndrome in rheumatoid arthritis. Rheumatol Rehabil 20: 148–150

Bazzi C, Pagani C, Sorgato G et al. (1991) Uremic polyneuropathy: a clinical and electrophysiological study in 135 short and long term haemodialysed patients. Clin Nephrol 35: 176–181

Beasley WC (1956) Influence of method on estimates of normal knee extensor force among normal and post-polio children. Phys Ther Rev 36: 21–41

Beasley WC (1961) Quantitative muscle testing: principles and applications to research and clinical services. Arch Phys Med Rehabil 42: 398–406

Becker KL, Titus JH, McConahey WM et al. (1964) Morphologic evidence of thyroiditis in myasthenia gravis. JAMA 187: 994–1000

Becker PE (1962) Two new families of benign sex-linked recessive muscular dystrophy. Rev Can Biol 21: 551–566

Becker PE (1971) Genetic approaches to the nosology of muscle disease: Myotonias and similar diseases. Birth Defects 7: 57–62

Becker PE (1977) Myotonia congenita and syndromes associated with myotonia. In: Becker PE, Lenz W, Vogel et al. (eds) Topics in human genetics, vol 3. Thieme, Stuttgart

Becker PE, Kiener F (1955) Eine neue X-chromosale Muskeldystrophie. Arch Psychiatr Nervenkr 193: 427–448

Beckett VL, Dinn JJ (1972) Segmental demyelination in rheumatoid arthritis. QJM 91: 71–80

Beckmann R (1977) Detection of preclinical Duchenne muscular dystrophy and its female carriers. Isr J Med Sci 13: 102–106

Beggs A H, Koenig M, Boyce FM et al. (1990) Detection of 98% of DMD/BMD gene deletions by polymerase chain reaction. Hum Genet 86: 45–48

Beggs AH, Neumann PE, Arahata K et al. (1992) Possible influences on the expression of X chromosome-linked dystrophin abnormalities by heterozygosity for autosomal recessive Fukuyama congenital muscular dystrophy. Proc Nat Acad Sci USA 89: 623–627

Behan AR, Perera T, Myles AB (1983) Polymyalgia rheumatica and corticosteroids: how much for how long? Ann Rheum Dis 42: 374–378

Behan WMH, Behan PO, Dick HA (1978) HLA B8 in polymyositis. N Engl J Med 298: 1260–1261

Behse F, Buchthal F (1977a) Alcoholic neuropathy: clinical, electrophysiological and biopsy findings. Ann Neurol 2: 95–110

Behse F, Buchthal F (1977b) Peroneal muscular atrophy (PMA) and related disorders. II. Histological findings in sural nerves. Brain 100: 67–85

Behse F, Buchthal F (1978) Sensory action potentials and biopsy of the sural nerve in neuropathy. Brain 101: 473–493

Behse F, Buchtal F, Carlsen F et al. (1972) Hereditary neuropathy with liability to pressure palsies. Brain 95: 777–794

Behse F, Buchtal F, Carlsen F (1977) Nerve biopsy and conduction studies in diabetic neuropathy. J Neurol Neurosurg Psychiatry 40: 1072–1082

Beighton P, Gumpel JM, Carnes NGM (1968) Prodromal trigeminal sensory neuropathy in progressive systemic sclerosis. Ann Rheum Dis 27: 367–369

Bejaoui K, Hirabayashi K, Heutati F et al. (1995) Linkage of Miyoshi myopathy (distal autosomal recessive muscular dystrophy) locus to chromosome 2p 12–14. Neurology 45: 768–772

Belanger AY, McComas AJ (1981) Extent of motor unit activation during effort. J Appl Physiol 51: 1131–1135

Belangra EA, Hedberg CW, Glenich JG et al. (1990) An investigation of the cause of the eosinophilia-myalgia syndrome associated with tryptophan use. N Engl J Med 323: 356–365

Bell CD, Conen PE (1968) Histopathological changes in Duchenne muscular dystrophy. J Neurol Sci 7: 529–544

Belsh JM, Schiffman PL (1990) Misdiagnosis in patients with amyotrophic lateral sclerosis. Arch Intern Med 150: 2301–2305

Bender AN, Willner JP (1978) Nemaline (rod) myopathy: the need for histochemical evaluation of affected families. Ann Neurol 4: 37–42

Benecke R, Conrad B (1980) The distal sensory nerve action potential as a diagnostic tool for differentiation of lesions in dorsal roots and peripheral nerves. J Neurol 223: 231–239

Bengtsson A (1986) Primary fibromyalgia: a clinical and laboratory study. Linköping, Sweden (Linköping University Medical Dissertations, no. 224).

Bengtsson A, Henriksson KJ, Larsson J (1986) Muscle biopsy in primary fibromyalgia. Scand J Rheumatol 15: 1–6

Ben-Hamida C, Doerflinger N, Belal S et al. (1994a) Localisation of Friedreich's ataxia with selective vitamin E deficiency to chromosome 8q by homozygosity mapping. Nature Genet 5: 195–200

Ben-Hamida C, Soussi-Yanicostas N, Butler-Browne GS et al. (1994b) Biochemical and histochemical analysis in chronic proximal spinal muscular atrophy. Muscle Nerve 17: 400–410

Ben-Hamida M, Hentati F (1984) Maladie de Charcot et sclerose laterale amyotrophique juvenile. Rev Neurol 140: 202–206

Ben-Hamida M, Hentati F (1989) Tunisian severe childhood muscular dystrophy: a normal spinal cord and anterior horn neurons. Muscle Nerve 12: 156

Ben-Hamida M, Belal S, Sirugo G et al. (1993) Friedreich's ataxia phenotype not linked to chromosome 9 and associated with selective autosomal recessive vitamin E deficiency in two inbred Tunisian families. Neurology 43: 2179–2183

Ben-Hamida M, Fardeau M, Attia N (1983) Severe childhood muscular dystrophy affecting both sexes and frequent in Tunisia. Muscle Nerve 6: 469–480

Ben Hamida M, Hentati F, Ben-Hamida C (1987) A case of multiminicore disease with rigid spine syndrome. Rev Neurol 143. 284

Ben Jelloun-Dellagi S, Chaffey S, Hentati F et al. (1990) Presence of normal dystrophin in Tunisian childhood autosomal recessive muscular dystrophy. Neurology 40: 1903

Bennett AE, Cash PJ (1943) Myasthenia gravis: curare sensitivity, a new diagnostic test and approach to causation. Arch Neurol Psychiatry 49: 537–547

Bennett WR, Huston BP (1984) Rhabdomyolosis in thyroid storm. Am J Med 77: 733–735

Ben Othmane K, Ben-Hamida M, Pericak-Vance MA et al. (1992) Linkage of Tunisian auosomal recessive Duchenne-like mucular dystrophy to the pericentromeric region of chromosome 13q. Nature Genetics 2: 315–317

Bensimon G, Lacanblez L, Meininger V (1994) A controlled trial of Riluzole in amyotrophic lateral sclerosis. N Engl J Med 330: 585–591

Ben-Tovim DI, Schwartz MS (1981) Hypoalgesia in depressive illness. Br J Psychiatry 138: 37–39

Beratis NG, Danesino C, Hirschhorn K (1975) Detection of homozygotes and heterozygotes for metachromatic leucodystrophy in lymphoid cell lines and peripheral leucocytes. Ann Hum Genet 38: 485–493

Berenberg RA Pollock JM, Di Mauro S et al. (1977) Lumping or splitting? "Opthalmoplegia plus" or Kearns–Sayre syndrome? Ann Neurol 1: 37–54

Berg BO, Rosenberg SH, Asbury AK (1972) Giant axonal neuropathy. Pediatrics 49: 894–899

Berger AR, Busis NA, Ligigian EL et al. (1985) Cervical root stimulation in radiculopathy. Neurology 35 [Suppl 1]: 68

Berger JR, Ayyar R, Sheremata WA (1981) Guillain–Barré syndrome complicating acute hepatitis B. Arch Neurol 38: 366–368

Bergeson PS, Singer SA, Kaplan AM (1982) Intramuscular injection in children. Pediatrics 70: 944–948

Bergmans J (1971) Computer-assisted on line measurement of motor unit potential parameters in human electromyography. Electromyography 11: 161–181

Bergmark J (1950) Intermittent spinal claudication. Acta Med Scand 246 [Suppl]: 30–36

Bergström J (1962) Muscle electrolytes in man. Scand J Clin Lab Invest 14 [Suppl 68]: 1–110

Bergström K, Franksson C, Mattel G et al. (1973) The effects of thoracic duct lymph drainage in myasthenia gravis. Eur Neurol 9: 157–167

Bernstein LP, Antel JP (1981) Motor neuron disease: decremental responses to repetitive nerve stimulation. Neurology 31: 202–204

Bernstein RM, Morgan SH, Chapman J et al. (1984) Anti Jo-1 antibody: a marker for myositis with interstitial lung disease. Br Med J 289: 151–152

Berry EM, Maunder CM, Wilson M (1974) Carcinoid myopathy and treatment with cyproheptadine (Periactin). Gut 15: 34–38

Berry H (1993) Traumatic peripheral nerve lesions. In: Brown WF, Bolton CF (eds) Clinical electromyography, 2nd edn. Butterworth-Heinemann, Boston, pp 323–368

Berry H, Richardson PM (1976) Common peroneal nerve palsy: a clinical and electrophysiological review. J Neurol Neurosurg Psychiatry 39: 1162–1171

Berry H, MacDonald EA, Mrazek AC (1991) Accessory nerve palsy: a review of 23 cases. Can J Neurol Sci 18: 337–341

Bertelson CJ, Pogo AO, Chaudhuri A et al. (1988) Localisation of the McLeod locus (XK) within Xp 21 by deletion analysis. Am J Hum Genet 42: 703–711

Bertorini TE, Igarashi M (1985) Postpoliomyelitis muscle pseudohypertrophy. Muscle Nerve 8: 644–649

Bertorini TE, Palmieri GMA, Griffin J et al. (1991) Effect of dantrolene in Duchenne muscular dystrophy. Muscle Nerve 14: 503–507

Berzelius J (1848) Jahres-Bericht über die Fortschritte der Chemie und Mineralogie 27: 586

Besser R, Vogt T, Gutmann L (1990) Pancuronium improves the neuromuscular transmission defect of human organophosphate intoxication. Neurology 40: 1275–1277

Bethlem J, van Wijngaarden GK (1976) Benign myopathy with autosomal dominant inheritance: a report on three pedigrees. Brain 99: 91–100

Bethlem J, Arts WF, Dingemans KP (1978) Common origin of rods, cores, miniature cores and focal loss of cross-striations. Arch Neurol 35: 555–566

Bethlem J, van Gool J, Hulsmann WC et al. (1966) Familial non-progressive myopathy with muscle cramps after exercise. Brain 89: 569–588

Bethlem J, van Wijngaarden GK, Meijer AEFH et al. (1969) Neuromuscular disease with Type 1 fibre atrophy, central nuclei and myotube-like structures. Neurology 19: 705–710

Better OS, Stern JH (1990) Early management of shock and prophylaxis of acute renal failure in traumatic rhabdomyolysis. N Eng J Med 322: 825–828

Bever CT Jr, Aquino AV, Penn AS (1983) Prognosis of ocular myasthenia. Ann Neurol 14: 516–519

Bever CT, Chang HW, Penn AS et al. (1982) Penicillamine-induced myasthenia gravis: effects of penicillamine on acetylcholine receptor. Neurology 32: 1077–1082

Bhan A, Baithun SI, Kopelman P et al. (1990) Fatal myocarditis with acute polymyositis in a young adult. Postgrad Med J 66: 229–231

Bialer MG, McDaniel NL, Kelly TE (1991) Progression of cardiac disease in Emery-Dreifuss muscular dystrophy. Clin Cardiol 14: 411–416

Bickerstaff ER (1978) Brainstem encephalitis (Bickerstaff encephalitis). In: Vinken PJ, Bruyn GW (eds) Handbook of neurology, vol 34. North Holland, Amsterdam, pp 605–609

Biemand A (1966) Myopathia distalis juvenilis. In: Kuhn E (ed) Symposium über progressive Muskeldystrophien. Springer, Berlin Heidelberg New York pp 95–100

Biemand A, Daniels AP (1934) Familial periodic paralysis and its transition into spinal muscular atrophy. Brain 57: 91–108

Bigland-Ritchie B, Woods JJ (1984) Changes in muscle contractile properties and neural control during human muscular fatigue. Muscle Nerve 7: 691–699

Bigland-Ritchie B, Carfarelli E, Vollestad NK (1986) Fatigue of submaximal static contractions. Acta Physiol Scand 128 [Suppl 556]: 137–148

Bigner DD, Olson WN, McFarlin DE (1971) Peripheral polyneuropathy: high and low molecular weight IgM and amyloidosis. Arch Neurol 24: 365–373

Billimoria JD, Gibberd FB, Clemens ME (1982) Metabolism of phytanic acid in Refsum's disease. Lancet i: 194–196

Birch R (1984) Traction lesions of the brachial plexus. Br J Hosp Med 32: 140–143

Birch R (1986) Lesions of peripheral nerves: the present position. J Bone Joint Surg (Br) 68: 108

Bird TD, Shaw CM (1978) Progressive myoclonus and epilepsy with dentatorubral degeneration. J Neurol Neurosurg Psychiatry 41: 140–149

Bischoff A (1966) Die diabetische Neuropathie. Thieme, Stuttgart

Bischoff A (1968) Diabetische Neuropathie. Pathologische Anatomie, Pathophysiologie und Pathogenese auf grund elektronon mikroskopischer Untersuchungen. Dtsch Med Wochenschr 93: 237–241

Bischoff A (1973) Ultrastructural pathology of peripheral nervous system in early diabetes. In: Lamerini-Davalos RA, Cole HS (eds) Advances in metabolic disorders, suppl 2. Academic Press, London, pp 441–449

Bischoff A (1975) Neuropathy in leucodystrophies. In: Dyck PJ, Thomas PK, Lambert EH (eds) Peripheral neuropathy, vol 2. Saunders, Philadelphia, pp 891–919

Bischoff C, Stålberg E, Falck B et al. (1994) Reference values of motor unit action potentials obtained with multi-MUAP analysis. Muscle Nerve 17: 842–851

Bithum S, Daeschaer CW, Travis LB et al. (1964) Dermatomyositis. J Pediatr 64 : 101–131

Bjelle A, Henriksson K-G, Hofer PA (1980) Polymyositis in eosinophilic fasciitis. Eur Neurol 19: 128–137

Black JT, Bhatt GP, De Jesus PV et al. (1974) Diagnostic accuracy of clinical data, quantitative electromyography and histochemistry in neuromuscular disease: a study of 105 cases. J Neurol Sci 21: 59–70

Black JT, Garcia-Mullen R, Good E et al. (1972) Muscle rigidity in a newborn due to continuous peripheral nerve hyperactivity. Arch Neurol 27: 413–425

Black JT, Judge O, Demers L et al. (1977) Ragged-red fibres: a biochemical and morphological study. J Neurol Sci 26: 479–488

Blackie JD, Lees AJ (1990) Botulinum toxin treatment in spasmodic torticollis. J Neurol Neurosurg Psychiatry 53: 640–643

Blau JN, Logue V (1961) Intermittent claudication of the cauda equina: an unusual syndrome resulting from central protrusion of a lumbar intervertebral disc. Lancet i: 1081–1086

Bleecker ML, Bohlman M, Marcland R et al. (1985) Carpal tunnel syndrome: role of carpal canal size. Neurology 35: 1599–1604

Bleehan SS, Lovelace RE, Cotton RE (1959) Mononeuritis multiplex in periarteritis nodosa. QJM 127: 193–209

Blom S, Zakrisson JE (1974) The stapedius reflex in the diagnosis of myasthenia gravis. J Neurol Sci 21: 71–76

Blomstrand E, Ekblom B (1982) The needle biopsy technique for fibre type determination in human skeletal muscle: a methodological study. Acta Physiol Scand 116: 437–442

Blomstrand E, Celsing F, Friden J et al. (1984) How to calculate human muscle fibre areas in biopsy samples: methodological considerations. Acta Physiol Scand 122: 545–551

Bodensteiner JB (1994) Congenital myopathies. Muscle Nerve 17: 131–144

Bodensteiner JB, Engel AG (1978) Intracellular calcium accumulation in Duchenne dystrophy and other myopathies: a study of 567 000 muscle fibres in 114 biopsies. Neurology 28: 439–446

Bohan A, Peter JB (1975) Dermatomyositis and polymyositis. In: Buchanan WW, Carson Dick W (eds) Recent advances in rheumatology, no. 1, part 1. Churchill Livingstone, London, pp 39–66

Bohan A, Peter JB, Bowman RL et al. (1977) A computer-assisted analysis of 153 patients with polymyositis and dermatomyositis. Medicine 56: 255–286

Boland BJ, Silbert PL, Groover RV et al. (1996) Skeletal cardiac and smooth muscle failure in Duchenne muscular dystraphy. Paediatr Neurol 14: 7–12

Bolger GB, Sullivan KM, Spense AM et al. (1986) Myasthenia gravis after allogenic bone marrow transplantation: relationship to chronic graft versus host disease. Neurology 36: 1087–1091

Bollaert PE, Robin-Lherbier B, Escanye JM et al. (1989) Phosphorus nuclear magnetic resonance evidence of abnormal skeletal muscle metabolism in chronic alcoholics. Neurology 39: 821–824

Bollen E, Den Heyer JC, Tolsma MHJ et al. (1992) Eye movements in myotonic dystrophy. Brain 115: 445–450

Bolthauser A, Spycher MA, Steinmann B (1982) Infantile phytanic acid storage disease: a variant of Refsum's disease? Eur J Paediatr 139: 317

Bolton CF (1976) Electrophysiological changes in uraemic neuropathy after renal transplantation. Neurology 26: 152–161

Bolton CF, Young GB (1990) In: Stoneham MA (ed) Neurological complications of renal disease. Butterworth, London, pp 1–256

Bolton CF, Gilbert JJ, Hahn AF et al. (1984) Polyneuropathy in critically ill patients. J Neurol Neurosurg Psychiatry 47: 1223–1231

Bolton CF, Young GB, Zochodne DW (1993) The neurological complications of sepsis. Ann Neurol 33: 94–100

Bonilla E, Schotland D (1970) Histochemical diagnosis of muscle phosphofructokinase deficiency. Arch Neurol 22: 8–12

Bonner D, Ron M, Chalder T et al. (1994) Chronic fatigue syndrome: a follow up study. J Neurol Neurosurg Psychiatry 57: 617–621

Bonnette H, Roeloff R, Olson WH (1974) Multicore disease: report of a case with onset in middle age. Neurology 24: 1039–1044

Bonney G (1986) Iatrogenic injuries of nerves. J Bone Joint Surg [Br] 68: 9–13

Booker H, Chun RW, Sanguino M (1970) Myasthenia gravis syndrome associated with trimethadione. JAMA 212: 2262–2263

Boone CM, Chen TR, Ruddle FG (1972) Assignment of CDHA locus in man to chromosome C11 using somatic cell hybrids. Proc Natl Acad Sci USA 69: 510–514

Boongird P, Vejjajiva A (1978) Electrophysiologic findings and prognosis in Bell's palsy. Muscle Nerve 1: 461–466

Borenstein S, Desmedt JE (1973) Electromyographical signs of collateral reinnervation. In: Desmedt JE (ed) New developments in electromyography and clinical neurophysiology, vol 1. Karger, Basel, pp 130–140

Borenstein S, Desmedt JE (1974) Temperature and weather correlates of myasthenic fatigue. Lancet II: 63–64

Borenstein S, Noel P, Jacquy J et al. (1977) Myotonic dystrophy with nerve hypertrophy. J Neurol Sci 34: 87–99

Borg K, Borg J, Linblom U (1987b) Sensory involvement in distal myopathy (Welander). J Neurol Sci 80: 323–332

Borg K, Sachs L, Kaijser L (1987a) Autonomic cardiovascular responses in distal myopathy (Welander). Acta Neurol Scand 76: 261–266

Borg K, Solders G, Borg J et al. (1989) Neurogenic involvement in distal myopathy (Welander). J Neurol Sci 91: 53–70

Borges J, Vincent A, Molinaar PC et al. (1994) Passive transfer of seronegative myasthenia gravis to mice. Muscle Nerve 17: 1393–1400

Borgi L, Savoldi F, Scelsi R et al. (1983) Nuclear magnetic resonance response of protons in normal and pathological human muscles. Exp Neurol 81: 89–96

Bosch EP, Pelham RW, Rasool CG et al. (1979) Animal models of alcoholic neuropathy: morphologic, electrophysiologic and biochemical models. Muscle Nerve 2: 133–144

Bosch EP, Yamada T, Kimura J (1985) Somatosensory evoked potentials in motor neuron disease. Muscle Nerve 8: 556–562

Bosches R, Sherman JC (1953) Variability of course of Guillain-Barré syndrome. Neurology 3: 789–799

Bosco C, Komi PV (1980) Influence of ageing on the mechanical behaviour of leg extensor muscles. Eur J Appl Physiol 45: 209–219

Boska MD, Moussavi RS, Carson PJ et al. (1990) The metabolic basis of recovery after fatiguing exercise of human muscle. Neurology 40: 240–244

Botney M, Fields HL (1983) Amitryptiline potentiates morphine analgesia by a direct action on the central nervous system. Ann Neurol 13: 160–164

Bouchard JP, Gagny F, Tomé FM et al. (1989) Nuclear inclusions in oculo-pharyngeal muscular dystrophy in Quebec. Can J Neurol Sci 16: 446–450

Bouché P, Gherardi R, Cathala HP et al. (1983) Peroneal muscular atrophy. I. Clinical and electro-physiological study. J Neurol Sci 61: 389–399

Bouché P, Leger JM, Travers MA et al. (1986) Peripheral neuropathy in systemic vasculitis: clinical and electrophysiological study of 22 patients. Neurology 36: 1598–1602

Boudin B, Mikol J, Guillard A et al. (1976) Fatal systemic carnitine deficiency with lipid storage in skeletal muscle, heart, liver and kidney. J Neurol Sci 30: 313–325

Boulton AJM, Drury C, Clarke B et al. (1982) Continuous subcutaneous insulin infusion in the management of painful diabetic neuropathy. Diabetes Care 5: 386–390

Bourel P, Reg A, Blanc JF et al. (1976) Syndrome du canal tarsien. Rev Rheumatol 43: 723–728

Bouwsma G, van Wijngaarden GK (1980) Spinal muscular atrophy and hypertrophy of the calves. J Neurol Sci 44: 275–279

Bove KE, Iannokone ST, Hilton PK et al. (1980) Cylindrical spirals, a familial neuromuscular disorder. Ann Neurol 7: 550–556

Bowden DH, Fraser D, Jackson SH et al. (1956) Acute recurrent rhabdomyolysis (paroxysmal myohemo-globinuria). Medicine 35: 335–353

Bowen J, Gregory R, Squier M et al. (1996) The post-irradiation lower motor neuron syndrome. Brain 119: 1429–1439

Bowles AP, Asher SW, Pickett JB (1982) Use of Tinel's sign in the carpal tunnel syndrome. Ann Neurol 13: 689–690

Bowles NE, Dubowitz V, Sewry CA et al. (1987) Dermatomyositis, polymyositis and Coxsackie B virus infection. Lancet i: 1004–1007

Boysen G, Galassi F, Kamieniecka Z et al. (1979) Familial amyloid neuropathy and corneal lattice dystrophy. J Neurol Neurosurg Psychiatry 42: 1020–1030

Braakhekke JP, De Bruyn MI, Sregeman DF et al. (1986) The second wind phenomenon in McArdles disease. Brain 109: 1087–1101

Braddom RI, Johnson EW (1974) Standardisation of H reflex and diagnostic use in SI radiculopathy. Arch Phys Med Rehabil 55: 161–166

Bradley DM, Parsons EP, Clarke AJ (1993) Experience with screening newborns for Duchenne muscular dystrophy in Wales. Br Med J 306: 357–360

Bradley WG (1969) Ultrastructural changes in adynamia episodica hereditaria and normokalaemic periodic paralysis. Brain 92: 379–390

Bradley WG (1979) The limb-girdle syndromes. In: Vinken PJ, Bruyn GW (eds) Handbook of clinical neurology, vol 40. North Holland, Amsterdam, pp 433–469

Bradley WG, Fulthorpe JJ (1978) Studies of sarcolemmal integrity in myopathic muscle. Neurology 28: 670–677

Bradley WG, Chad D, Verghese JP et al. (1984a) Painful lumbosacral plexopathy with elevated erythrocyte sedimentation rate: a treatable inflammatory syndrome. Ann Neurol 15: 457–464

Bradley WG, Hedhind W, Cooper C et al. (1984b) A double-blind controlled trial of bovine brain gangliosides in amyotrophic lateral sclerosis. Neurology 34: 1079–1082

Bradley WG, Hudgson P, Gardner-Medwin D et al. (1969) Myopathy associated with abnormal lipid metabolism in skeletal muscle. Lancet i: 495–498

Bradley WG, Hudgson P, Larson PF et al. (1972a) Structural changes in the early stages of Duchenne muscular dystrophy. J Neurol Neurosurg Psychiatry 35: 451–455

Bradley WG, Jenkinson M, Park DC et al. (1972b) A myopathy associated with lipid storage. J Neurol Sci 16: 137–154

Bradley WG, Jones MZ, Mussini JM et al. (1978) Becker-type muscular dystrophy. Muscle Nerve 1: 111–132

Bradley WG, Madrid R, Thrush DC et al. (1975) Recurrent brachial plexus neuropathy. Brain 98: 381–398

Bradley WG, Price DL, Watanabeck A (1970) Familial centronuclear myopathy. J Neurol Neurosurg Psychiatry 33: 687–693

Bradley WG, Taylor R, Rice DR et al. (1990) Progress in myopathy in hyperkalaemic periodic paralysis. Arch Neurol 47: 1013–1017

Bradshaw DY, Jones HR (1992) Guillain-Barré syndrome in children. Muscle Nerve 15: 500–506

Brain WR, Henson RA (1958) Neurological syndromes associated with carcinoma: the carcinomatous neuromyopathies. Lancet ii: 971–974

Brain WR, Norris F (1965) The remote effects of cancer on the nervous system. Grune and Stratton, New York

Brain WR, Wright AD, Wilkinson M (1947) Spontaneous compression of both median nerves in the carpal tunnel. Lancet i: 277–282

Bramwell E (1922) Observations of myopathy. Proc R Soc Med 16: 1–12

Brand PW (1964) Deformity in leprosy. In: Cochrane RG, Davey TF (eds) Leprosy in theory and practice, 2nd edn. John Wright, Bristol, p 447

Brandt IK, De Luca VA (1966) Type III glycogenosis: a family with an unusual tissue distribution of the enzyme lesion. Am J Med 40: 779–784

Brasher HR, Phillips LH (1991) Autoantibodies to GABAergic neurons and response to plasmapheresis in stiff man syndrome. Neurology 41: 1588–1592

Braun PE, Frail DE, Lator N (1982) Myelin-assisted glycoprotein is the antigen for a monoclonal IgM in polyneuropathy. J Neurochem 39: 1261–1265

Braun RM, Davidson K, Doehr S (1989) Provocative testing in the diagnosis of dynamic carpal tunnel syndrome. J Hand Surg 14A: 195–197

Bray GM, Kaarsow M, Ross RT (1965) Ocular myopathy with dysphagia. Neurology 15: 678–684

Brechenmacher C, Vital C, Deminaere C et al. (1987) Guillain-Barré syndrome: an ultrastructural study of peripheral nerve in 65 patients. Clin Neuropathol 6: 19–24

Brennan MF (1977) Uncomplicated starvation versus cancer cachexia. Cancer Res 37: 2359–2364

Brenner T, Shahin R, Steiner I et al. (1992) Presence of acetylcholine receptor antibodies in human milk. Autoimmunity 12: 315

Bresolin N, Miranda AF, Chang HW et al. (1984) Phosphoglycerate kinase deficiency myopathy: biochemical and immunological studies of the mutant enzyme. Muscle Nerve 7: 542–551

Brettle RP, Gross M, Legg NH et al. (1978) Treatment of acute polyneuropathy by plasma exchange. Lancet ii: 1100

Briani C, Brannigan TH, Trojaborg W et al. (1996) Chronic inflammatory demyelinating polyneuropathy. Neuromusc Disord 6: 311–325

Brigden W (1957) Uncommon myocardial diseases: the non-coronary cardio-myopathies. Lancet ii: 1179–1184, 1243–1249

Bril PLA, Cole G, Proctor NSF (1979) Centronuclear myopathy. J Neurol Neurosurg Psychiatry 42: 548–556

Briscoe DM, McMeneman JB, O'Donohue NV (1987) Prognosis in Guillain-Barré syndrome. Arch Dis Child 62: 733–735

Bristol LA, Rothstein JD (1996) Glutamate transporter gene expression in amyotrophic lateral sclerosis motor cortex. Ann Neurol 39: 676–679

Bristowe JS (1886) Cases of ophthalmoplegia complicated with various other affections of the nervous system. Brain 8: 313–344

Britt BA, Frodis W, Scott E et al. (1982) Comparison of the caffeine skinned fibre tension (CSFT) test with the caffeine-halothane contracture (CHC) test in the diagnosis of malignant hyperthermia. Can Anaesth Soc J 29: 550–562

Brodie MJ, Moore MR, Goldberg A (1977) Enzyme abnormalities in the porphyrias. Lancet ii: 699–701

Brody IA, Dudley AW (1969) Thyrotoxic hypokalaemic periodic paralysis. Arch Neurol 21: 1–6

Brody JA, Hirano A, Scott RM (1971) Recent neuropathologic observations in amyotrophic lateral sclerosis and Parkinson-dementia of Guam. Neurology 21: 528–536

Bromberg ME, Forshew DA, Nan KL et al. (1993) Motor unit number estimation, isometric strength and electromyographic measures in amyotrophic lateral sclerosis. Muscle Nerve 16: 1213–1219

Brook JD, McCurrach ME, Harley HG et al. (1992) Molecular basis of myotonic dystrophy: expansion of a trinucleotide (CTG) repeat at the 3′ end of a transcript encoding a protein kinase family member. Cell 68: 799–808

Brooke MH (1973) Congenital fibre type disproportion. In: Kakulas BA (ed) Clinical studies in myology. Excerpta Medica, Amsterdam, pp 147–159

Brooke MH (1977) A clinician's view of neuromuscular diseases. Williams & Wilkins, Baltimore

Brooke MH, Engel WK (1969a) The histographic analysis of human muscle biopsies with regard to fibre types. I. Adult male and female. Neurology 19: 221–233

Brooke MH, Engel WK (1969b) The histographic analysis of human muscle biopsies with regard to fibre types. II. Diseases of the upper and lower motor neuron. Neurology 19: 378–393

Brooke MH, Engel WK (1969c) The histographic analysis of human muscle biopsies with regard to fibre types. III. Myotonias, myasthenia gravis and hypokalaemic paralysis. Neurology 19: 469–477

Brooke MH, Engel WK (1969d) The histographic analysis of human muscle biopsies with regard to fibre types. IV. Children's biopsies. Neurology 19: 591–605

Brooke MH, Kaiser KK (1970) Muscle fiber types: how many and what kind? Arch Neurol 23: 369–379

Brooke MH, Carroll JE, Davis JE et al. (1979) The prolonged exercise test. Neurology 29: 636–643

Brooke MH, Fenichel GM, Griggs RC et al. (1983) Clinical investigation in Duchenne dystrophy. II. Determination of the "power" of therapeutic trials based on the natural history. Muscle Nerve 6: 91–103

Brooke MH, Griggs RC, Mendell DR et al. (1981) Clinical trials in Duchenne dystrophy. I. The design of the protocol. Muscle Nerve 4: 186–197

Brooke BR. World Federation of Neurology Research Group on Neuromuscular Diseases) (1994) El Escorial WFN criteria for the diagnosis of amyotrophic lateral sclerosis. J Neurol Sci 124: 965–1085

Brooks BR, Lewis D, Rawling J et al. (1994) The natural history of amyotrophic lateral sclerosis. In: Williams AC (ed) Motor neuron disease. Chapman and Hall, London, pp 131–169

Brooks BR, Sufit RL. De Paul R et al. (1991) Design of clinical therapeutic trials in amyotrophic lateral sclerosis. In: Rowland LP (ed) Advances in neurology, vol 56. Raven Press, New York, pp 521–546

Brooks JE (1969) Hyperkalemic periodic paralysis: intracellular EMG studies. Arch Neurol 20: 13–18

Brooks VD (1956) An intracellular study of the action of repetitive nerve volleys and of botulinum toxin on miniature endplate potentials. J Physiol (Lond) 134: 264–267

Brosnan JV, Craggs RI, King RHM (1984) Attempts to suppress experimental allergic neuritis in the rat by pretreatment with antigen. Acta Neuropathol 64: 153–160

Brossard J (1886) Etude clinique sur une forme héréditaire d'atrophie musculaire progressive débutant par members inférieurs. Steinheil, Paris.

Brown BI, Brown DH (1966) Lack of an α1,4 glucan: α1,4 glucan 6-glycosyl transferase in a case of Type IV glycogenosis. Proc Natl Acad Sci USA 56: 725–729

Brown GL, Harvey AM (1939) Congenital myotonia in the goat. Brain 62: 341–363

Brown JC (1974) Muscle weakness after rest in myotonic disorders: an electrophysiological study. J Neurol Neurosurg Psychiatry 37: 1336–1342

Brown JC, Johns RJ (1967) Nerve conduction in familial dysautonomia (Riley–Day syndrome). JAMA 201: 200–203

Brown JC, Charlton JE, White DJK (1975) A regional technique for study of the sensitivity to curare in human muscle. J Neurol Neurosurg Psychiatry 38: 18–26

Brown MJ, Martin J, Asbury AK (1976) Painful diabetic neuropathy: a morphometric study. Arch Neurol 33: 164–171

Brown MM, Thompson A, Goh BT et al. (1988) Bell's palsy and HIV infection. J Neurol Neurosurg Psychiatry 51: 42

Brown MS, Asbury AK (1984) Diabetic neuropathy. Ann Neurol 15: 2–12

Brown MS, Greene DA (1984) Diabetic neuropathy: pathophysiology and management. In: Asbury AK, Gilliatt RW (eds) Periphral nerve disorders. Butterworths, London, pp 126–153

Brown RH (1996) Dystrophin associated proteins and the muscular dystrophies. Brain Pathol 6 : 19–24

Brown WF, Bolton CF (1993) Clinical electromyography, 2nd edn. Butterworth-Heinemann, Bostons p 810

Brown WF, Feasby TE (1984) Conduction block and denervation in Guillain–Barré polyneuropathy. Brain 107: 219–239

Brown WF, Milner-Brown HS (1976) Some electrical properties of motor units and their effects on the methods of estimating motor unit numbers. J Neurol Neurosurg Psychiatry 39: 249–257

Brown WF, Yates SK (1982) Percutaneous localisation of conduction abnormalities in human entrapment neuropathies. Can J Neurol Sci 9: 391–400

Brown WF, Feasby TE, Hahn AF (1993) Electrophysiological changes in the acute "axonal" form of Guillain–Barré syndrome. Muscle Nerve 16: 200–205

Brown WF, Strong MJ, Snow R (1988) Methods for estimating numbers of motor units in biceps brachialis muscles and losses of motor units with ageing. Muscle Nerve 11: 423–432

Brownell AKW (1988) Malignant hyperthermia: relationship to other diseases. Br J Anaesth 60: 303–308

Brownell B, Oppenheimer DR, Hughes JT (1970) The central nervous system in motor neuron disease. J Neurol Neurosurg Psychiatry 33: 338–357

Brownell B, Oppenheimer DR, Spalding JMK (1972) Neurogenic muscle atrophy in myasthenia gravis. J Neurol Neurosurg Psychiatry 35: 311–322

Brubaker DB, Winkelstein A (1981) Plasma exchange in rheumatoid vasculitis. Vox Sang 41: 295–301

Brunberg JA, McCormick WF, Schochet SS (1971) Type III glycogenosis: an adult with diffuse weakness and muscle wasting. Arch Neurol 25: 171–178

Brunner HG, Jansen G, Nillesen W et al. (1993) Reverse mutation in myotonic dystrophy. N Engl J Med 328: 476–480

Brunner HG, Smeets HJM, Nillesen W et al. (1991) Myotonic dystrophy: predictive value of normal results on clinical examination. Brain 114: 2303–2311

Brunner NG, Berger CL, Namba T et al. (1976) Corticotropin and corticosteroids in generalised myasthenia gravis: comparative studies and role in management. Ann NY Acad Sci 274: 577–595

Bruno CS, Servidei S, Shanske S et al. (1993) Glycogen branching enzyme in adult polyglucosan body disease. Ann Neurol 33: 88–93

Brust JCM, List TA, Catalano LW et al. (1974) Ocular myasthenia gravis mimicking progressive external opthalmoplegia. Neurology 24: 755–760

Brust JCM, Lovelace RE, Devi S (1978) Clinical and electrodiagnostic features of Charcot–Marie–Tooth syndrome. Acta Neurol Scand 58 [Suppl. 68]: 1–142

Bryant SH (1969) Cable properties of external intercostal muscle fibres from myotonic and non-myotonic goats. J Physiol (Lond) 204: 539–550

Bryant SH (1977) The physiological basis of myotonia. In: Rowland LP (ed) Pathogenesis of human muscular dystrophies. Excerpta Medica, Amsterdam, pp 715–728 (Congress series 404)

Bryant SH, Morales-Aquilera A (1971) Chloride conductance in normal and myotonic muscle fibres and the action of monocarboxylic aromatic acids. J Physiol (Lond) 219: 367–383

Buchman AS, Cochran EJ (1992) Distal myopathies. In: Vinken PJ, Bruyn GW, Klawan SAL (eds) Handbook of clinical neurology, vol. 62, Myopathies. Elsevier, Amsterdam, pp 197–208

Buchthal F (1977) Diagnostic significance of the myopathic EMG. In: Rowland LP (ed) Pathogenesis of human muscular dystrophies. Excerpta Medica, Amsterdam, pp 205–218 (Congress series 404)

Buchthal F, Behse F (1977) Peroneal muscular atrophy (PMA) and related disorders. I. Clinical manifestations as related to biopsy findings, nerve conduction and electromyography. Brain 100: 41–46

Buchthal F, Behse F (1979) Nerve conduction, nerve biopsy and electromyography in men with increased blood levels of lead. In: Persson A (ed) Sixth international congress of electromyography: symposia. Caslon Press, Stockholm, pp 210–214

Buchthal F, Olsen PZ (1970) Electromyography and muscle biopsy in infantile spinal muscular atrophy. Brain 93: 15–30

Buchthal F, Pinelli L (1953) Analysis of muscle action potentials as a diagnostic aid in neuromuscular disorders. Acta Med Scand 142 [Suppl 226] 315–327

Buchthal F, Rosenfalck P (1963) Electrophysiological aspects of myopathy with particular reference to progressive muscular dystrophy. In: Bourne GH, Golarz MN (eds) Muscular dystrophy in man and animals. Karger, Basel, pp 193–262

Buchthal F, Rosenfalck A (1966) Evoked action potentials and conduction velocity in human sensory nerves. Brain Res 3: 1–122

Buchthal F, Rosenfalck A (1971) Sensory potentials in polyneuropathy. Brain 94: 241–262

Buchthal F, Guld C, Rosenfalck P (1957) Multi-electrode study of the territory of a motor unit. Acta Physiol Scand 39: 83–104

Buchthal F, Rosenfalck A, Trojaborg W (1974) Electrophysiological findings in entrapment of the median nerve at wrist and elbow. J Neurol Neurosurg Psychiatry 37: 340–360

Buchthal F, Schmalbruch H (1980) Motor units of mammalian muscle. Physiol Rev 60: 90–142

Buckingham JM, Howard FH, Bernatz PE et al. (1976) The value of thymectomy in myasthenia gravis. Ann Surg 184: 453–457

Buckley J, Warlow C, Smith P et al. (1983) Motor neuron disease in England and Wales, 1959–1979. J Neurol Neurosurg Psychiatry 46: 197–205

Bulcke JAL (1984) Commentary: ultrasound and CT scanning in the diagnosis of neuromuscular diseases. In: Gamstorp I,

Sarnat HB (eds) Progressive spinal muscular atrophies. Raven Press, New York, pp 153–161

Bulcke JAL, Baert A (1982) Clinical and idiological aspects of myopathies. Springer-Verlag, Berlin Heidelberg New York, p 187

Bullock G, White AM, Worthington J (1968) The effects of catabolic and anabolic steroids on amino acid incorporation by skeletal muscle ribosomes. Biochem J 108: 417–425

Bulman DE, Murphy EG, Zuorzycka-Gaarn EE et al. (1991) Differentiation of Duchenne and Becker muscular dystrophy phenotypes with amino and carboxy-terminal antisera specific for dystrophin. Am J Hum Genet 48: 295–304

Bunch TW (1981) Prednisone and azathioprine for polymyositis: long-term follow up. Arthritis Rheum 24: 45–48

Bunch TW (1990) Polymyositis. Mayo Clin Proc 65: 1480–1497

Bundey S (1972) A genetic study of infantile and juvenile myasthenia gravis. J Neurol Neurosurg Psychiatry 35: 41–51

Bundey S (1974) Detection of heterozygotes for myotonic dystrophy. Clin Genet 5: 107–109

Bundey S (1983) Clinical evidence for heterogeneity in myotonic dystrophy. J Med Genet 19: 341–348

Bundey S (1985) Genetics and neurology. Churchill Livingstone, Edinburgh, pp 340

Bundey S (1992) Genetics and neurology, 2nd edn. Churchill-Livingstone, Edinburgh, pp 459

Bundey S, Lovelace RE (1975a) A genetic study of chronic spinal muscular atrophy with onset in infancy or childhood (chronic spinal muscular atrophy). In: Bradley WG, Gardner-Medwin D, Walton JN (eds) Recent advances in myology. Excerpta Medica, Amsterdam, pp 506–570

Bundey S, Lovelace RE (1975b) A clinical and genetic study of chronic proximal spinal muscular atrophy. Brain 98: 455–472

Bundey S, Carter CO, Soothill JF (1970) Early recognition of heterozygotes for the gene of dystrophia myotonica. J Neurol Neurosurg Psychiatry 33: 279–293

Bunge RP, Bunge MB (1978) Evidence that contact with connective tissue matrix is required for normal interaction between Schwann cells and nerve fibres. J Cell Biol 78: 943–950

Bunn HF (1981) Evaluation of glycosylated hemoglobin in diabetic patients. Diabetes 30: 613–617

Burgen ASV, Dickens F, Zatman LJ (1949) Action of botulism toxin on the neuromuscular junction. J Physiol (Lond) 109: 10–24

Burges J, Vincent A, Molenaar PC et al. (1994) Passive transfer of sero-negative, myasthenia gravis to mice. Muscle Nerve 17: 1393–1400

Burke D, Mackenzie RA, Skuse NF et al. (1975) Cutaneous afferent activity in median and radial nerve fascicles: a microelectrode study. J Neurol Neurosurg Psychiatry 38: 855–864

Burke D, Skuse NF, Lethlean AK (1974a) Sensary conduction of the sural nerve in polyneuropathy. J Neurol Neurosurg Psychiatry 37: 647–652

Burke D, Skuse NF, Lethlean AK (1974b) An analysis of myotonia in paramyotonia congenita. J Neurol Neurosurg Psychiatry 37: 900–906

Burke RE, Fahn S, Mayon R et al. (1981) Neuroleptic malignant syndrome caused by dopamine-depleting drugs in a patient with Huntington disease. Neurology 31: 1022–1026

Burke RE, Levine DM, Zajac FE et al. (1971) Mammalian motor units: physiological-histochemical correlation in three types in cat gastrocnemius. Science 174: 709–712

Burke RE, Strick PL, Kanda K et al. (1977) Anatomy of medial gastrocnemius and soleus motor nuclei in cat spinal cord. J Neurophysiol 40: 667–680

Burke WE, Tuttle WW, Thompson CW et al. (1953) The relation of grip strength and grip strength endurance to age. J Appl Physiol 5: 618–630

Burley D, Stein J (1979) Drug-induced peripheral neuropathies (letter). Br Med J i: 1082

Burn DJ, Ball J, Lees AJ et al. (1991) A case of progressive encephalomyelitis with rigidity and positive antiglutamic acid dehydrogenase antibodies. J Neurol Neurosurg Psychiatry 54: 449–451

Burrows EH (1963) Sagittal diameter of the spinal cord in cervical spondylosis. Clin Radiol 14: 77–86

Buxton J, Shelbourne P, Davies J et al. (1992) Detection of an unstable fragment of DNA specific to individuals with myotonic dystrophy. Nature 355: 547–548

Buzzard EF (1905) The clinical history and post-mortem examination in five cases of myasthenia gravis. Brain 28: 438–483

Buzzard EF, Greenfield JB (1921) Pathology of the nervous system. Constable, London

Byrne E, Dennett X, Crotty B et al. (1986) Dominantly inherited cardio-skeletal myopathy with lysosomal glycogen storage and normal acid maltase levels. Brain 109: 523–536

Bywaters EGL (1957) Peripheral vascular obstruction in rheumatoid arthritis and its relationship to other vascular lesions. Ann Rheum Dis 16: 84–103

Cafario ALP, Rossi B, Risaliti R et al. (1989) Type 1 fibre abnormalities in the skeletal muscle of patients with hypertrophic and dilated cardiomyopathy. J Am Coll Cardiol 14: 1464–1473

Cafferty MS, Lovelace RE, Hayes AP et al. (1991) Polyglucosan body disease. Muscle Nerve 14: 102–107

Callaghan N (1966) Restless leg syndrome in uraemic neuropathy. Neurology 16: 359–361

Callen JP (1984) Myositis and malignancy. Clin Rheum Dis 10: 117–130

Callen JP (1988) Malignancy in polymyositis-dermatomyositis. Clin Dermatol 2: 55–63

Calne DB, Eisen A, McGeer E et al. (1986) Alzheimer's disease, Parkinson's disease and motoneuron disease: a biotrophic interaction between ageing and environment? Lancet ii: 1067–1070

Calo M, Crisi G, Martinelli C et al. (1986) CT and the diagnosis of myopathies. Neuroradiology 28: 53–57

Cammermeyer J (1956) Neuropathological changes in hereditary neuropathies: manifestation of the syndrome heredopathia atactica polyneuriformis in the presence of interstitial hypertrophic polyneuropathy. J Neuropathol Exp Neurol 15: 340–361

Campa JF, Sanders DB (1974) Familial hypokalemic periodic paralysis: local recovery after nerve stimulation. Arch Neurol 31: 110–115

Campbell CS, Wolf RF (1954) Lipoma producing a lesion of the deep branch of the ulnar nerve J Neurosurg 11: 310–311

Campbell H, Bramwell E (1900) Myasthenia gravis. Brain 23: 277–336

Campbell IW, Ewing DJ, Harrower BD et al. (1976) Peripheral and autonomic nerve function in diabetic ketoacidosis. Lancet ii: 167–169

Campbell MJ, Paty DW (1974) Carcinomatous neuromyopathy. I. Electrophysiological studies. J Neurol Neurosurg Psychiatry 37: 131–141

Campbell MJ, McComas AJ, Petito F (1973) Physiological basis of ageing in muscles. J Neurol Neurosurg Psychiatry 36: 174–182

Campbell MJ, Simpson E, Crombie AL et al. (1970) Ocular myasthenia: evaluation of tensilon tomography and electronystagmography as diagnostic tests. J Neurol Neurosurg Psychiatry 33: 639–646

Campbell WW, Ward LC, Swift TR (1981) Nerve conduction velocity varies inversely with height. Muscle Nerve 4: 520–523

Campuzano V, Montermini L, Malto MD et al. (1996) Friedreich's ataxia: autosomal recessive disease caused by an intrinsic GAA triplet repeat expansion. Science 271: 1423–1427

Camu W, Billiard M, Baldy-Moulinier M (1993) Fasting plasma and CSF amino acid levels in ALS. Acta Neurol Scand 88: 51–55

Canal N, Comi G, Saibene V et al. (1978) The relationship between peripheral and autonomic neuropathy in insulin dependent diabetes: a clinical and instrumental evaluation. In: Canal N, Pozza G (eds) Peripheral neuropathies. Elsevier, Amsterdam, p 247

Cancilla PA, Kalyananaman K, Verity MA et al. (1971) Familial myopathy with probable lysis of myofibrils in Type 1 fibres. Neurology 21: 579-

Cannieu JMA (1897) Recherches sur une anastomose entre la branche profonde de cubitale et le médian. Bull Soc d'Anat Physiol Bordeaux 18: 339

Cannon SC, Brown RH, Corey DP (1991) A sodium channel defect in hyperkalaemic episodic paralysis: potassium-induced failure of inactivation. Neuron 6: 619-626

Cao A, Cianchetti C, Calisti L et al. (1978) Schwartz–Jampel syndrome. J Neurol Sci 35: 175-187

Cappock SW, Watkins PT (1991) The natural history of diabetic femoral neuropathy. QJM 79: 307-313

Carey JS (1986) Motor neuron disease – a challenge to medical ethics: discussion paper. J R Soc Med 79: 216-220

Carfi J, Dong MA (1985) Posterior interosseus syndrome revisited. Muscle Nerve 8: 499-502

Carlson BM (1986) Regeneration of entire skeletal muscles. Fed Proc 45: 1456-1460

Caroff SN (1980) The neuroleptic malignant syndrome. J Clin Psychratry 41: 79-83

Caroscio JT, Calhoun WF, Yahr MD (1984) Prognostic factors in motor neuron disease: a prospective study of longevity. In: Rose FC (ed) Research progress in motor neuron disease. Pitman, London, pp 34-43

Carpenter S, Karpati G (1979) Duchenne muscular dystrophy: plasma membrane loss initiates muscle cell necrosis unless it is repaired. Brain 102: 147-161

Carpenter S, Karpati G (1984) Pathology of skeletal muscle. Churchill Livingstone, Edinburgh

Carpenter S, Karpati G, Andermann F et al. (1974) Giant axonal neuropathy. Arch Neurol 31: 312-316

Carpenter S, Karpati G, Heller I et al. (1978) Inclusion body myositis: a distinct variety of idiopathic inflammatory myopathy. Neurology 28: 8-17

Carpenter S, Karpati G, Rothman S et al. (1976) The childhood type of dermatomyositis. Neurology 26: 952-962

Carroll GJ, Will RK, Peter JB et al. (1987) Penicillamine-induced polymyositis and dermatomyositis. J Rheumatol 14: 995-998

Carroll JE, Brooke MH, De Vivo DC et al. (1978) Biochemical and physiologic consequences of carnitine palmitoyl transferase deficiency. Muscle Nerve 1: 103-110

Carry MR, Ringel SP, Starcevich JM (1986) Distribution of capillaries in normal and diseased human skeletal muscle. Muscle Nerve 9: 445-454

Carter ND, Heath R, Jeffrey S et al. (1983) Carbonic anhydrase III in Duchenne muscular dystrophy. Clin Chim Acta 133: 201-208

Carter ND, Morgan JE, Monaco AP et al. (1990) Dystrophin expression and genotypic analysis of two cases of benign X-linked myopathy (McLeod syndrome). J Med Genet 27: 345-347

Caruso C, Buchthal F (1965) Refractory period of muscle and electromyographic findings in relatives of patients with muscular dystrophy. Brain 88: 29-50

Caruso C, La Bianca O, Ferrannini E (1973) Effect of ischaemia on sensory potentials of normal subjects of different ages. J Neurol Neurosurg Psychiatry 36: 455-466

Casanova G, Jerusalem F (1979) Myopathology of myotonic dystrophy: a morphometric study. Acta Neuropathol (Berl) 45: 231-240

Case Records (1984) Case 39-1984. N Engl J Med 311: 839-847

Case Records (1992) Case 34-1992. N Engl J Med 337: 548-557

Caseli RJ, Daube JR, Hunder GG et al. (1988) Peripheral neuropathic syndromes in giant cell (temporal) arteritis. Neurology 38: 685-689

Casey EB, Harrison MJG (1972) Diabetic amyotrophy: A follow-up study. Br Med J i: 656-659

Casey EB, Le Quesne PM (1972) Electrophysiological evidence for a distal lesion in alcoholic neuropathy. J Neurol Neurosurg Psychiatry 35: 624-630

Casey EB, Jellife AM, Le Quesne PM et al. (1973) Vincristine neuropathy: clinical and electrophysiological observations. Brain 96: 69-86

Casier H, Merlevedi E (1962) On the mechanism of the disulfiram-ethanol intoxication symptoms. Arch Int Pharmacodyn Ther 139: 165-176

Castleman B (1966) The pathology of the thymus gland in myasthenia gravis. Ann NY Acad Sci 135: 496-503

Castleman B, Norris EH (1949) The pathology of the thymus in myasthenia gravis: a study of 35 cases. Medicine (Baltimore) 28: 27-58

Castro LH, Ropper AH (1993) Human immune globulin infusion in Guillain–Barré syndrome: worsening during and after treatment. Neurology 43: 1034-1036

Caswell AH, Baker SP, Boyd H et al. (1978) Beta adrenergic receptor and adenylate cyclase in transverse tubules of skeletal muscle. J Biol Chem 10: 3049-3054

Caughey JE, Myrianthopolous NC (1963) Dystrophia myotonica and related disorders. Thomas, Springfield

Cavanagh JB (1964) The significance of the "dying-back" process in experimental and human neurological disease. Int Rev Exp Pathol 7: 219-267

Cavanagh JB (1979) The "dying-back" process: a common denominator in many naturally occurring and toxic neuropathies. Arch Pathol Lab Med 103: 659-664

Cavanagh JB (1985) Mechanisms of damage by chemical agents. In: Swash M, Kennard C (eds) Scientific basis of clinical neurology. Churchill Livingstone, Edinburgh, pp 631-645

Cavanagh JB, Buxton PH (1989) Trichloroethylene cranial neuropathy: is it really a toxic neuropathy or does it activate latent herpes virus? J Neurol Neurosurg Psychiatry 52: 297-301

Cavanagh JB, Gysbers MF (1983) Ultrastructural features of the Purkinje cell damage caused by acrylamide in the rat. J Neurocytol 12: 413-437

Cavanagh JB, Jacobs JM (1964) Some quantitative aspects of diphtheritic neuropathy. Br J Exp Pathol 45: 309-322

Cavanagh JB, Mellick RS (1965) On the nature of the peripheral nerve lesions associated with acute intermittent porphyria. J Neurol Neurosurg Psychiatry 28: 320-327

Cavanagh JB, Fuller NH, Johnson HRH et al. (1974) The effects of thallium salts with particular reference to the nervous system changes. QJM 43: 293-319

Cavanagh NPC, Eames RA, Galvin RJ et al. (1979a) Hereditary sensory neuropathy with paraplegia. Brain 102: 79-84

Cavanagh NPC, Lake BD, McMeniman P (1979b) Congenital fibre type disproportion myopathy: a histological diagnosis with an uncertain clinical outlook. Arch Dis Child 54: 735-743

Cazzato G (1970) Myopathic changes in denervated muscle: a study of biopsy material in various neuromuscular diseases. In: Walton JW, Canal N, Scarlata G (eds) Muscle diseases. Excerpta Medica, Amsterdam, pp 392-401

CDC (1989) Eosinophilia-myalgia syndrome. New Mexico. MMWR 38: 765-767

Celsing F, Blomstrand E, Melichna J et al. (1986) Effect of hyperthyroidism on fibre type composition, fibre area, glycogen content and enzyme activity in human skeletal muscle. Clin Physiol 6: 171

Cenkovich F, Shih-Fong H, Gersten JW (1982) A quantitative electromyographic index that is independent of the force of contraction. Electroencephalogr Clin Neurophysiol 54: 79-86

Cervera R, Ramirez G, Fernandez-Sola J et al. (1991) Antibodies to endothelial cells in dermatomyositis: association with interstitial lung disease. Br Med J 302: 880-881

Ceston R, Lejonne U (1902) Une myopathie avec retractions familiales. Nouv Icanographie Salpetriere 15: 38–52

Chad DA, Lacomis D (1994) Critically ill patients with newly acquired weakness: the clinico-pathological spectrum. Ann Neurol 35: 257–259

Chad DA, Hammer K, Sargent J (1986) Slow resolution of multi-focal weakness and fasciculation: a reversible motor neuron syndrome. Neurology 36: 1260–1263

Chad DA, Smith TW, Blumenfeld A et al. (1990) Human immun-odeficiency virus (HIV) associated myopathy. Ann Neurol 28: 579–582

Chalikian D, Bardri R (1982) Sarcolemmal demosterol accumula-tion and membrane physical properties in 20 : 25 diazocholes-terol myotonia. Muscle Nerve 5: 118–124

Chaikin HL (1980) Rhabdomyolysis secondary to drug overdose and prolonged coma. South Med J 73: 990–994

Chalk CH, Dyck PT, Conn DL (1993) Vasculitic neuropathy. In: Dyck PJ, Thomas PK (eds) Peripheral neuropathy, 3rd edn, vol 2. WB Saunders, Philadelphia, pp 1424–1436

Chalk CH, Murray NM, Newsom-Davis J et al. (1990) Response of the Lambert–Eaton myasthenic syndrome to treatment of associated small cell lung carcinoma. Neurology 40: 1552–1556

Chalk CH, Windebank AT, Kimmel DW et al. (1992) The distinc-tive clinical features of paraneoplastic sensory neuronopathy. Can J Neurol Sci 19: 346–351

Challenor YB, Felton CP, Brust JCM (1984) Peripheral nerve involvement in sarcoidosis: an electrodiagnostic study. J Neurol Neurosurg Psychiatry 47: 1219–1222

Chalmers A, Sayson R, Walters K (1982) Juvenile dermatomyosi-tis: medical, focal and economic status in adulthood. Can Med Assoc J 126: 31–33

Chamberlain JS, Chamberlain JR, Fenwick RG et al. (1992) Diagnosis of Duchenne and Becker muscular dystrophies by polymerase chain reaction. JAMA 267: 2609–2615

Chamberlain MA, Bruckner FE (1970) Rheumatoid neuropathy: clinical and electrophysiological features. Ann Rheum Dis 29: 609–616

Chamberlain S, Farrel M, Shaw J et al. (1993) Genetic recombina-tion events which position the Friedreich's ataxia locus proxi-mal to the D 9S 15/D 9S 5 linkage group on chromosome 9q. Ann J Hum Genet 52: 99–109

Chamberlain S, Robinson N, Walker JL et al. (1980) Effect of lecithin on disability and on plasma-free choline levels in Friedreich's ataxia. J Neurol Neurosurg Psychiatry 43: 843–845

Chan RC, Hsu TC (1991) Quantitative comparison of motor unit potential parameters between monopolar and concentric needles. Muscle Nerve 14: 1028–1032

Chan YW, Kay R, Schwartz MS (1991) Juveline distal spinal mus-cular atrophy of upper extremities in Chinese males. J Neurol Neurosurg Psychiatry 54: 165–166

Chanard J, Bindi P, Lavand S et al. (1989) Carpal tunnel syn-drome and type of dialysis membrane. Br Med J 298: 867–869

Chance PF, Pleasure D (1993) Charcot-Marie-Tooth syndrome. Arch Neurol 50: 1180–1184

Chance PF, Alderson MK, Leppig KA et al. (1993) DNA deletion associated with hereditary neuropathy with liability to pres-sure palsies. Cell 72: 143–151

Chance PF, Matsunami N, Lensch W et al. (1992) Analysis of the DNA duplication 17p 11.2 in Charcot-Marie-Tooth neuropathy Type 1 pedigrees: additional evidence for a third autosomal CMT 1 locus. Neurology 42: 2037–2041

Chaney WC (1924) Tendon reflexes in myxoedema: a valuable aid in diagnosis. JAMA 82: 2013–2016

Chang L, Anderson T, Migneco A et al. (1993) Cerebral abnor-malities in myotonic dystrophy. Arch Neurol 50: 917–923

Chapoy PR, Angelini A, Brown WJ et al. (1980) Systemic carni-tine deficiency. N Engl J Med 303: 1389–1394

Charchaglie RJ, Fernandez BL, Perec CJ et al. (1974) Functional studies of the parotid and pancreas glands in amyotrophic lateral sclerosis. J Neurol Neurosurg Psychiatry 37: 863–867

Charcot JM (1869) Lectures on the diseases of the nervous system. Lecture XIII, 2nd series. New Sydenham Society, London 1881. Republished 1962, Hafner, New York, p 192

Chari VR, Katiyar BC, Rastogi BL (1977) Neuropathy in hepatic disorders. J Neurol Sci 31: 93–111

Charnas L. Trapp B, Griffin J (1988) Congenital absence of peripheral myelin: abnormal Schwann cell development causes lethal arthrogryposis multiplex congenita. Neurology 38: 966–974

Charness ME, Morady F, Scheinman MM (1984) Frequent neuro-logic toxicity associated with amiodarone therapy. Neurology 34: 669–671

Chandry V, Corse A, Carnblath DR et al. (1994) Multifocal mononeuropathy: electrodiagnostic features. Muscle Nerve 17: 198–205

Chazot G, Berger B, Carrier H et al. (1976) Manifestations neu-rologiques des gammopathies monoclonales. Rev Neurol (Paris) 132: 195–212

Cheah JS, Tock EPC, Tan SP (1975) The light and electron micro-scope changes in the skeletal muscles during paralysis in thy-rotoxic periodic paralysis. Am J Med Sci 269: 365–374

Chelmicka-Schorr E, Bernstein LP, Surbrugge EG et al. (1979) Eaton–Lambert syndrome in a 9-year-old girl. Arch Neurol 36: 572–574

Chen K-M (1994) Disappearance of amyotrophic lateral sclerosis and Parkinson dementia from Guam. In: Rose FC (ed) ALS – from Charcot to the present and into the future. Smith-Gordon, London, pp 49–57

Chen M (1986) The epidemiology of self-perceived fatigue among adults. Prev Med 15: 74–81

Cherington M (1974) Botulism: 10 years' experience. Arch Neurol 30: 432–437

Cherington M (1976) Guanidine and germine in Eaton–Lambert syndrome. Neurology 26: 944–946

Cherington M, Ryan DW (1970) Treatment of botulism with guanidine. N Engl J Med 282: 195–197

Cherington M, Snyder RD (1968) Tick paralysis: neurophysio-logic studies. N Engl J Med 278: 95–97

Cherington M, Lewin E, McCrimmon A (1968) Serum creatine phosphokinase changes following needle electromyographic studies. Neurology 18: 271–272

Chia L-G (1988) Pure trigeminal motor neuropathy. Br Med J 296: 609–610

Chiappa KH, Young RR (1985) Evoked responses: overused, underused or misused? Arch Neurol 42: 76–77

Chiba A, Kusonoki S, Shimuzu T et al. (1992) Serum IgG anti-body to ganglioside GQ16 is a possible marker of Miller Fisher syndrome. Ann Neurol 31: 677–679

Chiedozi LC (1979) Pyomyositis: review of 205 cases in 112 patients. Am J Surg 137: 255–259

Child JS, Perloff JK, Bach PM et al. (1986) Cardiac involvement in Friedreich's ataxia. J Am Coll Cardiol 7: 1370–1378

Choi DW (1992) Amyotrophic lateral sclerosis and glutamate – too much of a good thing? N Engl J Med 326: 1493–1495

Chokroverty S (1989) AAEE Case Report #13. Diabetic amyo-trophy. Muscle Nerve 10: 679–684

Chokroverty S, Reyes MG, Rubino FA et al. (1977) The syndrome of diabetic amyotrophy. Ann Neurol 2: 181–194

Chopra JS, Bannerjee JM, Murthi JMK et al. (1980) Paralytic rabies: a clinico-pathological study. Brain 103: 789–802

Chopra JS, Dhand UK, Meta S et al. (1986) Effect of protein-calorie malnutrition on peripheral nerves. Brain 109: 307–323

Chopra JS, Harwitz LJ, Montrgomary DAD (1969). The patho-gensis of sural nerve changes in diabetes millitus. Brain 92: 391–418

Chopra JS, Prabhakar S, Bannerjee AK (1984) The wasted leg syndrome: clinical electrophysiological and histopathological studies. In: Rose FC (ed) Research progress in motor neuron disease. Pitman, London, pp 422–431

Chou SM (1968) Myxovirus-like structures and accompanying nuclear changes in chronic polymyositis. Arch Pathol 86: 649–658

Chou SM (1986) Inclusion body myositis: a chronic persistent mumps myositis. Hum Pathol 17: 765–777

Chou S, Gutmann L (1970) Picornavirus-like crystals in subacute polymyositis. Neurology 20: 205–213

Chou SM, Hartmann HA (1965) Axonal lesions and waltzing syndrome after IDPN administration in rats, with a concept of "axostasis". Acta Neuropathol (Berl) 4: 590–603

Chou SM, Nouaka J (1978) Werdnig-Hoffmann disease: proposal of a pathogenetic mechanism. Acta Neuropathol (Berl) 41: 45–54

Chrissian SA, Stolov WC, Hongladarom T (1976) Needle electromyography: its effect on serum phosphokinase activity. Arch Phys Med Rehabil 57: 114–119

Christenssen F (1959) Topography of terminal motor innervation in striated muscles from stillborn infants. Am J Phys Med 38: 65–78

Christiansen FT, Houliston JB, Dawkins RL (1978) HLA, anti DNA and complement in myasthenia gravis. Muscle Nerve 1: 467–470

Christie BGB (1961) Electrodiagnostic features of Charcot-Marie-Tooth disease. Proc R Soc Med 54: 321–324

Chudley AE, Barunada MA (1979) Diaphragmatic elevation in neonatal myotonic dystrophy. Am J Dis Child 133: 1182–1185

Church SC (1967) The heart in myotonia atrophica. Arch Intern Med 119: 176–181

Churg J, Strauss L (1951) Allergic granulomatosis, allergic angiitis and periarteritis nodosa. Am J Pathol 27: 277–320

Cianchetti C, Abbritti G, Perticoni G et al. (1976) Toxic polyneuropathy of shoe industry workers. J Neurol Neurosurg Psychiatry 39: 1151–1161

Cioni R, Paradiso C, Battistini N et al. (1985) Automatic analysis of surface EMG (preliminary findings in healthy subjects and in patients with neurogenic motor diseases). Electroencephalogr Clin Neurophysiol 61: 243–246

Clancy RR, Kelts KA, Oehlert JW (1980) Clinical variability in congenital fiber type disproportion. J Neurol Sci 46: 257–266

Clark AF, Vignos PJ Jr (1979) Experimental corticosteroid myopathy: effect on myofibrillar ATPase activity and protein degradation. Muscle Nerve 2: 265–273

Clark DS, Meyerberg RJ, Morales RR et al. (1975) Heart block and Kearns–Sayres: electrophysiologic and pathologic correlation. Chest 68: 727–730

Clark JR, Carlson RD, Sasaki CT et al. (1985) Facial paralysis in Lyme disease.

Clark JR, Miller RG, Vidgoff JM et al. (1979) Juvenile-onset metachromatic leucodystrophy. Neurology 29: 346–353

Clarke E, Bearn JG (1972) The spiral nerve bands of Fontana. Brain 95: 1–20

Clarke FM, Masters CJ (1976) Interactions between muscle proteins and glycolytic enzymes. Int J Biochem 7: 359–365

Clarkson PM, Apple FS, Byrnes WC et al. (1987) Creatine kinase isoforms following isometric exercise. Muscle Nerve 10: 41–44

Claus D (1990) Central motor conduction. Muscle Nerve 13: 1125–1132

Clemens PR, Fenwick RG, Chamberlain JS et al. (1991) Carrier detection and prenatal diagnosis in Duchenne and Becker muscular dystrophy families using dinucleotide repeat polymorphisms. Am J Hum Genet 49: 951–960

Clemens PR, Yamamoto M, Engel AG (1990) Adult phosphorylase b kinase deficiency. Ann Neurol 28: 529–538

Clements PJ, First DE, Compton DS et al. (1978) Muscle disease in progressive systemic sclerosis. Arthritis Rheum 21: 62–71

Clements RS, Reynertson R (1977) Myoinositol metabolism in diabetes mellitus: effect of insulin treatment. Diabetes 26: 215–221

Clerk A, Sewry CA, Dubowitz V et al. (1992) Characterisation of dystrophin in fetuses at risk for Duchenne muscular dystrophy. J Neurol Sci 111: 82–91

Clinicopathological conference (1990) Case 39-1990. N Engl J Med 323: 895–908

Cobb CA, Moiel RG (1974) Ganglion of the peroneal nerve. J Neurosurg 41: 255–259

Cochrane P, Hughes RR, Buxton PH et al. (1973) Myophosphorylase deficiency (McArdle's disease) in two inter-related families. J Neurol Neurosurg Psychiatry 36: 217–224

Cochrane RG, Davey TF (1964) Leprosy in theory and practice. 2nd edn. John Wright, Bristol

Coërs C (1975) Motor innervation of myasthenic muscles related to age. Lancet ii: 555

Coërs C, Hildenbrand J (1965) Latent neuropathy in diabetes and alcoholism: electromyographic and histological study. Neurology 15: 19–38

Coërs C, Telerman-Toppet N (1977) Morphological changes of motor units in Duchenne's muscular dystrophy. Arch Neurol 34: 396–402

Coërs C, Woolf AL (1959) The innervation of muscle: a biopsy study. Blackwell Scientific Publications, Oxford

Coërs C, Woolf AL (1981) Pathological anatomy of the intramuscular motor innervation. In: Walton J (ed) Disorders of voluntary muscle, 4th edn. Churchill Livingstone, Edinburgh, pp 238–260

Coërs C, Telerman-Toppet N, Gerard JM (1973) Terminal innervation ratio in neuromuscular disease: disorders of lower motor neuron, peripheral nerve and muscle. Arch Neurol 29: 215–222

Cogan DG (1965) Myasthenia gravis: a review of the disease and description of lid twitch as a characteristic sign. Arch Ophthalmol 74: 217–221

Cohen LG, Starr A, Pratt H (1985) Cerebral somatosensory potentials evoked by muscle stretch, cutaneous taps and electrical stimulation of peripheral nerves in the lower limbs in man. Brain 108: 103–122

Cohen MS, Younger D (1981) Aspects of the natural history of myasthenia gravis: crisis and death. Ann NY Acad Sci 377: 670–677

Cohen P, Solomon NH (1955) Familial dysautonomia: case report with autopsy. J Pediatr 46: 663–670

Coimbra A, Andrade C (1971) Familial amyloid polyneuropathy: an electron microscopic study of the peripheral nerve in five cases. I. Interstitial changes. Brain 94: 199–206

Cole CG, Abbs SJ, Dubowitz V et al. (1992) Linkage of Emery–Dreifuss muscular dystrophy to the red-green cone pigment (RGCD) genes, proximal to factor VIII. Neuromusc Disord 2: 51–57

Coleman RA, Stajich JM, Pact VW et al. (1986) The ischaemic exercise test in normal adults and in patients with weakness and cramps. Muscle Nerve 9: 216–221

Colling-Saltin AS (1978) Enzyme histochemistry on skeletal muscle of the human fetus. J Neurol Sci 39: 169–185

Collins AF, Nulsen FE, Randt CT (1960) Relation of peripheral nerve fibre size and sensation in man. Arch Neurol 3: 381–385

Collins GH, Webster H de F, Victor M (1964) The ultrastructure of myelin and axonal alterations in sciatic nerves of thiamine deficient and chronically starved rats. Acta Neuropathol (Berl) 3: 511–521

Combarros O, Calleja J, Figols J et al. (1983) Dominantly inherited hereditary motor and sensory neuropathy Type 1. J Neurol Sci 61: 181–191

Compston DAS, Vincent A, Newsom-Davis J et al. (1980) Clinical, pathological HLA antigen and immunological evidence for disease heterogeneity in myasthenia gravis. Brain 103: 579–601

Conen PE, Murphy GE, Donaghue WL (1963) Light and electron microscopic studies of "myogranules" in a child with hypotonia and muscle weakness. Can Med Assoc J 89: 983–986

Conn JW, Knopt RF, Nesbit RM (1964) Clinical characteristics of primary aldosteronism from analysis of 145 cases. Am J Surg 107: 159–172

Connolly AM, Pestronk A, Trotter JZ et al. (1993) Anti β tubulin antibodies in chronic inflammatory demyelinating polyneuropathy. Neurology 43: 557–562

Conomy JP, Barnes KI, Conomy JM (1979) Cutaneous sensory function in diabetes mellitus. J Neurol Neurosurg Psychiatry 42: 656–661

Conrad B, Sindermann F, Prochazka VJ (1972) Interval analysis of repetitive denervation potentials of human skeletal muscle. J Neurol Neurosurg Psychiatry 35: 834–840

Conradi S, Ronnevi L-O (1985) Cytotoxic activity in the plasma of amyotrophic lateral sclerosis (ALS) patients against normal erythrocytes. J Neurol Sci 68: 135–145

Conradi S, Grimby L, Lundemo G (1982a) Pathophysiology of fasciculations studied by electromyography of single motor units. Muscle Nerve 5: 202–208

Conradi S, Ronnevi L-O, Norris FH (1982b) Motor neuron disease and toxic metals. In: Rowland LP (ed) Human motor neuron diseases. Raven Press, New York, pp 201–231

Consensus Development Statement: clinical use of botulinum toxin A (1991). Arch Neurol 48: 1294–1297

Conway MJ, Siebel JA, Eaton RP (1974) Thyrotoxicosis and periodic paralysis: improvement with beta blockade. Ann Intern Med 81: 332–336

Cook JD, Henderson-Tiltan AC (1984) Beneficial responses to a calcium channel antagonist in myotonic syndromes Neurology 34: 193–194

Coquet M, Degoul F, Vital A et al. (1993) MERFF family with 8344 mutation in tRNA$^{(lys)}$: evidence of a mitochondrial vasculopathy in muscle biopsies. Neuromusc Disord 3: 593–597

Coquet M, Vallat JM, Vital C et al. (1983) Nuclear inclusions in oculopharyneal dystrophy. J Neurol Sci 60: 151–156

Coquet M, Vital C, Julien J (1990) Presence of inclusion body myositis-like filaments in oculopharyneal muscular dystrophy. Neuropathol Appl Neurobiol 16: 393–400

Corfi J, Ma DM (1985) Posterior interosseous syndrome revisited. Muscle Nerve 8: 499–502

Cornblath DR, McArthur JC (1988) Predominatly sensory neuropathy in patients with AIDS and AIDS-related complex. Neurology 38: 794–796

Cornblath DR, Asbury AK, Albers JW et al. (1991a) Research criteria for diagnosis of chronic inflammatory demyelinating polyneuropathy (CIDP). Neurology 41: 617–618

Cornblath DR, McArthur JC, Kennedy PGE et al. (1987) Inflammatory demyelinating peripheral neuropathies associated with human T cell lymphotropic virus type III infection. Ann Neurol 21: 32–40

Cornblath DR, Sumner AJ, Danbe J et al. (1991b) Conduction block in clinical practice. Muscle Nerve 14: 869–871

Cornelio F, Di Donato S (1985) Myopathies due to enzyme deficiencies. J Neurol 232: 329–340

Cornelio F, Bresolin N, Singer A et al. (1984) Clinical varieties of neuromuscular disease in debrancher deficiency. Arch Neurol 41: 1027–1032

Cornelio F, Di Donato S, Peluchetti D et al. (1977) Fatal cases of lipid storage myopathy with carnitine deficiency. J Neurol Neurosurg Psychiatry 40: 170–178

Correlli J, Monteverde DA, Bueri JA et al. (1991) Peripheral nervous system and spinal cord involvement in lymphoma. Acta Neurol Scand 83: 45–51

Coulton GR, Morgan JE, Partridge TA et al. (1988) The mdx mouse skeletal muscle myopathy. 1. A histological, morphometric and biochemical investigation. Neuropath Exp Neurobiol 14: 53–70

Cowan JMA, Rothwell JC, Dick JPR et al. (1984) Abnormalities in central motor pathway conduction in multiple sclerosis. Lancet ii: 304–307

Cowen D, Olmstead EV (1963) Infantile neuroaxonal dystrophy. J Neuropathol Exp Neurol 22: 175–236

Cox B, Blaxter M, Buckle A et al. (1987) The health and lifestyle survey. Health Promotion Research Trust, London

Coxon A, Pallis CA (1976) Metronidazole neuropathy. J Neurol Neurosurg Psychiatry 39: 403–405

Cravens G, Kline DG (1990) Posterior interosseous nerve palsies. Neurosurgery 27: 397–402

Crerar MM, Hudson JW, Matthews KE et al. (1988) Studies on the expression and evolution of the glycogen phosphorylase gene family in the rat. Genome 30: 582–590

Creutzfeldt OD, Abbott BC, Fowler WM et al. (1963) Muscle membrane potentials in episodic adynamia. Electroencephalogr Clin Neurophysiol 15: 508–519

Crews J, Kaiser KK, Brooke MH (1976) Muscle pathology of myotonia congenita. J Neurol Sci 28: 449–457

Critchley EMR, Mitchell JD (1990) Human botulism. Br J Hosp Med 43: 290–292

Croft PB, Wilkinson M (1965) The incidence of carcinomatous neuromyopathy in patients with various types of carcinoma. Brain 88: 427–434

Croft PB, Wilkinson M (1969) The course and prognosis in some types of carcinomatous neuromyopathy. Brain 92: 1–8

Croft PB, Cutting JC, Jewesbury ECO et al. (1977) Ocular myopathy (progressive external ophthalmoplegia) with neuropathic complications. Acta Neurol Scand 55: 169–197

Croft PB, Henson RA, Urich H et al. (1965) Sensory neuropathy with bronchial carcinoma. Brain 88: 501–514

Croft PB, Urich H, Wilkinson M (1967) Peripheral neuropathy of sensorimotor type associated with malignant disease. Brain 90: 31–66

Crowe WE, Bove KE, Levinson JE et al. (1982) Clinical and pathogenic implication of histopathology in childhood polydermatomyositis. Arthritis Rheum 25: 126–139

Cruikshank JK, Corbin DOC, Bucher B (1992) HTLV-I and neurological disease. In: Rudge P (ed) Neurological aspects of human retroviruses. Bailliere, London, pp 61–81 (Bailliere's clinical neurology, vol 1)

Crutchfield CA, Gutmann L (1980) Hereditary aspects of median-ulnar nerve communications. J Neurol Neurosurg Psychiatry 43: 53–55

Cruz-Martinez A, Du Theil LA (1989) Electrophysiologic evaluation of Emery–Dreifuss muscular dystrophy. Electromyogr Clin Neurophysiol 29: 99–103

Cruz-Martinez A, Anciones B, Ferrer MJ et al. (1985) Electrophysiologic study in benign human botulism type B. Muscle Nerve 8: 580–585

Cruz-Martinez A, Ferrer MT, Lopez-Terradas JM et al. (1979) Single-fibre electromyography in central core disease. J Neurol Neurosurg Psychiatry 42: 662–666

Crymble B (1968) Brachial neuralgia and the carpal tunnel syndrome. Br Med J iii: 470–471

Culp WJ, Ochoa J, Cline M et al. (1989) Heat and mechanical hyperalgesia induced by capsacin. Brain 112: 1317–1331

Cumming WJK, Hardy M, Hudgson P et al. (1976) Carnitine palmitoyl transferase deficiency. J Neurol Sci 30: 247–258

Cumming WJK, Weiser R, Teoh R et al. (1977) Localised nodular myositis: a clinical and pathological variant of polymyositis. QJM 46: 531–546

Currie OB, Basten JF, Francis MJO et al. (1974) Calcium uptake by sarcoplasmic reticulum of muscle from vitamin D deficient rabbits. Nature 249: 83–84

Currie S, Henson RA, Morgan HG et al. (1970) The incidence of the non-metastatic neurological syndromes of obscure origin in the reticuloses. Brain 93: 629–640

Cushing H (1912) The pituitary body and its disorders. Lippincott, Philadelphia

Dalakas MC (1991) Polymyositis, dermatomyosiis and inclusion body myositis. N Engl J Med 325: 1487–1498

Dalakas MC (1992) Inflammatory myopathies. In: Rowland LP, Di Mauro S (eds) Handbook of clinical neurology, vol 62. Elsevier, Amsterdam, pp 369–390

Dalakas MC, Engel WK (1983) Treatment of "permanent" muscle weakness in familial hypokalaemic periodic paralysis. Muscle Nerve 6: 182–186

Dalakas MC, Pezeshkpour GH (1988) Neuromuscular diseases associated with human immunodeficiency virus infection. Ann Neurol 23: S34–S48

Dalakas MC, Elder G, Hallett M et al. (1986) A long-term follow up study of patients with post poliomyelitis neuromuscular symptoms. N Engl J Med 314: 959–963

Dalakas MC, Illa I, Pezeshkpour GH et al. (1990) Mitochondrial myopathy caused by longterm AZT (zidovudine) therapy. N Engl J Med 322: 1098–1105

Dalakas MC, Leon-Monzon M, Illa I et al. (1992) Immuno-pathology of HTLV-1 associated polymyositis (HTLV PM). Neurology 42: Suppl. 301–302

Dalakas MC, Pezeshkpour GH, Gravell M et al. (1986) Poly-myositis in patients with AIDS. JAMA 256: 2381–2383

Dalakas MC, Roze JW, Paul J et al. (1983) Increased circulation of T lymphocytes bearing surface thymosin α_1 in patients with myasthenia gravis. Neurology 33: 144–149

Dal Canto MC, Gurney ME (1995) Neuropathological changes in two lines of mice carrying a transgenic for mutant human Cu, Zn SOD, and in mice overexpressing wild type human SOD: a model of familial amyotrophic lateral sclerosis (FALS). Brain Res. 676: 25–40

Dalmau J, Graus F, Rosenblum MK et al. (1992) Anti-Hu associ-ated paraneoplastic encephalomyelitis sensory neuronopathy. Medicine 71: 59–72

Daniels CW (1906) Observations in the federated Malay States on beri-beri. Stud Inst Med Res Fed Malay States 4: 1

Danon M, Carpenter S (1991) Myopathy with thick filament (myosin) loss following prolonged paralysis with vecuronium during steroid treatment. Muscle Nerve 14: 1131–1139

Danon MJ, Oh SJ, Di Mauro S et al. (1981) Lysosomal glycogen storage disease with normal acid maltase. Neurology 31: 51–57

Danon MJ, Reyes MG, Perurena OH et al. (1982) Inclusion body myositis: a corticosteroid resistant idiopathic inflammatory myopathy. Arch Neurol 39: 760–764

Danta G, Hilton RC, Lynch PG (1975) Chronic progressive exter-nal ophthalmoplegia. Brain 98: 473–492

Dark AJ, Streeten BW (1977) Ultrastructural study of cataract in myotonia dystrophica. Am J Ophthalmol 84: 666–674

Darnell RB, DeAngelis LM (1993) Regression of small cell lung carcinoma in patients with paraneoplastic neuronal antibod-ies. Lancet 341: 21–22

Das PK, Bray GM, Agnayo AJ et al. (1976) Diminished onabath-sensitive Na/k ATPase activity in sciatic nerves of rats with streptozotocin-induced diabetes. Exper Neurol 53: 285–288

Dastur DK, Gagrat BM, Manghani DK (1979) Human muscle in disuse atrophy. Neuropathol Applied Neurobiol 5: 85–101

Dastur DK, Gagrat BM, Wadia NH et al. (1975) Nature of muscu-lar change in osteomalacia: light and electron microscope observations. J Pathol 117: 211–228

Dastur DK, Manghani DK, Osuntokun BO et al. (1982) Neuro-muscular and related changes in malnutrition. J Neurol Sci 55: 207–230

Dastur DK, Ramamohan Y, Shal JS (1973) Ultrastructure of lepromatous nerves: neural pathogenesis in leprosy. Int J Lepr 41: 47–80

Dau PC, Denys EH (1982) Plasmapheresis and immunosuppres-sive drug therapy in the Eaton-Lambert syndrome. Ann Neurol 11: 570–575

Dau PC, Lindstrom JM, Cassell JK et al. (1977) Plasmapheresis and immunosuppressive drug therapy in myasthenia gravis. N Engl J Med 297: 1134–1140

Daube JR (1978) The description of motor unit potentials in elec-tromyography. Neurology 28: 623–625

Daube JR (1979) Needle examination in electromyography. Muscle Nerve E (AAEE, minimonograph no. 11)

Daube JR (1988) Statistical estimates of number of motor units in thenar and foot muscles in patients with amyotrophic lateral sclerosis or the residue of poliomyelitis. Muscle Nerve 11: 957A

Dausset J, Degos L, Hors (1974) A review: the association of the HLA antigens with disease. Clin Immunol Immunopathol 3: 127–149

David A, McDonald E, Mann A et al. (1990) Tired, weak or in need of rest: fatigue among general practice attenders. Br Med J 301: 1199–1202

David AS, Gilham RA (1986) Neuropsychological study of motor neuron disease. Psychosomatics 27: 441–445

David AS, Wessely S, Pelosi AJ (1991) Chronic fatigue syndrome: signs of a new approach. Br J Hosp Med 45: 158–163

David CB, Tolayma A (1978) Typhoid fever: unusual presenta-tion. J Pediatr 93: 533

Davidenkow S (1927) Über die neurotische Muskelatrophie Charcot–Marie: klinisch-genetische Studien. Z Neurol 108: 344

Davidenkow S (1939) Scapuloperoneal amyotrophy. Arch Neurol Psychiatry 41: 694–701

Davidson DWW, Jellinek EH (1977) Hypertension and papill-loedema in the Guillian–Barré syndrome. J Neurol Neurosurg Psychiatry 40: 144–148

Davies CE, Copplestone JA, Oschier DG et al. (1985) Acute vin-cristine neurotoxocity. Lancet i: 637–638

Davies DM (1954) Recurrent peripheral nerve palsies in a family. Lancet ii: 266–268

Davies KE (1993) Meeting report of the Royal Society of Medicine. J R Soc Med 86: 189

Davies ER, Sutton D, Bly AJ (1966) Myelography in brachial plexus injury. Br J Radiol 39: 362–368

Davies KE, Jackson J, Williamson R et al. (1983) Linkage analysis of myotonic dystrophy and sequences on chromosome 19 using cloned complement 3 gene probe. J Med Genet 20: 259–263

Davies MJ (1984) The cardiomyopathies: a review of terminology, pathology and pathogenesis. Histopathology 8: 363–393

Davies MJ, Anderson RH, Becker AE (1985) The conduction system of the heart. Butterworth, London, pp 252–280

Davies-Jones GAB, Esiri MM (1971) Neuropathy due to amyloid in myelomatosis. Br Med J ii: 444

Davis GR, Brown IT, Schwartz MS et al. (1983) A dedicated microcomputer-based instrument for interval analysis of multicomponent waveforms in single-fibre EMG. Electroence-phalogr Clin Neurophysiol 56: 110–113

Davis LE, Drachman DB (1972) Myeloma neuropathy. Arch Neurol 27: 507–511

Dawkins RL, Mastaglia FL (1973) Cell-mediated cytotoxicity to muscle in polymyositis: Effective immunosuppression. N Engl J Med 228: 434–438

Dawson DM, Hallett M, Millender LH (1990) Entrapment neu-ropathies. Little Brown, Boston, p 434

Dawson GD (1954) A summation technique for the detection of small evoked potentials. Electroencephalogr Clin Neurophysiol 6: 65–84

Dayan AD (1967) Peripheral neuropathy of metachromatic leu-codystrophy. J Neurol Neurosurg Psychiatry 30: 311–318

Dayan AD, Williams R (1967) Demyelinating peripheral neuropathy in liver disease. Lancet ii: 13–134

Dayan AD, Croft PB, Wilkinson M (1965) Association of carcinomatous neuromyopathy with different histological types of carcinoma of the lung. Brain 88: 435–448

Dayan AD, Gardner-Thorpe C, Down PJ et al. (1970) Peripheral neuropathy in uremia. Neurology 20: 649–658

Dayan AD, Ogul E, Graveson GS (1972) Polyneuritis and herpes zoster. J Neurol Neurosurg Psychiatry 35: 170–175

Dayan AD, Urich H, Gardner-Thorpe C (1971) Peripheral neuropathy in myeloma. J Neurol Sci 14: 21–35

De Angelis MS, Palmucci L, Leone M et al. (1991) Centronuclear myopathy: clinical, morphological and genetic characteristic: a review of 288 cases. J Neurol Sci: 103: 2–9

de Belleroche J, Orrell R, King A (1995) Familial amyotrophic lateral sclerosis/motor neuron disease (FALS): a review of current developments. J Med Genet 32: 841–847

De Coster W, De Reuck I, Thierry E (1974) A late auosomal dominant form of limb-girdle muscular dystrophy. Eur Neurol 12: 159–172

De Gans J, Stam J, van Wijngaarden GK (1985) Rhabdomyolysis and concomitant neurological lesions after intravenous heroin abuse. J Neurol Neurosurg Psychiatry 48: 1057–1059

Degoul F, Nelson I, Lestienne P et al. (1991) Deletions of mitochondrial DNA in Kearns–Sayre syndrome and ocular myopathies. J Neurol Sci 101: 168–177

Dehaene I, Martin JJ, Geens K et al. (1986) Guillain–Barré syndrome with opthalmoplegia: clinico-pathologic study of the central and peripheral nervous systems including the oculomotor nerves. Neurology 36: 851–854

Dehkarghani F, Sarnat HB, Brewster MA et al. (1981) Congenital muscle fiber type disproportion in Krabbe's leucodystrophy. Arch Neurol 38: 585–587

De Jager AEJ, Meinesz AF (1983) Acid maltase deficiency: treatment of respiratory insufficiency with cuirass respirator. J Neurol 230: 105–110

DeJager AEJ, Minderhoud JM (1991) Residual signs in severe Guillain–Barré syndrome. J Neurol Sci 104: 151–156

Déjérine J, Sottas J (1893) Sur la neurité: interstitiale, hypertrophique et progressive de l'enfance. C R Soc Biol (Paris) 45: 63–96

De Jong JGY (1947) Dver families met hereditaire dispositie tot het optreden van neuritiden, gecorreleerd met migraine. Psychiatr Neurol B1 50: 60–76

Dekel S, Papaioannou T, Rushworth G et al. (1980) Idiopathic carpal tunnel syndrome caused by carpal stenosis. Br Med J 280: 1297–1299

De la Monte SM, Gabuzda DH, Ho DD et al. (1988) Peripheral neuropathy in the acquired immunodeficiency syndrome. Ann Neurol 23: 485–492

De la Monte SM, Ropper AH, Dickersin GR et al. (1986) Relapsing central and peripheral demyelinating disease. Arch Neurol 43: 626–629

Delaney P (1977) Neurologic manifestation of sarcoidosis: review of the literature with report of 23 cases. Ann Intern Med 87: 336–345

de Lateur BJ, Halliday WR (1978) Pentazocine fibrous myopathy: report of two cases and literature review. Arch Phys Med Rehabil 59: 394–397

Della-Guistina E, Ferriere G, Evrard PH et al. (1979) Progressive bulbar paralysis in childhood (Londi syndrome). Acta Paediatr Belg 32: 129–

De Lisa J, Saeed MA (1983) The tarsal tunnel syndrome. Muscle Nerve 6: 664–670

Delisle MB, Carpenter S (1984) Neurofibrillary axonal swellings and amyotrophic lateral sclerosis. J Neurol Sci 63: 241–250

Delman J, Gravis F, Fosenblum MK et al. (1992) Anti-Hu associated paraneoplastic encephalomyelitis/ sensory neuronopathy: a clinical study of 71 patients. Medicine 71: 59–72

Demakis JG, Proskey A, Rahimtoola SH et al. (1974) The natural course of alcoholic cardiomyopathy. Ann Intern Med 80: 293–

Denborough MA (1982) Heat stroke and malignant hyperpyrexia. Med J Aust 1: 204–205

Denborough MA, Lovell RRH (1960) Anaesthetic deaths in a family. Lancet ii: 45

Denborough MA, Dennet X, Anderson RM (1973) Central core disease and malignant hyperpyrexia. Br Med J : 272–273

Denborough MA, Galloway GJ, Hopkinson KC (1982) Malignant hyperpyrexia and sudden infant death. Lancet I: 1068–1069

Denfel T (1992) Evidence for genetic heterogeneity of a malignant hyperthermia susceptibility. Am J Hum Genet 50: 1151–1161

Denny-Brown DE (1939) Myopathic weakness of quadriceps. Proc R Soc Med 32: 867–869

Denny-Brown DE (1948) Primary sensory neuropathy with muscular changes associated with carcinoma. J Neurol Neurosurg Psychiatry 11: 73–87

Denny-Brown DE (1951) Hereditary sensory radicular neuropathy. J Neurol Neurosurg Psychiatry 14: 237–252

Denny-Brown DE (1953) Clinical problems in neuromuscular physiology. Am J Med 15: 368–390

Denny-Brown DE (1960) Experimental studies pertaining to hypertrophy, regeneration and degeneration. Assoc Res Neuromusc Dis 38: 147–196

Denny-Brown DE, Brenner C (1944) Paralysis of nerve induced by direct pressure and tourniquet. Arch Neurol Psychiatry 51: 1–26

Denny-Brown DE, Foley JM (1941) Evidence of a chemical mediator in myotonia. Trans Am Neurol Assoc 62: 187–191

Denny-Brown DE, Nevin S (1941) The phenomenon of myotonia. Brain 64: 1–18

Denny-Brown DE, Pennybacker JB (1938) Fibrillation and fasciculation in voluntary muscle. Brain 61: 311–334

Denys EH, Dau PC, Lindstrom JM (1979) Neuromuscular transmission before and after plasmapheresis in myasthenia gravis and the myasthenic syndrome. In: Dau PC (ed) Plasmapheresis and the immunobiology of myasthenia gravis. Houghton Mifflin, Boston, pp 248–257

Deschuytere J, Roselle N, De Keyser C (1976) Monosynaptic reflexes in the superficial forearm flexors in man and their clinical significance. J Neurol Neurosurg Psychiatry 39: 555–565

De Silva HJ, Goonetilleke AKE, Semaratha N et al. (1988). Skeletal muscle necrosis in severe falciparum malaria. Br Med J 296: 1039

Desmedt JE (1973) The neuromuscular disorder in myasthenia gravis. I. Electrical and mechanical responses to nerve stimulation in hand muscles. In: Desmedt JE (ed) New developments in electromyography and clinical neurophysiology, vol 1. Karger, Basel, pp 241–304

Desmedt JE, Borenstein S (1975) Spontaneous fibrillation potentials in human muscular dystrophy: relation to muscle fibre segmentation. Nature 258: 531–534

Desmedt JE, Borenstein S (1976a) Diagnosis of myathenia gravis by nerve stimulation. Ann NY Acad Sci 183: 207–302

Desmedt JE, Borenstein S (1976b) Regeneration in Duchenne muscular dystrophy: electromyographic evidence. Arch Neurol 33: 642–650

Desmedt JE, Borenstein S (1977) Double-step nerve stimulation test for myasthenic block: sensitisation of post-activation exhaustion by ischaemia. Ann Neurol 1: 55–64

Desnick RJ, Simmons RL, Allen KY et al. (1972) Correction of enzymatic deficiencies by renal transplantation: Fabry's disease. Surgery 72: 203–211

Devor M (1983) Nerve pathophysiology and mechanisms of pain in causalgia. J Auton Nerve Syst 7: 371

De Vere R, Bradley WG (1975) Polymyositis: its presentation, morbidity and mortality. Brain 98: 637–666

Devi S, Lovelace RE, Duarte N (1977) Proximal peroneal nerve conduction velocity: recording from anterior tibial and peroneus brevis muscles. Ann Neurol 2: 116–119

de Visser M, Verbeeten B Jr (1985) Computed tomography of the skeletal musculature in Becker-type muscular dystrophy and benign infantile spinal muscular atrophy. Muscle Nerve 8: 435–444

de Visser M, Scholte HR, Schutgens RBH et al. (1986) Riboflavin-responsive lipid storage myopathy and glutamic aciduria Type 2 of early adult onset. Neurology 36: 367–372

de Visser M, Ungerboer de Visser BM, Berbeeten B (1988) Electromyographic and computed tomographic findings in five patients with monomelic spinal muscular atrophy. Eur Neurol 28: 135–138

Dewhurst AG, Hall D, Schwartz MS et al. (1986) Kearns–Sayre syndrome, hypoparathyroidism and basal ganglion calcification. J Neurol Neurosurg Psychiatry 49: 1323–1324

De Wind LT, Jones RJ (1950) Cardio-vascular observations in dystrophia myotonica. JAMA 144: 299–303

Deyo RA, Tsui-Wu YJ (1987) Descriptive epidemiology of low back pain and its related medical care in the United States. Spine 12: 264–268

Deyo RA, Loeser JD, Bigos SJ (1990) Herniated lumbar intervertebral disc. Ann Intern Med 112: 598–603

Dickey BF, Myers AR (1984) Pulmonary disease in polymyositis/dermatomyositis. Semin Arthritis Rheum 14: 60–76

Dickoff DJ, Simpson DM, Wiley CA et al. (1993) HTLV-1 in acquired adult myopathy. Muscle Nerve 16: 162–165

Di Donato S (1994) Human defects of β oxidation: clinical and molecular aspects. In: Schapira AHV, Di Mauro SD (eds) Mitochondrial disorders in neurology. Butterworth-Heinemann, London, pp 145–165

Di Donato S, Frerman FE, Rimoldi M et al. (1986) Systemic carnitine deficiency due to a lack of electron transfer flavoprotein (ubiquinone oxidoreductase). Neurology 36: 957–963

Di Donato S, Garvaglia B, Remoldi M et al. (1992) Clinical and biomedical phenotypes of carnitine deficiencies. In: Ferrari R, Di Mauro S, Sherwood G (eds) L-Carnitine and its role in medicine. Academic Press, London, pp 81–98

Di Marco AF, Kellings JS, Di Marco MS et al. (1985) The effects of inspiratory resistive training on respiratory muscle function in patients with muscular dystrophy. Muscle Nerve 8: 284–290

Di Mauro S (1979) Metabolic myopathies. In: Vinken PJ, Bruyn GW (eds) Diseases of muscles, part II. North Holland, Amsterdam, pp 175–234 (Handbook of clinical neurology, vol 41)

Di Mauro S (1993) Mitochondrial encephalomyopathies. In: Rosenberg RN, Prusiner SB, Di Mauro S, Barchi RL, Kunkel LM (eds) Molecular and genetic basis of neurological disease. Butterworth-Heinemann, Boston, pp 665–694

Di Mauro S, Bresolin N (1986a) Phosphorylase deficiency. In: Engel AG, Banker BQ (eds) Myology. McGraw-Hill, New York, pp 1585–1601

Di Mauro S, Bresolin N (1986b) Newly recognised defects of terminal glycolysis. In: Engel AG, Banker BQ (eds) Myology. McGraw-Hill, New York, pp 1619–1628

Di Mauro S, Di Mauro PMM (1973) Muscle carnitine palmitoyl transferase deficiency and myoglobinuria. Science 18: 929–931

Di Mauro S, Hartlage PL (1978) Fatal infantile form of muscle phosphorylase deficiency. Neurology 28: 1124–1129

Di Mauro S, Servidei S (1993) Disorders of carbohydrate metabolism: glycogen storage diseases. In: Rosenberg RN, Prusiner SB, Di Mauro S, Barchi RL, Kunkel LM (eds) The molecular and genetic basis of neurological disease. Butterworth-Heinemann, Boston, pp 93–119

Di Mauro S, Arnold S, Miranda A et al. (1978a) McArdle's disease: the mystery of reappearing phosphorylase activity in muscle culture – a fetal isoenzyme. Ann Neurol 3: 60–66

Di Mauro S, Stern LZ, Mehler M et al (1978b) Adult onset maltase deficiency : a post mortem study. Muscle Nervel 1: 27–36

Di Mauro S, Barilla E, Lee CP et al. (1976) Luft's disease: further biochemical and ultrastructural studies of skeletal muscle in the second case. J Neurol 27: 217–232

Di Mauro S, Bonilla E, Zeviani M et al. (1985) Mitochondrial myopathies. Ann Neurol 17: 521–538

Di Mauro S, Bresolin N, Hays AP (1984) Disorders of glycogen metabolism of muscle. CRC Crit Rev Clin Neurobiol 1: 83–116

Di Mauro S, Dalakas M, Miranda AF (1983a) Phosphoglycerate kinase deficiency: another cause of recurrent myoglobinuria. Ann Neurol 13: 11–19

Di Mauro S, Hartnig QB, Hays AP et al. (1979) Debrancher deficiency: neuromuscular disorder in five adults. Ann Neurol 5: 422–436

Di Mauro S, Hays AP, Easwood AB (1983b) In: Scarlato G, Ceri C (eds) Mitochondrial pathology in muscle diseases. Piccin Medical Books, Padua, pp 111–129

Di Mauro S, Mehler M, Arnold S et al. (1977) Genetic heterogeneity of glycogen diseases. In: Pathogenesis of human muscular dystrophies. Excerpta Medica, Amsterdam, pp 506–517

Di Mauro S, Miranda AF, Kahn S et al. (1981) Human muscle phosphoglycerate mutase deficiency: newly discovered metabolic myopathy. Science 212: 1277–1279

Di Mauro S, Tonin P, Servidei S (1992) Metabolic myopathies. In: Rowland LP, Di Mauro S (eds) Handbook of clinical neurology, vol 62. Elsevier, Amsterdam, pp 479–526

Dinn JJ, Dinn EK (1985) Natural history of acromegalic peripheral neuropathy. QJM 57: 833–842

Docherty TJ, Brown WF (1993) The estimated numbers and relative sizes of thenar motor units as selected by multiple point stimulation in young and older adults. Muscle Nerve 16: 355–366

Doherty P, Dickson JG, Flanigan TP et al. (1986) Effects of amyotrophic lateral sclerosis serum on cultured chick spinal neurons. Neurology 36: 1330–1334

Donaghy M, Duchen LW (1986) Sera from patients with motor neuron disease and associated paraproteinaemia fail to inhibit experimentally induced motor sprouting of motor nerve terminals. J Neurol Neurosurg Psychiatry 49: 817–819

Donaghy M, Hakin RN, Bamford JM et al. (1987) Hereditary sensory neuropathy with neurotrophic keratitis. Brain 110: 563–583

Donaghy M, King RHM, McKeran RO et al. (1990) Cerebrotendinous xanthomatosis. J Neurol 237: 216–219

Donek A, Witt TN, Stockmann HB et al. (1990) Normal dystrophin in McLeod myopathy. Ann Neurol 28: 720–722

Dong MM, Wasserman EJL, Giebried J (1980) Repetitive stimulation of the trapezius muscle: its value in myasthenic testing. Muscle Nerve 3: 439

Donner M, Rapola J, Somer H (1975) Congenital muscular dystrophy: a clinico-pathological and follow up study of 15 patients. Neuropaediatrie 6: 239–258

Donofrio PD, Albers JW (1990) Polyneuropathy: classification by nerve conduction studies and electromyography. Muscle Nerve 13: 889–903

Donofrio PD, Alessi AJ, Albers JW et al. (1989) Electrodiagnostic evolution of carcinomatous neuronopathy. Muscle Nerve 12: 508–513

Dons B, Bollerup K, Bond-Petersen F et al. (1979) The effect of weight-lifting exercise related to muscle fibre composition and muscle cross-sectional area in humans. Eur J Appl Physiol 40: 95–106

Dorfman LJ (1984) The distribution of conduction velocities (DCV) in peripheral nerves: a review. Muscle Nerve 7: 2–11

Dorfman LJ, McGill KC (1988) Automatic quantitative electromyography. Muscle Nerve 11: 804–818 (AAEE minimonograph no. 29)

Dorfmann LJ, Cummins KL, Reaven GM et al. (1983) Studies of diabetic polyneuropathy using conduction velocity distribution (DCV) analysis. Neurology 33: 773–779

Dorfman LJ, McGill KC, Cummins KL (1985) Electrical properties of commercial concentric EMG electrodes. Muscle Nerve 8: 1–8

Douglas AC, MacLeod JG, Matthews JD (1973) Symptomatic sarcoidosis of skeletal muscle. J Neurol Neurosurg Psychiatry 36: 1034–1040

Dowling PC, Bosch VV, Cook SD et al. (1982) Serum immunoglobulins in Guillain–Barré syndrome. J Neurol Sci 57: 435–440

Dowling PC, Menonna JP, Cook SD (1977) Guillain–Barré syndrome in greater New York - New Jersey. JAMA 238: 317–318

Downie AW, Scott TR (1967) An improved technique for radial nerve conduction studies. J Neurol Neurosurg Psychiatry 30: 332–336

Drachman DA (1968) Ophthalmoplegia plus. The neurodegenerative disorders associated with progressive external ophthalmoplegia. Arch Neurol 21: 170–183

Drachman DB, Kuncl RW (1994) Myasthenia gravis. In: Hohlfeld R (ed) Immunology of neuromuscular disease. Kluwer, Dordrecht, pp 165–207

Drachman DB, Adams RN, Josifek LF et al. (1982) Functional activities of autoantibodies to acetylcholine receptors and the clinical severity of myasthenia gravis. N Engl J Med 307: 769–775

Drachman DB, De Silva S, Ramsay D et al. (1987) Humerol pathogenesis of myasthenia gravis. Ann NY Acad Sci 505: 90–105

Drachman DB, Kao I, Angus CW et al. (1977) Effect of myasthenic immunoglobulin on acetylcholine receptors of cultured muscle. Ann Neurol 1: 504

Drachman DB, Murphy JRN, Nigam MP et al. (1967) "Myopathic" changes in chronically denervated muscle. Arch Neurol 16: 14–24

Drachman DB, Toyka KB, Myer E (1974) Prednisone in Duchenne muscular dystrophy. Lancet ii: 1409–1412

Dreifuss FE, Hogan GR (1961) Survival in X-chromosomal muscular dystrophy. Neurology 11: 734–737

Dreyfus JC, Alexandre Y (1971) Immunological studies on glycogen storage disease Types III and V. Demonstration of the presence of an immunoreactive protein in one case of muscle phosphorylase deficiency. Biochem Biophys Res Commun 44: 1364–1370

Dreyfus P, Hakim S, Adams RD (1957) Diabetic ophthalmoplegia: report of a case, with postmortem study and comments on vascular supply of human oculomotor nerve. Arch Neurol 77: 337–349

Driedger H, Pruzanski W (1980) Plasma cell neoplasia with peripheral neuropathy. Medicine (Baltimore) 59: 301–310

Drury J, Boulton AJM, Hardisty CA et al. (1982) Glycosylated haemoglobin levels in diabetic neuropathy. Diabetologia 22: 385

Duboc C, Jehenson P, Dinh ST et al. (1987) Phosphorous NMR spectroscopy study of muscle enzyme deficiencies involving glycogenolysis and glycolysis. Neurology 37: 663–671

Dubois EL (1974) Lupus erythematosis, 2nd edn. Southern California Press, Los Angeles

Dubowitz V (1964) Infantile muscular atrophy: a prospective study with particular reference to a slowly progressive variety. Brain 87: 707–718

Dubowitz V (1965) Pseudo-muscular dystrophy. In: Research in muscular dystrophy. Proc IIIrd Symp Res Commun Musc Dystr Group (GB), Pitman, London, pp 57–73

Dubowitz V (1985) Muscle biopsy: a practical approach 2nd edn. Bailliere-Tindall. London pp 720

Dubowitz V (1980) The floppy infant. Heinemann, London, p 158

Dubowitz V (1991) Chaos in the classification of the spinal muscular atrophies of childhood. Neuromusc Disord 1: 77–80

Dubowitz V (1992) Transferring myoblasts in Duchenne dystrophy. Br Med J 305: 844–845

Dubowitz V (1995) Muscle disorders in childhood, Saunders, Philadelphia

Dubowitz V, Heckmatt J (1980) Management of muscular dystrophy: pharmacological and physical aspects. Br Med Bull 36: 139–144

Dubowitz V, Roy J (1970) Central core disease of muscle: clinical, histochemical and electron microscopic studies of an affected mother and child. Brain 93: 133–146

Dubowitz V, Heckmatt JZ, Hyde SA et al. (1986) Therapeutic trial of isaxonine in Duchenne muscular dystrophy. Muscle Nerve 9: 270

Dubrovsky A, Toratuto AL (1983) Reinnervation in Duchenne muscular dystrophy. Muscle Nerve 6: 299–302

Duc M, Duc ML, Mauary G (1970) Paralysies intermittentes pas hyperkalémie révèlatrices d'une maladie d'Addison. Ann Méd (Nancy) 9: 387–390

Duchen LW (1970) Changes in motor innervation and cholinesterase localisation induced by botulinum toxin in skeletal muscles of the mouse: Differences between fast and slow muscles. J Neurol Neurosurg Psychiatry 33: 40–54

Duchen LW, Anjorin A, Watkins PJ et al. (1980) Pathology of autonomic neuropathy in diabetes. Ann Intern Med 92: 301

Ducla-Soares J, Breitenfeld L. Povoa P et al. (1991) Plasma catacholamines and postural hypotension in familial amyloiditic polyneuropathy of the Portuguese type. Clin Autonomic Res 1: 271–274

Duffy P, Wolf J, Collins G, DeVoe AG et al. (1974) Possible person-to-person transmission of Creutzfeldt–Jakob disease. N Engl J Med 290: 692–693

Duncan D (1934) A determination of the number of nerve fibres in the eighth theracic and largest lumbar ventral roots of the albino rat. J Comp Neurol 59: 47–60

Duncan C, Strub R, McGarry P et al. (1970) Peripheral nerve biopsy as an aid to diagnosis in infantile neuro axonal dystrophy. Neurology 20: 1024–1032

Dunn HG, Daube JR, Gomez MR (1978) Heredofamilial brachial plexus neuropathy (hereditary neuralgic amyotrophy with brachial predilection) in childhood. Dev Med Child Neurol 20: 28–46

Dunn HG, Lake BD, Dolman CL et al. (1969) The neuropathy of Krabbe's infantile cerebral sclerosis (globoid cell leucodystrophy). Brain 92: 329–344

Durrleman S, Alperovitch A (1989) Increasing trend of ALS in France and elsewhere: are the changes real? Neurology 39: 768–773

Durnler FE, Benson MD (1984) Primary structure of an amyloid prealbumin and its plasma precursor in a heredo-familial plyneuropathy of Swedish origin. Proc Natl Acad Sci USA 81: 694–698

Dwarzak F, Casazza F, Mora M et al. (1994) Lysosomal glycogen storage with normal acid maltase: a familial study with successful heart transplant. Neuromusc Disord 4: 243–247

Dwyer JM (1992) Manipulating the immune system with immune globulin. N Engl J Med 326: 107–116

Dyck JD, Bushek W, Spring EM et al. (1987) Vibratory and cooling detection thresholds compared with other tests in diagnosing and staging diabetic neuropathy. Diabetes Care 10: 432–440

Dyck PJ (1975a) Quantitation and cutaneous sensation in man. In: Dyck PJ, Thomas PK, Lambert EM (eds) Peripheral neuropathy, vol. 1. Saunders, Philadelphia, chap 22

Dyck PJ (1975b) Inherited neuronal degeneration and atrophy affecting peripheral motor, sensory and autonomic neurons. In: Dyck PJ, 1 Lambert EH, Thomas PK (eds) Peripheral neuropathy, vol. 2. Saunders, Philadelphia, pp 825–867

Dyck PJ (1984) Inherited degeneration and atrophy affecting peripheral motor, sensory and autonomic neurons. In: Dyck PJ, Thomas PK, Lambert EH, Bunge PR (eds) Peripheral neuropathy. Saunders, Philadelphia, pp 1600–1655

Dyck PJ (1993) Quantitative sensory testing: a consensus report from the Peripheral Neuropathy Association. Neurology 43: 1050–1052

Dyck PJ, Lambert EH (1968a) Lower motor and primary sensory neuron diseases with peroneal muscular atrophy. I. Neurologic, genetic and electrophysiologic findings in hereditary polyneuropathies. Arch Neurol 18: 603–618

Dyck PJ, Lambert EH (1968b) Lower motor and primary sensory neuron diseases with peroneal muscular atrophy. II. Neurologic, genetic and electrophysiologic findings in various neuronal degenerations. Arch Neurol 18: 619–625

Dyck PJ, Lambert EH (1969) Dissociated sensation in amyloidosis. Compound action potential, quantitative histologic and teased fibre, and electron microscopic studies of sural nerve biopsies. Arch Neurol 20: 490–507

Dyck PJ, Lambert EH (1970) Polyneuropathy associated with hypothyroidism. J Neuropathol Exp Neurol 29: 631–658

Dyck PJ, Ohta M (1975) Neuronal atrophy and degeneration predominantly affecting peripheral sensory neurons. In: Dyck PJ, Thomas PK, Lambert EH (eds) Peripheral neuropathy, vol. 2. Saunders, Philadelphia, pp 791–824

Dyck PJ, Thomas PK (1993) Peripheral neuropathy, 3rd edn. Saunders, Philadelphia, p 1720 (2 vols)

Dyck PJ, Chance P, Lebo R et al. (1993) Hereditary motor and sensory neuropathies. In: Dyck PJ, Thomas PK (eds) Peripheral neuropathy, 3rd edn. Saunders, Philadelphia, pp 1094–1186

Dyck PJ, Conn DL, Okazaki H (1972) Necrotizing angiopathic neuropathy: three dimensional morphology of fiber degeneration related to sites of occluded vessels. Mayo Clin Proc 47: 461–475

Dyck PJ, Daube J, O'Brien P et al. (1986a) Plasma exchange in chronic inflammatory demyelinating polyradiculoneuropathy. N Engl J Med 314: 461–465

Dyck PJ, Giannini C, Lais A (1993) Pathologic alterations in nerves. In: Dyck PJ, Thomas PK (eds) Peripheral neuropathy. Saunders, Philadelphia, pp 514–595

Dyck PJ, Gutrecht JA, Bastron JA et al. (1968) Histologic and teased fiber measurements of sural nerve in disorders of lower motor and primary sensory neurons. Mayo Clin Proc 43: 81–123

Dyck PJ, Hansen S, Karns T et al. (1985a) Capillary number and percentage closed in human diabetic sural nerve. Proc Natl Acad Sci USA 82: 2513–2517

Dyck PJ, Karns J, Lais A et al. (1984a) Pathologic alteration of the peripheral nervous system of humans. In: Dyck PJ, Thomas PK, Lambert EH, Bunge R (eds) Peripheral neuropathy, 2nd edn. Saunders, Philadelphia, pp 760–870

Dyck PJ, Karns JL, Lambert EG (1989) Longitudinal study of neurologic deficits and nerve conduction abnormalities in hereditary motor and sensory neuropathy Type 1. Neurology 39: 1302–1308

Dyck PJ, Karns J, O'Brien PC et al. (1984b) Detection thresholds of cutaneous sensation in humans. In: Dyck PJ, Thomas PK, Lambert EH, Bunge R (eds) Peripheral neuropathy, vol. 1. Saunders, Philadelphia, pp 1103–1138

Dyck PJ, Karns J, O'Brien PC et al. (1986b) Neuropathy symptom profile in health, motor neuron disease, diabetic neuropathy and amyloidosis. Neurology 36: 1300–1308

Dyck PJ, Lais AC, Offero KP (1974) The nature of myelinated wave fiber degeneration in dominantly inherited hypertrophic neuropathy. Mayo Clin Proc 50: 621–637

Dyck PJ, Lais AC, Ohta M et al. (1975a) Chronic inflammatory polyradiculoneuropathy. Mayo Clin Proc 50: 621–637

Dyck PJ, Lambert EH, O'Brien PC (1976) Pain in peripheral neuropathy related to rate and kind of fiber degeneration. Neurology 20: 466–471

Dyck PJ, Lambert EH, Sanders K et al. (1971) Severe hypomyelination and marked abnormality of conduction in Déjérine-Sottas hypertrophic neuropathy: myelin thickness and compound action potential of sural nerve in vitro. Mayo Clin Proc 46: 432–436

Dyck PJ, Low PA, Windebank AJ et al. (1991) Plasma exchange in polyneuropathy associated with monoclonal gammopathy of undetermined significance. N Engl J Med 325: 1482–1486

Dyck PJ, Mellingen JF, Reaven TJ et al. (1983) Not "indifference" to pain but varieties of hereditary sensory and autonomic neuropathy. Brain 106: 373–380

Dyck PJ, O'Brien PC, Oviatt KF et al. (1982) Prednisone improves chronic inflammatory demyelinating polyradiculoneuropathy more than no treatment. Ann Neurol 11: 136–141

Dyck PJ, O'Brien PC, Swanson C et al. (1985b) Combined azathioprine and prednisone in chronic inflammatory demyelinating polyneuropathy. Neurology 35: 1173–1176

Dyck PJ, Oviatt KF, Lambert EH (1981) Intensive evaluation of unclassified neuropathies yields improved diagnosis. Ann Neurol 10: 222–226

Dyck PJ, Sherman WR, Hallcher LM et al. (1980) Human diabetic endoneurial sorbitol, fructose and myoinositol related to sural nerve morphometry. Ann Neurol 8: 590–596

Dyck PJ, Thomas PK, Lambert EH (1975b) Peripheral neuropathy, vols 1 and 2. Saunders, Philadelphia

Dyken MG, Smith OM, Peake RC (1967) An electromyographic diagnostic screening test in McArdle's disease and a case report. Neurology 17: 45–50

Dyro FM, Bauer SB, Hallett M et al. (1983) Complex repetitive discharges in the external urethral sphincter in a pediatric population. Neurourol Urodynam 2: 39–44

Eales L, Dowdel EB, Sweeney GD (1971) The electrolyte disorder of the acute porphyric attack and the possible role of delta amino-laevulinic acid. S Afr J Lab Clin Med 17: 89–97

Eames RA, Lange LS (1967) Clinical and pathological study of ischaemic neuropathy. J Neurol Neurosurg Psychiatry 30: 215–226

Earl CJ, Fullerton PM, Wakefield GS et al. (1964) Hereditary neuropathy with liability to pressure palsies. QJM 33: 481–498

Eaton LM (1943) Diagnostic tests for myasthenia gravis with prostigmine and quinine. Mayo Clin Proc 18: 230–236

Eaton LM, Lambert EH (1957) Electromyography and electric stimulation of nerves in diseases of motor units: observations on myasthenic syndrome associated with malignant tumours. JAMA 163: 1117–1124

Eberling P, Gilliatt RW, Thomas PK (1960) A clinical and electrical study of ulnar nerve lesions in the hand. J Neurol Neurosurg Psychiatry 23: 1–9

Ebers GC, George AL, Barchi RL et al. (1991) Paramyotonia congenita and hyperkalaemic periodic paralysis are linked to the adult muscle sodium channel gene. Ann Neurol 30: 810–816

Eberstein A, Beattie B (1985) Simultaneous measurement of muscle conduction velocity and EMG power spectrum changes during fatigue. Muscle Nerve 8: 768–773

Eckardt VF, Nix W (1991) The anal sphincter in patients with myotonic dystrophy. Gastroenterology 100: 424–430

Edds MV (1950) Collateral regeneration of residual motor axons in partially denervated muscles. J Exp Zool 113: 507–552

Editorial (1978) Dumb rabies. Lancet ii: 1031–1032

Editorial (1981) Human muscle fatigue. Lancet ii: 729–730

Editorial (1982a) Chemotherapy of leprosy. Lancet ii: 77–78

Editorial (1982b) Hypoglycaemic peripheral neuropathy. Lancet i: 1447–1448

Editorial (1985) Neurospinous claudication. Lancet ii: 704

Editorial (1990) Creatine deficiency. Lancet 335: 631–633

Editorial (1992) The heart in myotonic dystrophy. Lancet 339: 528–529

Edstrom L (1970) Selective atrophy of red muscle fibres in the quadriceps in long-standing knee joint dysfunction: Injuries to the anterior cruciate ligament. J Neurol Sci 11: 551–559

Edstrom L (1975) Histochemical and histopathological changes in skeletal muscle in late-onset hereditary distal myopathy. J Neurol Sci 26: 147–157

Edstrom L, Grimby L (1986) Effect of exercise on the motor unit. Muscle Nerve 9: 104–126

Edstrom L, Kugelberg E (1968) Histochemical composition distribution of fibres and fatiguability of single motor units. J Neurol Neurosurg Psychiatry 31: 424–433

Edstrom L, Thornell LE, Eriksson A (1980) A new type of hereditary distal myopathy with characteristic sarcoplasmic bodies and intermediate skeletin filaments. J Neurol Sci 47: 171–190

Edstrom L, Wroblewski R, Mair WGP (1982) Genuine myotubular myopathy. Muscle Nerve 5: 604–613

Edwards RHT (1971) Percutaneous needle-biopsy of skeletal muscle in diagnosis and research. Lancet ii: 593–596

Edwards RHT (1977) Energy metabolism in normal and dystrophic human muscle. In: Rowland LP (ed) Pathogenesis of human muscular dystrophies. Excerpta Medica, Amsterdam, pp 415–429

Edwards RHT (1986) Interaction of chemical with electromechanical factors in human skeletal muscle fatigue. Acta Physiol Scand 128 [Suppl 556]: 149–155

Edwards RHT, McDonnell M (1974) A hand-held clinical dynamometer for evaluating voluntary muscle function in patients. Lancet ii: 757–758

Edwards RHT, Dawson MJ, Wilkie DR et al. (1982) Clinical use of nuclear magnetic resonance in the investigation of myopathy. Lancet i: 725–731

Edwards RHT, Griffiths RD, Hayward M et al. (1986) Modern methods of diagnosis of muscle diseases. J R Coll Physicians Lond 20: 49–55

Edwards RHT, Round JM, Jones DA (1983) Needle biopsy of skeletal muscle: a review of 10 years experience. Muscle Nerve 6: 676–683

Edwards RHT, Wiles CM, Gohil K et al. (1982) Energy metabolism in human myopathy. In: Schotland DL (ed) Disorders of the motor unit. Wiley, New York, pp 715–726

Edwards RHT, Wiles CM, Round JM et al. (1979) Muscle breakdown and repair in polymyositis: a case study. Muscle Nerve 2: 223–228

Edwards RHT, Young A, Hosking GP et al. (1977) Human skeletal muscle function: description of tests and normal values. Clin Sci Mol Med 52: 283–290

Edwards WG, Lincoln CR, Bassett FH III et al. (1969) The tarsal tunnel syndrome. JAMA 207: 716–719

Edwards Y, Sakoda S, Schon EA (1989) The gene for human muscle-specific phsophoglycerate mutase PGAMM mapped to chromosome 7 by polymerase chain reaction. Genomics 5: 948–951

Eisen A (1974) Early diagnosis of nerve palsy. Neurology 24: 256–262

Eisen A (1988) Use of somatosensory evoked potentials for the evaluation of the peripheral nervous system. Neurol Clin 6: 825–838

Eisen A (1993) The electrodiagnosis of plexopathies. In: Brown WJ, Bolton CJ (eds) Clinical electromyography. Butterworth-Heinemann, Boston, pp 211–225

Eisen A, Danon J (1974) The mild cubital tunnel syndrome. Neurology 24: 609–613

Eisen A, Humphreys P (1974) The Guillain-Barré syndrome: a clinical and electro-diagnostic study of 25 cases. Arch Neurol 30: 438–443

Eisen A, Berry K, Gibson G (1983) Inclusion body myositis (IBM): myopathy or neuropathy? Neurology 33: 1109–1114

Eisen A, Hoirch M, Moll A (1983) Evaluation of radiculopathies by segmental stimulation and somatosensory evoked potentials. Can J Neurol Sci 10: 178–182

Eisen A, Schomer D, Melmed C (1977) An electrophysiological method for examining lumbosacral root compression. Can J Neurol Sci 4: 117–123

Eisen A, Schulzer M, MacNeil M et al. (1993) Duration of amyotrophic lateral sclerosis is age-dependent. Muscle Nerve 16: 27–32

Eisen A, Shytbel W, Murphy K et al. (1990) Cortical magnetic stimulation in amyotrophic lateral sclerosis. Muscle Nerve 13: 146–151

Ekbom KR, Hed LK, Astrom KE (1964a) Weakness of proximal limb muscles probably due to myopathy after partial gastrectomy. Acta Med Scand 174: 493–496

Ekbom KR, Hed R, Kirstein R et al. (1964b) Muscular affections in chronic alcoholism. Arch Neurol 10: 449–458

Eklund G (1975) A new electrodiagnostic method for reassessing sensory nerve conduction across the carpal tunnel. Ups J Med Sci 80: 63–64

Eksted J (1964) Human single muscle fiber action potentials. Acta Physiol Scand 61 [Suppl 226]: 1–96

Eksted J, Stålberg E (1969) Abnormal connections between skeletal muscle fibres. Electroencephalogr Clin Neurophysiol 27: 607–609

Eksted J, Nilsson G, Stålberg E (1974) Calculation of the electromyographic jitter. J Neurol Neurosurg Psychiatry 37: 526–539

Eldjorn C, Try K, Stokke O et al. (1966) Dietary effects on serum phytanic acid levels and on clinical manifestations in heredopathia atactica polyneurifirmis. Lancet i: 691–693

Elia M, Carter A, Bacon S et al. (1981) Clinical usefulness of urinary 3-methylhistidine excretion in indicating muscle protein breakdown. Br Med J 282: 351–354

Ellenberg M (1978) Diabetic truncal mononeuropathy: a new clinical syndrome. Diabetes Care 1: 10–13

Ellis FR, Halsall PJ (1980) Malignant hyperpyrexia. Br J Hosp Med 24: 318–327

Ellis FR, Heffron JJA (1985) Clinical and biochemical aspects of malignant hyperpyrexia. In: Atkinson RS, Adams AP (eds) Recent advances in anaesthesia and analgesia, vol 15. Churchill-Livingstone, Edinburgh, pp 173–207

Ellis FR, Keaney NP, Harriman DGF et al. (1972) Screening for malignant hyperpyrexia. Br Med J iii: 559–561

Elmqvist D, Lambert EH (1968) Detailed analysis of neuromuscular transmission in a patient with the myasthenic syndrome sometimes associated with bronchogenic carcinoma. Mayo Clin Proc 43: 689–713

Elmqvist D, Hofmann WW, Kugelberg J et al. (1964) An electrophysiological investigation of neuromuscular transmission in myasthenia gravis. J Physiol (Lond) 174: 417–434

El-Negamy E, Sedgwick EM (1979) Delayed cervical somatosensory potentials in cervical spondylosis. J Neurol Neurosurg Psychiatry 42: 238–241

Elston JS (1987) Long-term results of treatment of idiopathic belpharospasm with botulinum. Br J Ophthalmol 71: 664–668

Emery AEH (1971) Review: the nosology of the spinal muscular atrophies. J Med Genet 8: 481–495

Emery AEH (1977) Muscle histology and creatine kinase levels in the fetus in Duchenne muscular dystrophy. Nature 256: 472–473

Emery AEH (1980) Duchenne muscular dystrophy. Br Med Bull 36: 117–122

Emery AEH (1987) Duchenne muscular dystrophy. Oxford University Press, Oxford, p 317

Emery AEH (1989) Emery–Dreifuss mucular dystrophy and other related disorders. Br Med Bull 45: 772–787

Emery AEH, Burt D (1980) Intracellular calcium and pathogenesis and antenatal diagnosis of Duchenne muscular dystrophy. Br Med J 280: 355–357

Emery AEH, Dreifuss FE (1966) Unusual type of benign X-linked muscular dystrophy. J Neurol Neurosurg Psychiatry 29: 338–342

Emery AEH, Holloway S (1982) Familial motor neuron diseases. In: Rowland LP (ed) Human motor neuron diseases. Raven Press, New York, pp 139–147

Emery AEH, Skinner R (1976) Clinical studies in benign (Becker-type) X-linked muscular dystrophy. Clin Genet 10: 189–201

Emery AEH, Walton JN (1967) The genetics of muscular dystrophy. In: Steinberg AG, Bearn AG (eds) Progress in medical genetics, vol V. Academic Press, New York, pp 116–145

Emery AEH, Clark ER, Simon S et al. (1967) Detection of carriers of benign X-linked muscular dystrophy. Br Med J iv: 522–523

Emery ES, Fenichel GM, Eng G (1968) A spinal muscular atrophy with scapulo-peroneal distribution. Arch Neurol 18: 129–133

Emery PW, Edwards RHT, Rennie MJ et al. (1984) Protein synthesis in muscle measured in vivo in cachectic patients with cancer. Br Med J 289: 584–587

Emeryck B, Hausmanowa-Petrusewicz I, Nowak R (1974) Spontaneous volleys of high frequency potentials (BHFP) in neuromuscular diseases. Electromyography 14: 313–313 and 339–354

Emslie-Smith AM, Engel AG (1990) Microvascular changes in early and advanced dermatomyositis: a quantitative study. Ann Neurol 27: 343–356

Emslie-Smith AM, Engel AG (1991) Necrotizing myopathy with pipestem capillaries, microvascular deposition of the complement membrane attack complex (MAC) and minimal cellular infiltration. Neurology 41: 936–939

Emslie-Smith AM, Arahata K, Engel AG (1989) Major histocompatibility complex Class I antigen expression, immunolocalisation of interferon subtypes and T-cell mediated cytotoxicity in myopathies. Hum Pathol 20: 224–231

Enders V, Karch H, Toyka KV et al. (1993) The spectrum of immune responses to Campylobacter jejuni and glycoconjugates in Guillain-Barré syndrome and in other neuroimmunological disorders. Ann Neurol 34: 136–144

Engel AG (1966a) Late-onset rod myopathy (a new syndrome?): light and electron microscopic observations in two cases. Mayo Clin Proc 41: 713–741

Engel AG (1966b) Electron microscopic observations in thyrotoxic and corticosteroid-induced myopathies. Mayo Clin Proc 41: 785–796

Engel AG (1970a) Acid maltase deficiency in adults: studies in four cases of a syndrome which may mimic muscular dystrophy or other myopathies. Brain 93: 599–616

Engel AG (1970b) Evolution and content of vacuoles in primary hypokalalemic periodic paralysis. Mayo Clin Proc 45: 774–814

Engel AG (1972) Neuromuscular manifestations of Graves disease. Mayo Clin Proc 47: 919–925

Engel AG (1984) Myasthenia gravis and myasthenic syndromes. Ann Neurol 16: 519–534

Engel AG (1986) Carnitine deficiency syndromes and lipid storage myopathies. In: Engel AG, Banker BQ (eds) Myology. McGraw-Hill, New York, pp 1663–1696

Engel AG (1994) Quantitative morphological studies of muscle. In: Engel AG, Franzini-Armstrong C (eds) Myology, 2nd edn. McGraw-Hill, New York, pp 1018–1045

Engel AG, Angelini C (1973) Carnitine deficiency of human muscle with associated lipid storage myopathy: a new syndrome. Science 179: 899–902

Engel AG, Arahata K (1984) Monoclonal antibody analysis of mononuclear cells in myopathies. II. Phenotypes of autoinvasive cells in polymyositis and inclusion body myositis. Ann Neurol 16: 209–215

Engel AG, Arahata K (1986) Mononuclear cells in myopathies. Hum Pathol 17: 704–721

Engel AG, Gomez MR (1970) Acid maltase levels in muscle in heterozygous acid maltase deficiency and in non-weak and neuromuscular disease controls. J Neurol Neurosurg Psychiatry 33: 801–804

Engel AG, Lambert EH (1969) Calcium activation of electrically inexcitable muscle fibres in primary hypokalaemic periodic paralysis. Neurology 19: 857–858

Engel AG, Santa T (1971) Histometric analysis of the ultrastructure of the neuromuscular junction in myasthenia gravis and in the myasthenic syndrome. Ann N Y Acad Sci 183: 46–63

Engel AG, Siekert RG (1972) Lipid storage myopathy responsive to prednisone. Arch Neurol 27: 174–181

Engel AG, Angelini C, Gomez MR (1972) Fingerprint body myopathy. Mayo Clin Proc 47: 377–388

Engel AG, Banker BQ, Eiben RM (1977a) Carnitine deficiency: clinical, morphological and biochemical observations in a fatal case. J Neurol Neurosurg Psychiatry 40: 313–322

Engel AG, Gomez MR, Groover RV (1971) Multicore disease. Mayo Clin Proc 46: 666–681

Engel AG, Gomez MR, Seybold ME et al. (1973) The spectrum and diagnosis of acid maltase deficiency. Neurology 23: 95–106

Engel AG, Lambert EH, Howard FM Jr (1977c) Immune complexes (IgG and C₃) at the motor end-plate in myasthenia gravis. Mayo Clin Proc 52: 267–280

Engel AG, Lambert EH, Mulder DM et al. (1982) A newly recognized congenital myasthenic syndrome attributed to a prolonged open time of the acetylcholine-induced ion channel. Ann Neuro ii: 553–569

Engel AG, Lambert EH, Rosevar JW et al. (1965) Clinical and electromyographic studies in a patient with primary hypokalaemic periodic paralysis. Am J Med 38: 626–640

Engel AG, Lindstrom JM, Lambert EH et al. (1977d) Ultrastructural localization of the acetylcholine receptor in myasthenia gravis and its experimental autoimmune model. Neurology 27: 307–315

Engel AG, Sahashi K, Fumagalli G (1981b) The immunopathology of acquired myasthenia gravis. Ann NY Acad Sci 377: 158–174

Engel AG, Tsujihata M, Jerusalem F (1973) Quantitative asessment of motor end-plate ultrastructure in normal and diseased human muscle. In: Dyck PJ, Thomas PK, Lambert EH (eds) Peripheral neuropathy, vol 2. Saunders, Philadelphia pp 1404–1415

Engel AG, Tsujihata MT, Lambert EH et al. (1976) Experimental autoimmune myasthenia gravis: a sequential and quantitative study of the neuromuscular junction ultrastructure and electrophysiologic correlation. J Neurlpathol Exp Neurol 35: 569–587

Engel WK (1961) Muscle target fibres; a newly recognised sign of denervation. Nature 191: 389–390

Engel WK (1967) Focal myopathic changes produced by electromyographic and hypodermic needles. Arch Neurol 16: 509–513

Engel WK (1971) "Ragged-red fibres" in ophthalmoplegia syndromes and their differential diagnosis. In: Kakulas BA (ed) Muscle diseases (abstracts of papers presented at the 2nd International Congress on Muscle Diseases, Perth 1971). Excerpta Medica, Amsterdam, p 28 (International Congress Series 237)

Engel WK, Gold GN, Karpati G (1968) Type C fiber hypotrophy and central nuclei. Arch Neurol 18: 435–444

Engel WK (1973) Duchenne muscular dystrophy: a histologically based ischaemia hypothesis and comparison with experimental ischaemia myopathy. In: Pearson CM (ed) The striated muscle. Williams and Wilkins, Baltimore, pp 453–472

Engel WK (1977) Integrative histochemical approach to the defect of Duchenne muscular dystrophy. In: Rowland LP (ed) Pathogenesis of human muscular dystrophies. Excerpta Medica, Amsterdam, pp 277–309

Engel WK, Brooke MH (1966) Histochemistry of the myotonic disorders. In: Kuhn E (ed) Progressive Muskeldystrophic-Myotonie-Myasthenie. Springer, Berlin Heidelberg New York, p 203

Engel WK, McFarlin DE (1966) Discussion of paper by Fenichel. Ann NY Acad Sci 135: 68–77

Engel WK, Resnick JS (1966) Late-onset rod myopathy: a newly recognised acquired and progressive disease. Neurology 16: 308–309

Engel WK, Brooke MH, Nelson PG (1966) Histochemical studies of denervated or tenotomised cat muscle. Ann NY Acad Sci 138: 160–185

Engel WK, Eyerman EL, Williams HE (1963) Late onset type of skeletal muscle phosphorylase deficiency: a new familial variety with completely and partially affected subjects. N Engl J Med 268: 135–137

Engel WK, Lichter AS, Galdi HP (1981) Polymyositis: remarkable response to total body irradiation Lancet i: 658

Engel WK, Trotter JL, McFarlin DE (1977) Thymic epithelial cell contains Ach receptor. Lancet i: 1310–1311

Engel WK, Vick NA, Glueek CJ et al. (1970) A skeletal muscle disorder associated with intermittent symptoms and a possible defect of lipid metabolism. N Engl J Med 282: 697–704

Engel WK, Oberc MA (1975) Abundant nuclear rods in adult onset rod disease J Neuropathol Exp Neurol 34: 119–132

Engsner G, Woldemoriam T (1974) Motor nerve conduction velocity in marasmus and in kwashiorkor. Neuropäed 5: 34–48

Erb WH (1891) Dystrophia muscularis progressiva: klinische und pathologisch-anatomische Studien. Dtsch Nervenheil 1: 13–94, 173–261

Erbslöh F, Abel M (1970) Deficiency neuropathies. In: Vinken PJ, Bruyn GW (eds) Handbook of clinical neurology, vol 7. Elsevier, Amsterdam

Erminio F, Buchthal F, Rosenfalck P (1959) Motor unit territory and muscle fiber concentration in paresis due to peripheral nerve injury and anterior horn cell involvement. Neurology 9: 657–671

Errasti JM, Campbell KP (1993) Dystrophin and the membrane skeleton. Curr Opin Cell Biol 5: 82–87

Esiri M, MacLennan ICM (1974) Experimental myositis in rats. I. Histology and creatine phosphokinase changes, and passive transfer to normal syngeneic rats. Clin Exp Immonol 17: 139–150

Espir MLE, Matthews WB (1973) Hereditary quadriceps myopathy. J Neurol Neurosurg Psychiatry 36: 1041–1045

Esteban A, Molina-Negro P (1986) Primary hemifacial spasm: a neurophysiological study. J Neurol Neurosurg Psychiatry 49: 58–63

Estes D, Christian CL (1971) The natural history of systemic lupus erythematosus by prospective analysis. Medicine 50: 85–95

Estes JW, Morley TJ, Levine IM et al. (1967) A new hereditary acanthocytosis syndrome. Am J Med 42: 868–881

Eulenberg A (1886) Ueber eine familiäre durch 6 Generationen verfolgbare Form congenitaler Paramyotonie. Neurol Centrbl 55: 265–272

European MH Group (1984) A protocol for the investigation of malignant hyperpyrexia (MH) susceptibility. Br J Anaesth 56: 1267–1269

Evans BA, Daube JR, Litchy WJ (1990) A comparison of magnetic and electrical stimulation of spinal nerves. Muscle Nerve 13: 414–420

Evans BA, Stevens JC, Dyck PJ (1981) Lumbosacral plexus neuropathy. Neurology 31: 1327–1330

Evans BM, Kriss A, Jeffries D et al. (1993) British Society for Clinical Neurophysiology: guidelines for preventing transmission of infective agents and toxic substances by clinical neurophysiology procedures: an update. J Electrophysiol Technol 19: 129–135

Evans CC, Kaufman HD (1971) Unusual presentation of seminoma of the testis. Br J Surg 58: 703–704

Ewing DJ, Campbell IW, Clarke BF (1980) Assessment of cardiovascular effects in diabetic autonomic neuropathy and prognostic implications. Ann Intern Med 92: 308–311

Fagerberg SE (1959) Diabetic neuropathy: a clinical and histological study on the significance of vascular affections. Acta Med Scand 164 [Suppl 345]: 1–97

Fairfax AJ (1977) A survey of the prevalence of skeletal muscle dystrophies and other neuromuscular disorders as a cause of complete heart block. MD thesis, University of London

Falck B (1983) Automatic analysis of individual motor unit potentials recorded with a special two channel electrode. Academic dissertation. Univ of Turku

Falck B, Hurme M (1983) Conduction velocity of the posterior interosseous nerve across the Arcade of Frohse. Electromyogr Clin Neurophysiol 23: 565–576

Falck B, Hurme M, Hakkarainen S et al. (1984) Sensory conduction velocity of plantar digital nerves in Morton's metatarsalgia. Neurology 34: 698–701

Famborough DM, Drachman DM, Satyamurti S (1973) Neuromuscular junction in myasthenia gravis: decreased acetylcholine receptors. Science 182: 293–295

Fardeau M (1975) Pathology of Refsum's disease. In: Dyck PJ, Thomas PK, Lambert EM (eds) Peripheral neuropathy, vol 2. Saunders, Philadelphia, pp. 881–890

Fardeau M (1984) Pathology of Refsum's disease. In: Dyck PJ, Thomas PK, Lambert EG, Bunge R (eds) Peripheral neuropathy, 2nd edn. Saunders, Philadelphia pp 1693

Fardeau M, Engel WK (1969) Ultrastructural study of a peripheral nerve biopsy in Refsum's disease. J Neuropathol Neurol 28: 278–289

Fardeau M, Tomé FMS (1994) Congenital myopathies. In: Engel AG, Franzini-Armstrong C (eds) Myology, 2nd edn. McGraw-Hill, New York, pp 1487–1532

Fardeau M, Abelanet R, Laudat P et al. (1976) Maladie de Refsum. Etude histologique, ultrastructurale et biochemique d'une biopsie de nerf péripherique. Rev Neurol 12: 185–196

Fardeau M, Godet-Guillain J, Tomé FMS et al. (1978) Une nouvelle affection musculaire familiale, définé par l'accumulation intra-sarco-plasmique d'un matériel granulo-filamentaire dense en microscopie électronique. Rev Neurol 131: 411–425

Fardeau M, Harpey J-P, Caille B (1975) Disproportion congénitales de différentes types de fibre musculaire avec petitesse relative des fibres de Type 1: Documents morphologiques concernant les biopsies musculaires prélevées chez trois membrs d'une même famille. Rev Neurol 131: 745–766

Forfar JC, Brown GJ, Cull RE (1979) Proximal myopathy during beta blockade. Br Med J 279: 1331–1332

Fariello R, Meloff K, Murphy EG et al. (1978) A case of Schwartz-Jampel syndrome with unusual muscle biopsy findings. Ann Neurol 3: 93–96

Faris AA, Reyes MG (1971) Reappraisal of alcoholic myopathy. J Neurol Neurosurg Psychiatry 34: 86–92

Farrell SA, Davidson RG, Thorp P (1987) Neonatal manifestations of Schwartz-Jampel syndrome. Am J Med Genet 27: 799–805

Fauchald P, Rygvold O, Oystese B (1972) Temporal arteritis and polymyalgia rheumatica: clinical and biopsy findings. Ann Intern Med 77: 845–852

Fawcett PRW, McLachlan SM, Nicholson SM et al. (1982) D-Penicillamine associated myasthenia gravis: immunological and electrophysiological studies. Muscle Nerve 5: 328–334

Fazio M (1892) Ereditarieta della paralisi bulbare progressiva. Riforma Med 8: 327

Fealey RD, Low PA, Thomas JE (1989) Thermoregulatory sweating abnormalities in diabetes mellitus. Mayo Clin Proc 64: 617–628

Feasby TE (1992) Inflammatory demyelinating polyneuropathies. Neurol Clin 10: 651–670

Feasby TE, Gilbert JJ, Brown WF et al. (1986) An acute axonal form of Guillain–Barré polyneuropathy. Brain 109: 1115–1126

Feasby TE, Hahn AF, Brown WF (1983) Long-term plasmapheresis in chronic progressive demyelinating polyneuropathy. Ann Neurol 14: 122

Feasby TE, Hahn AF, Brown WF et al. (1993) Severe axonal degeneration in acute Guillain-Barré syndrome: evidence of two different mechanisms. J Neurol Sci 116: 185–192

Feer DWG, Wang J, Barany F et al. (1993) Hyperkalaemic periodic paralysis: rapid and molecular diagnosis and relationship of genotype to phenotype in 12 families. Neurology 43: 668–673

Feibel JH, Campa JF (1976) Thyrotoxic neuropathy: Basedow's paraplegia. J Neurol Neurosurg Psychiatry 39: 491–497

Feigenbaum JA, Munsat TL (1970) A neuromuscular syndrome of scapulo-peroneal distribution. Bull Los Angeles Neurol Soc 35: 47–57

Feigin RD, Barron KS (1986) Treatment of Kawasaki syndrome. N Engl J Med 315: 389–390

Feinglass EJ, Arnett FC, Dorsch CA et al. (1976) Neuropsychiatric manifestation of systemic lupus erythematosus: diagnosis, clinical spectrum and relationship to other features of the disease. Medicine 55: 323–339

Feit H, Brooke MH (1976) Myophosphorylase deficiency: two different molecular etiologies. Neurology 26: 963–967

Feldman RA, Morris JG, Pollard RA (1981) Epidemiological characteristics of botulism in the United States 1950-1979. In: Lewis GE (ed) Biomedical aspects of botulism. Academic Press, New York, pp 129–142

Felmus MT, Patten BM, Swanke L (1976) Antecedent events in amyotrophic lateral sclerosis. Neurology 26: 167–172

Feltkamp TEW, Van den Berg-Loonen PM, Nijenhuis CE et al. (1984) Myasthenia gravis, autoantibodies and HLA antigen. Br Med J i: 131–133

Feltkamp-Vroom T (1966) Myoid cells in human thymus. Lancet i: 1320–1321

Fenichel GM, Shy GM (1963) Muscle biopsy experience in myasthenia gravis. Arch Neurol 9: 237–243

Fenichel GM, Emery ES, Hunt P (1967) Neurogenic atrophy simulating facio-scapulo-humeral dystrophy: a dominant form. Arch Neurol 17: 257–260

Ferguson FR (1962) A critical review of the clinical features of myasthenia gravis. Proc R Soc Med 55: 49–52

Ferguson IT, Mahon M, Cumming WJK (1983) An adult case of Andersen's disease: Type IV glycogenosis. J Neurol Sci 60: 337–351

Fernandes J, Van de Kamer JH (1968) Hexose and protein tolerance tests in children with liver glycogenosis caused by a deficiency of the debranching enzyme system. Pediatrics 41: 935–944

Fernandes L, Swinson DR, Hamilton EDB (1977) Dermatomyositis complicating penicillamine treatment. Ann Rheum Dis 36: 94–95

Fernandez-Sola J, Campistol J, Casademont J et al. (1990) Reversible cyclosporin myopathy. Lancet 335: 362–363

Ferrara JCM, Deeg HJ (1991) Graft-versus-host disease. N Engl J Med 324: 667–674

Ferreiro JE, Arguelles DJ, Rams HJ (1986) Thyrotoxic periodic paralysis. Am J Med 80: 146–150

Ferrero B, Durelli L, Cavallo R et al. (1993) Therapies for exacerbation of myasthenia gravis. Ann NY Acad Sci 681: 563–566

Fidzianska A, Baduiska B, Ryniewicz B et al. (1981) Cap disease Neurology 31: 1113–1117

Fidzianska-Dolot A, Hausmanowa-Petrusewicz I (1984) Morphology of the lower motor neuron and muscle. In: Gamstorp I, Sarnat HB (eds) Progressive spinal muscular atrophies. Raven Press, New York, pp 55–89

Figorella-Branger D, Kozak-Ribbens G, Rodet L et al. (1993) Pathological findings in 165 patients explored for malignant hyperthermia susceptibility. Neuromusc Disord 3: 553–556

Fine EJ, Hallett M (1980) Neurophysiological study of subacute combined degeneration. J Neurol Sci 45: 331–336

Fine EJ, Saria E, Paroski MW et al. (1990) The neurophysiological profile of vitamin B_{12} deficiency. Muscle Nerve 13: 158–164

Fischbeck KH, Ionasescu V, Ritter AW et al. (1986) Localisation of the gene for X-linked spinal muscular atrophy. Neurology 36: 1595–1598

Fischbeck KH, Kamholz J, Shi YJ et al. (1988) X-linked myoglobinuria. Neurology 38 [Suppl 1]: 174 (abstr)

Fishbein DB, Robinson LE (1993) Rabies. N Engl J Med 329: 1632–1638

Fishbein WN (1985) Myoadenylate deaminase deficiency: inherited and acquired forms. Biochem Med 33: 158–169

Fisher CM (1956) An unusual variant of acute idiopathic polyneuritis: syndrome of ophthalmoplegia, ataxia and areflexia. N Engl J Med 225: 57–65

Fisher CM, Adams RD (1956) Diphtheritic polyneuritis: a pathological study. J Neuropathol Exp Neurol 15: 243–268

Fisher MA (1983) F response analysis of motor disorders of central origin. J Neurol Sci 62: 13–22

Fisher MA, Shivde AJ, Teixara C et al. (1979) The F wave: a clinically useful physiological parameter for the evaluation of radicular injury. Electromyogr Clin Neurophysiol 19: 65–75

Fisher MJ, Meyer RA, Adams GR et al. (1990) Direct relationship between proton T_2 and exercise intensity in skeletal muscle MR images. Invest Radiol 25: 480

Fisher MR, Dooms GC, Hricak H et al. (1986) Magnetic resonance imaging of the normal and pathologic muscular system. Magn Res Imag 4: 491–496

Fitch CW, Anger LE (1967) The Frank vectorcardiogram and the electrocardiogram in Duchenne's progressive muscular dystrophy. Circulation 35: 1124–1131

Fitch N, Karpati G, Pinsky L (1971) Congenital blepharophimosis, joint contractures and muscular hypotonia. Neurology 21: 1214–1220

Fitting JW, Bischoff A, Regli F et al. (1979) Neuropathy, amyloidosis and monoclonal gammapathy. J Neurol Neurosurg Psychiatry 42: 193–202

Fitzsimons R, Sewry CA (1985) Immunocytochemistry. In: Dubowitz V (ed) Muscle biopsy: a practical approach, 2nd edn. Balliere Tindall, London, pp 104–207

Fitzsimons RB, Tyer HDD (1980) A study of a myopathy presenting as idiopathic scoliosis: multicore disease or mitochondrial myopathy? J Neurol Sci 46: 33–48

Flaten TP (1989) Rising mortality from motor neuron disease. Lancet 335: 1018–1019

Fleckenstein JL, Canby RC, Parkey RW et al. (1988) Acute effects of exercise on MRI of skeletal muscle in normal volunteers. AJR 151: 231–237

Fleischer GA, McConahey M, Pankow M (1965) Serum creatine kinase, lactic dehydrogenase and glutamic oxaloacetic transaminase in thyroid disease and pregnancy. Mayo Clin Proc 40: 300–311

Folli F, Solimena M, Cofieli R et al. (1993) Autoantibodies to 128 kD synpatic protein in three women with the stiff man syndrome and breast cancer. N Engl J Med 328: 546–551

Fontaine B (1993) Periodic paralysis, myotonia congenita and sarcolemmal ion channels: a success of the candidate gene approach. Neuromusc Disord 3: 101–107

Fontaine B, Khurana TS, Hoffman EP et al. (1990) Hyperkalaemic periodic paralysis and the adult muscle sodium channel α subunit gene. Science 250: 1000–1002

Fontaine B, Vale-Santos J, Jurkat-Rott K et al. (1994) Mapping of the hypokalaemic periodic paralysis (hypo PP) locus to chromosome 1q 31-32 in three European families. Nature Genet 6: 267–272

Fontana AD, Vital-Brasilo (1985) Mode of action of phoneutria nigriventor spider venom at the isolated phrenic nerve diaphragm of the rat. Brasil J Med Biol Research 18: 557–565

Foote RA, Kimborough SM, Stevens JC (1982) Lupus myositis. Muscle Nerve 5: 65–68

Foraq TI, Teebi As (1990) Duchenne-like muscular dystrophy in the Arabs. Am J Med Genet 37: 290–295

Forfar JC, Brown GJ, Cull RE (1979) Proximal myopathy during betablockade. Br Med J 279: 1331–1332

Foster DB (1945) Degeneration of peripheral nerves in pernicious anaemia. Arch Neurol 54: 102–109

Foulis AK (1986) Class II major histocompatibility complex and organ-specific autoimmunity in man. J Pathol 150: 5–11

Fowler CJ, Carroll MB, Burns D et al. (1987) A portable system for measuring cutaneous thresholds for warming and cooling. J Neurol Neurosurg Psychiatry. 50: 1211–1215

Fowler CJ, Kilby RS, Harrison MJG (1985) Decelerating burst and complex repetitive discharges in the striated muscle of the urthral sphincter, associated with urinary retention in women. J Neurol Neurosurg Psychiatry 48: 1004–1009

Fowler TJ, Danta G, Gilliatt RW (1972) Recovery of nerve conduction after a pneumatic tourniquet: observation of the hind limb of the baboon. J Neurol Neurosurg Psychiatry 35: 638–647

Fowler WM, Layzer RB, Taylor RG et al. (1974) The Schwartz–Jampel syndrome. J Neurol Sci 22: 127–146

Fox MW, Harms RW, Davis DH et al. (1990) Selected neurologic complications of pregnancy. Mayo Clin Proc 65: 1595–1618

Frame B, Heinze EG, Block MA et al. (1968) Myopathy in primary hyperparathyroidism. Ann Intern Med 68: 1022–1027

Francke U, Ochs HD, DeMartinrille B et al. (1985) Minor Xp21 chromosome deletion in a male associated with expression of Duchenne muscular dystrophy, chronic granulomatous disease, retinitis pigmentosa and McLeod syndrome. Am J Hum Genet 37: 250–267

Frank A (1993) Low back pain. Br Med J 306: 901–909

Frank JP, Maroti Y, Butler IJ et al. (1980) Central core disease and malignant hyperthermia syndrome. Ann Neurol 7: 11–17

Fraser DM, Campbell IW, Ewing DJ et al. (1977) Peripheral and autonomic nerve function in newly diagnosed diabetes mellitus. Diabetes 26: 546–550

Frazer DD, Frank JA, Dalakas M et al. (1991) Magnetic resonance imaging in the idiopathic inflammatory myopathies. J Rheumatol 18: 1693–1700

Frdzranska A, Badurska B, Ryniewicz B et al. (1981) Cap disease. Neurology 31: 1113–1120

Frdzranska A, Goebel HH, Lenard HG et al. (1982) Congenital muscular dystrophy (CMD) – a collagen formative disease? J Neurol Sci 55: 79–90

Freddo L, Ariga T, Macala LC (1985) The neuropathy of plasma cell dyscrasia: binding of IgM M-proteins to peripheral nerve glycolipid. Neurology 35: 1420–1424

French Cooperative Group on Plasma Exchange in Guillain–Barré Syndrome (1987) Efficacy of plasma exchange in Guillain–Barré syndrome. Ann Neurol 22: 753–761

French Cooperative Group on Plasma Exchange in Guillain–Barré Syndrome – one year follow up (1992) Ann Neurol 32: 94–97

Freud S (1895) Uber die Bernhardt'sche sensibilitatstornung am Oberschenkel. Neurol Centralbl 14: 491–492

Freund H-J (1983) Motor unit and muscle activity in voluntary control. Rev Physiol 63: 387–436

Freund H-J, Büdingen HJ, Dietz V (1975) Activity of single motor units from human forearm muscles during voluntary isometric contractions. J Neurophysiol 38: 933–946

Friedman DP, Tortaglino LM (1993) Amyotrophic lateral sclerosis: hyperintensity of the corticospinal tracts on MR images of the spinal cord. AJR 160: 604–606

Friedreich N (1863) Ueber degenerative Atrophic der Spinalen Hinterstraenge. Arch Pathol Anat Physiol Klin Med 26: 391–419; 26: 433–459; 27: 1–26

Friedreich N (1976) Uebr Ataxie mit besonderer Beruchsichtigung der heriditären Formen. Virchows Arch Pathol Anat 68: 145–245

Frijns CJM, Deutekom IV, Frantz RR et al. (1994) Dominant congenital benign spinal muscular atrophy. Muscle Nerve 17: 192–197

Friman G (1976) Serum creative phosphokinase in epidemic influenza. Scand J Defect Dis. 8: 13–20

Friman G, Schiller HH, Schwartz MS (1977) Disturbed neuromuscular transmission in viral infections. Scand J Infect Dis 9: 99–103

Frizzera G, Banks PM, Massarelli G et al. (1983) A systemic lymphoproliferative disorder with morphologic features of Castleman's disease. Am J Surg Pathol 7: 211–231

Fross RD, Daube J (1987) Neuropathy in the Miller Fisher syndrome. Neurology 37: 1493–1498

Fry HJH (1986) Overuse syndrome in musicians: prevention and management. Lancet ii: 728–731

Fu R, DeLisa JA, Kraft GH (1980) Motor nerve latencies through the tarsal tunnel in normal adult subjects. Arch Phys Med Rehabil 61: 243–248

Fu YH, Pizzuti A, Fenwick RG Jr et al. (1992) An unstable triplet repeat in a gene related to myotonic muscular dystrophy. Science 255: 1256–1258

Fuglsang-Frederiksen A, Schell O, Buchthal F (1976) Diagnostic yield of analysis of the pattern of electrical activity and of individual motor unit potentials in myopathy. J Neurol Neurosurg Psychiatry 39: 742–750

Fuglsang-Frederiksen A, Dahl K, Lo Monaco M (1984a) Electrical muscle activity during a gradual increase in force in patients with neuromuscular diseases. Electroencephalogr Clin Neurophysiol 57: 320–329

Fuglsang-Frederiksen A, Lo Monaco M Dahl K, (1984b) Integrated electrical activity and number of zero crossings during a gradual increase in muscle force in patients with neuromuscular diseases. Electroencephalogr Clin Neurophysiol 58: 211–219

Fuglsang-Frederiksen A, Lo Monaco M, Dahl K (1985) Turns analysis (peak ratio) in EMG using the mean amplitude as a substitute of force measurement. Electroencephalogr Clin Neurophysiol 60: 225–227

Fujii J, Otsu K, Zorzato F et al. (1991) Identification of a mutation in porcine ryanodine receptor associated with malignant hyperthermia. Science 253: 448–451

Fujino H, Lobayashi T, Goto I et al. (1991) Diagnostic magnetic resonance imaging of the muscles in patients with polymyositis and dermatomyositis. Muscle Nerve 14: 716–720

Fukuhara N, Tokiguchi S, Shirakawa K et al. (1980) Myoclonus epilepsy associated with ragged-red fibres (mitochondrial abnormalities): disease entity or a syndrome? J Neurol Sci 47: 117–133

Fukunaga H, Engel AH, Osame M et al. (1982) Paucity and disorganisation of pre-synaptic membrane active zones in the Lambert–Eaton myasthenic syndrome. Muscle Nerve 5: 686–697

Fukuyama Y, Kawazura M, Haruna H (1960) A peculiar form of congenital progressive muscular dystrophy: report of 15 cases. Paediatr Univ Tokyo 4: 5–8

Fukuyama Y, Osawa M, Suzuki H (1981) Congenital progressive muscular dystrophy of the Fukuyama type: clinical, genetic and pathological considerations. Brain Development 3: 1–29

Fuller GN, Jacobs JM, Guiloff RJ (1990) Axonal atrophy in the painful peripheral neuropathy of AIDS. Acta Neuropathol 81: 198–203

Fullerton PM (1969) Toxic chemicals and peripheral neuropathy: clinical and epidemiological features. Proc R Soc Med 62: 201–204

Furukawa T, Peter JB (1977) X-linked muscular dystrophy. Ann Neurol 2: 414–416

Furukawa T, Toyokura Y (1976) Chronic spinal muscular atrophy of facio-scapulo-humeral type. J Med Genet 13: 285–289

Gaan D (1967) Chronic thyrotoxic myopathy with involvement of respiratory and bulbar muscles. Br Med J iii: 415–416

Gabbay KH, Merola LO, Field RA (1966) The sorbitol pathway: presence in nerve and cord with substrate accumulation in diabetes. Science 151: 209–210

Gabreels-Festen AAWM, Gabreels FJM, Jennekens FGI et al. (1992a) Autosomal recessive form of hereditary motor and sensory neuropathy Type I. Neurology 42: 1755–1761

Gabreels-Festen AAWM, Gabreels FJM, Jennekens FGI (1993) Hereditary motor and sensory neuropathies: present status of Types I, II and III. Clin Neurol Neurosurg 95: 93–107

Gabreels-Festen AAWM, Joosten EMG, Gabreels FJM et al. (1992b) Early morphological features in dominantly inherited demyelinating motor and sensory neuropathy (HMSN Type 1). J Neurol Sci 107: 145–154

Gadian DG, Radda GK, Ross BD et al. (1981) Examination of a myopathy by phosphorus nuclear magnetic resonance. Lancet ii: 774–775

Gajdusek DC (1984) Environmental factors provoking physiological changes which induce motor neuron disease and early neuronal ageing in high incidence foci in the Western Pacific. In: Rose FC (ed) Research progress in motor neuron disease. Pitman, London, pp 44–69

Gajdusek DC, Gibbs CJ, Asher DM et al. (1977) Precautions in medical care of, and in handling materials from, patients with transmissible virus dementia (Creutzfeldt–Jakob disease). N Engl J Med 297: 1253–1258

Gallai V, Hockaday HM, Hughes JT et al. (1981) Ponto-bulbar palsy with deafness (Brown–Vialetto-van Laere syndrome): a report on three cases. J Neurol Sci 50: 259–275

Gallant EM, Fletcher TF, Goettl VM et al. (1986) Porcine malignant hyperthermia: cell injury enhances halothane sensitivity of biopsies. Muscle Nerve 9: 174–184

Gamboa ET, Eastword AB, Hayes AS et al. (1979) Isolation of influenza virus from muscle in myoglobinuria polymyositis. Neurology 2: 1221–1235

Gamstorp I (1956) Adynamia episodica hereditaria. Acta Paediatr Scand [Suppl] 108: 1–126

Gan R, Jabre JF (1992) The spectrum of concentric macro EMG correlations. II. Patients with diseases of muscle and nerve. Muscle Nerve 15: 1085–1088

Gantel M, Lakey A, Barlow DP et al. (1993) Titin antibodies in myasthenia gravis. Neurology 43: 1581–1585

Gantayet M, Swash M, Schwartz MS (1992) Fiber density in acute and chronic inflammatory demyelinating polyneuropathy. Muscle Nerve 15: 168–171

Garcia W (1974) Elevated creative phosphokinase levels associated with large muscle mass: another pitfall in evaluating the clinical significance of total CPK activity JAMA 228: 1395–1396

Garcia CA, Fleming H (1977) Reversible corticospinal tract disease due to hyperthyroidism. Arch Neurol 34: 647–648

Gardner E (1940) Decrease in human neurones with age. Anat Rec 77: 529–536

Gardner WJ, Sava GA (1962) Hemifacial spasm: a reversible pathophysiologic state. J Neurosurg 19: 240–247

Gardner-Medwin D (1970) Mutation rate in Duchenne type of muscular dystrophy. J Med Genet 7: 334–337

Gardner-Medwin D (1977) Children with genetic muscular disorders. Br J Hosp Med 17: 314–340

Gardner-Medwin D (1980) Clinical features and classification of the muscular dystrophies. Br Med Bull 36: 109–115

Gardner-Medwin D, Walton JN (1969) Myokymia with impaired muscular relaxation. Lancet i: 127–130

Gardner-Medwin D, Hudgson P, Walton JN (1967) Benign spinal muscular atrophy arising in childhood and adolescence. J Neurol Sci 5: 121–158

Gardner-Medwin D, Pennington RJ, Walton JN (1971) The detection of carriers of X-linked muscular dystrophy genes. J Neurol Sci 13: 459–474

Gardner-Thorpe C, Foster JB, Barwick DD (1976) Unusual manifestations of Herpes zoster: a clinical and electrophysiological study. J Neurol Sci 28: 427–447

Garland H (1955) Diabetic amyotrophy. Br Med J ii: 1287–1290

Garland H, Moorhouse D (1952) Compressive lesions of the external popliteal (common peroneal) nerve. Br Med J ii: 1373–1378

Garlepp MJ, Dawkins RL (1984) Immunological aspects. In: Ansell BM (ed) Inflammatory disorders of muscle. Clin Rheum Dis 10: 35–51

Garlepp MJ, Dawkins RL, Christiansen FT (1983) HLA antigen and acetylcholine receptor antibodies in penicillamine-induced myasthenia gravis. Br Med J 286: 338–340

Garruto RM, Yase Y (1986) Neurodegenerative disorders of the Western Pacific: the search for mechanisms of pathogenesis. TINS 9: 368–374

Gaskell HS, Korb M (1946) Occurrence of multiple neuritis in cases of cutaneous diphtheria. Arch Neurol Psychiatry 55: 559–572

Gassel MM (1963) A study of femoral nerve conduction time. Arch Neurol 9: 607–614

Gassel MM, Trojaborg W (1964) Clinical and electrophysiological study of the pattern of conduction times in the distribution of the sciatic nerve. J Neurol Neurosurg Psychiatry 27: 351–357

Gastant JL, Pellissier JF (1985) Neuropathie en cisplatine: étude clinique, electrophysiologique et morphologique. Rev Neurol (Paris) 141: 614–626

Gath I, Sjaastad O, Løken AC (1969) Myopathic electromyographic changes correlated with histopathology in Wohlfart-Kugelberg–Welander disease. Neurology 19: 344–353

Gauthier G (1979) Thomas Morton's disease: a nerve entrapment syndrome. Clin Orthop 142: 90–92

Geenen EK, Bunker TD (1985) Anterior interosseous nerve syndrome. Br J Hosp Med 34: 235–236

Geiger LR, Mancall EL, Penn AS et al. (1974) Familial neuralgic amyotrophy: report of three families with review of the literature. Brain 97: 87–102

Gelberman RH, Aronson D, Weisner MH (1980) Carpal tunnel syndrome: results of a prospective trial of steroid injection and splinting. J Bone Joint Surg [Am] 62: 1181–1184

Gelberman RH, Hergenroeder PT, Hargens AR et al. (1981) The carpal tunnel syndrome - a study of carpal tunnel pressures. J Bone Joint Surg [Am] 63: 380–383

Genkins G, Sivak M, Tortter PI (1993) Treatment strategies in myasthenia gravis. Ann NY Acad Sci 681: 603–608

Genth E, Mierau R, Genetzky P et al. (1990) Immunogenetic associations of scleroderma-related antinuclear antibodies. Arthritis Rheum 33: 654–665

George TM, Burke JM, Sobotka PA et al. (1984) Resolution of stiff man syndrome with cortisol replacement in a patient with deficiencies of ACTH, growth hormone and prolactin. N Engl J Med 310: 1511–1513

Gevritsen van der Hoop R, Vecht CJ, Van der Burg MEL et al. (1990) Prevention of cisplatin neurotoxicity with an ACTH (4–9) analog in patients with ovarian cancer. N Engl J Med 322: 89–93

Gharbi Ben Ayed A, Samoud A, Ben Dridi MF (1993) The Stark-Kaeser type scapulo-peroneal amyotrophy of neurogenic origin: study of a familial case. Arch Francaises de Pediatrie 50: 135–137

Gherardi R, Bouché P, Escourolle R et al. (1983) Peroneal muscular atrophy. II. Nerve biopsy studies. J Neurol Sci 61: 401–416

Gherhardi R, Lebargy F, Banlard P et al. (1989) Necrotizing vasculitis and HIV replication in peripheral nerves. N Engl J Med 321: 685–686

Giannini F, Passero S, Cioni R et al. (1991) Electrophysiologic evaluation of local steroid injection in carpal tunnel syndrome. Arch Phys Med Rehabil 72: 738–742

Gibbels E, Schaefer HE, Runne U et al. (1985) Severe polyneuropathy in Tangier disease mimicking syringomyelia or leprosy. J Neurol 232: 283–294

Gibberd FB, Simmonds JP (1980) Neurological disease in ex Far East prisoners of war. Lancet ii: 135–137

Gibberd FB, Billimania JD, Page NGR et al. (1979) Heredipathia atactica polyneuriformis (Refsum's disease) treated by diet and plasma exchange. Lancet i: 575–578

Gibson JA, Halliday D, Morrison WL et al. (1987) Decrease in human quadriceps muscle protein turnover consequent upon leg immobilisation. Clin Sci 72: 503–509

Gibson JNA, Smith K, Rennie MJ (1988) Prevention of disuse muscle atrophy by means of electrical stimulation: maintenance of protein synthesis. Lancet ii: 767–770

Gilchrist J, Barkhaus P, Bril V et al. (1992) Single fiber EMG reference values: a collaborative effort. Muscle Nerve 15: 151–161

Gilchrist JM, Massey JM, Sanders DB (1994) Single fiber EMG and repetitive nerve stimulation of the same muscle in myasthenia gravis. Muscle Nerve 17: 171–175

Giles RE, Blanc H, Cann HM et al. (1980) Maternal inheritance of human mitochondrial DNA. Proc Natl Acad Sci USA 77: 6715–6719

Gilliatt RW (1966) Nerve conduction in human and experimental neuropathies. Proc R Soc Med 59: 989–993

Gilliatt RW (1976) Thoracic outlet compression syndrome. Br Med J I: 1274–1275

Gilliatt RW, Harrison MJG (1984) Nerve compression and entrapment. In: Asbury AK, Gilliatt RW (eds) Peripheral nerve disorders. Butterworths, London, pp 243–286

Gilliatt RW, Sears TA (1958) Sensory nerve action potentials in patients with peripheral nerve lesions. J Neurol Neurosurg Psychiatry 21: 109–118

Gilliatt RW, Willison RG (1962) Peripheral nerve conduction in diabetic neuropathies. J Neurol Neurosurg Psychiatry 25: 11–18

Gilliatt RW, Goodman HV, Willison RE (1961) The recording of lateral popliteal nerve action potentials in man. J Neurol Neurosurg Psychiatry 24: 305–318

Gilliatt RW, Le Quesne PM, Logue V et al. (1970) Wasting of the hand associated with a cervical rib or band. J Neurol Neurosurg Psychiatry 33: 615–624

Gillon KRW, Hawthorn JN (1983) Sorbitol, inositol and nerve conduction in diabetes. Life Sci 32: 1943–1947

Gillord EF, Ohtsu K, Fujii J et al. (1991) A substitution of cysteine for arginine 614 in the ryanodine receptor is potentially causative of human malignant hyperthermia. Genomics 11: 543–547

Glantz MJ, Burger PC, Friedman AH et al. (1994) Treatment of radiation induced nervous system injury with heparin and warfarin. Neurology 44: 2020–2027

Glaser GH (1966) Crisis, precrisis and drug resistance in myasthenia gravis. Ann NY Acad Sci 135: 335–345

Glenner GG (1983) Alzheimer's disease: the commonest form of amyloidosis. Arch Pathol Lab Med 107: 281–282

Glick B, Shapira Y, Stern A (1984) Congenital muscle fiber-type disproportion myopathy. Ann Neurol 16: 405–406

Godet-Guillain J, Fardeau M (1970) Hypothyroid myopathy: histological and ultrastructural study of an atrophic form. In: Walton JN, Canal N, Scarlato S (eds) Muscle diseases. Excerpta Medica, Amsterdam, pp 512–515 (ICS 199)

Goebel HH (1986) Neuropathological aspects of congenital myopathies. Prog Neuropathol 6: 231–262

Goebel HH, Lenard HG, Görke W et al. (1977) Fibre type disproportion in the rigid spine syndrome. Neuropädiatrie 8: 467–477

Goebel HH, Veits, Dyck PJ (1980) Confirmation of critical unmyelinated fiber absence in hereditary sensory neuropathy. J Neuropathol Exp Neurol 39: 670–675

Gold BJ, Price DL, Griffin JW et al. (1988) Neurofilament antigens in acrylamide neuropathy. J Neuropathol Exp Neurol 47: 145–157

Goldberg AL (1969) Protein turnover in skeletal muscle. I. Protein catabolism during work-induced hypertrophy and growth induced with growth hormone. J Biol Chem 244: 3217–3222

Goldberg AL, Goodman HM (1969) Relationship between cortisone and muscle work in determining muscle size. J Physiol (Lond) 200: 667–675

Goldenberg DL, Simms RW, Geiger A et al. (1990) High frequency of fibromyalgia in patients with chronic fatigue seen in a primary care practice. Arthritis Rheum 33: 381–385

Goldman JM, Clemens ME, Gibberd FB et al. (1985) Screening of patients with retinitis pigmentosa for heredopathia atactica polyneuritiformis (Refsum's disease). Br Med J 290: 1109–1110

Goldspink DF (1977) The influence of immobilisation and stretch on protein turnover of rat skeletal muscle. J Physiol 264: 267–273

Goldstein G, Mackay IR (1966) Contrasting abnormalities in the thymus in systemic lupus erythematosus and myasthenia gravis: a quantitative histological study. Am J Exp Biol Med Sci 43: 381–390

Gollnick PD, Armstrong RB, Saltin B et al. (1973) Effect of training on enzyme activity and fibre composition of human skeletal muscle. J Appl Physiol 34: 107–111

Gollnick PD, Armstrong RB, Saubert CW IV et al. (1972) Enzyme activity and fibre composition in skeletal muscle of untrained and trained men. J Appl Physiol 33: 312–319

Gombault M (1880–1881) Contribution à l'étude anatomique de la névrite parenchymateuse subaiguë et chronique. Névrite segmentaire péri-axile. Arch Neurol 1: 11

Gomez MR (1994) Motor neuron diseases in children. In: Engel AG, Franzini-Armstrong C (eds) Myology, 2nd edn. McGraw-Hill, New York, pp 1837–1853

Gomez MR, Clermont V, Bernstein J (1962) Progressive bulbar paralysis in childhood (Fazio-Londé disease): report of a case with pathologic evidence of nuclear atrophy. Arch Neurol 6: 317–323

Gonatas NK, Perez MC, Shy GM et al. (1965) Central "core" disease of skeletal muscle. Am J Pathol 47: 503–524

Good I (1948) Myocardial changes in fatal diphtheria: a summary of observations in 221 cases. Am J Med Sci 219: 257

Good JL, Khuvana RK, Mayer RF et al. (1993) Pathophysiological studies of neuromuscular function in subacute organophosphate poisoning induced by phosmet. J Neurol Neurosurg Psychiatry 56: 290–294

Goodall RJ (1956) Nerve injuries in fresh fractures. Tex Med 52: 93–95

Gooden DS, Rowley HA, Olney RK (1988) Magnetic resonance imaging in amyotrophic lateral sclerosis. Ann Neurol 23: 418–420

Goodgold J, Eberstein A (1983) Electrodiagnosis of neuromuscular diseases, 3rd edn. Williams and Wilkins, Baltimore

Goodman JJ (1954) Femoral neuropathy in relation to diabetes mellitus. Diabetes 3: 266–271

Goonatilleka A, Modarres-Sedeghi H, Guiloff RJ (1994) Accuracy, reproducibility and variability of hand-held dynamometry in motor neuron disease. J Neurol Neurosurg Psychiatry 57: 326–332

Gordon AM, Green JR, Lagunoff D (1970) Studies on a patient with hypokalaemic familial periodic paralysis. Am J Med 48: 185–195

Gordon EE, Januszko DM, Kaufman C (1967) A critical survey of stiff man syndrome. Am J Med 42: 582–599

Gordon RM, Silverstein A (1970) Neurological manifestation in progressive systemic sclerosis. Arch Neurol 22: 126–134

Goren H, Steinberg MC, Farbourg GH (1980) Familial oculoleptomeningeal amyloidosis. Brain 103: 473–478

Gorin F, Baldwin B, Tait R et al. (1990) Stiff man syndrome: a disorder with auto antigenic heterogenicity. Ann Neurol 28: 711–714

Gorman CA, Dyck PJ, Pearson JS (1965) Symptom of restless legs. Arch Intern Med 115: 155–160

Gospe SM, Lazaro RP, Lava NS et al. (1989) Familial X-linked myalgia and cramps. Neurology 39: 1277–1280

Gosselin S, Kyle RA, Dyck PJ (1991) Neuropathy associated with monoclonal gammopathies of undetermined significance. Ann Neurol 30: 54–61

Goto I, Kobayashi T, Autoku Y et al. (1986) Adrenoleukodystrophy and variants. J Neurol Sci 72: 103–112

Gottdiener JS, Sherber HS, Hawley RJ et al. (1978) Cardiac manifestation in polymyositis. Am J Cardiol 41: 1141–1149

Gould JS, Wissinger HA (1978) Carpal tunnel syndrome in pregnancy. South Med J 71: 144–145

Gowers WR (1886) A manual of diseases of the nervous system. Dawson, London

Gowers WR (1902) A lecture on myopathy and a distal form. Br Med J ii: 89–92

Goy JJ, Stauffer JC, Deruaz JP et al. (1989) Myopathy as possible side effect of cyclosporin. Lancet i: 1446–1447

Graf RJ, Halter JB, Halar E et al. (1979) Nerve conduction abnormalities in untreated maturity-onset diabetes: relation to levels of fasting plasma glucose and glycosylated haemoglobin. Ann Intern Med 90: 298–303

Graig FA, Smith JC (1965) Serum creatine phosphokinase activity in altered thyroid states. J Clin Endocrinol Metab 25: 723–731

Grant R, Sutton DL, Behan DO et al. (1987) Nifedipine in the treatment of myotonia in myotonic dystrophy. J Neurol Neurosurg Psychiatry 50: 199–206

Green DE (1983) Mitochondral structure, function and replication. N Engl J Med 309: 182–183

Green D, Joynt RJ, Van Allen MW (1964) Neuromyopathy associated with a malignant carcinoid tumour. Arch Intern Med 114: 494–496

Green DP (1984) Diagnostic and therapeutic value of carpal tunnel injection. J Hand Surg 9A: 850–854

Green H, Thomson J, Daub W et al. (1979) Fiber composition, fiber size and enzyme activities in vastus lateralis of elite athletes involved in high exercise. Eur J Appl Physiol 41: 109–117

Greenbaum AL, Young GG (1950) Distribution of protein in tissues of rats treated with anterior pituitary growth hormone. Nature 165: 521–522

Greenbaum D, Richardson PC, Salmon MW et al. (1964) Pathological observations on six cases of diabetic neuropathy. Brain 87: 201–214

Greene DA, De Jesus PV, Winegrad A (1975) Effects of insulin and dietary myoinositol on impaired peripheral motor nerve conduction velocity in acute streptozotocin diabetes. J Clin Invest 55: 1326–1336

Greenfield's Neuropathology (1976) Blackwood W, Corsellis JAN (eds) Edward Arnold, London

Greenfield JG, Shy GM, Alvard EC et al. (1957) In: An atlas of muscle pathology in neuromuscular diseases. Livingstone, Edinburgh, p 104

Greenwood RJ, Hughes RAC, Bowden N et al. (1984) Controlled trial of plasma exchange in acute inflammatory polyradiculoneuropathy. Lancet i: 877–879

Gregerson G (1967) Diabetic neuropathy: influence of age, sex, metabolic control and duration of diabetes on motor conduction velocity. Neurology 17: 972–980

Gregerson G (1968) Variation in motor conduction velocity produced by acute changes of the metabolic state in diabetic patients. Diabetologia 4: 273–277

Griep PAM, Gielen FLH, Boom HBK et al. (1982) Calculation and registration of the same motor unit action potential. Electroencephalogr Clin Neurophysiol 53: 388–404

Griffiths PD (1966) Serum levels of ATP: creatine phosphotransferase (creatine kinase). The normal range and effect of muscular activity. Clin Chim Acta 13: 413–420

Griffiths RD, Cady EB, Edwards RHT et al. (1985) Muscle energy metabolism in Duchenne dystrophy studied by ^{31}P-NMR: controlled trials show no effect of allopurinol or ribose. Muscle Nerve 8: 760–767

Grigor R, Edmunds J, Lewkonia R et al. (1978) Systemic lupus erythematosus: a prospective analysis. Ann Rheum Dis 37: 121–128

Griggs RC (1977) The myotonic disorders and the periodic paralyses. In: Griggs RC, Moxley RT III (eds) Advances in neurology: treatment of neuromuscular disorder, vol 17. Raven Press, New York, pp 143–159

Griggs RC, Donohoe KM, Utell MJ et al. (1981) Evaluation of pulmonary function in neuromuscular disease. Arch Neurol 38: 9–12

Griggs RC, Engel WK, Resnick JS (1970) Acetazolamide treatment of hypokalaemic paralysis. Ann Intern Med 73: 39–48

Griggs RC, Mendell JR, Brooke MH et al. (1985) Clinical investigation in Duchenne dystrophy. V. Use of creatine kinase and pyruvate kinase in carrier detection. Muscle Nerve 8: 60–67

Griggs RC, Moxley RT, Mendell JR et al. (1993) Duchenne dystrophy: randomised controlled trial of prednisone (18 months) and azathioprine (12 months). Neurology 43: 520–527

Griggs RC, Reeves W, Moxley RT (III) (1977) The heart in Duchenne dystrophy. In: Rowland LP (ed) Pathogenesis of human muscular dystrophies. Excerpta Medica, Amsterdam, pp 661–671

Grimby L, Hannerz J (1970) Difference in recruitment order of motor units in phasic and tonic flexion reflex in spinal man. J Neurol Neurosurg Psychiatry 33: 562–570

Grimby L, Hannerz J, Hedman B (1979) Contraction time and voluntary discharge properties of individual short toe extensor motor units in man. J Physiol (Lond) 289: 191–201

Grimby L, Hannerz J, Hedman B (1981) Fatigue and voluntary discharge properties of single motor units in man. J Physiol (Lond) 316: 545–554

Grob D, Namba T (1976) Characteristics and mechanism of neuromuscular block in myasthenia gravis. Ann NY Acad Sci 274: 143–173

Grob D, Arsura EL, Brunner NG et al. (1987) The course of myasthenia gravis and therapies affecting outcome. Ann NY Acad Sci 505: 472–499

Grob D, Brunner NG, Namba T (1981) The natural course of myasthenia gravis and the effect of various therapeutic measures. Ann NY Acad Sci 377: 652–669

Grob D, Liljestrand A, Johns PJ (1957) Potassium movement in patients with familial periodic paralysis. Am J Med 23: 356–375

Groen RJ, Sie OG, van Weerden TW (1993) Dominant inherited spinal muscular atrophy with atrophic and hypertrophic calves. J Neurol Sci 114: 81–84

Gross B, Ochoa J (1979) Trichinosis: a clinical report and histochemistry of muscle. Muscle Nerve 2: 394–398

Gross EG, Dexter JD, Roth RG (1966) Hypokalemic myopathy with myoglobinuria associated with licorice ingestion. N Engl J Med 274: 602–606

Gross MLP, Thomas PK (1981) The treatment of chronic relapsing and chronic progressive idiopathic inflammatory polyneuropathy by plasma exchange. J Neurol Sci 52: 69–78

Gruber W (1870) Über die Verbindung des Nervus medianus mit den Nervus ulnaris am Unterarme des Menschen und der Säugethiere. Arch Anat Physiol 37: 501–522

Gruener R, McArdle B, Ryman BE et al. (1968) Contracture of phosphorylase deficient muscle. J Neurol Neurosurg Psychiatry 31: 268–283

Grunfeld J-P, Ganeval D, Chanard J et al. (1972) Acute renal failure in McArdle's disease. N Engl J Med 286: 1237–1241

Gubbay SS, Kahana E, Zilber N et al. (1985) Amyotrophic lateral sclerosis: a study of its presentation and prognosis. J Neurol 232: 295–300

Guggenheim MA, Ringel SP, Silverman A et al. (1982) Progressive neuromuscular disease in children with chronic cholestasis and vitamin E deficiency: diagnosis and treatment with α-tocopherol. J Pediatr 100: 51–58

Guiheneuc P, Calamel J, Doncorli C et al. (1983) Automatic detection and pattern recognition of single motor unit potentials in needle EMG. In: Desmedt JE (ed) Computer-aided electromyography. Karger, Basel, pp 73–127 (Progress in Clinical Neurophysiology, vol 10)

Guiheneuc P, Jinet J, Grouleau J-Y et al. (1980) Early phase of vincristine neuropathy in man. J Neurol Sci 45: 355

Guiliano VJ (1974) Polymyositis in a patient with acquired hypogammaglobulinemia Am J Med Sci 268: 53–56

Guillain G (1938) Synthese générale de la discussion. J Belge Neurol Psychiatr 38: 323–329

Guillain G (1953) Considérations sur le syndrome de Guillain et Barré. Ann Med 545: 81–92

Guillain G, Barré JA, Strohl A (1916) Sur un syndrome de radiculo-névrite avec hyperalbuminose due liquede céphalo-rachidien sans un réaction cellulaire. Remarques sur les caractéres cliniques et graphiques des réflexes tendineuses. Bull Soc Med Hôp Paris 10: 146–147

Guillain–Barré Syndrome Study Group (1985) Plasmapheresis and acute Guillain–Barré syndrome. Neurology 35: 1096–1104

Guiloff R, Fuller GN (1992) Other neurological diseases in HIV-1 infection: clinical aspects. In: Rudge P (ed) Neurological aspects of human retroviruses. Ballière's Clinical Neurology 1, 175–209

Guiloff RJ, Modarres-Sedeghi H (1992) Voluntary activation and fibre density of fasciculations in motor neuron disease. Ann Neurol 31: 416–424

Guiloff RJ, Sheratt RM (1977) Sensory conduction in medial plantar nerve. J Neurol Neurosurg Psychiatry 40: 1168–1181

Guiloff RJ, Thomas PK, Contreras M et al. (1982) Evidence for linkage of Type 1 hereditary motor and sensory neuropathy with the Duffy locus on chromosome 1. Ann Hum Genet 46: 25–27

Gurney ME, Belton AC, Cashman N et al. (1984) Inhibition of terminal axonal sprouting by serum from patients with amyotrophic lateral sclerosis. N Engl J Med 311: 933–939

Gussoni E, Pavlath GK, Lantot AM et al. (1992) Normal dystrophin transcripts detected in Duchenne muscular dystrophy patients after myoblast transplantation. Nature 356: 435–438

Gustafsson R, Tata TR, Lindberg O et al. (1965) The relationship between the structure and activity of rat skeletal muscle mitochondria after thyroidectomy and thyroid hormone treatment. J Cell Biol 26: 555–578

Gutmann E, Hanzlikova V (1976) Fast and slow motor units and aging. Gerontology 22: 280–300

Gutmann L (1970) Atypical peroneal neuropathy. J Neurol Neurosurg Psychiatry 33: 453–456

Gutmann L (1977) Median-ulnar nerve communications and carpal tunnel syndrome. J Neurol Neurosurg Psychiatry 40: 982–986

Gutmann L (1991) Facial and limb myokymia. Muscle Nerve 14: 1043–1049 (AAEM minimonograph no. 37)

Gutmann L, Crosby TW, Takamari M et al. (1972) The Eaton–Lambert syndrome and autoimmune disorders. Am J Med 53: 354–356

Gutmann L, Fakadej A, Riggs JE (1983) Evolution of nerve conduction abnormalities in children with dominant hypertrophic neuropathy of the Charcot–Marie–Tooth type. Muscle Nerve 6: 515–519

Guy RJC, Richards F, Edmunds ME et al. (1984) Diabetic autonomic neuropathy and iritis. Br Med J 289: 343–346

Guzé BH, Baxter LR (Jr) (1985) Neuroleptic malignant syndrome. N Engl J Med 313: 163–166

Guzetta F, Ferriere G, Cyon F (1982) Congenital hypomyelination polyneuropathy: pathological findings compared with polyneuropathies starting later in life. Brain 105: 395–416

Haase GR, Engel AG (1960) Paroxysmal recurrent rhabdomyolysis. Arch Neurol 2: 410–419

Haffler DA, Johnson D, Kelly JJ et al. (1986) Monoclonal gammopathy and neuropathy: myelin-associated glycoprotein reactivity and clinical characteristics. Neurology 36: 75–78

Hagberg B, Westerberg B (1983) Hereditary motor and sensory neuropathy in Swedish children. Acta Paediatr Scand 72: 379–383

Hagberg JM, Coyle EF, Carroll JE et al. (1982) Exercise hyperventilation in patients with McArdle's disease. J Appl Physiol 52: 991–994

Hagert CG, Lundberg G, Hansen T (1977) Entrapment of the posterior interosseous nerve. Scand J Plast Reconstr Surg ii: 205–212

Hahn AF, Brown WF, Koopman WJ et al. (1990) X-linked dominant hereditary motor and sensory neuropathy. Brain 113: 1511–1525

Hahn AF, Parker AW, Bolton CF et al. (1991) Neuromyotonia in hereditary neuropathy. J Neurol Neurosurg Psychiatry 54: 230–235

Håkanson CH (1956) Conduction velocity and amplitude of the action potential as related to circumference in the isolated fibre of frog muscle. Acta Physiol Scand 37: 14–34

Hakelius L, Stålberg E (1974) EMG studies of free autogenous muscle transplants in man. Scand J Plast Reconstr Surg 8: 211–219

Häkkinen K, Komi PV (1983) Electromyographic and mechanical characteristics of human skeletal muscle during fatigue under voluntary and reflex conditions. Electroencephalogr Clin Neurophysiol 55: 436–444

Halban J (1894) Die dicke der Quergestreiften Muskelfasern und ihre Bedeutung. Anat Hefte 3: 267

Hall LW, Trim CM, Woolf N (1972) Further studies of porcine malignant hyperthermia. Br Med J ii: 145–148

Hall S, Bartelson JD, Onofrio BM et al. (1985) Lumbar spinal stenosis. Ann Interm Med 103: 271–275

Hallam PJ, Harding AE, Berciano J et al. (1992) Duplication of part of chromosome 17 is commonly associated with hereditary motor and sensory neuropathy Type 1. Ann Neurol 31: 570–572

Hall-Craggs ECB (1970) The longitudinal division of fibres in overloaded rat skeletal muscle. J Anat 107: 459–470

Hall-Craggs ECB (1971) Observation on the fate of muscle fibres temporarily isolated by transection of a muscle belly. Z Zellforsch Mikroskop Anat 119: 68–76

Hall-Craggs ECB, Lawrence CA (1970) Longitudinal fibre division in skeletal muscle: a light and electron-microscopic study. Z Zellforsch Mikroskop Anat 109: 481–494

Haller RG, Drachman DB (1976) Experimental alcoholic myopathy. Neurology 36: 370–371

Haller RG, Drachman DB (1980) Alcoholic rhabdomyolysis: an experimental model in the rat. Science 208: 412–415

Haller RG, Carter NW, Ferguson E et al. (1984) Serum and muscle potassium in experimental alcoholic myopathy. Neurology 34: 529–532

Haller RG, Lewis SF, Cook JD et al. (1985) Myophosphorylase deficiency impairs muscle oxidative metabolism. Ann Neurol 17: 196–199

Hallgren R, Lundin L, Roxin L-E et al. (1980) Serum and urinary myoglobin in alcoholics. Acta Med Scand 208: 33–39

Halonen JP, Falck B, Kalima H (1981) The firing rate of motor units in neuromuscular disorders. J Neurol 225: 269–276

Halter SK, De Lisa JA, Stolov WC et al. (1981) Carpal tunnel syndrome in chronic renal dialysis patients. Arch Phys Med Rehabil 62: 197–201

Hamid A, Slavin G, Mair WGP et al. (1981) Fibre type changes in striated muscle of alcoholics. J Clin Pathol 34: 991–995

Hamjian TA, Walker FO (1994) Serial neurophysiological studies of intramuscular botulinum A toxin in humans. Muscle Nerve 17: 1385–1392

Hammans SR, Morgan-Hughes JA (1994) Mitochondrial myopathies: clinical features, investigation, treatment and genetic counselling. In: Schapira AHV, Di Mauro S (eds) Mitochondrial disorders in neurology. Butterworth-Heinemann, London, pp 49–74

Hammans SR, Sweeney MG, Brockington M et al. (1991) Mitochondrial encephalopathies: molecular genetic analysis from blood samples. Lancet 337: 1311–1313

Hanauer A, Cheri M, Fuyita R et al. (1990) The Friedreich's ataxia gene is assigned to chromosome 9q 13–21 by mapping to tightly-linked markers and shows linkage disequilibrium with D9515. Am J Hum Genet 46: 133–137

Hankey GJ (1987) Guillain–Barré syndrome in Western Australia 1980–1985. Med J Austr 146: 130–133

Hannerz J (1974) Discharge properties of motor units in relation to recruitment order in voluntary contraction. Acta Physiol Scand 81: 374–384

Hanney DR (1978) Symptom prevalence in the community. JR Coll Gen Pract 28: 492–499

Hansen KN, Bjerre-Kundsen J, Brodthagen U et al. (1982) Muscle cell leakage due to long-distance training. Eur J Appl Physiol 48: 177–188

Hansen S, Ballantyne JP (1978) A quantitative electrophysiological study of motor neuron disease. J Neurol Neurosurg Psychiatry 41: 773–783

Hanson PA, Rowland LP (1971) Moebius syndrome and facio-scapulo-humeral muscular dystrophy. Arch Neurol 24: 31–39

Hanya N, Ikeda S, Nakadai A et al. (1989) Peripheral nerve pathological findings in familial amyloid polyneuropathy. Ann Neurol 25: 340–350

Hara H, Hagara H, Manatari S et al. (1987) Emery–Driefuss muscular dystrophy. J Neurol Sci 79: 23–31

Hardie RJ, Pullon HWH, Harding AE et al. (1991) Neuro-acanthocytosis. Brain 114: 13–49

Harding AE (1981) Friedreich's ataxia: a clinical and genetic study of 90 families with an analysis of early diagnostic criteria and intrafamilial clustering of clinical features. Brain 104: 589–620

Harding AE (1984) Inherited neuronal atrophy and degeneration predominantly of lower motor neurons. In: Dyck PJ, Thomas PK, Lambert EH, Bunge R (eds) Peripheral neuropathy, vol 2. Saunders, Philadelphia, pp 1537–1556

Harding AE (1995) From the syndrome of Charcot–Marie–Tooth to disorders of peripheral myelin protein. Brain 118: 809–818

Harding AE, Hewer RL (1983) The heart disease of Friedreich's ataxia. QJM 28: 489

Harding AE, Holt IJ (1989) Mitochondrial myopathies. Br Med Bull 45: 760–771

Harding AE, LeFanu J (1977) Carpal tunnel syndrome related to antebrachial Cimino - Breschia Fisula. J Neurol Neurosurg Psychiotry: 511–513

Harding AE, Thomas PK (1980a) The clinical features of hereditary motor and sensory neuropathy types I and II. Brain 103: 259–280

Harding AE, Thomas PK (1980b) Hereditary distal spinal muscular atrophy: a report on 34 cases and a review of the literature. J Neurol Sci 45: 337–348

Harding AE, Thomas PK (1980c) Autosomal recessive forms of hereditary motor and sensory neuropathy (types I and II). J Neurol Neurosurg Psychiatry 43: 669–678

Harding AE, Thomas PK (1984) Genetically determined neuropathies. In: Asbury AK, Gilliatt RW (eds) Peripheral nerve disorders. Butterworths, London, pp 205–242

Harding AE, Bradbury PG, Murray NMF (1983) Chronic asymmetrical spinal muscular atrophy. J Neurol Sci 59: 69–83

Harding AE, Matthews S, Jones S et al. (1985) Spino-cerebellar degeneration associated with a selective defect of vitamin E absorption. N Engl J Med 313: 32–35

Harding AE, Muller DPR, Thomas PK et al. (1982a) Spino-cerebellar degeneration secondary to chronic intestinal malabsorption: a vitamin E deficiency syndrome. Ann Neurol 12: 419–424

Harding AE, Thomas PK, Baraister M et al. (1982b) X-linked recessive bulbo-spinal muscular atrophy: a report of 10 cases. J Neurol Neurosurg Psychiatry 45: 1012–1019

Harley HG, Rundle SA, Rearden W et al. (1992) Unstable DNA sequence in myotonic dystrophy. Lancet 339: 1125–1128

Harman JB, Richardson AT (1954) Generalised myokymia in thyrotoxicosis. Lancet ii: 473–474

Harper PS (1975) Congenital myotonic dystrophy in Britain. II. Genetic basis. Arch Dis Child 50: 514–521

Harper PS (1989) Myotonic dystrophy, 2nd edn. Saunders, London

Harper PS (1996) New genes for old diseases. JR Coll Phys Lond 30: 221–231

Harper PS, Dyken PR (1972) Early-onset dystrophic myotonia: evidence supporting a maternal environmental factor. Lancet ii: 53–54

Harriman DGF, Reid R (1972) The incidence of lipid droplets in human skeletal muscle in neuromuscular disorders: a histochemical, electron microscopic and freeze-etch study. J Pathol 106: 1–24

Harriman DGF, Sumner DW, Ellis FR (1973) Malignant hyperpyrexia myopathy. QJM 42: 639–664

Harrington H, Hallett M, Tyler HR (1984) Ganglioside therapy for amyotrophic lateral sclerosis: a double-blind controlled trial. Neurology 34: 1083–1085

Harris CM, Tanner E, Goldstein MN et al. (1979) The surgical treatment of the carpal tunnel syndrome correlated with preoperative nerve conduction studies. J Bone Joint Surg [Am] 61: 93–98

Harrison BM, Hansen LA, Pollard JD et al. (1984) Demylination induced by serum from patients with Guillain–Barré syndrome. Ann Neurol 15: 163–170

Harrison GG (1971) Anaesthetic-induced malignant hyperpyrexia: a suggested method of treatment. Br Med J iii: 454–456

Harrison GG (1975) Control of a malignant hyperpyrexia syndrome in MHS swine by dantrolene sodium. Br J Anaesth 47: 62–65

Harrison MJG (1976) Muscle wasting after prolonged hypoglycemic coma: case report with electrophysiological data. J Neurol Neurosurg Psychiatry 39: 456–470

Harrison MJG (1978) Lack of evidence of generalised sensory neuropathy in patients with carpal tunnel syndrome. J Neurol Neurosurg Psychiatry 41: 957–959

Harrison MJG, Nurick S (1970) Results of anterior transposition of the ulnar nerve for ulnar neuritis. Br Med J i: 27–29

Hart Y, Schwartz MS, Bruckner F et al. (1988) Relapsing dermatomyositis associated with sarcoidosis. J Neurol Neurosurg Psychiatry 51: 311–315

Hartung HP, Toyka KV (1990) T cell and macrophage activation in experimental autoimmune neuritis and Guillain–Barré syndrome. Ann Neurol 27: 557–563

Hartung HP, Hughes RAC, Taylor WA et al. (1990) T cell activation in Guillain–Barré syndrome and in MS: elevated serum levels of soluble IL-2 receptors. Neurology 40: 215–218

Hartz CR, Linscheid RL, Gramse RR et al. (1981) The pronator teres syndrome: compressive neuropathy of the median nerve. J Bone Joint Surg 63A: 885–890

Harvey AM, Masland RL (1941a) A method for the study of neuromuscular transmission in human subjects. Johns Hopkins Med J 68: 81–93

Harvey AM, Masland RL (1941b) The electromyogram in myasthenia gravis. Johns Hopkins Med J 69: 1–13

Harvey DG, Toraile RM, Rosenbaum HE (1979) Amyotrophic lateral sclerosis with ophthalmoplegia – a clinico-pathological study. Arch Neurol 36: 615–617

Harvey JC, Sherbourne DH, Siegel CI (1965) Smooth muscle involvement in myotonic dystrophy. Am J Med 39: 81–90

Hasegawa H, Matsuoka T, Goto Y et al. (1991) Strongly succinate dehydrogenase reactive blood vessels in muscles from patients with mitochondrial myopathy, encephalopathy, lactic acidosis and stroke-like episodes. Ann Neurol 29: 601–605

Haslock DI, Wright V, Harriman DGF (1970) Neuromuscular disorders in rheumatoid arthritis: a motor point muscle biopsy study. Q J Med 39: 335–358

Hatfall SJ, Garland HG, Goldie W (1937) Gold treatment of arthritis: review of 900 cases. Lancet ii: 838–842

Hatt MU (1970) Hohen Lokalisation den cervicalen Diskushernie in Klinik Electromyographic (EMG) und Myelographie. Dtsch Z Nervenheilk 197: 56–65

Haughton JF, Little TW, Powers RK et al. (1994) M/RMS: an EEG method for quantifying upper motor neuron and functional weakness. Muscle Nerve 17: 936–942

Haupt HM, Hutchins GM (1982) The heart and cardiac conducting system in polymyositis/dermatomyositis. Am J Cardiol 50: 998–1006

Hauser WA, Karnes WE, Annis J et al. (1971) Incidence and prognosis of Bell's palsy in the population of Rochester Minnesota. Mayo Clin Proc 46: 258–262

Hausmanowa-Petrusewicz I (1978) Spinal muscular atrophy: infantile and juvenile type. US Dept of Commerce, Springfield Va, USA

Hausmanowa-Petrusewicz I, Karwanska A (1986) Electromyographic findings in different forms of infantile and juvenile proximal spinal muscular atrophy. Muscle Nerve 9: 37–46

Hausmanowa-Petrusewicz I, Fidzianska A, Niebroj-Dobosz I et al. (1980) Is Kugelberg-Welander spinal muscular atrophy a fetal defect? Muscle Nerve 3: 389–402

Hausmanowa-Petrusewicz I, Niebroj-Dobosz I, Borkowska J et al. (1977) Carrier detection in Duchenne dystrophy. In: Rowland LP (ed) Pathogenesis of human muscular dystrophies. Excerpta Medica, Amsterdam, pp 32–41

Hausmanowa-Petrusewicz I, Zaremba J, Barkowska J et al. (1984) Chronic proximal spinal muscular atrophy of childhood and adolescence: sex influence. J Med Genet 21: 447–450

Havard CWH (1979) Progress in endocrine exophthalmus. Br Med J i: 1001–1004

Haverkamp LJ, Appel V, Appel SH (1995) Natural history of amyotrophic lateral sclerosis in a database population Brain 118: 707–719

Haverkort-Poels PJE, Joosten EMG, Ruitenbeck WL (1987) Prevention of recurrent exertional rhabdomyolysis by dantrolene sodium. Muscle Nerve 10: 45–46

Hawkes CH, Fox J (1981) Motor neuron disease in leather workers. Lancet i: 507

Hawkes CH, Cavanagh JB, Mowbray S et al. (1984) Familial motor neuron disease: report of a family with five postmortem studies. In: Rose FC (ed) Recent progress in motor neuron disease. Pitman, London, pp 70–98

Hawley RJ, Cohen MH, Saini N et al. (1980) The carcinomatous neuromyopathy of oat cell lung carcinoma. Ann Neurol 7: 45–72

Hawley RJ, Milner MR, Gottdiener JS et al. (1991) Myotonic heart disease. Neurology 41: 259–262

Hawley RJ, Schellinger D, O'Doherty DS (1984) Computed tomographic patterns of muscles in neuromuscular disease. Arch Neurol 41: 383–387

Haymaker W, Kernohan JW (1949) Landry–Guillain–Barré syndrome: a clinico-pathologic report of 50 fatal cases and a critique of the literature. Medicine 28: 59–141

Haynes J, Thrush DC (1972) Paramyotonia congenita: An electrophysiological study. Brain 95: 553–558

Hayward M (1980) Electrodiagnosis of the muscular dystrophies. Br Med Bull 36: 127–132

Hayward M (1983) Quantification of interference patterns. In: Desmedt JE (ed) Computer aided electromyography. Karger, Basel, pp 128–149 (Progress in clinical neurology, vol 10)

Hayward M, Willison RG (1977) Automatic analysis of the electromyogram in patients with chronic partial denervation. J Neurol Sci 33: 415–423

Heads T, Pollock M, Robertson A et al. (1991) Sensory nerve pathology in amyotrophic lateral sclerosis. Acta Neuropathol 82: 316–320

Heath R, Schwartz MS, Brown IRF et al. (1983) Carbonic anhydrase III in neuromuscular disorders. J Neurol Sci 59: 383–388

Heathfield KWG, Williams JRB (1954) Peripheral neuropathy and myopathy associated with bronchogenic carcinoma. Brain 77: 122–135

Heckman R, Ludin HP (1982) Differentiation of spontaneous activity from normal and denervated electrical muscle. J Neurol Neurosurg Psychiatry 45: 331–336

Heckman JZ (1990) How to perform a muscle biopsy. Br J Hosp Med 43: 128–131

Heckmatt JZ, Dubowitz V (1988) Real-time ultrasound imaging of muscles. Muscle Nerve 11: 56–65

Heckmatt J, Hasson N, Saunders C et al. (1989) Cyclosporin in juvenile dermatomyositis. Lancet i: 1063–1066

Heckmatt JZ, Leeman S, Dubowitz V (1982) Ultrasound imaging in the diagnosis of muscle disease. J Paediatr 101: 656–660

Heckmatt JZ, Moosa A, Hutson C et al. (1984) Diagnostic needle muscle biopsy: a practical and reliable alternative to open biopsy. Arch Dis Child 59: 528–532

Heckmatt JZ, Pier N, Dubowitz V (1988) Real time ultrasound imaging of muscles. Muscle Nerve 11: 56–65

Heckmatt JZ, Sewry CA, Hodes D et al. (1985) Congenital centronuclear (myotubular) myopathy: a clinical, pathological and genetic study of eight children. Brain 108: 941–964

Hed R (1955) Myoglobinuria in man with special reference to familial forms. Acta Med Scand 151 [Suppl 303]: 1–100

Hed R, Lundmark C, Fahlgren H et al. (1962) Acute muscular syndrome in chronic alcoholism. Acta Med Scand 171: 585–599

Heene R (1973) Histological and histochemical findings in muscle spindles in dystrophia myotonica. J Neurol Sci 18: 369–372

Heffernan LP, Rewcastle NB, Humphrey JC (1968) The spectrum of rod myopathies. Arch Neurol 18: 529–542

Heffner RR(Jr), Armbrustmacher VW, Earlek M (1977) Focal myositis. Cancer 40: 301–306

Hegstrom RM, Murray JS, Pendras JP et al. (1961) Haemodialysis in the treatment of chronic uraemia. Trans Am Soc Artif Intern Organs 7: 136–152

Heimann-Patterson TD, Natter HN, Rosenberg HR et al. (1986) Malignant hyperthermia susceptibility in X-linked muscle dystrophies. Pediatr Neurol 2: 356–358

Helliwell TR, Nguyen TM, Morris GE et al. (1992) The dystrophin-related protein, utrophin, is expressed on the sarcolemma of regenerating human skeletal muscle fibres in dystrophies and inflammatory myopathies. Neuromusc Disord 2: 177–184

Hellmann DB, Laing TJ, Petri M et al. (1988) Mononeuritis multiplex: the yield of evaluations for occult diseases. Medicine 67: 145–153

Hellman ES, Tschudy DP, Bartter FC (1962) Abnormal electrolyte and water metabolissm in acute intermittent porphyria. Am J Med 32: 734–746

Helmholtz H (1850) Vorläufiger Bericht über die Fortpflanzungsgeschindigkeit der Nervenreizung. Arch Anat Physiol Wiss Med 71

Henneman E, Somjey G, Carpenter D (1965) Functional significance of cell size in spinal motoneurons. J Neurophysiol 28: 650–680

Henriksson K-G (1979) "Semiopen" muscle biopsy technique. Acta Neurol Scand 59: 317–323

Henriksson K-G, Stålberg E (1978) The terminal innervation pattern in polymyositis: A histochemical and single fibre EMG study. Muscle Nerve 1: 3–13

Henriksson K-G, Nilsson O, Rosén I et al (1977) Clinical, neurophysiological and morphological findings in Eaton–Lambert syndrome. Acta Neurol Scand 56: 117–140

Henry EW, Sidman RL (1988) Long lives for homozygous Trembler mutant mice despite virtual absence of peripheral nerve myelin. Science 241: 344–346

Henry MM, Swash M (1992) Coloproctology and the pelvic floor, 2nd edn. Butterworth-Heinemann, London.

Henson RA (1974) Neuromuscular disorders associated with malignant disease. In: Walton JN (ed) Disorders of voluntary muscle. Churchill Livingstone, Edinburgh, pp 760–774

Henson RA, Urich H (1970) Peripheral neuropathy associated with malignant disease. In: Vinken PJ, Bruyn GW (eds) Handbook of clinical neurology, vol 8. Elsevier, Amsterdam, pp 131–148

Henson RA, Urich H (1982) Cancer and the nervous system. Blackwell Scientific Publications, Oxford

Henson RA, Russell DS, Wilkinson M (1954) Carcinomatous neuropathy and myopathy. Brain 77: 82–121

Henson RA, Stern GM, Thompson VC (1965) Thymectomy for myasthenia gravis. Brain 88: 11–28

Henson TE, Muller J, De Myer WE (1967) Hereditary myopathy limited to females. Arch Neurol 17: 238–247

Hepp P (1887) Ueber einen Fall von acuter parenchysmatoeser Myositis, welche geschwinde Bilder und Fluctuation vortauschte. Berl Klin Wochenschr 22: 389–391

Herrington MS (1937) Successful treatment of two cases of familial periodic paralysis with potassium citrate. JAMA 108: 1339

Herrn CV, Master S (1968) Pyomyositis tropicans in Uganda. East Afr Med J 45: 463–471

Hers HG (1963) α-Glucosidase deficiency in generalised glycogen-storage disease (Pompe's disease). Biochem J 86: 11–16

Hertel G, Ricker K, Hirsch A (1977) The regional curare test in myasthenia gravis. J Neurol 214: 257–265

Hertzman PA, Blevins WL, Mayer J et al. (1990) Association of the eosinophilia-myalgia syndrome with the ingestion of tryptophan. N Engl J Med 322: 869–873

Hess CW, Mills KR, Murray NMF (1986) Measurement of central motor conduction in multiple sclerosis using magnetic brain stimulation. Lancet ii: 355–358

Hesselvik A (1969) Neuropathological studies on myelomatosis. Acta Neurol Scand 45: 91–108

Heuser JE, Reese TS, Dennis MJ et al. (1979) Synaptic vesicle exocytosis captured by quick freezing and correlated with quantal transmitter release. J Cell Biol 81: 275–300

Hewer RL (1968) Study of fatal cases of Friedreich's ataxia. Br Med J iii: 639–652

Hewlett RH, Brownell B (1975) Granulomatous myopathy: its relationship to sarcoidosis and polymyositis. J Neurol Neurosurg Psychiatry 38: 1090–1099

Heyck H, Landahn G, Carsten PM (1966) Enzymbestimmungen bei dystrophia musculorum progressiva. IV. Die Serumenzymkinetik im präklinischen Stadium des Typs Duchenne währund der ersten 2 Lebensjahre. Klin Wochenschr 44: 695–700

Heyland D, Souve M (1991) Neuroleptic malignant syndrome without the use of neuroleptics. Can Med Assoc J 145: 817–819

Hibi N, Shima K, Tashiro K et al. (1984) Development of a highly sensitive enzyme immunoassay for serum carbonic anhydrase III. J Neurol Sci 65: 333–340

Hicks EP (1972) Hereditary perforating ulcer of the foot. Lancet i: 319–321

Hicks JT, Korenyi-Bouth A, Utsinger PD et al. (1982) Neuromuscular and immunological abnormalities in an adult man with Kawasaki disease. Ann Intern Med 96: 607–610

Hickson RC, Davis JR (1981) Partial prevention of glucocorticoid-induced muscle atrophy by endurance training. Am J Physiol 241: E226–232

Hierons R (1957) Changes in the nervous system in acute porphyria. Brain 80: 176–192

Hierons R, Johnson MK (1978) Clinical and toxicological investigations of a case of delayed neuropathy in men after acute poisoning by an organophosphorus pesticide. Arch Toxicol (Berl) 40: 279–284

Higuchi I, Nakamara K, Nakagana M et al. (1993) Steroid-responsive myalgia in a patient with Becker muscular dystrophy. J Neurol Sci 115: 219–222

Hildebrand J, Coers C (1967) The neuromuscular function in patients with malignant tumours. Brain 90: 67–82

Hill NA, Howard FM, Huffer BR (1985) The incomplete anterior interosseous nerve syndrome. J Hand Surg 10A: 4–16

Hillaire D, Leclere A, Fauré S et al. (1994) Localisation of merosin negative congenital muscular dystrophy to chromosome 6q2 by homozygosity matching. Hum Mol Genet 3: 1651–1661

Hilton P, Spathis GS, Stanton SL (1983) Transient autonomic and sensory neuropathy in newly diagnosed insulin-dependent diabetes mellitus. Br Med J 286: 686

Hilton-Brown P, Stålberg E (1983a) The motor unit in muscular dystrophy: a single fibre EMG and scanning EMG study. J Neurol Neurosurg Psychiatry 46: 981–995

Hilton-Brown P, Stålberg E (1983b) Motor unit size in muscular dystrophy: a macro EMG and scanning EMG study. J Neurol Neurosurg Psychiatry 46: 996–1005

Hilton-Brown P, Stålberg E (1986) Size of motor units and firing rate in muscular dystrophy. In: Dimitrijevic MR, Kakulas BA, Vrobova G (eds) Recent achievements in restorative neurology, vol 2, Progressive neuromuscular diseases. Karger, Basel, pp 289–304

Hilton-Brown P, Stålberg E, Trontelj J et al. (1985) Causes of the increased fibre density in muscular dystrophies studied with single fibre EMG during electrical stimulation. Muscle Nerve 8: 383–388

Hinderks GJ, Frohlich J (1979) Low serum creatine kinase values associated with administration of steroids. Clin Chem 25: 2050–2051

Hirago T, Leipold HW, Cash WC et al. (1993) Reduced numbers and intense anti-ubiquitin immunostaining of bovine motor neurons affected with spinal muscular atrophy. J Neurol Sci 118: 43–47

Hirano A (1991) Cytopathology of amyotrophic lateral sclerosis. Adv Neurol 56: 91–101

Hirano A, Donnenfeld H, Sasaki S et al. (1984) The fine structure of motor neuron disease. In: Rose FC (ed) Research progress in motor neuron disease. Pitman, London, pp 328–348

Hirano M, Pavlakis SG (1994) Mitochondrial myopathy, encephalopathy, lactic acidosis and stroke-like episodes (MELAS): current concepts. J Child Neurol 9: 4–13

Hiyasaka K, Kumuro M. Sato W et al. (1993) Charcot–Marie-Tooth neuropathy Type 1B is associated with mutations of the myelin P_0 gene. Nature Genet 5: 31–34

Hjorth RJ, Walsh JC, Willison RG (1973) The distribution and frequency of spontaneous fasciculations in motor neuron disease. J Neurol Sci 18: 469–474

Ho K-J, Scully KT (1980) Acute rhabdomyolysis in renal failure in Weil's disease. Ala J Med Sci 17: 133–137

Ho KL (1989) Basophilic bodies of skeletal muscle in hypothyroidism. Hum Pathol 20: 1119–1124

Ho MF, Chalmers RM, Davis MB et al. (1996) A novel point mutation in the McLeod syndrome gene in neuroacanthocytosis. Ann Neurol 39: 672–675

Ho M, Chelly J, Carter N (1994) Isolation of the gene for McLeod syndrome that encodes a novel membrane transport protein: a 50kb deletion point mutation. Cell 77: 869–880

Ho TW, Mishu B, Li CY et al. (1995) Guillain–Barré syndrome in northern China. Brain 118: 597–605

Hodgkinsen SJ, Pollard JD, McLeod JG (1990) Cyclosporin A in the treatment of chronic demyelinating polyradiculoneuropathy. J Neurol Neurosurg Psychiatry 53: 327–330

Hodgson SV, Abbs S, Clark S et al. (1992) Correlation of clinical and deletion data in Duchenne and Becker muscular dystrophy with special reference to mental ability. Neuromusc Disord 2: 269–276

Hodgson SV, Hart K, Abbs S et al. (1989) Correlation of clinical and deletion data in Duchenne and Becker muscular dystrophy. J Med Genet 26: 682–693

Hoefer PFA, Aranow H, Rowland LP (1958) Myasthenia gravis and epilepsy. Arch Neurol Psychiatry 80: 10–17

Hoefsloot LH, van der Ploeg AT, Kroos MD et al. (1990) Adult and infantile glycogenosis Type 2 in one family explained by allelic diversity. Am J Hum Genet 46: 45–52

Hoeldtke RD, O'Dorisio TM, Boden G (1986) Treatment of autonomic neuropathy with a somatostatin analogue SMS-201-995. Lancet ii: 602–605

Hoffman EP (1991) Molecular diagnostics of Duchenne/Becker dystrophy. J Neurol Sci 101: 129–132

Hoffman EP, Brown H, Kunkel LM (1987a) Dystrophin: the protein product of the Duchenne muscular dystrophy locus. Cell 51: 919–928

Hoffman EP, Fischbeck KH, Brown RH et al. (1988) Characterisation of dystrophin in muscle biopsy specimens from patients with Duchenne's or Becker's muscular dystrophy. N Engl J Med 318: 1363–1368

Hoffman EP, Knudson CM, Campell KP et al. (1987b) Subcellular fractionation of dystrophin to the triads of skeletal muscle. Nature 330: 754–758

Hoffman EP, Kunkel LM, Angelini C et al. (1989) Improved diagnosis of Becker muscular dystrophy by dystrophin testing. Neurology 39: 1011–1017

Hogan GR, Gutmann L, Schmidt R et al. (1969) Pompe's disease. Neurology 19: 894–900

Hohlfeld R, Engel AG (1991) Coculture with autologous myotubes of cytotoxic T cells isolated from muscle in inflammatory myopathies. Ann Neurol 29: 498–507

Hohlfeld R, Engel AG, i K et al. (1991) Polymyositis mediated by T lymphocytes that express the acetylcholine receptor. N Engl J Med 324: 877–881

Hohlfeld R, Kalies I, Hohleisen B et al. (1986) Myasthenia gravis: stimulation of antireceptor autoantibodies by autoreactive T cell lines. Neurology 36: 618–621

Holme E, Gretter J, Jacobsen LE et al. (1989) Carnitine deficiency induced by pivampicillin and pivmecillinam therapy. Lancet ii: 469–473

Holmes GP, Kaplan JE, Gantz NM et al. (1988) Chronic fatigue syndrome: a working case definition. Ann Intern Med 108: 387–389

Holt IJ, Harding AE, Morgan-Hughes JA (1988) Deletion of mitochondrial DNA in patients with mitochondrial myopathies. Nature 331: 717–719

Holt IJ, Harding AE, Petty RKH et al. (1990) A new mitochondrial disease associated with mitochondrial DNA heteroplasmy. Am J Hum Genet 46: 428–433

Hongell A, Mattsson HS (1971) Neurographic studies before, after and during operation for median nerve compression in the carpal tunnel. Scand J Plast Reconstr Surg 5: 103–109

Hoogendijk JE, Hensels GW, Gabreels-Festem AAWM et al. (1992) De novo mutation in hereditary motor and sensory neuropathy Type 1. Lancet 339: 1081–1082

Hopf HC (1962) Untersuchungen über die Unterschiede in der Leitgeschwindigkeit motorischer Nervenfasern beim Menschen. Dtsch Z Nervenheilk 183: 579–588

Hopf HC (1963) Electromyographic study of so-called mononeuritis. Arch Neurol 9: 113–118

Hopf HC (1975) Peripheral neuropathy in acrodermatitis chronica atrophicans (Herxheimer). J Neurol Neurosurg Psychiatry 38: 452–468

Hopf HC, Gutmann L (1990) Diabetic third nerve palsy: evidence for a mesencephalic lesion. Neurology 40: 1041–1045

Hopkins AP, Morgan-Hughes JA (1969) The effect of local pressure in diphtheritic neuropathy. J Neurol Neurosurg Psychiatry 32: 614–623

Hopkins IJ, Lindsey JR, Ford FR (1966) Nemaline myopathy: a long-term clinico-pathologic study of affected mother and daughter. Brain 89: 299–310

Hopkins PM, Ellis FR, Halsall PJ (1991) Ryanodine contracture: a potentially specific in vitro diagnostic test for malignant hyperthermia. Br J Anaesth 66: 611–613

Hoppel C (1992) The physiological role of carnitine. In: Ferrari R, De Mauro S, Sherwood G (eds) L-carnitine and its role in medicine. Academic-Press, London, pp 5–19

Hoppel CL, Tomec RJ (1972) Carnitine palmitoyl transferase: location of two enzymatic activities in rat liver mitochondria. J Biol Chem 247: 832–841

Horikawa H, Konagaya M, Takayanangi T et al. (1986) The muscle CT of thigh in chronic Werdnig–Hoffman disease [in Japanese]. Clin Neurol 26: 490–497

Horoupion DS (1989) Hereditary sensory neuropathy with deafness: a familial multisystem atrophy. Neurology 39: 244–248

Horowitz M, McNeill JD, Maddern GJ et al. (1986) Abnormalities of gastric and esophageal emptying in polymyositis and dermatomyositis. Gastroenterology 90: 434–439

Horowitz SH, Genkins, G, Kornfield P et al. (1975) Regional curare test in evaluation of ocular myasthenia. Arch Neurol 32: 84–88

Horton WA, Eddridge R, Brody HA (1976) Familial motor neuron disease. Neurology 26: 460–465

Hosking GP, Bhat US, Dubowitz V et al. (1976) Measurement of muscle strength and performance in children with normal and diseased muscle. Arch Dis Child 51: 957–963

Houston ME, Bentzen H, Larson H (1979) Inter relationships between skeletal muscle adaptations and performance as studied by detraining and retraining. Acta Physiol Scand 105: 163–170

Howard BD, Gunderson CB (1980) Effects and mechanisms of polypeptide neurotoxins that act presynaptically. Ann Rev Pharmacol Toxicol 20: 307–336

Howard FM Jr (1963) A new and effective drug in the treatment of the stiff man syndrome: a preliminary report. Mayo Clin Proc 38: 203–212

Howard R (1908) A case of congenital defect of the muscular system (dystrophia muscularis congenita) and its association with congenital talipes equina varus. Proc Roy Soc Med 1: 157

Howard RS, Murray NMF (1992) Surface EMG in the recording of fasciculations. Muscle Nerve 15: 1240–1245

Howard RS, Wyles GM, Loh L (1989) Respiratory complications, and their management in motor neuron disease. Brain 112: 1155–1170

Howel D, Brunsdon C (1987) A simple test for the random arrangements of muscle fibres. J Neurol Sci 77: 49–57

Höweler CJ, Busch HFM, Bernini LF et al. (1980) Dystrophia myotonica and myotonia congenita concurring in one family: a clinical and genetic study. Brain 103: 497–514

Howell DA, Lees AJ, Toghill PJ (1979) Spinal internuncial neurons in progressive encephalomyelitis with rigidity. J Neurol Neurosurg Psychiatry 42: 773–785

Howes EL Jr, Price HM, Pearson CM et al. (1966) Hypokalaemic periodic paralysis: electron microscope changes in the sarcoplasm. Neurology 16: 242–256

Howlett SA (1975) Renal failure associated with actazolamide therapy for glaucoma. South Med J 65: 504–506

Howse AJG, Seddon H (1966) Ischaemic contracture of muscle associated with carbon monoxide and barbiturate poisoning. Br Med J i: 192–195

Hu X, Ray PN, Murphy EG et al. (1990) Duplication or mutation at the Duchenne muscular dystrophy locus. Am J Hum Genet 46: 682–695

Huard J, Bouchard JP, Roy R et al. (1992) Human myoblast transplantation: preliminary results of 4 cases. Muscle Nerve 15: 550–560

Huber SJ, Kissel JT, Shuttleworth EC et al. (1989) Magnetic resonance imaging and clinical correlates of intellectual impairment in myotonic dystrophy. Arch Neurol 46: 536–537

Hudgson P, Peter JB (1984) Classification. Clin Rheum Dis 10: 3–8

Hudgson P, Gardner-Medwin D, Fulthorpe JL et al. (1967) Nemaline myopathy. Neurology 17: 1125–1142

Hudgson P, Gardner-Medwin D, Worsfold M et al. (1968) Adult myopathy from glycogen storage disease due to acid maltase deficiency. Brain 91: 435–462

Hudson AJ (1981) Amyotrophic lateral sclerosis and its association with dementia. parkinsonism and other neurological disorders: a review. Brain 104: 217–247

Huff TA, Horton ES, Lebovitz HE (1967) Abnormal insulin secretion in myotonic dystrophy. N Engl J Med 277: 837–841

Hug G, Soukup S, Ryan M (1984) Rapid prenatal diagnosis of glycogen storage disease Type 2 by electron microscopy of cultured amniotic fluid cells. N Engl J Med 310: 1018

Hughes BP (1962) A method for the estimation of serum creatine kinase and its use in comparing serum creatine kinase and aldolase activity in normal and pathological stages. Clin Chim Acta 7: 597–603

Hughes BP (1971) Creatine phosphokinase in facio-scapulo-humeral muscular dystrophy. Br Med J iii: 464–465

Hughes DTD, Swann JC, Gleeson JA et al. (1965) Abnormalities in swallowing associated with dystrophic myotonica. Brain 88: 1037–1041

Hughes JT, Brownell B (1972) Pathology of peroneal muscular atrophy (Charcot–Marie–Tooth disease). J Neurol Neurosurg Psychiatry 35: 648–657

Hughes JT, Esiri M, Oxbury JM et al. (1971) Chloroquine myopathy. Q J Med 40: 85–93

Hughes RAC (1990) Guillain–Barré syndrome. Springer, London, pp 308

Hughes RAC (1991) Ineffectiveness of high-dose intravenous methylprednisolone in Guillain–Barré syndrome. Lancet 338: 1142

Hughes RAC, Newsom-Davis JM, Perkin GD et al. (1978) Controlled trial of prednisolone in acute polyneuropathy. Lancet ii: 750–753

Hughes RC, Matthews WB (1969) Pseudomyotonia and myokymia. J Neurol Neurosurg Psychiatry 32: 11–14

Hugon J, Labeau M, Tabaraud F et al. (1987) Central motor conduction in motor neuron disease. Ann Neurol 22: 544–546

Hunsacker RH, Fulkerson PK, Baary FJ et al. (1982) Cardiac function in Duchenne muscular dystrophy: results of 10-year follow up study and non-invasive tests. Am J Med 73: 235–238

Hunter D, Bomford RR, Russell DS (1940) Poisoning by methyl mercury compounds. QJM 9: 193–213

Hurst LC, Weissberg D, Carroll RE (1985) The relationship of the double crush to carpal tunnel syndrome: an analysis of 1000 cases of carpal tunnel syndrome. J Hand Surg 10B: 202–204

Hurwitz LJ,. McCormick D, Allen IV (1970) Reduced muscle alphaglucosidan (acid maltase) activity in hypothyroid myopathy. Lancet i: 67–69

Husby G, Ranlov PJ, Sletten K et al. (1985) The amyloid in familial amyloid cardiomyopathy of Danish origin is related to prealbumin. Clin Exp Immunol 60: 207–216

Huxley AF (1986) Discoveries on muscle: observation, theory and experiment. Br Med J 293: 115–118

Hyde SA, Scott OM, Goddard CH et al. (1982) Prolongation of ambulation in Duchenne muscular dystrophy by appropriate arthroses. Physiotherapy 68: 105–108

Iaizzo PA, Lehmann-Horn F (1990) The correlation between electrical after-activity and slowed relaxation in myotonia. Muscle Nerve 13: 240–246

Ibraghimov-Beskrovnaya O, Ervasti JM et al. (1992) Primary structure of dystrophin associated glycoproteins linking dystrophin to the extracellular matrix. Nature 355: 696–702

Igarashi S, Tanno Y, Onodera O (1992) Strong correlation between the number of CAG repeats in androgen receptor genes and the clinical onset of features of spinal and bulbar muscular atrophy. Neurology 42: 2300–2302

Ikeda S, Hanyu N, Hongo M et al. (1987) Hereditary generalised amyloidosis with polyneuropathy: clinico-pathological study of 65 Japanese patients. Brain 110: 315–337

Illa I, Nath A, Dalakas MC (1991) Immunocytochemical and virological characteristics of HIV-associated inflammatory myopathies. Ann Neurol 29: 474–481

Illingworth B, Cori GT, Cori CF (1956) Amylo-1,6 glucosidase in muscle tissue in generalised glycogen storage disease. J Biol Chem 218: 123–129

Ilyas AA, Mithen FA, Dalakas MC et al. (1992) Antibodies to acidic glycolipids in Guillain–Barré syndrome and chronic inflammatory demyelinating polyneuropathy. J Neurol Sci 107: 111–121

Ingall TJ, McLeod JG (1991) Autonomic function in hereditary motor and sensory neuropathy (Charcot–Marie–Tooth disease). Muscle Nerve 14: 1080–1083

Inglis AE, Straub LR, Williams CS (1972) Median nerve neuropathy at the wrist. Clin Orthop 83: 48–54

Ingram DA, Swash M (1987) Central motor conduction is abnormal in motor neuron disease. J Neurol Neurosurg Psychiatry 50: 159–166

Ingram DA, Davis GR, Schwartz MS et al. (1984) Cancer associated myasthenic (Eaton–Lambert) syndrome: distribution of abnormality and effect of treatment. J Neurol Neurosurg Psychiatry 47: 806–812

Ingram DA, Davis GR, Schwartz MS et al. (1985) The effect of continuous voluntary activation on neuromuscular transmission: a SF EMG study of myasthenia gravis and anterior horn cell disorders. Electroencephalogr Clin Neurophysiol 60: 207–213

Ingram DA, Davis GR, Swash M (1987a) The double collision technique: a new method for measurement of the motor nerve refractory period distribution in man. Electroencephalogr Clin Neurophysiol 66: 225–234

Ingram DA, Davis GR, Swash M (1987b) Motor nerve conduction velocity distributions in man: results of a new computer-based collision technique. Electroencephalogr Clin Neurophysiol 66: 235–243

Inoue A, Tsukada N, Koh C-S et al. (1987) Chronic relapsing demyelinating polyneuropathy associated with hepatitis B infection. Neurology 37: 1663–1666

Ionanescu V (1995) Charcot–Marie–Tooth neuropathies from clinical description to molecular genetics. Muscle Nerve 18: 267–275

Ionanescu V, Radu H, Nicolescu P (1975) Identification of Duchenne muscular dystrophy carriers. Arch Pathol 99: 436–441

Ionanescu VV, Searby CC, Ionanescu R (1989) Manifesting carrier of Becker muscular dystrophy (BMD): clinical and recombinant DNA studies. Acta Neurol Scand 79: 500–503

Ionanescu VV, Ionanescu R, Searby C (1993) Screening of dominantly inherited Charcot–Marie–Tooth neuropathies. Muscle Nerve 16: 1232–1238

Ionanescu V, Searby C, Ionanescu R et al. (1995) New point mutations and deletion of the connexion 32 gene in X-linked Charcot–Marie–Tooth neuropathy. Neuromusc Disord 5: 297–299

Irani DN, Cornblath DR, Chaudhry V et al. (1993) Relapse in Guillain–Barré syndrome after treatment with human immune globulin. Neurology 43: 872–875

Irvine AT, Tibbles J (1981) Treatment of Fisher's variant of Guillain–Barré syndrome by exchange transfusion. Can J Neurol Sci 8: 49–50

Isaacs GR, Bradley WG, Henderson G (1973) Longitudinal fibre splitting in muscular dystrophy: a serial cinematographic study. J Neurol Neurosurg Psychiatry 36: 813–819

Isaacs H (1961) A syndrome of continuous muscle fibre activity. J Neurol Neurosurg Psychiatry 24: 319–325

Isaacs H, Badenharst M (1993) False negative results with muscle caffeine, halothane for malignant testing hyperthermia. Anaesthesiology 79: 5–9

Isaacs H, Barlow MB (1974) Central core disease associated with elevated creatine phosphokinase levels: two members of a family known to be associated with malignant hypertheramia. S Afr Med J 48: 640–642

Isaacs H, Frere G (1974) Syndrome of continuous muscle fibre activity: histochemical, nerve terminal and end-plate study of two cases. S Afr Med J 10: 1601–1607

Isaacs H, Heffron JJA (1974) The syndrome of continuous muscle fibre activity cured: further studies. J Neurol Neurosurg Psychiatry 37: 1231–1235

Isaacs H, Heffron JJA, Badenhorst M (1975) Central core disease. J Neurol Neurosurg Psychiatry 38: 1177–1186

Isenberg D (1984) Myositis in other connective tissue disorders. In: Ansell BM (ed) Clinics in rheumatic disease, vol 10. Saunders, London, pp 151–174

Isenberg D, Snaith ML (1981) Muscle disease in systemic lupus erythematosus: a study of its nature, frequency and cause. J Rheumatol 8: 917–924

Ishikawa K, Engelhardt JK, Fujisawa T et al. (1977) A neuromuscular transmission block produced by a cancer tissue extract derived from a patient with the myasthenic syndrome. Neurology 27: 140–143

Ishimoto S, Goto I, Ohta M et al. (1983) A quantitative study of the muscle satellite cell in various neuromuscular disorders. J Neurol Sci 62: 303–314

Ito Y, Yagishita S, Nakajima S et al. (1986) Congenital insensitivity to pain with anhidrosis. Neuropediatrics 17: 103–110

Itoh J, Akiguchi I, Midorikawa R et al. (1980) Sarcoid myopathy with typical rash of dermatomyositis. Neurology 30: 1118–1121

Iwashita H, Ohnishi A, Asada M et al. (1977) Polyneuropathy, skin hyperpigmentation, edema and hypertrichosis in localised osteosclerotic myeloma. Neurology 27: 657–681

Iyer G, Taari GM, Kapadia CR et al. (1973) Neurological manifestations in tropical spruce: a clinical and electro-diagnostic study. Neurology 23: 959–966

Iyer V, Fenichel GM (1976) Normal median nerve proximal latency in carpal tunnel syndrome: a clue to co-existing Martin–Gruber anastomosis. J Neurol Neurosurg Psychiatry 39: 449–452

Jabre JF (1980) Ulnar nerve lesions at the wrist: new technique for recording from the sensory dorsal branch of the ulnar nerve. Neurology 30: 873–876

Jabre JF (1981) Surface recording of the H reflex of the flexor carpi radialis. Muscle Nerve 4: 435–438

Jabre JF, Wilbourn AJ (1979) The EMG findings in 100 consecutive ulnar neuropathies. Acta Neurol Scand 60 [Suppl 73]: 91

Jackson CE, Barohn RJ (1992) Improvement of the exercise test after therapy in thyrotoxic periodic paralysis. Muscle Nerve 15: 1069–1071

Jackson CE, Strehler DA (1968) Limb-girdle muscular dystrophy. Pediatr 41: 495–502

Jacobs C, Bozian D, Heffner RR(Jr) et al. (1981) An eye movement disorder in amyotrophic lateral sclerosis. Neurology 31: 1282–1287

Jacobs PA, Hunt PA, Mayer M et al. (1981) Duchenne muscular dystrophy (DMD) in a female with an X autosome translocation: further evidence that the DMD locus is at Xp 21. Am J Hum Genet 33: 513–518

Jacobson RR, Trantman JR (1971) The treatment of leprosy with the sulphones. I. Faget's original 22 patients: a 30-year follow up on sulphone therapy for leprosy. Int J Lepr 39: 726–737

Jagganathan K (1973) Juvenile motor neuron disease. In: Spillane JD (ed) Tropical neurology. Oxford University Press, London, pp 127–130

Jakobsen J (1979) Early and preventable changes of peripheral nerve structure and function in insulin-deficient diabetic rats. J Neurol Neurosurg Psychiatry 42: 509–518

Jamal GA, Hansen S (1985) Electrophysiological studies in the post-viral fatigue syndrome. J Neurol Neurosurg Psychiatry 48: 691–694

Jamal GA, Weir AI, Hansen S et al. (1986) Myotonic dystrophy. Brain 109: 1279–1296

Jamil S, Keer JT, Lucas SB et al. (1993) Use of polymerase chain reaction to assess efficacy of leprosy chemotherapy. Lancet 342: 264–268

James NT (1973) Compensatory hypertrophy in the extensor digitorum longus muscle of the rat. J Anat 116: 57–65

Jammes Y, Ponget J, Grimand C et al. (1985) Pulmonary function and electromyographic study of respiratory muscles in myotonic dystrophy. Muscle Nerve 8: 586–594

Janiszewski DW, Caroscio JT, Wishman LH (1983) Amyotrophic lateral sclerosis: a comprehensive rehabilitation approach. Arch Phys Med Rehabil 64: 304–307

Janeway R, Kelly DC (1966) Papilloedema and hydrocephalus associated with recurrent polyneuritis. Arch Neurol 15: 507–514

Janko M, Trontelj JV, Gersak K (1989) Fasciculations in motor neuron disease: discharge rate reflects extent and recency of collateral sprouting. J Neurol Neurosurg Psychiatry 52: 1357–1381

Jankovic J, Schwartz K, Donovan DT (1990) Botulinum toxin treatment of cranio-cervical dystonia, spasmodic dysphonia and other focal dystonias and hemifacial spasms. J Neurol Neurosurg Psychiatry 53: 633–639

Jannetta PJ, Abbasy M, Maroon KC et al. (1977) Etiology and definitive microsurgical treatment of hemifacial spasm. J Neurosurg 47: 321–338

Janssen RS, Kaye AD, Lisak RP et al. (1983) Radiologic evaluation of the mediastinum in myasthenia gravis. Neurology 33: 534–539

Jansson E, Kaijser L (1977) Muscle adaption to extreme endurance training in man. Acta Physiol Scand 100: 315–324

Jaspan JB, Herold K, Maselli R et al. (1983) Treatment of severely painful diabetic neuropathy with an aldolase reductase inhibitor: relief of pain and improved somatic and autonomic function. Lancet ii: 758–762

Jaspan JB, Wallman RL, Bernstein I et al. (1982) Hypoglycaemic peripheral neuropathy in association with insulinoma. Medicine 61: 33–44

Jean WC, Dalman J, Ho A et al. (1994) Analysis of the IgG subclass distribution and inflammatory infiltrates in patients with anti-Hu associated paraneoplastic encephalomyelitis. Neurology 44: 140–147

Jebsen RH, Tenckhoff H, Honet TC (1967) Natural history of uraemic polyneuropathy and effects of dialysis. N Engl J Med 277: 327–333

Jefferson D, Eames RA (1979) Subclinical entrapment of the lateral femoral cutaneous nerve: an autopsy study. Muscle Nerve 2: 145–154

Jefferson D, Neary D, Eames RA (1981) Renaut body distribution at sites of human peripheral nerve entrapment. J Neurol Sci 49: 19–29

Jeffery S, Edwards Y, Carter N (1980) Distribution of CAIII in fetal and adult human tissue. Biochem Genet 18: 843–849

Jelenson P. Duboc D, Bloch G et al. (1991) Diagnosis of muscular glycogenoses by in vivo natual abundance ^{13}C NMR spectroscopy. Neuromusc Disord 1: 99–101

Jenkins P, Emerson PA (1981) Myopathy induced by rifampicin. Br Med J 283: 105-

Jennekens FGI, Maijer AEFH, Bethlem J et al. (1974) Fibre hybrids in type groups. J Neurol Sci 23: 337–352

Jennekens FGI, Roovd JJ, Veldman H et al. (1983) Congenital nemaline myopathy. I. Defective organisation of alpha actinin is restricted to muscle. Muscle Nerve 6: 61–68

Jennekens FGI, Tomlinson BE, Walton JN (1971) Data on the distribution of fibre types in five human limb muscles: an autopsy study. J Neurol Sci 14: 245–257

Jensen KE, Jakobsen J, Thomsen C et al. (1990) Improved energy kinetics following high protein diet in McArdle's syndrome. Acta Neurol Scand 81: 499–503

Jerusalem F, Steb SP (1992) The limb girdle syndromes. In: Vinken PJ, Bruyn GW, Klawans HL (eds) Myopathies. Elsevier, Amsterdam, pp 179–196 (Handbook of clinical neurology, vol 68.)

Jerusalem F, Engel AG, Gomez MR (1973) Sarcotubular myopathy: a newly recognised benign congenital, familial muscle disease. Neurology 23: 897–906

Jerusalem F, Rakusa M, Engel AG et al. (1974) Morphometric analysis of skeletal muscle: capillary ultrastructure in inflammatory myopathies. J Neurol Sci 23: 391–402

Jerusalem F, Spiess H, Baumgartner G (1975) Lipid storage myopathy with normal carnitine levels. J Neurol Sci 24: 273–282

Job CK (1973) Mechanisms of nerve destruction in tuberculoid borderline leprosy: an electron microscope study. J Neurol Sci 20: 25–38

Johns TR, Crowley WJ, Miller JQ et al. (1971) The syndrome of myasthenia and polymyositis with comments on therapy. Ann NY Acad Sci 183: 64–71

Johnsen T (1981) Familial periodic paralysis with hypokalaemia. Dan Med Bull 28: 1–27

Johnsen T, Beck-Nielsen H (1979) Insulin receptors, insulin secretion and glucose disappearance rate in patients with periodic hypokalaemic paralysis. Acta Endocrinol 90: 272–282

Johnson EW, Melvin JL (1971) Value of electromyography in lumbar radiculopathy. Arch Phys Med Rehabil 52: 239–243

Johnson MA, Polger J, Weightman D et al. (1973) Data on the distribution of fibre types in 36 human muscles: an autopsy study. J Neurol Sci 18: 111–129

Johnson MA, Turnbull DM, Dick DJ et al. (1983) A partial deficiency of cytochrome C oxidase in chronic progressive external ophthalmoplegia. J Neurol Sci 60: 31–53

Johnson RH, Spalding JMK (1974) Disorders of the autonomic nervous system. Blackwell Scientific Publication, Oxford

Johnson RL, Smyth CJ, Holt GW et al. (1959) Steroid therapy and vascular lesions in rheumatoid arthritis. Arthritis Rheum 2: 224–249

Johnson RT, Richardson EP (1968) The neurological manifestations of systemic lupus erythematosus. Medicine (Baltimore) 47: 333–369

Johnston CLW, Schwartz MS, Wansborough-Jones MH (1981) Acute inflammatory polyradiculoneuropathy following Type A viral hepatitis. Postgrad Med J 57: 647–648

Johnstone AP, Nussey SS (1994) Direct evidence for limited clonality of antibodies to glutamic acid decarboxylase (GAD) in stiff man syndrome using baculovirus-expressed GAD. J Neurol Neurosurg Psychiatry 57: 659

Jokelainen M (1977a) Amyotrophic lateral sclerosis in Finland. I. An epidemiologic study. Acta Neurol Scand 56: 185–193

Jokelainen M (1977b) Amyotrophic lateral sclerosis in Finland. II. Clinical characteristics. Acta Neurol Scand 56: 194–204

Joliffe DS (1977) Leprosy reactional states and their treatment. Br J Dermatol 97: 345–352

Jolly F (1895) Über myasthenia gravis pseudoparalytica. Klin Wochenschr 32: 1–7

Jones CT, Swingler RJ, Simpson SA et al. (1995) Superoxide dysmutase mutations in an unselected cohort of Scottish amyotrophic lateral sclerosis. J Med Genet 32: 290–292

Jones GE, Witkowski JA (1983) Membrane abnormalities in Duchenne muscular dystrophy. J Neurol Sci 58: 159–174

Jones HE (1947) Sex differences in physical abilities. Hum Biol 19: 12–19

Jones SJ (1979) Investigation of brachial plexus traction lesions by peripheral and spinal sensory evoked potentials. J Neurol Neurosurg Psychiatry 42: 107–116

Jones SJ, Wynn Parry CB, Landi A (1981) Diagnosis of brachial plexus traction lesions by sensory nerve action potentials and somatosensory evoked potentials. Injury 12: 376–382

Jopling WH, Morgan-Hughes JA (1965) Pure neural tuberculoid leprosy. Br Med J ii: 788–790

Josselson J, Pula T, Sadler JH (1980) Acute rhabdomyolysis associated with an Echo virus infection. Arch Intern Med 140: 1671–1672

Joy JL, Oh SH, Baysal AI (1990) Electrophysiological spectrum of inclusion body myositis. Muscle Nerve 13: 949–951

Juergens SM, Kurland LT, Okazata H et al. (1980) ALS in Rochester Minnesota 1925–1977. Neurology 30: 463–470

Julien J, Vital CL, Aupy G et al. (1980) Guillain–Barré syndrome and Hodgkin's disease – ultrastructural study of a peripheral nerve. J Neurol Sci 45: 23–27

Julien J, Vital CL, Vallat JM et al. (1974) Oculo-pharyngeal muscular dystrophy: a case with abnormal mitochondria and finger print inclusions. J Neurol Sci 21: 165–169

Kadrie HA, Yates SK, Milner-Brown HS et al. (1976) Multiple point electrical stimulation of ulnar and median nerves. J Neurol Neurosurg Psychiatry 39: 973–985

Kaeser HE (1965) Scapulo-peroneal muscular atrophy. Brain 88: 407–418

Kaeser HE (1970) Nerve conduction velocity measurements. In: Vinken PJ, Bruyn G (eds) Handbook of clinical neurology, vol 7. Elsevier, Amsterdam, pp 116–196

Kaeser HE (1984a) Drug-induced myasthenic syndromes. Acta Neurol Scand 70 [Suppl 100]: 39–47

Kaeser HE (1984b) Transient global amnesia due to clioquinol Acta Neurol Scand 70 [Suppl 100]: 175–179

Kagen LJ (1977) Myoglobinuria in inflammatory myopathies. JAMA 237: 1448–1452

Kagen LJ (1984) Dermatomyositis and polymyositis. Clin Exp Rheumatol 2: 271–277

Kahlke W, Richterich R (1965) Refsum's disease (heredopathia atactica polyneuritiformis). An inborn error of lipid metabolism with storage of 3,7,11,15-tetramethylhexadecanoic acid. II. Isolation and identification of a storage product. Am J Med 39: 237–241

Kaji R, Nobuyuki O, Tsuji I et al. (1993) Pathological findings at the site of condution block in multifocal motor neuropathy. Ann Neurol 33: 152–158

Kaji R, Shibasaki H, Kimura J (1992) Multifocal demyelinating motor neuropathy. Neurology 42: 506–509

Kakulas BA, Mastaglia FL (1992) Drug-induced toxic and nutritional myopathies. In: Mastaglia FL, Lord Walton (eds) Skeletal muscle pathology. Churchill Livingstone, Edinburgh, pp 511–540

Kalow W, Britt BA, Terreau ME et al. (1970) Metabolic error of muscle metabolism after recovery from malignant hyperpyrexia. Lancet ii: 895–898

Kaltreider HB, Talal N (1969) The neuropathy of Sjogren's syndrome. Ann Intern Med 70: 751–762

Kamakura K, Kawai M, Arahata K et al. (1990) A manifesting carrier of Duchenne muscular dystrophy with severe myocardial symptoms. J Neurol 237: 483–485

Kamieniecka Z (1977) Myopathies with abnormal mitochondria: a clinical, histological and electrophysiological study. Acta Neurol Scand 55: 57–75

Kamieniecka Z, Schmalbruch H (1978) Myopathies with abnormal mitochondria. Muscle Nerve 1: 413–415

Kamoshita S, Konishi Y, Sagawa M et al. (1976) Congenital muscular dystrophy as a disease of the central nervous system. Arch Neurol 33: 513–516

Kankeleit H (1916) Über primäre nicht eiterige Polymyositis Deutsch. Arch Klin Med 120: 335–349

Kannot, Sudo K, Takeuchi I et al. (1980) Hereditary deficiency of lactate dehydrogenase M subunit. Clin Chim Acta 108: 267–276

Kao I, Drachman DB, Price DL (1976) Botulinum toxin: mechanism of presynaptic blockade. Science 193: 1256–1258

Kaldor J, Speed BR (1984) GBS and *Campylobacter jejuni*: a serological study. Br Med J 288: 1867–1870

Kaplan JG, Rosenberg R, Reinitz E et al. (1990) Peripheral neuropathy in Sjogren's syndrome. Muscle Nerve 13: 570–579

Kaplan PE (1984) Posterior interosseous neuropathies: natural history. Arch Phys Med Rehabil 65: 399–400

Kaplan PE, Kernohan WT (1981) Tarsal tunnel syndrome: an electrodiagnostic and surgical correlation. J Bone Joint Surg [Am] 63: 96–99

Kaplan SJ, Glickel SZ, Eaton RG (1990) Predictor factors in the non-surgical treatment of carpal tunnel syndrome. J Hand Surg 15 106–108

Karch S, Urich H (1975) Infantile polyneuropathy with defective myelination: an autopsy study. Dev Med Child Neurol 17: 504–511

Karli P, Bergstrom L (1974) Effect of baclofen on myotonia. Lancet i: 1285–1286

Karlsberg RP, Roberts R (1978) Effect of altered thyroid function on plasma creatine kinase clearance in the dog. Am J Physiol 235: E614–618

Karnegay JN, Tuler SM, Miller DM et al. (1988) Muscular dystrophy in a litter of golden retriever dogs. Muscle Nerve 11: 1056–1064

Karno T, Sudo K, Takeuchi I et al. (1980) Hereditary deficiency of lactate dehydrogenase M subunit. Clin Chim Acta 108: 267–276

Karpawich PP, Hart ZH, Perry BL et al. (1987) Childhood periodic paralysis with dysrhythmias. Am Heart J 114: 186–187

Karpati G, Carpenter C (1992) Skeletal muscle pathology in neuromuscular diseases. In: Rowland LP, Di Mauro S (eds) Myopathies. Elsevier, Amsterdam, pp 1–48 (Handbook of clinical neurology, vol 62.)

Karpati G, Engel WK (1968) "Type grouping" in skeletal muscles after experimental reinnervation. Neurology 18: 447–451

Karpati G, Carpenter S, Andermann F (1971) A new concept of childhood nemaline myopathy. Arch Neurol 24: 291–304

Karpati G, Carpenter S, Engel AG et al. (1975) The syndrome of systemic carnitine deficiency: clinical, morphological, biochemical and pathophysiologic features. Neurology 25: 16–24

Karpati G, Carpenter S, Morris GE et al. (1993) Localisation and quantitation of the chromosome 6-encoded dystrophin-related protein in normal and pathological human muscle. J Neuropathol Exp Neurol 52: 119–128

Karpati G, Carpenter S, Watters GV et al. (1973) Infantile myotonic dystrophy. Neurology 23: 1066–1077

Karttinen A, Härttel G, Lauhija A (1970) Multiple serum enzyme analyses in chronic alcoholics. Acta Med Scand 188: 257–264

Kasai K (1979) Serum myoglobin level in altered thyroid states. J Clin Endocrinol Metab 48: 1–4

Kasperek S, Zebrowski S (1971) Stiff man syndrome and encephalomyelitis. Arch Neurol 24: 22–31

Katirji MB, Wilbourn AJ (1988) Common peroneal mononeuropathy: a clinical and electrophysiologic study of 116 lesions. Neurology 38: 1723–1728

Katrak SM, Pollack M, O'Brien GP et al. (1980) Clinical and morphological features of gold neuropathy. Brain 103: 671–693

Katz AL, Pate D (1980) Floppy head syndrome. Arthritis Rheum 23: 131–132

Katz B, Miledi R (1964) The development of acetylcholine sensitivity in nerve-free segments of skeletal muscle. J Physiol (Lond) 170: 389–396

Katz JS, Wolfe GI, Burns DK (1996) Isolated weak extensor myopathy: a common cause of dropped head syndrome. Neurology 46: 917–921

Kaufman L (1960) Anaesthesia in dystrophia myotonica. Proc R Soc Med 53: 183–188

Kaufman LD, Gruber BL, Gregersen PK (1991) Clinical follow-up and immunogenetic studies of 32 patients with eosinophilia-myalgia syndrome. Lancet 337: 1071–1074

Kausch K. Lehmann-Horn F, Janka M et al. (1991) Evidence for linkage of the central core disease locus to the proximal long arm of human chromosome 19. Genomics 10: 765–769

Kausch K, Miller CR, Grimm T et al. (1991) No evidence for linkage of autosomal dominant proximal spinal muscular atrophies to chromosome 5q markers. Hum Genet 86: 317–318

Kawamura Y, Dyck PJ, Shimono M et al. (1981) Morphometric comparison of the vulnerability of peripheral motor and sensory neurons in amyotrophic lateral sclerosis. J Neuropathol Exp Neurol 40: 667–675

Kawamura Y, O'Brien PC, Okazaki H et al. (1977) Lumbar motoneurons of man. II. The number and diameter distribution of large and intermediate diameter cytons in "motor neuron columns" of spinal cord of man. J Neuropathol Exp Neurol 36: 861–870

Kay R, Chan YW, Schwartz MS (1994) The wasted leg syndrome. Neuromusc Disord 4: 521–525

Kearns TP, Sayre GP (1958) Retinitis pigmentosa, external ophthalmoplegia and complete heart block: an unusual syndrome with histologic study in one of two cases. Arch Ophthalmol 60: 280–289

Kellam AMP (1987) The neuroleptic malignant syndrome, so called: a survey of the world literature. Br J Psychiatry 150: 752–759

Kellerman J, Hedlund W, Orlin JB et al. (1983) Plasmapheresis with immunosuppression in amyotrophic lateral sclerosis. Arch Neurol 40: 752–753

Kelly JJ Jr (1983) The electrodiagnostic findings in peripheral neuropathies associated with monoclonal gammopathies. Muscle Nerve 6: 504–509

Kelly JJ Jr (1985) Peripheral neuropathies associated with monoclonal proteins: a clinical review. Muscle Nerve 8: 138–150

Kelly JJ Jr, Adelman LS, Barkman E (1988) Polyneuropathies associated with IgM monoclonal gammopathies. Arch Neurol 45: 1355–1359

Kelly JJ Jr, Kyle RA, Miles JM et al. (1981a) The spectrum of peripheral neuropathy in myeloma. Neurology 31: 24–31

Kelly JJ Jr, Kyle RA, Miles JM et al. (1983) Osteosclerotic myeloma and peripheral neuropathy. Neurology 33: 202–210

Kelly JJ Jr, Kyle RA, O'Brien PC et al. (1979) The natural history of peripheral neuropathy in primary systemic amyloidosis. Ann Neurol 6: 1–7

Kelly JJ Jr, Kyle RA, O'Brien PC et al. (1981b) The prevalence of monoclonal gammopathy in peripheral neuropathy. Neurology 31: 1480–1483

Kemble F (1968) Electrodiagnosis of the carpal tunnel syndrome. J Neurol Neurosurg Psychiatry 31: 23–27

Kendall D (1960) Aetiology, diagnosis and treatment of paraesthesia in the hand. Br Med J ii: 1633–1640

Kennard C, Newland AC, Ridley A (1982) Treatment of Guillain-Barré syndrome by plasma exchange. J Neurol Neurosurg Psychiatry 42: 847–850

Kennard C, Swash M, Henson RA (1980) EACA myapathy: a toxic effect of epislon aminocaproic acid. Muscle Nerve 3: 202–206

Kennedy PGE (1987) Neurological complications of Varicella zoster virus. In Kennedy PG, Johnson RT (eds) Infections of the nervous system. Butterworth, London, pp 177–208

Kennedy WR, Alter M, Song JH (1968) Progressive proximal spinal and bulbar muscular atrophy of late onset: a sex-linked recessive trait. Neurology 18: 677–680

Kennedy WR, Navarro X, Goetz FC et al. (1990) The effect of pancreatic transplantation on diabetic neuropathy. N Engl J Med 322: 1031–1037

Kennett RP, Fawcett PRW (1993) Repetitive nerve stimulation of anconeus in the assessment of neuromuscular transmission disorders. Electroenceph Clin Neurophysiol 89: 170–176

Kennett RP, Harding AE (1986) Peripheral neuropathy associated with the sicca syndrome. J Neurol Neurosurg Psychiatry 49: 90–92

Kessler HA, Trenholme GM, Harris AA et al. (1980) Acute myopathy associated with Influenza A/Texas/1/77 infection. JAMA 243: 461–462

Khaledi AA, Griffith DG, Edwards RHT (1983) The clinical presentation of hypothyroid myopathy and its relationship to abnormalities in structure and function of skeletal muscle. Clin Endocrinol 19: 365–376

Khurana TS, Watkins SG, Chafey P et al. (1991) Immunolocalisation and developmental expression of dystrophin-related protein in skeletal muscle. Neuromusc Disord 1: 185–194

Kiers L, Altermatt HJ, Lennon VA (1991) Paraneoplastic antineuronal nuclear IgG and autoantibodies (Type 1) localise antigen in small cell lung carcinoma. Mayo Clin Proc 66: 1209–1216

Kiessling WR, Ricker K, Pflughaupt KW et al. (1981) Serum myoglobin in primary and secondary skeletal muscle disorders. J Neurol 224: 229–233

Killian JM, Wilfong AA, Burnett L et al. (1994) Decremental motor responses to repetitive nerve stimulation in ALS. Muscle Nerve 17: 747–754

Kiloh LG, Nevin S (1952) Progressive dystrophy of the external ocular muscles (ocular myopathy). Brain 74: 115–143

Kim RC, Collins GH (1980) The neuropathology of rheumatoid disease. Hum Pathol 12: 5–15

Kimura J (1974) F wave velocity in the central segment of the median and ulnar nerves: a study in normal subjects and patients with Charcot-Marie-Tooth disease. Neurology 24: 539–546

Kimura J (1978) Proximal versus distal slowing of motor nerve conduction velocity in the Guillain-Barré syndrome. Ann Neurol 3: 344–350

Kimura J (1979) The carpal tunnel syndrome: localisation of conduction abnormalities within the distal segment of the median nerve. Brain 102: 619–635

Kimura J (1984) Principles and pitfalls of nerve conduction studies. Ann Neurol 16: 415–429

Kimura J (1989) Electrodiagnosis in diseases of nerve and muscle: principles and practice, 2nd edn. Davis, Philadelphia

Kimura J (1993) Consequences of peripheral nerve demyelination: basic and clinical aspects. Can J Neurol Sci 20: 263–270

Kimura J, Giron LT, Young JM (1976) Electrophysiological study of Bell's palsy – electrically elicited blink reflex in asessment of prognosis. Arch Otolaryngol 102: 140–143

Kimura J, Rodnitzky RL, Okawara S (1975) Electrophysiologic analysis of aberrant regeneration after facial nerve paralysis. Neurology 25: 898–993

Kimura J, Sakimura Y, Machida M et al. (1988) Effects of desynchronised inputs on compound sensory and muscle action potentials. Muscle Nerve 11: 694–702

King AB (1950) Neurologic conditions occurring as complications of pregnancy. Arch Neurol Psychiatry 63: 611–614

King JO, Denborough MA (1973) Malignant hyperpyrexia in Australia and New Zealand. Med J Aust 1: 525–528

Kinoshita M, Satayoshi E, Kumagai M (1975) Familial Type 1 fibre atrophy. J Neurol Sci 25: 11–17

Kiprov DB, Miller RG (1984) Polymyositis associated with monoclonal gammopathy. Lancet ii: 1183–1186

Kissel JJ, Mendell JR (1996) Neuropathies associated with monoclonal gammopathies Neuromusc. Disord. 6: 3–18

Kissel JT, Beam W, Bresolin N et al. (1985) Physiologic assessment of phosphoglycerate mutase deficiency. Neurology 35: 828–833

Kissel JT, Holterman RK, Rammohan KW et al. (1991) The relationship of complement-mediated microvasculopathy to the histologic features and clinical duration of disease in dermatomyositis. Arch Neurol 48: 26–30

Kissel JT, Lynn DJ, Rammohan KW et al. (1993) Mononuclear cell analysis of muscle biopsies in prednisone and azathioprine-treated Duchenne muscular dystrophy. Neurology 43: 532–536

Kissel JT, Mendell JR, Rammohan KW (1986) Microvascular deposition of complement membrane attack complex in dermatomyositis. N Engl J Med 314: 329–334

Kissel P, Schmitt J, Duc M et al. (1970) Myasthenia and thyrotoxicosis. In: Walton JN, Canal N, Scarlato G (eds) Muscle diseases. Excerpta Medica, Amsterdam, pp 464–481 (ICS 199)

Kissel JT, Slivka AP, Wormolts JR et al. (1985) The clinical spectrum of necrotizing angiopathy of the peripheral nervous system. Ann Neurol 18: 251–257

Kite JH (1966) Morton's toe neuroma. South Med J 59: 20–25

Kjeldsen K, Braengdgaard H, Sidenius P et al. (1987) Diabetes decreases Na/K pump concentration in skeletal muscles, heart ventricular muscle and peripheral nerves of rat. Diabetes 36: 842–848

Kjeldsen K, Gøtzsche CO, Nørgaard A et al. (1984) Effect of thyroid function on number of Na-K pumps in human skeletal muscle. Lancet ii: 8–10

Kjellin KG, Stibler H (1976) Isoelectric focussing and electrophoresis of cerebrospinal fluid protein in muscular dystrophies and spinal muscular atrophies. J Neurol Sci 27: 45–57

Klein D (1958) La dystrophie myotonique (Steinert) et la. myotonie congénitale (Thomsen) en Suisse. J Genet Hum 7 [Suppl]: 1–328

Klein I, Mantell P, Parker M et al. (1980) Resolution of abnormal muscle enzyme studies in hypothyroidism. Am J Med Sci 279: 159–162

Kline DG, De Jonge BR (1968) Evoked potentials to evaluate peripheral nerve injury. Surg Gynecol Obstet 127: 1239–1248

Klinkerfuss GH (1967) An electron microscopic study of myotonic dystrophy. Arch Neurol 16: 181–193

Klinkerfuss G, Bleisch V, Dioso MM et al. (1967) A spectrum of myopathy associated with alcoholism. II. Light and electron microscopic observations. Ann Intern Med 67: 493–510

Knill-Jones RP, Goodwill CJ, Dayan AD et al. (1972) Peripheral neuropathy in chronic liver disease: clinical, electrodiagnostic and nerve biopsy findings. J Neurol Neurosurg Psychiatry 35: 22–30

Knochel JP (1982) Rhabdomyolysis and myoglobinuria. Ann Rev Med 33: 435–443

Knuttson B (1961) Comparative value of electromyographic, myelographic and clinical neurological examination in diagnosis of lumbar root compression syndrome. Acta Orthop Scand [Suppl 49]: 1–135

Kobayashi S, Tanaka M, Tamura N et al. (1992) Serum cardiac troponin T in polymyositis/dermatomyositis. Lancet 340: 726

Kocen RS, Thomas PK (1970) Peripheral nerve involvement in Fabry's disease. Arch Neurol 22: 81–88

Kocen RS, King RHM, Thomas PK et al. (1973) Nerve biopsy findings in two cases of Tangier disease. Acta Neuropathol (Berl) 26: 317–327

Koch MC, Grimm T, Harley GH et al. (1991) Genetic risks for children of women with myotonic dystrophy. Am J Genet 48: 1084–1091

Koenig M, Beggs AH, Moyer H et al. (1989) The molecular basis for Duchenne versus Becker muscular dystrophy: correlation of severity with type of deletion. Am J Hum Genet 45: 498–506

Koenig M, Hoffman EP, Bertelson CJ et al. (1987) Complete cloning of the Duchenne muscular dystrophy (DMD) cDNA and preliminary genomic organisation of the DMD gene in normal and affected individuals. Cell 50: 509–517

Kolb ME, Horne ML, Mortz R (1982) Dantrolene in human malignant hyperthemia: a multicenter study. Anesthesiology 56: 254–262

Kolb WP, Haxby JA, Arroyare CM et al. (1972) Molecular analysis of the membrane attack mechanism of complement. J Exp Med 135: 549–566

Kolodny EH (1993) Metachromatic leucodystrophy and multiple sulphatase deficiency: sulphatide lipidosis. In: Rosenberg RN, Pruisner SB, Di Mauro S, Barchi RL, Kunkel LM (eds) The molecular and genetic basis of neurological disease, Butterworth, Boston

Kolodny RC, Kahn CB, Goldstein HH et al. (1974) Sexual function in diabetic man. Diabetes 23: 396–309

Komar J, Varga B (1975) Syndrome of the rectus abdominis muscle. J Neurol 210: 121–125

Komi PV, Viitasalo JHT, Havu M et al. (1977) Skeletal muscle fibres and muscle enzyme activities in monozygous and dizygous twins of both sexes,. Acta Physiol Scand 100: 385–392

Kondo K (1978) Motor neuron disease: changing population patterns and clues for etiology. In: Schoenberg BS (ed) Neurological epidemiology: principles and clinical applications. Raven Press, New York, pp 509–543 (Advances in neurology 19)

Kondo K, Horikawa Y (1974) Genetic heterogeneity of hereditary sensory neuropathy. Arch Neurol 30: 336–337

Kondo K, Yussa T (1980) Genetics of congenital nemaline myopathy. Muscle Nerve 3: 308–315

Konotey-Ahulu FID, Baillod R, Comty CM et al. (1965) Effect of periodic dialysis on the peripheral neuropathy of end-stage renal failure. Br Med J ii: 1212–1215

Koo B, Becker LE, Chang S et al. (1993) Mitochondrial encephalomyopathy, lactic acidosis, stroke-like episode (MELAS). Ann Neurol 34: 25–32

Kopec J, Hausmanowa-Petrusewicz I (1976) On-line computer application in clinical quantitative electromyography. Electromyogr Clin Neurophysiol 16: 49–64

Kopec J, Hausmanowa-Petrusewicz I (1983) Computer Analyse des EMG und klinische Ergebnisse. Z EEG-EMG 1: 28–35

Korczyn AD (1971) Bell's palsy and diabetes mellitus. Lancet i: 108–109

Kori SH, Fuley KM, Posner JB (1981) Brachial plexus lesions in patients with cancer: 100 cases. Neurology 31: 45–50

Kornberg AJ, Pestronk A, Bieser K et al. (1994) The clinical correlates of high titer IgG anti GM$_1$ antibodies. Ann Neurol 35: 234–237

Kornfeld P, Nail J, Smith H et al. (1981) Acetylcholine receptor antibodies in myasthenia gravis. Muscle Nerve 4: 413–419

Korobkin R, Asbury AK, Sumner AJ et al. (1975) Glue sniffing neuropathy. Arch Neurol 32: 158–162

Korsan-Bengsten K, Ysander L, Blohme G et al. (1969) Extensive muscle necrosis after long-term treatment with *epsilon* aminocaproic acid (EACA) in a case of hereditary periodic oedema. Acta Med Scand 185: 341–346

Koski CL (1990) Characterisation of complement fixing antibodies to peripheral nerve myelin in Guillain-Barré syndrome. Ann Neurol 27: 544–547

Koski CL, Gratz E, Sutherland J et al. (1986) Clinical correlation with anti-peripheral nerve myelin antibodies in Guillain-Barré syndrome. Ann Neurol 19: 573–577

Koustros A (1982) Myositis with Kawasaki's disease. Am J Dis Child 136: 78–79

Kraft GH (1990) Fibrillation potential amplitude and muscle atrophy following peripheral nerve injury. Muscle Nerve 13: 814–821

Kramer LD, Ruth RA, Johns ME et al. (1981) A comparison of stapedial reflex fatigue with repetitive stimulation and single-fibre EMG in myasthenia gravis. Ann Neurol 9: 531–536

Krarup C, Stewart JD, Sumner AJ et al. (1990) A syndrome of asymmetric limb weakness with motor conduction block. Neurology 40: 118–127

Krause KH, Witt T, Ross A (1977) The anterior tarsal tunnel syndrome. J Neurol 217: 67–74

Krendel DA, Sanders DB, Massey JM (1987) Single fiber electromyography in chronic progressive external ophthalmoplegia. Muscle Nerve 10: 299–320

Kristensson K, Ollson Y, Sourander P (1967) Peripheral nerve change in Tay-Sachs' and Batten-Spielmeyer-Vogt disease. Acta Pathol Microbiol Scand 70: 630–632

Kristoferitsch W, Sluga E, Graf M et al. (1988) Neuropathy associated with acrodermatitis chronica atrophicans. Ann NY Acad Sci 539: 35–45

Krivit W, Shapiro E, Kennedy W et al. (1990) Treatment of late infantile metachromatic leucodystrophy by bone marrow transplantation. N Engl J Med 372: 28–32

Krivit W, Shapiro E, Lockman L et al. (1992) see Kolodny (1993)

Krolick KA, Thompson PA, Zoda TE et al. (1993) Influence of immunological fine specificity on the induction of experimental myasthenia gravis. Ann NY Acad Sci 681: 179–197

Krugliak I, Gathoth N, Behar AJ (1978) Neuropathic form of arthrogryposis multiplex congenita: report of 3 cases with complete necropsy including the first reported case of agenesis of muscle spindles. J Neurol Sci 37: 179–185

Kruse R, Scheunemann W, Baier W et al. (1982) Hypocalcaemic myopathy in idiopathic hypoprathyroidism. Eur J Pediatr 138: 280–282

Ku DY, Yen CK, Li CC (1943) Acute poisoning by common salt containing barium chloride. Chin Med J 51: 303–304

Kucera J, Dorovini-Zis K (1979) Types of human intrafusal muscle fibers. Muscle Nerve 2: 437–451

Kugelberg E (1949) Electromyography in muscular dystrophies: differentiation between dystrophies and chronic lower motor neuron lesions. J Neurol Neurosurg Psychiatry 12: 19–136

Kugelberg E, Edstrom L (1968) Differential histochemical effects of muscle contractions on phosphorylase and glycogen in various types of fibres: relation to fatigue. J Neurol Neurosurg Psychiatry 31: 415–423

Kugelberg E, Petersen I (1949) Insertion activity in electromyography. J Neurol Neurosurg Psychiatry 12: 268–273

Kugelberg E, Welander L (1956) Heredo-familial juvenile muscular atrophy simulating muscular dystrophy. Arch Neurol Psychiatry 75: 500–509

Kuhn E, Fiehn W. Seiler D et al. (1979) The autosomal recessive (Becker) form of myotonia congenita. Muscle Nerve 2: 109–117

Kuncl RW, Pestronk A, Drachman DB et al. (1986) The pathophysiology of penicillamine-induced myasthenia gravis. Ann Neurol 20: 740–744

Kunkel LM, Beggs AH, Hoffman EP (1989) Molecular genetics of Duchenne and Becker muscular dystrophy. Clin Chem 35: 21–24

Kurdi A, Abdul-Kader M (1979) Clinical and electrophysiological studies of diphtheritic neuritis in Jordan. J Neurol Sci 42: 243–250

Kuribayashi T, Kurihara T, Tanaka M et al. (1982) Diabetic neuropathy and electrophysiological studies: evoked potentials, nerve conduction and short-latency SEP. In: Goto Y,

Huriuchi A, Kogure K (eds) Diabetic neuropathy. Excerpta Medica, Amsterdam, p 120

Kurland LT, Faro SN, Sielder H (1960) Minamata disease. World Neurol 1: 370

Kurland LT, Radhakrishnan K, Williams DB et al. (1994) Amyotrophic lateral sclerosis–Parkinson-Dementia complex on Guam: epidemiologic and aetiological perspectives. In: Williams AC (ed) Motor neuron disease. Chapman and Hall, London, pp 109–130

Kurtonen P, Rapola J, Noponen AL et al. (1972) Nemaline myopathy: report of four cases and review of the literature. Acta Paed Scand 61: 353–361

Kurtzke JF (1982) Motor neuron disease. Br Med J 284: 141–142

Kurtzke JF (1985) Neurological system. In: Holland WW, Detels R, Knox G (eds) Oxford textbook of public health, vol 4. Oxford University Press, Oxford, pp 203–249

Kusumi RK, Plouffe JE, Wyatt RH et al. (1980) Central nervous system toxicity associated with metronidazole therapy. Ann Intern Med 93: 59–60

Kuzuhara S, Kanazawa I, Nakanishi T et al. (1983) Ethylene oxide polyneuropathy. Neurology 33: 377–380

Kwaan JHM, Rapopart I (1970) Postoperative brachial plexus palsy: a study on the mechanism. Arch Surg 101: 612–615

Kyle RA, Bayard ED (1975) Amyloidosis: review of 236 cases. Medicine (Baltimore) 54: 271–299

Kyle RA, Dyck PJ (1992) Amyloidosis and neuropathy. In: Dyck PJ, Thomas PK (eds) Peripheral Neuropathy, 3rd edn. Saunders, Philadelphia, pp 1294–1309

Kyle RA, Dyck PJ (1993) Neuropathy associated with monoclonal gammopathies. In: Dyck PJ, Thomas PK (eds) Peripheral Neuropathy, 3rd edn. Saunders, Philadelphia, pp 1275–1287

Kyle RA, Greipp PR (1983) Amyloidosis (AL): clinical and laboratory features in 229 cases Mayo Clin Proc 58: 665–683

Kyle RA, Finkelstein S, Elvebach LR et al. (1972) Incidence of monoclonal proteins in a Minnesota community with a cluster of multiple myeloma. Blood 40: 719–724

Lachman T, Shahani BT, Young RR (1980) Late responses as aids to diagnosis in peripheral neuropathy. J Neurol Neurosurg Psychiatry 43: 156–162

Lacomblez L, Bensiman G, Leigh PN et al. (1996) Dose-ranging study of rilazole in amyotrophic lateral sclerosis. Lancet 347: 1425–1431

Lafontaine S, Rasminsky M, Saida T et al. (1982) Conduction block in rat myelinated fibres following acute exposure to anti-galactocerebroside serum. J Physiol (Lond) 323: 287–306

Lagier R, Cox JN (1975) Pseudomalignant myositis ossificans. Hum Pathol 6: 653–665

Lagueny A, Deliac MM, Deliac P et al. (1991) Diagnostic and prognostic value of electrophysiological tests in meralgia paresthetica. Muscle Nerve 14: 51–56

Laing N, Majda B, Akkari P et al. (1992) Assignment of a gene (NEM-1) for autosomal dominant nemaline myopathy to chromosome 1. Am J Hum Genet 50: 576–583

Lake BD, Wilson J (1975) Zebra body myopathy: clinical, histochemical and ultrastructural studies. J Neurol Sci 24: 437–446

Lakhanpal S, Bunch TW, Ilstrup DM et al. (1986) Polymyositis-dermatomyositis and malignant lesions: does an association exist? Mayo Clin Proc 61: 645–653

Lambert CD, Fairfax AJ (1977) Skeletal muscle pathology in chronic heart block. J Clin Pathol 30: 467–472

Lambert EH (1962) Diagnostic value of electrical stimulation of motor nerves. Electroencephalogr Clin Neurophysiol 22: 9–16

Lambert EH (1966) Defects of neuromuscular transmission in syndromes other than myasthenia gravis. Ann NY Acad Sci 135: 367–386

Lambert EH, Dyck PJ (1975) Compound action potentials of sural nerve in vitro in peripheral neuropathy. In: Dyck PJ, Thomas

PK, Lambert EH (eds) Peripheral neuropathy. Saunders, Philadelphia, pp 427–441

Lambert EH, Elmqvist D (1971) Quantal components of endplate potentials in myasthenic syndrome. Ann NY Acad Sci 183: 183–199

Lambert EH, Mulder DW (1964) Nerve function studies in experimental polyneuritis. Electroencephalogr Clin Neurophysiol 22: 29–35

Lambert EH, Rooke GD (1965) Myasthenic state and lung cancer. In: Lord Brain, Norris FH (eds) Remote effects of cancer on the nervous system. Grune and Stratton, New York, pp 67–80

Lambert EH, Eaton LM, Rooke ED (1956) Defect of neuromuscular transmission associated with malignant neoplasm. Am J Physiol 187: 612–613

Lambert EH, Sayre GP, Eaton LM (1954) Electrical activity of muscle in polymyositis. Trans Am Neurol Assoc 79: 64–69

Lambert EH, Underdahl CD Beckett S et al. (1951) A study of the ankle jerk in myxoedema. J Clin Endocrinol Metab 11: 186–1205

Lance JW, Burke D, Pollard J (1979) Hyperexcitability of motor and sensory neurons in myotonia. Ann Neurol 5: 523–532

Landau WM (1952) The essential mechanism in myotonia: An electromyographic study. Neurology 2: 369–388

Landay AL, Jessop C, Lennette ET et al. (1991) Chronic fatigue syndrome: clinical condition associated with immune activation. Lancet 338: 707–715

Landi G, D'Alessandro R, Dassi BC et al. (1993) Guillain–Barré syndrome after exogenous gangliosides in Italy. Br Med J 307: 1463–1464

Landon DN (1985) Structure and function of nerve fibres. In: Swash M, Kennard C (eds) Scientific basis of clinical neurology. Churchill Livingstone, Edinburgh, pp 375–389

Landouzy L, Déjerine J (1885) De la myopathie atrophique progressive: myopathie sans neuropathie, débutante d' ordinaire dans l'enfance, par la face. Rev Méd (Paris) 5: 81–117, 253–366

Landrieu P, Sard G, Allaire C (1990) Dominantly transmitted congenital indifference to pain. Ann Neurol 27: 574–578

Landry O (1859) Note sur la paralysie ascendante aiguë. Gazette Hebdomadaire Med Chir 6: 472–474

Lane RJM, Mastaglia FL (1978) Drug-induced myopathies in man. Lancet ii: 562–566

Lane RJM, Radoff FM (1981) Alcohol and serum creatine kinase levels. Ann Neurol 10: 581–582

Lane RJM, Bandopadhyay R, de Belleroche J (1993) Abnormal glycine metabolism in motor neuron disease. J R Soc Med 86: 501–505

Lane RJM, Emslie-Smith A, Mosquera IE et al. (1989) Clinical, biochemical and histological responses to treatment in polymyositis: a prospective study. J R Soc Med 82: 333–338

Lane RJM, Gardiner-Medwin D, Roses AD (1980) Electrocardiographic abnormalities in carriers of Duchenne muscular dystrophy. Neurology 30: 499–501

Lane RJM, McLelland NJ, Martin AM et al. (1979) Epsilon amino caproic acid (EACA) myopathy. Postgrad Med J 55: 282–285

Lang AH, Falck B (1980) A two channel method for sampling, averaging and quantifying motor unit potentials. J Neurol 223: 199–206

Lang AH, Portanen VSG (1976) Satellite potentials and the duration of motor unit potentials in normal, neuropathic and myopathic muscles. J Neurol Sci 27: 513–524

Lang AH, Forström SF, Björkqvist SE et al. (1977) Statistical variation of nerve conduction velocity: an analysis in normal subjects and uraemic patients. J Neurol Sci 33: 229–241

Lang AH, Prusa A, Hynninen P et al. (1985) Evolution of nerve conduction velocity in later childhood and adolescence. Muscle Nerve 8: 38–43

Lang B, Johnston I, Leys R et al. (1993) Autoantibody specificities in Lambert-Eaton myasthenic syndrome. Ann NY Acad Sci 681: 382–393

Lang BA, Laxer RM, Murphy G et al. (1991) Treatment of dermatomyositis with intravenous immunoglobulin. Am J Med 91: 169–171

Lang B, Molenaar PL, Newsom-Davis J et al. (1984) Passive transfer of Lambert–Eaton myasthenic syndrome in mice: decreased rates of resting and evoked release of acetylcholine from skeletal muscle. J Neurochem 42: 658–662

Lang B, Newsom-Davis J, Wray D et al. (1981) Autoimmune aetiology for myasthenic (Eaton–Lambert) syndrome. Lancet ii: 224–226

Lange DJ, Trojaborg W (1994) Do GM$_1$ antibodies induce demyelination? Muscle Nerve 17: 105–107

Langmuir AD, Bregman DJ, Kurland LT et al. (1984) An epidemiologic and clinical evaluation of Guillain–Barré syndrome reported in association with the administration of swine influenza vaccines. Am J Epidemiol 119: 842–879

Lango FM (1994) Will ciliary neurotrophic factor slow progression of motor neuron disease? Ann Neurol 36: 125–126

Lapresle J, Salisachs P (1973) Onion bulbs in a nerve biopsy specimen from an original case of Roussy–Levy disease. Arch Neurol 29: 346–348

Larach MG (1989) Standardisation of the caffeine/halothane muscle contracture test. Anesth Analg 59: 511–515

Larsson L-E (1975) On the relation between the EMG frequency spectrum and the duration of symptoms in lesions of the peripheral motor neuron. Electroencephalogr Clin Neurophysiol 38: 69–78

Larsson L-E (1978) Morphological and functional characteristics of aging skeletal muscle in man: a cross-sectional study. Acta Physiol Scand [Suppl 457]: 1–36

Larsson L-E (1982) Physical training effects on muscle morphology in sedentary males at different ages. Med Sci Sports Exercise 14: 203–206

Larsson L-E, Ansved T (1985) Effects of long-term physical training and detraining on enzyme histochemical and functional skeletal muscle characteristics in man. Muscle Nerve 8: 714–722

Larsson L-E, Sjodin B, Karlsson J (1978) Histochemical and biochemical changes in human skeletal muscle with age in sedentary males aged 22 to 65 years. Acta Physiol Scand 103: 31–39

Lascelles RG, Mohr PD, Neary D et al. (1977) The thoracic outlet syndrome. Brain 100: 601–612

La Spada AR, Rolling DB, Harding AE et al. (1992) Meiotic stability and genotype/phenotype correlation of the trinucleotide repeat in X-linked spinal and bulbar muscular atrophy. Nature Genet 2: 301–303

La Spada AR, Wilson EM, Lubahn DB et al. (1991) Androgen receptor gene mutations in X-linked spinal and bulbar muscular atrophy. Nature 352: 77–79

Latov N, Gross RB, Kastelman J et al. (1981) Complement fixing anti-peripheral nerve myelin antibodies in patients with inflammatory polyneuritis and with polyneuropathy and paraproteinaemia. Neurology 31: 1530–1534

Latov N, Hays AP, Sherman WH (1988) Peripheral neuropathy and anti MAG antibodies. CRC Crit Rev Neurobiol 3: 301–332

Lauritzen M, Liguari R, Trojaborg W (1991) Orthodromic sensory conduction along the ring finger in normal subjects and in patients with carpal tunnel syndrome. Electroencephalogr Clin Neurophysiol 81: 18–23

Lawrence DG, Locke S (1963) Neuropathy in children with diabetes mellitus. Br Med J i: 784–785

Lawson DH, Henry DA, Lowe JM et al. (1979) Severe hypokalemia in hospitalised patients. Arch Intern Med 139: 978–980

Lawyer T, Netsky MG (1953) Amyotrophic lateral sclerosis: a clinico-anatomic study of 53 cases. Arch Neurol Psychiat 69: 171–172

Layzer RB (1982) Neurological progress: periodic paralysis and the Na:K pump. Ann Neurol 11: 547–552

Layzer RB (1985a) McArdle's disease in the 1980s. N Engl J Med 312: 370–371

Layzer RB (1985b) Neuromuscular manifestations of systemic disease. Davis, Philadelphia, p 434

Layzer RB (1994) The origin of muscle fasciculations and cramps. Muscle Nerve 17: 1243–1249

Layzer RB, Goldfield E (1974) Periodic paralysis caused by abuse of thyroid hormone. Neurology 24: 949–952

Layzer RB, Lovelace RE, Rowland LP (1967a) Hyperkalaemic periodic paralysis. Arch Neurol 16: 455–472

Layzer RB, Rowland LP, Ranney HM (1967b) Muscle phosphofructokinase deficiency. Arch Neurol 17: 512–523

Layzer RB, Shearn MA, Satya Murti S (1977) Eosinophilic polymyositis. Ann Neurol 1: 65–71

Lazaro RP, Dettinger MP, Rodichok LD et al. (1986) Muscle pathology in Bassen–Kornzweig syndrome and vitamin E deficiency. Am J Clin Pathol 86: 378–387

Lebo CP, Sang KU, Norris FH(Jr) (1976) Cricopharyngeal myotomy in amyotrophic lateral sclerosis. Laryngoscope 86: 862–868

Lebo RV, Anderson LA, Di Mauro S et al. (1990) Rare McArdle's disease locus: polymorphic site on 11q13 contains CpG sequence. Hum Genet 86: 17–24

Lebo RV, Chance PF, Dyck PJ et al. (1991) Chromosome 1 Charcot–Marie–Tooth disease (CMT1B) locus in the Fc γ receptor gene region. Hum Genet 88: 1–12

Lederman RS, Calabrese LH (1986) Overuse syndromes in instrumentalists. Med Prob Perform Artists I: 7–11

Lee EL, Oh GC, Lam KL et al. (1976) Congenital sensory neuropathy with anhidrosis. Pediatrics 57: 259–262

Lee S, Ho S (1987) Acute effects of verapamil on neuromuscular transmission in patients with myasthenia gravis. Proc Nat Sci Council Rep China 811: 307–312

Leff RL, Love LA, Miller FW et al. (1992) Viruses in the idiopathic inflammatory myopathies: absence of candidate viral genomes in muscle. Lancet 339: 1192–1195

Lefvert AK, Osterman PO (1983) Newborn infants to myasthenic mothers: a clinical study and an investigation of acetylcholine receptor antibodies in 17 children. Neurology 33: 133–138

Leger JM, Bouche P, Bolgert F et al. (1989) The spectrum of polyneuropathies in patients infected with HIV. J Neurol Neurosurg Psychiatry 52: 1369–1374

Lehesjoki AE, Sankila EM, Miao J et al. (1990) X-linked neonatal myotubular myopathy: one recombination detected from four polymorphic DNA markers from Xq 28. J Med Genet 27: 288–291

Lehmann-Horn F, Iazzo PA, Hart H et al. (1991) Altered gating and conductance of Na$^+$ channels in hyperkalaemic periodic paralysis. Pfleuger's Arch 418: 297–299

Lehmann-Horn F, Rüdel R, Dengler R et al. (1981) Membrane defects in paramyotonia congenita with and without myotonia in a warm environment. Muscle Nerve 4: 396–406

Lehmann-Horn F, Rüdel R, Ricker K et al. (1983) Two cases of adynamia episodica hereditaria: in vitro investigation of muscle cell membrane and contraction parameters. Muscle Nerve 6: 113–121

Lehmann-Horn F, Rüdel R, Ricker K (1987) Membrane defects in paramyotonia congenita. Muscle Nerve 12: 281–287

Leibowitz U (1966) Bell's palsy – two disease entities? Neurology 16: 1105–1109

Leibowitz U (1969) Epidemic incidence of Bell's palsy. Brain 92: 109–114

Leigh PN, Roy-Chaudhuri K (1994) Motor neuron disease. J Neurol Neurosurg Psychiatry 55: 886–896

Leigh PN, Swash M (1991) Cytoskeletal pathology in motor neuron diseases. Adv Neurol 56: 115–124

Leigh PN, Anderton BH, Dodson A et al. (1988) Ubiquitin deposits in anterior horn cells in motor neuron disease. Neuro Sci Lett 93: 197–203

Leigh PN, Rothwell JC, Traub M et al. (1980) A patient with reflex myoclonus and muscle rigidity: jerking stiff man syndrome. J Neurol Neurosurg Psychiatry 43: 1135–1141

Lemann J, Donatelli AA (1964) Calcium intoxication due to primary hyperparathyroidism: a medical and surgical emergency. Ann Intern Med 60: 447–461

Lenard HG, Schaub J, Kentel J et al. (1974) Electromyography in Type II glycogenosis. Neuropaediatrie 5: 410–424

Lennon VA, Lambert EH, Palmer AC et al. (1981) Acquired and congenital myasthenia gravis in dogs – a study of 20 cases. In: Satoyoshi E (ed) Myasthenia gravis – pathogenesis and treatment. Tokyo University Press, Tokyo, pp 41–54

Lennon VA, Lambert EH, Whittingham S et al. (1982) Autoimmunity in the Lambert-Eaton myasthenic syndrome. Muscle Nerve 5: 521–525

Lennon VA, Lindstrom JM, Seybold ME (1975) Experimental autoimmune myasthenia: a model of myasthenia gravis in rats and guinea pigs. J Exp Med 141: 1365–1375

Lennon VA, Sas DF, Busk MF et al. (1991) Enteric neuronal autoantibodies in pseudoobstruction with small cell lung carcinoma. Am Gastroenterol Assoc 100: 127–142

Leon-Monzan M, Lamperth L, Dalakas MC (1993) Search for HIV proviral DNA and amplified sequences in the muscle biopsies of patients with HIV polymyositis. Muscle Nerve 16: 408–413

Leovey A, Szobor A, Szegedi G et al. (1975) Myasthenia gravis: ALG treatment of seriously ill patients. Eur Neurol 13: 422–432

Le Quesne PM (1984) Toxic neuropathies. In: Asbury AK, Gilliatt RW (eds) Peripheral nerve disorders. Butterworth, London, pp 184–204

Le Quesne PM, McLeod JG (1977) Peripheral neuropathy following single exposure to arsenic. J Neurol Sci 32: 437–451

Lerrick AJ, Wray D, Vincent A et al. (1982) Electrophysiological effects of serum factors in myasthenia gravis studied in mouse diaphragm. Ann Neurol 13: 186–191

Lester JM, Silber DI, Cohen MH et al. (1983) The co-dispersion index for the measurement of fibre type distribution patterns. Muscle Nerve 6: 581–587

Lester JM, Soule NW, Bradley WG et al. (1993) An augmented computer model of motor unit reorganisation in neurogenic diseases of skeletal muscle. Muscle Nerve 16: 43–56

Leth A, Wulff K, Carfitsen M et al. (1985) Progressive muscular dystrophy in Denmark. Acta Paediatr Scand 74: 881–885

Levin B, Engel WK (1975) Iatrogenic muscle fibrosis: arm levitation as an initial sign. JAMA 234: 621–624

Levin KH, Maggiano HJ, Wilbourn AJ (1996) Cervical radiculopathies: comparison of surgical and EMG localization of single root lessons. Neurology 46: 1022–1025

Levitt LP, Rose LI, Dawson DM (1972) Hypokalaemic periodic paralysis with arrhythmia. N Engl J Med 286: 253–254

Levitt RC, Nouri N, Jedlicka AE et al. (1991) Evidence for genetic heterogeneity in malignant hypethermia susceptibility. Genomics 11: 543–547

Levy E, Haltia M, Fernandez-Madrid I et al. (1990) Mutation in gelsolin gene in Finnish hereditary amyloidosis. J Exp Med 172: 1865–1867

Lewis MH (1969) Median nerve decompression after Colles' fracture. J Bone Joint Surg 60B: 195–196

Lewis RA, Sumner AJ (1982) The electrodiagnostic distinction between chronic familial and acquired demyelinative neuropathies. Neurology 32: 592–596

Lewis RA, Grunnet ML, Zimmerman AW (1982) Peripheral nerve demyelination in Cockayne's syndrome. Muscle Nerve 5: 557

Lewis RA, Sumner AJ, Brown MH et al. (1982) Multifocal demyelinating neuropathy with persistent conduction block. Neurology 32: 958–964

Lexell J, Downham DW (1991) The occurrence of fibre type grouping in healthy human muscle. Acta Neuropathol 81: 377–381

Lexell J, Taylor C (1991) Fiber density: a fast and accurate way to estimate human muscle fiber areas. Muscle Nerve 14: 476–477

Lexell J, Taylor CC, Sjostrom M (1988) What is the cause of the ageing atrophy? J Neurol Sci 84: 275–294

Leys K, Lang B, Johnston T et al. (1991) Calcium channel autoantibodies in the Lambert-Eaton myasthenic syndrome. Ann Neurol 29: 307–314

Lhermitte F, Chain F, Escourolle R et al. (1973) Un nouveau cas de contracture tétaniforme distinct du "stiff man syndrome"; étude pharmacologique et neuropathologique d' un cas d'encéphalomyélite a prédominance médullaire. Rev Neurol (Paris) 128: 3–21

Li T-M, Alberman E, Swash M (1988) Comparison of sporadic and familial disease amongst 580 cases of motor neuron disease. J Neurol Neurosurg Psychiatry 51: 778–784

Li T-M, Swash M, Alberman E (1985) Morbidity and mortality in motor neuron disease: comparison with multiple sclerosis and Parkinson's disease; age and sex specific rates and cohort analysis. J Neurol Neurosurg Psychiatry 48: 320–327

Libbey CA, Rubinow A, Shirahama T et al. (1984) Familial amyloid polyneuropathy: demonstration of prealbumin in a kinship of German/English ancestry with onset in the seventh decade. Am J Med 76: 18–24

Lichtenfield P (1971) Autonomic dysfunction in the Guillain-Barré syndrome. Am J Med 50: 772–780

Lightfoot RW(Jr) (1979) The vasculitis syndromes. In: McCarthy DJ (ed) Arthritis and allied conditions, 9th edn. Lea and Febiger, Philadelphia, pp 723–736

Liguari R, Dahl K. Fuglsang-Frederiksen A (1992a) Turns-amplitude analysis of the electromyographic recruitment pattern disregarding force measurement. I. Method and reference values in healthy subjects. Muscle Nerve 15: 1314–1318

Liguari R, Dahl K. Fuglsang-Frederiksen A et al. (1992b) Turns-amplitude analysis of the electromyographic recruitment pattern disregarding force measurement. II. Findings in patients with neuromuscular disorders. Muscle Nerve 15: 1319–1324

Lilienfeld DE, Chan E, Ehland J et al. (1989) Rising mortality from motor neuron disease in the USA 1962–1984. Lancet 335: 710–712

Limburg PC, The TH, Hummel-Tappel E et al. (1983) Acetylcholine receptor antibodies in myasthenia gravis. J Neurol Sci 58: 357–370

Lindberg C, Borg K, Edstrom L et al. (1991) Inclusion body myositis and Welander distal myopathy: a clinical neurophysiological and morphological comparison. J Neurol Sci 103: 76–81

Lindholm T (1967) Electromyographic changes after nitrofurantion (Furantoin) therapy in non-uraemic patients. Neurology 17: 1017–1020

Lindstrom J (1980) Experimental auto-immune myasthenia gravis. J Neurol Neurosurg Psychiatry 43: 568–576

Lindstrom JM, Seybold M, Lennon VA et al. (1976) Antibody to acetylcholine receptor in myasthenia gravis: prevalence, clinical correlates and diagnostic value. Neurology 26: 1054–1059

Lindstrom L, Petersen I (1983) Power spectrum analysis of EMG signals and its applications. In: Desmedt JE (ed) Computer-aided electromyography. Karger, Basel, pp 1–51

Links TP, Zwarts MJ, Wilmink JT et al. (1990) Permanent muscle weakness in familial hypokalaemic periodic paralysis. Brain 113: 1873–1889

Linnt PW, Harper PS (1991) Genetic counselling in facio-scapulo-humeral muscular dystrophy. J Med Genet 28: 655–664

Linscheid RL, Burton RC Frederichs EJ (1970) Tarsal tunnel syndrome. South Med J 63: 1313–1323

Lipicky RJ, Bryant SH, Salman JH (1971) Cable parameters: sodium chloride and water content and potassium efflux in isolated external intercostal muscle of normal volunteers and patients with myotonia congenita. J Clin Invest 50: 2091–2103

Lipkin WI, Parry G, Kiprov D et al. (1985) Inflammatory neuropathy in homosexual men with lymphadenopathy Neurology 35: 1479–1483

Lisak RP, Abdou NI, Zweiman B et al. (1976) Aspects of lymphocyte function in myasthenia gravis. Ann NY Acad Sci 274: 402–410

Lisak RP, Lebeau J, Tucker SH et al. (1972) Hyperkalaemic periodic paralysis and cardiac arrhythmia. Neurology 22: 810–815

Lisak RP, Mitchell M, Zweiman B et al. (1977) Guillain–Barré syndrome and Hodgkin's disease: three cases with immunological studies. Ann Neurol 1: 72–78

Lishman WA, Russell WR (1961) The brachial neuropathies. Lancet ii: 941–947

Little BW, Perl DP (1982) Oculo-pharyngeal muscular dystrophy: an autopsied case from the French-Canadian kindred. J Neurol Sci 53: 145–158

Littler WA (1970a) Peripheral sensorimotor neuropathy in association with a seminoma of an undescended testicle. Postgrad Med J 46: 166–167

Littler WA (1970b) Heart block in peroneal muscular atrophy. QJM 39: 431–440

Littlewood R, Bajada S (1981) Successful plasmapheresis in the Miller–Fisher syndrome. Br Med J i: 778

Liveson JA (1984) Nerve lesions associated with shoulder dislocation: an electrodiagnostic study of 11 cases. J Neurol Neurosurg Psychiatry 47: 742–744

Lloyd AR, Gandewa SC, Hales JP (1991) Muscle performance, voluntary activation, twitch properties and perceived effort in normal subjects and patients with the chronic fatigue syndrome. Brain 114: 85–98

Lloyd AR, Hickier I, Boughton CR et al. (1990) Prevalence of chronic fatigue syndrome in an Australian population. Med J Austr 153: 522–528

Lockman JA, Kennedy WR, White JG (1967) The Chediak-Higashi syndrome: electrophysiological and electron microscopic observations on the peripheral neuropathy. J Pediatrics 70: 942–951

Lockman LA, Krivit W, Desnick RJ (1971) Relief of the painful crises of Fabry's disease by diphenylhydantoin. Neurology 21: 423

Logigian EL, Kaplan RF, Steere AC (1990) Chronic neurologic manifestations of Lyme disease. N Engl J Med 323: 1438–1444

Loizou LA, Small M, Dalton GA (1980) Cricopharyngeal myotomy in motor neuron disease. J Neurol Neurosurg Psychiatry 43: 42–45

London SF, England JD (1991) Dynamic F waves in neurogenic claudication. Muscle Nerve 14: 457–461

London SF, Gross KF, Ringel SP (1991) Cholesterol-lowering agent myopathy (CLAM). Neurology 41: 1159–1160

Louwese ES, Vianney de Jong JMB, Kuether G (1990) Critique of assessment methodology in amyotrophic lateral sclerosis. In: Rose FC (ed) Amyotrophic lateral sclerosis. Demos, New York, pp 11–179

Loonen MCB, Busch HFM, Koster JF et al. (1981a) A family with different clinical forms of acid maltase deficiency (glycogenosis Type II): biochemical and genetic studies. Neurology 31: 1209–1216

Loonen MCB, Schram AW, Kosier JF et al. (1981b) Identification of heterozygotes for glycogenosis Type 2 (acid maltase deficiency). Clin Genet 19: 55–63

Lopez-Adaros H, Held JR (1971) Guillain-Barré syndrome associated with immunisiation against rabies: epidemiological aspects. Res Publ Assoc Res Nerve Ment Dis 49: 178–186

Lotti M Becker CE, Aminoff MJ (1984) Organophosphate polyneuropathy: pathogenesis and prevention. Neurology 34: 658–662

Lotz BP, Engel AG, Nishino H et al. (1989) Inclusion body myositis. Brain 112: 727–747

Lovelace RE, Horwitz SJ (1968) Peripheral neuropathy in long-term diphenylhydantoin therapy. Arch Neurol 18: 69–77

Low PA (1987) Recent advances in the pathogenesis of diabetic neuropathy. Muscle Nerve 10: 121–128

Low PA, Burke WJ, McLeod SG (1978) Congenital sensory neuropathy with selective loss of small myelinated nerve fibers. Ann Neurol 3: 179–182

Low PA, McLeod JG, Turtle JR et al. (1974) Peripheral neuropathy in acromegaly. Brain 97: 139–152

Low PA, Walsh JC, Huang CY et al. (1975) The sympathetic nervous system in diabetic neuropathy – a clinical and pathological study. Brain 98: 357–364

Low PK, Goodwin TG, Fang Q et al. (1992) Feasibility, safety and efficacy of myoblast transfer therapy on Duchenne muscular dystrophy boys. Cell Transplant 1: 235–244

Lowe DR, Hill DF, Dickson G et al. (1989) An autosomal transcript in skeletal muscle with homology to dystrophin. Nature 339: 44–58

Lowe J (1994) New pathological findings in amyotrophic lateral sclerosis. J Neurol Sci 124: 538–551

Lowe J, Lennox G, Jefferson D et al. (1988) A filamentous inclusion body within anterior horn neurons in motor neuron disease defined by immunocytochemical localisation of ubiquitin. Neuro Sci Lett 94: 203–210

Luchetti R, Schönhuber R, Alfarano M et al. (1990) Carpal tunnel syndrome: correlations between pressure measurement and intra-operative electrophysiological nerve study. Muscle Nerve 13: 1164–1168

Ludgate M, Swillens S, Mercken L et al. (1986) Homology between thyroglobulins and acetylcholinesterase: an explanation for pathogenesis of Graves ophthalmology? Lancet ii 219–220

Ludin HP (1980) Electromyography in practice. Thieme, Stuttgart, p 173

Ludin HP, Beyeler F (1977) Temperature dependence of normal sensory nerve action potentials. J Neurol 216: 173–180

Ludin HP, Lütsche J, Valsangiocomo F (1977) Vergleichende Untersuchung orthochromer und antichromer sensibiler Nervenleitgeschwindigkeiten. II. Befunde bei Polyneuropathien und bei Status nach Polyradiculitis. Z EEG-EMG 8: 180

Ludman H (1981) Facial palsy. Br Med J 282: 545–547

Lueck CJ, Trend P, Swash M (1991) Cyclosporin in the management of polymyositis and dermatomyositis. J Neurol Neurosurg Psychiatry 54: 1007–1008

Luft R, Ikkos D, Palmieri G et al. (1962) A case of severe hypermetabolism of non-thyroid origin with a defect in the maintenance of mitochondrial respiratory control. J Clin Invest 41: 1776–1804

Lugnegard H, Walheim G. Wennberg A (1977) Operative treatment of ulnar neuropathy in the elbow region: a clinical and electrophysiological study. Acta Orthop Scand 48: 168–176

Lund N, Bengtsson A, Thorborg P (1986) Muscle tissue oxygen pressure in patients with primary fibromyalgia. Scand J Rheumatol 15: 165–173

Lundberg A, Lilja LG, Lundberg PO et al. (1972) Heredepathia atactica polyneuriformis (Refsum's disease): experience of dietary treatment and plasmapheresis. Eur Neurol 8: 301–309

Lundberg P, Harmsen E, Ho C et al. (1990) Nuclear magnetic resonance studies of cellular metabolism. Ann Biochem 191: 193–198

Lundberg PO, Osterman PO, Stålberg E (1970) Neuromuscular signs and symptoms in acromegaly. In: Walton JN, Canal N, Scarlato G (eds) Muscle diseases. Excerpta Medica, Amsterdam, pp 531–534

Lundberg PO, Stålberg E, Thiele B (1974) Paralysis periodica paramyotonica. J Neurol Sci 21: 309–321

Lundborg G (1987) Nerve regeneration and repair. Acta Orthop Scand 58: 145–169

Lundborg G, Myers R, Powell H (1983) Nerve compression injury and increase in endoneurial fluid pressure: a miniature compartment syndrome. J Neurol Neurosurg Psychiatry 46: 1119–1124

Lundh H, Nilsson O, Rosén I (1977) 4-Aminopyridine: a new drug tested in the treatment of Eaton–Lambert syndrome. J Neurol Neurosurg Psychiatry 40: 1109–1112

Lundh H, Nilsson O, Rosén I (1984) Treatment of Lambert-Eaton syndrome: 3, 4 diaminopyridine and pyridostigmine. Neurology 34: 1324–1330

Lundholm K, Holm G, Schersten T (1978) Insulin resistance in patients with cancer. Cancer Res 38: 4665–4670

Lunsford LD, Bissonette DJ, Jannetta PJ et al. (1980) Anterior surgery for cervical disc disease I. Treatment of lateral cervical disc herniation in 253 cases. J Neurosurg 53: 1–11

Lunt PW, Harper PS (1991) Genetic counselling in facio scapulo humeral muscular dystrophy. J Med Genet 28: 655–664

Lunt PW, Meredith AL, Harper PS (1986) First trimester prediction in fetus-at-risk for myotonic dystrophy. Lancet ii: 350–351

Lupski JR, Wise CA, Kuwano A et al. (1992) Gene dosage is a mechanism for Charcot-Marie-Tooth disease Type IA. Nature (Genet) 1: 29–33

Lutschg J, Jerusalem F Ludin HP et al. (1978) The syndrome of "continuous muscle fibre activity". Arch Neurol 35: 198–205

Lyon G (1969) Ultrastructural study of a nerve biopsy from a case of early infantile chronic neuropathy. Acta Neuropathol (Berl) 13: 131–142

Mabry CC Roeckel IE, Munich RL et al. (1965) X-linked pseudohypertrophic muscular dystrophy with a late onset and slow progression. N Engl J Med 273: 1062–1070

Macalpine I, Hunter R (1967) A clinical reassessment of the insanity of George III and some of its historical implications. Bull Inst Hist Res 40: 166–185

Macalpine I, Hunter R (1969) Porphyria and King George III. Sci Am 221: 38–46

Macdonald RD, Engel AG (1969) The cytoplasmic body. Acta Neuropathol 14: 99

Macdonell RAL, Schwartz MS, Swash M (1990) Carpal tunnel syndrome: which finger should be tested? Muscle Nerve 13: 601–606

MacDougall B, Weeks PM, Wray RC (1977) Median nerve compression and trigger finger in the mucopolysaccharidoses and related diseases. Plast Reconstr Surg 59: 260–263

MacFadzean AJ, Yeung R (1967) Periodic paralysis complicating thyrotoxicosis in Chinese. Br Med J i: 451–455

Machlin LJ, Gabriel E, Spiegel HE et al. (1978) Plasma activity of pyruvate kinase and glutamic oxaloacetic transaminase as indices of myopathy in the vitamin E deficient rat. J Nutrition 108: 163–168

Mackenzie AE, Allen G, Lahey D et al. (1991) A comparison of the caffeine-halothane muscle contracture test with the molecular genetic diagnosis of malignant hyperthermia. Anesthesiology 75: 4–8

Macklem PT (1986) Muscular weakness and respiratory function. N Engl J Med 314: 775–776

Maclean G, Wessely S (1994) Professional and popular views of chronic fatigue syndrome. Br Med J 308: 776–777

MacLennan DH, Duff C, Zorzato F et al. (1990) Ryanodine receptor gene is a candidate for predisposition to malignant hyperthermia. Nature 343: 559–561

MacNicol MF (1979) The results of operation for ulnar neuritis. J Bone Joint Surg [Br] 61: 159–164

Maertens de Nordhout A, Rothwell JC, Thompson PD et al. (1988) Percutaneous electrical stimulation of lumbosacral roots in man. J Neurol Neurosurg Psychiatry 51: 174–181

Magee KE, De Jong RN (1965) Hereditary distal myopathy with onset in infancy. Arch Neurol 13: 387–390

Magid SK, Kagen LJ (1983) Serologic evidence for acute toxoplasmosis in polymyositis/dermatomyositis. Am J Med 75: 313–320

Magistris MR, Roth G (1985) Long-lasting conduction block in hereditary neuropathy with liability to pressure palsies. Neurology 35: 1639–1641

Magladery JW, McDougal DB (1950) Electrophysiological studies of nerve and reflex activity in normal man. Bull J Hopkins Hosp 86: 265–290

Magladery JW, Porter WE, Park AM et al. (1951) Electrophysiological studies of nerve and reflex activity in normal man. Bull Johns Hopkins Hosp 88: 499–519

Magora A, Sheskin J, Sagher F et al. (1971) The conduction of the peripheral nerve in leprosy under various forms of treatment. Int J Lepr 39: 639–652

Magyar E, Talerman A, Mohacsy J et al. (1977) Muscle changes in rheumatoid arthritis. Virchows Arch (Pathol Anat) 373: 267–278

Mahjneh I, Vannelli G, Bushby K et al. (1992) A large inbred Palestinian family with two forms of muscular dystrophy. Neuromusc Disord 2: 277–283

Mahloudji M, Teasdale RD, Adamkiewicz JJ et al. (1969) The genetic amyloidoses with particular reference to hereditary neuropathic amyloidosis, Type 2 (Indiana or Rukavina type). Medicine (Baltimore) 48: 1–37

Mahon M, Toman A, Willan PLT et al. (1984) Variability of histochemical and morphometric data from needle biopsy specimens of human quadriceps femoris muscle. J Neurol Sci 63: 85–100

Mahoney FI, Barthel DW (1965) Functional evaluation: the Barthel index. Maryland State Med J 14: 61–65

Mahoney MJ, Haseltine FP, Hobbins JC (1977) Prenatal diagnosis of Duchenne's muscular dystrophy. N Engl J Med 297: 968–973

Malamud M (1968) Infantile progressive muscular atrophy (Werdnig–Hoffman disease – amyotonia congenita of Oppenheim). In: Minckler J (ed) Pathology of the nervous system, vol 1. McGraw Hill, New York, pp 725–730

Mair WGP, Tomé FMS (1972) Atlas of the ultrastructure of diseased human muscle. Churchill Livingstone, Edinburgh

Malleson P (1982) Juvenile dermatomyositis: a review. J R Soc Med 75: 33–37

Mallette LE, Patten BM, Engel WK (1975) Neuromuscular disease in secondary hyperparathyroidism. Ann Intern Med 82: 474–483

Mandelli M, Rossi A, Passero F et al. (1993) Involvement of peripheral sensory fibres in amyotrophic lateral sclerosis: electrophysiological study of 64 cases. Muscle Nerve 16: 166–172

Manji H, Schwartz MS, McKeran RO (1990) Lambert–Eaton syndrome, autonomic neuropathy and inappropriate antidiuretic hormone secretion in a patient with small cell carcinoma of the lung. J Neurol 237: 324–325

Mann DMA, Yates PO (1974) Motor neuron disease: the nature of the pathogenic mechanisms. J Neurol Neurosurg Psychiatry 37: 1036–1046

Mannen T, Iwata M, Toyokura Y et al. (1977) Preservation of a certain motor neurone group of the sacral cord in amyotrophic lateral sclerosis: Its clinical significance. J Neurol Neurosurg Psychiatry 40: 464–469

Manning JJ, Adour KK (1972) Facial paralysis in children. Pediatrics 49: 102–109

Maranon G, Richet C (1937) Les syndromes neuromusculaires. Bull NY Acad Med 118: 293–298

Marconi G, Pizzi A, Arimondi CG et al. (1991) Limb-girdle muscular dystrophy with autosomal dominant inheritance. Acta Neurol Scand 83: 234–238

Marie P (1886) Sur deux cas d'acromegalie: hypertrophie singulaire non-congenitale, des extremités superieures, inférieures et ophaliques. Rev Méd (Paris) 6: 297–333

Marin EL, Vernick S, Friedmann LW (1983) Carpal tunnel syndrome: median nerve stress test. Arch Phys Med Rehabil 64: 206–208

Markesbery WR, Griggs RC, Hew B (1977) Distal myopathy: electron microscopic and histochemical studies. Neurology 27: 727–735

Markesbery WR, McQuillen MP, Procopis EG et al. (1974) Muscle carnitine deficiency: association with lipid myopathy, vacuolar neuropathy and vacuolated leucocytes. Arch Neurol 31: 320–324

Marotte LR (1974) An electron microscope study of chronic median nerve compression in the guinea pig. Acta Neuropathol (Berl) 27: 69–82

Mars H, Lewis LA, Robertson AL et al. (1969) Familial hypo β-lipoproteinaemia. Am J Med 46: 886–900

Marshall A, Duchen LW (1975) Sensory system involvement in infantile spinal muscular atrophy. J Neurol Sci 26: 349–359

Marsh GG, Munsat TL (1974) Evidence for early impairment of verbal intelligence in Duchenne muscular dystrophy. Arch Dis Child 49: 118–122

Marshall J (1959) Observations on endocrine function in dystrophia myotonica. Brain 82: 221–231

Marson MH, Hughes JM, Dowell VR et al. (1974) Current trends in botulism The United States JAMA 229: 1305–1308

Martin DT, Swash M (1987) Muscle pathology in the neuroleptic malignant syndrome. J Neurol 235: 120–121

Martin JB, Craig JM, Eckol RE et al. (1971) Hypokalaemic myopathy in chronic alcoholism. Neurology 21: 1160–1168

Martin J, Tomkin GH, Hutchinson M (1983) Peripheral neuropathy in hypothyroidism – an association with spurious polycythaemia (Gaisbock's syndrome). J R Soc Med 76: 187–189

Martin JE, Mather K, Swash M et al. (1991) Expression of heat shock protein epitopes in tubular aggregates. Muscle Nerve 14: 219–222

Martin JJ, Bruylend M, Busch HFM et al. (1986) Pleocore disease, multiminicore disease and focal loss of cross striations. Acta Neuropathol 72: 142–146

Martin JJ, Clara R, Centerick C et al. (1976) Is congenital fibre type disproportion a true myopathy? Acta Neurol Belg 76: 335

Martin JJ, Centerick CM, Mercelis RJ (1982) Nuclear inclusions in oculopharyngeal muscular dystrophy. Muscle Nerve 5: 735–737

Martin P (1763) Tal on Nervus Allmanna Egenskaper; Manniskans Kropp. Lars Salvius, Stockholm

Martin RJ, Sufit RL, Ringel SP et al. (1983) Respiratory improvement by muscle training in adult-onset acid maltase deficiency. Muscle Nerve 6: 201–203

Martin RW, Duffy J, Engel AG et al. (1990) The clinical spectrum of the eosinophilia-myalgia syndrome associated with L-tryptophan ingestion. Ann Intern Med 113: 124–134

Martinez AC (1986) Spinal evoked potentials and SFEMG in diabetic neuropathy. Electromyogr Clin Neurophysiol 26: 499–511

Martinez AJ, Hooshmand H, Faris AA (1973) Acute alcoholic myopathy. J Neurol Sci 20: 245–252

Martoni F, Catani G, Mateddu A et al. (1994) Familial cardiomyopathy, mental retardation and myopathy-associated with desmin type intermediate filaments. Neuromusc Disord 4: 233–241

Martyn C, Jellinek EH, Webb JN (1981) Lipid storage myopathy: successful treatment with propranolol. Br Med J 282: 1999–2000

Martyn CN, Barker DJP, Osmond C (1988) Motoneuron disease and past poliomyelitis in England and Wales. Lancet i: 1319–1321

Marx A, O'Connor R, Gender KI et al. (1990) Characterisation of a protein with acetylcholine receptor epitope form myasthenia gravis-associated thymomas. Lab Invest 62: 279–286

Maselli RA, Cashman NR, Wollman RL et al. (1992) Neuromuscular transmission as a function of motor unit size in patients with prior poliomyelitis. Muscle Nerve 15: 648–655

Maselli RA, Wollman RL, Leung C et al. (1993) Neuromuscular transmission in amyotrophic lateral sclerosis. Muscle Nerve 16: 1193–1203

Massey EW, Pleet AB (1978) Handcuffs and cheiralgia paresthetica. Neurology 28: 1312–1313

Mastaglia FL (1973) Pathological changes in skeletal muscle in acromegaly. Acta Neuropathol (Berl) 27: 273–286

Mastaglia FL, Kakulas BA (1969) Regeneration in Duchenne muscular dystrophy: a histological and histochemical study. Brain 92: 809–818

Mastaglia FL, Ojeda VJ (1985a) Inflammatory myopathies, I. Ann Neurol 17: 215–227

Mastaglia FL, Ojeda VJ (1985b) Inflammatory myopathies; II. Ann Neurol 17: 317–323

Mastaglia FL, Walton JN (1971a) An electron microscopic study of skeletal muscle from cases of the Kugelberg–Welander syndrome. Acta Neuropathol (Berl) 17: 201–219

Mastaglia FL, Walton JN (1971b) Histological and biochemical changes in skeletal muscle from cases of chronic juvenile and early adult spinal muscular atrophy (Kugelberg–Welander syndrome). J Neurol Sci 12: 15–44

Mastaglia FL, Barwick DD, Hall R (1970a) Myopathy in acromegaly. Lancet ii: 907–909

Mastaglia FL, Papadimitriou JM, Hawkins RL et al. (1977) Vacuolar myopathy associated with chloroquine, lupus erythematosus and thymoma. J Neurol Sci 34: 315–328

Mastaglia FL, Papadimitriou JM, Kakulas BA (1970b) Regeneration of muscle in Duchenne muscular dystrophy: an electron microscope study. J Neurol Sci 11: 425–444

Masters CL, Dawkins RL, Zilki PJ et al. (1977) Penicillamine-associated myasthenia gravis: anti-acetylcholine receptor and anti-striational antibodies. Am J Med 63: 689–694

Masuda T, Sadoyama T (1986) The propagation of single motor unit action potentials detected by a surface electrode assay. Electroencephalogr Clin Neurophysiol 63: 590–598

Mateer JE, Gutmann L, McComas CF (1983) Myokymia in Guillain-Barré syndrome. Neurology 33: 374–376

Mathew P, Todd NV (1993) Intradural conus and cauda equina tumours. J Neurol Neurosurg Psychiatry 56: 69–74

Matsuishi T, Hirata K, Terasawa K et al. (1985) Successful carnitine treatment in two siblings having lipid storage myopathy with hypertrophic cardiomyopathy. Neuroped 16: 6–12

Matsuishi T, Yoshimo M, Terasawa K et al. (1984) Childhood acid maltase deficiency – a clinical biochemical and morphologic study of three patients. Ann Neurol 41: 47–52

Matsumara K, Ivonaka I, Campbell KP (1993) Abnormal expression of dystrophin-associated proteins in Fukuyama-type congenital muscular dystrophy. Lancet 341: 521–522

Matsumara K, Tomé FMS, Collin H et al. (1992) Deficiency of the 50 kDa dystrophin-associated glycoprotein in severe childhood autosomal recessive muscular dystrophy. Nature 359: 320–322

Matsunaga M, Inokudi T, Ohnishi A et al. (1973) Oculopharyngeal involvement in familial neurogenic muscular atrophy. J Neurol Neurosurg Psychiatry 36: 104–111

Mattell G, Bergstrom K, Eranksen C et al. (1976) Effects of some immunosuppressive procedures on myasthenia gravis. Ann NY Acad Sci 274: 659–676

Mattell G, Wedlund JE, Osterman PO et al. (1981) Effect of long-term azathioprine alone and combined with steroids in the course of myasthenia gravis. In: Satayoshi E (ed) Myasthenia gravis – pathogenesis and treatment. Tokyo University Press, Tokyo, pp 373–382

Matthews WB (1965) Sarcoidosis of the nervous system. J Neurol Neurosurg Psychiatry 28: 23–29

Matthews WB (1966) Facial myokymia. J Neurol Neurosurg Psychiatry 29: 35–39

Matthews WB (1975) Spongiform encephalopathies. In: Matthews WB (ed) Recent advances in clinical neurology, vol 1. Churchill Livingstone, Edinburgh, pp 172–186

Matthews WB (1984) Sarcoid neuropathy. In: Dyck PJ, Thomas PK, Lambert EH, Bunge R (eds) Peripheral neuropathy, vol 2. Saunders, Philadelphia, pp 2018-2026

Matthews WB, Esiri MM (1983) The migrant sensory neuritis of Wartenberg. J Neurol Neurosurg Psychiatry 46: 1-4

Matthews WB, Beauchamp M, Small DG (1974) Cervical somatosensory evoked response in man. Nature 252: 230-231

Maunder-Sewry CA, Dubowitz V (1981) Needle muscle biopsy for carrier detection in Duchenne muscular dystrophy. J Neurol Sci 49: 305-324

Maurice-Williams RS (1981) Spinal degenerative disease. John Wright, Bristol

Mauro A (1961) Satellite cell of skeletal muscle fibers. J Biophys Biochem Cytol 9: 493-495

Mawdsley C, Mayer RF (1965) Nerve conduction in alcoholic polyneuropathy. Brain 88: 335-356

Max MB, Kishore-Kumar R, Schäferse et al. (1991) Effect of desipramine in painful diabetic neuropathy. Pain 45: 3-9

Mayer RF (1965) Peripheral nerve function in Vitamin B$_{12}$ deficiency. Arch Neurol 13: 355-362

Mayer RF (1966) Peripheral nerve conduction in alcoholics. Psychosom Med 28: 475-483

Mayer RF, Williams IR (1974) Incrementing responses in myasthenia gravis. Arch Neurol 31: 24-26

McArdle B (1951) Myopathy due to a defect in muscle glycogen breakdown. Clin Sci Mol Med 10: 13-33

McArdle B (1962) Adynamia episodica hereditaria and its treatment. Brain 85: 121-148

McArdle B (1974) Metabolic and endocrine myopathies. In: Walton JN (ed) Disorders of voluntary muscle. Churchill Livingstone, Edinburgh, pp 726-759

McCarthy TV, Healy JMS, Heffron JJA et al. (1990) Localisation of the malignant hyperthermia susceptibility locus to human chromosome 19q 12-13.2. Nature 343: 562-564

McComas AJ (1977) Neuromuscular function and disorders. Butterworth, London

McComas AJ (1995) Motor unit estimation: anxieties and achievements. Muscle Nerve 18: 369-379

McComas AJ, Fawcett PRW, Campbell MJ et al. (1971a) Electrophysiological estimation of the number of motor units within a human muscle. J Neurol Neurosurg Psychiatry 34: 121-131

McComas AJ, Sica REP, Campbell MJ et al. (1971b) Functional compensation in partially denervated muscles. J Neurol Neurosurg Psychiatry 34: 453-460

McComas AJ, Sica REP, Currie S (1971c) An electrophysiological study of Duchenne dystrophy. J Neurol Neurosurg Psychiatry 34: 461-468

McComas AJ, Campbell MJ, Sica REP (1971d) Electrophysiological study of dystrophia myotonica. J Neurol Neurosurg Psychiatry 34: 132-139

McComas AJ, Sica REP, McNabb AR et al. (1974) Evidence for reversible motor neurone dysfunction in thyrotoxicosis. J Neurol Neurosurg Psychiatry 37: 548-558

McComas AJ, Upton ARM, Sica REP (1973) Motor neurone disease and ageing. Lancet ii: 1474-1480

McComas CF, Schochet SS (Jr), Morris HH (III) et al. (1983) The constellation of adult acid maltase deficiency: clinical, electrophysiologic and morphologic features. Clin Neuropathol 2: 182-187

McCombe PA, Pollard JD, McLeod JG (1987) Chronic inflammatory demyelinating radiculopolyneuropathy. Brain 110: 1617-1630

McDaniel HG, Pittman CS, Oh SJ et al. (1977) Carbohydrate metabolism in hypothyroid myopathy. Metabolism 26: 867-873

McDonald WI (1963) The effects of experimental demyelination on conduction in peripheral nerve: a histological and electrophysiologial study. I. Clinical and histological observations. Brain 86: 481-500

McEvoy KM, Windebank AJ, Daube JR et al. (1989) 3-4 diaminopyridine in the treatment of Lambert-Eaton myasthenic syndrome. N Engl J Med 321: 1567-1571

McGuigan L, Burke D, Fleming A (1983) Tarsal tunnel syndrome and peripheral neuropathy in rheumatoid disease. Ann Rheum Dis 42: 128-131

McKeran RO, Halliday D, Purkiss P et al (1979) 3-Methylhistidine excretion as an index of myofibrillar protein catabolism in neuromuscular disease. J Neurol Neurosurg Psychiatry 42: 536-541

McKeran RO, Slavin G, Andrews TM et al. (1975) Muscle fibre type changes in hypothyroid myopathy. J Clin Pathol 28: 659-663

McKeran RO, Slavin G, Ward P et al. (1981) Hypothyroid myopathy - a clinical and pathological study. J Pathol 132: 35-54

McKhann GM, Cornblath DR, Griffin JW et al. (1993) Acute motor axonal neuropahy: a frequent cause of acute flaccid paralysis in China. Ann Neurol 33: 333-342

McKhann GM, Cornblath DR, Ho T et al. (1991) Clinical and electrophysiological aspects of acute paralytic disease of children and young adults in Northern China. Lancet 338: 593-597

McKusick VA (1982) The human gene map 20 October 1982. Clin Genet 22: 359-391

McKusick VA, Norum RA, Farkas JH et al. (1967) The Riley-Day syndrome. Isr J Med Sci 3: 372-378

McLean I (1979) Nerve root stimulation to evaluate conduction across the lumbosacral plexus. Acta Neurol Scand 60[Suppl 73]: 270

McLellan DL, Swash M (1976) Longitudinal sliding of the median nerve during movement. J Neurol Neurosurg Psychiatry 39: 566-570

McLeod JG (1971) An electrophysiological and pathological study of peripheral nerves in Friedreich's ataxia. J Neurol Sci 12: 333-349

McLeod JG (1984) Carcinomatous neuropathy. In: Dyck PJ, Thomas PK, Lambert EH, Bunge R (eds) Peripheral neuropathy, vol 2. Saunders, Philadelphia, pp 2180-2191

McLeod JG (1992) Autonomic dysfunction in peripheral nerve disease. Muscle Nerve 15: 3-13

McLeod JG, Evans WZ (1981) Peripheral neuropathy in spinocerebellar degeneration. Muscle Nerve 4: 51-61

McLeod JG, Walsh JC (1975) Peripheral neuropathy associated with lymphoma and other reticuloses In Dyck PJ, Thomas PK, Lambert EH Peripheral Neuropathy Saunders, Philadelphia, pp 1314-1325

McLeod JG, Baker W de C, Lethlean AK et al. (1972) Centronuclear myopathy with autosomal dominant inheritance. J Neurol Sci 15: 375-387

McLeod JG, Hargrave JC, Gye RS et al. (1975) Nerve grafting in leprosy. Brain 98: 203-212

McLeod JG, Walsh JC Little JM (1969) Sural nerve biopsy. Med J Aust 2: 1092-1096

McLeod JG, Walsh JC, Prineas JW et al. (1976) Acute idiopathic polyneuritis: a clinical and electrophysiological follow up study. J Neurol Sci 27: 145-162

McMannis P, Lambert EH, Daube J (1986) The exercise test in periodic paralysis. Muscle Nerve 9: 704-710

McMaster KR, Powers JM, Hennigar GR et al. (1979) Nervous system involvement in Type IV glycogenosis. Arch Pathol Lab Med 103: 105-111

McPherson EW, Taylor CA(Jr) (1981) The King syndrome: malignant hyperthermia, myopathy and multiple anomalies. Am J Med Genet 8: 159-165

McQuillen MP (1971) Idiopathic polyneuritis: serial studies of nerve and immune functions. J Neurol Neurosurg Psychiatry 34: 607-615

McQuillen MP, Engback L (1973) Mechanism of antibiotic-induced neuromuscular block. Trans Am Neurol Soc 98: 86-89

McQuillen MP, Johns RJ (1967) The nature of the defect in the Eaton–Lambert syndrome. Neurology 17: 527–533

McQuillen MP, Cantor HE, O'Rourke JR (1968) Myasthenic syndrome associated with antibiotics. Arch Neurol 18: 402–415

McQuillen MP, Tucker K, Pellagrina ED (1967) Syndrome of subacute generalised muscular stiffness and spasm. Arch Neurol 16: 165–174

Meadows JC, Marsden CD (1969) A distal form of chronic spinal muscular atrophy. Neurology 19: 53–58

Meadows JC, Marsden CD, Harriman DGF (1969) Chronic spinal muscular atrophy in adults. II. Other forms. J Neurol Sci 9: 551–566

Mebs D (1989) Snake venoms: toolbox of the neurologist. Endeavour 13: 157–161

Mechler F (1974) Changing electromyographic findings during the chronic course of polymyositis. J Neurol Sci 23: 237–242

Medical Research Council (1943) Aids to the investigation of peripheral nerve injuries. Her Majesty's Stationery Office, London

Medical Research Council (1983) Aids to the investigation of peripheral nerve injuries. Her Majesty's Stationery Office, London

Medical Staff of the Royal Free Hospital (1957) An outbreak of encephalomyelitis in the Royal Free Hospital Group, London in 1955. Br Med J ii: 895–904

Medsgar TA Jr (1990) Tryptophan-induced eosinophilia-myalgia syndrome. N Engl J Med 322: 926–928

Medsgar TA, Dawson WN(Jr), Masi AT (1970) The epidemiology of polymyositis. Am J Med 48: 715–723

Mehler M, Di Mauro S (1976) Late onset acid maltase deficiency: detection of patients and heterozygotes by urinary enzyme assay. Arch Neurol 33: 692–695

Mehler M, Di Mauro S (1977) Residual acid maltase activity in late onset acid maltase deficiency. Neurology 27: 178–184

Meier C, Gertsch M, Zimmerman A et al. (1983) Nemaline myopathy presenting as cardiomyopathy. N Engl J Med 38: 1536–1537

Meier C, Roberts K, Steck A et al. (1984) Polyneuropathy in Waldenstrom's macroglobulinaemia: reduction of endoneurial IgM deposits after treatment with chlorambucil and plasmapheresis. Acta Neuropathol (Berl) 64: 297–307

Meier C, Voellmy W, Gertsch M et al. (1984) Nemaline myopathy appearing in adults as cardiomyopathy. Arch Neurol 41: 443–445

Meinck HM (1992) Stiff man syndrome (SMS) and progressive encephalomyelitis with rigidity and myoclonus. Mov Disord 7 [Suppl 1]: 164

Meinck HM, Conrad B (1986) Neuropharmacological investigation in the stiff man syndrome. J Neurol 233: 340–347

Meinck HM, Ricker K, Conrad B (1984) The stiff man syndrome: new pathophysiological aspects from abnormal exteroceptive reflexes and the response to clomipramine, clonidine and tizanidine. J Neurol Neurosurg Psychiatry 47: 280–287

Mejlszenkier JD, Safran AP, Hersly SS et al. (1973) The myositis of influenza. Arch Neurol 29: 441–443

Melamed NB, Satya-Murti S (1983) Obturator neuropathy after total hip replacement. Ann Neurol 13: 578–579

Melki J, Abdelhak S, Sheth P et al. (1990) Gene for chronic proximal spinal muscular atrophies maps to chromosome 5q. Nature 344: 767–768

Mellgren SI, Conn DL, Stevens JC et al. (1989) Peripheral neuropathy in primary Sjogren's syndrome. Neurology 39: 390–394

Melsom R (1983) Serodiagnosis of leprosy: the past, the present and some prospects for the future. Int J Lepr 51: 235–252

Meltzer HY, Holy PA (1974) Black–white differences in serum creatine phosphokinase (CPK) activity. Clin Chim Acta 54: 215–224

Meltzer HY, McBride E, Poppei RW (1973) Rod (nemaline) bodies in the skeletal muscle of an acute schizophrenic patient. Neurology 23: 769–780

Meltzer HY, Mrozak S, Boyer M (1970) Effect of intramuscular injections on serum phosphocreatine kinase activity. Am J Med Sci 259: 42–48

Melzack M, Wall PD (1965) Pain mechanisms: a new therapy. Science 150: 971–979

Ménard DB, Haddad H, Blain JG et al. (1976) Granulomatous myositis and myopathy associated with Crohn's colitis. N Engl J Med 295: 818–819

Mendell JR, Moxley RT, Griggs RC et al. (1989) Randomised double-blind six month trial of prednisone in Duchenne's muscular dystrophy. N Engl J Med 320: 1592–1597

Mendell JR, Sahenk Z, Gales T et al. (1991) Amyloid filaments in inclusion body myositis. Arch Neurol 48: 1228–1234

Menkes JH (1985) Textbook of child neurology, 3rd edn. Lea and Febiger, Philadelphia

Meretoja J, Teppo L (1971) Histopathological findings of familial amyloidosis with cranial neuropathy as principal manifestation. Report of three cases. Acta Pathol Microbiologica Scand 79: 432–440

Merlini L, Granata C, Dominici P et al. (1986) Emery–Dreifuss muscular dystrophy. Muscle Nerve 9: 481–485

Mertens HG, Zschoke S (1965) Neuromyotonie. Klin Wochenschr 43: 917–925

Mertens HG, Balzereit F, Leipert M (1969) The treatment of severe myasthenia gravis with immunosuppressive agent. Eur Neurol 2: 321–339

Mertens HG, Hertel G, Reuther P et al. (1981) Effect of immunosuppressive drugs (azathioprine). Ann NY Acad Sci 377: 691–698

Merton PA, Morton HB (1980) Stimulation of the cerebral cortex in the intact human subject. Nature 285: 227

Merton PA, Hill DK, Morton HB (1981) Indirect and direct stimulation of fatigued human muscle. In: Porter R, Whelan J (eds) Human muscle fatigue: physiological mechanisms. Pitman, London, pp 128–129

Merton PA, Morton HB, Hill DK et al. (1982) Scope of a technique for electrical stimulation of the human brain, spinal cord and muscle. Lancet ii: 596–600

Meryon E (1852) On the granular and fatty degeneration of the voluntary muscles. Med Chir Trans 35: 73–85

Mesgarzadeh M, Schneck CD, Bonarkdarpour A (1989) Carpal tunnel: MR imaging. Radiology 171: 743–748, 749–755

Metheny JA (1978) Dermatomyositis, a vocal and swallowing disease entity. Laryngoscope 88: 147–161

Metzger AC, Behan A, Goldberg LS et al. (1974) Polymyositis and dermatomyositis: combined methotrexate and corticosteroid therapy. Ann Intern Med. 81: 182–189

Meyer JG, Neudorfer B, Rethel R et al. (1981) Über die Beziehung zwischen alcoholische Polyneuropathie und Vitamin B_1, B_{12} und Folsaure. Nervenartz 52: 329–332

Meyer M, Hilfiker P (1983) Computerised motor neuropathy. In: Desmedt JE (ed) Computer aided electromyography. Karger, Basel, pp 242–257

Meyers KR, Gilden DH, Renaldi FJ et al. (1972) Periodic muscle weakness, normokalaemia and tubular aggregates. Neurology 22: 269–279

Mhiri C, Baudrimont M, Bonne G et al. (1991) Zidovudine myopathy. Ann Neurol 29: 606–614

Middleton LT, Moser H (1994) Workshop Report: 23rd ENMC Workshop on rare neuromuscular diseases. Neuromusc Disord 4: 273–275

Mikol F, Stagel M, Mikol J (1976) Etude de cinq cas des myopathies oculaires. Rev Neurol 132: 325–341

Miledi R (1962) Induced innervation of end-plate free muscle segments. Nature 193: 281–282

Milhorat AT, Wolff AG (1943) Studies in diseases of muscle. XII. Progressive muscular dystrophy of atrophic distal type. Arch Neurol Psychiatry 49: 655–664

Miller F, Korsvick H (1981) Baclofen in the treatment of stiff man syndrome. Ann Neurol 9: 511–512

Miller FW, Leitman SF, Cronin ME et al. (1992) A randomised double-blind controlled trial of plasma exchange and leucopheresis in patients with polymyositis/dermatomyositis. N Engl J Med 326: 1380–1384

Miller G, Wessel HB (1993) Diagnosis of dystrophinopathies: review for the clinician. Ped Neurol 9: 3–9

Miller JR, Gunaka RV, Myers JC (1980) Amyotrophic lateral sclerosis: search for polio virus by nucleic acid hybridisation. Neurology 30: 884–886

Miller RG (1979) The cubital tunnel syndrome: diagnosis and precise localisation. Ann Neurol 6: 56–59

Miller RG (1991) AAEM case report no. 1: Ulnar neuropathy at the elbow. Muscle Nerve 14: 97–101

Miller RG, Camp PE (1979) Post-operative ulnar neuropathy. JAMA 242: 1636–1639

Miller RG, Hummel EE (1980) The cubital tunnel syndrome: treatment with simple decompression. Ann Neurol 7: 567–569

Miller RG, Kuntz NL (1986) Nerve conduction studies in infants and children. J Child Neurol 1: 22

Miller RG, Olney RK (1982) Persistent conduction block in compression neuropathy. Muscle Nerve 5: 5154–5156

Miller RG, Davis CJF, Illingworth DR et al. (1980) The neuropathy of abetalipoproteinaemia. Neurology 30: 1286–1291

Miller RG, Giannini D, Milner-Brown HS et al. (1987) Effects of fatiguing exercise on high energy phosphates force and EMG. Muscle Nerve 10: 810

Miller RG, Layzer RB, Mellenthin MA et al. (1985) Emery-Dreifuss muscular dystrophy with autosomal dominant transmission. Neurology 35: 1230–1233

Miller RG, Peterson GW, Daube JR et al. (1988) Prognostic value of electrodiagnosis in Guillain-Barré syndrome. Muscle Nerve 11: 769–774

Miller RG, Storey J, Greco C (1990) Ganciclovir in the treatment of aggressive AIDS-related polyradiculopathy. Neurology 40: 569–574

Millikan CH, Haines SF (1953) The thyroid gland in relation to neuromuscular disease. Res Publ Assoc Res Nerv Ment Dis 32: 87–98

Mills KR, Murray NMF (1985a) Proximal conduction in early Guillain-Barré syndrome. Lancet ii: 659

Mills KR, Murray NMF (1985b) Corticospinal tract conduction time in multiple sclerosis. Ann Neurol 18: 601–605

Mills KR, Murray NMF (1986) Electrical stimulation over the human vertebral column: which neural elements are excited? Electroencephalogr Clin Neurophysiol 63: 582–589

Milner-Brown HS, Stein RB, Lee RG (1974) Contractile and electrical properties of human motor units in neuropathies and motor neurone disease. J Neurol Neurosurg Psychiatry 37: 670–676

Milner-Brown HS, Stein RB, Yemm R (1973) The orderly recruitment of human motor units during voluntary isometric contractions. J Physiol (Lond) 230: 359–370

Mineo I, Kono N, Shimizu T et al. (1984) A comparative study on glucagon effect between McArdle disease and Torui disease. Muscle Nerve 7: 552–559

Miralles GD, O'Fallon JR, Talley NJ (1992) Plasma cell dyscrasia with polyneuropathy. N Eng J Med 327: 1919–1923

Miranda A, Di Mauro S, Eastwood A et al. (1979) Lipid storage myopathy, ichthyosis and steatorrhoea. Muscle Nerve 2: 1–13

Miranda AF, Nette EG, Harlage PL et al. (1979) Phosphorylase isoenzymes in normal and myophosphorylase deficient human heart. Neurology 29: 1538–1541

Misgorzadch M, Schneck CD, Bonakdarpour A (1989) Carpal tunnel syndrome. Radiology 171: 743–748, 749–775

Misra VP, King RHM, Harding AE et al. (1991) Peripheral neuropathy in Chediak-Higashi syndrome. Acta Neuropathol 81: 354–358

Mitsumoto H (1979) McArdle's disease: phosphorylase activity in regenerating muscle fibres. Neurology 29: 258–262

Mitsumoto H, Ikeda K, Holmlund T et al. (1994) The effects of ciliary neurotrophic factor on motor dysfunction in Wobbler mouse motor neuron disease. Ann Neurol 36: 142–148

Mitsumoto H, Ikeda K, Wang V et al. (1993) Ciliary neurotrophic factor (CNTF) improves neuromuscular function and muscle strength following onset of motor neuron disease in the Wobbler mouse. Neurology 43: A415

Mitsumoto H, Sliman RH, Schafer IA et al. (1985) Motor neuron disease and adult hexosaminidase – a deficiency in two families: evidence for multisystem degeneration. Ann Neurol 17: 378–385

Mittag T, Kornfeld P, Tormay A et al. (1976) Detection of anti-acetylcholine receptor factors, in serum and thymus from patients with myasthenia gravis. N Engl J Med 294: 691–694

Mittelbach F (1966) Die Begleitmyopathie bei Neurogenen Atrophien. Springer, Berlin Heidelberg New York

Miyoshi K, Kawai H, Ewasa M et al. (1986) Autosomal recessive distal muscular dystrophy as a new type of progressive muscular dystrophy. Brain 109: 31–54

Mizoguchi T (1976) Division of the pyriformis muscle for the treatment of sciatica. Arch Surg 111: 719–720

Mizuno Y, Otsuka S. Takano Y et al. (1979) Giant axonal neuropathy: combined central and peripheral nervous system disease. Arch Neurol 36: 107–108

Mizuno Y, Yoshida M, Nonaka I et al. (1994) Expression of entrophin (dystrophin-related protein) and dystrophin-associated glycoproteins in muscles from patients with Duchenne muscular dystrophy. Muscle Nerve 17: 206–216

Mizusawa H, Ohkoshi N, Watanabe M et al. (1991) Peripheral neuropathy of mitochondrial myopathies. Rev Neurol 147: 501–507

Mizusawa H, Takagi A, Sugita H et al. (1983) Mounding phenomena: an experimental study in vitro. Neurology 33: 90–93

Mizutani T, Sakamaki S, Tsuchiya N et al. (1992) Amyotrophic lateral sclerosis with ophthalmoplegia and multisystem degeneration in patients on long-term use of respirators. Acta Neuropathol 84: 372–377

Moersch FP. Woltman MW (1956) Progressive fluctuating muscular rigidity and spasm (stiff man syndrome): report of a case and some observations in 13 other cases. Mayo Clin Proc 31: 421–427

Mohire MD, Tandan R, Fries TJ et al. (1988) Early onset benign autosomal dominant limb girdle myopathy with contractures (Bethlem myopathy). Neurology 38: 573–580

Mokri B, Engel AG (1975) Duchenne dystrophy: electron microscopic findings pointing to a basic or early abnormality in the plasma membrane of the muscle fiber. Neurology 25: 1111–1120

Mokri B, Ohnishi A, Dyck PH (1981) Disulfisam neuropathy. Neurology 31: 730–735

Mokuno K, Riku S, Matsucho Y et al. (1984) Serum muscle specific enolase in progressive muscular dystrophy and other neuromuscular diseases. J Neurol Sci 63: 345–352

Mokuno K, Riku S, Matsuoka Y et al. (1985) Serum carbonic anhydrase III in progressive muscular dystrophy. J Neurol Sci 67: 223–228

Mokuno K, Riku S, Matsuoka Y et al. (1986) Serum carbonic anhydrase III in myotonic dystrophy. Muscle Nerve 9: 256–260

Moldaver J (1954) Tourniquet paralysis syndrome. Arch Surg 68: 136–144

Mollman JE (1990) Cisplatin neurotoxicity. N Engl J Med 322: 126–127

Mollman JE, Glover DJ, Hogan WM et al. (1988) Cisplatin neuropathy, risk factors, prognosis and protection by WR2721. Cancer 61: 2192–2195

Monaco AP, Birtelson CT, Liechti-Gallati S et al. (1988) An explanation for the phenotype differences between patients bearing partial deletions of the DMD locus. Genomics 2: 90–95

Monden Y, Nakahara K, Kagatoni K et al. (1984) Myasthenia gravis with thymoma: analysis of perioperative prognosis for 465 patients with myasthenia gravis. Ann Thor Surg 38: 46–52

Mongini T, Dariguzzi C, Palmucci L et al. (1991) Myoglobinuria and palmitoyl transferase deficiency in father and son. J Neurol 238: 323–324

Moody JF (1965) Electrophysiological investigation into the neurological complication of carcinoma. Brain 88: 1033–1035

Moore MJ, Rebeiz JJ, Holden M et al. (1971) Biometric analyses of normal skeletal muscle. Acta Neuropathol (Berl) 19: 51–56

Moore PM, Cupps TR (1983) Neurological complication of vasculitis. Ann Neurol 14: 155–167

Moosa A, Dubowitz V (1970) Peripheral neuropathy in Cockayne's syndrome. Arch Dis Child 45: 674–677

Moosa A, Dubowitz V (1971) Slow nerve conduction velocity in cretins. Arch Dis Child 46: 852–854

Moosa A, Dubowitz V (1976) Motor nerve conduction velocity in spinal muscular atrophy of childhood. Arch Dis Child 51: 974–977

Moosa A, Brown BH, Dubowitz V (1972) Quantitative electromyography: carrier detection in Duchenne type muscular dystrophy using a new automatic technique. J Neurol Neurosurg Psychiatry 35: 841–844

Moraes CT, DiMacro S, Zeviani M et al. (1989) Mitochondrial DNA deletions in progressive external ophthalmoplegia and Kearns-Sayre syndrome. N Engl J Med 330: 1293–1299

Moraes CR, Ciacci F, Silvestri G et al. (1993) A typical clinical presentation with a MELAS mutation at position 3243 of human mtDNA. Neuromusc Disord 3: 43–53

Morgan GT(Jr), McGuire JL, Ochoa J (1981) Penicillamine-induced myositis in rheumatoid arthritis. Muscle Nerve 4: 137–140

Morgan O St C, Mara C, Rodgers-Johnson P et al. (1989) HTLV-1 and polymyositis in Jamaica. Lancet ii: 1184–1187

Morgan-Hughes JA, Brett EM, Lake BD et al. (1973) Central core disease or not? Brain 96: 527–536

Morgan-Hughes JA, Darveniza P, Kahn SN et al. (1977) A mitochondrial myopathy characterised by a deficiency in reducible cytochrome-b. Brain 100: 616–640

Morgan-Hughes JA, Darveniza P, Landon DN et al. (1979) A mitochondrial myopathy with a deficiency of respiratory chain NADH-CoQ reductase activity. J Neurol Sci 43: 27–46

Morgan-Hughes JA, Hayes DJ, Clark JB et al. (1982) Mitochondrial encephalomyopathies: biochemical defects in two cases revealing defects in the respiratory chain. Brain 105: 553–582

Morgan-Hughes JA, Hayes DJ, Clarke JB et al. (1984) Mitochondrial myopathies: results of exploratory therapeutic trials. Biochemical and clinical aspects of co-enzyme Q TINS 4: 417–424

Morgan-Hughes JA, Lecky BRF, Landon DN et al. (1981) Alterations in the number and affinity of junctional acetylcholine receptors in a myopathy with tubular aggregates. Brain 104: 279–295

Morgan-Hughes JA, Mair WPG, Lascelles PT (1970) A disorder of skeletal muscle associated with tubular aggregates. Brain 93: 873–880

Morita H, Kando K, Hoshiaok et al. (1990). Rigid spine syndrome with respiratory failure. J Neurol Neurosurg Psychiatry 53: 782–784

Morita H, Ohco S, Fukunaga M et al. (1989) Increased accumulation of n isopropyl p (121_I) iodo-amphetamine in two cases with mitochondrial encephalomyopathy with lactic acidosis and stroke-like episodes (MELAS). Neuroradiology 31: 358–361

Morley GK Mooradian AD, Levine AL et al. (1984) Mechanism of pain in diabetic peripheral neuropathy: effect of glucose on pain perception in humans. Am J Med 77: 79–82

Morris EP, Nheji G, Squire JM (1990) The three-dimensional structure of the nemaline rod Z band. J Cell Biol 111: 2961–2978

Morris HH, Peters BH (1976) Pronator syndrome: clinical and electrophysiological features in 7 cases. J Neurol Neurosurg Psychiatry 39: 4461–4464

Mortara P, Chio A, Rossa MG et al. (1984) Motor neuron disease in the province of Turin, Italy, 1966–1980. J Neurol Sci 66: 165–173

Morton NE, Chung CS, Peters HA (1963) Genetics of muscular dystrophy. In: Bourne GM, Golarz MN (eds) Muscular dystrophy in man and animals. Karger, Basel, pp 323–365

Morton TG (1876) A peculiar and painful affliction on the fourth metatarsophalangeal articulation. Am J Med Sci 71: 37–45

Moser H, Emery AE (1974) The manifesting carrier in Duchenne muscular dystrophy. Clin Genet 5: 271–284

Moser HW, Moser AB, Kawamura N et al. (1980) Adreno-leucodystrophy: elevated C26 fatty acid in cultured skin fibroblasts. Ann Neurol 7: 542–549

Moser HW, Naidu S, Kumar AJ et al. (1987) The adrenoleucodystrophies. CRC Crit Rev Neurobiol 3: 29

Moss HH, Casey P, Stocking CB et al. (1993) Home ventilation for amyotrophic lateral sclerosis patients. Neurology 43: 438–443

Motomura M, Johnston I, Lang B et al. (1995) An improved diagnostic assay for Lambert-Eaton myasthenic syndrome. J Neurol Neurosurg Psychiatry 58: 85–87

Moulds RFW, Denborough MA (1974a) Identification of susceptibility to malignant hyperpyrexia. Br Med J ii: 245–247

Moulds RFW, Denborough MA (1974b) Biochemical basis of malignant hyperpyrexia. Br Med J ii: 241–244

Moxley RT (III) (1992) Myotonic muscular dystrophy. In: Vinken AJ Bruyn CW, Klawans HL (eds) Handbook of clinical neurology. Elsevier, Amsterdam, pp 209–259

Moxley RT (III) (1996) Proximal myotonic myopathy. Neuromusc Disord 6: 87–93

Moxley RT, Levenson M, Griggs RC et al. (1990) Decreased breakdown of muscle protein after prednisone therapy in Duchenne dystrophy. J Neurol Sci 98 [Suppl]: 419

Mueller EA, Hettinger T (1953) Ueber Unterschiede der Trainingsgeschwindigkeit atrophierter und normalen Muskeln. Arbeits Physiol 15: 223–230

Mukano K (1969) Electron microscopic studies on human extraocular muscles under pathologic conditions. I. Rod formation in normal and diseased muscles (polymyositis and ocular myasthenia). Jpn J Ophthalmol 13: 35–51

Mulder DW (1982) Clinical limits of amyotrophic lateral sclerosis. In: Rowland LP (ed) Human motor neuron diseases. Raven Press, New York, pp 15–29

Mulder DW, Espinoza RE (1969) Amyotrophic lateral sclerosis: Comparison of the clinical syndrome in Guam and the United States. In: Norris FH, Kurland LT (eds) Motor neurone diseases. Grune & Stratton, New York, pp 12–19

Mulder DW, Howard FM (1976) Patient resistance and prognosis in amyotrophic lateral sclerosis. Mayo Clin Proc 51: 537–541

Mulder DW, Kurland LT, Offord KP et al. (1986) Familial adult motor neuron disease. Neurology 36: 511–517

Mulder DW, Lambert EH, Bashon JA et al. (1961) The neuropathies associated with diabetes: a clinical and electromyographic study of 103 unselected diabetic patients. Neurology 11: 275–284

Mulder DW, Lambert EH, Eaton LM (1959) Myasthenic syndrome in patient with amyotrophic lateral sclerosis. Neurology 9: 627–631

Muller B, Melki J, Burlet P et al. (1992) Proximal spinal muscular atrophy (SMA) Type II and III in the same sibship are not caused by different alleles at the SMA locus on 5q. Am J Hum Genet 50: 892–895

Muller DPR (1986) Vitamin E: its role in neurological function. Postgrad Med J 62: 107–112

Muller DPR, Lloyd JK (1982) Effect of large oral doses of Vitamin E on the neurological sequelae of abetalipoproteinaemia. Ann NY Acad Sci 393: 133–144

Muller DPR, Lloyd JK, Wolff OH (1983) Vitamin E and neurological function. Lancet i: 225–228

Multicenter Group (1992) Diagnosis of Duchenne and Becker muscular dystrophies by polymerase chain reaction. JAMA 267: 2609–2615

Mumenthaler M, Narakas A, Gilliatt RW (1984) Brachial plexus disorders. In: Dyck PJ, Thomas PK, Lambert EH, Bunge R (eds) Peripheral neuropathy, 2nd edn. Saunders, Philadelphia, pp 1382–1424

Münchhoff P, Wilske B, Preac-Mursic V et al. (1986) Antibodies against *Borrelia burgdorfri* in Bavarian forest workers. Zentralbl Bakteriol Hejg (A) 263: 412–419

Munsat TL (1967) Therapy of myotonia: a double-blind evaluation of diphenylhydantoin, procainamide and placebo. Neurology 17: 359–367

Munsat TL (1970) A standardized forearm ischaemic exercise test. Neurology 20: 1171–1178

Munsat TL (1977) The classification of human dystrophies. In: Rowland LP (ed) Pathogenesis of human muscular dystrophies. Excerpta Medica, Amsterdam, pp 21–31

Munsat TL (1991a) Workshop report: International SMA collaboration. Neuromusc Disord 1: 81

Munsat TL (1991b) Poliomyelitis – new problems with an old disease. N Engl J Med 324: 1206–1207

Munsat TL, Barnes JE (1965) Relation of multiple cranial nerve dysfunction to the Guillain–Barré syndrome. J Neurol Neurosurg Psychiatry 28: 115–120

Munsat TL, Bradley WG (1977) Serum creatine phosphokinase levels and prednisone treated muscle weakness. Neurology 27: 96–97

Munsat TL, Serratrice G (1992) Facio-scapulo-humeral and scapulo-peroneal syndromes. In: Vinken PJ, Bruyn GW Klawans HL (eds) Handbook of clinical neurology, vol 62. Elsevier Amsterdam, pp 161–177

Munsat TL, Andries PL, Finison L et al. (1988) The natural history of motor neuron loss in amyotrophic lateral sclerosis. Neurology 38: 409–413

Munsat TL, Piper O, Cancilla P et al. (1972) Inflammatory myopathy with facio-scapulo-humeral distribution. Neurology 22: 335–347

Munsat TL, Skerry L, Korf B et al. (1990) Phenotypic heterogenity of spinal muscular atrophy mapping to chromosome 5q 11.2–13.3 (SMA 5q). Neurology 40: 1831–1836

Munsat TL, Thompson LR, Coleman RF (1969a) Centronuclear (myotubular) myopathy. Arch Neurol 20: 120–131

Munsat TL, Woods R, Fowler W (1969b) Neurogenic muscular atrophy of infancy with prolonged survival. Brain 29: 9–24

Muntoni F, Cau M, Ganau A et al. (1993) Brief report: deletion of the dystrophin muscle promoter region associated with X-linked dilated cardiomyopathy. N Engl J Med 329: 921–925

Murase T, Ikeda H, Muro T et al. (1973) Myopathy associated with Type III glycogenosis. J Neurol Sci 20: 287–295

Murray IPC, Simpson JA (1958) Acroparaesthesiae in myxoedema: a clinical and electromyographic study. Lancet i: 1360–1363

Murray NMF, Wade DT (1980) The sural sensory action potential in Guillain–Barré syndrome. Muscle Nerve 3: 444

Mussini E, Cornelio F, Colombo L et al. (1984) Increased myofibrillar protein catabolism in Duchenne muscular dystrophy measured by 3-methylhistidine excretion in the urine. Muscle Nerve 7: 388–391

Mussini I, Di Mauro S, Angelini C (1970) Early ultrastructural and biochemical changes in muscle, in dystrophia myotonica. J Neurol Sci 10: 585–604

Mustasoki P (1980) Variegate porphyria. AJM 49: 191–203

Myllydla VV, Toivakka E, Ala-Hurltla V et al. (1979) Juvenile amyotrophic lateral sclerosis: a report of two cases in a single family. Acta Neurol Scand 60: 170–177

Nadkarni N, Prior TW, Mendell JR (1994) The impact of molecular genetics on the care of patients with muscle disease. Curr Opin Neurol 7: 435–447

Nagler W (1971) Peripheral neuropathy in acute intermittent porphyria. Arch Phys Med Rehabil 51: 426–430

Nagulesparen M, Trickey R, Davies MJ et al. (1976) Muscle changes in acromegaly. Br Med J ii: 914–915

Nair KR (1976) Acrodystrophic neuropathy. Neurology (India) 25: 94–99

Nair KR (1978) Acrodystrophic neuropathy. J Assoc Phys Ind 26: 347–353

Najjar SS (1974) Muscular hypertrophy in hypothyroid children: the Kocher–Debré syndrome. J Pediatr 85: 236–239

Nakanishi T, Sohue I, Toyokura Y et al. (1984) The Crow–Fukase syndrome: a study of 102 cases in Japan. Neurology 34: 712–720

Nakano KK (1978) The entrapment neuropathies. Muscle Nerve 1: 264–279

Nakano KK, Lundergan C, Okihiro MM (1977) Anterior interosseous nerve syndromes: diagnostic methods and alternative treatments. Arch Neurol 34: 477–488

Namba T, Grob D (1970) Familial occurrence of myasthenia gravis and rheumatoid arthritis. Arch Intern Med 125: 1056–1058

Namba T, Aberfeld DL, Grob D (1970) Chronic proximal spinal muscular atrophy. J Neurol Sci 11: 401–423

Namba T, Brown SB, Grob D (1970) Neonatal myasthenia gravis: report of two cases and review of the literature. Pediatrics 45: 488–504

Namba T, Brunner NG, Brown SB et al. (1971) Familial myasthenia gravis. Arch Neurol 25: 49–60

Namba T, Brunner NG, Grob D (1974) Idiopathic giant cell polymyositis. Arch Neurol 31: 27–30

Namba T, Brunner NG, Grob D (1978) Myasthenia gravis in patients with thymoma with particular reference to onset after thymectomy. Medicine (Baltimore) 57: 411–433

Nandedkar S, Stålberg E (1983) Simulation of macro EMG motor unit potentials. Electroencephalogr Clin Neurophysiol 56: 52–62

Nandedkar SD, Barkhaus PE, Saunders DB et al. (1988b) Analysis of amplitude and area of concentric needle EMG motor unit action potentials. Electroencephalogr Clin Neurophysiol 69: 561–567

Nandedkar SD, Sanders DB, Stålberg EV (1985) Selectivity of electromyographic recording techniques: a simulation study. Med Biol Eng Comp 23: 536–540

Nandedkar SD, Sanders DB, Stålberg EV (1986) Simulation and analysis of the electromyographic interference pattern in normal muscle. I. Turns and amplitude measurements. Muscle Nerve 9: 423–430

Nandedkar SD, Sanders DB, Stålberg EV et al. (1988a) Simulation of concentric needle EMG motor unit action potentials. Muscle Nerve 11: 151–159

Nandedkar SD, Stålberg EV, Sanders DB (1985) Simulation techniques in electromyography. IEEE Trans Biomed Eng BME-32: 775–784

Nanji AA (1983) Serum creatine kinase isoenzymes: a review. Muscle Nerve 6: 83–90

Narakas A (1978) Surgical treatment of traction injuries of the brachial plexus. Clin Orthop 133: 71–90

Narakas A (1984) Operative treatment for radiation-induced and metastatic brachial plexopathy in 45 cases, 15 having an omentoplasty. Bull Hosp Joint Dis 44: 354–375

Narunan A, Coakley J, Thomas V et al. (1989) Distinction of Becker from limb-girdle muscular dystrophy by means of dystrophin cDNA probes. Lancet i: 466–468

Nassanova VA, Ivanova MM, Alchnzarova VD et al. (1979) Diffuse faciitis with eosinophilia (pseudo-sclerodermic syndrome). Therap Arkh 50: 7–14

Nathan PW (1976) The gate control theory of pain: a critical review. Brain 99: 123–158

Nattrass FJ (1954) Recovery from "muscular dystrophy". Brain 77: 549–570

Navarro X, Miralles R, Espadaler JM et al. (1993) Comparison of sympathetic sudomotor and skin responses in alcoholic neuropathy. Muscle Nerve 16: 404–407

Ndraye-Niang M, Diagne M, Ndraye IP et al. (1986) The value of electromyographic studies in leprosy. Acta Leprol 100: 51–56

Neary D, Eames RA (1975) The pathology of ulnar nerve compression in man. Neuropathol Appl Neurobiol 1: 69–88

Neary D, Ochoa J, Gilliatt RW (1975) Sub-clinical entrapment neuropathy in man. J Neurol Sci 24: 283–298

Neary D, Snowden JS, Mann DMA et al. (1990) Frontal lobe dementia and motor neuron disease. J Neurol Neurosurg Psychiatry 53: 23–32

Neilson S, Robinson I, Alperovitch A (1994) Rising amyotrophic lateral sclerosis mortality in France 1968–1990. J Neurol 241: 448–455

Nelson RM, Soderberg GL (1983) Laser-etched bifilar fine wire electrode for skeletal muscle motor unit recording. Electroencephalogr Clin Neurophysiol 55: 238–239

Nelson TE, Butler IJ (1992) Malignant hyperthermia: skeletal muscle defect(s) predisposing to labile calcium regulation. J Child Neurol 7: 329–331

Nelson TE, Flewellen EH (1983) The malignant hyperthermia syndrome. N Engl J Med 309: 416–418

Nelson TE, Flewellen EH, Gloyna DF (1983) Spectrum of susceptibility to malignant hyperthermia: diagnostic dilemma. Anesth Analg Cleveland 62: 545–552

Nemmi R, Foltri ML, Fazio R et al. (1990) Axonal neuropathy with monoclonal IgG kappa that binds to a neurofilament protein. Ann Neurol 28: 361–364

Nemmi R, Galassi G, Cohen M et al. (1981) Symmetrical sarcoid polyneuropathy: analysis of a sural nerve biopsy. Neurology 31: 1217–1223

Neville HE, Brooke MH (1973) Central core fibres: central and unstructured. In: Kakulas BA (ed) Basic research in myology. Excerpta Medica, Amsterdam, pp 497–511 (International Congress Series 294)

Neville HE, Harrold S (1985) Protein degradation in cultured skeletal muscle from Duchenne muscular dystrophy patients. Muscle Nerve 8: 253–257

Nevin S (1936) Two cases of muscular degeneration occuring in late adult life with a review of the recorded cases of late progressive muscular dystrophy (late progressive myopathy). QJM 5: 51–68

Newburger JW, Takahashi M, Burns JC et al. (1986) The treatment of Kawasaki syndrome with intravenous gammaglobulin. N Engl J Med 315: 341–347

Newham D, Edwards RHT (1979) Effort syndromes. Physiotheraphy 65: 52–56

Newham DJ, Johns DA, Edwards RHT (1983) Large delayed plasma creatine kinase changes after stopping exercise. Muscle Nerve 6: 380–385

Newman RJ, Bone PJ, Chan L et al. (1982) Nuclear magnetic resonance studies of forearm muscle in Duchenne dystrophy. Br Med J 284: 1027–1074

Newrick PG, Langton-Hewer R (1984) Motor neurone disease: can we do better? A study of 42 patients. Br Med J 289: 539–542

Newrick PG, Langton-Hewer R (1985) Pain in motor neurone disease. J Neurol Neurosurg Psychiatry 48: 838–840

Newrick PG, Wilson AJ, Jakubowski J et al. (1986) Sural nerve oxygen tension in diabetes. Br Med J 293: 1053–1054

Newsom-Davis J (1979a) Plasma exchange in myasthenia gravis. Plasma Therapy 1: 17–31

Newsom-Davis J (1979b) Anti-acetylcholine receptor antibody in myasthenia gravis. In: Rose FC (ed) Clinical neuroimmunology. Blackwell Scientific Publications, Oxford, pp 128–136

Newsom-Davis J (1993) Myasthenia gravis and the Lambert-Eaton myasthenic syndrome. Prescriber's J 33: 205–212

Newsom-Davis J, Mills KR (1993) Immunological associations of acquired neuromyotonia (Isaac's syndrome). Brain 116: 453–469

Newsom-Davis J, Murray NMF (1984) Plasma exchange and immunosuppressive drug treatment in the Lambert-Eaton myasthenic syndrome. Neurology 34: 480–485

Newsom-Davis J, Vincent A (1979) Combined plasma-exchange and immunosuppression in myasthenia gravis. Lancet ii: 688

Newsom-Davis J, Goldman M, Lohn L et al. (1976) Diaphragm function and alveolar hypoventilation. QJM 45: 87–100

Newsom-Davis J, Vincent A, Wilcox N (1982) Acetylcholine receptor antibody: clinical and experimental aspects. In: Evered DC Whalen J (eds) Receptors, antibodies and disease. Pitman, London, pp 225–247 (Ciba Foundation symposium no. 90)

Newsom-Davis J, Vincent A, Wilson SG et al. (1978) Long term effects of repeated plasma exchange in myasthenia gravis. Lancet i: 464–468

Newsom-Davis J, Willcox N, Schluep M et al. (1987) Immunological heterogeneity and cellular mechanisms in myasthenia gravis. Ann NY Acad Sci 505: 12–26

Nguyen HH, Wolfe JT, Holmes DR Jr et al. (1988) Pathology of the cardiac conducting system in myotonic dystrophy. J Am Coll Cardiol 11: 662–671

Niakan E, Berorini TE, Acchiarde SR et al. (1981) Procainamide induced myasthenia-like weakness in a patient with peripheral neuropathy. Arch Neurol 38: 378–379

Nichols WC, Gregg RE, Bryan Brewer H et al. (1990) A mutation in apoprotein A_1 in the Iowa type of familial amyloidotic polyneuropathy. Genomics 8: 318–323

Nicholson GA, Appel SA (1977) Is there acetylcholine receptor in human thymus? J Neurol Sci 34: 101–108

Nicholson GA, Valention LJ, Cherryson AK et al. (1994) A frame shift mutation in the PMP22 gene in a hereditary neuropathy with liability to pressure palsies. Nature Genet 6: 263–266

Nicholson LVB, Walls TJ (1983) Variation of serum myoglobin levels in normal individuals J Neurol Sci 62: 41–58

Nicholson LVB, Johnson MA, Gardner-Medwin D et al. (1990) Heterogeneity of dystrophin expression in patients with Duchenne and Becker muscular dystrophy. Acta Neuropathol 80: 239–250

Nickel SN, Frame B, Bevin J et al. (1961) Myxoedema neuropathy and myopathy: a clinical and pathologic study. Neurology 11: 125–137

Nielsen VK (1971a) The peripheral nerve function in chronic renal failure. I. Clinical signs and symptoms. Acta Med Scand 190: 105–111

Nielsen VK (1971b) The peripheral nerve function in chronic renal failure. II. Intercorrelation of clinical symptoms and signs and clinical grading of neuropathy. Acta Med Scand 190: 113–117

Nielsen VK (1973) The peripheral nerve function in chronic renal failure. V. Sensory and motor conduction velocity. Acta Med Scand 194: 445–454

Nielsen VK (1974) The peripheral nerve function in chronic renal failure. IX. Recovery after renal transplantation: electrophysiological aspects (sensory and motor nerve conduction). Acta Med Scand 195: 171–180

Nielsen VK (1984a) Pathophysiology of hemifacial spasm. I. Ephaptic transmission and ectopic excitation. Neurology 34: 418–426

Nielsen VK (1984b) Pathophysiology of hemifacial spasm. I. Lateral spread of the supraorbital nerve reflex. Neurology 34: 427–431

Nielsen VK, Friis ML, Johnsen T (1982) Electromyographic distinction between paramyotonia congenita and myotonia congenita: effect of cold. Neurology 32: 827–832

Nienhuis AW, Coleman RF, Brown WJ et al. (1967) Nemaline myopathy: a histopathologic and histochemical study. Am J Clin Pathol 48: 1–13

Nigst H, Dick W (1979) Syndromes of compression of the median nerve in the proximal forearm (pronator teres syndrome and anterior interosseous syndrome). Arch Orthop Trauma Surg 93: 307–312

Nigro G, Comi LI, Politano L et al. (1990) The incidence and evolution of cardiomyopathy in Duchenne muscular dystrophy. Int J Cardiol 26: 271–277

Nigro G, Comi LI, Politano L et al. (1995) Evaluation of the cardiomyopathy in Beckers muscular dystrophy Muscle Nerve 18: 283–291

Nimelstein SH, Brody S, McShane D et al. (1980) Mixed connective tissue disease: a subsequent evaluation of the original 25 patients. Medicine (Baltimore) 59: 239–248

Nishiskai M, Homma M (1977) Circulating autoantibody against human myoglobin in polymyositis. JAMA 237: 1842–1844

Nishikai M, Reichlin M (1980) Radioimmunoassay of serum myoglobin in polymyositis and other conditions. Arthritis Rheum 20: 1514–1518

Nishino H, Engel AG, Rima BK (1989) Inclusion body myositis: the mumps hypothesis. Ann Neurol 25: 260–264

Nissen-Petersen H, Guld C, Buchthal F (1969) A delay line to record random action potentials. Electroencephalogr Clin Neurophysiol 26: 100–106

Nixon JC, Hobbs WK, Greenblatt J (1966) Myoglobinuria and skeletal muscle phosphorylase deficiency: report of a case of McArdle's disease. Can Med Assoc J 94: 977–985

Nobel W, Black D, Johnson P et al. (1974) Effect of chronic compression on the microcirculation and function of peripheral nerves. In: Cervos-Navarros O (ed) Pathology of cerebral microcirculation. Walter de Gruyter, New York, p 483

Nobile-Orazio E (1996) Multifocal motor neuropathy. J Neurol Neurosurg Psychiatry 60: 599–603

Nobile-Orazio E, Carpo M, Meucci N et al. (1992) Guillain-Barré syndrome associated with high titres of anti GM$_1$ antibodies. J Neurol Sci 109: 200–206

Nobile-Orazio E, Meucci N, Barbieri S et al. (1993) High dose intravenous immunoglobulin therapy in multifocal motor neuropathy. Neurology 43: 537–544

Noël P (1973) Sensory nerve conduction in the upper limbs at various stages of diabetic neuropathy. J Neurol Neurosurg Psychiatry 36: 786–796

Noël P, Desmedt JE (1980) Cerebral and far field somatosensory evoked pootentials in neurologic disorders involving the cervical spinal cord, brainstem, thalamus and cortex. In: Desmedt JE (ed) Clinical uses of cerebral brainstem and spinal somatosensory evoked potentials in clinical neurophysiology, vol 7. Karger, Basel, pp 205–230

Nonaka I, Sunohara N, Ishiura S et al. (1981) Familial distal myopathy with rimmed vacuole and lamellar (myeloid) body formation. J Neurol Sci 51: 141–155

Nonaka I, Sunohara N, Satoyoshi E et al. (1985) Autosomal recessive distal muscular dystrophy. Ann Neurol 17: 51–59

Nonaka I, Takagi A, Sugita H (1981) The significance of Type 2C muscle fibres in Duchenne muscular dystrophy. Muscle Nerve 4: 326–333

Norris FH (1975) Recent advances in motor neurone diseases. In: Bradley WG, Gardner-Medwin D, Walton JN (eds) Recent advances in myology. Excerpta Medica, Amsterdam, pp 522–536

Norman A, Thomas N, Coackley J et al. (1989) Distinction of Becker from limb-girdle muscular dystrophy by means of dystrophin aDNA probes. Lancet i 466–468

Norris FH Jr, Panner BJ (1966) Hypothyroid myopathy. Arch Neurol 14: 574–589

Norris FH, Smith RA, Denys EH (1985) Motor neurone disease: towards better care. Br Med J 291: 259–262

Northfield DWC (1973) The surgery of the central nervous system. Blackwell, Oxford

Novak DJ, Victor M (1974) Affection of the vagus and sympathetic nerves in alcoholic polyneuropathy. Arch Neurol 30: 273–284

Nudel V, Zuk D, Einat P et al. (1989) Duchenne muscular dystrophy gene product is not identical in muscle and brain. Nature 337: 76–78

Nukada H, Pollock M, Haas LF (1982) The clinical spectrum of Type II hereditary sensory neuropathy. Arch Neurol 30: 336–340

Nyland H, Matre R, Mark S (1981) Immunological characterisation of sural nerve biopsies from patients with Guillain-Barré syndrome. Ann Neurol 9: 580–586

Oakley CM (1984) The heart in the Guillain-Barré syndrome. Br Med J 288: 94

O'Brien MD, Upton ARM (1972) Anterior interosseous nerve syndrome: a case report with neurophysiological investigation. J Neurol Neurosurg Psychiatry 35: 531–536

O'Brien T, Kelly M, Saunders C (1992) Motor neurone disease: a hospice perspective. Br Med J 304: 471–473

Ochoa J (1970) Isoniazid neuropathy in man: quantitative electron microscope study. Brain 93: 831–850

Ochoa J (1982) Pain in local nerve lesions. In: Culp WJ, Ochoa J (eds) Abnormal nerves and muscles as impulse generators. Oxford University Press, New York, pp 560–587

Ochoa J (1986) The newly recognised painful ABC syndrome: thermographic aspects. Thermology 2: 65–66, 101–107

Ochoa J, Mair WGP (1969) The normal sural nerve in man. II. Changes in the axons and Schwann cells due to ageing. Acta Neuropathol (Berl) 13: 217–239

Ochoa J, Marotte LR (1973) The nature of the nerve lesion caused by chronic entrapment in the guinea pig. J Neurol Sci 19: 491–495

Ochoa JL, Torebjork HE (1980) Parasthesiae from ectopic impulse generation in human sensory nerves. Brain 103: 835–853

Ochoa J, Torebjork E (1989) Sensations evoked by intraneural microstimulation of identified C nociceptor fibres in human skin nerves. J Physiol 415: 583

Ochoa J, Danta G, Fowler TJ et al. (1971) Nature of the nerve lesion caused by a pneumatic tourniquet. Nature 233: 265–266

Ochoa J, Fowler TJ, Gilliatt RW (1972) Anatomical changes in peripheral nerves compressed by a pneumatic tourniquet. J Anat 113: 433–455

Oda K (1993) Differences in acetylcholine receptor antibody interactions between extraocular and extremity muscle fibres. Ann NY Acad Sci 681: 238–255

O'Duffy JD, Randall RV, MacCarty CS (1973) Median neuropathy (carpal tunnel syndrome) in acromegaly. Ann Intern Med 78: 379–383

Odusok K, Eisen A (1979) An electrophysiological quantitation of the cubital tunnel syndrome. Can J Neurol Sci 6: 403–410

Oertel G (1986) Changes in human skeletal muscles due to ageing. Acta Neuropathol (Berl) 69: 309–313

Oh SJ (1987) Overlap myasthenic syndrome. Neurology 37: 1411–1414

Oh SJ (1988) Electromyography: neuromuscular transmission studies. Williams and Wilkins, Baltimore, p 304

Oh SJ (1989) Diverse electrophysiological spectrum of the Lambert-Eaton myasthenic syndrome. Muscle Nerve 12: 464–469

Oh SJ, Cho HK (1990) Edrophonium responsiveness not necessarily diagnostic of myasthenia gravis. Muscle Nerve 13: 187–191

Oh SJ, Danon MJ (1983) Non progressive congenital neuromuscular disease with uniform type 1 fibre Arch Neurol 40: 147–150

Oh SJ, Arnold TW, Park KH et al. (1991a) Electrophysiological improvement following decompression surgery in tarsal tunnel syndrome. Muscle Nerve 14: 407–410

Oh SJ, Claussen GC, Odabasiz et al. (1995) Multifocal demyelinating motor neuropathy: pathological evidence of inflammatory demyelinating polyradiculoneuropathy Neurology 45: 1828–1832

Oh SJ, Kim DE, Kuruoglu R et al. (1992) Diagnostic sensitivity of the laboratory tests in myasthenia gravis. Muscle Nerve 15: 720–724

Oh SJ, Meyers GJ, Wilson ER et al. (1983) A benign form of reducing body myopathy. Muscle Nerve 6: 278–282

Oh SJ, Sarala PK, Kuba T et al. (1979) Tarsal tunnel syndrome: electrophysiological study. Ann Neurol 5: 327–330

Oh SJ, Slaughter R, Hawell L (1991b) Paraneoplastic vasculitic neuropathy: a treatable neuropathy. Muscle Nerve 14: 152–156

Ohama E, Ohara S, Ikuta F et al. (1987) Mitochondrial angiopathy in cerebral blood vessels of mitochondrial encephalomyopathy. Acta Neuropathol 74: 226–233

Ohlendieck K, Campbell KP (1991) Dystrophin constitutes 5% of membrane cytoskeleton in skeletal muscle. FEBS Lett 283: 230–234

Ohlendieck K, Matsumara K, Ionasescu VV et al. (1993) Duchenne muscular dystrophy: deficiency of dystrophin-associated proteins in the sarcolemma. Neurology 43: 795–800

Ohnishi A, Dyck PJ (1974) Loss of small peripheral neurons in Fabry's disease. Histologic and morphometric evaluation of cutaneous nerves, spinal ganglia and posterior columns. Arch Neurol 31: 120–127

Ohnishi A, Schilling K, Brimijoin WS et al. (1977) Lead neuropathy. I. Morphometry, nerve conduction and choline-transference transport. J Neuropathol Exp Neurol 36: 499–518

Ohnishi A, Yamashita Y, Goto I et al. (1979) De- and remyelination, and onion bulbs in cerebrotendinous xanthomatosis. Acta Neuropathol 45: 43–45

Ohno K, Tanaka M, Sahashi K et al. (1991) Mitochondrial DNA deletions in inherited recurrent myoglobinuria. Ann Neurol 29: 364–369

Ohta M, Eleffson RD, Lambert EH et al. (1973) Hereditary sensory neuropathy, Type II. Clinical, electrophysiologic, histologic and biochemical studies of a Quebec kinship. Arch Neurol 29: 23–37

Ohtani Y, Matsuda I, Iwamasa T et al. (1982) Infantile glycogen storage myopathy in a girl with phosphorylase kinase deficiency. Neurology 32: 833–838

Ohtani Y, Miike T, Ishitsu T et al. (1985) A case of malignant hyperthermia with mitochondrial dysfunction. Brain Dev 7: 249–251

Okinaka S, Shizumi K, Iino S et al. (1957) The association of periodic paralysis and hyperthyroidism in Japan. J Clin Endocrinol Metab 17: 1454–1457

Olarte M, Adams D (1977) Accessory nerve palsy. J Neurol Neurosurg Psychiatry 40: 1113–1116

Oldstone MBA, Wilson CG, Perrin LH et al. (1976) Evidence for immune complex formation in patients with amyotrophic lateral sclerosis. Lancet ii: 169–172

O'Leary PA, Waisman M (1946) Dermatomyositis: a study of 50 cases. Arch Dermatol Syph 41: 1001–1014

Olney RK, Wilbourn AJ (1985) Ulnar nerve conduction study of the first dorsal interosseous muscle. Arch Phys Med Rehabil 66: 16–18

Olney RK, Aminoff MJ, Gelb DJ et al. (1988) Neuromuscular effects distant from the site of botulinum neurotoxin injection. Neurology 38: 1780–1783

Olson W, Engel WK, Walsh GO et al. (1972) Oculocraniosomatic neuromuscular disease with "ragged-red fibres". histochemical and ultrastructural changes in limb muscles of a group of patients with idiopathic progressive external ophthalmoplegia. Arch Neurol 26: 193–211

O'Neill JH, Murray NM, Newsom-Davis J (1988) The Lambert-Eaton syndrome: a review of 50 cases. Brain 11: 577–596

Ono S, Nagao K, Yamanchi M (1994) Amorphous material of the skin in amyotrophic lateral sclerosis. Neurology 44: 537–540

Oosterhuis HJGH (1981) Observations of the natural history of myasthenia gravis and of effect of thymectomy. Ann NY Acad Sci 377: 678–690

Oosterhuis HJGH (1983) Myasthenia gravis. Churchill Livingstone, Edinburgh, p 269

Oosterhuis HJGH, Limburg PC, Hummel-Tappel E et al. (1983) Anti-acetylcholine receptor antibodies in myasthenia gravis. II. Clinical and serological followings of individual patients. J Neurol Sci 58: 371–385

Oosterhuis HJGH, Ritsuna RJ, Horst JW (1985) Failure of stapedius reflexometry in the diagnosis of myasthenia gravis. Ann Neurol 18: 519–520

Oppenheimer DR (1976) Diseases of the basal ganglia, cerebellum and motor neurons. In: Blackwood W, Corsellis JAN (eds) Greenfield's neuropathology. Edward Arnold, London, pp 608–651

Oppenheimer DR, Spalding JMK (1973) Late residue of acute idiopathic polyneuritis. J Neurol Neurosurg Psychiatry 36: 978–988

Oram S (1981) Clinical heart disease, 2nd edn. Blackwell Scientific Publications, Oxford, pp 711–747

Oram S, Stokes W (1961) The heart in scleroderma. Br Heart J 23: 243–259

Ørding H, Hedengrau AM, Skøvgaard LT (1991) Evaluation of 119 anaesthetics received after investigation for susceptibility to malignant hyperthermia. Acta Anaesth Scand 35: 711–716

Ormerod IEC, Harding AE, Miller DH (1994) Magnetic resonance imaging in degenerative ataxic disorders. J Neurol Neurosurg Psychiatry 57: 51–57

Ortman JA, Sahenk Z, Mendell JR (1983) The experimental production of Renaut bodies in response to mechanical stress. J Neurol Sci 62: 233–241

Osborn M, Goebel HH (1983) The cytoplasmic bodies in a congenital myopathy can be stained with antibodies to desmin, the muscle-specific intermediate protein. Acta Neuropathol 62: 149–152

Osserman KE (1958) Myasthenia gravis. Grune and Stratton, New York

Osserman KE, Genkins G (1971) Critical reappraisal of the use of edrophonium (Tensilon) chloride test in myasthenia gravis and significance of clinical classification. Ann NY Acad Sci 135: 312–326

Osserman KE, Kaplan LT (1952) Rapid diagnostic test for myasthenia gravis: increased muscular strength without fasciculations, after intravenous administration of edrophonium (Tensilon) chloride. JAMA 150: 265–268

O'Sullivan DJ, McLeod JG (1978) Distal chronic spinal muscular atrophy involving the hands. J Neurol Neurosurg Psychiatry 41: 653–658

Osuntokun BO (1971) Motor nerve conduction in Kwashiorkor (protein-calorie deficiency) before and after treatment. S Afr J Med Sci 2: 109–119

Osuntokun BO (1981) Cassava diet, chronic cyanide intoxication and neuropathy in Nigerian Africans. World Rev Nutr Diet 36: 141–173

Otsuka M, Endo M (1960) The effect of guanidine on neuromuscular transmission. J Pharmacol Exp Ther 128: 273–282

Ouahchi K, Anita M, Kayden IJ et al. (1995) Atresia and isolated vitamin E deficiency is caused by mutations on the α tocopherol transfer protein. Nature Genet 9: 141–145

Ozdemir C, Young RR (1976) The results to be expected from electrical testing in the diagnosis of myasthenia gravis. Ann NY Acad Sci 274: 203–222

Paasuke RT, Brownell AKW (1986) Serum creatine kinase level as a screening test for susceptibility to malignant hyperthermia. JAMA 255: 769–771

Pachman LM, Cooke N (1980) Juvenile dermatomyositis: a clinical and immunologic study. J Pediatr 96: 226–234

Pachman LM, Maryjowski MC (1984) Juvenile dermatomyositis and polymyositis. Clin Rheum Dis 10: 95–115

Pachner AR, Steere AC (1985) The triad of neurologic manifestations of Lyme disease. Neurology 35: 47–53

Packer JW, Foster RR, Garcia A et al. (1972) The humeral fracture with radial nerve palsy: is exploration warranted? Clin Orthop 88: 34–38

Padberg GW, Lunt PW, Koch M et al. (1991) Diagnostic criteria for facio-scapulo-humeral muscular dystrophy. Neuromusc Disord 1: 231–234

Paine RS (1957) Facial paralysis in children. Pediatrics 19: 303–316

Palace J, Wiles CM, Newsom-Davis J (1991) 3–4 diaminopyridine in the treatment of congenital (hereditary) myasthenia. J Neurol Neurosurg Psychiatry 54: 1069

Pallis C, Scott JT (1965) Peripheral neuropathy in rheumatoid arthritis. Br Med J i: 1141–1147

Palmer MS, Dryden AJ, Hughes JT et al. (1991) Homozygous prion protein epitope predisposes to sporadic Creutzfeld-Jakob disease. Nature 352: 340–342

Palmucci L, Doraguzzi C, Mangini T et al. (1992) Dilating cardiomyopathy as the expression of Xp-21 Becker-type muscular dystrophy. J Neurol Sci 111: 218–221

Panayiotopoulos CP (1978) F wave conduction velocity in the deep peroneal nerve: Charcot–Marie–Tooth disease and dystrophia and dystrophia. Muscle Nerve 1: 37–44

Panayiotopoulos CP (1979) F chronodispersion: a new electrophysiological method. Muscle Nerve 2: 68–72

Panayiotopoulos CP, Scarpalezos S (1976) Dystrophia myotonica: peripheral nerve involvement and pathogenetic implications. J Neurol Sci 27: 1–16

Panayiotopoulos CP, Scarpalezos S, Papapetropoulos T (1974) Electrophysiological estimation of motor units in Duchenne muscular dystrophy. J Neurol Sci 23: 89–98

Pancrazio JJ, Oie HK, Kim YK (1992) Voltage sensitive calcium channels in a human small cell lung cancer line. Acta Physiol Scand 144: 463–468

Panegyres PK, Mastaglia FL, Kakulas BA (1990) Limb-girdle syndromes: clinical, morphological and electrophysiological studies. J Neurol Sci 95: 201–218

Panegyres PK, Moore N, Gibson R et al. (1993) Thoracic outlet syndromes and magnetic resonance imaging. Brain 116: 823–841

Pang KA, Schwartz MS (1993) Guillain-Barré syndrome following jellyfish stings (Pelagia noctiluca). J Neurol Neurosurg Psychiatry 56: 1133

Papatestas AE, Genkins G, Horowitz SH et al. (1976) Thymectomy in myasthenia gravis: pathologic, clinical and electrophysiologic correlations. Ann NY Acad Sci 274: 535–543

Papilion JD, Neff RS, Shall LM (1988) Compression neuropathy of the radial nerve as a complication of elbow arthroscopy. Arthroscopy 4: 284–286

Paramesh K, Smith BH, Kalyanaraman K (1975) Early onset myotonic dystrophy in association with polyneuropathy. J Neurol Neurosurg Psychiatry 38: 1136–1139

Parhad IM, Clark AW Barron KD et al. (1978) Diaphragmatic paralysis in motor neuron disease: report of 2 cases and review of the literature. Neurology 28: 18–22

Park HW, Watkins AL (1949) Facial paralysis: analysis of 500 cases. Arch Phys Med Rehabil 30: 749–761

Parks BJ (1973) Post-operative peripheral neuropathies. Surgery 74: 348–357

Parry GJG (1985) Mononeuropathy multiplex. Muscle Nerve 8: 493–498

Parry GJG (1988) Peripheral neuropathies associated with human immunodeficiency virus infection. Ann Neurol 23: 549–553

Parry GJG, Clarke S (1988) Multifocal acquired demyelinating neuropathy masquerading as motor neuron disease. Muscle Nerve 11: 102–107

Parry GJG, Holtz SJ, Ben-Zeev D et al. (1986) Gammopathy with proximal motor axonopathy simulating motor neuron disease. Neurology 36: 273–286

Partanen JV, Nousiainen U (1983) End-plate spikes in electromyography are fusimotor unit potentials. Neurology 33: 1039–1043

Partanen VSJ (1978) Double discharges in neuromuscular diseases. J Neurol Sci 36: 377–382

Partanen VSJ, Lang AH (1982) An analysis of double discharges in the human electromyogram. J Neurol Sci 36: 363–375

Partridge TA (1991) Invited review. Myoblast transfer: a possible therapy for inherited myopathies? Muscle Nerve 14: 197–212

Partridge T (1993) Pathophysiology of muscular dystrophy. Br J Hosp Med 49: 26–36

Partridge TA, Morgan JE, Coulton GR et al. (1989) Conversion of mdx myofibres from dystrophin negative to positive by injection of normal myoblasts. Nature 337: 176–179

Pascuzzi RM, Coslett MB, Johns TR (1983) Long-term corticosteroid treatment of myasthenia gravis: report of 116 patients. Ann Neurol 15: 291–298

Pascuzzi RM, Roos KL, Phillips LH (1986) Granulomatous inflammatory myopathy associated with myasthenia gravis. Arch Neurol 43: 621–623

Patel AN, Swami RK (1969) Muscle percussion and neostigmine test in the clinical evaluation of neuromuscular disorders. N Engl J Med 281: 523–526

Patel H, Berry K, MacLeod P et al. (1983) Cytoplasmic body myopathy: report on a family and review of the literature. J Neurol Sci 60: 281

Patel K, Voit T, Dunn MJ et al. (1988) Dystrophin and nebulin in the muscular dystrophies. J Neurol Sci 87: 315–326

Paterson IS (1962) Generalized myotonia following suxamethonium. Br J Anaesth 34: 340–342

Patrick J, Lindstrom JM (1973) Autoimmune response to acetylcholine receptor. Science 180: 871–872

Patten BM (1975) A hypothesis to account for the Mary Walker phenomenon. Ann Intern Med 82: 411–415

Patten BM (1984) Neuropathy and motor neuron syndromes associated with plasma cell disease. Acta Neurol Scand 70: 47–61

Patten BM, Bilezikian JP, Mallette LE et al. (1974) Neuromuscular disease in primary hyperparathyroidism. Ann Intern Med 80: 182–193

Patten BM, Hart A, Lovelace R (1972) Multiple sclerosis associated with defects in neuromuscular transmission. J Neurol Neurosurg Psychiatry 35: 385–394

Patten BM, Oliver KL, Engel WK (1974) Serotonin-induced muscle weakness. Arch Neurol 31: 347–349

Patten BM, Zito G, Harati Y (1979) Histologic findings in motor neuron disease. Arch Neurol 36: 560–564

Patterson FP, Morton KS (1973) Neurological complication of fractures and dislocations of the pelvis. J Trauma 12: 1013–1023

Patterson VH, Hill TRG, Fletcher PJH et al. (1979) Central core disease: clinical and pathological evidence of progression within a family. Brain 102: 581–594

Paty DW, Campell MJ, Hughes D (1974) Carcinomatous neuromyopathy. II. Immunological studies. J Neurol Neurosurg Psychiatry 37: 142–151

Pavlakis SG, Phillips PC, Di Mauro S et al. (1984) Mitochondrial myopathy, encephalopathy, lactic acidosis and stroke-like episodes – a distinctive clinical syndrome. Ann Neurol 16: 481–488

Pavlides NA, Karsh J, Moutsopoulos HM (1982) The clinical picture of primary Sjögren's syndrome. J Rheumatol 9: 685–690

Pavy FW (1887) Address on diabetes. Washington International Congress. Medical News, Philadelphia, 24 Sept 1887

Pawlikawsska T, Chalder T, Hirsch SR et al. (1994) Population-based study of fatigue and psychological distress. Br Med J 308: 763–766

Payan J (1969) Electrophysiological localization of ulnar nerve lesions. J Neurol Neurosurg Psychiatry 32: 208–220

Payan J (1978) The blanket principle: a technical note. Muscle Nerve 1: 423–426

Payne EE, Spillane JD (1957) The cervical spine: an anatomico-pathological study of 70 specimens with particular reference to the problems of cervical spondylosis. Brain 80: 571–596

Payton OD, Poland JL (1983) Aging process: implications for clinical practice. Phys Ther 63: 41–48

Pearce LR, Wysowski DK, Gross TP (1990) Myopathy and rhabdomyolysis associated with Lovastatin-Gemfibrozil combination therapy. JAMA 264: 71–75

Pearn JH (1973) The gene frequency of acute Werdnig-Hoffman's disease (SMA Type I): a total population survey in north east England. J Med Genet 10: 260–265

Pearn JH (1978) Incidence, prevalence and gene frequency studies of chronic childhood spinal muscular atrophy. J Med Genet 15: 409–413

Pearn JH (1980) Classification of spinal muscular atrophies. Lancet i: 919–921

Pearn JH (1982) Infantile motor neuron diseases. In: Rowland LP (ed) Human motor neuron diseases. Raven Press, New York, pp 121–130

Pearn J, Hudgson P (1979) Distal spinal muscular atrophy. J Neurol Sci 43: 183–191

Pearn JH, Wilson J (1973) Acute Werdnig–Hoffman's disease: acute infantile spinal muscle atrophy. Arch Dis Child 48: 425–530

Pearn JH, Hudgson P, Walton JN (1978) A clinical and genetic study of spinal muscular atrophy of adult onset. Brain 101: 591–606

Pearson CM (1963) Pathology of human muscular dystrophy. In: Bourne GH, Golarz MN (eds) Muscular dystrophy in man and animals. Karger, Basel, pp 1–45

Pearson CM (1964) The periodic paralyses: differential features and pathological observations in permanent myopathic weakness. Brain 87: 341–354

Pearson CM, Bohan A (1977) The spectrum of polymyositis and dermatomyositis. Med Clin North Am 61: 439–457

Pearson CM, Curries S (1974) Polymyositis and related disorders. In Walton JN (ed). Disorders of Voluntary muscle. Churchill Livingstone London, pp 614–652

Pearson J, Pytel BA (1978) Quantitative studies of sympathetic ganglia and spinal cord intermediolateral gray columns in familial dysautonmia. J Neurol Sci 39: 47–59

Pearson J, Budzilovich G, Fringold MJ (1971) Sensory, motor and autonomic dysfunction: The nervous system in familial dysautonomia. Neurology 21: 486–493

Pe Benito R, Sher JH, Cracco JB (1978) Centro nuclear myopathy: clinical and pathologic features. Clin Pediatr 17: 259–265

Pedersen L, Trojaborg W (1981) Visual, auditory and somatosensory pathway involvement in hereditary cerebellar ataxia. Friedreich's ataxia and familial spastic paraplegia. Electroencephalogr Clin Neurophysiol 52: 283–297

Peet RM, Hendricksen JD, Gunderson TP et al. (1956) Thoracic outlet syndrome: evaluation of a therapeutic exercise program. Mayo Clin Proc 31: 281–287

Pellisier JF, Ponget J, Charpin C et al. (1989) Myopathy associated with desmin-type intermediate filaments. J Neurol Sci 89: 49–61

Pellock JM, Behrens M, Lewis L et al. (1989) Kearns–Sayre syndrome and hypoparathyroidism. Ann Neurol 3: 455–458

Pennington RJT (1981) Biochemical aspects of muscle disease. In: Walton JN (ed) Disorders of voluntary muscle, 4th edn. Churchill Livingstone, Edinburgh, pp 417–447

Penrose LS (1948) The problem of anticipation in pedigrees of dystrophia myotonica. Ann Eugen 14: 125–232

Pentland B, Fox KAA (1983) The heart in Friedreich's ataxia. J Neurol Neurosurg Psychiatry 46: 1138–1142

Percy AK, Kaback MM, Herndon RM (1977) Metachromatic leucodystrophy: comparison of early and late onset forms. Neurology 27: 933–941

Perkoff GT (1972) Alcoholic myopathy. Ann Rev Med 22: 125–132

Perkoff GT, Hardy P, Velez-Garcia E (1966) Reversible acute muscular syndrome in chronic alcoholism. N Engl J Med 274: 1277–1285

Perkoff GT, Silber R, Tyler FH et al. (1959) Studies in disorders of muscles. XII. Myopathy due to administration of therapeutic amounts of 17-OH corticosteroids. Am J Med 26: 891–898

Perlo VP. Polkanzer DC, Schwab RS et al. (1966) Myasthenia gravis: evaluation of treatment in 1355 patients. Neurology 16: 431–439

Perlo VP, Shahani BT, Huggins CE et al. (1981) Effect of plasmapheresis in myasthenia gravis. Ann NY Acad Sci 377: 709–724

Perloff JK (1981a) Pathogenesis of hypertrophic cardiomyopathy hypotheses and speculation. Am Heart J 101: 219–226

Perloff JK (1981b) Neurological disorders and heart diseases. In: Braunwald E (ed) Heart disease Saunders, Philadelphia, pp 1803–1845

Perloff JK (1984) Cardiac rhythm and conduction in Duchenne's muscular dystrophy. J Am Coll Cardiol 3: 1263–1267

Perloff JK, de Leon AC, O'Docherty D (1966) The cardiomyopathy of progressive muscular dystrophy. Circulation 33: 625–648

Perloff JK, Roberts WL, de Leon AC et al. (1967) The distinctive electrocardiogram of Duchenne's progressive muscular dystrophy. Am J Med 42: 179–188

Perloff JK, Stevenson WG, Roberts NK et al. (1984) Cardiac involvement in myotonic dystrophy; a prospective study of 25 patients. Am J Cardiol 54: 1074–1081

Pernow BB, Havel RJ, Jennings DB (1967) The second wind phenomenon in McArdle's syndrome. Acta Med Scand 142[Suppl 472]: 294–307

Perry SV (1992) The Xp21 myopathies: current research and the prospect for treatment. Neuromusc Disord 2: 137–141

Perry TL, Krieger C, Hansen S et al. (1991) Amyotrophic lateral sclerosis: fasting levels of cysteine and organic sulfate are normal as are brain contents of cysteine. Neurology 41: 487–490

Pestronk A (1991) Motor neuropathies, motor neuron disorders and antiglycolipid antibodies. Muscle Nerve 14: 927–936

Pestronk A, Drachman DB (1978) A new stain for quantitative measurement of sprouting at neuromuscular junctions. Muscle Nerve 1: 70–74

Pestronk A, Drachman DB (1985) Polymyositis: reduction of acetylcholine receptors in skeletal muscle. Muscle Nerve 8: 233–239

Pestronk A, Chaudhry V, Feldman EL et al. (1990) Lower motor neuron syndromes defined by patterns of weakness, nerve conduction abnormalities and high titers of antiglycolipid antibodies. Ann Neurol 27: 316–326

Pestronk A, Drahman DB, Griffin JW (1980) The effects of aging on sprouting and regeneration. Exp Neurol 70: 65–82

Pestronk A, Drachman DB, Self SG (1985) Measurement of junctional acetylcholine receptors in myasthenia gravis: clinical correlates. Muscle Nerve 8: 245–251

Petajan JH (1991) Motor unit recruitment. Muscle Nerve 14: 489–502 (AAEM minimonograph no. 13.)

Peterson K, Rosenblum MK, Kotanides H et al. (1992) Paraneoplastic cerebellar degeneration. 1. A clinical analysis of 55 anti-Yo antibody positive patients. Neurology 42: 1931–1937

Petty RKH, Duncan R, Jamal GA et al. (1993) Brain stem encephalitis and the Miller Fisher syndrome. J Neurol Neurosurg Psychiatry 56: 201–203

Petty RKH, Harding AE, Morgan-Hughes JA (1986a) The clinical features of mitochondrial myopathy. Brain 109: 915–938

Petty RKH, Thomas PK, Landon DN (1986b) Emery–Dreiffuss syndrome. J Neurol 233: 108–114

Pfister HW, Kristoferitsch W, Skoldenberg B (1993) Therapy of Lyme neuroborreliosis. In: Weber K, Burgdorfer W (eds) Aspects of Lyme borreliosis. Springer, Berlin Heidelberg New York, pp 328–339

Pfister HW, Wilske B, Weber K (1994) Lyme borreliosis: basic science and clinical aspects. Lancet 343: 1013–1016

Phalen GS (1966) The carpal tunnel syndrome: 17 years experience in diagnosis and treatment of 654 hands. J Bone Joint Surg [Am] 48: 211–228

Phalen GS (1972) The carpal tunnel syndrome: clinical evaluation of 598 hands. Clin Orthop 83: 29–40

Phillips MS, Steward S, Anderson JR (1984) Neuropathological findings in Miller-Fisher syndrome. J Neurol Neurosurg Psychiatry 47: 492–495

Phillips OC, Ebner H, Nelson AT et al. (1969) Neurologic complications following spinal anaesthesia with lidocaine: a prospective review of 10,440 cases. Anaesthesiology 30: 289

Philpot J, Sewry CA, Pennock J et al. (1995) Clinical phenotype in congenital muscular dystrophy correlation with expression of merosin in skeletal muscle Neuromusc Dis 35: 301–305

Pickett JB III (1988) Botulism. Muscle Nerve 11: 1201–1205 (AAEE Case Report no. 16.)

Pickett JB, Schmidley JW (1980) Sputtering positive potentials in the EMG: an artefact resembling positive waves. Neurology 30: 215–218

Pickett JBE, Layzer RB, Levin SR et al. (1975) Neuromuscular complications of acromegaly. Neurology 25: 638–645

Pierach CA (1982) Haematin therapy for the acute porphyric attack. Semin Liver Dis 2: 125–128

Pierobon-Bormioli S, Armani M, et al. (1985) Familial neuromuscular disease with tubular aggregates. Muscle Nerve 8: 291–294

Pierobon-Bormioli S, Sartore S, Dalla Libera L et al. (1981) "Fast" isomyosins and fiber types in mammalian skeletal muscle. J Histochem Cytochem 29: 1179–1188

Pillay PK, Russell WG, Wilbourn AJ et al. (1988) Solitary primary lymphoma of the sciatic nerve. Neurosurgery 23: 370–371

Pimstone N, Marine N, Pimstone B (1968) Beta-adrenergic blockade in thyrotoxic myopathy Lancet ii: 1219–1220

Pinching AJ, Peters DK, Newsom-Davis J (1976) Remission of myasthenia gravis following plasma exchange. Lancet ii: 1373–1376

Pinelli P, Arrigo A, Moglia A (1975) Myasthenic decrement and myasthenic myopathy: a study of the effects of thymectomy. J Neurol Neurosurg Psychiatry 38: 525–532

Piper H (1909) Weitere Mitteilungen über die Geschwindigkeit der Enrugungsleitung im markhaltigen menschlichen Nerven. Pflugers Arch Ges Physiol 127: 474–480

Pirart J (1978) Diabetes mellitus and its degenerative complications: a prospective study of 4400 patients observed between 1947 and 1973. Diabetes Care 1: 168–188, 252–263

Pirskanen R (1977) Genetic aspects of myasthenia gravis: a family study of 264 Finnish patients. Acta Neurol Scand 56: 365–388

Pirskanen R, Tillikainen A, Hokkanen E (1972) Histocompability (HLA) antigens associated with myasthenia gravis. Ann Clin Res 4: 304–306

Pitkeathley DA, Cromes EN (1966) Polymyositis in rheumatoid disease. Ann Rheum Dis 25: 127–132

Pittman JG, Decker JW (1971) Acute and chronic myopathy associated with alcoholism. Neurology 21: 293–296

Pleasure DE (1975) A-beta lipoproteinaemia and Tangier disease. In: Dyck PJ, Thomas PK, Lambert EH (eds) Peripheral neuropathy, vol 2. Saunders, Philadelphia, pp 928–941

Pleasure DE, Feldman B, Prokop DJ (1973) Diphtheria toxin inhibits the synthesis of myelin proteolipid and basic proteins by peripheral nerve in vitro. J Neurochem 20: 81

Pleasure DE, Walsh GO, Engel WK (1970) Atrophy of skeletal muscles in patients with Cushing's syndrome. Arch Neurol 22: 118–125

Pleasure DE, Wyszynski B, Sumner D et al. (1979) Skeletal muscle calcium metabolism and contractile force in vitamin D deficient chicks. J Clin Invest 64: 1157–1167

Plotz PH, Dalakas M, Leff RL et al. (1989) Current concepts in the idiopathic inflammatory myopathies: polymyositis, dermatomyositis and related disorders. Ann Intern Med 111: 143–154

Plowman PN, Stableforth DE (1977) Dermatomyositis with fibrosing alveolitis: response to treatment with cyclophosphamide. Prod R Soc Med 70: 738–740

Poewe W, Willeit H, Sluga E et al. (1985) The rigid spine syndrome – a myopathy of uncertain nosological position. J Neurol Neurosurg Psychiatry 48: 887–893

Polans AS, Buczylko J, Crabb J et al. (1991) A photoreceptor calcium-binding protein is recognised by autoantibodies obtained from patients with cancer-associated retinopathy. J Cell Biol 112: 981–989

Polgar JG, Bradley WG, Upton ARM et al. (1972) The early detection of dystrophia myotonica. Brain 95: 761–776

Polgar J, Johnson MA, Weightman D et al. (1973) Data on fibre size in 36 human muscles. J Neurol Sci 19: 307–318

Pollard JD, McLeod JG, Angel Honnibal TG et al. (1982) Hypothyroid polyneuropathy: clinical, electrophysiological and nerve biopsy findings in two cases. J Neurol Sci 53: 461–471

Pollock M, Nukada H, Frith RW et al. (1983a) Peripheral neuropathy in Tangier disease. Brain 106: 911–928

Pollock M, Nukada H, Taylor P et al. (1983b) Comparison between fascicular and whole sural nerve biopsy. Ann Neurol 13: 65–68

Polson MJR, Barker AT, Freeston IL (1982) Stimulation of nerve trunks with time-varying magnetic fields. Med Biol Eng Comp 20: 243–244

Pons F, Léger JOC, Chevrallay M et al. (1986) Immunocytochemical analysis of myosin heavy chains in human fetal skeletal muscles. J Neurol Sci 76: 151–163

Ponsford SN (1988) Sensory conduction in medial and lateral plantar nerves. J Neurol Neurosurg Psychiatry 51: 188–191

Porter GA, Dmytrenko GK, Winkelmann JC et al. (1992) Dystrophin colocalises with spectrin in distinct subsarcolemmal domains in mammalian skeletal muscle. J Cell Biol 117: 997–1005

Portwood MM, Wicks JJ, Leiberman JS et al. (1986) Intellectual and cognitive function in adults with myotonic muscular dystrophy. Arch Phys Med Rehabil 67: 299–303

Posas HN, Rivner MH, Meador KJ (1990) Stimulation single fiber EMG abnormalities induced by megadose thiamine. Muscle Nerve 13: 879

Poskanzer DC, Kerr DNS (1961) A third type of periodic paralysis with normokalaemia and favourable response to sodium chloride. Am J Med 31: 328–342

Poskanzer DC, Cantor HM, Kaplan GS (1969) The frequency of preceding poliomyelitis in amyotrophic lateral sclerosis. In: Norris FH, Karland LT (eds) Motor neuron diseases. Grune & Stratton, New York, p 286

Poulos A, Pollard AC, Mitchell JD et al. (1984) Pattern of Refsum's disease. Arch Dis Child 59: 222–229

Poulton J (1996) New genetics of mitochondrial DNA diseases. Br J Hosp Med 55: 712–716

Poulton J, Deadman ME, Bindoff L et al. (1993) Families of mtDNA rearrangements can be detected in patients with mtDNA deletions Hum Mol Genet 2: 23–30

Pourmand R, Saunders DB, Corwin HM (1983) Late onset McArdle's disease with unusual electromyographic features. Arch Neurol 40: 374–377

Prasher D, Smith A, Findlay L (1990) Sensory and cognitive event-related potentials in myalgic encephalomyelitis. J Neurol Neurosurg Psychiatry 53: 247–253

Pratt H, Starr A (1981) Mechanically and electrically evoked somatosensory potentials in humans: scalp and neck distributions of short latency components. Electroencephalogr Clin Neurophysiol 51: 138–147

Pratt H, Amlie RN, Starr A (1979a) Short-latency mechanically evoked somatosensory potentials in humans. Electroencephalogr Clin Neurophysiol 47: 524–531

Pratt H, Starr A, Amlie RN et al. (1979b) Mechanically and electrically evoked somatosensory potentials in normal humans. Neurology 29: 1236-1244

Prelle A, Moggio M, Comi GP et al. (1992) Congenital myopathy associated with abnormal accumulation of desmin and dystrophin. Neuromusc Disord 2: 169-175

Preston DC, Logigian EL (1992) Lumbrical and interossei recording in carpal tunnel syndrome. Muscle Nerve 15: 1253-1257

Pridmore C, Baraitser M, Brett EM et al. (1992) Distal spinal muscular atrophy with vocal cord paralysis. J Med Genet 29: 197-199

Prier S, Gibbert C, Bodros A et al. (1979) Neurophysiological changes in non-vaccinated rabies patients. Lancet i: 620

Prineas J (1970) Peripheral nerve changes in thiamine-deficient rats. Arch Neurol 23: 541-548

Prineas JW (1981) Pathology of the Guillain-Barré syndrome. Ann Neurol 9: S6-S19

Prineas JW, McLeod JG (1976) Chronic relapsing polyneuritis. J Neurol Sci 27: 427-458

Prineas J, Hall R, Barwick DD et al. (1968) Myopathy associated with pigmentation following adrenalectomy for Cushing's syndrome. QJM 37: 63-77

Prineas JW, Mason AS, Henson RA (1965) Myopathy in metabolic bone disease. Br Med J i: 1034-1036

Propp RP, Means E, Deibel R et al. (1975) Waldenströms macroglobulinaemia and neuropathy: deposition of M component of myelin sheaths. Neurology 25: 980-988

Prusiner SB (1982) Novel proteinaceous infection particles cause scrapie. Science 215: 136-144

Prusiner SB (1991) Molecular biology of prion diseases. Science 252: 1515-1522

Pruzanski W (1966) Variants of myotonic dystrophy in preadolescent life (the syndrome of myotonic dysembryoplasia). Brain 89: 563-568

Pryse-Phillips WEM (1984) Validation of a diagnostic sign in carpal tunnel syndrome. J Neurol Neurosurg Psychiatry 47: 870-872

Pryse-Phillips W, Johnson GJ, Larsen B (1982) Incomplete manifestations of myotonic dystrophy in a large kinship in Labrador. Ann Neurol 11: 582-591

Ptacek LJ, Johnson KJ, Griggs RC (1993) Genetics and physiology of the myotonic muscle disorders. N Engl J Med 328: 482-489

Ptacek LJ, Tawil R, Griggs RC et al. (1992) Linkage of atypical myotonia congenita to a sodium channel locus. Neurology 42: 431-433

Ptacek LJ, Tawil R, Griggs RC et al. (1994a) Sodium channel mutations in acetazolamide-responsive myotonia congenita, paramyotonia congenita, and hyperkalaemic periodic paralysis. Neurology 44: 1500-1503

Ptacek LJ, Tawil R, Griggs RC et al. (1994b) Dihydropyridine receptor mutations cause hypokalaemic periodic paralysis. Cell 77: 863-868

Pullen H, Doig A, Lambie AT (1967) Intensive intravenous potassium replacement therapy. Lancet ii: 809-811

Pumplin DW, Reese TS, Llinas R (1981) Are the pre-synaptic membrane particles calcium channels? Proc Natl Acad Sci USA 78: 7201-7213

Puvanendran K, Cheah JS, Naganathan N et al. (1979a) Thyrotoxic myopathy: a clinical and quantitative analytic electromyographic study. J Neurol Sci 42: 441-451

Puvanendran K, Cheah JS, Naganathan N et al. (1979b) Neuromuscular transmission in thyrotoxocosis. J Neurol Sci 43: 47-57

Quadiri MR, Church SE, McColl KEL et al. (1986) Chester porphyria: a clinical study of anew form of acute porphyria. Br Med J 292: 455-459

Quane KA, Healy JMS, Keating KE et al. (1993) Mutations in the ryanodine receptor gene in central core disease and malignant hyperthermia. Nature (Genet) 5: 51-55

Quick DT (1969) Pancreatic dysfunction in amyotrophic lateral sclerosis. In: Norris FH, Kurland LT (eds) Motor neuron diseases. Grune & Stratton, New York, pp 189-198

Quick DT, Greer M (1966) Pancreatic dysfunction in amyotrophic lateral sclerosis. Neurology 17: 112-116

Quinlivan RM, Dubowitz V (1992) Cardiac transplantation in Becker muscular dystrophy. Neuromusc Dis 2: 165-167

Rabinbach A (1991) The human motor: energy, fatigue and the origins of modernity. Basic Books, New York

Rabizadeh S, Gralla EB, Borchelt DR et al. (1995) Mutations associated with amyotrophic lateral sclerosis convert superoxide dismutase from an antiapoptotic gene to a proapoptotic gene; studies in yeast and neural cells. Proc Natl Acad Sci USA 92: 3024-3028

Radu EW, Skarpil V, Kaeser HE (1975) Facial myokymia. Eur Neurol 13: 499-512

Raff MC, Asbury AK (1968) Ischaemic mononeuropathy and mononeuropathy multiplex in diabetes mellitus. N Engl J Med 279: 17-22

Raff MC, Sangalong V, Asbury AK (1968) Ischaemic mononeuropathy multiplex associated with diabetes mellitus. Arch Neurol 18: 487-499

Rail D, Stark R, Sirash M et al. (1980) Improvement in nerve conduction after plasma exchange for Guillain-Barré syndrome. J Neurol Neurosurg Psychiatry 43: 1147

Ramanathan J, Sibai BM, Pillai R et al. (1988) Neuromuscular transmission studies in pre-eclamptic women receiving magnesium sulphate. Am J Obst Gynecol 158: 40-46

Ramsay A (1986) Post-viral fatigue syndrome: the saga of Royal Free Disease. Gower Medical Publications, London

Ramsay ID (1965) Electromyography in thyrotoxicosis. QJM 34: 255-267

Ramsay ID (1966) Muscle dysfunction in hyperthyroidism. Lancet ii: 931-935

Ramsay ID (1974) Thyroid disease and muscle dysfunction. Year Book, Chicago

Ramsay RB, McGowry JD, Fischer VW et al. (1978) Alteration of developing and adult rat muscle membranes by zuclomiphene and other hypocholesterolemic agents. Acta Neuropathol (Berl) 44: 15-19

Ranvier L (1873) Propriétés et structures différentes des muscles rouges et des muscles blancs chez les lapins et chez les raies. CR Hebd Séances Acad Sci (Paris) 77: 1030-1035

Rao SN, Katiyar BC, Nair KRP et al. (1980) Neuromuscular status in hypothyroidism. Acta Neurol Scand 61: 167-177

Rao VR (1971) Muscle function in thyroid disease. Leda Press, Kakinada, India

Rappaport L, Coutard F, Samuel JL et al. (1988) Storage of phosphorylated desmin in a familial myopathy. FEBS Lett 231: 421-425

Raskin NH, Fishman RA (1969) Pyridoxine deficiency neuropathy due to hydralazine. N Engl J Med 273: 1182-1185

Rasminsky M (1985) Conduction in normal and pathological nerve fibres. In: Swash M, Kennard C (eds) Scientific basis of clinical neurology. Churchill Livingstone, Edinburgh, pp 390-399

Raukler E, Fletcher R, Krantz P (1985) Malignant hyperpyrexia and sudden death. Am J Forensic Med Pathol 6: 149-153

Ravits J, Hallett M, Baker M et al. (1990) Clinical and electromyographic studies of post poliomyelitis muscular atrophy. Muscle Nerve 13: 667-674

Rayman G, Hassan A. Tooke JE (1986) Blood flow in the skin of the foot related to posture in diabetes mellitus. Br Med J 292: 87-90

Read D, Warlow C (1978) Peripheral neuropathy and solitary plasmacytoma. J Neurol Neurosurg Psychiatry 41: 177-184

Rebouche CJ, Engel AG (1983) Carnitine metabolism and deficiency syndromes. Mayo Clin Proc 58: 533-540

Read DJ, Feest TG, Nassim MA (1981) Clonazepam: effective treatment for restless legs syndrome in uraemia. Br Med J 283: 885–886

Redmond JNT, McKenna MJ, Feingold M et al. (1992) Sensory testing versus nerve conduction velocity in diabetic polyneuropathy. Muscle Nerve 15: 1334–1339

Reeback J, Benton S, Swash M et al. (1979) Penicillamine-induced neuromyotonia. Br Med J i: 1464–1465

Reed DM, Kurland LT (1963) Muscle fasciculations in a healthy population. Arch Neurol 9: 363–367

Reed RJ, Bliss BO (1973) Morton's neuroma: regressive and productive intermetatarsal elastofibroma. Arch Pathol Lab Med 95: 123–129

Rees JH, Soudain SE, Gregson NA et al. (1995) *Campylobacter jejuni* infection and Guillain–Barré syndrome. N Eng J Med 333: 1374–1379

Reeves WC, Griggs RC, Nanda NC et al. (1980) Echocardiographic evaluation of cardiac abnormalities in Duchenne's dystrophy and myotonic muscular dystrophy. Arch Neurol 37: 273–277

Refsum S (1946) Heredopathia atactica polyneuritiformis: a familial syndrome not hitherto described. Acta Psychiatr Scand [Suppl] 38: 1–303

Refsum S (1981) Heredopathia atactica polyneuritiformis: phytanic acid storage disease (Refsum's disease): a biochemical well-defined disease with a specific dietary treatment. Arch Neurol 38: 605–606

Refsum S (1984) Heredopathia atactica polyneuritiformis (Refsum disease). In: Dyck PJ, Thomas PK, Lambert EH, Bunge R (eds) Peripheral neuropathy, vol 2. Saunders, Philadelphia, pp 1680–1703

Refsum S, Lonnum A. Sjaastad D et al. (1967) Dystrophia myotonica: repeated pneumoencephalographic studies in ten patients. Neurology 17: 345–348

Regan TJ (1973) Alcoholic cardiomyopathy. In: Fowler NG (ed) Myocardial disease. Grune and Stratton, New York

Reilly MM, King RHM (1993) Familial amyloid polyneuropathy. Brain Pathology 3: 165–170

Reimers CD, Schedel H Fleckenstein JL et al. (1994) Magnetic resonance imaging of skeletal muscles in idiopathic inflammatory myopathies of adults. J Neurol 241: 306–314

Reinstein L (1981) Hand dominance in carpal tunnel syndrome. Arch Phys Med Rehabil 62: 202–203

Reinstein L, Ostrow SS, Wiernik PH (1980) Peripheral neuropathy after cis-platinum (II) (DDP) therapy. Arch Phys Med Rehab 61: 280–282

Reiss GK, Desmoulin F, Martin CF et al. (1991) In vitro correlation between force and energy metabolism in porcine hyperthermic muscle studied by ^{31}P NMR. Arch Biochem Physiol 287: 312

Reitan J, Pape E, Fossa SD et al. (1980) Osteosclerotic myeloma with polyneuropathy. Acta Med Scand 208: 137–144

Remen L (1932) Zur Pathogenese und Therapie der Myasthenia Gravis psuedoparalytica. Dtsch Z Nervenheil 128: 66–78

Remlinger P (1928) Les paralysies du traitement antirabique. Ann Inst Pasteur 42: 71–78

Rennels GD, Ochoa J (1980) Neuralgic amyotrophy manifesting as anterior interosseous nerve palsy. Muscle Nerve 3: 160–164

Rennie MJ, Edwards RHT, Milward DJ et al. (1982) Effect of Duchenne muscular dystrophy on muscle protein synthesis. Nature 296: 165–167

Renwick D, Chandraker A, Bannister P (1992) Missed neuroleptic malignant syndrome. Br Med J 304: 831–832

Resnik JS, Engel WK (1967) Myotonic lid-lag in hypokalaemic periodic paralysis J Neurol Neurosurg Psychiatry 30: 47–51

Resnick JS, Dorman JD, Engel WK (1969) Thyrotoxic periodic paralysis. Am J Med 47: 831–836

Reuther P, Fulpius BW, Mertens HG et al. (1979) Anti-acetylcholine receptor antibody under long-term azathioprine treatment in myasthenia gravis. In: Dau PC (ed) Plasmapheresis and the immunobiology of myasthenia gravis. Houghton-Mifflin, Boston, pp 329–342

Reyes MG, Goldberg H, Fesco K et al. (1987) Zebra body myopathy. J Child Neurol 2: 307

Reyes MG, Norowha P, Thomas WJr et al. (1983) Myositis of chronic graft versus host disease. Neurology 33: 1222–1224

Reznik M (1973) Current concepts of skeletal muscle regeneration. In: Pearson CM (ed) The striated muscle. Williams and Wilkins, Baltimore, pp 185–225

Reznik M, Engel WK (1970) Ultrastructural and histochemical correlations of experimental muscle regeneration. J Neurol Sci 11: 167–185

Reznik M, Hansen JL (1969) Mitochondria in degenerating and regenerating skeletal muscle. Arch Pathol 57: 601–608

Rhodes KM, Tattersfield AE (1982) Guillain–Barré syndrome associated with campylobacter infection. Br Med J 285: 173–174

Riche P (1897) Le nerf anbitale et les muscles de l'eminence thenar. Bull Mem Soc (Anat) Paris 5: 251

Richter RB (1954) Peripheral neuropathy and connective tissue disease. J Neuropathol Exp Neurol 13: 168–180

Rickards D, Isherwood I, Hutchinson R et al. (1982) Computed tomography in dystrophia myotonica. Neuroradiology 24: 27–31

Ricker K, Mertens HG (1968) The differential diagnosis of the myogenic (facio-) scapulo-peroneal syndrome. Eur Neurol 1: 275–307

Ricker K, Camacho L, Grafe P et al. (1989) Adynamia episodica hereditaria: what causes the weakness? Muscle Nerve 12: 883–891

Ricker K, Herte G, Stokieck S (1977) Influence of temperature on neuromuscular transmission in myasthenia gravis. J Neurol 216: 273–282

Ricker K, Koch MC, Lehmann-Horn F et al. (1994) Proximal myotonic myopathy: a new dominant disorder with myotonia, muscle weakness and cataracts. Neurology 44: 1448–1452

Ricker K, Koch MC, Lehmann-Horn F et al. (1995) Proximal myotonic myopathy Arch Neurol 52: 25–31

Ricker K, Lehmann-Horn F, Moxley R (1990) Myotonia fluctuans. Arch Neurol 47: 268–272

Ricker K, Moxley RT (III), Heine R et al. (1994) Myotonia fluctuans: a third type of muscle sodium channel disease. Arch Neurol 51: 1095–1102

Ricker K, Moxley RT, Rohkamm R (1989) Rippling muscle disease. Arch Neurol 46: 405–408

Ricker K, Rohkamm R, Böhlen R (1986) Adynamia episodica and paralysis periodica paramyotonica. Neurology 36: 682–686

Riddoch D, Morgan-Hughes JP (1975) Prognosis in adult polymyositis. J Neurol Sci 26: 71–80

Rideau Y, Glorion B, Delanbier A et al. (1984) The treatment of scoliosis in Duchenne muscular dystrophy. Muscle Nerve 7: 281–286

Rideau Y, Jankowski LW, Grellet J (1981) Respiratory function in the muscular dystrophies. Muscle Nerve 4: 155–164

Ridley A (1969) The neuropathy of acute intermittent porphyria QJM 38: 307–333

Ridley A (1975) Porphyric neuropathy. In: Dyck PJ, Thomas PK, Lambert EH (eds) Peripheral neuropathy, vol 2. Saunders, Philadelphia, pp 942–955

Ridley A, Cavanagh JB (1972) Exercise as a factor in the neuropathy of porphyria. Lancet ii: 87–88

Ridley DS (1969) Reactions in leprosy. Lepr Rev 40: 77–81

Rietschel M, Rudnik-Schoneberg S, Zerres K (1992) Clinical variability of autosomal dominant spinal muscular atrophy. J Neurol Sci 107: 65–73

Riley CM, Moore RH (1966) Familial dysautonomia differentiated from related disorders: case reports and discussions of current concepts. Pediatrics 37: 435–446

Riley CM, Day RL, Greely DM et al. (1949) Central autonomic dysfunction with defective lacrimation. I. Report of 5 cases. Pediatrics 3: 468–478

Rimma NA, Cork LC (1993) Alterations in neurofilament mRNA in hereditary canine spinal muscular atrophy. Lab Invest 69: 436–442

Ringel SP, Bender AN, Engel WK (1976) Extrajunctional acetylcholine receptors: alterations in human and experimental neuromuscular diseases. Arch Neurol 33: 751–758

Ringel SP, Carrole JE, Schold C (1977) The spectrum of mild X-linked recessive muscular dystrophy. Arch Neurol 34: 408–416

Ringel SP, Kenny CE, Neville HE et al. (1987) Spectrum of inclusion body myositis. Arch Neurol 44: 1154–1157

Ringel SP, Murphy JR, Alderson K et al. (1993) The natural history of amyotrophic lateral sclerosis. Neurology 43: 1316–1322

Ringel SP, Neville HE, Duster MC et al. (1978) A new congenital neuromuscular disease with trilaminar muscle fibers. Neurology 28: 282–289

Ringel SP, Thorne G, Phanupak P et al. (1979) Immune complex vasculitis, polymyositis and hyperglobulinemic purpura. Neurology 29: 682–689

Risk WS, Bosch EP, Kimura J et al. (1981) Chronic tetanus: clinical report and histochemistry of muscle. Muscle Nerve 4: 363–366

Rives KL, Furth ED, Becker DV (1965) Limitations of the ankle jerk test: intercomparison with other tests of thyroid function. Ann Intern Med 62: 1139–1146

Roa BB Garcia CA, Suter V et al. (1993) Charcot–Marie–Tooth type 1a: association with a spontaneous point mutation in the PMP22 gene. N Engl J Med 329: 96–101

Robb SA, Fielder AHL, Saunders CE et al. (1988) C4 complement allotypes in juvenile dermatomyositis. Hum Immunol 22: 31–38

Roberts AH, Bamforth J (1968) The pharynx and esophagus in ocular muscular dystrophy. Neurology 18: 645–652

Roberts CJ (1990) Single fibre EMG in the chronic fatigue syndrome. J Neurol Sci 98: Suppl 97.

Roberts M, Willison H, Vincent A et al. (1994) Serum factor in the Miller Fisher variant of Guillain–Barré syndrome and neurotransmitter release. Lancet 343: 454–455

Roberts M, Willison HJ, Vincent A et al. (1995) Multifocal motor neuropathy: human sera block distal motor conduction in mice. Ann Neurol 38: 111–118

Roberts NK (1981) The prevalence of conduction defects and cardiac arrhythmias in progressive systemic sclerosis. Ann Intern Med 94: 38–40

Roberts RG, Bobrow M, Bentley DR (1992) Point mutations in the dystrophin gene. Proc Natl Acad Sci USA 89: 2331–2335

Robillard RB, Hilsinger RL, Adour KK (1986) Ramsay Hunt facial paralysis: clinical analysis of 185 patients. Otolaryngol Head Neck Surg 95: 292–297

Robinson DR (1947) Pyriformis syndrome in relation to sciatic pain. Am J Surg 73: 355–358

Robson JS (1968) Uraemic neuropathy. In: Robertson RF (ed) Symposium: Some aspects of neurology. Royal College of Physicians of Edinburgh, Edinburgh pp 74–84

Roden DM, Woosley RL (1986) Drug therapy: tocainide. N Engl J Med 315: 41–45

Roelofs RI, Engel WK, Chanvin PB (1972) Histochemical phosphorylase activity in regenerating muscle fibers from myophosphorylase-deficient patients. Science 177: 795–797

Roelofs RI, Hrushesky W, Rogin J et al. (1984) Peripheral sensory neuropathy and cisplatin chemotherapy. Neurology 34: 934–938

Roessler KM, Hess CW, Schmidt UD (1989) Investigation of facial motor pathways by electrical and magnetic stimulation: sites and mechanism of excitation. J Neurol Neurosurg Psychiatry 52: 1149–1156

Rohkamm R Boxler K, Ricker K et al. (1983) A dominantly inherited myopathy with excessive tubular aggregates. Neurology 33: 331–336

Roisen F, Bartfeld H, Donenfeld D et al. (1982) Neuron-specific in vitro cytotoxicity of sera from patients with amyotrophic lateral sclerosis. Muscle Nerve 5: 48–53

Rolleston JD (1925) Acute infectious diseases. Heinemann, London

Román GC, Spencer PS, Schoenberg BS (1985) Tropical myeloneuropathies: the hidden endemics. Neurology 35: 1158–1170

Romero NB, Nivoche Y, Lunardi J et al. (1993) Malignant hyperthermia and central core disease: analysis of two families with heterogenous clinical expression. Neuromusc Disord 3: 547–551

Ronnevi L-O, Conradi S, Karlsson E (1984) Cytotoxic effect of immunoglobulins in amyotrophic lateral sclerosis (ALS). Acta Neurol Scand 69 [Suppl 98]: 181–183

Roos RP, Viola MV, Wallmann R et al. (1980) Amyotrophic lateral sclerosis with antecedent poliomyelitis. Arch Neurol 37: 312–313

Ropert A, Metral S (1990) Conduction block in neuropathies with necrotizing vasculitis. Muscle Nerve 13: 102–105

Ropes MW (1976) Systemic lupus erythematosis. Harvard University Press. Cambridge, Mass

Ropper AH (1986) Unusual clinical variants and signs in Guillain–Barré syndrome. Arch Neurol 43: 1150–1152

Ropper AH (1992) The Guillain–Barré syndrome. N Engl J Med 326: 1130–1136

Ropper AH, Marmaron A (1984) Mechanism of pseudotumour in Guillain–Barré syndrome. Arch Neurol 41: 259–261

Ropper AH, Shahani BT (1983) Proposed mechanism of ataxia in Fisher syndrome. Arch Neurol 40: 537–538

Ropper AH, Shahani BT (1984) Diagnosis and management of acute areflexic paralysis with emphasis on Guillain–Barré syndrome. In: Asbury AK, Gilliatt RW (eds) Peripheral nerve disorders. Butterworth, London, pp 21–45

Ropper AH, Albers WJ, Addison R (1988) Limited relapse in Guillain–Barré syndrome after plasma exchange. Arch Neurol 45: 314–315

Ropper AH, Wijdicks EFM, Shahani BT (1990) Electrodiagnostic changes in early Guillain–Barré syndrome: a prospective study in 113 patients. Arch Neurol 47: 881–887

Ropper AH, Wijdicks EFM, Truax BT (1991) Guillain–Barré syndrome. Davis, Philadelphia.

Rosati G, Pinna L, Granieri E et al. (1977) Studies on epidemiological, clinical and etiological aspects of ALS disease in Sardinia, Southern Italy. Acta Neurol Scand 55: 231–244

Rose AL, Walton JN (1966) Polymyositis: a survey of 89 cases with particular reference to treatment and prognosis. Brain 89: 747–768

Rose AL, Willison RG (1967) Quantitative electromyography using automatic analysis: studies in healthy subjects and patients with primary muscle disease. J Neurol Neurosurg Psychiatry 30: 403–410

Rosen DR, Siddique T, Patterson D et al. (1993) Mutations in Cu-Zn superoxide dismutase gene are associated with familial amyotrophic lateral sclerosis. Nature 362: 59–62

Rosen I (1984) Neurophysiological aspects of organic solvent toxicity. Acta Neurol Scand 70 [Suppl 100]: 101–106

Rosen I, Werner CO (1980) Neurophysiological investigation of posterior interosseous nerve entrapment causing lateral elbow pain (abstract). Electroencephalogr Clin Neurophysiol 50: 125

Rosen I, Haeger-Aronsen B, Rhenstrom S et al. (1978) Neurophysiological observations after chronic styrene exposure. Scand J Work Environ Health 4 [Suppl 2]: 104–105

Rosenberg NL, Neville HE, Ringel SP (1985) Tubular aggregates: their association with neuromuscular diseases including the syndrome of myalgia/cramps. Ann Neurol 42: 973

Rosenberg NL, Rotbart HA, Abzug MJ et al. (1989) Evidence for a novel picorna virus in human dermatomyositis. Ann Neurol 26: 204–209

Rosenberg RN (1982) Amyotrophy in multisystem genetic diseases. In: Rowland LP (ed) Human motor neuron diseases. Raven Press, New York, pp 149–158

Rosenberg RN (1994) Mitochondria in evolution and disease. J Child Neurol 9: 1–3

Rosenberg RN, Lovelace RE (1968) Mononeuritis multiplex in lepromatous leprosy. Arch Neurol 19: 310–314

Rosenblum JL, Leating JP, Prensky AL et al. (1981) A progressive neurologic syndrome in children with chronic liver disease. N Engl J Med 304: 503–508

Rosenfalck P (1969) Intra and extracellular potential fields of active nerve and muscle fibres. Acta Physiol Scand [Suppl] 321: 1–168

Rosenfalck P (1975) Electromyography. Sensory and motor conductions: findings in normal subjects. Laboratory of Clinical neurophysiology, Rikshospitalet, Copenhagen

Rosenow EC, Engel AG (1978) Acid maltase deficiency in adults presenting as respiratory failure. Am J Med 64: 485–491

Roses AD, Pericak-Vance MA, Yamaoka LH et al. (1983) Recombinant DNA strategies in genetic neurological diseases. Muscle Nerve 6: 339–355

Rosing HS, Hopkins LC, Wallace DC et al. (1985) Maternally inherited mitochondrial myopathy and myoclonic epilepsy. Ann Neurol 17: 228–237

Rosman NP, Kakulas BA (1966) Mental deficiency associated with muscular dystrophy: a neuropathological study. Brain 89: 769–787

Ross BD, Radda GK, Godian DG et al. (1981) Examination of a case of suspected McArdle's syndrome by ^{31}P nuclear magnetic resonance. N Engl J Med 304: 1338–1342

Ross DR, Varipapa RJ (1989) Treatment of painful diabetic neuropathy with capsaicin. N Engl J Med 321: 474–475

Ross JS, Masaryk TJ, Schraeder M et al. (1990) MR imaging of the post-operative lumbar spine. AJNR 11: 771–776

Roth G (1982) The origin of fasciculations. Ann Neurol 12: 542–547

Roth G (1984) Fasciculations and their F response. J Neurol Sci 63: 299–306

Roth G (1985) Mid motor axonal re-excitation in human peripheral nerve. Electromyogr Clin Neurophysiol 25: 401–411

Rothig H-J, Bernhardt W, Afting E-G (1984) Excretion of total and muscular N^T- methylhistidine and creatinine in muscle disease. Muscle Nerve 7: 374–379

Rothrock JF, Johnson PC, Rothrock SM et al. (1984) Fulminant polyneuritis after overdose of disulfiram and ethanol. Neurology 34: 357–359

Rothstein J, Martin IJ, Kuncl RW (1992) Decreased glutonate transport by the brain and spinal cord in ALS. N Engl J Med 326: 1464–1468

Rothstein JD, van Kammen M, Levey AT et al. (1995) Selective loss of glial glutamate transporter GLT-1 in amyotrophic lateral sclerosis. Ann Neurol 38: 73–84

Rothstein TL, Carlson CB, Sumi SM (1971) Polymyositis with facio-scapulo-humeral distribution. Arch Neurol 25: 313–319

Rotthauwe HW, Kowaleweski S, Mumenthaler M (1969) Congenitale Muskeldystrophie. Z Kinderheilk 106: 131–162

Rotthauwe HW, Martier W, Beyer H (1972) Neuer Typ einer recessiv X-chromosomal verebten Muskeldystrophie: scapulo-humero-distale Muskeldystrophie mit frühzeitigen Kontrakturen und Herzrhythmusstörungen. Humangenetik 16: 181–200

Rouleau G, Karpati G, Carpenter S et al. (1987) Glucocorticoid excess induces preferential depletion of myosin in denervated skeletal muscle fibres. Muscle Nerve 10: 428–438

Round JM, Jones DA, Edwards RHT (1982) A flexible microprocessor system for the measurement of cell sizes. J Clin Pathol 35: 620–624

Roussy G, Lévy G (1926) Sept cas d'une maladie familiale particuliere: trouble de la march pieds bots et aréflexie tendineuse généralisé avec accessoirement, légère maladresse des mains. Rev Neurol 1: 427–450

Rowland LP (1980a) Biochemistry of muscle membranes in Duchenne muscular dystrophy. Muscle Nerve 3: 3–20

Rowland LP (1980b) Controversies about the treatment of myasthenia gravis. J Neurol Neurosurg Psychiatry 43: 644–659

Rowland LP (1984) Myoglobinuria. Can J Neurol Sci 11: 1–13

Rowland LP (1992a) Amyotrophic lateral sclerosis and auto immunity. N Engl J Med 327: 1752–1753

Rowland LP (1992b) Progressive external ophthalmoplegia and ocular myopathies. In: Rowland LP, Di Mauro S (eds) Handbook of clinical neurology, vol 62. Elsevier, Amsterdam, pp 287–329

Rowland LP (1994a) Mitochondrial encephalomyopathies: lumping, splitting and melding. In: Schapira AHV, Di Mauro S (eds) Mitochondrial disorders in neurology. Butterworth-Heinemann, Oxford, pp 116–129

Rowland LP (1994b) Riluzole for amyotrophic lateral sclerosis: too soon to tell. N Engl J Med 330: 636–637

Rowland LP, Layzer RB (1975) Muscular dystrophies, atrophies and related diseases. In: Baker AB, Baker LH (eds) Clinical neurology, vol 3. Harper & Row, New York

Rowland LP, Penn AS (1972) Myoglobinuria. Med Clin North Am 56: 1233–1256

Rowland LP, Blake DM, Hirano M et al. (1991) Clinical syndromes associated with ragged-red fibres. Rev Neurol 147: 467–473

Rowland LP, Clarke C, Olarte M (1977) Therapy for dermatomyositis and polymyositis. In: Griggs RC, Moxley RT (III) (eds) Advances in neurology, vol 17. Raven Press, New York

Rowland LP, Defendiui R, Sherman W et al. (1982) Macroglobulinemia with peripheral neuropathy simulating motor neuron disease. Ann Neurol 11: 532–536

Rowland LP, Fahn S, Schotland DL (1963) McArdle's disease. Arch Neurol 9: 325–342

Rowland LP, Hoefer PFA, Aranow H(Jr) et al. (1956) Fatalities in myasthenia gravis. Neurology 6: 306–326

Roy N, Mahadevan MS, McLean M et al. (1995) The gene for neuronal apoptosis inhibitary protein is partially deleted in individuals with spinal muscular atrophy. Cell 80: 167–178

Rubenstein AE, Horowitz SH, Bender AN (1979) Cholinergic dysautonomia and Eaton-Lambert syndrome. Neurology 29: 720–723

Rubenstein AE, Weinapel SF (1977) Acute hypokalaemic myopathy in alcoholism: a clinical entity. Arch Neurol 34: 553–555

Rubin E (1979) Alcoholic myopathy in heart and skeletal muscle. N Engl J Med 301: 28–33

Rubin E, Katz AM, Lieber C et al. (1976) Muscle damage produced by chronic alcohol consumption Am J Physiol 83: 499–516

Rubin RH, Hattwick MAW, Jones S et al. (1973) Adverse reaction to duck embryo rabies vaccine. Arch Intern Med 78: 643–647

Rubinstein LJ (1960) Ageing changes in muscle. In: Bourne GH (ed) Structure and function of muscle, vol 3. Academic Press, London, pp 209–226

Rüdel R, Lehmann-Horn F (1985) Membrane changes in myotonia. Physiol Rev 65: 310–356

Rüdel R, Dengler R, Ricker K et al. (1980) Improved therapy of myotonia with the lidocaine derivative tocainide. J Neurol 222: 275–278

Rüdel R, Ruppersberg JP, Spittelmeister W (1989) Abnormalities of the fast sodium current in myotonic dystrophy, recessive, generalised myotonia and adynamia episodica. Muscle Nerve 12: 281–286

Rudge P (1974) Tourniquet paralysis with prolonged conduction block. J Bone Joint Surg [Br] 56: 716–720

Rudge P, Ochoa J, Gilliatt RW (1974) Acute peripheral nerve compression in the baboon. J Neurol Sci 23: 403–420

Rudnicki S, Vriesendorp F, Koski CL et al. (1992) Electrophysiologic studies in the Guillain–Barré syndrome: effects of plasma exchange and antibody rebound. Muscle Nerve 15: 57–62

Rudolph JA, Spier SJ, Byrns G et al. (1992) Periodic paralysis in quarter horses: a sodium channel mutation disseminated by selective breeding. Nature Genet 2: 144–147

Ruff RL, Martyn D, Gordon AL (1982) Glucocorticoid-induced atrophy is not due to impaired excitability in rat muscle. Am J Physiol 243: E512

Rukavina JG, Block WD, Jackson CE et al. (1956) Primary systemic amyloidosis. Medicine (Baltimore) 35: 239–334

Rundles RW (1945) Diabetic neuropathy: general review with report of 125 cases. Medicine (Baltimore) 24: 111

Russell AS, Lindstrom JM (1978) Penicillamine-induced myasthenia gravis associated with antibodies to acetylcholine receptor. Neurology 28: 847–849

Russell DS (1953) Histological changes in the striped muscles in myasthenia gravis. J Pathol 65: 279–289

Russell WR (1952) Poliomyelitis. Edward Arnold, London, p 84

Sabin TD, Swift TR (1975) Leprosy. In: Dyck PJ, Thomas PK, Lambert EH (eds) Peripheral neuropathy, vol 2. Saunders, Philadelphia, pp 1166–1198

Sabin TD, Hackett ER, Brand PW (1974) Temperatures along the course of certain nerves affected in leprosy. Int J Lepr 42: 38–42

Sabina RL, Fishbein WN, Pezeshkpour G et al. (1992) Molecular analysis of the myoadenylate deaminase deficiencies. Neurology 42: 170–179

Sabina RL, Morisaki T, Clarke P et al. (1990) Characterisation of the human and rat myoadenylate deaminase genes. J Biol Chem 265: 9423–9433

Sabina RL, Swain JL, Holmes EW (1989) Myoadenylate deaminase deficiency. In: Scriber C, Beaudet AL, Sly WS, Valle D (eds) The metabolic basis of inherited disease. McGraw-Hill, New York, pp 1077–1084

Sachdev KK, Taori GM, Pereira SM (1971) Neuromuscular states in protein-calorie malnutrition. Neurology 21: 801–805

Sachs JA (1979) The relevance of HLA antigens in some neurological disorders. In: Rose FC (ed) Clinical neuroimmunology. Blackwell Scientific Publications, Oxford, pp 42–52

Sack GH, Cork LC, Morris JM et al. (1984) Autosomal dominant inheritance of hereditary canine spinal muscular atrophy. Ann Neurol 15: 369–393

Sadowsky CH, Sacks E, Ochoa J (1976) Post-radiation motor neuron syndrome. Arch Neurol 33: 786–787

Sagawa M (1970) Clinical studies of congenital muscular dystrophy. Brain Dev 2: 439–451

Sahgal V, Sahgal S (1977) A new congenital myopathy. Acta Neuropathol 37: 225–230

Said G (1978) Perhexiline neuropathy: a clinicopathological study. Ann Neurol 3: 259–266

Said G, Ropert A, Faux N (1984) Length-dependent degeneration of fibres in Portuguese amyloid polyneuropathy. Neurology 34: 1025–1032

Said G, Slama G, Selva J (1983) Progressive centripetal degeneration of axons in small fibre diabetic polyneuropathy. Brain 106: 791–807

Saida T, Saida K, Lisak RP et al. (1982) In vivo demyelinating activity of sera from patients with Guillain–Barré syndrome. Ann Neurol 11: 69–75

Sakoda S, Shanske S, Di Mauro S et al. (1988) Isolation of acDNA encoding the B isoenzyme of human phosphoglycerate mutase (PGAM) and characterization of the PGAM gene family. J Biol Chem 263: 16899–16905

Sakuta R, Nonaka I (1989) Vascular involvement in mitochondrial myopathy. Ann Neurol 25: 594–601

Salazar AM (1982) Discussion. In: Rowland LP (ed) Human motor neuron diseases. Raven Press, New York, pp 179–180

Salih MAM, Omer MIA, Biyoumi RA et al. (1983) Severe autosomal recessive muscular dystrophy in an extended Sudanese kindred. Dev Med Child Neurol 25: 43–52

Salisachs P (1982) Ataxia and other data reviewed in Charcot-Marie-Tooth and Refsum's disease. J Neurol Neurosurg Psychiatry 45: 1085–1091

Salmon MA, Esiri MM, Ruderman NB (1971) Myopathic disorder associated with mitochondrial abnormalities, hyperglycaemia and hyperketonaemia. Lancet ii: 290–293

Salmons S, Henriksson J (1981) The adaptive response of skeletal muscle to increased use. Muscle Nerve 4: 94–105

Saltin B, Nazar K, Costill DL et al. (1976) The nature of the training response: peripheral and central adaptations to one-legged exercise. Acta Physiol Scand 96: 289–305

Salviati G, Pierobon-Bormioli S, Betto R et al. (1985) Tubular aggregates: sarcoplasmic reticulum origin, calcium storage ability and functional implications. Muscle Nerve 8: 299–305

Samaha FJ, Gergely J (1969) Biochemical abnormalities of sarcoplasmic reticulum in muscular dystrophy. N Engl J Med 280: 184–188

Samaha FJ, Schroeder JM, Rebeiz JJ et al. (1967) Studies on myotonia: biochemical and electron microscope studies on myotonia congenita and myotonia dystrophica. Arch Neurol 17: 22–33

Samanta A, Burden AC (1985) Painful diabetic neuropathy. Lancet i: 348–349

Sander JE, Sharp FR (1981) Lumbosacral plexus neuritis. Neurology 31: 470–473

Sanders DB, Howard JF (1986) Single fibre EMG in myasthenia gravis. Muscle Nerve 9: 809–819 (AAEE minimonograph no. 25)

Sanders DB, Howard JF Jr, Johns TR (1979) Single fibre electromyography in myasthenia gravis. Neurology 29: 68–76

Sanders EA, Peters AC, Gratana JW et al. (1987) Guillain–Barré syndrome after Varicella zoster infection. J Neurol 234: 437–440

Sanders KA, Rowland LP, Younger DS et al. (1993) Motor neuron diseases and ALS: GM_1 antibodies and paraproteinemia. Neurology 43: 418–420

Sandro S, Novarro C, Fernandez JM et al. (1990) Skin biopsy findings in glycogenosis III. Ann Neurol 27: 480–486

Sandstedt P (1981) Effects of a previous electromyographic examination studied by frequency analysis, muscle biopsy and creatine kinase. Acta Neurol Scand 64: 303–309

Sandstedt P, Henriksson K-G, Larsson L-E (1982a) Quantitative electromyography in polymyositis and dermatomyositis – a long-term study. Acta Neurol Scand 65: 110–121

Sandstedt P, Nordell LE, Henriksson K-G (1982b) Quantitative analysis of muscle biopsies from volunteers and patients with neuromuscular disorders. Acta Neurol Scand 66: 130–144

Sanes JR (1987) Cell lineage and the origin of muscle fibre types. Trends in Neurological Sciences 10: 463–466

Santa T, Engel AG, Lambert EH (1972) Histometric study of neuromuscular junction. I. Myasthenia gravis. Neurology 22: 71–82

Sanyal SK, Johnson WW, Dische MR et al. (1980) Dystrophic degeneration of papillar muscle and ventricular myocardium; a structural basis for mitral valve prolapse in Duchenne's muscular dystrophy. Circulation 62: 430–439

Sargeant AJ, Davies CTM, Edwards RHT et al. (1977) Functional and structural changes after disuse of human muscle. Clin Sci Mol Med 52: 337–342

Saraiva MJM, Costa PP, Goodman DS (1993) Transthyretin and familial amyloidotic polyneuropathy. In: Rosenberg RN, Prusiner SB, Di Mauro S, Barchi RL, Kunkel LM (eds) The molecular and genetic basis of neurological disease. Butterworth, Boston, pp 889–894

Sarnat HB (1990) Myotubular myopathy: arrest of morpho-genesis of myofibers associated with persistence of fetal vimentin and desmin. Can J Neurol Sci 17: 109–123

Sarnat HB (1993) Does increased desmin in myofibres constitute a storage disease? Neuromusc Disord 3: 3–4

Sasaski T, Shikura K, Sugai K et al. (1989) Muscle histochemistry in myotubular (centronuclear) myopathy. Brain Dev 11: 26–32

Sato T, Walker DL, Peters HA et al. (1971) Chronic polymyositis and myxovirus-like inclusions: electron microscopic and viral studies. Arch Neurol 24: 409–418

Satoyoshi E, Kinoshita M (1970) Some aspects of thyrotoxic and steroid myopathy. In: Walton JN, Canal N, Scarlato G (eds) Muscle diseases. Excerpta Medica, Amsterdam, pp 454–463 (ICS 199)

Sauron B, Bouche P, Cathala HP et al. (1984) Miller-Fisher's syndrome: clinical and electrophysiologic evidence of peripheral origin in 10 cases. Neurology 34: 953–956

Savage DCL, Forbes M, Pearce GW (1971) Idiopathic rhabdo-myolysis. Arch Dis Child 46: 594–607

Savage G (1875) Overwork as a cause of insanity. Lancet ii: 127

Savazzi GM, Migone L, Cambi V (1980) The influence of glo-merular filtration rate on uremic polyneuropathy. Clin Nephrol 13: 64–72

Savino PJ, Sergott RC, Bosley TM et al. (1985) Hemifacial spasm treated with botulinum toxin A injection. Arch Opthalmol 103: 1305–1306

Sayeed ZA, Velmurugendran CU, Arjunds G et al. (1975) Anterior horn cell disease seen in South India. J Neurol Sci 26: 484–498

Scadding GK, Vincent A, Newsom-Davis J et al. (1981) Acetyl-choline receptor antibody synthesis by thymic lymphocytes: correlation with thymic histology. Neurology 31: 935–943

Scappetta C, Vaccario ML, Casali C et al. (1984) Distal muscular dystrophy with autosomal recessive inheritance. Muscle Nerve 7: 478–481

Scarlato G, Spinnler H (1967) La miopatica ipotiroidea. Systema Nerv 19: 96

Schapira AHV, Di Mauro S (1994) Mitochondrial disorders in neurology. Butterworth-Heinemann, London, p 254

Schapira AHV, Thomas PK (1986) A case of recurrent idiopathic opthalmoplegic neuropathy (Miller Fisher syndrome). J Neurol Neurosurg Psychiatry 49: 463–464

Schapira D, Swash M (1985) Neonatal spinal muscular atrophy presenting as respiratory distress: a clinical variant. Muscle Nerve 8: 661–663

Schatz G (1991) The mitochondrial protein import machinery. In: Sato T, Di Mauro S (eds) Mitochondrial encephalomy-opathies. Raven, New York, pp 57–74

Schaumberg HH, Spencer PS (1984) Human toxic neuropathy due to industrial agents. In: Dyck PJ, Thomas PK, Lambert EH, Bunge R (eds) Peripheral neuropathy. Saunders, Philadelphia, pp 2115–2132

Schaumberg HH, Kaplan J, Windebank A et al. (1983a) Sensory neuropathy from pyridoxine abuse – a new megavitamin syn-drome. N Engl J Med 309: 445–448

Schaumberg HH, Spencer PS, Thomas PK (1983b) Disorders of peripheral nerves. FA Davies, Philadelphia, pp 145–146

Schedel H, Reimers CD, Naegele M et al. (1992) Imaging tech-niques in myotonic dystrophy. Eur J Radiol 15: 230–238

Schielker E, Pfister HW, Einhaupl KM (1989) Peripheral facial nerve palsy associated with HIV infection. Lancet i: 553

Schiffer D, Brignolio F, Chio A et al. (1986) Clinico-anatomic study of a family with bulbo-spinal muscular atrophy in adults. J Neurol Sci 73: 11–22

Schiller HH, Mair WGP (1974) Ultrastructural changes of muscle in malignant hyperthermia. J Neurol Sci 21: 93–100

Schiller HH, Stålberg E (1976) Human botulism studied with single fibre electromyography. Arch Neurol 35: 346–349

Schiller JH, Jones JC (1993) Paraneoplastic syndromes associated with lung cancer. Curr Opin Oncol 5: 335–342

Schimseiden RJ, Onjerboen de Vision BM, Kemp B (1985) The flexor carpi radialis H reflex in lesions of the sixth and seventh cervical roots. J Neurol Neurosurg Psychiatry 48: 445–449

Schmalbruch H (1976) Muscle fibre splitting and regeneration in diseased human muscle. Neuropathol Appl Neurobiol 2: 3–20

Schmalbruch H (1992) The muscular dystrophies. In: Mastaglia FL, Lord Walton (eds) Skeletal muscle pathology, 2nd edn. Churchill Livingstone, Edinburgh, pp 283–318

Schmalbruch H, Hellhammer V (1976) The number of satellite cells in normal human muscle. Anat Rec 185: 279–288

Schmalbruch H, Jensen HJ, Bjaerg M et al. (1991) A new mouse mutant with progressive motor neuronopathy. J Neuropathol Exp Neurol 50: 192–197

Schmalbruch H, Kamienecka Z, Arroc M (1987) Early fatal nema-line myopathy: case report and review. Dev Med Child Neurol 29: 800–804

Schmid R, Mahler R (1959) Chronic progressive myopathy with myoglobinuria: demonstration of a glycogenolytic defect in the muscle. J Clin Invest 38: 2044–2058

Schmidt B, Servidei S. Gabbai AA et al. (1987) McArdle's disease in two generations: autosomal recessive transmission with manifesting heterozygote. Neurology 37: 1558–1561

Schmidt-Achert M, Fischer P, Pongratz D (1992) Myocardial evidence of dystrophin mosaic in a Duchenne muscular dys-trophy carrier. Lancet 340: 1235–1236

Schmitt H-P, Krause KH (1981) An autopsy study of a familial oculo-pharyngeal muscular dystrophy (OPMD) with distal spread and neurogenic involvement. Muscle Nerve 4: 296–305

Schmitt H-P, Volk B (1975) The relationship between target, targetoid and targetoid-core fibres in severe neurogenic mus-cular atrophy. J Neurol 210: 167–181

Schneiderman LJ, Sampson WI, Schoene WC et al. (1969) Genetic studies of a family with two unusual autosomal dominant conditions, muscular dystrophy and Pelger–Huet anomaly. Am J Med 46: 380–393

Schoene WC, Asbury AK, Åstrom KE et al. (1970) Hereditary sensory neuropathy. J Neurol Sci 11: 463–472

Scholte HR, Jennekens FGI, Bouvy JJBJ (1979) Carnitine palm-itoyl transferase II deficiency with normal carnitine palmitoyl transferase I in skeletal muscle and leucocytes. J Neurol Sci 40: 39–51

Scholz W (1925) Klinische, pathologisch-anatomische und erbiologische Untersuchungen bei familiarer Hirnsklerose im kindersalter. Z Ges Neurol Psychiatr 99: 651

Schotland DL, Bonilla E, Wakayama Y (1979) Pathogenesis of muscle cell damage in the dystrophies: morphologic aspects including freeze-fracture studies. In: Aguayo AJ, Karpati G (eds) Current topics in nerve and muscle research. Excerpta Medica, Amsterdam, pp 29–37

Schotland DL, Bonilla E, Wakayama Y (1980) Application of the freeze-fracture technique to the study of human neuromuscu-lar disease. Muscle Nerve 3: 21–27

Schotland DL, Di Mauro S, Bonilla E et al. (1976) Neuromuscular disorder associated with a defect in mitochondrial energy supply. Arch Neurol 33: 475–479

Schott GD, Wills MR (1975) Myopathy in hypophosphataemic osteomalacia presenting in adult life. J Neurol Neurosurg Psychiatry 38: 297–304

Schott GD, Wills MR (1976) Muscle weakness in osteomalacia. Lancet i: 626–629

Schott K, Koenig E (1991) T-wave response in cervical root lesions. Acta Neurol Scand 84: 273–276

Schraeder PL, Peters HA, Dahl DS (1972) Polymyositis and pena-cillamine. Arch Neurol 27: 456–457

Schröder JM (1993) Neuropathy associated with mitochondrial disorders. Brain Pathol 3: 177–190

Schröder JM, Adams RD (1968) The ultrastructural morphology of the muscle fiber in myotonic dystrophy. Acta Neuropathol (Berl) 10: 218–241

Schröder JM, Becker PE (1972) Anomalien des T systems und des sarkoplasmitischen Reticulums beider Myotonie, Paramyotonie und Adynamie. Virchows Arch [Path Anat] 357: 319–344

Schultze FR (1895) Beiträge zur Muskelpathologies. Dtsch Z Nervenheilk 6: 65

Schumm F, Stöhr M (1984) Accessory nerve stimulation in the assessment of myasthenia gravis. Muscle Nerve 7: 147–151

Schumm F, Weithölter H, Fatch-Moghadam A et al. (1985) Thymectomy in myasthenia with pure ocular symptoms. J Neurol Neurosurg Psychiatry 48: 332–337

Schwab RS, Leland CC (1953) Sex and age in myasthenia gravis as critical factors in incidence and remissions. JAMA 153: 1270–1273

Schwartz JF, Rowland LP, Eder H et al. (1963) Bassen–Kornzweig syndrome: deficiency of serum beta lipoprotein. Arch Neurol 8: 438–454

Schwartz JP, Breakfield XO (1980) Altered nerve growth faster in fibroblasts from patients with familial dysautonomia. Proc Natl Acad Sci (USA) 77: 1154–1158

Schwartz L, Rockoff MA, Koka BV (1984) Masseter spasm with anaesthesia: incidence and implications. Anesthesiology 61: 772–775

Schwartz MS, Moosa A (1977) Sensory nerve conduction in spinal muscular atrophy. Dev Med Child Neurol 19: 50–53

Schwartz MS, Stålberg E (1975a) Single fibre electromyographic studies in myasthenia gravis with repetitive nerve stimulation. J Neurol Neurosurg Psychiatry 38: 678–682

Schwartz MS, Stålberg E (1975b) Myasthenia gravis with features of the myasthenic syndrome. Neurology 25: 80–84

Schwartz MS, Stålberg E (1975c) Myasthenic syndrome studied with single fibre electromyography. Arch Neurol 32: 815–817

Schwartz MS, Swash M (1975) Scapulo-peroneal atrophy with sensory involvement: Davidenkow's syndrome. J Neurol Neurosurg Psychiatry 38: 1063–1067

Schwartz MS, Swash M (1982) Pattern of involvement in the cervical segments in the early stage of motor neuron disease: a single fibre EMG study. Acta Neurol Scand 65: 424–431 (see Swash M, Schwartz MS [1991])

Schwartz MS, Gordon JA, Swash M (1980a) Slowed nerve conduction with wrist flexion in carpal tunnel syndrome. Ann Neurol 8: 69–71

Schwartz MS, Mackworth-Young CG, McKeran RO (1983) The tarsal tunnel syndrome in hypothyroidism. J Neurol Neurosurg Psychiatry 46: 440–442

Schwartz MS, Moosa A, Dubowitz V (1977a) Correlation of single fibre EMG and muscle histochemistry using an open biopsy recording technique. J Neurol Sci 31: 369–378

Schwartz MS, Sargeant M, Swash M (1976a) Longitudinal fibre splitting in neurogenic muscular disorders: its relation to the pathogenesis of "myopathic" change. Brain 99: 617–636

Schwartz MS, Sargeant MK, Swash M (1977b) Neostigmine-induced end-plate proliferation in the rat. Neurology 27: 289–293

Schwartz MS, Stålberg E, Schiller H et al. (1976b) The reinnervated motor unit in man. J Neurol Sci 27: 303–312

Schwartz MS, Stålberg E, Swash M (1980b) Pattern of segmental motor involvement in syringomyelia: a single fibre EMG study. J Neurol Neurosurg Psychiatry 43: 150–155

Schwartz MS, Swash M, Gross M (1978) Benign post-infection polymyositis. Br Med J ii: 1256–1257

Schwartz MS, Swash M, Ingram DA et al. (1988) Patterns of selective involvement of thigh muscles in neuromuscular disease. Muscle Nerve 11: 1240–1245

Schwartz O, Jampel RS (1962) Congenital blepharophimosis associated with a unique generalised myopathy. Arch Ophthalmol 68: 52–57

Schwartzman WA, Lampertis MS, Kennedy CA et al. (1991) Staphylococcal pyomyositis in patients infected by the human immunodeficiency virus. Am J Med 90: 595–600

Schwimmbeck PL, Dyrberg T, Drachman DB et al. (1989) Molecular mimicry and myasthenia gravis. J Clin Invest 84: 1174–1180

Scott JM, Weir DG (1981) The methyl folate trap. Lancet ii: 337–340

Scott JM, Wilson P, Dinn JJ et al. (1981) Pathogenesis of subacute combined degeneration: a result of methyl group deficiency. Lancet ii: 334–337

Scott OM, Hyde SA, Goddard C et al. (1982) Quantitation of muscle function in children: a prospective study in Duchenne muscular dystrophy. Muscle Nerve 5: 291–301

Seay AR, Ziter FA, Hill HR (1978) Defective neutrophil function in myotonic dystrophy. J Neurol Sci 35: 25–30

Sebille A, Gray F (1979) Electromyographic recording and muscle biopsy in lepromatous leprosy. J Neurol Sci 40: 3–10

Sedal L. McLeod JG, Walsh JC (1973) Ulnar nerve lesions associated with the carpal tunnel syndrome. J Neurol Neurosurg Psychiatry 36: 118–123

Seddon HJ (1943) Three types of nerve injury. Brain 66: 237–288

Segal AW, Peters TJ (1976) Characterisation of the enzyme defect in chronic granulomatous disease. Lancet 1: 1363–1364

Segura RP, Petajan JH (1979) Neural hyperexcitability in hyperkalaemic periodic paralysis. Muscle Nerve 2: 245–249

Segura RP. Sahgal V (1981) Hemiplegic atrophy: electrophysiological and morphological studies. Muscle Nerve 4: 246–248

Seigel RS, Seeger JF, Gabrielsen TO et al. (1979) Computerised tomography in oculo-craniosomatic disease (Kearns–Sayre syndrome). Radiology 130: 159–164

Seiler D, Fiehn W, Kuhn E (1975) Disturbances in cholesterol biosynthesis as a cause of experimental myotonia. In: Bradley WG, Gardner-Medwin D, Walton JN (eds) Recent advances in myology. Excerpta Medica, Amsterdam, pp 429–433

Senanayake N, Johnson NK (1982) Acute polyneuropathy after poisoning by a new organophosphate insecticide. N Engl J Med 306: 155–157

Selby RC (1974) Neurosurgical aspects of leprosy – Surg Neurol 2: 165–177

Seppalainen AM, Hernberg S, Kock B (1979) Relationship between blood lead levels and nerve conduction velocities. Neurotoxicology 1: 313–332

Seppalainen AM, Lindstrom K. Martelin T (1980) Neurophysiological and psychological picture of solvent poisoning. Ann J Ind Med 1: 31–42

Serratrice G, Pellisier JF (1987) Les myopathies oculaires; études nosologiques en 48 cas. Presse Med 16: 1969–1974

Serratrice G, Gastaut JL, Dubois-Gambenelli D (1973) Amyotrophie necrogene périphique au cours du syndrome de Maninesco-Sjojren. Rev Neurol 128: 432–441

Serratrice G, Pellissier JF, Cros D (1978a) Les atteintes musculaires des ostéomalacies: étude clinique, histoenzymologiques et ultrastructurales de 10 cas. Rev Rheumat 45: 621–626

Serratrice G, Pellissier JF, Faugere MC et al. (1978b) Centronuclear myopathy: possible central nervous system origin. Muscle Nerve 1: 62–69

Serratrice G, Pellissier JF, Ponget J et al. (1982) Les syndromes scapulo-peronieres. Rev Neurol 138: 691–711

Serratrice G, Pellissier JF, Roux H et al. (1990) Fasciitis, perimyositis, myositis, polymyositis and eosinophilia. Muscle Nerve 13: 385–395

Serratrice G, Roux H, Aquaron R et al. (1969) Myopathie scapulo-peronières. Sem Hôp (Paris) 45: 2678–2683

Serratrice G, Salaman G, Jiddane M et al. (1985) Résultats du scanner X musculaire dans 145 cas de maladies neuromusculaires. Rev Neurol 141: 404–412

Servo C, Palo J, Pikanën E (1977) Polyols in the cerebrospinal fluid and plasma of neurological, diabetic and uraemic patients. Acta Neurol Scand 56: 111–116

Seybold NE, Drachman DB (1974) Gradually increasing doses of prednisone in myasthenia gravis. N Engl J Med 290: 81–84

Seybold NE, Lindstrom JM (1979) Serial anti Ach receptors antibody titres in patients with myasthenia gravis: effects of steroid therapy In Dow PC (ed) Plasmapheresis and the Immunobiology of myasthenia gravis Houghton Mifflin, Boston, 307–314

Sghirlanzoni A, Peluchetti D, Montegazza R et al. (1984) Myasthenia gravis: prolonged treatment with steroids. Neurology 34: 170–174

Shafiq SA, Dubowitz V, Petersen H de C et al. (1967) Nemaline myopathy: report of a fatal case with histochemical and electron microscopical studies. Brain 90: 817–828

Shafiq SA, Gorycki MA, Asiedu SA et al. (1969) Tenotomy: effect on the fine structure of the soleus of the rat. Arch Neurol 20: 625–633

Shah AJ, Sahgal V, Muschler G et al. (1982) Morphogenesis of the mitochondrial alterations in muscle diseases. J Neurol Sci 55: 25–37

Shahani BT (1970) The human blink reflex. J Neurol Neurosurg Psychiatry 33: 792–800

Shahani BT (1985) Modern approach to nerve conduction studies. In: Delwaide PJ, Gorio A (eds) Clinical neurophysiology in peripheral neuropathies. Elsevier, Amsterdam, pp 103–124

Shahani BT, Russell WR (1969) Motor neuron disease: an abnormality of nerve metabolism. J Neurol Neurosurg Psychiatry 32: 1–5

Shahani BT, Goodgold J, Spielholtz NI (1967) Sensory nerve action potential in the radial nerve. Arch Phys Med Rehabil 48: 602–607

Shahani BT, Halperin JJ, Boulu P et al. (1984) Sympathetic skin response. J Neurol Neurosurg Psychiatry 47: 536–542

Shahani M, Dastur FD, Dastoor DH et al. (1979) Neuropathy in tetanus. J Neurol Sci 43: 173–182

Shalanski ML, Wisniewski H (1969) Neurofibrillary degeneration induced by vincristine neuropathy. Arch Neurol 20: 199–206

Shanske S, Moraes CT, Lombes A et al. (1990) Widespread tissue distribution of mitochondrial DNA deletions in Kearns–Sayre syndrome. Neurology 40: 24–28

Shapira Y, Harel S, Russel A (1977) Mitochondrial encephalomyopathies: a group of neuromuscular disorders with defects in oxidative metabolism. Isr J Med Sci 13: 161–164

Shapiro F, Bresnan MJ (1982) Orthopedic management of childhood neuromuscular disease. II. Peripheral neuropathies. Friedreich's ataxia, and arthrogryposis multiplex congenita. J Bone Joint Surg [Am] 64: 949–953

Shapiro F, Specht LA (1991) Orthopedic deformities in Emery-Dreifuss muscular dystrophy. J Pediatr Orthop 11: 336–340

Sharief MK, Hentges R, Liardi M (1991) Intrathecal immune response in patients with the post-polio syndrome. N Engl J Med 325: 749–755

Sharma AK, Thomas PK (1974) Peripheral nerve structure and function in experimental diabetes. J Neurol Sci 23: 1–15

Sharma KR, Minhier MA, Miller RG (1993) Cyclosporin increases muscular force generation in Duchenne muscular dystrophy. Neurology 43: 527–532

Sharp GC (1981) Mixed connective tissue disease and overlap syndromes. In: Kelly WN, Harris ED Jr, Ruddy S, Sledge P (eds) Textbook of rheumatology. Saunders, Philadelphia, pp 1151–1161

Sharp GC, Irvine WS, Tan EM et al. (1972) Mixed connective tissue disease: apparently distinct rheumatic disease syndrome associated with a specific antibody to an extratable nuclear antigen (ENA). Am J Med 52: 148–159

Sharpe MC, Archard LC, Banatrala JE et al. (1991) Chronic fatigue syndrome: guidelines for research. J R Soc Med 84: 118–122

Sharrard WJW (1964) The segmental innervation of the lower limb muscles in man. Ann R Coll Surg Engl 35: 106–122

Shaunak S, Aug L, Colston K et al. (1987) Muscle strength in healthy white and Asian subjects. Clin Sci 73: 541–546

Shaw DJ, Meredith AL, Sarfarazi M et al. (1985) The apolipoprotein C11 gene: subchromosomal localisation and linkage to the myotonic dystrophy locus. Hum Genet 70: 271–273

Shaw PJ (1994) Excitotoxicity and motor neurone disease: a review of the evidence. J Neurol Sci 124: S6–S13

Shea JD, McClain EJ (1969) Ulnar nerve compression syndromes at and below the wrist. J Bone Joint Surg [Am] 51: 1095–1103

Shelbourne P, Davies J, Buxton J et al. (1993) Direct diagnosis of myotonic dystrophy with a disease specific DNA marker. N Engl J Med 328: 471–475

Shellock FG, Fokunaga T, Mink JH et al. (1991) Acute effects of exercise on MR imaging of skeletal muscle and concentric and eccentric actions. AJR 156: 765–768

Shepherd JJ (1983) Tropical myositis: is it an entity and what is its cause? Lancet ii: 1240–1242

Sher E, Canal N, Piccolo G et al. (1989) Specificity of calcium channel auto antibodies in Lambert-Eaton myasthenic syndrome. Lancet ii: 640–643

Sher JH, Rimalovski AB, Athanassiades TJ et al. (1967) Familial centronuclear myopathy: a clinical and pathological study. Neurology 17: 727–742

Sher JH, Shafiq SA, Schutta HS (1979) Acute myopathy with selective lysis of myosin filaments. Neurology 29: 100–106

Sheramata W, Kott S, Cyr DP (1971) The Chediak-Higashi-Steinbrinck syndrome. Arch Neurol 25: 289–294

Sheth KJ, Swick HM (1980) Peripheral nerve conduction in Fabry's disease. Ann Neurol 7: 319–323

Shields RW (1984) Single fiber electromyography in the differential diagnosis of myopathic limb girdle syndromes and chronic spinal muscular atrophy. Muscle Nerve 7: 265–272

Shields RW (1986) Limb-girdle syndromes. In: Engel AG, Banker BQ (eds) Myology. McGraw Hill, New York, pp 1349–1365

Shilito P, Mulenaar PC, Vincent A et al. (1995) Acquired neuromyotonia. Evidence for auto-antibodies against K$^+$ channels of peripheral nerves. Ann Neurol 38: 714–722

Shima K, Tashiro K, Hibi N et al. (1983) Carbonic anhydrase III: immunohistochemical localization in human skeletal muscle. Acta Neuropathol 5: 237–239

Shimomura C Nonaka I (1989) Nemaline myopathy: comparative muscle histochemistry in the severe neonatal, moderate congenital and adult onset forms. Pediatr Neurol 5: 25–31

Shirabe T, Tawara S, Terao A et al. (1975) Myxoedematous polyneuropathy. J Neurol Neurosurg Psychiatry 38: 241–247

Shokeir MHK, Kobrinsky NL (1976) Autosomal recessive muscular dystrophy in Manitoba Hutterites. Clin Genet 9: 197–202

Shuaib A, Martin JM, Mitchell LB et al. (1988) Multicore myopathy: not always a benign entity. Can J Neurol Sci 15: 10–14

Shulman LE (1975) Diffuse fasciitis with eosinophilia: a new syndrome? Trans Assoc Am Physicians 88: 70–86

Shumate JB, Brooke MH, Camell JE et al. (1979) Increased serum CK after exercise: a sex-linked phenomenon. Neurology 29: 902–904

Shurin SB, Rekate HL, Annable W (1982) Optic atrophy induced by vincristine. Paediatrics 70: 288–291

Shy GM, Magee KR (1956) A new congenital non-progressive myopathy. Brain 79: 610–621

Shy GM, McEachern D (1951) The clinical features and response to cortisone of menopausal muscular dystrophy. J Neurol Neurosurg Psychiatry 14: 101–107

Shy GM, Engel WK, Somers JE et al. (1963) Nemaline myopathy: a new congenital myopathy. Brain 86: 793–810

Shy GM, Gonatas NK, Perez M (1966) Two childhood myopathies with abnormal mitochondria I, Megaconial myopathy. II. Pleoconial myopathy. Brain 89: 133–147

Shy GM, Wanko T, Rowley PB et al. (1961) Studies in familial periodic paralysis. Exp Neurol 3: 53–121

Shy ME, Rowland LP, Smith T et al. (1986) Motor neuron disease and plasma cell dyscrasia. Neurology 36: 1429–1436

Sibert JR, Williams V, Burkinshaw R et al. (1987) Swivel workers in Duchenne muscular dystrophy. Arch Dis Child 62: 741–742

Siddique T, Pericak-Vance MA, Brooks BR et al. (1989) Linkage analysis in familial amyotrophic lateral sclerosis. Neurology 39: 919–925

Siegel IM (1972) Pathogenesis of stance in Duchenne muscular dystrophy. Arch Phys Med Rehabil 53: 403–406

Siegel IM (1977) The clinical management of muscle disease. Heinemann, London

Siegel IM (1978) The management of muscular dystrophy: a clinical review. Muscle Nerve 1: 453–460

Sigurgeirsson B, Lindelof B, Edhag O et al. (1992) Risk of cancer in patients with dermatomyositis or polymyositis. N Engl J Med 326: 363–367

Silver RM, Heyes MP, Maize JL et al. (1990) Scleroderma, fasciitis, and eosinophilia associated with the ingestion of tryptophan. N Engl J Med 322: 874–881

Silverman L, Mendell G, Saheuk Z (1976) Significance of CPK isoenzymes in Duchenne muscular dystrophy. Neurology 26: 561–564

Silverstein A, Siltzback LE (1969) Muscle involvement in sarcoidosis. Arch Neurol 21: 235–241

Sima AAF, Briff V, Nathaniel V et al. (1988) Regeneration and repair of myelinated fibres in sural nerve biopsy specimens from patients with diabetic neuropathy treated with sorbinil. N Engl J Med 319: 548–555

Simkin AP (1982) Simian stance: a sign of spinal stenosis. Lancet ii: 652–653

Simmonds Z, Albers JW, Bromberg MB et al. (1993a) Presentation and initial clinical course in patients with chronic inflammator demyelinating polyradiculopathy: comparison of patients without and with monoclonal gammopathy. Neurology 43: 2202–2209

Simmonds Z, Bromberg MB, Feldman EL et al. (1993b) Polyneuropathy associated with IgA monoclonal gammopathy of undetermined significance. Muscle Nerve 16: 77–83

Simos RW, Goldenberg DL (1988) Symptoms mimicking neurologic disorders in fibromyalgia syndrome. J Rheumatol 15: 1271–1273

Simon GS, Dewey WL (1981) Narcotics and diabetes. I. The effect of streptozotocin-induced diabetes on the anti-nociceptive potency of morphine. J Pharmacol Exp Ther 218: 318–323

Simpson DM, Bender AN (1988) Human immunodeficiency virus-associated myopathy: analysis of 11 patients. Ann Neurol 24: 79–84

Simpson JA (1958) An evaluation of thymectomy in myasthenia gravis. Brain 81: 112–144

Simpson JA (1960) Myasthenia gravis: a new hypothesis. Scott Med J 5: 419–436

Simpson JA (1966) Myasthenia gravis as an autoimmune disease. Ann NY Acad Sci 135: 506–516

Simpson JA (1978) Myasthenia gravis: a personal view of pathogenesis and mechanism. Muscle Nerve 1: 45–56, 151–156

Simpson JA (1981) Myasthenia gravis and myasthenic syndromes. In: Walton JN (ed) Disorders of voluntary muscle, 4th edn. Churchill Livingstone, Edinburgh, pp 585–624

Sinaki M, Wood MB, Mulder DW (1984) Rehabilitative operation for motor neuron disease: tendon transfer for segmental muscular atrophy of the upper extremities. Mayo Clin Proc 59: 338–342

Sinclair D (1967) Cutaneous sensation. Oxford University Press, London

Singh A, Jolly SS (1963) Wasted leg syndrome: a compressive neuropathy of lower limb. J Assoc Phys India 11: 1031–1037

Singh N, Behse F, Buchthal F (1974) Electrophysiological study of peroneal palsy. J Neurol Neurosurg Psychiatry 37: 1202–1213

Singh N, Kumor A, Ghai OP (1976) Conduction velocity of motor nerves in children suffering from protein-calorie malnutrition and marasmus. Electromyogr Clin Neurophysiol 16: 381–392

Singh N, Sachdev KK, Susheela AK (1980) Juvenile muscular atrophy localised to arms. Arch Neurol 40: 297–299

Singsen BH, Bernstein BH, Karnrcich HK et al. (1977) Mixed connective tissue disease in childhood J Pediatr 90: 893–900

Sinha S, Newsom-Davis J, Miles K et al. (1991) Autoimmune aetiology for acquired neuromyotonia (Isaac's syndrome). Lancet 338: 75–77

Sinkeler SPT, Daanen HAM, Wevers RA et al. (1985) The relation between blood lactate and ammonia in ischaemic handgrip exercise. Muscle Nerve 8: 523–527

Sivak ED, Streib EW (1980) Management of hypoventilation in motor neuron disease presenting with respiratory insufficiency. Ann Neurol 7: 188–191

Sivak ED, Gipson WT, Hanson MR (1982) Long-term management of respiratory failure in amyotrophic lateral sclerosis. Ann Neurol 12: 18–23

Sivak ED, Salanga VD, Wolbourn AT et al. (1981) Adult-onset acid maltase deficiency presenting as diaphragmatic paralysis. Ann Neurol 9: 613–615

Sjostrom M, Downham DY, Lexell J (1986) Distribution of different fiber types in human skeletal muscles: why is there a difference within a fascicle? Muscle Nerve 9: 30–36

Skaria JB, Katiyar B, Srivastara T et al. (1975) Myopathy and neuropathy associated with osteomalacia. Acta Neurol Scand 51: 37–58

Skjeldaal OH, Stokke O, Refsum S (1987) Clinical and biochemical heterogeneity in conditions with phytanic acid accumulation. J Neurol Sci 77: 87–96

Skjeldaal OH, Stolce O, Refsum S et al. (1992) Phytanic acid storage disease. In: Dyck PJ, Thomas PK (eds) Peripheral neuropathy, 3rd edn. Saunders, Philadelphia, pp 1149–1160

Slavin G, Martin F, Ward K et al. (1983) Chronic alcohol excess is associated with selective, but reversible injury to Type 2B muscle fibres. J Clin Pathol 36: 772–777

Slavin G, Sowter C, Ward P et al. (1982) Measurement of striated muscle fibre diameters using interactive computer-aided microscopy. J Clin Pathol 35: 1268–1271

Slonim AE, Goans PJ (1985) Myopathy in McArdle's syndrome: improvement with a high protein diet. N Engl J Med 312: 355–359

Slonim AE, Coleman RA, McElligot J et al. (1983) Improvement of muscle function in acid maltase deficiency by high protein therapy. Neurology 33: 34–38

Slucka C (1968) The electrocardiogram in Duchenne's progressive muscular dystrophy. Circulation 38: 933–940

Slutsker L. Hoesig FC, Miller L et al. (1990) Eosinophilia myalgia syndrome associated with exposure to tryptophan from a single manufacturer. JAMA 264: 213–217

Small DG, Matthews WB, Small M (1978) The cervical somatosensory evoked potential (SEP) in the diagnosis of multiple sclerosis. J Neurol Sci 35: 211–224

Smit GPA, Fernandes J, Leonard JV et al. (1990) The long-term outcome of patients with glycogen storage diseases. J Inherit Metab Dis 13: 411–418

Smith AF, MacFie WG, Oliver MF (1970) Clofibrate, serum enzymes and muscle pain. Br Med J ii: 26–28

Smith B (1969) Skeletal muscle necrosis associated with carcinoma. J Pathol 97: 207–210

Smith BE, Dyck PJ (1990) Peripheral neuropathy in the eosinophilia-myalgia syndrome associated with L-tryptophan ingestion. Neurology 40: 1035–1040

Smith I, Elton RA, Thomson WHS (1979) Carrier detection in X-linked recessive (Duchenne) muscular dystrophy: serum creatine phosphokinase values in premenarchal, menstruating, post-menopausal and pregnant normal women. Clin Chim Acta 98: 207–216

Smith IS, Kahn SN, Lacey BW et al. (1983) Chronic demyelinating neuropathy associated with benign paraproteinaemia. Brain 106: 169–196

Smith PEM, Calverly PMA, Edwards RHT et al. (1987) Practical problems in the respiratory care of patients with muscular dystrophy. N Engl J Med 316: 1197–1205

Smith R, Stern G (1967) Myopathy, osteomalacia and hyperparathyroidism. Brain 90: 593–602

Smith RG, Hamilton S, Hofmann F et al. (1992) Serum antibodies to L-type calcium channels in patients with amyotrophic lateral sclerosis. N Engl J Med 327: 1721–1728

Smith SA, Miller RG, Murphy JR et al. (1994) Treatment of ALS with high dose pulse cyclophosphamide. J Neurol Sci 124: 584–587

Smith T, Trojaborg W (1986) Clinical and electrophysiological recovery from peroneal palsy. Acta Neurol Scand 74: 328–335

Snape WJ, Battle WM, Schwartz SS et al. (1982) Metoclopramide to treat gastroparesis due to diabetes mellitus: a double-blind controlled trial. Ann Intern Med 96: 444–446

Sneddon J (1980) Myasthenia gravis: the difficult diagnosis. Br J Psychiatry 136: 92–93

Snider WD, Harris GL (1979) A physiological correlate of disuse-induced sprouting at the neuromuscular junction. Nature 281: 69–71

Snooks SJ, Swash M (1985) Motor conduction velocity in the human spinal cord: slowed conduction in multiple sclerosis and radiation myelopathy. J Neurol Neurosurg Psychiatry 48: 1135–1139

Snooks SJ, Swash M (1986) Slowed motor conduction in lumbosacral nerve roots in cauda equina lesions: a new diagnostic technique. J Neurol Neurosurg Psychiatry 49: 808–816

Snooks SJ, Setchell M, Swash M et al. (1984) Injury to innervation of pelvic floor sphincter musculature in childbirth. Lancet ii: 546–550

Snowdon JA, MacFie AC, Pearce JB (1976) Hypocalcaemic myopathy with paranoid psychosis. J Neurol Neurosurg Psychiatry 39: 48–52

So YT, Aminoff MJ, Olney RK (1989a) The role of thermography in the evaluation of lumbosacral radiculopathy. Neurology 39: 1154–1158

So YT, Holtzman DM, Abrams DI et al. (1988) Peripheral neuropathy associated with acquired immunodeficiency syndrome. Arch Neurol 45: 945–948

So YT, Olney RK, Aminoff MJ (1989b) Evaluation of thermography in the diagnosis of selected entrapment neuropathies. Neurology 39: 1–5

Soares VM, Brzustowicz LM, Kleyn PW et al. (1993) Refinement of the spinal muscular atrophy locus to the interval between D55435 and MAP1b. Genomics 15: 365–371

Sobrevilla LA, Goodman ML, Kane CA (1964) Demyelinating central nervous system disease, macular atrophy and acanthocytosis (Bassen-Kornzweig syndrome). Am J Med 37: 821–828

Sobue G, Hashizume Y Mukai E et al. (1989) X-linked recessive bulbo-spinal neuronopathy. Brain 112: 209–232

Sobue G, Nakao N, Morakami K et al. (1990) Type 1 familial amyloid polyneuropathy. Brain 113: 903–919

Sobue I, Saito N, Iida M et al. (1978) Juvenile type of distal and segmental muscular atrophy of upper extremities. Ann Neurol 3: 429–432

Sohi AS, Kandheri KC, Singh N (1971) Motor nerve conduction studies in leprosy. Int J Dermatol 10: 151–155

Sokol RJ, Guggenheim MA, Henbi JE et al. (1985) Frequency and clinical progression of the vitamin E deficiency neurological disorder in children with prolonged neonatal cholestasis. N Engl J Med 313: 1580–1583

Sokoloff MC, Goldberg LS, Pearson CM (1971) Treatment of corticosteroid-resistant polymyositis with methotrexate. Lancet i: 1416

Solders G (1988) Discomfort after fascicular sural nerve biopsy. Acta Neurol Scand 77: 503–504

Solders G, Nennesmo I, Persson A (1989) Diphtheritic neuropathy: an analysis based on muscle and nerve biopsy and repeated neurophysiological and autonomic function tests. J Neurol Neurosurg Psychiatry 52: 876–880

Solimena M, Folli F, Morello F et al. (1990) Autoantibodies to GABA-ergic neurons and pancreatic beta cells in stiff man syndrome. N Engl J Med 322: 1555–1560

Solomon E, Swallow D, Burgess S et al. (1979) Assignment of the human acid α-glucosidase gene (αGLV) to chromosome 17 using somatic cell hybrids. Ann Hum Genet 42: 273–281

Somer H, Dubowitz V, Donner M (1976) Creatine kinase isoenzymes in neuromuscular diseases. J Neurol Sci 29: 129–136

Song SK, Rubin E (1972) Ethanol produces muscle damage in human volunteers. Science 175: 327–328

Sørensen AWS, With TK (1971) Persistent paresis with porphyric attacks. Acta Med Scand 190: 219–222

Sorensen RS (1993) Double crush syndrome: what is the evidence? J Neuromusculoskeletal System 1: 23–29

Sories BC, Dalakas MC (1991) Dysphagia with the post polio syndrome. N Engl J Med 324: 1162–1167

Sourander P, Olsson Y (1968) Peripheral neuropathy in globoid cell leucodystrophy (Morbus Krabbe). Acta Neuropathol (Berl) 11: 69–81

Spaans F (1970) Occupational nerve lesions. In: Diseases of nerves. North-Holland, Amsterdam, pp 326–343 (Handbook of clinical neurology, vol 7, part 1)

Spaans F (1985) Guillain–Barré syndrome with exclusively motor involvement. Electroencephalogr Clin Neurophysiol 61: 15–16

Spaans F, Wilts G (1982) Denervation due to lesions of the central nervous system. J Neurol Sci 57: 291–305

Spaans F, Jennekens FGI, Mirandolle JF et al. (1986) Myotonic dystrophy associated with hereditary motor and sensory neuropathy. Brain 109: 1149–1168

Spaans F, Theunissen P, Reekers AD et al. (1990) Schwartz–Jampel syndrome. 1. Clinical, electromyographic and histologic studies. Muscle Nerve 13: 516–527

Spargo E (1984) The acute effects of alcohol on plasma creatine kinase (CK) activity in the rat. J Neurol Sci 63: 307–316

Spehlmann R, Norcross K, Rasmus SC et al. (1981) Improvement of stiff man syndrome with sodium valproate. Neurology 31: 1162–1163

Spencer CH, Jordan SC, Hanson V (1979) Circulating immune complexes in juvenile dermatomyositis. Clin Res 27: 808A

Spencer GE, Vignos PJ (Jr) (1962) Bracing for ambulation in childhood progressive muscular dystrophy. J Bone Joint Surg (Am) 44: 234–242

Spencer PS, Schaumberg HH (1977a) Ultrastructural studies of the dying-back process. III. The evolution of experimental peripheral giant axonal degeneration. J Neuropathol Exp Neurol 36: 276–299

Spencer PS, Schaumberg HH (1977b) Central-peripheral-distal axonopathy: the pathology of dying-back neuropathies. In: Zimmerman H (ed) Progress in neuropathology, vol 3. Grune and Stratton, New York, pp 253–259

Spencer PS, Schaumberg HH (1980) Classification of neurotoxic disease: a morphological approach. In: Spencer PS, Schaumberg HH (eds) Experimental and clinical neurotoxicology Williams and Wilkins, Baltimore, p 92

Spencer PS, Roy DN, Ludoff A et al. (1987) Lathyrism: evidence for a role of the neuroexcitatory amino acid BOAA. Lancet ii: 1066–1068

Spencer PS, Schaumberg HH, Rayleigh RA et al. (1975) Nervous system degeneration produced by the industrial solvent methyl n-butyl ketone. Arch Neurol 32: 219–222

Spillane JD (1947) Nutritional disorders of the nervous system. Livingstone, Edinburgh

Spillane JD, Urich H (1976) Trigeminal neuropathy with nasal ulceration: report of two cases and one necropsy. J Neurol Neurosurg Psychiatry 39: 105–113

Spillane JD, Wells CEC (1969) Acrodystrophic neuropathy: a critical review of the syndrome of trophic ulcers, sensory neuropathy and bony erosion, together with an account of 16 cases in South Wales. Oxford University Press, London

Spillane JD, Nathan PW, Kelly RE et al. (1971) Painful legs and moving toes. Brain 94: 541–556

Spindler H, Felsenthal G (1978) Sensory conduction in the musculocutaneous nerve. Arch Phys Med Rehabil 59: 20–23

Spinner M (1968) The arcade of Frohse and its relationship to posterior interosseous nerve paralysis. J Bone Joint Surg [Br] 50: 809–812

Spiro AJ, Kennedy C (1965) Hereditary occurrence of nemaline myopathy. Arch Neurol 13: 155–159

Spiro AJ, Moore CL, Prineas JW et al. (1970) A cytochrome-related inherited disorder of the nervous system and muscle. Arch Neurol 23: 103–112

Spiro AJ, Shy GM, Gonatas NK (1966) Myotubular myopathy. Arch Neurol 14: 1–14

Stadhouders A, Jap P, Walliman TH (1990) Biochemical nature of mitochondrial crystals. J Neurol Sci 98S: 304–305

Stålberg E (1977) Electrogenesis in human dystrophic muscle. In: Rowland LP (ed) Pathogenesis of human muscular dystrophies. Excerpta Medica, Amsterdam, pp 570–587

Stålberg E (1980) Macro EMG, a new recording technique. J Neurol Neurosurg Psychiatry 43: 475–482

Stålberg E (1982a) Electrophysiological studies of reinnervation in ALS. In: Rowland LP (ed) Human motor neuron diseases. Raven Press, New York, pp 47–59

Stålberg E (1982b) Macroelectromyography in reinnervation. Muscle Nerve 5: S135–S138

Stålberg E (1983) Macro EMG Muscle Nerve 6: 619–630

Stålberg E (1985) The motor unit: electromyography. In: Swash M, Kennard C (eds) Scientific basis of clinical neurology. Churchill Livingstone, Edinburgh, pp 458–462

Stålberg E, Antoni L (1980) Electrophysiological cross section of the motor unit. J Neurol Neurosurg Psychiatry 43: 469–474

Stålberg E, Antoni L (1983) Computer-aided analysis. In: Desmedt JE (ed) Computer-aided electromyography. Karger, Basel, pp 186–234

Stålberg E, Droszeghy P (1991) Scanning EMG in normal muscle and in neuromuscular disorders. Electroencephalogr Clin Neurophysiol 81: 403–416

Stålberg E, Fawcett PRW (1982) Macro EMG in healthy subjects of different ages. J Neurol Neurosurg Psychiatry 45: 870–878

Stålberg E, Thiele B (1973) Discharge pattern of motoneurones in humans. In: Desmedt JE (ed) New developments in electromyography and clinical neurophysiology, vol 3. Karger, Basel, pp 234–241

Stålberg E, Thiele B (1975) Motor unit fibre density in the extensor digitorum communis muscle. J Neurol Neurosurg Psychiatry 38: 874–880

Stålberg E, Trontelj JV (1982) Abnormal discharges generated within the motor unit as observed with single fibre EMG. In: Culp WJ, Ochoa J (eds) Abnormal nerves and muscles as impulse generators. Oxford University Press, Oxford, pp 443–474

Stålberg E, Trontelj JV (1994) Single fibre electromyography, 2nd edn. Raven Press, New York

Stålberg E, Andreassen S, Falck B et al. (1986) Quantitative analysis of individual motor unit potentials: a proposition for standardised terminology and criteria for measurement. J Clin Neurophysiol 3: 1–36

Stålberg E, Bischoff C, Falck B (1994) The jiggle, a way to detect abnormality in quantitative EMG. Muscle Nerve 17: 392–399

Stålberg E, Borges O, Ericsson M et al. (1989) The quadriceps femoris muscle in 20–70-year-old subjects. Muscle Nerve 12: 382–389

Stålberg E, Chu J, Bril V et al. (1983) Automatic analysis of the EMG interference pattern. Electroencephalogr Clin Neurophysiol 56: 672–681

Stålberg E, Mihelin M, Trontelj JV (1992) Electrical microstimulation with single fiber electromyography. J Clin Neurophysiol 9: 105–119

Stålberg E, Schiller HH, Schwartz MS (1975a) Safety factor in single human motor end-plates studied in vivo with single fibre electromyography. J Neurol Neurosurg Psychiatry 38: 799–804

Stålberg E, Schwartz MS, Thiele B et al. (1976a) The normal motor unit in man. J Neurol Sci 27: 291–301

Stålberg E, Schwartz MS, Trontelj JV (1975b) Single fibre electromyography in various processes affecting the anterior horn cell. J Neurol Sci 24: 403–415

Stålberg E, Trontelj JV, Janko M (1974) Single fibre EMG findings in muscular dystrophy. In: Hausmanowa-Petrusewicz I, Jedrzejowska H (eds) Structure and function of normal and diseased muscle and peripheral nerve. Polish Medical Publishers, Warsaw, pp 185–190

Stålberg E, Trontelj JV, Schwartz MS (1976b) Single muscle fibre recording of the jitter phenomenon in patients with myasthenia gravis and in members of their families. Ann NY Acad Sci 274: 189–202

Stanwood SE, Kraft GH (1971) Diagnosis and management of brachial plexus injuries. Arch Phys Med Rehabil 52: 52–60

Stark RJ (1978) Polymyositis presenting with severe weakness involving only one arm. Aust NZ J Med 8: 544–546

Stark RJ (1979) Eosinophilic polymyositis. Arch Neurol 36: 721–722

Staunton H, Davis MB, Guiloff RT et al. (1991) Irish (Donegal) amyloidosis associated with the transthyretin ALA 60 (Appalachian) variant. Brain 114: 2675–2679

Staunton H, Dervan P, Kale R et al. (1987) Hereditary amyloid polyneuropathy in northwest Ireland. Brain 110: 1231–1245

Steare SE, Dubowitz V, Benatar A (1992) Subclinical cardiomyopathy in Becker muscular dystrophy. Br Heart J 68: 304–308

Steinberg D, Mize C, Avigan J et al. (1966) On the metabolic error in Refsum's disease. Trans Am Neurol Assoc 91: 168–172

Steiner I, Argov Z, Cahan C et al. (1985) Guillain–Barré syndrome after epidural anaesthesia. Neurology 35: 1473–1475

Steiner WR (1903) Dermatomyositis, with report of a case which presented with a rare muscle anomaly but once described in man. J Exp Med 6: 407–442

Steinmeyer K, Klocke R, Ortland C et al. (1991b) Inactivation of muscle chloride channel by transposon insertion in myotonic mice. Nature 354: 304–308

Steinmeyer K, Ortland C, Jeutsch TJ (1991a) Primary structure and functional expression of a developmentally regulated skeletal muscle chloride channel. Nature 354: 301–304

Stenman AB, Schaumberg HH, Asbury AK (1980) Acute sensory neuronopathy: a distinct clinical entity. Ann Neurol 7: 354–360

Stephan DA, Buish NRM, Chittenden AB et al. (1994) A rippling muscle disease gene is localised to Ch 19.41 Neurology 44: 1915–1920

Stern BJ, Krumholtz A, Johns C et al. (1985) Sarcoidosis and its neurological manifestations. Arch Neurol 42: 909–917

Stern GM, Hall JM, Robinson DC (1964) Neonatal myasthenia gravis. Br Med J ii: 284–286

Stern GM, Hoffrand AV, Urich H (1965) The peripheral nerves and skeletal muscles in Wegener's granulomatosis. Brain 88: 151–164

Stern LM, Caudrey DJ, Perrett LV et al. (1984) Progression of muscular dystrophy assessed by computed tomography. Dev Med Child Neurol 26: 569–573

Stern MB (1984) The anterior interosseous nerve syndrome (the Kiloh–Nevin syndrome). Clin Orthop 187: 223–227

Stevens JC (1987) The electrodiagnosis of carpal tunnel syndrome. Muscle Nerve 10: 99–113 AAEE minimonograph no. 26

Stevens A, Rosellen (1970) Sensory nerve conduction velocity of n. cutaneus femoris lateralis. Electromyography 10: 397–402

Steventon G, Williams AC, Waring RH et al. (1988) Xenobiotic metabolism in motor neuron disease. Lancet ii: 644–647

Stewart BM (1966) The hypertrophic neuropathy of acromegaly. Arch Neurol 14: 107–110

Stewart JD (1994) Focal peripheral neuropathies 2nd. Ed. Elsevier, New York

Stewart JD, Angus E, Gendron D (1983) Sciatic neuropathies. Br Med J 287: 1108–1109

Stöthr M (1977) Benign fibrillation potentials in normal muscle and their correlation with end-plate and denervation potentials. J Neurol Neurosurg Psychiatry 40: 765–768

Stöhr M (1978) Low frequency bizarre discharges. Electrograph Clin Neurophysiol 18: 147–156

Stokes M, Young A (1984) The contribution of reflex inhibition to arthrogenous muscle inhibition. Clin Sci 67: 7–14

Stokke O, Skrede S, Ek J et al. (1984) Refsum's disease, adrenoleucodystrophy and Zellweger's syndrome. Scand J Clin Lab Invest 44: 463

Stoner GL (1979) Importance of the neural predilection of Mycobacterium leprae in leprosy. Lancet ii: 993–996

Stranock SD, Newsom-Davis J (1978) Ultrastructure of the muscle spindle in dystrophia myotonica. II. The sensory and motor nerve terminals. Neuropathol Appl Neurobiol 4: 407–418

Straus S, Dale JK, Tobi M et al. (1988) Acyclovir treatment of the chronic fatigue syndrome: lack of efficacy in a placebo-controlled trial. N Engl J Med 319: 1692–1698

Straus S, Tosato G, Armstrong G et al. (1985) Persisting illness and fatigue in adults with evidence of Epstein-Barr virus infection. Ann Intern Med 102: 7–16

Strauss MB (1935) Etiology of "alcoholic" polyneuritis. Am J Med Sci 189: 378–382

Streib EW (1977) Adverse effects of magnesium salt cathartics in patients with the myasthenic syndrome (Lambert–Eaton syndrome). Ann Neurol 2: 175–176

Streib EW (1986) Successful treatment with tocainide of recessive generalised congenital myotonia. Ann Neurol 19: 501–504

Streib EW, Rothner DA (1980) Eaton–Lambert myasthenic syndrome: long-term treatment of three patients with prednisone. Ann Neurol 8: 121–122

Streib EW, Sun SF (1983) Distribution of electrical myotonia in myotonic muscular dystrophy. Ann Neurol 14: 80–82

Streib EW, Meyers DG, Sun SF (1985) Mitral valve prolapse in myotonic dystrophy. Muscle Nerve 8: 650–653

Streib EW, Sun SF, Yarkowsky T (1982) Transient paresis in myotonic syndromes: a simplified electrophysiologic approach. Muscle Nerve 5: 719–723

Streib EW, Wilbourn AJ, Mitsumoto H (1979) Spontaneous electrical muscle fibre activity in polymyositis and dermatomyositis. Muscle Nerve 2: 14–18

Strichartz G, Hahin R, Cahalan M (1982) Pharmacological models for sodium channels producing abnormal impulse activity. In: Culp W, Ochoa J (eds) Abnormal nerves and muscles as impulse generators. Oxford University Press, Oxford, pp 98–129

Strickland GT, Moser KM (1967) Sarcoidosis with Landry-Guillain-Barré syndrome and clinical response to corticosteroids. Am J Med 43: 131–135

Stromer MH, Tabatabai LB, Robson RM et al. (1976) Nemaline myopathy, an integrated study: selective extraction. Exp Neurol 50: 402–421

Strunk S, Smith CW, Blumberg JM (1967) Ultrastructural studies on the lesion produced in skeletal muscle fibres by crude type A Clostridium perfringens toxin and its purified alpha fraction. Am J Pathol 50: 89

Stuart CA, Armstrong RM, Provow SA et al. (1983) Insulin resistance in patients with myotonic dystrophy. Neurology 33: 679–685

Stuhmer W, Conti F, Suzuki H et al. (1989) Structural parts involved in activation and inactivation of the sodium channel. Nature 339: 597–603

Suarez GA, Kelly JJ (1992). The dropped head syndrome. Neurology 42: 1625–1627

Subramony SH (1988). Neuralgic amyotrophy (acute brachial neuritis). Muscle Nerve 11: 39–44 (AAEE case report no. 14)

Subramony SH, Malhotra CP, Mishra SK (1983) Distinguishing paramyotonia congenita and myotonia congenita by electromyography. Muscle Nerve 6: 374–379

Sugie H, Russin R, Verity M (1984) Emetine myopathy: two case reports with pathobiochemical analysis. Muscle Nerve 7: 54–59

Sulaiman AR, Kinder DS (1989) Vascularized muscle fibres: etiopathogenesis and clinical significance. J Neurol Sci 92: 37–54

Summers BA, Swash M, Schwartz MS et al. (1987) Juvenile-onset bulbo-spinal muscular atrophy with deafness: Vialetto–van Laere syndrome or Madras-type motor neuron disease? J Neurol 34: 440–442

Sumner AJ (1981) The physiological basis for symptoms in Guillain-Barré syndrome. Ann Neurol 9: S28–S30

Sun KO, Chan YW, Cheung RTF et al. (1994) Management of tentanus: a review of 18 cases. J R Soc Med 87: 135–137

Sun SF, Streib EW (1983) Autosomal recessive generalised myotonia. Muscle Nerve 6: 143–148

Sunderland S (1953) The relative susceptibility to injury of the medial and lateral popliteal divisions of the sciatic nerve. Br J Surg 41: 300–302

Sunderland S (1978) Nerves and nerve injuries, 2nd edn. Churchill Livingstone, Edinburgh

Sunderland S (1991) Nerve injuries and their repair. Churchill Livingstone, Edinburgh, p 538

Sung JH, Park SH, Mastri AR et al. (1980) Axonal dystrophy in the gracile nucleus and congenital biliary atresia and cystic fibrosis (Mucoviscidosis): beneficial effect of vitamin E therapy. J Neuropathol Exp Neurol 39: 584–597

Sunohara N, Arahata K, Hoffman EP et al. (1990) Quadriceps myopathy: forme fruste of Becker muscular dystrophy. Ann Neurol 28: 634–639

Sunohara N, Nonaka I, Kamei N et al. (1989) Distal myopathy with rimmed vacuole formation. Brain 112: 65–83

Suomalainen A, Kankonen J, Amati S et al. (1995) An autosomal locus predisposing to deletions of mitochondrial DNA Nature Genet. 9: 146–151

Suomalainen A, Paltan A, Leinonen H et al. (1992) Inherited dilated cardiomyopathy with multiple deletions of mitochondrial DNA. Lancet 340: 1319–1320

Suput D, Zripan A, Sepe A et al. (1993) Discrimination between neuropathy and myopathy by use of magnetic resonance imaging. Acta Neurol Scand 87: 118–123

Sutherland SK (1978) The management of bites by the Sydney funnel web spider (Atrax robustus). Med J Austr 1: 148–150

Suzuki S, Kobayashi T, Goto I et al. (1986) Dietary treatment of adrenoleukodystrophy. Neurology 36: 104–106

Swan CHJ, Wharton BA (1963) Polyneuritis and renal carcinoma. Lancet ii: 383–384

Swash M (1972) The morphology and innervation of the muscle spindle in dystrophia myotonica. Brain 95: 357–368

Swash M (1974) Acute fatal carcinomatous neuromyopathy. Arch Neurol 30: 324–326

Swash M (1980) Vulnerability of lower brachial myotomes in motor neurone disease: a clinical and single fibre EMG study. J Neurol Sci 47: 59–68

Swash M, Fox KP (1972) The effect of age on human skeletal muscle: studies of the morphology and innervation of muscle spindles. J Neurol Sci 16: 417–432

Swash M, Fox KP (1974) The pathology of the human muscle spindle: effect of denervation. J Neurol Sci 22: 1–24

Swash M, Fox KP (1975a) Abnormal intrafusal muscle fibres in myotonic dystrophy: a study using serial sections. J Neurol Neurosurg Psychiatry 30: 71–99

Swash M, Fox KP (1975b) The fine structure of the spindle abnormality in myotonic dystrophy. Neuropathol Appl Neurobiol I: 171–187

Swash M, Fox KP (1975c) Pathology of the muscle spindle in myasthenia gravis. J Neurol Sci 26: 39–47

Swash M, Fox KP (1976) The pathology of the muscle spindle in Duchenne muscular dystrophy. J Neurol Sci 29: 17–32

Swash M, Heathfield KWG (1983) Quadriceps myopathy: a variant of the limb-girdle dystrophy syndrome. J Neurol Neurosurg Psychiatry 46: 355–357

Swash M, Rowan AJ (1972) EEG criteria of hypocalcemia and hypercalcemia. Arch Neurol 26: 218–228

Swash M, Schwartz MS (1977) Implication of longitudinal muscle fibre splitting in neurogenic and myopathic disorders. J Neurol Neurosurg Psychiatry 40: 1152–1159

Swash M, Schwartz MS (1981) Familial multicore disease with focal loss of cross striations and ophthalmoplegia. J Neurol Sci 52: 1–10

Swash M, Schwartz MS (1982) A longitudinal study of changes in motor units in motor neurone disease. J Neurol Sci 56: 185–197

Swash M, Schwartz MS (1983a) Iatrogenic neuromuscular disorders: a review. J R Soc Med 26: 149–151

Swash M, Schwartz MS (1983b) Normal muscle spindle morphology in myotonic dystrophy is not due to myotonia alone. Clin Neuropathol 2: 75–78

Swash M, Schwartz MS (1984) Staging motor neuron disease: single fibre EMG studies of asymmetry, progression and compensatory reinnervation. In: Rose FC (ed) Research progress in motor neuron disease. Pitman, London, pp 123–140

Swash M, Schwartz MS (1991) Motor neuron disease. In: Oxbury J, Swash M (eds) Clinical neurology. Churchill Livingstone, Edinburgh, pp 1356–1366

Swash M, Schwartz MS (1992) What do we really know about ALS? J Neurol Sci 113: 4–16

Swash M, Schwartz MS (1993) Malaria myositis. J Neurol Neurosurg. Psychiatry 56: 1328

Swash M, Snooks SJ (1986) Slowed motor conduction in lumbosacral nerve roots in cauda equina lesions. J Neurol Neurosurg Psychiatry 49: 808–816

Swash M, Brown MM, Thakkar C (1995) CT muscle imaging on the clinical assessment of neuromuscular disease. Muscle Nerve 18: 708–714

Swash M, Fox KP, Davidson A (1975) Carcinoid myopathy: serotonin-induced muscle weakness in man? Arch Neurol 32: 572–574

Swash M, Leader M, Brown A et al. (1986) Focal loss of anterior horn cells in the cervical cord in motor neuron disease. Brain 109: 939–952

Swash M, Perrin J, Schwartz MS (1979a) Significance of immunoglobulin deposition in peripheral nerve in neuropathies associated with paraproteinaemia. J Neurol Neurosurg Psychiatry 42: 179–183

Swash M, Scholtz CL, Vowels G et al. (1988) Selective and asymmetric vulnerability of corticospinal and spinocerebellar tracts in motor neuron disease. J Neurol Neurosurg Psychiatry 51: 785–789

Swash M, Schwartz MS, Apps MCP (1985) Adult onset acid maltase deficiency. J Neurol Sci 68: 61–74

Swash M, Schwartz MS, Carter ND et al. (1983) Benign X-linked myopathy with acanthocytosis (McLeod's syndrome): its relationship to X-linked muscular dystrophy. Brain 106: 717–733

Swash M, Schwartz MS, Li T-M (1989) Trends in mortality from motor neuron disease. Lancet 335: 958

Swash M, Schwartz MS, Sargeant MK (1978a) Pathogenesis of longitudinal splitting of muscle fibres in neurogenic disorders and in polymyositis. Neuropathol Appl Neurobiol 4: 99–115

Swash M, Schwartz MS, Sargeant MK (1987b) The significance of ragged-red fibres in neuromuscular disease. J Neurol Sci 36: 347–355

Swash M, Schwartz MS, Sargeant MK (1979b) Osteomalacic myopathy: an experimental approach. Neuropathol Appl Neurobiol 5: 295–302

Swash M, Schwartz MS, Thompson A et al. (1988) Distal myopathy with focal granular degenerative change in vacuolated Type 2 fibres. Clin Neuropathol 7: 249–253

Swash M, Schwartz MS, Van den Berg MJ et al. (1977) Myopathy in Whipples disease Gut 18: 800–804

Swash M, Thompson A, Ingram DA et al. (1988) Polysaccharide (amylopectin) storage myopathy. Muscle Nerve 11: 1–17

Swash M, van den Noort S, Craig JW (1970) Late-onset proximal myopathy with diabetes mellitus in four sisters. Neurology 20: 694–699

Sweeney VP, Pathak MH, Asbury AK (1970) Acute intermittent porphyria: increased ALA synthetase activity during an acute attack. Brain 93: 369–380

Swift TR (1979) Weakness from magnesium-containing cathartics. Muscle Nerve 2: 295–298

Swift TR, Ignacio OJ (1975) Tick paralysis. Neurology 25: 1130–1133

Swift TR, Gross JA, Ward LC et al. (1981) Peripheral neuropathy in epileptic patients. Neurology 31: 826–831

Swift TR, Hackett ER, Shipley DE et al. (1973) Peroneal and tibial nerves in lepromatous leprosy: clinical and electrophysiologic observations. Int J Lepr 41: 25–34

Swift TR, Leshner RT, Gross JA (1980) Arm diaphragm synkinesis: electrodiagnostic studies of aberrant regeneration of phrenic motor neurons. Neurology 30: 339–344

Swillons S, Ludgate M, Mercken L et al. (1986) Analysis of sequence and structure homologies between thyroglobulin and aectylcholinesterase: possible functional and clinical significance. Biochem Biophys Res Commun 137: 142–148

Sydow O Stibler H, Hast R (1985) Abnormal erythrocyte survival in patients with myotonic dystrophy. Acta Neurol Scand 22: 522–524

Synek VM (1986) Validity of median nerve somatosensory evoked potentials in the diagnosis of supraclavicular brachial plexus lesions. Electroencephalogr Clin Neurophysiol 65: 27–35

Sazbo RM, Chodgey LK (1989) Stress carpal tunnel pressures in patients with carpal tunnel syndrome and normal patients. J Hand Surg (Am) 14: 624

Tabuenca JM (1981) Toxic-allergic syndrome caused by ingestion of rape seed oil denatured with aniline. Lancet ii: 567–568

Tackman W, Lehmann HJ (1974a) Refractory period in human sensory nerve fibres. Eur Neurol 12: 277–292

Tackman W, Lehmann HJ (1974b) Relative refractory period of median nerve sensory fibres in the carpal tunnel syndrome. Eur Neurol 12: 309–316

Tahmoush AJ, Shaller KC, Zhang P et al. (1994) Muscle sodium channel inactivation defect in paramyotonia congenita with the thr 1313 met mutation. Neuromusc Disord 4: 447–454

Takahashi K, Nakamora H (1976) Axonal degeneration in beriberi neuropathy. Arch Neurol 33: 836–841

Takahashi M, Ohara T, Hashimoto K (1971) Electrophysiological study of nerve injuries in workers handling acrylamide. Int Arch Arbeits Med 28: 1–11

Takamori M, Gutmann L (1971) Intermittent defect of acetylcholine release in myasthenia gravis. Neurology 21: 47–54

Takeshita K, Yoshino K, Kitahara T et al. (1977) Survey of Duchenne-type and congenital type of muscular dystrophy in Shimani, Japan. Jpn J Hum Genet 22: 43

Takeuchi A, Kodama M, Takatsu M et al. (1989) Mono-neuropathy multiplex in incomplete Behcet's disease. Clin Rheumatol 8: 375–380

Takeuchi T, Marikawa N, Matzumoto H et al. (1962) A patho-logical study of Minamata disease in Japan. Acta Neuropathol 2: 40–57

Tamai H, Nakagawa T, Osako N et al. (1980) Changes in thyroid function in patients with euthyroid Grave's disease. J Clin Endocrinol Metab 50: 108–112

Tan CT (1985) Juvenile muscular atrophy of distal upper extrem-ities. J Neurol Neurosurg Psychiatry 48: 285–286

Tan E, Lynn DJ, Amato HA et al. (1994) Immunosuppressive treatment of motor neuron syndromes. Arch Neurol 51: 194–200

Tanado H, Shibasaki H, Hirata I et al. (1988) Central vs peri-pheral nerve conduction before and after treatment of sub-acute combined degeneration. Arch Neurol 45: 526–529

Tanaka H, Vemura N, Toyama Y et al. (1976) Cardiac involve-ment in the Kugelberg–Welander syndrome. Ann J Cardiol 38: 528–532

Tandon R, Bradley WG (1985) Amyotrophic lateral sclerosis. II. Etiopathogenesis. Ann Neurol 18: 419–431

Tang I, Sedmak GV, Siegesmund KA et al. (1975) Chronic myopathy associated with Coxsackie virus type A9. N Engl J Med 292: 608–611

Tang L-M, Swash M (1986) Significance of small muscle fibres in neuromuscular disease. Virchows Arch Pathol Anat 410: 113–118

Tang L-M, Schwartz MS, Swash M (1988) Postural effects on F-wave in lumbosacral root compression and canal stenosis. Brain 111: 207–213

Tanhehco JL, Wiechers DO, Golbus J et al. (1992) Eosinophilia-myalgia syndrome. Muscle Nerve 15: 561–567

Tanin P, Lewis P, Servidei S et al. (1990) Metabolic causes of myoglobinuria. Ann Neurol 27: 181–185

Tanin P, Shanske S, Brownell AK et al. (1989) Phosphoglycerate kinase deficiency: a third case with recurrent myoglobinuria. Neurology 39: 359–360

Tanji J, Kato M (1973) Firing rate of individual motor units in voluntary contraction of abductor digiti minimi muscle in man. Exp Neurol 40: 771–783

Tanner MH, Pierce BJ, Hall DC (1981) Toxic shock syndrome. West J Med 134: 477–484

Tanphaichitr V, Broquist HP (1974) Site of carnitine biosynthesis in the rat. J Nutr 104: 1669–1673

Tanzi F, Taglietti V (1981) Spectral analysis of surface motor unit action potentials and surface interference electromyogram. IEEE Trans Biomed Eng 28: 318–324

Tanzi F, Taglietti V, Zugga G et al. (1979) Computerized EMG analysis. Electromyogr Clin Neurophysiol 19: 495–503

Tarui S, Okuno G, Ikura Y et al. (1965) Phosphofructokinase deficiency in skeletal muscle: a new type of glycogenosis. Biochem Biopsy Res Commun 19: 517–523

Tasker W, Chutorian AM (1969) Chronic polyneuritis of child-hood. J Pediatr 74: 699–708

Taubin JA, Hejtmancik JF, Brink P et al. (1993) X-linked dilated cardiomyopathy. Circulation 87: 1854–1865

Taverner D (1955) Bell's palsy: a clinical and electromyographic study. Brain 78: 209–232

Taverner D, Cohen SB, Hutchinson BC (1971) Comparison of corticotrophin and prednisolone in treatment of idiopathic facial paralysis (Bell's palsy). Br Med J iv: 20–22

Tawil R, Forester J, Griggs RC et al. (1996) Evidence for antici-pation and association of deletion size with severity in facioscapulohumeral muscular dystrophy. Ann Neurol 39: 744–748

Tawil R, Storvick D, Feasby TE et al. (1993) Extreme variability of expression in monozygotic twins with FSH muscular dystro-phy. Neurology 43: 345–348

Taylor DJ, Styles P, Matthews PM et al. (1986) Energetics of human muscles: exercise-induced ATP depletion. Magn Res Med 3: 44

Taylor RO (1960) Heredofamilial mononeuritis multiplex with brachial predilection. Brain 83: 113–137

Tazelaar HD, Viggiano RW, Pickersgill J et al. (1990) Interstitial lung disease in polymyositis and dermatomyositis. Ann Rev Respir Dis 141: 727–733

Telerman-Toppet H, Gérard JM, Coërs C (1973) Central core disease: a study of clinically unaffected muscle. J Neurol Sci 19: 207–223

Telstaad W, Sorensen O, Larsen S et al. (1984) Treatment of the restless leg syndrome with carbamazepine: a double-blind study. Br Med J 288: 444–446

Tenser RB, Corbett JJ (1974) Myokymia and facial contraction in brain stem glioma. Arch Neurol 30: 425–427

Teoh R, McGuire L, Wong K et al. (1989) Increased incidence of thymoma in Chinese myasthenia gravis: possible relationship with Epstein–Barr virus. Acta Neurol Scand 80: 221–225

Terao S, Sobue G, Hashizume Y et al. (1994) Disease-specific patterns of neuronal loss in the spinal ventral horn in amyo-trophic lateral sclerosis, multiple system atrophy and X-linked recessive bulbospinal neuronopathy. J Neurol 241: 196–203

Terasawa K (1986) Muscle regeneration and satellite cells in Fukuyama type congenital muscular dystrophy. Muscle Nerve 9: 465–470

Teravainen H, Larsen A (1977) Some features of the neuromus-cular complications of pulmonary carcinoma. Ann Neurol 2: 495–502

Teravainen H, Juntunen J, Erikson K et al. (1978) Myopathy asso-ciated with chronic alcohol drinking: histological and electro-physiological study. Virchows Arch Pathol Anat 378: 45–53

Testa GF, Angelini C (1979) Assessment of the value of thymic scan in myasthenia gravis. J Neurol 220: 21–29

Thiele B, Stålberg E (1975) Single fibre EMG findings in polyneu-ropathies of different aetiology. J Neurol Neurosurg Psychiatry 38: 881–887

Thomas JE, Colby MY Jr (1972) Radiation induced or metastatic brachial plexopathy. JAMA 222: 1392–1395

Thomas JE, Howard FM Jr (1972) Segmental zoster paresis: a disease profile. Neurology 22: 459–466

Thomas PK (1971) Morphological basis for alterations in nerve conduction in peripheral neuropathies. Proc R Soc Med 64: 295–298

Thomas PK (1974) The anatomical substructure of pain: evidence derived from morphometric studies on peripheral nerve. Can J Neurol Sci 1: 92–97

Thomas PK (1978) Screening for peripheral neuropathy in patients treated by chronic haemodialysis. Muscle Nerve 1: 396–399

Thomas PK (1987) Post viral fatigue syndrome. Lancet ii: 218–219

Thomas PK, Eliasson SG (1975) Diabetic neuropathy. In: Dyck PJ, Thomas PK, Lambert EH (eds) Peripheral neuropathy, vol 2. Saunders, Philadelphia, pp 966–981

Thomas PK, Holdorff B (1993) Neuropathy due to physical agents. In: Dyck PJ, Thomas PK (eds) Peripheral neuropathy, 3rd edn. Saunders, Philadelphia, pp 990–1013

Thomas PK, Lascelles RG (1965) Schwann cell abnormalities in diabetic neuropathy. Lancet i: 1355–1357

Thomas PK, Lascelles RG (1966) The pathology of diabetic neuropathy. QJM [NS] 35: 489–509

Thomas PK, Sharma AK (1976) Neuropathy in experimental dia-betes. Br Med J ii: 478

Thomas PK, Walker JG (1965) Xanthomatous neuropathy in primary biliary cirrhosis. Brain 88: 1079–1088

Thomas PK, Ward JD (1975) Diabetic neuropathy. In: Keen H, Jarrett J (eds) Complications of diabetes. Edward Arnold, London, pp 151–177

Thomas PK, Calne DB, Elliott CF (1972) X-linked scapulo-peroneal syndrome. J Neurol Neurosurg Psychiatry 35: 208–215

Thomas PK, Hollinrake K, Lascelles RG et al. (1971) The polyneuropathy of chronic renal failure. Brain 94: 761–780

Thomas PK, King RHM, Kocen RS et al. (1977) Comparative ultrastructural observations on peripheral nerve abnormalities in late infantile, juvenile and late onset forms of metachromatic leucodystrophy. Acta Neuropathol 29: 237

Thomas PK, Lascelles RG, Hallpike JF et al. (1969) Recurrent and chronic relapsing Guillain–Barré polyneuritis. Brain 72: 589–606

Thomas PK, Ochoa J, Berthold CH et al. (1993) Microscopic anatomy of the peripheral nervous system. In: Dyck PJ, Thomas PK (eds) Peripheral neuropathy, 3rd edn. Saunders, Philadelphia, pp 28–92

Thomas PK, Schott GD, Morgan-Hughes JA (1975) Adult-onset scapulo-peroneal myopathy. J Neurol Neurosurg Psychiatry 38: 1008–1015

Thomas PK, Sears T, Gilliatt RW (1959) The range of conduction velocity in normal motor nerve fibres to the small muscles of the hand and foot. J Neurol Neurosurg Psychiatry 22: 175–181

Thomas PK, Walker RWH, Rudge P et al. (1987) Chronic demyelinating peripheral neuropathy associated with multifocal central nervous system demyelination Brain 110: 53–76

Thomas PK, Workman JM, Thage O (1984) Behr's syndrome. J Neurol Sci 64: 137–148

Thomasen E (1948) Myotonia, Thomsen's disease (myotonia congenita), paramyotonia and dystrophia myotonica. Universitets Forlaget, Aarhus

Thomashefsky AJ, Horwitz SJ, Feingold MH (1972) Acute autonomic neuropathy. Neurology 22: 251–255

Thompson AJ, Hutchinson M (1984) Myopathy in hypokalaemic periodic paralysis: reversal with metazolamide. Irish Med J 77: 171–172

Thompson MW (1985) Genetic management of pregnancies of carriers and possible carriers of Duchenne muscular dystrophy. (Unpublished)

Thompson PD (1993) Stiff muscles. J Neurol Neurosurg Psychiatry 56: 121–124

Thorburn W (1907) The symptoms due to cervical ribs. Med Chron (4th series) 14: 165–192

Thormell L-E, Edstrom L, Billeter R et al. (1984) Muscle fibre type composition in distal myopathy (Welander). J Neurol Sci 65: 269–292

Thornell L-E, Edstrom L, Eriksson A et al. (1980) The distribution of intermediate filament protein (skeletin) in normal and diseased human skeletal muscle. J Neurol Sci 47: 153–170

Thornell L-E, Eriksson A, Edstrom L (1983) Intermediate filaments in human myopathies. In: Dowben RM, Schay JW (eds) Cell and muscle motility, vol 4. Plenum Press, New York, pp 84–136

Thornton CA, Griggs RC (1994) Plasma exchange and intravenous immunoglobulin treatment of neuromuscular disease. Ann Neurol 35: 260–268

Thornton CA, Griggs RC, Moxlen RT (1994) Myotonic dystrophy with no trinucleotide repeat expansion Ann Neurol 35: 269–272

Thrush D (1992) Investigation of peripheral neuropathy. Br J Hosp Med 48: 133–22

Thrush DC, Holt IG, Bradley WG et al. (1974) Neurological manifestations of xeroderma pigmentosum in two siblings. J Neurol Sci 22: 91–104

Thrush DC, Morris CJ, Salman MV (1972) Paramyotonia congenita: A clinical histochemical and pathological study. Brain 95: 537–552

Timperley WR, Boulton, AJM, Davies-Jones GAB et al. (1985) Small vessel disease in progressive diabetic neuropathy associated with good diabetic control. J Clin Pathol 38: 1030–1038

Tindall RA, Phillips JT, Rawlins JA et al. (1993) A clinical therapeutic trial of cyclosporin in myasthenia gravis. Ann NY Acad Sci 681: 539–551

Tindall RJA, Rollins JA, Phillips JT et al. (1987) Preliminary results of a double-blind randomised placebo-controlled trial of cyclosporin in myasthenia gravis. N Engl J Med 316: 719–724

Tinel J (1917) Nerve wounds. Bailliére, Tindall & Cox, London

Tinsley JM, Blake DJ, Roche A et al. (1992) Primary structure of dystrophin-related protein. Nature 360: 591–593

Toda T, Segawa M, Nomura Y et al. (1993) Localisation of a gene for Fukuyama type congenital muscular dystrophy to chromosome 9Q31–33. Nature Genet 5: 283–286

Todorov A, Jéquier M, Klein D et al. (1970) Analyse de la segregation dans la dystrophie myotonique. J Genet Hum 18: 387–392

Tomanga M (1977) Histochemical and ultrastructural changes in senile human skeletal muscle. J Am Geriatr Soc 25: 125–131

Tomasi LG (1979) Reversibility of human myopathy caused by vitamin E deficiency. Neurology 29: 1182–1186

Tomé FMS, Fardeau M (1972) "Finger-print inclusions" in muscle fibres in dystrophia myotonica. Acta Neuropathol (Berl) 24: 62–67

Tomé FMS, Fardeau M (1975) Congenital myopathy with "reducing bodies" in muscle fibres. Acta Neuropathol (Berl) 31: 207–217

Tomé FMS, Fardeau M (1980) Nuclear inclusions in oculopharyngeal dystrophy. Acta Neuropathol (Berl) 49: 85–87

Tomé FMS, Evangelista T, Lecule A et al. (1994) Congenital muscular dystrophy with merosin deficiency. Cr Acad Sci (Paris) Life Sciences 317: 351–357

Tomlinson BE, Walton JN, Irving D (1974) Spinal cord limb motor neurones in muscular dystrophy. J Neurol Sci 22: 305–327

Tomlinson BE, Walton JN, Rebeiz JJ (1969) The effects of ageing and of cachexia upon skeletal muscle: a histopathological study. J Neurol Sci 9: 321–346

Tonin P, Lewis P, Servidei S et al. (1990) Metabolic causes of myoglobinuria. Ann Neurol 27: 181–185

Tonin P, Shanskes S, Miranda AF et al. (1993) Phosphoglycerate kinase deficiency Neurology 43: 387–391

Tonzola RF, Ackil AA, Shahani BT et al. (1981) Usefulness of electrophysiological studies in the diagnosis of lumbosacral root disease. Ann Neurol 9: 305–308

Torbergson T (1975) A family with dominant hereditary myotonia muscular hypertrophy and increased muscular irritability distinct from myotonia congenita (Thomsen) Acta Neurol Scand 51: 225–232

Torda C, Wolff HG (1951) Effects of administration of adrenocorticotrophic hormone on patients with myasthenia gravis. Arch Neurol 66: 163–170

Torebjork HE, Ochoa J, McCann FV (1979) Paresthesiae: abnormal impulse generation in sensory nerve fibres in man. Acta Physiol Scand 105: 518–520

Tornvall G (1963) Assessment of physical capabilities with special reference to the evaluation of maximal voluntary isometric muscle strength and maximal working capacity. Acta Physiol Scand 58 [Suppl 201]: 1–102

Toulouse P, Coatrieux JL, Le Marec B (1985) An attempt to differentiate female relatives of Duchenne type dystrophy from healthy subjects using an automatic EMG analysis. J Neurol Sci 67: 45–55

Toyka KV, Drachman DB, Griffin DE et al. (1977) Myasthenia gravis: a study of humoral immune mechanisms by passive transfer to mice. N Engl J Med 296: 125–131

Toyka KV, Drachman DB, Pestronk A et al. (1975) Myasthenia gravis: passive transfer from man to mouse. Science 190: 397–399

Traber MG, Sokol RJ, Ringel SP et al. (1987) Lack of tocopherol in peripheral nerves of vitamin E deficient patients with peripheral neuropathy. N Engl J Med 317: 262–265

Treem WR, Stanley CA, Finegold DN et al. (1988) Primary carnitine deficiency due to a failure of carnitine transport in kidney, muscle and fibroblasts. N Engl J Med 319: 1331–1336

Trend P St J, Wiles CM, Spencer GT et al. (1985) Acid maltase deficiency in adults: diagnosis and management in five cases. Brain 108: 845–860

Trojaborg W (1970) Rate of recovery in motor and sensory fibres of the radial nerve: clinical and electrophysiological aspects. J Neurol Neurosurg Psychiatry 33: 625–638

Trojaborg W (1976) Motor and sensory conduction in the musculo-cutaneous nerve. J Neurol Neurosurg Psychiatry 39: 890–899

Trojaborg W (1977) Electrophysiological findings in pressure palsy of the brachial plexus. J Neurol Neurosurg Psychiatry 40: 1160–1167

Trojaborg W (1990) Quantitative electromyography in polymyositis: a reappraisal. Muscle Nerve 13: 964–971

Trojaborg W, Buchthal F (1965) Malignant and benign fasciculation. Acta Neurol Scand 41 [Suppl 13]: 251–254

Trojaborg W, Frantzen E, Andersen I (1969) Peripheral neuropathy and myopathy associated with carcinoma of the lung. Brain 92: 71–82

Trokel SL, Hilal SK (1979) Recognition and differential diagnosis of enlarged extra-ocular muscles in computed tomography. Am J Ophthalmol 87: 503–512

Troni W, Corta Q, Contello R et al. (1984) Peripheral nerve function and metabolic control in diabetes mellitus. Ann Neruol 16: 178–183

Trontelj JV (1973) A study of the H reflex by single fibre EMG. J Neurol Neurosurg Psychiatry 36: 951–959

Trontelj J, Stålberg E (1983a) Responses to electrical stimulation of denervated human muscle fibres recorded with single fibre EMG. J Neurol Neurosurg Psychiatry 46: 305–309

Trontelj J, Stålberg E (1983b) Bizarre repetitive discharges recorded with single fibre EMG. J Neurol Neurosurg Psychiatry 46: 310–316

Trontelj JV, Stålberg E (1991) Single motor end plates in myasthenia gravis and LEMS at different firing rates. Muscle Nerve 14: 226–232

Trounce I, Byrne E, Marsuki S (1989) Decline in skeletal muscle mitochondrial respiratory chain function: possible factor in ageing. Lancet i: 637–639

Troutman JR (1984) Epidemiological aspects of Hansen's disease. Bull NY Acad Med 60: 722–731

Tsairis P, Dyck PJ, Mulder DW (1972) Natural history of brachial plexus neuropathy: report on 99 patients. Arch Neurol 27: 109–117

Tsairis P, Engel WK, Kark P (1973) Familial myoclonic epilepsy syndrome associated with skeletal muscle mitochondrial abnormalities. Neurology 23: 408

Tsujino S, Shanske S, Brownell AKW et al. (1994) Molecular genetic studies of muscle lactate dehydrogenase deficiency in white patients. Ann Neurol 36: 661–665

Tsujino S, Shanske S, Di Mauro S (1993a) Molecular genetic heterogeneity of myophosphorylase deficiency (McArdle's disease). N Engl J Med 329: 241–245

Tsujino S, Shanske S, Sakoda S et al. (1993b) The molecular genetic basis of muscle phosphoglycerate mutase (PGAM) deficiency. Am J Hum Genet 52: 472–477

Tsukagoshi H, Shoji H, Furukawa T (1970) Proximal neurogenic muscular atrophy in adolescence and adulthood with X-linked recessive inheritance. Neurology 20: 1188–1193

Tsukamoto H, Inagaki M, Tomita Y et al. (1992) Congenital cauda spinal atrophy: a case report. Neuropediatrics 23: 260–262

Tu PH, Raju P, Robinson KA et al. (1996) Transgenic mice carrying a human mutant superoxide dismutase transgene develop cytoskeletal pathology resembling human amyotrophic lateral sclerosis. Proc Natl Acad Sci USA 93: 3155–3160

Tuck RR, Schmelzer JD, Low PA (1984) Endoneurial blood flow and oxygen tension in the sciatic nerves of rats with experimental diabetic neuropathy. Brain 107: 935–950

Tugwell P, James SL (1972) Peripheral neuropathy with ethambutol. Postgrad Med J 48: 667–670

Turken SA, Cafferty M, Silverberg SJ et al. (1989) Neuromuscular involvement in mild asymptomatic primary hyperparathyroidism. Am J Med 87: 553–557

Turner HD, Bret EM, Bilbert RJ et al. (1978) Infant botulism in England. Lancet i: 1277–1278

Turner JWA, Heathfield KWG (1961) Quadriceps myopathy occuring in middle age. J Neurol Neurosurg Psychiatry 24: 18–21

Turner JWA, Lees F (1962) Congenital myopathy: a 50 year follow up. Brain 85: 733–740

Turner JWA, Parsonage M (1957) Neuralgic amyotrophy (paralytic brachial neuritis) with special reference to prognosis. Lancet ii: 209–212

Turnbull DM, Bartlett K, Stevens DL et al. (1984) Short chain acyl CoA dehydrogenase deficiency associated with a lipid storage myopathy and secondary carnitine deficiency. N Engl J Med 311: 1232–1236

Tyler FH, Stephens FE (1950) Studies in disorders of muscle. II. Clinical manifestations and inheritance of facio-scapulo-humeral dystrophy in a large family. Ann Intern Med 32: 640–660

Tyler FH, Stephens FE, Gunn FD et al. (1951) Studies in disorders of muscle. J Clin Invest 30: 492–502

Tylleskår T, Bonea M, Bikangi N et al. (1992) Cassava cyanogens and konzo, an upper motor neurone disease found in Africa. Lancet 339: 208–211

Tytel M, Black MM, Garner J et al. (1981) Axonal transport: each rate component reflects the movement of distinct macromolecular complexes. Science 214: 179–181

Tzall S, Martiniuk F, Adler A (1990) Identification of an RaS1 RFLP at the alpha acid glucosidase (GAA) locus. Nucleic Acid Res 18: 1661

Tzartos SJ, Efthimiadis A, Morel E et al. (1990) Neonatal myasthenia gravis: antigenic specifities of antibodies in sera from mothers and their infants. Clin Exp Immunol 30: 376

Uchino M, Araki S, Yoshida O et al. (1985) Structural proteins of the opaque muscle fibres in Duchenne muscular dystrophy. Neurology 35: 1364–1367

Ugawa Y, Inoue K, Takemura T et al. (1986) Accumulation of glycogen in sural nerve axons in adult onset Type III glycogenosis. Ann Neurol 19: 294–297

Uncini A, Di Muzio A, Sabatelli M et al. (1993) Sensitivity and specificity of diagnostic criteria for conduction block in chronic inflammatory demyelinating polyneuropathy. Electroencephalogr Clin Neurophysiol 89: 161–169

Uncini A, Lange DJ, Lovelace RE et al. (1990) Long duration polyphasic motor unit potentials in myopathies. Muscle Nerve 13: 263–267

Uncini A, Pullman SL, Lovelace RE et al. (1988) The sympathetic skin response. J Neurol Sci 87: 299–306

Unverricht H (1891) Dermatomyositis acuta. Dtsch Med Wochenschr 17: 41–44

Upton ARM, McComas AJ (1973) The double crush in nerve entrapment syndromes. Lancet ii: 359–362

Upton ARM, McComas AJ, Bianchi AF (1973) Neuropathy in McArdle's syndrome. N Engl J Med 289: 750–51

Urbanic RC, George JM (1981) Cushing's disease: 18 years' experience. Medicine (Baltimore) 60: 14–24

Urbano-Marquez A, Estruch R, Grau JM et al. (1986) Inflammatory myopathy associated with chronic graft-vs-host disease. Neurology 36: 1091–1093

Urbano-Marquez A, Estruch R, Novarro-Lopez A et al. (1989) The effects of alcoholism on skeletal and cardiac muscle. N Engl J Med 320: 409–414

Urihurne IJF, Morchio FT, Marin JC (1976) Compression syndrome of the deep motor branch of the ulnar nerve (pisohamate hiatus syndrome). J Bone Joint Surg [Am] 58: 145–147

Urich H (1974) Patterns of diffuse infiltration of the nervous system in leukaemias and lymphomas. Proc R Soc Med 67: 17–23

Urich H, Wilkinson M (1970) Necrosis of muscle with carinoma: myositis or myopathy? J Neurol Neurosurg Psychiatry 33: 398–407

Vainzoff M, Pavannello RCM, Pavannello I et al. (1991) Dystrophin immunofluorescence patterns in manifesting and asymptomatic carriers of Duchenne and Becker muscular dystrophies of different ages. Neuromusc Disord 1: 177–183

Vainzhoff M, Zubrycka-Gaarn EE, Rapaport D et al. (1991) Immunofluorescence dystrophin study in Duchenne muscular dystrophy through the concomitant use of two antibodies directed against the carboxy terminal and amino terminal region of the protein. J Neurol Sci 101: 141–147

Valentijn LJ, Baas F, Wolteman RA et al. (1992a) Identical point mutations of the peripheral myelin protein 22 in Trembler J mouse and a family with Charcot–Marie–Tooth disease. Nature Genet 2: 288–291

Valentijn LJ, Bolhuis PA, Zorn I et al. (1992b) The peripheral myelin gene PMP-22/GAS-3 is duplicated in Charcot–Marie–Tooth disease Type 1A. Nature Genet 1: 166–170

Valentine BA, Cooper BJ (1991) Canine X-linked muscular dystrophy: selective involvement of muscles in neonatal dogs. Neuromusc Disord 1: 31–38

Valeriano J, Tucker P, Kattah J (1983) An unusual cause of hypokalaemic muscle weakness. Neurology 33: 1242–1244

Vallat J-M, Desproges-Getteran R, Lebouter MJ et al. (1980) Cryoglobulinemic neuropathy: a pathologic study. Ann Neurol 8: 179–185

Vallat J-M, De Lumley L. Loubet A et al. (1982) Co-existence of minicores, cores and rods in the same muscle biopsy. Acta Neuropathol 58: 229–232

Vallat J-M, Dumas M, Giordano C et al. (1987a) Histologic study of peripheral nerve biopsies from 20 patients with tropical ataxic neuropathy. Neurology 33 [Supppl 1]: 255

Vallat J-M, Hugon M, Lubeau M et al. (1987b) Tick bite meningo radiculo neuritis: clinical, electrophysiological and histologic findings in 10 cases. Neurology 37: 749–753

Valli G, Barbiere S, Cappa S et al. (1983) Syndromes of abnormal muscular activity: overlap between continuous muscle fibre activity and the stiff man syndrome. J Neurol Neurosurg Psychiatry 46: 241–247

Valls-Sole J, Tolosa ES, Pujol M (1992) Myokymic discharges and enhanced facial nerve reflex responses after recovery from idiopathic facial palsy. Muscle Nerve 15: 37–42

Van den Berg LH, Karkhoff H, Oey PL et al. (1995) Treatment of multifocal motor neuropathy with high dose intravenous immunoglobulins. J Neurol Neurosurg Psychiatry 59: 248–252

Van der Berg IET, Berger R (1990) Phosphorylase b kinase deficiency in man. J Inherit Metab Dis 13: 442–451

Van der Does de Willebois AEM, Bethlem J, Meyer AEFH et al. (1968) Distal myopathy with onset in early infancy. Neurology 18: 383–390

Van der Geld H, Feltkamp TEW, Oosterhuis HJGH (1964) Reactivity of myasthenia gravis serum gammaglobulin with skeletal muscle and thymus demonstrated by immunofluorescence. Proc Soc Exp Biol Med 115: 782–785

Van der Hoeven JH, Links TP, Zwaris MJ et al. (1994) Muscle fibre conduction velocity in the diagnosis of familial hypokalaemic periodic paralysis: invasive vs surface determination. Muscle Nerve 17: 898–905

Van der Meche FGA et al. (1992) A randomized trial comparing intravenous immune globulin and plasma exchange in Guillain–Barré syndrome. N Engl J Med 326: 1123–1129

Van der Meulen JP, Gilbert GJ, Kane CA (1961) Familial hyperkalaemic paralysis with myotonia. N Engl J Med 264: 1–7

Van der Ploeg AT, Bolhuis PA, Wolterman RA et al. (1988) Prospects for enzyme therapy in glycogenosis Type 2 variants: a study on cultured muscle cells. J Neurol 235: 392–396

Van der Ploeg AT, Kroos MA, Swallow DM et al. (1989) An investigation of the possible influence of neutral alphaglucosidases on the clinical heterogeneity of glycogenosis Type 2. Ann Hum Genet 53: 185–192

van der Pleog RJO, Oosterhuis HJGH (1991) The "make/break test" as a diagnostic tool in functional weakness. J Neurol Neurosurg Psychiatry 54: 248–251

van der Pleog RJO, Fidler V, Oosterhuis HJGH (1991) Hand held myometry: reference values. J Neurol Neurosurg Psychiatry 54: 244–247

van der Ploeg RJO, Oosterhuis HJGH, Reuvekamp J (1984) Measuring muscle strength. J Neurol 231: 200–203

Van der Pool DW et al. (1968) Peripheral compression lesions of the ulnar nerve. J Bone Joint Surg [Br] 50: 792–803

Van der Vliet JA, Navarro X, Kennedy WR et al. (1988) Long-term follow up of polyneuropathy in diabetic kidney transplant recipients. Diabetes 37: 1247–1252

Van der Walt J, Swash M, Leake J et al. (1987) The pattern of involvement of acid maltase deficiency at autopsy. Muscle Nerve 10: 272–281

van Doorn PA, Brand A, Strengers PFW et al. (1990) High dose intravenous immunoglobulin treatment in chronic inflammatory demyelinating polyneuropathy: a double-blind, placebo-controlled cross-over study. Neurology 40: 209–212

van Dyck DH, Griggs RC, Markesbery W et al. (1975) Hereditary carnitine deficiency of muscle. Neurology 25: 154–159

van Graefe A (1856) Verhandlungen ärztlicher Gesellschaften. Berl Klin Wochenschr 5: 125–127

Van Laere JE (1966) Paralysie bulbo-pontine chronique progressive familiale avec surdité: un cas de syndrome de Klippel-Trenaunay dans la même fratrie: problèms diagnostiques et génétiques. Rev Neurol 115: 289–295

Van Munster ETL, Joosten EMG, Van Muster-Vijtde Haage MAM et al. (1986) The rigid spine syndrome J Neurol Neurosurg Psychiatry 49: 1292–1297

van Wensen PJM (1991) Heredo-familial plexus brachialis neuropathy. In: Winken PJ, Bruyn GW, Klawans HL (eds) Hereditary neuropathies and spinocerebellar atrophies. Elsevier, Amsterdam, pp 71–73 (Handbook of neurology, vol 60)

van Wijngaarden GK, Bethlem J (1971) The facio-scapulo-humeral syndrome. In: Kakulas BA (ed) Clinical studies in myology, 2nd International Congress on Muscle Diseases, Perth. Excerpta Medica, Amsterdam, pp 498–501 (International congress series 295)

van Wijngaarden GK, Bethlem J, Dingemans KP et al. (1977) Familial focal loss of cross striations. J Neurol 216: 163–172

van Wijngaarden GK, Fleury P, Bethlem J et al. (1969) Familial "myotubular" myopathy. Neurology 19: 901–908

van Wijngaarden GK, Hagen CJ, Bethlem J et al. (1968) Myopathy of the quadriceps muscle. J Neurol Sci 7: 201–206

Vasilescu C, Alexianu M, Dan A (1984) Neuronal type of Charcot–Marie–Tooth disease with the syndrome of continuous motor unit activity. J Neurol Sci 63: 11–25

Vasilescu C, Bucur G, Petrovici A et al. (1978a) Myasthenia in patients with dermatomyositis. J Neurol Sci 38: 129–144

Vasilescu C, Florescu A, Balta N (1978b) Electroneurographic evidence of polyneuropathy in chronic liver disease. Arch Psychiatr Nervenkr 225: 87–96

Vbrova G (1983) Duchenne dystrophy viewed as a disturbance of nerve–muscle interactions. Muscle Nerve 6: 671–675

Veda T (1993) Possible linkage between ALS and PDC on Guam. Wakayama Med Rep 34: 35–51

Veltana AN (1975) The case of the saltimbanque Prosper Laconte, a contribution to the study of the history of progressive muscular atrophy (Aran Duchenne) and amyotrophic lateral sclerosis (Charcot). Clin Neurol Neurosurg 78: 204–209

Veltana AN, Verjaal A (1961) Surgical d'heredopathic ataxique polynevritique. Rev Neurol 104: 15–23

Venables GS, Bates D, Cartlidge NEF et al. (1982) Acute polymyositis with subcutaneous oedema. J Neurol Sci 55: 161–164

Verbiest H (1955) Further experiences on the pathologic influence of a developmental narrowness of the bony lumbar vertebral canal. J Bone Joint Surg [Br] 37: 576–583

Vercolen JHMM, Swanink CMA, Fennis JFM et al. (1996) Prognosis in chronic fatigue syndrome. J Neurol Neurosurg Psychiatry 60: 489–494

Vercruysseen A, Martin JT, Marcelis R (1982) Neurophysiological studies in adrenomyeloneuropathy. J Neurol Sci 56: 327–336

Verdugo R, Ochoa JL (1992) Quantitiative somatosensory thermo test. Brain 115: 893–913

Verghese M, Ithnimani KV, Satranarayan KR et al. (1970) A study of conduction velocity of ulnar and median nerves in leprosy. Int J Lepr 38: 271–277

Verhagen WIM, Gabreels-Festen AAWM, van Wensen PJM et al. (1993) Hereditary neuropathy with liability to pressure palsies: a clinical, electroneurophysiological and morphological study. J Neurol Sci 116: 176–184

Verhiest W, Brucher JM, Gardderis P et al. (1976) Familial centronuclear myopathy associated with cardiomyopathy. Br Heart J 38: 504–509

Vermeulen M, van Doorn PA, Brand A et al. (1993) Intravenous immunoglobulin treatment in patients with chronic inflammatory demyelinating polyneuropathy: a double-blind, placebo-controlled study. J Neurol Neurosurg Psychiatry 56: 36–39

Vetters JM (1965) Immunofluorescence staining patterns in skeletal muscle using serum of myasthenic patients and normal controls. Immunology 9: 93–95

Vialetto E (1936) Contributo alla forina ereditaria della paralisi bulbare progressiva. Riv Sper Frevi 40: 1–24

Victor M (1984) Polyneuropathy due to nutritional deficiency and alcoholism. In Dyck PJ, Thomas PK, Lambert EH, Bunge R (eds). Peripheral neuropathy 2nd edn. Saundles, Philadelphra, RP 1899–1940

Victor M, Adams RD (1953) The effect of alcohol on the nervous system. Res Publ Assoc Res Nerv Ment Dis 32: 526–573

Victor M, Adams RD, Collins GH (1971) The Wernicke-Korsakoff syndrome: a clinical and pathological study of 245 patients, 82 with post-mortem examinations. Blackwell Scientific Publications, Oxford (Contemporary neurology series, vol 7).

Victor M, Banker BQ, Adams RD (1958) The neuropathy of multiple myeloma. J Neurol Neurosurg Psychiatry 21: 73–88

Victor M, Hayes R, Adams RD (1962) Oculopharyngeal muscular dystrophy. A familial disease of late life characterised by dysphagia and progressive ptosis of the eyelids. N Engl J Med 267: 1267–1272

Viets HR, Schwab RS (1935) Prostigmin in the diagnosis of myasthenia gravis. N Engl J Med 213: 1280

Vigliani EC (1954) Carbon disulphide poisoning in viscose rayon factories. Br J Ind Med 11: 235–244

Vignos PJ Jr, Kirby AC, Marsalis PH (1976) Contractile properties of rabbit fast and slow muscles in steroid myopathy. Exp Neurol 53: 444–453

Vignos PJ, Spencer GE, Archibald KC (1963) Management of progressive muscular dystrophy in childhood. JAMA 184: 89–96

Vincent A, Li Z, Hart A et al. (1993) Seronegative myasthenia gravis. Ann NY Acad Sci 681: 529–538

Vincent A, Newland C, Brueton L et al. (1995) Arthrogryposis multiple congenita with maternal auto antibodies specific to a fetal antigen. Lancet 346: 24–25

Vincent A, Newsom-Davis J (1980) Anti-acetylcholine receptor antibodies. J Neurol Neurosurg Psychiatry 43: 590–600

Vincent A, Newsom-Davis J, Martin V (1978a) Anti-acetylcholine receptor antibodies in D-penicillamine associated myasthenia gravis. Lancet i: 1254

Vincent A, Newsom-Davis J, Newton P et al. (1983) Acetylcholine receptor antibody and clinical response to thymectomy in myasthenia gravis. Neurology 33: 1276–1282

Vincent A, Scadding GK, Clarke C et al. (1979) Anti-acetylcholine receptor antibody synthesis in culture. In: Dau PC (ed) Plasmapheresis and the immunobiology of myasthenia gravis. Houghton Mifflin, Boston, pp 59–71

Vincent A, Scadding GK, Thomas HC et al. (1978b) In vitro synthesis of anti-acetylcholine receptor antibody by thymic lymphocytes in myasthenia gravis. Lancet i: 305–307

Vincent A, Whiting PJ, Schloep M et al. (1987) Antibody heterogeneity and specificity in myasthenia gravis. Ann NY Acad Sci 505: 106–120

Virmani V, Mohan PK (1985) Non-familial, spinal segmental muscular atrophy in juvenile and young subjects. Acta Neurol Scand 72: 336–340

Vita G, Harris JB (1981) The uptake of 99m-technetium diphosphonate into degenerating and regenerating muscle. J Neurol Scsi 51: 339–354

Vita G, Migliorato A, Toscano A et al. (1994) Immunocytochemistry of muscle cytoskeletal proteins in acid maltase deficiency. Muscle Nerve 17: 655–661

Vita G, Toscano A, Bresolin N et al. (1994) Muscle phosphoglycerate mutase (PGAM) deficiency in the first caucasian patient. J Neurol 241: 284–294

Vital A, Vital C, Riviere JP et al. (1987) Variability of morphological features in early infantile polyneuropathy with defective myelination. Acta Neuropathol 73: 295–300

Vliset AM vd, Thijssen HOM, Joosten E et al. (1988) CT in neuromuscular disorders: a comparison of CT and histology. Neuroradiology 30: 421–425

Voitk AS, Mueller JC, Farlinger DE et al. (1983) Carpal tunnel syndrome in pregnancy. Can Med Assoc J 128: 277–279

von Scheele C (1986) Levodopa in restless legs. Lancet ii: 426–427

Vracko R (1974) Basal lamina scaffold: anatomy and significance for maintenance of orderly tissue structure. Am J Pathol 77: 314–346

Vriesendrop FJ, Mishu B, Blaser MJ et al. (1993) Serum antibodies to GM_1, GD_{1B}, peripheral nerve myelin and Campylobacter jejuni in patients with Guillain–Barré syndrome and controls: correlation and prognosis. Ann Neurol 34: 130–135

Vukanovic S, Hanser H, Wettstein P (1980) CT localisation of myonecrosis for surgical decompression. Am J Radiol 135: 1298–1299

Waal Manning HT (1969) Effect of propranolol on the duration of the Achilles reflex. Clin Pharmacol Ther 10: 199–206

Wackenheim A, Babin E (1980) The narrow lumbar canal. Springer, Berlin Heldelberg New York, pp 91–95

Wada K, Veno S, Hazama T et al. (1983) Radioimmunoassay for antibodies to human skeletal muscle myosin in serum from patients with polymyositis. Clin Exp Immunol 52: 297–304

Waddell G (1982) An approach to backache. Br J Hosp Med 37: 187–219

Waddy H, Wessely S, Murray NMF (1990) Central motor conduction studies in chronic post viral fatigue syndrome. Electroencephalogr Clin Neurophysiol 75: Suppl S160

Wade D (1993) Assessment of motor function: impairment and disability. In: Greenwood R, Barnes MP, McMillan TM, Ward CD (eds) Neurological rehabilitation. Churchill Livingstone, Edinburgh, pp 147–160

Wade DT, Langton-Hewer R (1987) Functional abilities after stroke. J Neurol Neurosurg Psychiatry 50: 177–182

Wadia NH (1984a) SMON as seen from Bombay. Acta Neurol Scand 70 [Suppl 100]: 159–164

Wadia NH (1984b) Geographical patterns of neuropathy: India. In: Asbury AK, Gilliatt RW (eds) Peripheral nerve disorders. Butterworth, London, pp 287–302

Wadia RS, Shitra S, Amin RB et al. (1987) Electrophysiological studies in acute organophosphate poisoning. J Neurol Neurosurg Psychiatry 50: 1442–1448

Wagen BD, Gutmann L (1974) Wound botulism. JAMA 227: 1416–1417

Wagman IH, Lesse H (1952) Maximum conduction velocities of motor fibres of ulnar nerve in human subjects of various ages and sizes. J Neurophysiol 15: 235–244

Wagner AL, Buchthal F (1972) Motor and sensory conduction in infancy and childhood: a reappraisal. Dev Med Child Neurol 14: 189–216

Wagner E (1863) Fall einer seltenen Muskelkrankheit. Arch Heilkunde 4: 282–283

Wahren J, Felig P, Havel RJ et al. (1973) Amino acid metabolism in McArdle's syndrome. N Engl J Med 288: 774–777

Wakai S, Minami R, Kameda K et al. (1988) Electron microscopic study of the biopsied cardiac muscle in Duchenne's progressive muscular dystrophy. J Neurol Sci 84: 167–176

Wakayama Y, Fischbeck K, Bonilla E et al. (1982) Erythrocyte membrane studies. Neurology 32: 917

Wakayama Y, Schotland DL, Bonilla E et al. (1979) Quantitative ultrastructural study of muscle satellite cells in Duchenne dystrophy. Neurology 29: 401–407

Waksman BH, Adams RD (1956) A comparative study of experimental allergic neuritis in the rabbit, guinea pig and mouse. J Neuropathol Exp Neurol 15: 293–334

Waldenström J (1939) Neurological symptoms caused by so-called acute porphyria. Acta Psychiatr Neurol 14: 375–379

Waldstein SS, Bronsky D, Shrifter HB et al. (1958) The electromyogram in myxedema. Arch Intern Med 101: 97–102

Walker MB (1934) Treatment of myasthenia gravis with physostigmine. Lancet i: 1200

Walker MB (1938) Myasthenia gravis: a case in which fatigue of the forearm muscles could induce paralysis of the extra-ocular muscles. Proc R Soc Med 31: 722

Wall PD (1985) Pain. In: Swash M, Kennard (eds) The scientific basis of clinical neurology. Churchill Livingstone, Edinburgh, pp 163–171

Wallace SL, Lattis R, Ragan C (1958) Diagnostic significance of the muscle biopsy Am J Med 25: 600–610

Waller A (1850) Experiments on the section of the glossopharyngeal and hypoglossal nerves of the frog, and observations on the alterations produced thereby in the structure of their primitive fibres. Philos Trans R Soc London [Biol] 140: 423

Wallgren-Patterson C, Sainio K, Salmi T (1989) Electromyography in congenital nemaline myopathy. Muscle Nerve 12: 587–593

Wallis WE, van Poznak A, Plum F (1970) Generalised muscular stiffness, fasciculations and myokymia of peripheral nerve origin. Arch Neurol 22: 430–439

Walsh JC (1971) The neuropathy of multiple myeloma. Arch Neurol 25: 404–414

Walsh JC, Conomy AB (1977) The effect of ethyl alcohol on striated muscle: some clinical and pathological observations. Aust NZ J Med 7: 485–490

Walsh JC, McLeod JG (1970) Alcoholic neuropathy. An electrophysiological and histological study. J Neurol Sci 10: 457–469

Walton JN (1952) The electromyogram in myopathy: analysis with audiofrequency spectrometer. J Neurol Neurosurg Psychiatry 15: 219–226

Walton JN (1956) Amyotonia congenita: a follow-up study. Lancet i: 1023–1027

Walton JN (1963) Clinical aspects of human muscular dystrophy. In: Bourne GH, Golarz MN (eds) Muscular dystrophy in man and animals. Karger, Basel, pp 263–321

Walton JN (1973) Progressive muscular dystrophy: structural alteration in various stages and in carriers of muscular dystrophy. In: Pearson CM (ed) The striated muscle. Williams and Wilkins, Baltimore, pp 263–291

Walton JN (1983) The inflammatory myopathies. J R Soc Med 76: 998–1010

Walton JN, Nattress FJ (1954) On the classification, natural history and treatment of the myopathies. Brain 77: 169–231

Walton JN Warrick CK (1954) Osseous changes in myopathy. Br J Radiol 27: 1–15

Wang P, Clausen T (1976) Treatment of attacks in hyperkalaemic periodic paralysis by inhalation of salbutamol. Lancet i: 221–223

Ward JD, Barnes CG, Fisher DJ et al. (1971) Improvement in nerve conduction following treatment in newly diagnosed diabetes. Lancet i: 428–430

Ward JD, Simms JM, Knight G et al. (1983) Venous distension in the diabetic neuropathic root (physical sign of arterio-venous shunting). J R Soc Med 76: 1011–1014

Warmolts JR, Engel WK (1972a) Open biopsy electromyography. Arch Neurol 27: 512–517

Warmolts JR, Engel WK (1972b) Benefit from alternate day prednisone in myasthenia gravis. N Engl J Med 286: 17–20

Warmolts JR, Mendell JR (1980) Neurotonia: impulse-induced repetitive discharges in motor nerves in peripheral neuropathy. Ann Neurol 7: 245–250

Warner CL, Servidei S, Lange DJ (1990) X-linked spinal muscular atrophy (Kennedy's syndrome). Arch Neurol 47: 1117–1120

Warner TT, Mossman S, Murray NMF (1993) Hypokalaemia mimicking Guillain–Barré syndrome. J Neurol Neurosurg Psychiatry 56: 1134–1135

Warrel DA, Godfrey S, Olsen EGJ (1968) Giant cell arteritis with peripheral neuropathy. Lancet i: 1010–1013

Warren JD (1963) Anterior interosseous nerve palsy as a complication of forearm fractures. J Bone Joint Surg 45B: 511–512

Warszanski M, Telerman-Tappet N, Durdu J et al. (1975) The early stages of neuromuscular regeneration after crushing the sciatic nerve in the rat. J Neurol Sci 24: 21–32

Wartenberg R (1958) Neuritis, sensory neuritis, neuralgia. Oxford University Press, New York

Warton RG, Gillard EF (1993) Duchenne muscular dystrophy. In: Conneally PM (ed) Molecular basis of neurology. Blackwell Scientific Publications, Boston, pp 73–112

Waters DD, Nutter DO, Hopkins LD et al. (1975) Cardiac features of an unusual X-linked humero-peroneal neuromuscular disease. N Engl J Med 293: 1017–1020

Watkins H, Rosenzweig A, Hwang D-S et al. (1992) Characteristics and prognostic implications of myosin mis-sense mutations in familial hypertrophic cardiomyopathy. N Engl J Med 326: 1108–1114

Watkins PJ (1991) Diabetic autonomic neuropathy. N Engl J Med 322: 1078–1079

Watkins SM, Griffin JP (1978) High incidence of vincristine-induced neuropathy in lymphomas. Br Med J i: 610–612

Watts RA, Hoffbrand BI, Patton DF et al. (1987) Pyomyositis associated with human immunodeficiency virus infection. Br Med J 294: 1524–1525

Weber ER, Daube JR, Coventry MB (1976) Peripheral neuropathies associated with total hip arthroplasty. J Bone Joint Surg [Am] 58: 66–69

Weber K, Pfister HW (1994) Clinical management of Lyme borreliosis. Lancet 343: 1017–1020

Weber LD, Nashel DJ, Mellow MH (1981) Pharyngeal dysphagia in alcoholic myopathy. Ann Intern Med 95: 189–191

Wecker L, Laskowski MB, Dettborn W-D (1978) Neuromuscular dysfunction induced by acetylcholinesterase inhibition. Fed Proc 37: 2818–2822

Weiffenback B, Bagley RG, Falls K et al. (1992) Linkage analyses of 5 chromosome 4 markers localize the facio-scapulo-humeral muscular dystrophy (FSHD) gene to distal 4q 35. Am J Hum Genet 51: 416–423

Weinshilbourn RM, Axelrod S (1971) Reduced plasma dopamine β hydroxylase activity in familial dysautonomia. N Engl J Med 285: 938

Weinstein R, Schwartzman R, Levey GS (1975) Propranolol reversal of bulbar dysfunction and proximal myopathy in hyperthyroidism. Ann Intern Med 82: 540–541

Weiss DH, Walker MD, Wiernick PH (1974) Neurotoxicity of commonly used antineoplastic agents. N Engl J Med 291: 127–133

Weiss GM, Nelson RL, O'Neill BP et al. (1980) Use of adrenal biopsy in diagnosing adrenoleukomyeloneuropathy. Arch Neurol 37: 634–636

Welander L (1951) Myopathia distalis tarda hereditaria. Acta Med Scand 141 [Suppl 265]: 1–124

Welch LK, Appenzeller O, Bicknell JM (1972) Peripheral neuropathy with myokymia: sustained muscular contraction and continuous motor unit activity. Neurology 22: 161–169

Weller RO, McArdle B (1971). Calcification within muscle fibres in the periodic paralyses Brain 94: 263–272

Wells JW, Wells KE, Walsh FS et al. (1992) Human dystrophin expression corrects myopathic phenotype on transgenic mdx mice. Hum Mol Genet 1: 35–40

Wennberg A (1984) A neuropathy index based on motor-sensory electroneurography (ENeG). Acta Neurol Scand 70 [Suppl 100]: 107–111

Werdnig G (1891) Zwei fruhinfantile hereditäre Falle von progressiver Muskelatrophie unter den Bilde der Dystrophic aber auch mit neurotischer Grundlage. Arch Psychiatr Nervenkr 22: 437–481

Werk EE(Jr), Sholitan LJ, Marnell RT (1961) The stiff man syndrome and hyperthyroidism. Am J Med 31: 647–653

Werner CO (1979) Lateral elbow pain and posterior interosseous nerve entrapment. Acta Orthop Scand [Suppl 174]

Wessely S (1990) Old wine in new bottles: neurasthenia and ME. Psychol Med 20: 35–53

Wessely S, Powell R (1989) Fatigue syndromes. J Neurol Neurosurg Psychiatry 52: 940–948

Wessely S, Thomas PK (1990) The chronic fatigue syndrome: myalgic encephalomyelitis or postural fatigue. In: Kennard C (ed) Recent advances in clinical neurology, vol 6. Churchill Livingstone, Edinburgh, pp 85–131

Westphal C (1885) Über einen merkwurdigen Fall von periodische Lähmung. Berl Klin Wochenschr 22: 489

Wexler I (1983) Sequence of demyelination-remyelination in Guillain–Barré syndrome. J Neurol Neurosurg Psychiatry 46: 168–174

Wheatley LM, Urso D, Tumas K et al. (1992) Molecular evidence for the expression of nicotinic acetylcholine receptor α chain in mouse thymus. J Immunol 148: 3105–3109

Whitaker JN (1982) Inflammatory myopathy: a review of etiologic and pathogenetic factors. Muscle Nerve 3: 573–592

Whitaker JN, Engel WK (1972) Vascular deposits of immunoglobulin and complement in idiopathic inflammatory myopathy. N Engl J Med 286: 333–338

Whiteley AM, Swash M, Urich H (1976) Progressive encephalomyelitis with rigidity: its relation to subacute myoclonic spinal neuronitis and to the stiff man syndrome. Brain 99: 27–42

WHO Study Group (1982) Chemotherapy of leprosy for control programs. WHO Technical Reports Series, no 675

Wiechers DO, Hubbell SL (1981) Late changes in the motor unit after acute poliomyelitis. Muscle Nerve 4: 524–528

Wiechers DO, Johnson EW (1979) Diffuse abnormal electromyographic insertional activity. Arch Phys Med Rehabil 60: 419–422

Wiechers DO, Stow R, Johnson EW (1977) Electromyographic insertional activity mechanically provoked in biceps brachii. Acta Phys Med Rehabil 58: 573–578

Wiechers NJ, Mattson RH (1969) Acute paralytic brachial neuritis: a clinical and electrodiagnostic study. Neurology 19: 1153–1157

Wiederholt WC (1970) "End-plate noise" in electromyography. Neurology 21: 214–224

Wiederholt WC, Mulder DW, Lambert EH (1964) The Landry–Guillain–Barré–Strohl syndrome, or polyradiculoneuropathy: historical review, report on 97 patients and present concepts. Mayo Clin Proc 39: 427–451

Wiener LP, Stohlman SA, Davis RL (1980) Attempts to demonstrate virus in amyotrophic lateral sclerosis. Neurology 30: 1319–1322

Wijdicks EFM Ropper AH (1990) Acute relapsing Guillain–Barré syndrome after long asymptomatic intervals. Arch Neurol 47: 82–84

Wijmenga C, Frants RR, Brouwer OF et al. (1990) Location of facio-scapulo-humeral muscular dystrophy gene on chromosome 4. Lancet ii: 651–653

Wilbourn AJ, Aminoff MJ (1988) The electrophysiological examination in patients with radiculopathies. Muscle Nerve 11: 1099–1114 (AAEE minimonograph no.32)

Wiles CM, Karni Y (1983) The measurement of muscle strength in patients with peripheral neuromuscular disorders. J Neurol Neurosurg Psychiatry 46: 1006–1013

Wiles CM, Karni Y, Nicklin J (1990) Laboratory testing of muscle function in the management of neuromuscular disease. J Neurol Neurosurg Psychiatry 53: 384–387

Wiles CM, Young A, Jones DA et al. (1979) Muscle relaxation rate, fibre-type composition and energy turnover in hyper- and hypothyroid patients. Clin Sci 57: 375–384

Wilkie DR (1981) Shortage of chemical fuel as a cause of fatigue: studies by nuclear magnetic resonance and bicycle ergometry. In: Parter R, Whelan J (eds) Human muscle fatigue: physiological mechanisms. Pitman, London, pp 102–119

Wilkinson PC (1964) Serological findings in carcinomatous neuropathy. Lancet i: 1301–1303

Wilkinson PC, Zeromski J (1965) Immunofluorescent detection of antibodies against neurones in sensory carcinomatous neuropathy. Brain 88: 529–538

Williams DB, Windebank AJ (1991) Motor neuron disease (amyotrophic lateral sclerosis). Mayo Clin Proc 66: 54–82

Williams DB, Floate DA, Leicester J (1988) Familial motor neuron disease: differing patterns in large pedigrees. J Neurol Sci 86: 215–230

Williams IR, Jefferson D, Gilliatt RW (1980) Acute nerve compression during limb ischaemia. J Neurol Sci 46: 199–207

Williams LL, O'Dougherty MM, Wright FS et al. (1986) Dietary essential fatty acids, vitamin E and Charcot-Marie-Tooth disease. Neurology 36: 1200–1205

Williams PH, Trzil KP (1991) Management of meralgia paresthetica. J Neurosurg 74: 76–80

Willis T (1672) De arimi brutorum. Theatro Sheldoniana, Oxford, pp 404–406

Willison HJ, Chancellor AM, Patterson G et al. (1993) Anti glycolipid antibodies, immunoglobulins and paraproteins in motor neurone disease. J Neurol Sci 114: 209–215

Willison RG (1964) Analysis of electrical activity in healthy and dystrophic muscle in man. J Neurol Neurosurg Psychiatry 27: 386–394

Willison RG (1980) Arrangement of muscle fibres of a single motor unit in mammalian muscle. Muscle Nerve 3: 360–361

Willison RG (1982) Spontaneous discharges in motor nerve fibres. In: Culper J, Ochoa J (eds) Abnormal nerves and muscles as impulse generators. Oxford University Press, Oxford, pp 383–392

Willner J, Di Mauro S, Eastwood A et al. (1979) Muscle carnitine deficiency: genetic heterogeneity. J Neurol Sci 41: 235–246

Wilshe KR, Healey LA (1971) Clinical manifestation of biopsy-proven temporal arteritis. Arthritis Rheum 14: 424 (abstract)

Wilson A, Hickie S, Lloyd A et al. (1994) Longitudinal study of outcome of chronic fatigue syndrome. Br Med J 308: 756–759

Wilson DL, Stone GC (1979) Axoplasmic transport of proteins. Annu Rev Biophys Bioeng 8: 27–45

Wilson J, Walton JN (1959) Some muscular manifestations of hypothyroidism. J Neurol Neurosurg Psychiatry 22: 320–324

Wilson-MacDonald J, Caughey MA, Myers DB (1984) Diurnal variation in nerve conduction, hand volume and grip strength in the carpal tunnel syndrome. Br Med J 289: 1042

Windebank AJ, Bankovsky HL (1993) Porphyric neuropathy. In: Dyck PJ, Thomas PK (eds) Peripheral neuropathy, 3rd edn. Saunders, Philadelphia, pp 1161–1168

Windebank AJ, Daube JR, Litchy WJ et al. (1987) Late sequelae of paralytic poliomyelitis in Olmstead County, Minnesota. In: Halstad LS, Wiechers DO (eds) Research in clinical aspects of the late effects of poliomyelitis. March of Dimes, White Plains, pp 27–38

Winer JB, Hughes RAC (1988) Identification of patients at risk of arrhythmia in Guillain–Barré syndrome. QJM 68: 735–739

Winer JB, Hughes RAC, Anderson MJ et al. (1988) A prospective study of acute idiopathic neuropathy. II. Antecedent events. J Neurol Neurosurg Psychiatry 51: 613–618

Winer JB, Hughes RAC, Greenwood RJ et al. (1985) Prognosis in Guillain–Barré syndrome. Lancet i: 1202–1203

Winer JB, Hughes RAC, Osmond C (1988) A prospective study of acute idiopathic neuropathy. I. Clinical features and their prognostic value. J Neurol Neurosurg Psychiatry 51: 605–612

Winer N, Klachko DM, Baer RD et al. (1966) Myotonic response induced by inhibitors of cholesterol biosynthesis. Science 153: 312–313

Winkelmann RD, Mulder DW, Lambert EH et al. (1968) Course of dermatomyositis-polymyositis: comparison of untreated and cortisone-treated patients. Mayo Clin Proc 43: 545–556

Winkelmann RK (1982) Dermatomyositis in childhood. In: Callen JP (ed) Clinics in rheumatic diseases, vol 8. Saunders, London, pp 353–368

Wise RP, McDermot V (1962) A myasthenic syndrome associated with bronchial carcinoma. J Neurol Neurosurg Psychiatry 25: 31–39

Witt NJ, Zochodne DW, Bolton CF et al. (1991) Peripheral nerve function in sepsis and multiple organ failure. Chest 99: 176–184

Witte AS, Cornblath DR, Parry GJ et al. (1986) Azathioprine in the treatment of myasthenia gravis. Ann Neurol 15: 602–605

Wochner RD, Drews G, Strober W et al. (1966) Accelerated breakdown of immunoglobulin G (IgG) in myotonic dystrophy: an hereditary error of immunoglobulin catabolism. J Clin Invest 45: 321–329

Wochnik-Dyjas D, Niewiadomska-Wolska MT, Kostrzewska E (1978) Porphyric polyneuropathy and its pathogenesis in the light of electrophysiological investigations. J Neurol Sci 35: 243–256

Wohlfart G (1939) Histopathological studies on muscular atrophy. In: Winther K, Krabbe KH (eds) Proceedings of the 3rd International Congress of Neurology. Munksgaard, Copenhagen, pp 465–473

Wohlfart G (1957) Collateral regeneration from residual motor nerve fibres in amyotrophic lateral sclerosis. Neurology 7: 124–134

Wohlfart G (1958) Collateral regeneration in partially denervated muscle. Neurology 8: 175–180

Wohlfart G, Fixe U, Eliasson S (1955) Hereditary proximal spinal muscular atrophy: a clinical entity simulating progressive muscular dystrophy. Acta Psychiatr Neurol 30: 395–406

Wohlfart S, Wohlfart G (1935) Mikroskopische Untersuchungen an progressiven Muskelatrophien. Acta Med Scand [Suppl] 63: 1–137

Wolfe F, Smythe HA, Yunus MB et al. (1990) The American College of Rheumatology 1990 criteria for the classification of fibromyalgia. Arthritis Rheum 33: 160–172

Woltmann HW (1919) The nervous system in pernicious anaemia: an analysis of 150 cases. Am J Med Sci 173: 400–409

Woltmann HW, Wilder RM (1929) Diabetes mellitus. Arch Int Med 44: 576–603

Wong V, Hawkins BR, Yu YL (1992) Myasthenia gravis in Hong Kong Chinese. II. Paediatric disease. Acta Neurol Scand 86: 68–72

Woodall CJ, Riding MH, Graham DI et al. (1994) Sequences specific for enterovirus detected in spinal cord from patients with motor neurone disease. Br Med J 308: 1541–1543

Woolf AL (1960) Muscle biopsy in the diagnosis of the "floppy baby": Infantile hypotonia. Cerebral Palsy Bull 2: 19–27

Worden DK, Vignos PJ(Jr) (1962) Intellectual function in childhood progressive muscular dystrophy. Pediatrics 29: 968–977

Workshop (1995) The limb girdle muscular dystrophics. Neuromusc Disord 5: 337–348

World Federation of Neurology Research Committee Research Group on Neuromuscular Diseases (1988). J Neurol Sci 86: 333–360

World Health Organization (1988) A guide to leprosy control, 2nd edn. WHO, Geneva

Wyburn-Mason R (1941) Brachial neuritis occurring in epidemic form. Lancet ii: 662–663

Wynn-Parry CB (1980) Pain in avulsion lesions of the brachial plexus. Pain 9: 41–43

Wynn-Parry CB (1984) Brachial plexus injuries Br J Hosp Med 34: 130–139

Wulff CH, Gilliatt RW (1979) F waves in patients with hand wasting caused by a cervical rib and band. Muscle Nerve 2: 452–457

Yamanuchi Y, Arikawa E, Arahata K et al. (1995) Limb girdle muscular dystrophy: clinical and pathologic re-evaluation. J Neurol Sci 129: 15–20

Yang B-Z, Ding JH, Brown BI et al. (1990) Definitive prenatal diagnosis for Type 3 glycogen storage disease. Am J Hum Genet 47: 735–739

Yang B-Z, Stewart C, Ding JH et al. (1991) Type III glycogen storage disease: an adult case with mild disease but complete absence of debrancher protein. Neuromusc Disord 1: 173–176

Yao JK, Ellefson RD, Dyck PJ (1976) Lipid abnormalities in hereditary neuropathy. I. Serum non-polar lipids. J Neurol Sci 29: 161–175

Yasaki S, Dyck PJ (1991) Spatial distribution of fiber degeneration in acute hypoglycemic neuropathy in rat. J Neuropathol Exp Neurol 50: 681–692

Yase Y (1972) The pathogenesis of amyotrophic lateral sclerosis. Lancet ii: 292–293

Yase Y (1984) Environmental contribution to the amyotrophic lateral sclerosis process. In: Serratrice G, Desnuelle C, Pallissier JF et al. (eds) Neuromuscular disease. Raven Press, New York, pp 335–339

Yasuda T, Sobue G, Doyu M et al. (1994) Familial amyloidotic polyneuropathy with late onset and well preserved autonomic function: a Japanese kindred with novel mutant transthyretin (ALA 97 to GLY). J Neurol Sci 121: 97–102

Yates JR, Emery AEH (1985) A population study of adult-onset limb girdle muscular dystrophy. J Med Genet 22: 250–257

Yates SK, Hurst LN, Brown WF (1981) Physiological observation in the median nerve during carpal tunnel surgery. Ann Neurol 10: 227–229

Yau SC, Roberts RG Bobrow M et al. (1993) Direct diagnosis of carriers of point mutations in Duchenne muscular dystrophy. Lancet 341: 272–275

Yiannikas C, Shahani BT (1984) Painful sequelae of injuries to peripheral nerves. Am J Phys Med 63: 53–83

Yiannikas C, Walsh JC (1983) Somatosensory evoked responses in the diagnosis of thoracic outlet syndrome. J Neurol Neurosurg Psychiatry 46: 234–240

Yiannikas C, McLeod JG, Pollard JD et al. (1986) Peripheral neuropathy associated with mitochondrial myopathy. Ann Neurol 20: 249–257

Yiannikas C, Shahani BT, Young RR (1983) The investigation of traumatic lesions of the brachial plexus by electromyography and short latency somatosensory potentials evoked by stimulation of multiple peripheral nerves. J Neurol Neurosurg Psychiatry 46: 1014–1022

Ymard B, Morel D, Dulac O (1989) Myasthenie et grossesse: une étude clinique et immunologique de 42 cas (21 myasthénies néonatales). Rev Neurol 145: 696–701

Yokoyama K, Araki S, Abe H (1990) Distribution of nerve conduction velocities in acute thallium poisoning. Muscle Nerve 13: 117–120

Yoshida S, Akizuki M, Mimori T et al. (1983) The precipitating antibody to an acidic nuclear protein antibody, the J0-1, in connective tissue disease. Arthritis Rheum 26: 604–611

Yoshida T, Tsuchiya M, Ono A et al. (1977) HLA antigens and myasthenia gravis in Japan. J Neurol Sci 32: 195–201

Yoshizumi MO, Asbury AK (1974) Intra-axonal bacilli in lepromatous leprosy: a light and electron microscopic study. Acta Neuropathol (Berl) 27: 1–10

Yoss RE, Corbin KB MacCarthy CS et al. (1957) Significance of signs and symptoms in localisation of involved roots in cervical disc protrusion. Neurology 7: 673–683

Young HA, Hardy DG (1983) Thoracic outlet syndrome. Br J Hosp Med 33: 457–461

Young ID, Harper PS (1980) Hereditary distal spinal muscular atrophy with vocal cord paralysis. J Neurol Neurosurg Psychiatry 43: 413–418

Young RJ, Ewing DJ, Clarke BF (1985) Painful diabetic neuropathy. Lancet i: 349

Young RR, Asbury AK, Adams RD et al. (1969) Pure pan dysautonomia with recovery. Trans Am Neurol Assoc 94: 355–357

Young RR, Asbury AK, Corbett JL et al. (1975) Pure pan dysautonomia with recovery. Brain 98: 613–636

Young DS, Chou S, Hayes AP et al. (1988) Primary lateral sclerosis: a clinical diagnosis reemerges. Arch Neurol 45: 1304–1307

Yu NL, Jones SJ (1985) Somatosensory evoked potentials in cervical spondylosis: correlation of median, ulnar and posterior tibial nerve responses with clinical and radiological findings. Brain 108: 273–300

Yu YL, Murray NMF (1984) A comparison of concentric needle electromyography, quantitative EMG and single fibre EMG in the diagnosis of neuromuscular diseases. Electroencephalogr Clin Neurophysiol 58: 220–225

Yue KTN, Fritz IB (1962) Fate of tritium-labelled carnitine administered to dogs and rats. Am J Physiol 202: 122–128

Yuki N, Yoshino H, Sato S et al. (1990) Acute axonal polyneuropathy associated with anti GM_1 antibodies following *Campylobacter* enteritis. Neurology 40: 1900–1902

Yuki N, Yoshino H, Sato S et al. (1992) Severe acute axonal form of Guillain–Barré syndrome associated with IgG anti BD_{1A} antibodies. Muscle Nerve 15: 899–903

Yunus M (1983) Fibromyalgia syndrome: a need for uniform classification. J Rheumatol 10: 841–844

Yunus M, Massi AT, Calabro JJ et al. (1981) Primary fibromyalgia (fibrositis): a clinical study of 50 patients with matched normal controls. Semin Arthritis Rheum 11: 151–171

Zacks SI, Shields DR, Steinberg SA (1966) A myasthenic syndrome in the dog: a case report with electron microscopic observations on motor end-plates, and comparison with the fine structure of end-plates in myasthenia gravis. Ann NY Acad Sci 135: 79–97

Zaiwalla Z, Gawell MJ, Markwick J et al. (1984) Histocompatibility typing in amyotrophic lateral sclerosis. In: Rose FC (ed) Research progress in motor neurone disease. Pitman, London, pp 384–387

Zander Olsen P (1975) Prediction of recovery in Bell's palsy. Acta Neurol Scand [Suppl] 61: 52–90

Zappra M, Valentino P, Marchello LP et al. (1993) F-wave normative studies in different nerves of healthy subjects. Electroencephalogr Clin Neurophysiol 89: 67–72

Zatz M, Vianna-Morgante AM, Campos P et al. (1981) Translocation (X:6) in a female with Duchenne muscular dystrophy: implications for the localisation of the DMD locus. J Med Genet 18: 442–447

Zellweger H, Antonik A (1975) Newborn screening for Duchenne muscular dystrophy. Pediatrics 55: 30–34

Zellweger H, Afifi A, McCormick WF et al. (1967) Benign congenital muscular dystrophy: a special form of congenital hypotonia. Clin Pediatr 6: 655–663

Zellweger H, Pavone L, Biondi A et al. (1980) Autosomal recessive generalised myotonia. Muscle Nerve 3: 176–180

Zellweger H, Simpson J, McCormick WF et al. (1972) Spinal muscular atrophy with autosomal dominant inheritance. Neurology 22: 957–963

Zeviani M, Gallera C, Antozzi C et al. (1991) Maternally inherited myopathy and cardiomyopathy. Lancet 338: 143–147

Zeviani M, Servidei S, Bresolin N et al. (1991) Rapid detection of the A→G^{8344} mutation of mtDNA in Italian families with myoclonus epilepsy and RRF (MERRF). Am J Hum Genet 48: 203–211

Zhang Y, Chen HS, Khanna VK et al. (1993) A mutation in the human ryanodine receptor gene associated with central core disease. Nature Genet 5: 46–50

Zhao B, Yang T, Huang H et al. (1981) Acute polyradiculitis (Guillain–Barré syndrome): an epidemiological study of 156 cases observed in Beijing. Ann Neurol 9: S146–148

Zierz S (1994) Carnitine palmitoyl transferase deficiency. In: Engel AG, Franzini-Armstrong (eds) Myology, 2nd edn. McGraw-Hill, New York, pp 1577–1586

Zilkha KJ (1962) Discussion on motor neurone disease. Proc R Soc Med 55: 1028

Zimmerman EA, Lovelace RE (1968) The etiology of the neuropathy in acute intermittent porphyria. Trans Am Neurol Assoc 93: 294–296

Zinn AB, Kerr DW, Hoppel CL (1986) Fumarase deficiency: a new cause of mitochondrial encephalomyopathy. N Engl J Med 315: 469–473

Zorilla E, Kozak GP (1967) Ophthalmoplegia in diabetes mellitus. Ann Intern Med 67: 968–976

Zwarts MJ, van Weerden TW (1989) Transient paresis in myotonic syndromes. Brain 112: 665–680

Zwarts MJ, van Weerden TW, Links P et al. (1988) The muscle fibre conduction velocity and power spectra in familial hypokalaemic periodic paralysis. Muscle Nerve 11: 166–173

Zweig MH, Adornato B, van Steirtghem AC et al. (1980) Serum creatine kinase BB and MM concentrations determined by radioimmunoassay in neuromuscular disorders. Ann Neurol 7: 324–328

Subject Index

Acetylcholine receptor antibody 263–4, 271
Acid maltase deficiency 378–81
  cardiomyopathy 437
  electrophysiological assessment 379–80
  genetics 381
  laboratory investigations 379
  management 381
  muscle biopsy 380
  pathology 380–1
Acid phosphatase 45, 56
Acromegalic neuropathy 213–14
Acromegaly 421–3
  cardiomyopathy 439
  course 423
  electrophysiological assessment 422–3
  laboratory investigations 422
  muscle biopsy 423
  nerve biopsy 423
Acrylamide neuropathy 252–3
Activities of Daily Living scales 6
Acute pandysautonomia 231
Acute paralytic disease of Northern China 230–1
Addison's disease 421
Adrenal disorders 420–1
Adrenoleukodystrophy 197, 199
Adrenomyeloneuropathy 199
Adson's manoeuvre 167
Adynamia episodica hereditaria 405–6
Age, effects on muscles 50–1
Ageing 448–9
  electrophysiological assessment 448–9
  muscle biopsy 449
  nerve changes 449
Alcoholic myopathy 429–30
  cardiomyopathy 439
  management 430
  pathogenesis 429–30
Alcoholic neuropathy 73, 209–10
  electrophysiological assessment 209–10
  management 210
  pathological considerations 210
Allodynia 127
Alzheimer's disease 113
Amantadine 282
Amiodorone 252
Amphotericin 250
Amyloidosis 221
  causes of neuropathy in 192
Amyotrophic lateral sclerosis 103
  motor unit counts 33
  muscular strength assessment 5–6
Angiokeratoma corporis diffusum 197
Anterior horn cell disorders 89–120
  see also individual disorders
Anterior interosseous syndrome 145

Anticholinesterases 271–2
Anticonvulsant drugs, peripheral neuropathy 252
Antimicrobial drugs, peripheral neuropathy 251
Antineoplastic drugs, peripheral neuropathy 250–1
Antirheumatic drugs, peripheral neuropathy 251–2
Appel scale 6
Arsenic neuropathy 253, 254
Arthrogryposis multiplex congenita 375
  absence of muscle spindles 62
Ataxia telangiectasia 197, 200
ATPase 45
Autoimmune myositis 288
Autonomic neuropathy 202
Autosomal recessive muscular dystrophy of childhood 330–1
Axillary nerve 165
Axonal degeneration 67
Axonotmesis 134

Bassen–Kornzweig syndrome 197, 198, 199, 212
Batten–Bielschowsky syndrome 199
Becker muscular dystrophy 321–3
  cardiomyopathy 435, 440
  electrophysiological assessment 322
  genetic correlations 321–2
  management and carrier detection 323
  muscle biopsy 322–3
  onset and progression 1
  pseudohypertrophy in 9
Behçet's disease 224
Behr's syndrome 187, 188
Bell's palsy 156–8
  blink reflex 41, 158
  electrophysiological assessment 157–8
  management 158
  pathology 158
  prognosis 158
Bethlem myopathy 329–30
Biochemical tests 12–15
Bizarre high-frequency potentials 25–6
Black widow spider venom 282
Blink reflex 41
Blocking agent myopathy 428
Borrelia burgdorfi 306
Borreliosis *see* Lyme disease
Botulism 280–1
  electrophysiological assessment 281
  end-plate disorder 75
  management 281
  pathophysiology 280–1
  respiratory weakness in 7
  therapeutic use of botulinum toxin 281
Brachial neuritis 165
Brachial plexus lesions 164–7
  brachial neuritis 165

Brachial plexus lesions – *cont.*
classification 164
clinical features 164–5
electrophysiological assessment 165–6, 167
imaging 167
malignant infiltration/radiation injury 165
management 167
thoracic outlet syndrome 166–7
treatment 166
Brachial plexus palsies, hereditary 183–4
α–Bungarotoxin 282
Bunina bodies 113

Cachexia 447–8
Cap disease 374
Carbon disulphide neuropathy 253
Carbonic anhydrase III (CAIII) 14
Carcinoid syndrome 423–4
cardiomyopathy 439
Carcinomas *see* Malignant disease
Cardiomyopathy 433–40
clinical classification 433
endocrine myopathies 439
muscle disorders 434–8
neurogenic disorders 438–9
skeletal muscle 439–40
Cardiovascular drugs, peripheral neuropathy 252
Carnitine deficiency syndromes 393–5
Carnitine metabolism 391, 393
Carnitine palmityl transferase (CPTase) 396
Carnitine utilisation defects 391, 393–5
Carpal tunnel syndrome 124–34, 140–4, 208
acute 144–5
electrophysiological assessment 141–4
management 144
rheumatoid arthritis in 11
Castleman's disease 222
Cauda equina lesions 171
Central core disease 363–5
causation and associated features 365
electrophysiological assessment 364
laboratory investigations 364
management 366
muscle biopsy 364–5
Central cores 57
Central nucleation 55
Cerebro–tendinous xanthomatosis 197, 199
Cervical root lesions 161–4
causes 161
clinical features 162
electrophysiological assessment 162–3
imaging 164
Cervical spondylosis 161
Charcot–Marie–Tooth syndrome 69, 86, 175
diagnosis 181–2
electromyography 70, 73
fibre splitting 80
genetic studies 130
management 181
motor symptoms 127
nerve biopsy 67
nerve hypertrophy in 11, 123
prevalence 124
pseudomyotonia in 26
see also Hereditary motor and sensory neuropathies
Chediak-Higashi syndrome 189, 197, 200
Chemical–induced myopathy 430
Chemical–induced neuropathies 252–4

Chloramphenicol 250
Chloroquine myopathy 428–9
Cholinergic crisis 272
Chorea–acanthocytosis syndromes 189
Chronic distal motor neuropathy 202
Chronic fatigue syndrome 444–6
associated features 445
management 446
neurophysiological assessment 446
neuropsychiatric features 445–6
Chronic painless myopathy 428–9
Churg–Strauss syndrome 300
Chvostek's sign 420
Ciguatoxin 282
Cisplatin 251
Clinical assessment 1–17
biochemical tests 12–15
blood creatine kinase 12–14
general laboratory tests 15
urinary protein excretion tests 14–15
findings 2–11
fasciculation, myotonia, myokymia and myoedema 10
fatiguability 7–8
involvement of other systems 11
pain and cramps 9–10
peripheral nerves 11
sensory disturbances 10–11
tone and reflexes 9
wasting and hypertrophy 8–9
weakness 2–7
quantitative assessment of muscular strength 4–7
genetic aspects 11–12
imaging 15–17
magnetic resonance spectroscopy 16–17
investigational approach 12
onset and progression 1–2
Clioquinol 250
Clostridium botulinum see Botulism
Cockayne's syndrome 197, 200
Coeliac disease 431
Colistin 250
Collagen vascular disease 222–5
electrophysiological assessment 225
laboratory assessment 225
management 225
neuropathies associated with 222–5
pathology 225
Common peroneal syndromes 153–4
electrophysiological assessment and management 154
Compensatory mechanisms 76–84
electromyographic evidence 80–1
fibre splitting in disease 77–80
implications of fibre splitting 81–4
Complex repetitive discharges 25–6
Compression neuropathies 137–9
clinical implications 139
electrophysiological assessment 139
pathophysiology 138–9
Computed tomography 15–16
Concentric needle electromyography 22–33
clinical technique 22
electrodes 20
motor unit potential analysis 27–31
amplitudes 27
complexity 28
double discharges 30–1
duration 27–8
recruitment 28–30
abnormal 30

quantitative studies 31–3
  automatic analysis of interference pattern 32
  automatic analysis of motor unit potentials 31
  motor unit counts 32–3
relaxed muscle 22–7
  complex repetitive discharges 25–6
  end-plate noise 23
  end-plate spikes 23
  fasciculation potentials 24
  fibrillation potentials 23–4
  insertional activity 23
  insertional positive waves 23
  myokymia 26
  myotonia 26–7
  neuromyotonia 26
  positive sharp waves 25
Conchotome biopsy 44
Conduction block 37–8
Congenital fibre-type disproportion 371–2
  differential diagnosis 372
  electrophysiological assessment 371
  laboratory investigations 371
  management 372
  muscle biopsy 371–2
Congenital myasthenic syndromes 279–80
Congenital universal insensitivity to pain 186–7
Connexin 32 177
Conn's syndrome 421
Continuous muscle fibre activity syndrome 442–4
Conus medullaris lesions 171
Corticosteroid myopathy 428
Cramp 10
Cranial arteritis 224
Cranial mononeuropathies 203
Creatine kinase 12–14
  Kugelberg–Welander syndrome 13
  neuromuscular disease 13–14
  spinal muscular atrophy 95
Creutzfeldt–Jakob disease 86, 119–20
  spread by contaminated electrodes 21
Critical care neuropathies 238–9
  differential diagnosis 239
  electrophysiological assessment 238–9
  prognosis and treatment 239
Crotoxin 282
Cryoglobulinaemias 222
Cubital tunnel syndrome 146
Curare 282
Cushing's syndrome 420
Cysticercosis 305
Cytochrome oxidase 45
Cytoplasmic bodies 59
Cytoplasmic body myopathy 373

Dapsone 245
Debrancher enzyme deficiency 381–2
Decelerating bursts 25–6
Degenerative changes in muscle 55–60
  central cores 57
  cytoplasmic bodies 59
  fibre splitting 56
  moth-eaten fibres 56–7
  necrosis 55–6
  ragged-red fibres 58–9
  ring fibres 60
  rod bodies 57–8
  target fibres 57
  tubular aggregates 59

Déjérine–Sottas syndrome 86, 122, 182, 195
Demyelinating neuropathies 67, 68, 160
Dermatomyositis 285, 286–8
  clinical features 286
  cutaneous manifestations 287
  idiopathic 298
  juvenile 288, 302–3
  magnetic resonance imaging 16
  myopathy 286–7
  paraneoplastic 290–1
  systemic features 287–8
Desmin storage myopathies 373
Diabetic amyotrophy 172, 202–3
Diabetic neuropathy 201–7
  classification 201
  electrophysiological assessment 204–5
  focal and multifocal neuropathies 202–3
  laboratory investigations 203–4
  management 207
  nerve biopsy 68
  pathogenesis 206
  pathological considerations 205–6
  symmetrical polyneuropathy 201–2
Diastase 45
Digital neuropathy 223
Diphtheria 239–40
  cardiomyopathy 439
Disseminated neurogenic atrophy 54
Distal muscular dystrophy 338
Distal myopathy 336–8
  with rimmed vacuoles 337–8
Distal sensory neuropathy 238
Distal spinal muscular atrophy 93–4, 181
Distal symmetrical sensory neuropathy 223
Disulfiram 252
Disuse 447
Double-crush syndrome 136, 155–6
Dropped head syndrome 341
Drug-induced myopathies 425–9
  acute hypokalaemic paralysis 427–8
  acute rhabdomyolysis 425–6
  blocking agent/corticosteroid myopathy 428
  chronic painless myopathy 428–9
  inflammatory 426–7
  injection (focal) myopathy 428
  mitochondrial myopathy *see* Mitochondrial myopathies
  muscle cramp 425
  subacute/acute painful myopathy 428
  tryptophan-induced eosinophilia–myalgia syndrome 427
Drug-induced neuropathies 247–50
  peripheral 250–2
Duchenne muscular dystrophy 74, 75, 307–21
  cardiomyopathy 11, 434–5, 440
  carrier detection and genetic counselling 318–19
  diagnosis 318
  drug therapy 320–1
  electrophysiological assessment 312–13
  elevated creatine kinase in 13, 14
  fibre splitting 56, 80, 82
  genetic defect and dystrophin 309–11
  Gowers' manoeuvre 2, 3
  incidence and inheritance 308–9
  laboratory investigations 311–12
  magnetic resonance imaging 16
  management 320
  muscle biopsy 313–17
  myoblast transfer and gene therapy 321
  neonatal screening and fetal/neonatal diagnosis 319–20
  onset and progression 1

Duchenne muscular dystrophy – *cont.*
  pathological features in other organs   317–18
  pseudohypertrophy   9
  pseudomyotonia   26
  red blood cell abnormalities   14
Dying back distal axonopathies   249
Dynamometry   5
Dysaesthesiae   11, 127
Dysproteinaemias, neuropathies associated with   214–18
Dystrophin   309–11

Eaton–Lambert syndrome *see* Lambert–Eaton myasthenic
  syndrome
Ehlers–Danlos syndrome, tone and reflexes   9
Ehrlich's haematoxylin   45
Ekbom's syndrome   444
Elastin–van Gieson stain   45
Electrocardiography, in inflammatory myopathies   293
Electrodes *see* Electromyography
Electromyography   19–22
  acid maltase deficiency   379–80
  acromegaly   422–3
  ageing   448–9
  alcoholic neuropathy   209–10
  anterior interosseous syndrome   145
  Becker muscular dystrophy   322
  Bell's palsy   157–8
  brachial plexus lesions   165–6, 167
  carpal tunnel syndrome   141–4
  central core disease   364
  cervical root lesions   162–3
  Charcot–Marie–Tooth syndrome   177–8, 180
  chronic fatigue syndrome   446
  concentric needle *see* Concentric needle electromyography
  congenital fibre-type disproportion   371
  critical care neuropathies   238–9
  debrancher enzyme deficiency   382
  diabetic neuropathy   204–5
  Duchenne muscular dystrophy   312–13
  electrodes
    concentric needle   20
    macro   21
    monopolar   20
    single-fibre   20–1
    sterilisation   21
    surface   19–20
    wire   21
  entrapment neuropathies   136–7
  facio–scapulo–humeral muscular dystrophy   334
  Guillain–Barré syndrome   231–2
  hemifacial spasm   159
  hypokalaemic periodic paralysis   403, 406
  hypothyroidism   418–19
  inflammatory myopathies   293–5
  Isaacs' syndrome   443–4
  Kennedy syndrome   102
  Lambert–Eaton myasthenic syndrome   278
  leprosy   244–5
  limb–girdle muscular dystrophy   327
  lumbo–sacral disc prolapse   169–70
  Lyme disease   247
  McArdle's syndrome   385
  macro   34–5
  malignant disease   217–18
  malignant hyperpyrexia syndrome   410
  motor neuron disease   107–11
  multi-electrode studies   35–6
  multifocal motor neuropathy   237

myasthenia gravis   269–70
myeloma   221
myoglobinuria   412
myotonia   358–9
myotonic dystrophy   349–51
nerve conduction   36–42
  blink reflex   41
  F response   39–40
  H reflex   38–9
  mixed nerve action potential recording   38
  motor conduction block   38
  motor conduction velocity   37
  motor nerve conduction velocity distribution   40
  motor/sensory nerve refractory period   40–1
  sensory conduction   38
  somatosensory evoked responses   41–2
  stimulation of central motor pathways   42
neuropathies   128–9
osteomalacic myopathy   432
polyneuropathies   130–1
progressive external ophthalmoplegia   399
radial nerve syndromes   150
Refsum's disease   196
repetitive stimulation   36
scanning   35
scapulo–peroneal muscular dystrophy   335
Schwartz–Jampel syndrome   26
signal amplification   21–2
single-fibre   33–4
spinal muscular atrophy   96–7
steroid myopathy   420
stiff man syndrome   442
surface   36
syringomyelia   118
ulnar nerve syndromes   147, 148
Emery–Dreifuss muscular dystrophy   325
  cardiomyopathy   435, 440
Encephalomyopathies   400–1
End-plate disorders   62
End-plate noise   23
End-plate spikes   23
Endocrine myopathies   415–24
Endoneurium   63
Entrapment neuropathies   134–7, 203
  common sites of   135
  electrophysiological assessment   136–7, 156
  pathogenesis   135–6
Envenomation myopathies   430
Eosinophilic fasciitis   300
Eosinophilic myositis   300
Epineurial sheath   63
Erb's point   41
Erb's scapulo–humeral myopathy   329
Esterase   45
Ethambutol   250
Ethionamide   250
Ethylene oxide neuropathy   253
Exercise, effects on muscles   49–50
External ocular nerve syndromes   159–60

F chronodispersion   40
F response   39–40
Fabry's disease   197, 198–9
Facial myokymia   159
Facial nerve syndromes   159
Facio–scapulo–humeral muscular dystrophy   332–5
  differential diagnosis   334–5
  electrophysiological assessment   334

laboratory investigations 334
management 335
muscle biopsy 334
Familial amyloid polyneuropathy 189–92
cardiomyopathy 438–9
type I 190
type II 191
type III 191
type IV 191
Familial amyloidosis 192
Familial dysautonomia *see* Riley–Day syndrome
Familial motor neuron disease 106
Fasciculation 10
Fasciculation potentials 24
Fatiguability 7–8
Fazio–Londé syndrome 86, 95
Femoral mononeuropathy 152
Femoral neuropathy 172
Fibre splitting 56, 77–80
implications of 81–4
splitting as compensatory process 82
splitting and fibre–type grouping 81–2
Kugelberg–Welander syndrome 56, 78, 79, 80, 81, 82, 83
relation of splitting to myopathic changes in denervated
muscle 83–4
Fibrillation potentials 23–4
Fingerprint body myopathy 374
Fisher syndrome 229–30
management 236
Floppy infant syndrome 9
Fontana's spiral bands 136
Friedreich's ataxia 86, 123, 187, 188, 195
cardiomyopathy 11, 438, 440
electrophysiological assessment 188
management 188
pathology 188
Frozen shoulder 2
Fukuyama muscular dystrophy 332
Fumarase deficiency 397
Functional rating scales of muscular strength 6–7

Gangliosidosis 199
Gene therapy, Duchenne muscular dystrophy 321
Genetic counselling
Duchenne muscular dystrophy 318–19
mitochondrial myopathies 401–2
myotonic dystrophy 355
spinal muscular atrophy 101
Genetically determined neuropathies *see* Hereditary
neuropathies
Genetics
acid maltase deficiency 381
Becker muscular dystrophy 321–2
Duchenne muscular dystrophy 318–19
McArdle's syndrome 383–4
myotonic dystrophy 348–9
neuromuscular disease 11–12
Gerstmann–Straussler–Scheinker syndrome 120
Giant axonal neuropathy 86, 189
Giant cell arteritis 306
Globoid cell leukodystrophy 197
Glycogen storage diseases 377–86
acid maltase deficiency 378–81
Debrancher enzyme deficiency 381–2
lactate dehydrogenase deficiency 386
lysosomal with normal acid maltase activity 381
myophosphorylase deficiency 382–5
phosphofructokinase deficiency 385–6

phosphoglycerate kinase deficiency 386
phosphoglycerate mutase deficiency 386
phosphorylase b kinase deficiency 386
type IV glycogenosis 382
Glycogenoses
cardiomyopathy 437
type II *see* Acid maltase deficiency
type III 381–2
type IV 382
type IX 386
type V *see* McArdle's syndrome
type VII 17, 385–6
type VIII 386
type X 386
type XI 386
Golgi tendon organ 47
Gomori trichrome stain 45
Gowers' manoeuvre 2, 3
Graft versus host myositis 306
Granulomatous myositis 301, 303
Grouped denervation atrophy 54
Guillain–Barré syndrome 86, 121, 225–36
acute 226–7
acute axonal 230
antecedent events 227–8
blink reflex 41
cardiomyopathy 439, 440
chronic progressive 229
chronic relapsing 228
classification 226
CSF protein level 130
electromyography 70, 73, 231–2
management 234–6
myokymia 26
nerve biopsy 68
nerve conduction block 42
nerve hypertrophy 123
onset and progression 1
outcome 236
pathogenesis 233–4
pathology 232–3
pure form 230
respiratory weakness in 7
segmental demyelination 125
tone and reflexes 9
Guyon's canal 148

H reflex 38–9
Haematoxylin and eosin stain 45
Heavy metal intoxication 120
Hemifacial spasm 158–9
electrophysiological assessment 159
management 159
Hepatic neuropathy 209
Hereditary motor and sensory neuropathies 173, 174–84
brachial plexus palsies 183–4
with liability to pressure palsies 183
migrant sensory neuritis of Wartenberg 184
type 1 174–6, 181
type 1A 176–7
type 1B 177
type 2 179–81
type 3 *see* Déjérine–Sottas syndrome
type 5 182
type 6 182
X–linked phenotypes 177–9
Hereditary neuropathies 173–200
classification 173

Hereditary neuropathies – *cont.*
　hereditary sensory and autonomic neuropathies　184–8
　peroneal muscular atrophy　174–84
　with specific metabolic defects　189–200
Hereditary sensory and autonomic neuropathies　173, 184–9
　clinical features　184
　congenital universal insensitivity to pain　186–7
　management　187
　sensory neuropathy in hereditary ataxias　187–8
　type I　184–5
　type II　185
　type III *see* Riley–Day syndrome
　type IV　186
　type V　186
　see also Friedreich's ataxia　188
Herpes simplex　241
Herpes zoster　119, 241
Hexacarbon neuropathy　253
Hexosaminidase deficiency　107
HIV-related neuropathies　237–8
HMSN *see* Hereditary motor and sensory neuropathies
Hoffmann's syndrome　418
Holmes–Adie syndrome　186
Horner's syndrome　117, 164–5, 183
HSAN *see* Hereditary sensory and autonomic neuropathies
Hyaline body myopathy　374
Hydralazine　252
Hyperadrenalism　420–1
Hyperkalaemic periodic paralysis　357–8
Hyperparathyroidism　107, 419
Hyperpathia　11
Hypersensitivity vasculitis　224
Hyperthyroid bulbar myopathy　416
Hyperthyroid myopathy　107, 416–17
　cardiomyopathy　439
　investigations　417
　management　417
　muscle biopsy　417
　pathophysiology　417
Hypertrophy　8–9
Hypoadrenalism　421
Hypokalaemic periodic paralysis　402–5, 416
　biochemical features　405
　electrophysiological assessment　403
　muscle biopsy　403–5
　and paramyotonia congenita　405–6
　　DNA analysis　405–6
　　electrophysiological assessment　406
　　laboratory assessment　405
　　muscle biopsy　406
Hypoparathyroidism　419–20
Hypothyroid neuropathy　213
Hypothyroidism　418–19
　cardiomyopathy　439
　electrophysiological assessment　418–19
　laboratory investigations　418
　management and course　419
　muscle biopsy　419
　nerve biopsy　419
　pseudomyotonia in　26
Hypovitaminosis　211–13

Iatrogenic nerve injuries　134
Idiopathic inflammatory myopathies　285–91
Imaging　16–17
　brachial plexus lesions　167
　cervical root lesions　164
　inflammatory myopathies　293

Immunoglobulin therapy
　Guillain–Barré syndrome　235
　myasthenia gravis　275
Immunosuppressant drug therapy
　Guillain–Barré syndrome　236
　inflammatory myopathies　303
　myasthenia gravis　273–4
Inclusion body myositis　289–90
　cardiomyopathy　438
　muscle biopsy　298–300
Infantile distal myopathy　337
Infection-induced neuropathy　237–47
Inflammatory demyelinating neuropathy　238
Inflammatory myopathies　285–306
　aetiology　291–2
　cardiomyopathy　437–8
　drug-induced　306, 426–7
　electrocardiography　293
　electrophysiological assessment　293–5
　laboratory investigations　292–3
　muscle biopsy　295–300
　muscle imaging　293
　treatment and prognosis　302–3
　see also individual conditions
Inflammatory polyradiculoneuropathy *see* Guillain–Barré
　syndrome
Injection (focal) myopathy　428
Intercostal mononeuropathies　203
Isaacs' syndrome　10, 26, 127, 442–4
　electrophysiological assessment　443–4
　management　444
　muscle and nerve biopsy　444
　terminology　443
Ischaemic mononeuropathy　172
Isoniazid　250

Juvenile distal myopathy　337

Kawasaki syndrome　305–6
Kearns–Sayre syndrome　387, 398, 420
Kennedy syndrome　101–3
　electrophysiological assessment　102
　gynaecomastia　102
　inheritance and pathogenesis　102
　management　102–3
　pathology　102
α-Ketoglutarate dehydrogenase deficiency　397
Kocher–Debré–Semelaigne syndrome　418, 419
Konzo　115
Krabbe's disease　197, 198
Krebs cycle defects　397
Kugelberg–Welander syndrome　86, 99, 100
　clinical presentation　92–3
　compensatory mechanisms　76
　creatine kinase　13
　electromyography　70, 96
　fibre splitting　56, 78, 79, 80, 81, 82, 83
　muscle fibre hypertrophy　54
Kurtzke scale　6
Kuru　120

Lactate dehydrogenase deficiency　386
Lambert–Eaton myasthenic syndrome　87, 276–9
　differential diagnosis　279
　laboratory investigations　277–8
　management　278–9

muscle biopsy 278
pathophysiology 277
repetitive stimulation 36
Large fibre neuropathy 201
Late-onset dominant limb-girdle dystrophy 329
Lathyrism 115, 120
Lead neuropathy 253, 254
Legionella 306
Leprosy 124, 127, 242–6
diagnosis 245
dimorphous 244
electrophysiological assessment 244–5
indeterminate 242–3
laboratory assessment 244
management 245–6
outcome 242
pathology 245
tuberculoid 243–4
Leyden–Möbius pelvi-femoral myopathy 329
Limb-girdle muscular dystrophy 74, 325–31
clinical syndromes 326
differential diagnosis 328–9
electrophysiological assessment 327
fibre splitting 56, 80
laboratory investigations 326
management 329
muscle biopsy 327–8
pseudohypertrophy in 9
see also individual types
Limit dextrinosis 381–2
Localised nodular myositis 300
Lower limb syndromes 151–5
common peroneal syndromes 153–4
Morton's metatarsalgia 155
pelvic girdle nerves 151–2
sciatic nerve syndromes 152–3
tarsal tunnel syndrome 154–5
tibial nerve syndrome 154
Lumbo-sacral canal stenosis 170–1
Lumbo-sacral root/plexus lesions 167–72
cauda equina 171
causes 168
conus medullaris 171
disc prolapse 168–70
electrophysiological assessment 169–70
investigation 169
management 170
lumbo-sacral canal stenosis 170–1
lumbo-sacral plexus 171–2
Lyme disease 246–7
antibody tests 15
cranial neuropathies 246
electrophysiological assessment 247
laboratory diagnosis 247
peripheral neuropathy 247
radiculoneuritis 246
treatment and outcome 247

Mabry syndrome 324
McArdle's syndrome 382–5
biochemical basis 384
cardiomyopathy 437
electrophysiological assessment 385
elevated creatine kinase in 13
fatiguability in 7, 8
genetic basis 383–4
laboratory investigations 384
lactate levels in 14

magnetic resonance spectroscopy 17
management 385
muscle biopsy 385
pain in 10
standardised ischaemic lactate test 384–5
McLeod's syndrome 189, 324–5
elevated creatine kinase in 13
red blood cell abnormalities in 14
Macro electromyography 34–5
electrodes 21
Maghreb myopathy 46
Magnesium 282
Magnetic resonance spectroscopy 16–17
Malignant disease
electrophysiological assessment 217–18
laboratory investigations 217
management 218
nerve root and nerve infiltration 218
neuropathies associated with 214–18
incidence of 216
pathogenesis 216–17
types of 216
Malignant fasciculation 108
Malignant hyperpyrexia syndrome 407–10
associated disorders 409
electrophysiological assessment 410
elevated creatine kinase in 13
management 410
muscle biopsy 410
pathophysiology 409
screening for susceptibility 408–9
Malnutrition 210–11
Marinesco–Sjögren syndrome 187, 188–9
Martin–Gruber anastomosis 144
Median nerve syndromes 139–46
anterior interosseous syndrome 145
carpal tunnel syndrome 140–4
acute 144–5
pronator teres syndrome 145
MELAS 400–1
Meralgia paraesthetica 151–2
Mercury neuropathy 255
Merosin deficiency myopathy 331–2
MERRF 400
Metabolic myopathies 377–413
Metachromatic leukodystrophy 86, 197–8
electrophysiological assessment 198
pathology 197
Metal neuropathies 254–5
3-Methylhistidine 15
Metronidazole 250
Microbial toxic myopathy 430
Miller–Fisher syndrome 86
Mitochondrial myopathies 387–402
cardiomyopathy 436, 440
clinical syndromes 398–400
diagnosis 397–8
drug-induced 427
encephalomyopathies 400–1
fatty acid transport defects 391–6
genetic counselling 401–2
genetic defects 389
mitochondrial genetics 388–9
mitochondrial metabolism 388
ragged-red fibres 389–91
substrate utilisation defects 396–7
Mixed connective tissue disease 224
muscle biopsy 300
myositis and 288–9

Monoclonal gammopathies, neuropathies associated with 218–20
   electrophysiological assessment 219
   management 220
   pathology 219–20
Monomelic spinal muscular atrophy 94
Mononeuritis multiplex 121, 160, 203, 223, 238
Mononeuropathies 86–7, 121, 133–60
   causes **133**
   see also individual conditions
Monopolar electrodes 20
Myophosphorylase 45
Morton's metatarsalgia 155
Moth-eaten fibres 56–7
Motor double-crush syndrome 156
Motor end-plates 62
Motor nerve roots, disorders of 86
Motor nerves
   central, stimulation 42
   conduction block 37–8
   conduction velocity 37
      distribution 40
   refractory period 40–1
Motor neuron disease 86, 103–17
   aetiology 113–15
   clinical features 104–6
   differential diagnosis 106–7
   electrophysiological assessment 107–11
   epidemiology 103–4
   familial 106
   imaging 111
   laboratory investigations 111
   management 115–17
   muscle atrophy 55
   muscle biopsy 111–12
   pathology 112–13
Motor unit potential analysis 27–31
   amplitudes 27
   automatic 31
   complexity 28
   double discharges 30–1
   duration 27–8
   recruitment 28–30
      abnormal 30
Motor units 47–8
MRC scale 4–5
Multicore disease 365–6
Multifocal motor neuropathy 107, 236–7
Multiple mononeuropathies 121, 160
Multiple sclerosis 26
Muscle biopsy 43–63
   acid maltase deficiency 380
   acromegaly 423
   ageing 449
   Becker muscular dystrophy 322–3
   blood vessels 62–3
   central core disease 364–5
   Charcot-Marie-Tooth syndrome 178–9, 180
   conchotome biopsy 44
   congenital fibre-type disproportion 371–2
   debrancher enzyme deficiency 382
   Duchenne muscular dystrophy 313–17
   facio-scapulo-humeral muscular dystrophy 334
   histological methods 45–6
   histology 55–62
      degenerative changes 55–60
      regenerative changes 60–2
   hyperthyroid myopathy 417
   hypokalaemic periodic paralysis 403–5, 406

hypothyroidism 419
idiopathic dermatomyositis 298
idiopathic polymyositis 295–8
inclusion body myositis 298–300
indications for 51–2
Isaacs' syndrome 444
Lambert-Eaton myasthenic syndrome 278
limb-girdle muscular dystrophy 327–8
McArdle's syndrome 385
malignant hyperpyrexia syndrome 410
motor end-plates 62
motor neuron disease 111–12
muscle spindles 62
muscle structure *see* Skeletal muscle structure
myoglobinuria 412–13
myotonic dystrophy 351–4
myotubular myopathy 370
needle biopsy 43–4
nemaline myopathy 367–9
neuroleptic-malignant syndrome 411
open biopsy 44
osteomalacic myopathy 432
poliomyelitis 119
preparation of 44–5
progressive external ophthalmoplegia 399
Refsum's disease 196
scapulo-peroneal muscular dystrophy 336
Schwartz-Jampel syndrome 361
statistics 52–5
   central nucleation 55
   fibre hypertrophy 53–4
   fibre size 52–3
   fibre-type atrophy 53
   fibre-type grouping 54
   fibre-type predominance 52
steroid myopathy 420–1
terminal motor innervation 62
Muscle disorders *see* Myopathies
Muscle fibres 46–7
   atrophy *53*
   central cores 57
   distribution 48–9
   effects of age 50–1
   effects of training and exercise 49–50
   hypertrophy 53–4
   moth-eaten 56–7
   necrotic 55–6
   ragged-red 58–9, 389–91, 392
   ring fibres 60
   rod bodies 57–8
   size 52–3
   splitting *see* Fibre splitting
   target 57
   tubular aggregates 59
   type atrophy 53
   type grouping 54–5
     and fibre splitting 81–2
   type predominance 52
   types of 47–8
Muscle spindles 51, 62
Muscle-specific enolase 14
Muscular dystrophies 307–41
   autosomal recessive of childhood 330–1
   Becker *see* Becker muscular dystrophy
   congenital 331–5
   distal 338
   distal myopathies 336–8
   Duchenne *see* Duchenne muscular dystrophy
   Emery-Dreifuss 325

facio-scapulo-humeral 332-5
facio-scapulo-humeral, wasting in 9
Fukuyama 332
limb-girdle *see* Limb-girdle muscular dystrophy
ocular myopathies 338-41
oculo-pharyngeal 95, 339-41
scapulo-humeral *see* Scapulo-humeral muscular dystrophies
scapulo-peroneal *see* Scapulo-peroneal muscular dystrophy
X-linked 307-25
    cardiomyopathy in 434-5
Musculocutaneous nerve syndromes 150
Myasthenia gravis 87, 107, 257-83
    acetylcholine (ACh) receptor antibody 263-4, 271
    adult-onset 258-61
        generalised myasthenia 259-60
        ocular myasthenia 258-9
        physical examination 260-1
        weakness and course 258
    antibody-negative 265
    associated disorders 261
    autoimmune causation 261-2
    classification 258
    diagnosis 266-71
    drugs enhancing neurotransmission in 283
    electrophysiological tests 268-71
    end-plate disorder 75, 76
    experimental autoimmune 264
    management 271-5
        anticholinesterase drugs 271-2
        immunosuppressant therapy 273-4
        intravenous immunoglobulin therapy 275
        plasma exchange 274-5
        recommended 275
        thymectomy 272-3
    muscle pathology 266
    neonatal 261
    Osserman clinical severity classification 258
    pathogenesis 265
    pathophysiology 262
    penicillamine-induced 275-6
    pharmacological tests 267-8
    respiratory weakness in 7
    thymic pathology in 265-6
    with thymoma 261
Myasthenic crisis 259
Myasthenic syndrome 75
Mycobacterium leprae see Leprosy
Myelin 63
Myeloma, neuropathy associated with 220-2
    course and prognosis 222
    electrophysiological assessment 221
    laboratory investigations 221
    nerve biopsy 221
Myoadenylate deaminase 45
    deficiency 386-7
Myoedema 10
Myofibrillar adenosine triphosphatase 45
Myoglobinuria 411-13
Myokymia 10, 26
    complex repetitive discharges 25
Myopathic facies 266
    childhood 363-75
Myopathies 87
    childhood 363-75
    with cylindrical spirals 374
    drug-induced 425-9
    endocrine 415-24
    inflammatory *see* Inflammatory myopathies
    with lysis of myofibrils in type 1 fibres 373-4

metabolic 377-413
mitochondrial *see* Mitochondrial myopathies
nutritional 430-1
osteomalacic 431-2
toxic 429-30
with tubular aggregates 372-3
see also individual conditions
Myophosphorylase 45
Myophosphorylase deficiency *see* McArdle's syndrome
Myotonia 10, 26-7, 343-62
    chloride channel 345
    clinical tests 343-5
    differential diagnosis 360
    drug-induced 361-2
    electrophysiological findings 358-9
    exercise-induced 362
    laboratory investigations 358
    muscle pathology 359-60
    pathophysiology 345
    protein kinases 346
    sodium channel 345-6
    treatment 360
Myotonia congenita
    autosomal dominant 356
    autosomal recessive 356-7
Myotonia fluctuans 358
Myotonic dystrophy 346-55
    cardiomyopathy 435-6, 440
    congenital 348
    electrophysiological assessment 349-51
    genetic aspects 348-9
    genetic counselling 355
    laboratory investigations 349
    management 354-5
    muscle biopsy 351-4
    and protein kinases 346
    proximal 355
Myotubular myopathy 369-71
    aetiology 371
    investigations 370
    muscle biopsy 370
    outcome 370

Nalidixic acid 250
Necrosis 55-6
    subendomysial 56
Needle biopsy 43-4
Nemaline myopathy 58, 366-9
    investigations 367
    management 369
    muscle biopsy 367-9
Neonatal myasthenia 261
Nerve 63-4
Nerve biopsy 64-8
    acromegaly 423
    hypothyroidism 419
    identification of neuropathy 67-8
    indications for 67
    Isaacs' syndrome 444
    myeloma 221
    polyneuropathies 131
    progressive external ophthalmoplegia 400
Nerve conduction studies 36-42
    blink reflex 41
    F response 39-40
    H reflex 38-9
    mixed nerve action potential recording 38
    motor conduction block 37-8

Nerve conduction studies – *cont.*
  motor conduction velocity 37
  motor nerve conduction velocity distribution 40
  motor/sensory nerve refractory period 40–1
  sensory conduction 38
  somatosensory evoked responses 41–2
  stimulation of central motor pathways 42
Nerve entrapment syndromes 127
Nerve injuries 133–9
  compression neuropathies 137–9
  entrapment neuropathies 134–7
  functional classification 134
Nesting fibres 77
Neuralgic amyotrophy 165
Neuro-axonal dystrophy, infantile and juvenile 189
Neurogenic disorders, pathophysiological correlations 69–72
Neuroleptic–malignant syndrome 410–11
Neuromuscular jitter 33
Neuromuscular transmission disorders 87
Neuromuscular transmission, drugs affecting 282–4
Neuromyotonia *see* Isaacs' syndrome
Neuronopathy 121, 125
Neuropathies
  autonomic 121
  chronic hereditary sensory 127
  clinical approach 121–32
  clinical evaluation 122–3
  clinical features 122–4
  clinico-pathological correlations 127–8
  electromyography 128–9
  genetically determined *see* Hereditary neuropathies
  hypertrophic 121, 126
  motor symptoms 127
  peripheral 121
  positive/negative symptoms 126–9
  prevalence 123–4
  progression 123
  sensory symptoms 126–7
  see also Mononeuropathies; Polyneuropathies
Neuropraxia 134
Neurotmesis 134
Nicotine adenine dinucleotide (NADH) tetrazolium reductase
      technique 45
Niemann–Pick disease 199
Nitrofurantoin 250
Nodes of Ranvier 63, 64, 66
Norris scale 6
Notalgia paraesthetica 150
Nutritional myopathies 430–1

Obturator mononeuropathy 152
Ocular myasthenia 258–9
Ocular myopathies 338–41
Oculo-cranio-somatic neuromuscular disease 341
Oculo-cranio-somatic syndrome *see* Kearns–Sayre syndrome
Oculo-pharyngeal muscular dystrophies 95, 339–40, 339–41
  investigations 340–1
  management 341
Oil red O stain 45
Olivo-ponto-cerebellar atrophy 187
Onion bulb formation 68, 126
Open biopsy 44
Opportunistic radiculopathies 238
Organophosphate neuropathy 253, 254
Osteolytic myeloma 220
Osteomalacic myopathy 431–2
  clinical features 431
  electrophysiological assessment 432

laboratory investigations 431–2
  management 432
  muscle biopsy 432
Osteosclerotic myeloma 220
Overuse syndromes 446–7
Oxidation/phosphorylation coupling defects 397

Pain 9–10
Pain insensitivity, congenital 186–7
Paradoxical myotonia 357
Paraesthesiae 11
Paramyotonia congenital 357
Paraneoplastic autonomic neuropathy 215–16
Paraneoplastic mixed sensory neuropathy 215
Paraneoplastic sensory neuropathy 214–15
Paraneoplastic vasculitic neuropathy 216
Parathyroid disorders 419–20
Pathophysiological correlations 69–76
  acute neurogenic disorders 69–70
  axonal and demyelinating neuropathies 72–3
  chronic neurogenic disorders 70–1
  end-plate disorders 75–6
  myopathic disorders 73–5
  rapidly and slowly progressing neurogenic disorders 71–2
Pellagra 212
Pelvic girdle nerve syndromes 151–2
  femoral mononeuropathy 152
  meralgia paraesthetica 151–2
  obturator mononeuropathy 152
Penetration wounds 133
Penicillamine-induced myasthenia 275–6
Penicillin 250
Perhexilene maleate 252
Perineural cells 63
Periodic acid Schiff stain 45
Periodic paralysis 402–7
  cardiomyopathy 436–7
  hypokalaemic 402–5
    drug-induced 427–8
    and paramyotonia congenita 405–6
  management 406–7
  normokalaemic 406
  thyrotoxic 407
Peripheral nerve biopsy
  Charcot–Marie–Tooth syndrome 179, 180
  porphyria 194
  Refsum's disease 196
Peripheral nerves
  disorders 86
  examination 11
Peripheral neuropathies 124–6
  axonal transection 124–5
  distal axonopathy 125
  myelinopathy 125–6
  neuronopathy 125
Peroneal muscular atrophy *see* Hereditary motor and sensory
      neuropathies
Phalen's sign 143
Phosphofructokinase deficiency 17, 385–6
Phosphoglycerate kinase deficiency 17, 386
Phosphoglycerate mutase deficiency 386
Phosphorylase b kinase deficiency 386
Phytanic acid *see* Refsum's disease
Pituitary disorders 421–3
Plasma exchange therapy
  Guillain–Barré syndrome 236
  myasthenia gravis 274–5
POEMS 221

Poliomyelitis 118–19
Polyarteritis nodosa 222–3
  muscle biopsy 300
Polymyalgia rheumatica 306
Polymyositis 56, 76, 107, 285, 286–8
  cardiomyopathy 440
  clinical features 286
  cutaneous manifestations 287
  diagnosis 301–2
  fibre-type grouping 81
  HIV-1 304
  HTLV-1 304–5
  idiopathic 295–8
  myopathy 286–7
  paraneoplastic 290–1
  systemic features 287–8
Polyneuropathies 86, 121
  acquired 201–55
  clinical investigation 129–30
  electromyography 130–1
  management 131–2
  nerve biopsy 131
  outcome of investigation 131
  see also Neuropathies; and individual conditions
Pompe's disease see Acid maltase deficiency
Porphyria 86, 192–5
  acute intermittent 193
  classification 192
  course and management 194–5
  electrophysiological assessment 194
  haem synthesis in 193
  laboratory investigations 194
  nerve biopsy 194
Positive sharp waves 25
Post-irradiation syndromes 120
Post-polio syndrome 118–19
Pressure palsies, hereditary liability to 183
Primary fibromyalgia 446–7
Primary lateral sclerosis 106
Progressive external ophthalmoplegia 338–9, 398–400
  electrophysiological assessment 399
  genetics 399
  muscle biopsy 399
  myopathies 399
  nerve biopsy 400
Progressive muscular atrophy 106
Pronator teres syndrome 145
Protein-calorie malnutrition 431
Proximal motor neuropathy 202–3
Pseudo-tabetic neuropathy 202
Pseudohypertrophic muscular dystrophy see Duchenne
  muscular dystrophy
Pseudomyotonia 25–6
Pulmonary function tests 6–7
Pyomyositis 305
Pyridoxine deficiency 212
Pyruvate carboxylase deficiency 396–7
Pyruvate decarboxylase deficiency 396

Quadriceps myopathy 323

Rabies 241–2
Radial nerve syndromes 148–50
  compression injuries in upper arm 149
  posterior interosseous nerve lesions 149–50
  superficial branch 150
Radiculoneuritis 246

Ragged–red fibres 58–9, 389–91, 392
Ramsay–Hunt syndrome 187
Rankin scale 6
Rectus abdominis syndrome 150–1
Reducing body myopathy 374
Refsum's disease 86, 123, 195–6
  antibody tests 15
  cardiomyopathy 438, 440
  electrophysiological assessment 196
  laboratory investigations 195–6
  nerve and muscle biopsy 196
  pathology 196
  screening for susceptibility 196
  treatment and outcome 196
Regenerative changes in muscle 60–2
Renaut bodies 63, 136
Respiratory chain defects 397
Restless legs syndrome 444
Retinitis pigmentosa 123
Rhabdomyolysis 411–13, 425–6
Rheumatoid arthritis 223
  muscle biopsy 300
  and myositis 289
Rigid spine syndrome 330, 374–5
Riley–Day syndrome 185–6
  treatment 187
Ring fibres 60
Ringbinden 60
Rippling muscle disease 444
Rod bodies 57–8
Root compression syndromes 70
Roussy–Levy syndrome 175

Sarcoid myopathy 301
Sarcoidosis 224–5
Sarcoplasmic masses 60
Sarcotubular myopathy 374
Scanning electromyography 21, 35
Scapulo–humeral muscular dystrophy 95, 335–6
Scapulo–peroneal muscular dystrophy 94–5, 335–6
  cardiomyopathy 436
  differential diagnosis 336
  electrophysiological assessment 335
  laboratory investigations 335
  muscle biopsy 336
Schmidt–Lanterman incisures 63, 64
Schwartz–Jampel syndrome 361
  neuromyotonia 26
  pseudomyotonia in 26
Sciatic nerve syndromes 152–3
Scleroderma 224
  muscle biopsy 300
  myositis and 289
Scoliosis 101
Segmental demyelination 125
Sensory disturbances 10–11
Sensory double-crush syndrome 156
Sensory nerves
  conduction 38
  refractory period 40–1
Severe mixed sensorimotor neuropathy 223
Signal amplification in electromyography 21–2
Single-fibre electromyography 33–4
  electrodes 20–1
Sjögren's syndrome 224, 289
  antibody tests 15
Skeletal muscle structure 46–51
  distribution of muscle fibres 48–9

Skeletal muscle structure – *cont.*
  effects of age 50
  fibre types and motor units 47–8
  muscle fibres 46–7
  muscle spindles 51
  training and exercise 49–50
Small fibre neuropathy 201–2
Solitary plasmacytoma 220
Soman 282
Somatosensory evoked responses 41–2
Spheroid body myopathy 373
Spielmeyer–Vogt syndrome 199
Spinal accessory nerve syndromes 159
Spinal muscular atrophy 85–6, 89–103
  bulbar of childhood *see* Fazio–Londé syndrome
  bulbar with deafness *see* Vialetto–van Laere syndrome
  chronic asymmetrical 94
  classification 90
  clinical investigation 95–6
  clinical presentation 90–5
  distal 93–4
  electrophysiological investigation 96–7
  genetics and counselling 101
  management and treatment 101
  monomelic 94
  oculo-pharyngeal 95
  pathology 97–101
  pseudomyotonia in 26
  rare forms 94
  scapulo–humeral 95
  scapulo–peroneal 94–5
  type 1 *see* Werdnig–Hoffmann disease
  type 2 86
    clinical presentation 91–2
  type 3 *see* Kugelberg–Welander syndrome
  type 4 86
    clinical presentation 93–5
  X-linked recessive bulbospinal *see* Kennedy syndrome
Steroid myopathy 420–1
Stiff man syndrome 26, 441–2
Streptomycin 250
Stretch injuries of nerves 133
Subacute necrotising myopathy 291
Subacute/acute painful myopathy 428
Succinic dehydrogenase 45
Sudan black stain 45
Surface electromyography 36
  electrodes 19–20
Symmetrical sensorimotor neuropathy 220
Syringomyelia 117–18
Systemic lupus erythematosus 224
  muscle biopsy 300
  and myositis 289

Tabes dorsalis 68
Tangier disease 195, 197, 198, 199
Target fibres 57
Tarsal tunnel syndrome 154–5
  electrophysiological assessment 155
  management 155
Taxol 251
Tay–Sach's disease 198
Tennis elbow 150
Tetanus 240–1
Tetrodotoxin 282
Thallium neuropathy 253, 255
Thiamine deficiency 211

Thoracic outlet syndrome 166–7
Thymectomy 272–3
Thymoma 261, 265–6
Thyroid eye disease 416
Thyroid myopathies 415–19
Thyrotoxic periodic paralysis 407
Tibial nerve syndrome 154
Timed function tests 6
Tinel's sign 11, 128
  carpal tunnel syndrome 141, 143
  cervical root lesions 162
  common peroneal syndromes 154
  tarsal tunnel syndrome 155
  thoracic outlet syndrome 167
  ulnar nerve lesions 146
Tolosa–Hunt syndrome 203
Tone and reflexes 9
Toxic myopathies 429–30
Toxic neuropathies 247–50
  clinical features 248–9
  mechanisms of 249–50
Toxic oil syndrome 254
Toxins affecting neuromuscular transmission 282–4
Toxoplasmosis 305
Traction injuries of nerves 133
Training, effects on muscles 49–50
Trichlorethylene neuropathy 253–4
Trigeminal nerve syndromes 159
Trilaminar disease 374
Tropical ataxia neuropathy 213
Tropical sprue 431
Tryptophan–induced eosinophilia–myalgia syndrome 427
Tubular aggregates 59
Tufts Quantitative Neuromuscular Examination 5–6

Ulnar nerve syndromes 146–8
  electrophysiological assessment 147
  lesions at wrist and hand 148
  management 147–8
Upper limb syndromes 139–51
  median nerve 139–46
  musculocutaneous nerve 150
  notalgia paraesthetica 150
  radial nerve 148–50
  rectus abdominis syndrome 150–1
  ulnar nerves 146–8
Uraemic neuropathy 207–9
  electrophysiological assessment 208
  management 208–9
  pathological considerations 208

Vacuoles, in muscle disease 338
Vialetto–van Laere syndrome 86, 95
Vincristine 251
Viral myositis 303–5
Vitamin B12 deficiency 211–12
Vitamin E deficiency 212–13, 430–1
Von Recklinghausen's disease, nerve hypertrophy in 11

Waldenström's macroglobulinaemia 222
Wartenberg's migrant sensory neuritis 184
Wasted leg syndrome 94
Wasting 8–9
Weakness 2–7
  quantitative assessment of muscular strength 4–7

dynamometry 5
Functional Rating Scales 6–7
Medical Research Council Scale 4–5
Tufts Quantitative Neuromuscular Examination
5–6
Wegener's granulomatosis 224
Welander's distal myopathy 337
Werdnig–Hoffmann disease 85–6, 98, 100
clinical presentation 90–1
Wernicke–Korsakoff syndrome 209
Western Pacific ALS 117
Whipple's disease 305

Wire electrodes 21
Wright's manoeuvre 167

X–linked myalgia 323
X–linked myoglobinuria 323–4
X–linked myotubular myopathy 325
Xeroderma pigmentosum 197, 200

Zebra body myopathy 374
Zidovudine myopathy 304, 427